Equine Emergency and Critical Care Medicine

LOUISE L. SOUTHWOOD, BVSc, PhD, DACVS, DACVECC

Associate Professor of Large Animal Emergency and Critical Care
Department of Clinical Studies – New Bolton Center
University of Pennsylvania School of Veterinary Medicine
Kennett Square, Pennsylvania, USA

and

PAMELA A. WILKINS, DVM, MS, PhD, DACVIM, DACVECC

Professor, Veterinary Clinical Medicine
College of Veterinary Medicine
University of Illinois at Urbana-Champaign
Urbana, Illinois, USA

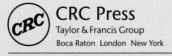

CRC Press
Taylor & Francis Group
Boca Raton London New York

CRC Press is an imprint of the
Taylor & Francis Group, an **informa** business

CRC Press
Taylor & Francis Group
6000 Broken Sound Parkway NW, Suite 300
Boca Raton, FL 33487-2742

© 2015 by Taylor & Francis Group, LLC
CRC Press is an imprint of Taylor & Francis Group, an Informa business

Printed and bound in India by Replika Press Pvt. Ltd.

No claim to original U.S. Government works

Printed on acid-free paper
Version Date: 20140715

International Standard Book Number-13: 978-1-84076-194-8 (Hardback)

10 0767039X

Library of Congress Cataloging-in-Publication Data

Equine emergency and critical care medicine / editors, Louise L. Southwood, Pamela Wilkins.
  p. ; cm.
Includes bibliographical references and index.
ISBN 978-1-84076-194-8 (hardcover : alk. paper)
  I. Southwood, Louise L., editor. II. Wilkins, Pamela, editor.
  [DNLM: 1. Horse Diseases--therapy. 2. Emergency Treatment--veterinary. SF 951]

SF951
636.1'08928--dc23   2014025991

Visit the Taylor & Francis Web site at
http://www.taylorandfrancis.com

and the CRC Press Web site at
http://www.crcpress.com

CONTENTS

Preface		18
Contributors		19
Abbreviations		21
Dedication		23
PART 1	**EMERGENCY MEDICINE**	**25**
CHAPTER **1**	**DIGESTIVE SYSTEM AND PERITONEAL DISEASE** *Louise L. Southwood*	**27**
	GENERAL APPROACH TO THE HORSE WITH DIGESTIVE SYSTEM AND PERITONEAL DISEASE	27
	COMMON PROCEDURES PERFORMED ON HORSES WITH DIGESTIVE SYSTEM AND PERITONEAL DISEASE	30
	Nasogastric intubation	30
	Abdominal palpation per rectum	32
	Abdominocentesis and peritoneal fluid analysis	35
	Abdominal ultrasonographic examination	39
	Intravenous catheterization	40
	Exploratory abdominal surgery (general surgical technique)	40
	DIGESTIVE SYSTEM DISEASES	47
	Oral cavity	47
	Esophagus	47
	Esophageal obstruction (choke)	47
	Stomach	51
	Equine gastric ulcer syndrome	51
	Gastric impaction	57
	Gastric neoplasia	58
	Gastric rupture	60
	Small intestine	62
	Strangulating lesions	62
	Epiploic foramen entrapment	64
	Gastrosplenic ligament entrapment	66
	Inguinal hernia	66
	Intussusception	66

Strangulation through a mesenteric rent	69
Strangulating pedunculated lipoma	71
Small intestinal volvulus	73
Non-strangulating lesions	75
Functional obstruction	76
Primary ileus	76
Equine grass sickness	78
Mechanical obstruction	80
Ileal impaction	80
Ileal muscular hypertrophy	82
Diverticula	84
Ascarid impaction	86
Neoplasia	88
Inflammatory lesions	90
Proximal enteritis (duodenitis–proximal jejunitis)	90
Inflammatory or infiltrative bowel disease	93
Proliferative enteropathy	96
Cecum	98
Cecal impaction	98
Cecocecal and cecocolic intussusception	101
Cecal infarction	104
Large colon	104
Strangulating or ischemic lesions	104
Large colon volvulus	104
Infarction	108
Non-strangulating lesions	108
Gas or spasmodic colic	109
Large colon impaction	110
Sand impaction	113
Enterolithiasis	115
Nephrosplenic ligament entrapment of the large colon	118
Right dorsal displacement of the large colon	122
Colitis	124
Right dorsal colitis	127
Small colon	129
Small colon impaction	130
Fecalith obstruction	132
Intestinal concretions and foreign body obstruction	133
Small colon strangulating pedunculated lipoma	135
Rectum	135

Rectal tear 135
Rectal prolapse 138
Perirectal abscess 140
Hernias 141
Inguinal and scrotal hernias 141
Strangulating umbilical hernia 144
Diaphragmatic hernia 145
Liver 146
Acute hepatic disease 146
PERITONEAL CAVITY 148
Peritonitis 148
Hemoperitoneum 152

CHAPTER **2**   **MUSCULOSKELETAL SYSTEM** *Liberty M. Getman and Troy N. Trumble* **155**

GENERAL APPROACH TO THE HORSE WITH A MUSCULOSKELETAL EMERGENCY 155
COMMON PROCEDURES PERFORMED ON HORSES WITH MUSCULOSKELETAL
    EMERGENCIES 157
Diagnostic procedures 157
Physical examination 157
Diagnostic imaging 158
Synoviocentesis and synovial fluid analysis 159
Therapeutic procedures 170
Splinting and casting 170
Regional limb perfusion 176
Antimicrobial-impregnated polymethylmethacrylate 179
MUSCULOSKELETAL EMERGENCIES 180
Bone 180
Fractures 180
Distal phalanx fracture 180
Middle phalanx facture 182
Proximal phalanx fracture 184
Third metacarpus/metatarsus fracture 186
Carpal fractures and luxations 189
Tarsal fractures and luxations 191
Olecranon fractures 194
Radial fractures 196
Tibial fractures 198
Humeral fractures 201
Femoral fractures 203
Pelvic fractures 207

Skull fractures   210
Infection   213
Septic physitis and epiphysitis   213
Septic osteomyelitis of the third phalanx   214
Tendons and ligaments   217
Traumatic disruption of the suspensory apparatus   217
Flexor tendon disruption   219
Extensor tendon disruption   222
Synovial structures   224
Articular luxations   224
Septic arthritis and wounds involving joints   227
Septic tenosynovitis and wounds involving tendon sheaths   234
Septic navicular bursitis   238
Hoof   242
Subsolar abscess   242
Hoof puncture wounds   242
Laminitis   245
Muscle disorders   247
Clostridial myositis   247
Rhabdomyolysis ('tying-up')   250
Hyperkalemic periodic paralysis   252

CHAPTER **3**   **RESPIRATORY TRACT** *Mathew P. Gerard and Pamela A. Wilkins*   **253**

GENERAL CONSIDERATIONS   253
COMMON PROCEDURES PERFORMED ON HORSES WITH RESPIRATORY TRACT
DISEASE   254
Intranasal oxygen administration   254
Endotracheal intubation   256
Temporary tracheostomy   258
Arterial blood gas collection and analysis   260
Transtracheal wash/tracheal fluid analysis   262
Thoracocentesis/pleural fluid analysis   264
Chest tube placement   265
UPPER RESPIRATORY TRACT DISEASES ASSOCIATED WITH OBSTRUCTION
AND RESPIRATORY DISTRESS   267
Severe arytenoid chondritis   267
Cicatrix   270
Bilateral laryngeal paresis   271
Strangles (*Streptococcus equi* subsp. *equi* lymphadenopathy)   274
Guttural pouch tympany   276

Snake bite   280
Clostridial myositis   282
Tracheal trauma   284
UPPER AIRWAY DISEASES ASSOCIATED WITH EPISTAXIS   286
Longus capitis and rectus capitis muscle rupture/basi-sphenoid/
  occipital fracture   286
Head trauma (sinus and nasal passage)   288
Foreign body obstruction   289
LOWER AIRWAY DISEASES   291
Pulmonary edema   291
Smoke inhalation   292
Pneumonia/pleuropneumonia   294
Pneumothorax/hemothorax   296
Heaves/recurrent airway obstruction   298
Equine multinodular pulmonary fibrosis   300
RESPIRATORY NEOPLASIA   302

CHAPTER 4   **CARDIOVASCULAR SYSTEM**   **305**
             Melinda Frye, Vanessa L. Cook, Louise L. Southwood, and Pamela A. Wilkins

GENERAL APPROACH TO THE HORSE WITH CARDIOVASCULAR DISEASE   305
COMMON PROCEDURES PERFORMED ON HORSES WITH CARDIOVASCULAR
  DISEASE   306
Base-apex electrocardiography   306
Echocardiography   308
Resuscitation following hemorrhage and hemolysis   311
Cardiopulmonary resuscitation – foals   312
Cardiopulmonary resuscitation – adults   315
CARDIOVASCULAR DISEASE   316
Cardiac diseases   316
Congestive heart failure   316
Inflammatory diseases   319
Endocarditis   320
Pericarditis   322
Myocarditis and myocardial degeneration   324
Arrhythmias   326
Atrial fibrillation   326
Third-degree atrioventricular block   329
Premature ventricular contractions   331
Ventricular tachycardia   333
Ventricular fibrillation   335
Asystole   337

Congenital cardiac defects	338
Ventricular septal defect	338
Tetralogy or pentalogy of Fallot	339
Patent ductus arteriosus	340
Vascular diseases	341
Hemorrhage	341
Post-castration hemorrhage	341
Peripheral artery/vein hemorrhage	342
Guttural pouch mycosis	343
Uterine artery rupture	347
Aortic aneurysm or rupture	350
Inflammatory	351
Thrombophlebitis and septic thrombophlebitis	351
Thromboembolic disease	354

CHAPTER **5**   **UROGENITAL SYSTEM** *Barbara L. Dallap Schaer and Dietrich H. Volkmann*   **357**

GENERAL APPROACH TO MARES WITH UROGENITAL PROBLEMS	357
GENERAL APPROACH TO STALLIONS WITH UROGENITAL PROBLEMS	358
COMMON PROCEDURES PERFORMED IN MARES AND STALLIONS WITH UROGENITAL PROBLEMS	358
REPRODUCTIVE TRACT PROBLEMS	358
Mares	358
Dystocia	358
Post-parturient shock	366
Uterus	369
Retention of fetal membranes and metritis	369
Uterine tear	373
Uterine prolapse	376
Uterine artery hemorrhage	377
Uterine torsion	377
Cervix, vagina/vestibule region, and perineum	379
Vaginal and cervical lacerations	379
Perineal lacerations	382
Bladder eversion, prolapse, or rupture	384
Rupture of the abdominal wall during pregnancy	386
Stallion	390
Post-castration complications	390
Priapism	393
Paraphimosis	394
Torsion of the spermatic cord	398

Penile and testicular trauma 400
URINARY TRACT 401
Urolithiasis 401
Acute kidney injury (previously known as acute renal failure) 404

CHAPTER 6 **SKIN** *Troy N. Trumble and Louise L. Southwood* **407**

GENERAL APPROACH TO THE HORSE WITH LACERATIONS AND PUNCTURE
WOUNDS 407
COMMON PROCEDURES PERFORMED ON HORSES WITH LACERATIONS AND
PUNCTURE WOUNDS 409
Abaxial sesamoid and low 4-point nerve blocks 409
Wound preparation 412
Synoviocentesis and synovial fluid analysis 412
Suturing techniques 412
Skin staples 414
Wound drains 415
Bandaging 416
Cast application 420
Regional limb perfusion 420
Skin scraping 420
Skin biopsy 421
SKIN PROBLEMS 421
Lacerations and puncture wounds 421
Distal limb 421
Upper limb and body 430
Head and neck 437
Cellulitis 440
Thermal and chemical injuries 442
Burns 442
Frostbite 446
Other skin diseases 446
Pruritus 446
Photosensitization 450
Pemphigus foliaceus 451
Toxic epidermal necrolysis 452

CHAPTER 7 **NEUROLOGY** *Pamela A. Wilkins* **453**

GENERAL APPROACH TO THE HORSE WITH NEUROLOGIC PROBLEMS 453
COMMON PROCEDURES PERFORMED ON HORSES WITH NEUROLOGIC
PROBLEMS 455

Neurologic examination — 455
Cerebrospinal fluid collection and analysis — 456
    Cerebrospinal fluid collection — 456
    Cerebrospinal fluid analysis — 459
DISEASE OF THE NERVOUS SYSTEM — 460
    Diseases producing cortical signs — 460
        Equine herpesvirus type 1 myeloencephalopathy — 460
        West Nile virus encephalomyelitis — 462
        Alphaviruses — 463
        Bacterial meningitis/encephalitis and brain abscess — 465
        Rabies — 466
        Equine protozoal myeloencephalitis — 467
        Head trauma — 468
        Temporohyoid osteoarthropathy — 472
        Hepatic encephalopathy — 474
    Diseases producing cerebellar signs — 476
        Parasitic encephalitis — 476
    Diseases producing spinal cord or peripheral nerve signs — 477
        Equine protozoal myeloencephalitis — 477
        Vertebral trauma — 477
        Botulism — 478
        Tetanus — 480
        Spinal cord abscess/vertebral osteomyelitis — 481
    Neoplastic disease producing cerebral, cerebellar, spinal cord, or peripheral nerve signs — 481

CHAPTER 8   **EYE AND ASSOCIATED STRUCTURES** — **483**
Elizabeth J. Davidson and Mary Lassaline-Utter

GENERAL APPROACH TO THE HORSE WITH AN INJURY INVOLVING THE EYE OR ASSOCIATED STRUCTURES — 483
DEFINITIONS — 483
COMMON PROCEDURES PERFORMED ON HORSES WITH OPHTHALMIC EMERGENCIES — 484
    Ophthalmic nerve blocks — 484
    Subpalpebral lavage catheter placement — 484
    Conjunctival graft — 486
    Tarsorrhaphy — 488
    Enucleation — 488
LESIONS AND DISEASES AFFECTING THE EYE AND ASSOCIATED STRUCTURES — 490
    Eyelid — 490
        Eyelid laceration — 490

Entropion	492
Orbital fracture	494
Cornea	495
Corneal ulceration	495
Corneal burns	498
Corneal laceration	499
Corneal stromal abscess	500
Immune-mediated keratitis	502
Intraocular	504
Equine recurrent uveitis	504
Hyphema	505
Retinal detachment	506
Glaucoma	508
Acute blindness	510

CHAPTER 9 **NEONATOLOGY** *Jane E. Axon, Catherine M. Russell, and Pamela A. Wilkins* **511**

GENERAL APPROACH TO THE CRITICALLY ILL EQUINE NEONATE	511
COMMON PROCEDURES PERFORMED ON HORSES WITH NEONATAL EMERGENCIES	511
Respiratory support	511
Cardiovascular support	513
Glucose support	515
Electrolyte therapy	515
Acid–base disturbances	516
Immune therapy	516
Antimicrobial therapy	516
Nutritional support	517
Temperature	517
Eyes	518
Umbilicus	518
DISEASES OF THE EQUINE NEONATE	518
Failure of passive transfer	518
Neonatal isoerythrolysis	520
Sepsis	523
Prematurity	528
Urinary tract disruption	532
Hypoxic ischemic syndrome	535
Pneumonia	540
Rib fractures	543

Meconium impaction/retention   545
Diarrhea/enterocolitis   547
Limb deformities   551

CHAPTER **10**   **TOXICOLOGY** *Robert H. Poppenga*   **555**

GENERAL CONSIDERATIONS FOR HORSES WITH INTOXICATION   555
GENERAL APPROACH TO TREATING HORSES WITH INTOXICATION   558
   Stabilize vital signs   558
   Obtain a history and clinically evaluate the patient   559
   Prevent continued systemic absorption of the toxicant   559
   Antidote administration   560
   Enhance elimination of absorbed toxicant   560
   Provide symptomatic and supportive care and closely monitor   562
COMMON PROCEDURES PERFORMED IN HORSES WITH INTOXICATION   562
   Gastrointestinal tract decontamination   562
TOXICITIES   565
   Naturally occurring toxins   565
     Plants   565
       Alsike clover   565
       Cyanogenic glycoside-containing plants   566
       Black walnut   570
       Locoweeds   571
       Maples   573
       Oleander   574
       Pyrrolizidine alkaloids   576
       White snakeroot (*Eupatorium rugosum*)   578
       Yellow-star thistle and Russian knapweed   579
     Mycotoxins   581
       Aflatoxins   581
       Ergot alkaloids   582
       Fumonisin mycotoxins   585
       Slaframine   586
       Tremorgenic mycotoxins   587
     Algal toxins   588
     Zootoxins   591
       Cantharidin   591
       Snake venoms   592
     Botulism   594
     Metals   596
       Iron   596

Lead 598

Mercury 600

Selenium 600

Non-steroidal anti-inflammatory drugs 602

Feed additives (ionophores) 603

Cholinesterase-inhibiting insecticides 605

Other toxic plants potentially affecting horses 606

Other potential causes of intoxication in horses 606

PART 2   **CRITICAL CARE**   **621**

CHAPTER **11**   **MONITORING** *K. Gary Magdesian and Louise L. Southwood*   **623**

GENERAL APPROACH TO MONITORING 623

MONITORING 624

Patient examination 624

Hematology 625

Plasma proteins 631

Serum or plasma biochemistry 633

Blood gas analysis 635

Coagulation profile 638

Urine output and urinalysis 642

Arterial blood pressure 645

Central venous pressure 646

Cardiac output 648

CHAPTER **12**   **FLUID THERAPY** *Vanessa L. Cook and Louise L. Southwood*   **653**

GENERAL APPROACH TO FLUID THERAPY 653

COMMON PROCEDURES PERFORMED FOR FLUID THERAPY 653

Intravenous catheterization 653

FLUIDS 658

Crystalloids 658

Isotonic crystalloids 658

Hypertonic saline 662

Colloids 664

Synthetic colloids 666

Hydroxyethyl starch 666

Dextrans 668

Gelatins 669

Naturally occurring colloids 669

Plasma and albumin   669
Blood and oxygen carrying solutions   671

CHAPTER **13**   **INOTROPE AND VASOPRESSOR THERAPY**   **675**
Brett S. Tennent-Brown and Janyce Seahorn

GENERAL APPROACH TO USE OF INOTROPE AND VASOPRESSOR THERAPY   675
PREPARATION AND ADMINISTRATION   676
INOTROPES AND VASOPRESSORS   678
   Dobutamine   678
   Norepinephrine   679
   Dopamine   680
   Vasopressin   681
   Phenylephrine   683
   Epinephrine   684

CHAPTER **14**   **SEDATION AND ANALGESIA** *Janyce Seahorn*   **685**

GENERAL APPROACH FOR USING SEDATION AND ANALGESIA   685
COMMON PROCEDURES PERFORMED WHEN USING SEDATION
   AND ANALGESIA   685
   Epidural catheterization   685
   Constant rate infusion   686
      Example   686
SEDATIVES AND ANALGESICS   687
   Alpha-2 agonists   687
   Opioids   689
   Acepromazine   692
   Benzodiazepines   692
   Ketamine   693
   Lidocaine   694
   Non-steroidal anti-inflammatory drugs   695
   Gabapentin   696

CHAPTER **15**   **NUTRITIONAL SUPPORT** *Brett S. Tennent-Brown*   **697**

GENERAL APPROACH TO PROVIDING NUTRITIONAL SUPPORT   697
COMMON PROCEDURES PERFORMED FOR PROVIDING NUTRITIONAL SUPPORT   697
   Body condition scoring   697
   Placement of an esophagostomy feeding tube   698
   Calculations of parenteral nutrition formulation   700

NUTRITIONAL SUPPORT 701
    Nutritional requirements 701
    Enteral nutrition 703
    Parenteral nutrition 706

CHAPTER **16**   **ANTIMICROBIAL DRUGS** *James A. Orsini*   **711**

GENERAL CONSIDERATIONS FOR ANTIMICROBIAL DRUG USE 711
GENERAL APPROACH TO ANTIMICROBIAL DRUG USE 712
    Prophylactic antimicrobial drug use 712
    Therapeutic antimicrobial drug use 714
    Adjunctive immunotherapy 717
    Alternative modes of delivery 718
ANTIMICROBIAL DRUGS 719
    Aminoglycosides 719
    Cephalosporins 721
    Chloramphenicol 724
    Enrofloxacin 724
    Imipenem (with cilastatin) 725
    Macrolides 726
    Metronidazole 727
    Penicillins 728
    Rifampin 729
    Tetracycline 730
    Trimethoprim-sulfonamides (potentiated sulfonamides) ... 731
    Vancomycin 731

CHAPTER **17**   **THE SYSTEMIC INFLAMMATORY RESPONSE**   **733**
    Michelle H. Barton and K. Gary Magdesian

GENERAL APPROACH TO THE SYSTEMIC INFLAMMATORY RESPONSE ... 733
SYSTEMIC INFLAMMATORY RESPONSE 733
    Endotoxemia 733
    Systemic inflammatory response syndrome 737
    Multiple organ dysfunction syndrome 740
    Sepsis and severe sepsis 744
    Septic shock 747
    Shock 749
    Disseminated intravascular coagulation 752

CHAPTER **18**   **POSTOPERATIVE COLIC PATIENT** *Louise L. Southwood*   **757**

GENERAL APPROACH TO THE POSTOPERATIVE COLIC PATIENT   757
MONITORING   758
    Patient observation   758
    Physical examination   759
    Incisional care   761
    Intravenous catheter   762
    Laboratory data   764
    Hemodynamic monitoring   765
BASIC MANAGEMENT   767
    Fluid and electrolyte therapy   767
        Crystalloids   767
        Colloids   768
    Antimicrobial drugs   768
    Anti-inflammatory drugs and analgesics   769
    Postoperative feeding   770
POSTOPERATIVE COMPLICATIONS   772
    Fever   772
    Incisional infection   773
    Shock   776
    Endotoxemia   779
    Postoperative ileus and motility modification   780
    Postoperative intra-abdominal adhesions   784

CHAPTER **19**   **THE PREGNANT MARE** *Pamela A. Wilkins*   **789**

INTRODUCTION   789
PREPARTUM PROBLEMS   789
    Placentitis   789
    Body wall hernia and prepubic tendon rupture   790
    Hydrops conditions   792
PERIPARTUM PROBLEMS   792
    Bleeding   792
GASTROINTESTINAL PROBLEMS   793
    Rectal prolapse   793
    Small colon trauma   793
    Small intestine trauma   794
    Large colon volvulus   794
PROBLEMS AT PARTURITION   795
    Dystocia   795
POSTPARTUM PROBLEMS   796
    Metritis–laminitis syndrome   796

CHAPTER **20**   **THE NEONATE** *Jane E. Axon and Pamela A. Wilkins*   **797**

INTRODUCTION   797
NURSING CARE   797
    Restraint of the foal   797
    Care of the recumbent foal   797
    Care of the standing foal   798
    Feeding the foal   799
    The mare   799
MONITORING   800
    Weight   800
    Body temperature   800
    Body systems   800
    Laboratory data   802
    The mare   802
FLUID AND ELECTROLYTE THERAPY   802
    Fluid therapy in the first 24 hours   803
    Fluid therapy after the first 24 hours   803
ANTIMICROBIAL THERAPY   806
    Instigation of antimicrobial therapy   806
    Route of administration   806
    Length of treatment   806
    Classes of commonly used antimicrobials   806

CHAPTER **21**   **THE RECUMBENT HORSE** *Pamela A. Wilkins*   **809**

GENERAL CONSIDERATIONS   809
MONITORING AND NURSING CARE   810
SPECIAL CONSIDERATIONS   812
APPENDIX: RESOURCES FOR DEVICES FOR MOVING, LIFTING, AND 'SLINGING'
    RECUMBENT HORSES (USA ONLY)   812
    Glides   812
    Slings   812
ADDITIONAL READING   812

References   **813**
Index   **863**

THE survival of horses requiring emergency management and critical care has improved considerably, even in the last 15 years. Major reasons for this improvement are early recognition of problems by owners, appropriate first aid, and timely referral by field veterinarians. Veterinarians at equine tertiary care facilities are now presented with horses that are cardiovascularly stable and with disease still in the early stages of progression. Diseases that historically required humane euthanasia are now often treatable. It is only through an ongoing team approach with owners, field and specialist veterinarians, and clinical and basic science researchers that we can continue to improve the care of our equine patients.

Recently, we reported an overall 76% survival rate of all emergency cases presented to our hospital. The survival for horses treated surgically was 80% with 70% survival in horses medically treated.[1] While these survival rates are good, there is room for improvement. Geriatric horses and neonates had the lowest survival (60% and 59%, respectively) as did horses with strangulating intestinal lesions (<60%), neurologic disease (54%), and laminitis (46%). These areas require our ongoing attention with regard to clinical and basic science investigation as well as owner education about the potential for a positive outcome for their horse. As was appropriately stated by Fessler and Adams[2]: 'The philosophic mind-set of the veterinarian and the aura of confidence, or lack thereof, that is portrayed to a client can set the tone for the decisions to be made … a veterinarian that is interested [in treating the horse] and willing to take risks can lead a client to invest in surgical repair [or other treatment]. A discouraging, disinterested professional viewpoint can lead a client to request euthanasia'.

As with anything that we do in equine medicine, the focus of this book is to improve the outcome of our patients. The chapters have been written by young and enthusiastic as well as experienced (and *still* enthusiastic) equine specialists and we are very thankful for their hard work and expertise. We would also like to thank Jill Northcott, our commissioning editor, who has been extremely patient and provided exceptional guidance. This book would not have been completed without the assistance of Peter Beynon, who undertook the copyediting, and Kate Nardoni at Cactus Design, who was project manager and provided the artwork. Most importantly, we need your feedback to continue to make this book as useful as possible for the equine veterinarian. If there is anything that has not been included or that is not particularly well explained, please contact us because your input is invaluable for future editions. It is an honor and pleasure to have had the opportunity to put this book together.

Louise L. Southwood
Pamela A. Wilkins

1 Southwood LL, Dolente BA, Russell G *et al.* (2009) Survival of equine emergency admissions to a large animal tertiary referral hospital. *Equine Vet J* **41**:459–464.
2 Fessler JF, Adams SB (1996) Decision making in ruminant orthopedics. *Vet Clin N Am Food Anim Pract* **12**:1–18.

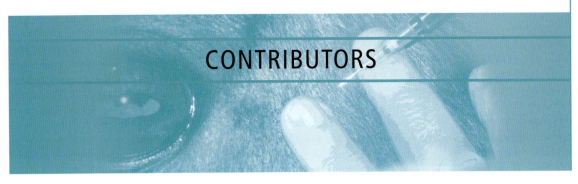

Jane E. Axon
BVSc, MANZCVSc, DACVIM,
    CMAVA
Clovelly Intensive Care Unit
Scone Equine Hospital, Scone
New South Wales, Australia

Michelle H. Barton
DVM, PhD, DACVIM
Fuller E. Callaway Endowed Chair
Professor of Large Animal Medicine
Josiah Meigs Distinguished Teaching
    Professor
Department of Large Animal
    Medicine
College of Veterinary Medicine
University of Georgia
Athens, Georgia, USA

Vanessa L. Cook
VetMB, MS, PhD, DACVS,
    DACVECC
Associate Professor - Large Animal
    Surgery and Emergency Critical
    Care
College of Veterinary Medicine
Michigan State University
East Lansing, Michigan, USA

Elizabeth J. Davidson
DVM, DACVS, DACVSMR
Associate Professor of Large
    Animal Sports Medicine and
    Imaging
Department of Clinical Studies –
    New Bolton Center
University of Pennsylvania School of
    Veterinary Medicine
Kennett Square, Pennsylvania, USA

Melinda Frye
DVM, MS, PhD, DACVIM
Associate Dean for Veterinary
    Academic and Student Affairs
Colorado State University
Fort Collins, Colorado, USA

Mathew P. Gerard
BVSc, PhD, DACVS
Clinical Associate Professor, Equine
    Surgery
College of Veterinary Medicine
North Carolina State University
Raleigh, North Carolina, USA

Liberty M. Getman
DVM, DACVS
Tennessee Equine Hospital
Thompson's Station, Tennessee, USA

K. Gary Magdesian
DVM, DACVIM, DACVECC,
    DACVCP, CVA
Henry Endowed Chair in
    Emergency Medicine and Critical
    Care
Professor, Department of Medicine
    and Epidemiology
School of Veterinary Medicine
University of California-Davis
Davis, California, USA

James A. Orsini
DVM, DACVS
Associate Professor of Surgery
Department of Clinical Studies –
    New Bolton Center
University of Pennsylvania School of
    Veterinary Medicine
Kennett Square, Pennsylvania, USA

Robert H. Poppenga
DVM, PhD, DABVT
CAHFS Toxicology Laboratory
School of Veterinary Medicine
University of California-Davis,
California, USA

Catherine M. Russell
BVSc, FANZCVSc
Clovelly Intensive Care Unit
Scone Equine Hospital, Scone
New South Wales, Australia

Barbara L. Dallap Schaer
VMD, DACVS, DACVECC
Associate Professor of Large Animal
    Emergency and Critical Care
Department of Clinical Studies –
    New Bolton Center
University of Pennsylvania School of
    Veterinary Medicine
Kennett Square, Pennsylvania, USA

Janyce Seahorn
DVM, MS, DACVA, DACVIM-LA,
    DACAVECC
Lexington Equine Surgery and
    Sports Medicine
Lexington, Kentucky, USA

Louise L. Southwood
BVSc, PhD, DACVS, DACVECC
Associate Professor of Large Animal
    Emergency and Critical Care
Department of Clinical Studies –
    New Bolton Center
University of Pennsylvania School of
    Veterinary Medicine
Kennett Square, Pennsylvania, USA

Brett S. Tennent-Brown
BVSc, MS, DACVIM, DACVECC
Senior Lecturer in Equine Medicine
Equine Center
University of Melbourne Veterinary
    Hospital
Werribee, Victoria, Australia

Troy N. Trumble
DVM, PhD, DACVS
Associate Professor
College of Veterinary Medicine
Veterinary Medical Center
University of Minnesota
St. Paul, Minnesota, USA

Mary Lassaline-Utter
DVM, PhD, DACVO
Department of Surgical and
    Radiological Sciences
School of Veterinary Medicine
University of California-Davis
Davis, California, USA

Dietrich H. Volkmann
BVSc, MMedVet, DACT
Professor in Theriogenology
College of Veterinary Medicine
University of Missouri
Columbia, Missouri, USA

Pamela A. Wilkins
DVM, MS, PhD, DACVIM,
    DACVECC
Professor, Veterinary Clinical
    Medicine
College of Veterinary Medicine
University of Illinois at Urbana-
    Champaign
Urbana, Illinois, USA

AAA	aromatic amino acid	COX	cyclooxygenase
ABG	arterial blood gas	CPD-A	citrate-phosphate-dextrose with adenine
ACE	angiotensin-converting enzyme	CRI	constant rate infusion
ACT	activated clotting time	CRT	capillary refill time
ACTH	adrenocorticotropic hormone	CSF	cerebrospinal fluid
ADH	antidiuretic hormone	CT	computed tomography
AF	atrial fibrillation	cTnI	cardiac troponin I
AIPM	antimicrobial-impregnated polymethylmethacrylate	CVP	central venous pressure
AKI	acute kidney injury	DAP	diastolic arterial pressure
ALD	angular limb deformity	DIC	disseminated intravascular coagulation
ALI	acute lung injury	DMSO	dimethylsulfoxide
ALP	alkaline phosphatase		
ALT	alanine aminotransferase	ECG	electrocardiogram
AO	atlanto-occipital (space)	EDTA	ethylenediamine tetra-acetic acid
aPTT	activated partial thromboplastin time	EEE	Eastern equine encephalomyelitis
ARDS	acute respiratory distress syndrome	EFE	epiploic foramen entrapment
AST	aspartate aminotransferase	EHM	equine herpesvirus myeloencephalopathy
ATIII	antithrombin III	EHV	equine herpesvirus
ATP	adenosine triphosphate	EMPF	equine multinodular pulmonary fibrosis
AVB	atrioventricular block	EPM	equine protozoal myeloencephalitis
		ERU	equine recurrent uveitis
BAL	bronchoalveolar lavage		
BALF	bronchoalveolar lavage fluid	Fab	fragment antigen binding (fragment)
BCCA	branched chain amino acid	FDPs	fibrin/fibrinogen degradation products
bpm	beats per minute	FE	fractional excretion
BUN	blood urea nitrogen	FIO_2	fraction of inspired O_2
		FLASH	fast localized abdominal sonography of horses
$CaNa_2EDTA$	calcium disodium versenate		
CARS	compensatory anti-inflammatory response syndrome	FPT	failure of passive transfer
CBC	complete blood count	GABA	gamma-aminobutyric acid
CHF	congestive heart failure	G-CSF	granulocyte colony-stimulating factor
CI	coagulation index	GFR	glomerular filtration rate
CK	creatine kinase	GGT	gamma glutamyltransferase
CN	cranial nerve	GI	gastrointestinal
CNS	central nervous system		
CO_2	carbon dioxide	Hb	hemoglobin (concentration)
COP	colloid osmotic pressure	HBOC	hemoglobin-based oxygen carrying (solution)
COPD	chronic obstructive pulmonary disease		

HE	hepatic encephalopathy
HIE	hypoxic–ischemic encephalopathy
HIS	hypoxic ischemic syndrome
HMPAO	(technetium-99m) hexamethylpropyleneamine oxime
HPA	hypothalamus–pituitary–adrenal (axis)
HYPP	hyperkalemic periodic paralysis
ICP	intracranial pressure
ICS	intercostal space
ICU	intensive care unit
IFAT	indirect immunofluorescent antibody test
IFN	interferon
IHC	immunohistochemistry
IL	interleukin
IM	intramuscular/intramuscularly
IMK	immune-mediated keratitis
INO_2	intranasal oxygen (insufflation)
IO	intraosseous
IOP	intraocular pressure
IT	intratracheal/intratracheally
IV	intravenous/intravenously
JFA	jaundiced foal agglutination (assay)
LCV	large colon volvulus
LDH	lactate dehydrogenase
LRT	lower respiratory tract
LS	lumbosacral (space)
MAP	mean arterial pressure
MCH	mean corpuscular hemoglobin
MCHC	mean corpuscular hemoglobin concentration
MCV	mean corpuscular volume
MIC	minimum inhibitory concentration
MODS	multiple organ dysfunction syndrome
MRI	magnetic resonance imaging
MRSA	methicillin-resistant *Staphylococcus aureus*
NE	neonatal encephalopathy
NI	neonatal isoerythrolysis
NMDA	N-methyl-D-aspartate
NO	nitric oxide
NPPE	negative pressure pulmonary edema
NSAID	non-steroidal anti-inflammatory drug
NSLE	nephrosplenic ligament entrapment
O_2ER	oxygen extraction ratio
OP	organophosphorus/organophosphate

P_ACO_2	partial alveolar pressure of carbon dioxide
P_aCO_2	arterial carbon dioxide tension
PAWP	pulmonary arterial wedge pressure
$PcvCO_2$	central venous carbon dioxide tension
$PvCO_2$	venous carbon dioxide tension
PaO_2	arterial oxygen tension
$PcvO_2$	central venous oxygen tension
PvO_2	venous oxygen tension
PCO_2	partial pressure of carbon dioxide
PCR	polymerase chain reaction
PCV	packed cell volume
PDA	patent ductus arteriosus
PEEP	positive end expiratory pressure
PFL	peritoneal fluid lactate
PGE2	prostaglandin E2
PMMA	polymethylmethacrylate
PO	per os/orally
PO_2	partial pressure of oxygen
PPN	partial parenteral nutrition
PPV	positive pressure ventilation
PT	prothrombin time
PTE	pulmonary thromboembolism
PVC	premature ventricular contraction
qs	quantum satis (as much as is enough)
RABV	rabies virus
RAO	recurrent airway obstruction
RBC	red blood cell
RER	resting energy requirements
RFM	retained fetal membranes
SAA	serum amyloid A
SaO_2	arterial oxygen saturation
SAP	systolic arterial pressure
$S_{cv}O_2$	central venous oxygen saturation
S_vO_2	venous oxygen saturation
SC	subcutaneous/subcutaneously
SCC	squamous cell carcinoma
SDH	sorbitol dehydrogenase
SG	specific gravity
SIRS	systemic inflammatory response syndrome
SPAOD	summer pasture-associated obstructive pulmonary disease
SV	stroke volume
SVR	systemic vascular resistance
TEG	thromboelastography
TEN	toxic epidermal necrolysis
THO	temporohyoid osteoarthropathy

TNF-α	tumor necrosis factor-α		VEE	Venezuelan equine encephalomyelitis
TPN	total parenteral nutrition		VSD	ventricular septal defect
TPP	total plasma protein			
TP	total protein		WBC	white blood cell
			WEE	Western equine encephalomyelitis
URT	upper respiratory tract		WNV	West Nile virus

Dedication

To Eric, Aiden, Kody, Kylie, and Bianca

PART 1

EMERGENCY
MEDICINE

CHAPTER **1** Digestive system and peritoneal disease

CHAPTER **2** Musculoskeletal system

CHAPTER **3** Respiratory tract

CHAPTER **4** Cardiovascular system

CHAPTER **5** Urogenital system

CHAPTER **6** Skin

CHAPTER **7** Neurology

CHAPTER **8** Eye and associated structures

CHAPTER **9** Neonatology

CHAPTER **10** Toxicology

DIGESTIVE SYSTEM AND PERITONEAL DISEASE

Louise L. Southwood

GENERAL APPROACH TO THE HORSE WITH DIGESTIVE SYSTEM AND PERITONEAL DISEASE

- The gastrointestinal (GI) tract is the most common source of digestive system and peritoneal disease. Horses with GI tract disease most commonly present on emergency with signs of abdominal pain (colic). Typical signs of colic include: pawing, flank staring, lying down, inappetence (mild); rolling intermittently (moderate); and persistently rolling with self-trauma to the head, limbs, and tuber coxae (severe).
- Dull demeanor, inappetence, diarrhea, and weight loss are also seen in horses with GI disease. Horses with esophageal (p. 47) and some gastric (p. 51) problems can present with excessive salivation (ptyalism) and/or drainage of feed and saliva from the nares.
- Signs can be mild to severe and can present acutely or as recurrent and intermittent signs of several days to months duration.
- A thorough history for a horse with suspected GI disease should include that listed in *Box 1.1*.
- Initial examination should involve general observations such as demeanor, signs of pain, evidence of trauma, sweating, abdominal distension, and any fecal staining on hindlimbs.
- Heart rate, respiratory rate, rectal temperature, mucous membrane color and moistness, capillary refill time (CRT), GI borborygmi, and digital pulses should be assessed.
- A nasogastric tube should be passed (p. 30) in any horse showing signs of colic or salivation to check for reflux or esophageal obstruction (choke), respectively, and to administer fluids if indicated.

Box 1.1 Pertinent history for horses with gastrointestinal disease

- Patient signalment
- Specific signs shown
- Duration of signs
- Reproductive history, if mare or stallion
- Pre-existing disease or lesion and current medication
- Previous episodes of colic or colic surgery
- Medication administered
- Vaccination and deworming history
- Recent change in housing, feeding, exercise regimen, or transportation
- Current feeding regimen and appetite, water consumption, as well as fecal and urine output

- Depending on the veterinarian's ability and experience, abdominal palpation per rectum can be performed (p. 32).
- Initial treatment of colic and some cases of diarrhea involves administration of flunixin meglumine as well as enteral water, with or without electrolytes (4–6 liters/500 kg), and/or mineral oil (colic only) via a nasogastric tube. Cyclo-oxygenase (COX)-I sparing non-steroidal anti-inflammatory drugs (NSAIDs) such as firocoxib or meloxicam may be used as an alternative to flunixin meglumine. If the horse does not respond to treatment with an NSAID, an alpha-2 agonist (xylazine or detomidine), with or without an opiate (butorphanol), can be used. While the majority of horses with colic recover with minimal treatment, 20–30% will require additional analgesia and/or IV fluid therapy and 4–6% will require surgery. Dose rates of drugs used in the initial management of colic are listed in *Box 1.2*.
- Indications for emergency referral of horses with GI disease are shown in *Box 1.3*.

Box 1.2 Dose rates of drugs used in the initial management of colic

DRUG	DOSE RATE (AMOUNT FOR A 500 KG HORSE)
Flunixin meglumine	1.1 mg/kg IV q12h (500 mg or 10 ml) (also available as an oral paste)
	0.25–0.5 mg/kg IV q6–8h (125–250 mg or 2.5–5.0 ml) (anti-inflammatory dose)
Firocoxib	0.27 mg/kg IV (loading dose) (135 mg or 6.75 ml)
	0.09 mg/kg IV q24h (45 mg or 2.25 ml)
Meloxicam	0.6 mg/kg IV or IM q24h (300 mg)
Xyalzine HCl	0.3–0.4 mg/kg IV (150–200 mg or 1.5–2.0 ml)
Detomidine HCl	0.01–0.02 mg/kg IV or IM (5–10 mg or 0.5–1.0 ml)
Butorphanol	0.01–0.02 mg/kg IV (5–10 mg or 0.5–1.0 ml) (with xylazine or detomidine)
N-butylscopolammonium bromide	0.3 mg/kg IV once (150 mg or 7.5 ml)

Box 1.3 Indications for referral of a horse with gastrointestinal disease

- Persistent, severe or recurrent pain
- Persistent or severe diarrhea
- Unresolved esophageal obstruction
- Shock (cool extremities, tachycardia, injected/toxic membranes)
- Abdominal distension
- Persistently absent borborygmi
- Reflux following nasogastric tube passage
- Abnormal findings on palpation per rectum (e.g. small intestinal distension, cecal or small colon impaction)

- Information that should be provided to the veterinarian at the referral hospital is shown in *Box 1.4*.
- Procedures performed at a referral hospital include physical examination, nasogastric intubation, abdominal palpation per rectum, and abdominocentesis and peritoneal fluid analysis. Hematology and plasma chemistry is typically evaluated. Transabdominal ultrasonographic examination is performed, if indicated.

- The main indication for emergency abdominal surgery is persistent or severe pain. Postoperative care of the colic patients is discussed in Chapter 18, Postoperative colic patient.
- The prognosis for horses with GI disease, particularly colic, has improved dramatically over the past 15 years and, in general, the survival rate is good to excellent for horses with most lesions following early and appropriate treatment.

Box 1.4 Minimum data base provided to the veterinarian at the referral hospital

- Signalment (age, breed, gender)
- Severity of signs (specific signs that the horse is showing)
- Duration of signs
- Recent reproductive history, if mare or stallion
- Any underlying disease and/or current medication
- Heart rate
- Respiratory rate
- Rectal temperature
- Oral mucous membrane color and capillary refill time
- Borborygmi (hypermotile, normal, hypomotile, absent)
- Fecal production (normal, none, diarrhea)
- Nasogastric reflux
- All drugs administered and time of administration
- Any financial constraints
- Insurance information
- Contact person and telephone number

COMMON PROCEDURES PERFORMED ON HORSES WITH DIGESTIVE SYSTEM AND PERITONEAL DISEASE

Nasogastric intubation

Indications

Nasogastric intubation should be performed as part of every colic examination (1) to remove accumulations of gastric fluid and gas that can lead to gastric rupture, (2) to gain information regarding the lesion site (i.e. a small intestinal obstruction should be suspected in horses with reflux), and (3) to give enteral fluids and electrolytes, mineral oil, or other laxatives. A nasogastric tube should also be passed in a horse with saliva and ingesta at the nares to check for and relieve an esophageal obstruction (choke) (p. 47).

Technique

- Passage of a nasogastric tube is performed with the horse standing and restrained with a halter and lead rope. A nose twitch is often required. Stocks may be used, but are not always necessary. While some horses may require sedation, this can make nasogastric tube passage more challenging because of difficulty in having the horse swallow the tube.
- A medium or large bore nasogastric tube should be used in adult horses, a small or medium nasogastric tube in weanlings, and a stallion catheter or similar sized tube can be used in neonates and small foals (**1.1A–C**).
- The left hand should be used if passing the tube from the left side and the right hand if passing the tube from the right side to avoid standing directly in front of the horse (**1.2**). Occasionally, a horse will strike with its forelimbs during nasogastric tube passage and standing directly in front of the horse could lead to serious injury.
- The tube should be lubricated with water prior to passage. The nasogastric tube is passed through the ventral nasal meatus into the pharynx. When initially placed into the nasal passage, the tube should be pushed ventrally and medially so that it enters the ventral meatus and avoids passage into the middle meatus and trauma to the ethmoid turbinates. Some resistance to passage will usually be felt when the tube is in the pharynx. Marking the tube with a permanent marker, using the

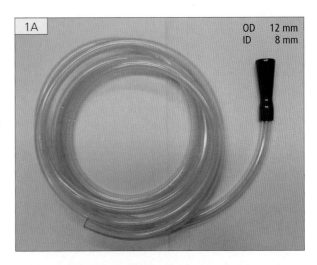

1A | OD 12 mm | ID 8 mm

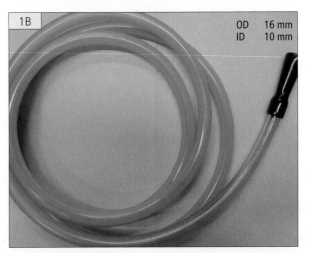

1B | OD 16 mm | ID 10 mm

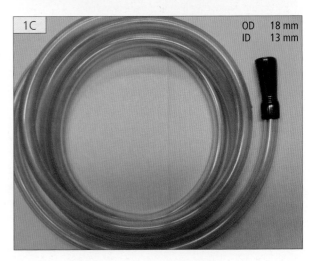

1C | OD 18 mm | ID 13 mm

1.1A–C Small (A), medium (B), and large (C) nasogastric tubes.

medial canthus of the eye as an estimate of the pharynx location prior to nasogastric tube passage, can assist with recognizing when the tube is in the pharynx (**1.3**). The horse's neck should be ventroflexed to facilitate passage of the tube into the esophagus rather than the trachea when the horse swallows.

- If the tube passes easily without resistance and there is no negative pressure created when sucking on the tube, it is likely to be in the trachea. The horse may also cough. The tube should be drawn back into the pharynx and another attempt made to pass the tube into the esophagus. when the horse swallows

- Rotating the tube, changing to the opposite nares, and blowing air through the tube will help facilitate swallowing of the tube.

- When the tube is in the esophagus, there should be a slight resistance to passage, which can be somewhat reduced by dilating the esophagus with air. Negative pressure should be created with sucking and the tube should be observed and palpated in the cervical esophagus. When air is blown down the tube while it is in the cervical esophagus, esophageal dilation should be seen.

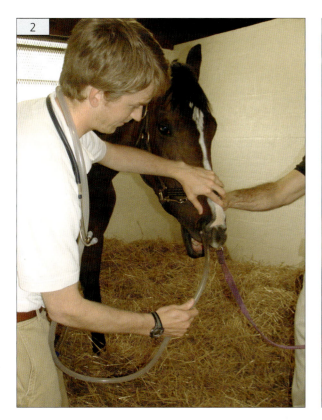

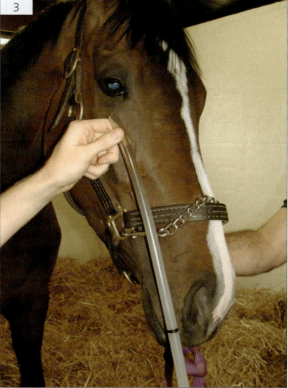

1.2 Position for placing a nasogastric tube. When standing on the right side of the horse, the tube is passed with the right hand and the left hand is used to steady the horse's head and create ventroflexion of the neck, which should facilitate nasogastric tube passage into the esophagus and not the trachea. Care should be taken to avoid occluding the contralateral naris.

1.3 Measuring the distance from the medial canthus of the eye to the nares. The tube can be permanently marked to determine when the tube is in the pharynx. This avoids having to repeatedly pass the tube through the nares, which is usually resented by the horse.

- The tube should be passed all the way through the cardia and into the stomach to relieve gas and fluid accumulations in the stomach and prevent aspiration of administered fluids, lubricants, and laxatives. Aspiration can occur when these are administered through a tube that remains in the esophagus.
- Horses and foals should always be checked for reflux prior to administering fluids via a nasogastric tube in order to prevent gastric rupture. Reflux is checked by infusing 500–1,000 ml of warm water through the tube and then holding the end of the tube in an empty bucket below the level of the horse's stomach to create a siphon. The net reflux is calculated by subtracting the volume of water infused to create the siphon from the total volume of reflux obtained.

Complications

Complications associated with nasogastric intubation include nasal hemorrhage, pharyngeal and esophageal trauma, aspiration pneumonia or inadvertent tracheal intubation and fluid administration, and, rarely, having problems with tube removal. Hemorrhage usually stops and the horse's head should be held in a normal position (not low or high) to facilitate clotting. Holding the horse's head high can cause aspiration of blood and pneumonia. The amount of blood loss should be monitored. Severe pharyngeal and esophageal trauma can be treated with oral sucralfate if the horse is inappetent as a consequence of the mucosal injury. Aspiration should be treated as for other cases of aspiration pneumonia (see Chapter 3). Aspiration of mineral oil and other lubricants or laxatives is typically fatal. Problems with nasogastric tube removal are extremely rare and reasons can be identified using endoscopy.

Abdominal palpation per rectum
Indications

While palpation per rectum is used most commonly for examination of the female reproductive tract, it is also used for examination of the caudal abdomen in horses with colic, fever of unknown origin, weight loss, inappetence, and inadequate fecal production.

Technique

- The horse is restrained in stocks or a stall with a halter and lead rope. The use of a nose twitch, with or without sedation (see Chapter 14), is recommended.
- A rectal sleeve with ample lubrication should be used. Topical lidocaine (2%) or systemic N-butylscopolammonium bromide (Buscopan®) can be used to lessen straining. Lidocaine can be mixed with the lubricant or placed in the rectum using a 60 ml syringe and extension tubing following removal of feces.
- Normal structures (**1.4**) that can be palpated in the caudal abdomen are the ventral band of the cecum coursing cranioventrally from the right caudodorsal abdomen towards the midline; aorta and iliac vessels lying dorsally; caudal pole of the left kidney dorsally and to the left of the midline; nephrosplenic space/ligament lateral to the left kidney; caudodorsal aspect of the spleen lying adjacent to the left body wall; fecal balls in the small colon; left ventral colon tenia; bladder with its round ligaments on the midline within the pelvic canal; ovaries and uterus; and inguinal rings.
- Abnormalities that can be palpated include duodenal (**1.5**) or jejunal distension (**1.6**) suggestive of a small intestinal lesion, ileal impaction (**1.7**), cecal impaction (**1.8**), large colon distension suggestive of a large intestinal lesion, pelvic flexure/left ventral colon impaction (**1.9**), right dorsal displacement of the large colon (**1.10**), entrapment of the large colon over the nephrosplenic ligament (**1.11**), and small colon impaction (**1.12**).

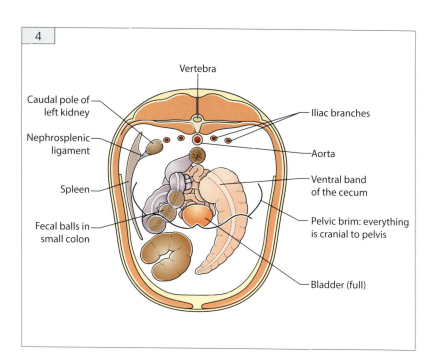

1.4 Schematic illustration of the normal anatomy per rectum.

Vertebra

Caudal pole of left kidney

Nephrosplenic ligament

Spleen

Fecal balls in small colon

Iliac branches

Aorta

Ventral band of the cecum

Pelvic brim: everything is cranial to pelvis

Bladder (full)

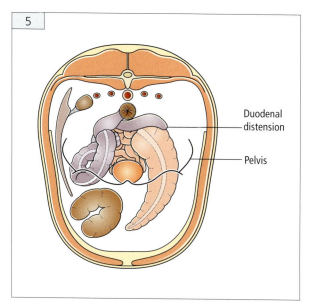

1.5 Schematic illustration of duodenal distension per rectum. The distended duodenum can be palpated coursing right to left around the base of the cecum.

Duodenal distension

Pelvis

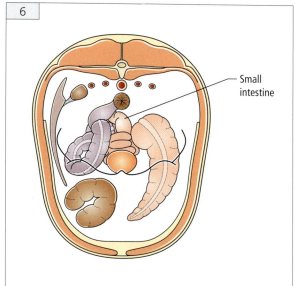

1.6 Schematic illustration of jejunal distension per rectum. Either one or several loops of small intestine can be palpated throughout the abdomen.

Small intestine

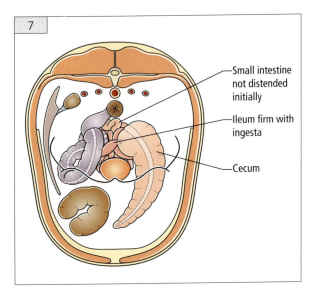

1.7 Schematic illustration of ileal impaction per rectum. A firm, 5–8 cm diameter smooth-surfaced ileum may be palpated in the mid-abdominal region adjacent to the cecal base coursing in a cranioventral direction towards the left abdomen.

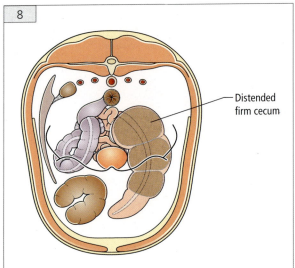

1.8 Schematic illustration of cecal impaction per rectum. The large and distended impacted cecum is found on the right side of the abdomen.

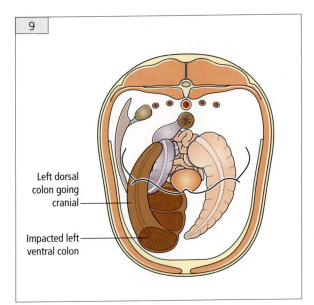

1.9 Schematic illustration of pelvic flexure/left ventral colon impaction per rectum. The impacted left ventral colon is identified in the left caudal abdomen and usually courses in a cranial direction. The impacted colon may be found in the ventral aspect of the left caudal abdomen or pushed back into the pelvic inlet.

1.10 Schematic illustration of right dorsal displacement of the large colon per rectum. The displaced colon can be palpated coursing around the base of the cecum. The cecum can not be palpated in most cases and the colon is distended.

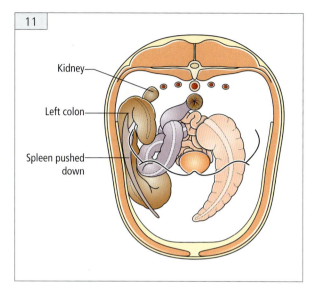

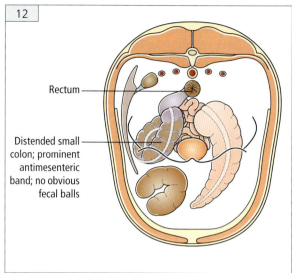

1.11 Schematic illustration of entrapment of the large colon over the nephrosplenic ligament per rectum. The large colon can be palpated coursing through the nephrosplenic space between the caudal pole of the left kidney and the dorsal aspect of the spleen. The spleen is usually pushed ventrally.

1.12 Schematic illustration of small colon impaction per rectum. The impacted small colon can be identified based on its small size, location, and the prominent antimesenteric (and mesenteric) bands.

Complications

Complications associated with abdominal palpation per rectum include rectal tear (p. 135) and trauma to the veterinarian.

Abdominocentesis and peritoneal fluid analysis

Indications

Abdominocentesis is performed in cases of colic or enterocolitis to assess intestinal injury, and in horses with a fever of unknown origin to diagnose peritonitis. In approximately 50% of GI neoplasia cases, neoplastic cells can be seen on cytologic evaluation of the peritoneal fluid. Abdominocentesis is not typically performed during the initial examination for colic in the field.

Technique

Abdominocentesis

• Abdominocentesis is performed with the horse restrained in stocks or in a stall with a halter and lead rope.

• A 10 cm × 10 cm area to the right of the midline at the most dependent aspect of the ventral abdomen is clipped and aseptically prepared. Alternatively, the area on the cranial midline where the pectoral muscles create a V-shape can be used. Ultrasonographic examination can be used to identify an area of peritoneal fluid accumulation; however, this is not particularly sensitive. Abdominocentesis should not be performed to the left of the midline because of the potential for splenic injury. Large subcutaneous vessels should be avoided to prevent sample contamination with blood and continued bleeding after the procedure.

- Abdominocentesis can be performed using an 18-gauge needle or a teat cannula. The use of an 18-gauge needle is easier and quicker. If an enterocentesis is accidentally performed, the hole into the intestine is likely to be smaller. However, fluid is obtained more often with a teat cannula because of the more appropriate length and larger bore. Teat cannula proponents suggest that enterocentesis is less likely because of the blunt tip.

- Abdominocentesis using an 18-gauge needle is performed by carefully inserting the needle through the skin, subcutaneous tissue, body wall (external or ventral rectus sheath, rectus abdominis muscle, and internal or dorsal rectus sheath), and into the peritoneal cavity (**1.13A, B**). It can be difficult to determine when the tip of the needle is within the peritoneal cavity and in some cases an 18-gauge 1½ inch needle may be of insufficient length. Spontaneous movement of the needle is associated with intestinal movement and can be an indication that the needle is correctly positioned. Multiple needles are often needed to obtain a sample.

- Abdominocentesis using a teat cannula requires infiltration of the subcutaneous tissue and body wall with 3 ml of 2% lidocaine. A stab incision is made using a #15 blade through the skin and body wall. Gauze sponge is wrapped around the teat cannula to prevent sample contamination (**1.14**). The teat cannula is pushed through the body wall and into the peritoneal cavity; considerable force is usually necessary. Correct positioning of the teat cannula within the peritoneal cavity can be confirmed by filling a 10 ml syringe with air and injecting the air through the teat cannula. If the teat cannula is not in the peritoneal cavity, the air will be heard rushing back out through the teat cannula.

- The needle or teat cannula is manipulated for several minutes in an attempt to obtain a sample from an area of fluid accumulation.

- The sample is collected into an EDTA (purple top) tube for cytology and a sterile plain (red top) tube, syringe, or culture vial for bacterial culture and sensitivity testing. Lactate concentration can be measured from a plain or lithium heparin (green top) tube.

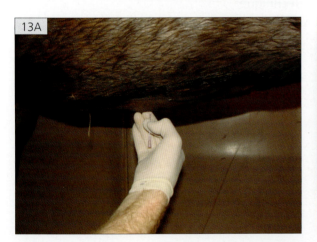
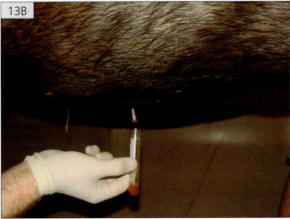

1.13A, B Abdominocentesis using an 18-gauge needle. (A) Needle insertion on the most ventral aspect of the abdomen to the right of the midline. (B) Collection of peritoneal fluid into an EDTA tube for cytology and a plain tube for bacterial culture and sensitivity testing. Note that the gross appearance of the fluid is consistent with peritonitis.

Peritoneal fluid analysis

- The gross appearance of normal peritoneal fluid is clear pale to dark yellow (**1.15A, B**). Cloudiness indicates a high nucleated cell count. Serosanguineous fluid is consistent with intestinal injury and the necessity for an abdominal exploration. Care should be taken during abdominocentesis to avoid blood contamination; however, with close observation during sample collection, blood contamination as opposed to serosanguineous or sanguineous peritoneal fluid can be differentiated. Splenic blood can be differentiated from a hemoabdomen by measuring packed cell volume (PCV) because the PCV of splenic blood is higher than that of the horse's peripheral blood. Green or brown fluid is consistent with peritoneal contamination with

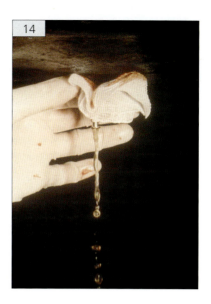

1.14 Abdominocentesis using a teat cannula. Note the gauze sponge around the teat cannula to prevent blood contamination of the sample from the skin and subcutaneous tissue. (Courtesy Dr Josie Traub-Dargatz)

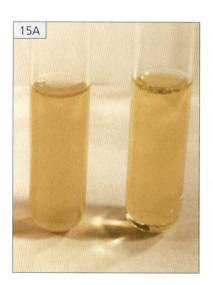 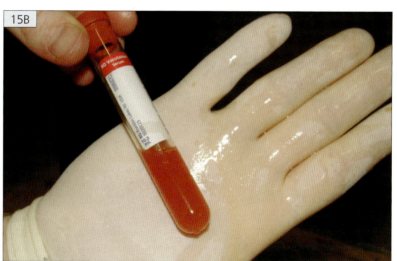

1.15A, B Peritoneal fluid. (A) Normal, (B) serosanguineous. (Courtesy Dr Josie Traub-Dargatz)

ingesta or an enterocentesis. Ingesta-contaminated peritoneal fluid and intraluminal fluid can be differentiated cytologically because intracellular bacteria (**1.16**) are observed with ingesta contamination of the peritoneal cavity.

- Normal total protein (TP) is <25 g/l (2.5 g/dl). A high TP concentration is indicative of intestinal damage and/or peritoneal inflammation.
- Normal total nucleated cell count is <10 × 10^9/l (10,000/µl), with approximately 50% neutrophils and 50% mononuclear cells. A high nucleated cell count is diagnostic for peritonitis, which can be primary or idiopathic, or secondary to intestinal injury, intestinal perforation, abscessation, or neoplasia.
- Peritoneal fluid lactate (PFL) is being used more frequently as an indication of strangulating intestinal lesions. Normal concentration of PFL is <1 mmol/l. There is an increased likelihood that a horse would require surgery or have a strangulating lesion as PFL concentration increases.[1] PFL concentration greater than that of plasma may suggest intestinal compromise; horses with a strangulating obstruction had a mean PFL concentration of 8.45 mmol/l compared with 2.1 mmol/l in horses with a non-strangulating obstruction.[2] Serial PFL measurements have also

been used to determine the need for surgery; a positive increase in PFL concentration over time ($[PFL]_2 - [PFL]_1 > 0$) and particularly an increase in PFL over time in horses with an admission PFL <4 mmol/l were useful for predicting whether a horses had a strangulating lesion.[3]

- It is important to recognize that PFL concentrations have not been investigated in horses with acute inflammatory intestinal disease or septic peritonitis.
- Cytology (hematoxylin and eosin; Gram stain) should be performed to identify any abnormal cells or intracellular bacteria.
- Culture and sensitivity testing should be performed in any case of septic peritonitis that is not associated with GI perforation.

Complications

Complications associated with abdominocentesis include enterocentesis and omental herniation in foals. If enterocentesis occurs, prophylactic treatment with antimicrobial drugs may be indicated. Omental herniation can be treated by resecting the herniated omentum, which often requires sedation and placing the foal in dorsal recumbency. Occasionally, a suture may need to be placed across the defect where abdominocentesis was performed.

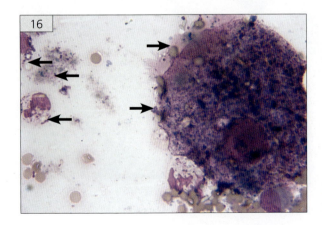

1.16 Intracellular bacteria and degenerate cells from a horse with a septic abdomen. (Courtesy Dr Raquel Walton)

Abdominal ultrasonographic examination

Indications

Abdominal ultrasonographic examination[3a] is not necessarily indicated in every horse presenting on an emergency basis with signs of GI tract disease. The major decision to be made on emergency admission of a horse with abdominal pain is whether or not abdominal surgery is indicated and this decision is primarily based on the persistence and severity of the horse's pain and other historical and physical examination findings.

Abdominal ultrasonographic examination can be useful when examining a horse with colic that is not particularly painful or the clinical signs are not necessarily consistent with a particular disease process. Ultrasonography can be used instead of palpation per rectum in small patients. Types of clinical situations in which abdominal ultrasonographic examination can be useful include:

- Identifying an area of peritoneal fluid accumulation for abdominocentesis (e.g. in a late-term pregnant mare). However, it is important to recognize that ultrasonography is not particularly sensitive for identifying small volumes of peritoneal fluid.
- Evaluating the volume and type of peritoneal fluid (e.g. hemoabdomen and peritonitis including ruptured viscus).
- Identifying distended and/or thickened loops of small intestine. In some cases, ultrasonography can be used to differentiate a strangulating from a non-strangulating obstruction (e.g. ultrasonographic examination can be used to differentiate primary ileus [p. 76] or proximal enteritis [p. 90] from a strangulating obstruction [p. 62]). Ultrasonography can also be used to identify thickened small intestine in cases of inflammatory or infiltrative bowel disease (p. 93) and proliferative enteropathy (uncommon) (p. 96).
- Diagnosis of jejunal, ileocecal (p. 66), and cecocecal/cecocolic intussusceptions (p. 101)

- Differentiating cecal (p. 98) from colonic impaction (p. 110).
- Identifying intraluminal sand (p. 113).
- Diagnosing nephrosplenic entrapment (p. 118) and right dorsal displacement (p. 122) of the large colon.
- Diagnosing large colon volvulus (LCV) (p. 104). A colon wall thickness ≥9 mm had a sensitivity of 67% and a specificity of 100% for diagnosis of a LCV[4], and finding a non-sacculated large colon ultrasonographically in the left ventral abdominal quadrant was consistently indicative of LCV in four horses.[5] Ultrasonographic evaluation is usually unnecessary in horses with a LCV because surgery or euthanasia is indicated based on the severity of pain and the author has found it insensitive for differentiating a LCV from colitis.
- Diagnosis of right dorsal colitis as a result of NSAID toxicity (p. 127).
- Evaluating the size of the stomach and wall thickness and irregularity (e.g. gastric outflow obstruction in foals [p. 51] and gastric impaction [p. 57]).
- Diagnosing diaphragmatic hernia.

Abdominal ultrasonographic examination can also be useful for evaluating the postoperative colic patient who is developing complications such as fever, colic, or persistent reflux.

Technique

As with any ancillary test, the value of the results are dependent on the skill of the operator and the experience of the clinician interpreting the findings, and they should be interpreted in conjunction with other clinical findings. Abdominal ultrasonographic examination is performed with the horse restrained and using a low frequency (2.5–3.5 MHz) curvilinear transducer.[6,7] The procedure can be performed without clipping the hair; however, if image quality is poor or the hair is long, clipping may be necessary. The skin or hair should be wetted with alcohol and ultrasound coupling gel used. The appropriate program for abdominal ultrasonography should be selected if necessary. Topographical locations for a complete examination include:[6–8]

- Left and right ventral abdomen from the sternum to the inguinal area to identify free fluid and distended small intestinal loops.
- Left and right paralumbar fossa or flank region.
- Left and right intercostal spaces from the ventral lung border to the costochondral junctions.

Recently, a procedure called fast localized abdominal sonography of horses (FLASH) has been described and the topographical areas included:[7]

- Ventral abdomen.
- Gastric window (left): examine the stomach at the 10th intercostal space (ICS) in the middle third (dorsoventrally) of the abdomen and then move the probe cranially and caudally for 2–3 ICSs. The normal adult horse stomach location is between the 7th and 10th or 11th and 13th ICS.[6]
- Splenorenal window (left): probe is placed at the dorsal and middle third of the abdomen at the 17th ICS to evaluate the nephrosplenic space for colonic entrapment (p. 118).
- Left middle third of the abdomen.
- Duodenal window (right): probe is placed in the 14th to 15th ICS in the dorsal part of the middle third (dorsoventrally) of the abdomen.
- Right middle third of the abdomen.
- Cranial ventral thorax just caudal to the triceps muscle to detect pleural effusion.

The normal duodenal, jejunal, cecal, and colon wall thicknesses are <3 mm. The normal stomach should be <7.5 mm thick. A small volume of anechoic peritoneal fluid is considered normal. Ultrasonographic findings are outlined under the specific diseases.

Complications
There are no recognized complications with abdominal ultrasonographic examination.

Intravenous catheterization
See Chapter 12, Fluid therapy.

Exploratory abdominal surgery (general surgical technique)
Indications
The most important factor that goes into making the decision for abdominal surgery in horses with colic is the duration and degree of the animal's signs of abdominal pain. If a horse's condition is deteriorating despite medical management and/or is non-responsive to analgesics (flunixin meglumine, xylazine, and butorphanol or detomidine), surgery or euthanasia is indicated. If the horse is not painful, emergency surgery is generally not indicated despite other abnormal findings on examination. It is important to distinguish dull demeanor from colic, because horses with enteritis or colitis are often dull, whereas horses with a surgical lesion usually demonstrate signs of abdominal pain. As with referral, the owner's decision as to whether or not they wish to pursue surgery for their horse is the overriding consideration.

Other factors that influence the decision for surgery include: tachycardia or an increasing heart rate; abnormal palpation per rectum findings; increasing abdominal distension; absent or decreasing borborygmi; and an absence of fecal production. Abnormal peritoneal fluid may influence the duration of medical management prior to surgery.

Additional diagnostic tests that may be considered in certain cases include: radiography in foals (see Chapter 9) and to diagnose enteroliths or sand impaction in adults; ultrasonographic examination to evaluate peritoneal fluid, intestinal distension, or masses; endoscopy to evaluate gastric ulceration; and laparoscopy in horses with low-grade recurrent or chronic colic.

Technique

The horse is anesthetized and positioned in dorsal recumbency and the ventral abdomen is clipped, aseptically prepared, and draped.

Ventral midline incision

- A 20–30-cm incision is made on the ventral midline from the umbilicus cranially through the skin, subcutaneous tissue, and linea alba (**1.17A, B**). An incision through the skin and subcutaneous tissue should be made initially, then a new blade used for the linea alba because the blade becomes dull during skin incision.
- Hemorrhage is usually controlled using mosquito or Kelly hemostats; alternatively, electrocautery can be used.
- Creation of 'score' lines (partial incision) through the linea alba or external rectus sheath should be avoided. If the linea alba or external rectus sheath is partially incised, the incision through the abdominal wall should be continued through these 'score' lines rather than making a separate incision immediately adjacent to it; this prevents weakening of the abdominal wall closure.

- Following the incision through the subcutaneous tissue, the abdominal wall can be entered through the linea alba, initially at or immediately cranial to the umbilicus. The linea alba is thickest, most distinct, and easily palpated at this location. An initial 2-cm incision is made by using the belly of the blade in a gentle backwards and forwards motion until the body wall is penetrated. Using the gripping end of the forceps to guard the abdomen from the blade, the abdominal cavity can be entered. Care must be taken not to cut onto the metal forceps as this will dull the blade.
- The peritoneal cavity is then entered bluntly using digital manipulation through the retroperitoneal adipose tissue and peritoneum.

Abdominal exploration

- It is important to keep the intestine moist during abdominal exploration and particularly during manipulation. Avoid unnecessary handling of the intestine. One method of abdominal exploration is described.

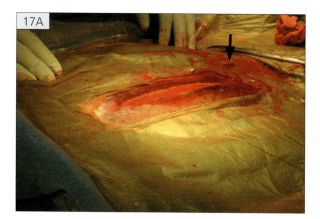
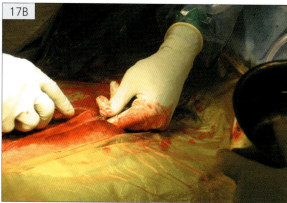

1.17A, B Ventral midline incision through the skin and subcutaneous tissue (A) and then extending through the body wall (B). Arrow, umbilicus. (Cranial is to the left.) (Courtesy Dr Samantha Hart)

- The first part of the GI tract identified in the normal horse is the cecal apex (**1.18A, B**), which lies along the ventral aspect of the abdomen. The cecum has a dorsally located base (cranial part or cupula, and caudal part), body, and apex. The base of the cecum cannot be exteriorized. The cecum has four tenial bands: (1) the lateral band on the right side of the abdomen giving rise to the cecocolic ligament, which attaches to the lateral free band of the right ventral colon; (2) the dorsal band, which gives rise to the ileocecal fold, which attaches the cecum to the antimesenteric border of the ileum; and (3) the medial and (4) ventral bands, which unite at the apex. The ileum enters the ventromedial aspect of the cecal base through the ileocecal orifice. The lateral and medial cecal arteries (veins) that branch from the ileocolic artery (vein) course within the lateral and medial bands. Common surgical disorders of the cecum include: impaction (p. 98); rupture (p. 98); infarction (p. 104); and cecocolic, cecocecal, and ileocecal intussusception (p. 89). Surgical procedures include partial typhlotomy, typhlectomy, and ileo- and jejunocecostomy.[8a]

- The cecum empties into the right ventral colon at the cecocolic orifice. The ascending or large colon (**1.19**) can be found by first identifying the cecocolic ligament and following the ventral colon to the pelvic flexure, which should lie in the left caudal abdomen. Alternatively, the pelvic flexure can be identified first. The large colon is evaluated by first exteriorizing the pelvic flexure and then gently lifting the remaining large colon from the abdomen. The large colon is attached to the dorsal body wall at the right dorsal colon only.

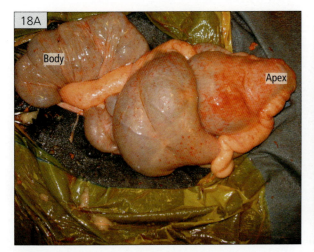
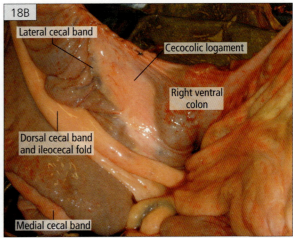

1.18A, B Cecal apex and body identified lying along the ventral body wall (A) and cecal bands with their respective folds and ligaments (B). (Cranial is to the right.) (Courtesy Dr Samantha Hart)

- Parts of the large colon to be identified (proximal to distal) are the right ventral colon, the sternal flexure, the left ventral colon, pelvic flexure, left dorsal colon, diaphragmatic flexure, and the right dorsal colon. The ventral colons have sacculations (haustra coli) and the dorsal colons do not. The right and left ventral colons have four tenial bands, the pelvic flexure and left dorsal colon have one antimesenteric band, and the right dorsal colon has three tenial bands. The right dorsal colon enters the transverse colon near the cecal base. The ventral colons are supplied by the colic branch of the ileocolic artery (vein) and the dorsal colons by the right colic artery (vein), which is a branch of the cranial mesenteric artery. The mesocolon attaches the dorsal and ventral colons.
- The large colon and cecum are commonly decompressed using a 14-gauge needle (18-gauge needle in foals) and suction (**1.20**). The needle is tunneled in the submucosa or subserosally before entering the intestinal lumen. A moist gauze swab is placed over the penetration site prior to removing the needle. Generally, if the needle is tunneled prior to penetration into the intestinal lumen, there is no intestinal leakage. If there is leakage or hemorrhage at the needle puncture site, an interrupted suture (3-0 synthetic absorbable suture material) should be placed across the needle hole. Surgical disorders of the large colon include impaction (p. 98), sand impaction (p. 101), enterolithiasis (p. 115), right dorsal displacement (p. 110), left dorsal displacement or nephrosplenic entrapment of the large colon (p. 106), tympany, infarction (p. 108), and volvulus (p. 104). Surgical procedures include enterotomy, resection and anastomosis, and colopexy.[8a]

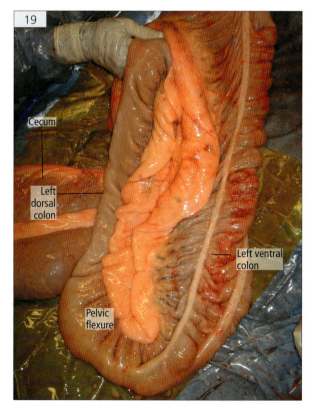

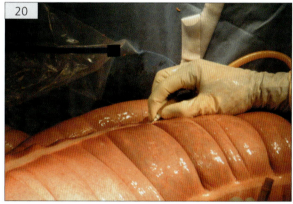

1.20 Colonic decompression using a 14-gauge needle and suction. (Courtesy Dr Samantha Hart)

1.19 Ascending or large colon with the left dorsal and ventral colon and pelvic flexure exteriorized from the abdomen. Note the tenia (bands) and haustra (sacculations) on the ventral colon and the lack of haustra on the dorsal colon. (Cranial is toward the top of the image.) (Courtesy Dr Samantha Hart)

- Enterotomy is commonly performed to evacuate the contents of the large colon. The colon is positioned on a colon tray (**1.21A, B**) or, less commonly, between the horse's hindlimbs. A 10–15-cm incision is made at the pelvic flexure and ingesta is softened and evacuated using water delivered via a hose placed into the dorsal and ventral colons. The enterotomy is closed in two layers using 2-0 synthetic absorbable suture material in a simple continuous pattern oversewn with a Cushing suture pattern.
- The right dorsal colon empties into the transverse colon, which cannot be exteriorized because of the short mesocolon; however, it can be palpated on the dorsal aspect of the abdomen as it courses right to left cranial to the root of the mesentery. It is important to carefully palpate the transverse colon as it can be a site for obstruction caused by enteroliths and sand.
- The transverse colon empties into the small or descending colon (**1.22**), which can be identified by its size, its location in the caudal aspect of the abdomen, a broad thick band on the antimesenteric border, sacculations, and the presence of fecal balls. There is also a mesenteric band. The small colon can be exteriorized by identifying a fecal ball in the colon, usually lying in the left caudal abdomen, and then gently

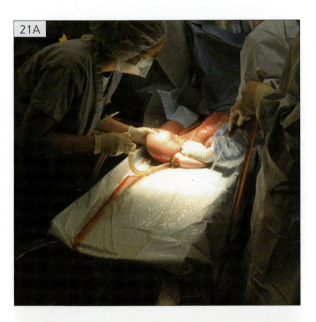

1.21A, B Large colon positioned on a colon tray (A) and pelvic flexure enterotomy (B). (Courtesy Dr Samantha Hart)

1.22 Descending or small colon. Note the prominent antimesenteric band and the fatty mesocolon. (Courtesy Dr Samantha Hart)

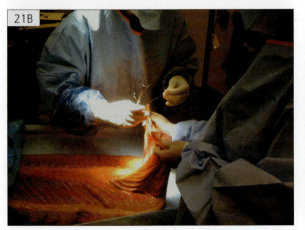

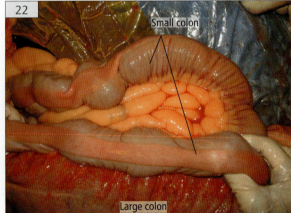

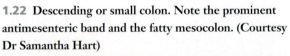

exteriorizing the proximal and distal aspects of the small colon from the abdomen. The proximal and distal 30 cm cannot be exteriorized; however, this can be followed in a proximal direction to the transverse colon and then in a distal direction to the rectum. The small colon is supplied by the middle colic artery, a branch of the cranial mesenteric artery, and the caudal mesenteric artery that branches into the left colic and cranial rectal arteries. Surgical disorders of the transverse and small colon are impaction (p. 130), fecaliths (p. 132), enteroliths (p. 115) and other intestinal concretions (e.g. trichobezoars, p. 133), foreign bodies (p. 133), meconium impaction, and atresia coli (see Chapter 9). Surgical procedures include enterotomy and resection and anastomosis.[8a]

- Following palpation and exteriorization of the colon, the small intestine can be identified by following the ileocecal fold to the ileum (**1.23**). The entire ileum cannot be exteriorized, but it can be followed in a distal direction to its opening into the cecum through the ileocecal orifice. The ileum is supplied by the ileocolic artery, a branch of the cranial mesenteric artery. The ileum is then followed in a proximal direction to the jejunum (**1.24**), which can be identified by its thinner wall and large arcuate vessels. Approximately 17–28 meters of jejunum can be followed in an proximal

direction to the duodenum. The jejunum is supplied by branches of the cranial mesenteric artery, which can be identified as large vascular arcades in the mesentery. When manipulating the small intestine it is important not to pull on the mesentery, because this can damage the arcuate vessels. Damage to an arcuate vessel results in ischemia of the intestinal segment supplied by the vessel, often requiring resection and anastomosis.

- The duodenum cannot be exteriorized because of its short mesentery, but it can be palpated. Once the jejunum is exteriorized, the duodenum is identified by first locating the duodenocolic ligament that attaches the antimesenteric border of the duodenum to the transverse colon at the duodenojejunal flexure. Beginning at the duodenocolic ligament and moving in a proximal direction, the duodenum courses from left to right caudal to the root of the mesentery and around the base of the cecum to the caudal duodenal flexure. The duodenum then courses in a cranial direction on the right side of the abdomen to the duodenal ampulla and cranial duodenal flexure (S-shaped sigmoid ansa) and then towards midline to the gastric pylorus. The stomach can be palpated in the left cranial abdomen. It cannot be exteriorized, but the greater curvature can be seen in horses with gastric distension.

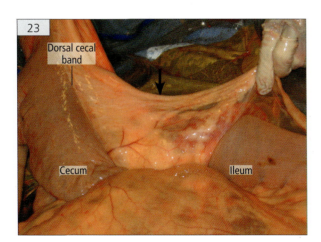

1.23 Ileum and ileocecal fold (arrow). (Cranial is to the right.) (Courtesy Dr Samantha Hart)

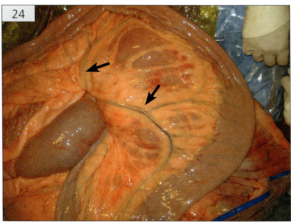

1.24 Jejunum with arcuate blood supply (arrows). (Courtesy Dr Samantha Hart)

- Surgical disorders of the small intestine include epiploic foramen entrapment (EFE) (p. 64), gastrosplenic ligament entrapment (p. 66), intussusception (ileocecal, and ileoileal and jejunojejunal) (p. 66), strangulation through a mesenteric rent (p. 69), strangulating pedunculated lipoma (p. 71), volvulus (p. 73), inguinal (p. 66) and other hernias (p. 141), ileal impaction (p. 80), ileal muscular hypertrophy (p. 88), ascarid impactions (p. 86), neoplasia (p. 88), and duodenal outflow obstruction (p. 56). Surgical procedures include jejunojejunostomy and jejuno- or ileocecostomy[8a] and, less commonly, duodenal/pyloric bypass techniques.
- Additional abdominal structures that should be palpated include: the liver in the cranial abdomen; the diaphragm; left and right kidneys dorsally; uterus and ovaries (females); inguinal rings (males); spleen adjacent to the left body wall; the nephrosplenic space between the spleen and the left kidney; and the epiploic foramen.

Body wall closure

- A visceral retainer may be used to keep the intestines in the abdomen and help to avoid inadvertent bowel penetration with the needle during abdominal wall closure. However, this is usually not necessary.

- The peritoneum is not sutured in the horse.
- The linea alba is usually closed in adult horses with #2 or #3 polyglactin 910 in a simple continuous pattern (**1.25A**). Bites should be placed 12–15 mm from the incision edge and approximately 10 mm apart. The subcutaneous tissue is closed using 2-0 synthetic absorbable suture (e.g. polyglactin 910 or polydioxanone), also in a continuous pattern. Staples or a simple continuous suture pattern with synthetic absorbable suture (**1.25B**) are used to appose the skin. Skin glue can be used for the skin if the skin is in close apposition following completion of the subcutaneous layer.

Complications

With early referral and surgical intervention the occurrence rate of postoperative complications decreases dramatically. Postoperative complications include colic, fever, incisional infection, shock, endotoxemia, diarrhea, salmonellosis, postoperative reflux or postoperative ileus, and adhesions. (See also Chapter 18.)

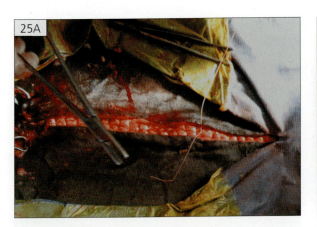
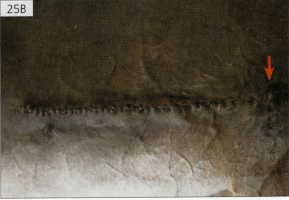

1.25A, B Linea alba closure using #2 polyglactin 910 in a simple continuous pattern (A) and skin closure using 2-0 poliglecaprone 25 (B). Arrow, umbilicus. (Courtesy Dr Samantha Hart)

DIGESTIVE SYSTEM DISEASES

Oral cavity

See Chapter 2 for mandibular and maxillary fractures and Chapter 6 for head and neck lacerations and puncture wounds.

Esophagus

- Esophageal lesions requiring emergency care are uncommon. Primary or secondary esophageal obstructions (choke) is the most common indication.

Esophageal obstruction (choke)
Key points

- Esophageal obstruction should be suspected in any horse with saliva and/or ingesta at the nares.
- A simple esophageal obstruction is relieved either spontaneously or with nasogastric tube passage (p. 30). Horses have an excellent prognosis.
- Underlying disease should be suspected in cases of recurrent esophageal obstruction.
- Horses with esophageal obstruction are at risk of aspiration pneumonia, esophageal perforation, and esophageal stricture. Early and appropriate treatment is necessary for a favorable outcome.

Definition/overview

Esophageal obstruction or 'choke' refers to an intraluminal obstruction of the cervical, thoracic, or abdominal esophagus. The obstruction most commonly occurs immediately caudal to the pharynx or at the thoracic inlet.[9] Other common sites are the mid-cervical region and cardia; however, obstruction can occur anywhere along the esophagus.

Etiology/pathogenesis

Esophageal obstruction occurs when feed is improperly masticated because of poor dentition, dehydration, sedation, the type of feed (e.g. apple, carrot, dry cubed or pelleted feed, inadequately soaked beet pulp), or behavioral reasons (i.e. greedy eater). Foreign body ingestion can also cause obstruction.[10] Poor dentition and inadequate dental care were identified in more than 90% of cases.[11] Sedated horses and horses recovering from general anesthesia are prone to esophageal obstruction and should not be fed until fully awake. Some horses are prone to choke during trailering. Choke was reported as a medical complication in an endurance horse during competition.[12]

Recurrent esophageal obstruction is more likely to be associated with a morphologic or functional lesion compared to a single episode of esophageal obstruction.[9] Horses or foals with any type of extra- or intramural or intraluminal esophageal space-occupying lesion, such as a vascular ring anomaly, ingested foreign body, granulation tissue, neoplasia, or stricture, are predisposed to obstruction. Obstruction has been associated with megaesophagus and esophageal diverticula.[9] Pharyngeal and esophageal dysfunction, such as that caused by guttural pouch mycoses or a brain lesion, can cause esophageal obstruction. Horses with gastric lesions, such as gastric impaction or gastric squamous cell carcinoma, can have secondary esophageal obstruction. In 34 cases of esophageal obstruction, 28 were due to ingesta impaction with no other lesion identified.[9]

Geriatric horses anecdotally appear to be predisposed with 40 out of 60 cases being more than 19 years old[11]; however, this may be a consequence of poor dentition. Ponies were reported to be predisposed to esophageal obstruction and this may reflect management.[11]

Clinical features

Horses with esophageal obstruction present with nasal discharge containing saliva and ingesta and excessive salivation (**1.26**).[9,11] Repeated attempts to swallow and muscle spasms in the area of the obstruction are commonly observed.[9,11] Horses may be dull or anxious. Some horses extend their head and neck, cough, show signs of colic, or sweat.[9,11] Eighty-eight percent of horses with choke had a palpable mass on the left lateroventral aspect of the neck.[11]

Heart rate, respiratory rate, rectal temperature, oral mucous membrane color and moistness, CRT, and intestinal borborygmi should be within normal limits in horses with simple esophageal obstruction. Heart and respiratory rates vary depending on the level of distress, the extent of fluid and electrolyte abnormalities, and esophageal damage. Oral mucous membranes will be dry with a prolonged CRT if the obstruction has been ongoing. Occasionally, esophageal perforation can occur if the obstruction is prolonged (**1.27**). An increase in respiratory rate and effort and fever may be observed in horses with severe aspiration pneumonia or intrathoracic esophageal perforation. Oral mucous membranes may be bright pink (injected), toxic or, rarely, cyanotic, with extensive pulmonary damage in severe cases of aspiration pneumonia or esophageal perforation.

Differential diagnosis

Guttural pouch mycosis; strangles; guttural pouch empyema; oral or pharyngeal lesion; pharyngeal dysfunction or foreign body; grass sickness; botulism; esophageal or gastric neoplasia; gastric impaction; vascular ring anomaly (foal); cleft palate (foal).

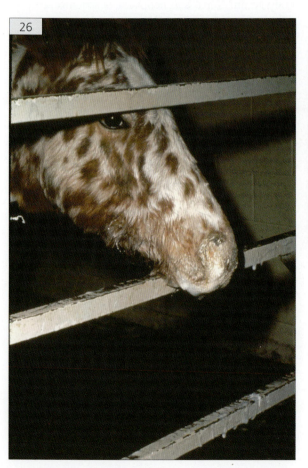

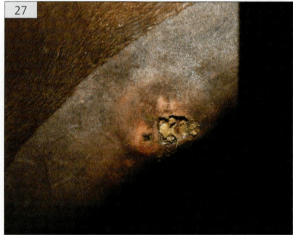

1.27 Esophageal perforation. Rupture of the esophagus has caused accumulation of ingested feed and saliva in the subcutaneous tissue and a severe necrotizing cellulitis. (Courtesy Dr Dean Hendrickson)

1.26 A horse with choke showing nasal discharge with saliva and ingesta. (Courtesy Dr Josie Traub-Dargatz)

Diagnosis

A diagnosis of esophogeal obstruction is usually based on a history of the horse being previously normal and then the finding of often profuse nasal discharge containing saliva and ingesta. A history of previous episodes of esophageal obstruction can aid in the diagnosis and may indicate an underlying disease. Knowledge of recent sedation or ingestion of carrots, apples, or pelleted or cubed feed can also help with making a diagnosis. Passage of a nasogastric tube into the esophagus is used to further support the diagnosis and estimate the location of the obstruction.

Esophageal endoscopy using a 1- or 3-meter video endoscope in foals and horses, respectively, can be used to obtain a definitive diagnosis (**1.28**), confirm the location of the obstruction, identify the obstructing material, and assess esophageal damage following relief of the obstruction (**1.29A, B**). The degree of the esophageal injury was associated with the development of complications.[10] While endoscopy and radiography are generally not required to obtain a diagnosis

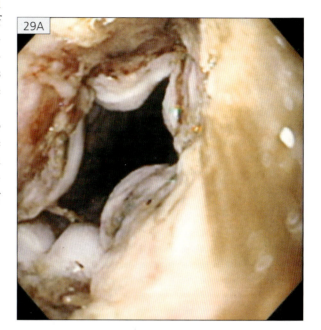

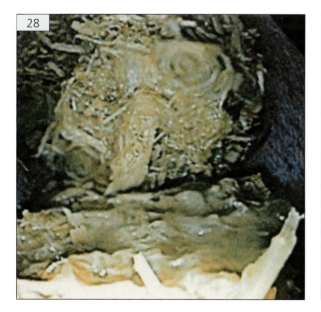

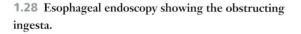

1.28 **Esophageal endoscopy showing the obstructing ingesta.**

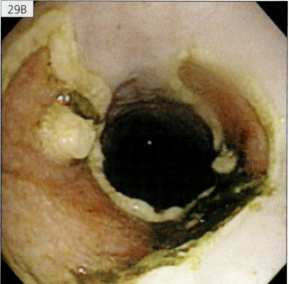

1.29A, B **(A) Esophageal endoscopy showing marked esophageal erosions following relief of a choke. (B) The same horse 12 days later. (Courtesy Dr Betina Dunkel)**

of esophageal obstruction,[9] plain and contrast cervical radiography can be used to confirm the diagnosis as well as diagnose esophageal perforation and any underlying disease. A diagnosis of underlying esophageal disease can be made endoscopically or radiographically following relief of the obstruction, particularly in cases of recurrent esophageal obstruction.

Tracheal endoscopy can be performed to identify tracheal contamination with ingesta. The likelihood that horses with moderate to severe tracheal contamination would develop aspiration pneumonia was higher than in horses with no tracheal contamination.[10]

Thoracic radiographic and/or ultrasonographic examination can be performed to diagnose aspiration pneumonia, which was reported to occur in 24–36% of cases.[9,10] Aspiration pneumonia was associated with a prolonged duration of obstruction; horses that had aspiration pneumonia had a median duration of obstruction of 18 hours compared with 4 hours in horses without aspiration pneumonia.[9] Male horses, horses <1 or >15 years old, and horses requiring general anesthesia to relieve the obstruction were also more likely to develop aspiration pneumonia.

Hematology and plasma biochemistry should be performed in horses with prolonged obstruction to evaluate for evidence of infection, electrolyte abnormalities, and azotemia.

Management/treatment

Many horses will resolve the obstruction without intervention. Initial treatment should involve sedation with xylazine and butorphanol, acepromazine (0.02–0.05 mg/kg IV), or detomidine and passage of a nasogastric tube. With the horse heavily sedated, lavage of the mass using tap water via the nasogastric tube can be performed. The nasogastric tube can be used to gently push the obstructing mass into the stomach. Some veterinarians recommend against lavage and manipulation of the obstructing mass with a tube and report that it is unnecessary and may be associated with aspiration pneumonia and esophageal damage.[11] If this is unsuccessful, the horse should be confined to a stall, sedated, treated with IV fluids and electrolytes, and have feed and water withheld. Flunixin meglumine should be administered to reduce inflammation at the site of obstruction. The horse should be muzzled or bedding removed from the stall. It is important to remember that anything given per os could be aspirated. The use of lubricants such as mineral oil and sodium carboxymethylcellulose to relieve the obstruction is not recommended because of the severity of pulmonary damage if aspirated. Oxytocin (0.11–0.22 IU/kg) is reported to cause esophageal relaxation and has been used to relieve the obstruction with variable success.[13]

The majority of obstructions (>80%) will resolve with sedation, rehydration, and withholding feed, either spontaneously[11] or with a single esophageal lavage.[9] If the obstruction does not resolve, general anesthesia with placement of an endotracheal tube and cuff inflation to prevent aspiration and resolution of the obstruction using endoscopic biopsy forceps, more aggressive lavage and manipulation, or, rarely, surgery is indicated. Feed should be gradually reintroduced, once the obstruction is relieved, with initial feeding of slurry and soft feed.

Any horse with signs of esophageal obstruction should be treated for aspiration pneumonia (see Chapter 3) with broad-spectrum antimicrobial drugs (see Chapter 16). The prognosis was good for horses with aspiration pneumonia with early treatment.[9] No problems with aspiration pneumonia were reported in 60 horses with esophageal obstruction.[11]

Esophageal stricture can occur in cases with extensive circumferential esophageal erosions (**1.30A, B**). Strictures can be managed medically[14,15] by feeding a soft diet or nasogastric tube feeding. Maximum stricture was observed 30 days following obstruction and the esophageal diameter increased rapidly thereafter and was normal 60 days following obstruction.[14]

An important part of management is to perform an oral examination with particular attention to the dentition. Recommendations with regard to feeding should also be discussed with the owner or manager.

The prognosis for horses with esophageal obstruction is excellent (>80%)[9-11] particularly if there is a short duration of signs, no complications, and no underlying disease. Aspiration pneumonia is the most common complication. Complications in addition to aspiration pneumonia include: esophageal stenosis/stricture, diverticula formation, necrosis, and rupture; esophagitis; diarrhea; renal failure; laryngeal hemiplegia; and laminitis.[10]

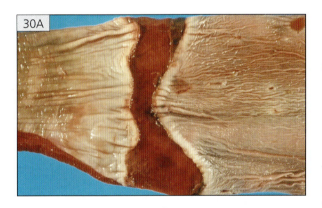

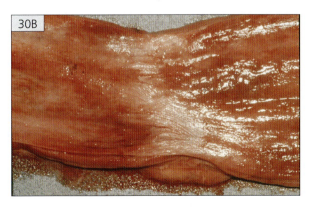

1.30A, B Circumferential, deep esophageal injury (A) and stricture (B). (Courtesy Dr Josie Traub-Dargatz)

Stomach

- Horses with gastric lesions can present on emergency with a variety of clinical signs ranging from acute colic to chronic dull demeanor, lethargy, anorexia, and weight loss. Bruxism, ptyalism, and dysphagia may also be clinical features. Gastric lesions are most often diagnosed using gastroscopy. Abdominal ultrasonographic examination can also be used to evaluate the size of the stomach and wall thickness and any irregularity.
- Gastric lesions requiring emergency management are uncommon.
- Treatment is usually medical and prognosis varies depending on the lesion.

Equine gastric ulcer syndrome
Key points
- Gastric ulceration is not a common cause of colic in adult horses and is rarely the primary lesion of horses presenting on an emergency basis with signs of colic. Gastric ulceration can occur secondary to other GI tract diseases.
- Foals with pyloric and duodenal ulcers can develop a gastric outflow obstruction and present with signs of bruxism, ptyalism, spontaneous reflux, diarrhea, postprandial colic, and lack of fecal production. Surgery may be necessary to manage these foals.

Definition/overview
Equine gastric ulcer syndrome refers to 'the disease complex that is associated with ulceration of the esophageal, gastric or duodenal mucosa'.[15a] Ulceration occurs on the non-glandular (squamous) and glandular gastric mucosa.[15b]

Etiology/pathogenesis
Gastric ulceration occurs when there is an imbalance between the protective and destructive mechanisms in the stomach.[16] Protective mechanisms include bicarbonate and mucous secretion and destructive mechanisms include hydrochloric acid, pepsin, bile acids, and organic acids. Prostaglandin E_2 promotes protective mechanisms including: (1) secretion of bicarbonate and mucous (glandular mucosa); (2) blood flow;

(3) production of surface-active phospholipids; (4) mucosal repair; and (5) sodium transport, which inhibits cell swelling.[16] Inhibition of prostaglandin can also increase gastric acid secretion. Therefore, inhibition of prostaglandin synthesis is thought to be one important factor in the development of equine gastric ulcer syndrome. Causes of prostaglandin inhibition are outlined in *Table 1.1*.

Ulceration of the glandular part of the stomach is thought to occur as a result of exposure to acid and concurrent loss of protective mechanisms. Non-glandular or squamous mucosal ulceration is thought to be caused by exposure to hydrochloric acid, pepsin, bile acids, volatile fatty acids, and other organic acids.[16–19] The squamous mucosa does not have a bicarbonate and mucous protective layer and responds to chronic exposure to acid by increasing the keratin layer thickness.[16,19] Causes of gastric acidity are listed in *Table 1.1*. Electrolyte supplementation can also damage the gastric mucosa, as can an indwelling large-bore nasogastric tube.

Clinical features

There are four clinical syndromes associated with gastric ulcers:[19a]
- Subclinical gastric ulcers.
- Clinical gastric ulcers.
- Perforating gastric ulcers with diffuse septic peritonitis.
- Pyloric and duodenal ulcers with stricture and gastric outflow obstruction.

Foals: Subclinical gastric ulcers are common, usually occur in foals <4 months of age, and are most often seen in the non-glandular mucosa along the greater curvature of the stomach adjacent to the margo plicatus.

Clinical ulcers usually occur in foals <9 months of age and are most often seen in the non-glandular mucosa adjacent to the margo plicatus or in the glandular mucosa. Diarrhea, inappetence, failure to thrive, rough hair coat, pot belly, and colic are common

Table 1.1 Factors that can inhibit prostaglandin synthesis and prolong exposure of the gastric mucosa to acid

FACTOR	MECHANISM
Inhibition of prostaglandin synthesis	
Parturition	↑ Endogenous corticosteroids
Stress associated with training or critical illness	↑ Endogenous corticosteroids
Stall confinement	↑ Endogenous corticosteroids
Non-steroidal anti-inflammatory drugs	Inhibition of cyclooxygenase
Gastric acid exposure	
Infrequent nursing	Milk is thought to buffer gastric acid
Recumbency	↑ Exposure of non-glandular mucosa to acid
Delayed gastric emptying	↑ Exposure of non-glandular mucosa to acid
Infrequent feed consumption/feed deprivation	↓ Absorption of acid and ↓ salivary bicarbonate
High concentrate diet	Carbohydrate fermentation with production of volatile fatty acids; ↑ exposure of mucosa to bile salts and pepsin
Low roughage diet	Roughage stimulates bicarbonate-rich saliva; alfalfa hay has high calcium and protein concentration, which is thought to be protective

clinical signs. Larger ulcers are associated with more severe signs of colic including rolling and lying in dorsal recumbency.

Foals with perforating gastric ulcers often do not present until signs of septic peritonitis and shock become apparent.

Pyloric and duodenal ulcers can cause stricture with subsequent gastric outflow obstruction and are seen most often in foals 3–6 months of age. Bruxism and ptyalism are the most common clinical signs.[20,21] Drooling of milk, spontaneous reflux, diarrhea, post-prandial colic, and lack of fecal production are also seen. Concurrent diseases include aspiration pneumonia, cholangitis, and esophagitis.[20]

Horses: Subclinical gastric ulcers are probably most common.[16] They occur most often in the non-glandular mucosa adjacent to the margo plicatus. Clinical signs include acute and recurrent colic, weight loss and poor condition, inappetence, and poor performance. While there is no correlation between ulcer severity and clinical signs, horses with clinical signs usually have more severe ulcers compared with horses without clinical signs.[16]

Gastric ulceration can occur secondary to other GI tract diseases: 49% of horses admitted for colic to a referral hospital had gastric ulceration and horses that were managed medically were more likely to have gastric ulcers (63%) than surgical cases (37%). Sixty-eight percent of horses diagnosed with proximal enteritis, 32% with a large colon impaction, and 14% with LCV had gastric ulceration.[22] Gastric ulceration in colic patients can be attributed to many of the factors listed in *Table 1.1*.

Differential diagnosis

Jejunal intussusception (foals); enteritis or enterocolitis (foals); ileocecal intussusception (young horses); infiltrative or inflammatory bowel disease; gas or spasmodic colic; large colon impaction; right dorsal displacement of the large colon; nephrosplenic ligament entrapment (NSLE) of the large colon.

Diagnosis

A diagnosis of equine gastric ulcer disease is made based on clinical signs, endoscopy, and response to treatment.[16]

Gastric ulcers are diagnosed using gastroscopy. A 3-meter video endoscope is required to assess the stomach of adult horses; a 1-meter endoscope is usually adequate for neonatal foals. Feed should be withheld for 18–24 hours in adult horses and for 4 hours in foals to allow adequate visibility of the gastric mucosa. A scoring system for gastric ulcers is shown in *Table 1.2*

SCORE	DESCRIPTION
Table 1.2 **Practitioner's simplified scoring system for gastric ulcers**[19a]	
0	Intact mucosal epithelium. Mild reddening or mild hyperkeratosis
1	Small single or small multifocal lesions
2	Large single or large multifocal lesions or extensive superficial lesions
3	Extensive and often coalescing lesions with areas of deep ulceration

(**1.31A-D–1.34**). Lesions are seen most commonly on the non-glandular or squamous mucosa in both adult horses and foals.[16] The location, severity, and response to treatment are assessed with gastroscopy.

Serum sucrose concentration has also been described as a potential screening test for gastric ulcers. Feed is withheld for 20 hours. A sample of blood is collected prior to sucrose administration. Horses are

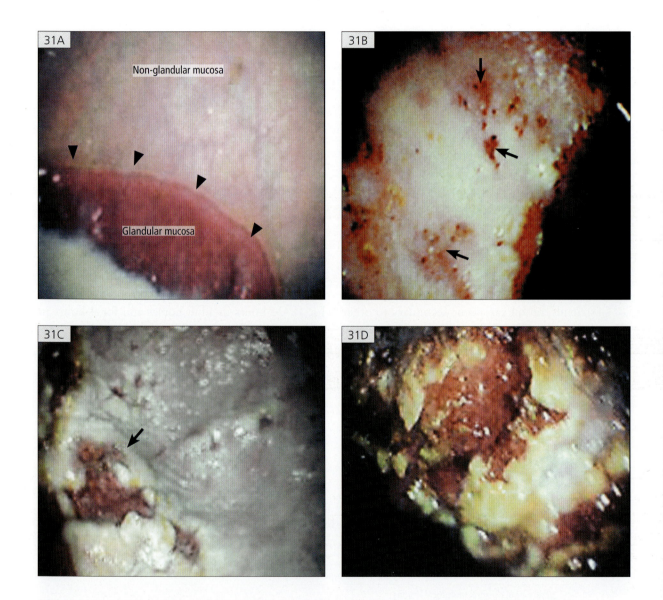

1.31A–D Gastroscopic images of the practitioner scoring system for gastric ulcers. (A) grade 0, no gastric ulceration; (B) grade 1, small ulcers; (C) grade 2, large ulcers; (D) grade 3, extensive, coalescing, and deep ulcers. Arrows, ulcers; arrowheads, margo plicatus. (Courtesy Dr James Orsini)

administered 250 g of table sugar (sucrose) as a 10% solution in tap water (i.e. 2.5 liters tap water) via a nasogastric tube. Serum sucrose concentration was increased at 30–90 minutes following sucrose administration and peaked at 45 minutes. Horses with no ulceration had a serum sucrose concentration of 0.30 +/− 0.43 mmol/l (103 +/− 146 pg/ml), horses with grade 1 ulcers 1.57 +/− 1.34 mmol/l (537 +/− 459 pg/ml), horses with grade 2 ulcers 4.17 +/− 0.46 mmol/l (1,427 +/− 157 pg/ml), and horses with grade 3 ulcers 9.92 +/− 1.1 mmol/l (3,394 +/− 368 pg/ml), all 45 minutes after sucrose administration.[23] While this test is not routinely performed, it could be considered where gastroscopic examination is unavailable.

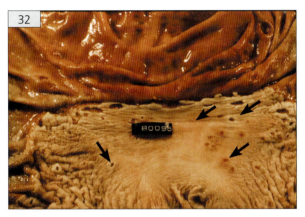

1.32 Small (grade 1) gastric ulcers identified at necropsy (arrows).

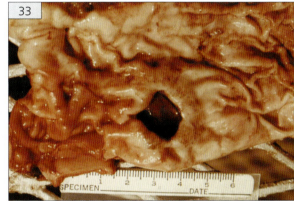

1.33 Large single ulcer in the non-gladular or squamous mucosa identified at necroscopy.

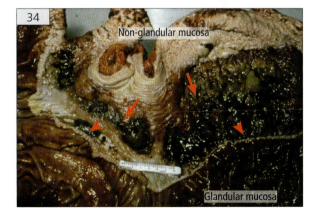

1.34 Extensive, coalescing, and deep gastric ulcers (grade 3) identified at necropsy (arrows). Arrowheads, margo plicatus.

Pyloric and duodenal ulcers with subsequent gastric outflow obstruction in foals can be tentatively diagnosed based on the age of the foal and clinical signs. The diagnosis can be confirmed using abdominal ultrasonographic examination, endoscopic examination of the esophagus, stomach, and duodenum, and upper GI contrast radiography (**1.35**).[20] Abdominal ultrasonography can be used to identify gastric distension and, rarely, duodenal abnormalities. In addition to gastric ulceration, esophageal mucosal ulceration viewed endoscopically is indicative of reflux esophagitis, which is consistent with the syndrome. Delayed gastric emptying is diagnosed with upper GI contrast radiography.[20]

Management/treatment of gastric ulcers

Gastric ulcer medication includes proton pump inhibitors, histamine (H2) receptor antagonists, prostaglandin analogs, and sucralfate.

Omeprazole: Omeprazole is a proton pump inhibitor that acts by blocking secretion of H+ at the parietal cell membrane H+–K+ pump. The current recommended dosage of omeprazole is 4 mg/kg PO q24h for treatment of gastric ulcers and 1 mg/kg PO q24h to prevent recurrence of gastric ulcers. Omeprazole paste was more effective than a compounded omeprazole suspension[24] and more effective than ranitidine for treating gastric ulcers.[25] Indiscriminate use of omeprazole in hospitalized horses with GI disease could potentially increase the risk of nosocomial infection because the higher gastric pH may alter the immune barrier provided by an acidic gastric environment. Use of omeprazole in critically ill patients, particularly those with GI tract disease, is only recommended following definitive diagnosis of gastric ulceration with gastroscopy.

Pantoprazole is a second-generation proton pump inhibitor. It may be used at 1.5 mg/kg IV in foals that are unable to tolerate oral drug administration.[16]

H2-receptor antagonists: H2-receptor antagonists act by binding to and competitively inhibiting parietal cell histamine receptors and consequently blocking hydrochloric acid secretion. Ranitidine and cimetidine are the two drugs commonly used in horses; however, cimetidine did not heal gastric ulcers in horses even at high doses and its use is currently not recommended.[16] The recommended dosage for ranitidine is 6.6 mg/kg PO q8h or 1.5 mg/kg IV q8h.[16]

Prostaglandin analogs: Prostaglandin analogs (prostaglandin E_1) enhance mucosal protection by stimulating mucus and bicarbonate production. The recommended dosage for prostaglandin analogs is 1–4 μg/kg PO q24h.[16] Complications may include colic and diarrhea.

Sucralfate: Sucralfate is a sulfated polysaccharide, which is a combination of octasulfate and aluminium hydroxide.[16] Sucralfate adheres to the ulcerated mucosa and forms a proteinacious bandage, stimulates prostaglandin E2 and mucus secretion, inactivates pepsin, and adsorbs bile acids. The current recommended dosage is 20–40 mg/kg PO q8h. Sucralfate can be used to manage horses with underlying GI disease that are suspected of having esophageal or gastric ulcers, particularly horses undergoing repeated nasogastric tube passage or those that have an indwelling nasogastric tube.

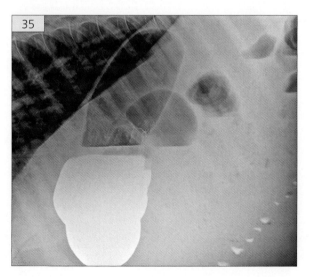

1.35 Upper gastrointestinal contrast radiography showing retention of barium in the stomach at 1 hour. The foal was found to have a duodenal stricture at surgery.

Management/treatment of pyloric and duodenal ulcers with stricture and gastric outflow obstruction

Gastric outflow obstruction in foals can be managed medically initially with antiulcer medication (i.e. sucralfate, omeprazole, ranitidine, prostaglandin analogues), withholding feed or providing small frequent feedings of milk, IV fluids (see Chapter 12), and total parenteral nutrition (see Chapter 15). Pain management can be provided as needed with butorphanol or alpha-2 agonists (see Chapter 14). NSAIDs should be avoided. Nasogastric tube passage is necessary to relieve gastric accumulation of water, milk, or feed if the foal is allowed to ingest anything and is always indicated when the foal shows signs of colic. Gastric rupture (p. 60) can occur in these foals.

Foals presenting with gastric outflow obstruction secondary to pyloric and duodenal ulcers may require surgical management with gastroduodenostomy or gastrojejunostomy, with or without jejunojejunostomy.[20,21] The decision to perform surgery can be difficult and is based on failure to respond to medical management over 1–3 weeks (i.e. persistent postprandial colic), retention of contrast material within the stomach for longer than 1 hour, or endoscopic evidence of duodenal stricture.

The overall short-term survival for horses with gastric outflow obstruction undergoing gastroduodenostomy or gastrojejunostomy, with or without jejunojejunostomy, was recently reported to be 92–100%[20,21] and 50–69% survived more than 2 years or to racing age.[20,21] All foals with pyloric obstruction, 52% foals with duodenal obstruction, and 75% of foals with obstruction of the pylorus and duodenum survived more than 2 years postoperatively. Obstruction of the duodenum, adhesions to the duodenum, and postoperative ileus were significantly associated with decreased long-term survival.[20]

Gastric impaction
Key points
- Gastric impaction is an uncommon cause of colic in horses.
- Gastric impaction should be considered as a differential diagnosis for persistent colic particularly if there are concurrent signs of anorexia, lethargy, weight loss, ptyalism, and/or spontaneous reflux.

Definition/overview
Gastric impaction refers to accumulation of ingesta in the stomach (**1.36**) and can be primary or secondary.

Etiology/pathogenesis
Primary gastric impaction occurs as a result of accumulation of dry, fibrous ingesta.[26–28] Proposed causes include poor hay quality, irregular feeding, ingestion of feeds that tend to swell (e.g. wheat, barley, and sugar beet pulp), and dental disease.[29] A disturbance of gastric function is a likely cause in horses with an extremely large and chronic gastric impaction. Recently, some horses with gastric impaction were found to have gross

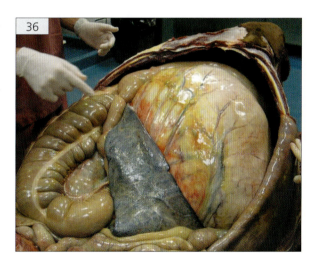

1.36 Gastric impaction. (Courtesy Dr Perry Habecker)

muscular thickening of the stomach wall and histologically focal fibrosis or myositis; however, whether these findings were a cause or an effect of the gastric impaction was not assertained.[29a] Persimmon seeds and mesquite beans have been identified as causes of gastric impaction.[30–32]

Pyloric stenosis can cause secondary gastric impaction. Causes of pyloric stenosis include congenital hypertrophic pyloric stenosis and acquired pyloric stenosis, most commonly from gastroduodenal ulceration and chronic inflammation, or neoplasia.[29] Other gastrointestinal disease (e.g. epiploic foramen entrapment) can also cause secondary gastric impaction.[29a] Gastric impaction has been associated with primary hepatic disease[33] and ragwort (*Senecio jacobaea*) or pyrrolizidine alkaloid (*Crotalaria* spp.) (see Chapter 10) poisoning, which primarily cause chronic liver disease.[34,35]

Clinical features
Horses with gastric impaction can present with clinical signs including colic, which may be acute and mild to severe, or chronic and intermittent. Other clinical features include anorexia, lethargy, weight loss, bruxism, ptyalism, and dysphagia. Gastronasal reflux with secondary aspiration pneumonia (see Chapter 3) can also be a feature. These horses are predisposed to gastric rupture (p. 60) and can present with signs of severe shock secondary to rupture.[29a]

Differential diagnosis
Esophageal obstruction; gastric neoplasia; gastroduodenal ulceration; gastric outflow obstruction; diaphragmatic hernia.

Diagnosis
Gastric impaction can be definitively diagnosed with gastroscopy and abdominal ultrasonography or at surgery or necropsy.[29a]

Management/treatment
Medical treatment includes gastric lavage using a nasogastric tube with warm water with or without mineral oil (2–4 ml/kg) or dioctyl sodium sulfosuccinate (0.2 g/kg in approximately 2–4 liters water for a 500 kg horse). Surgery is indicated if medical management is unsuccessful. In most cases the impaction can be resolved at surgery with instillation of water via an indwelling stomach tube or sterile isotonic fluid via a needle inserted adjacent to the greater curvature, and massage of the impacting mass. Gastric impaction can also be relieved rarely via a gastrotomy. Analgesia can be provided with flunixin meglumine. Intravenous fluid therapy (see Chapter 12) is often necessary. Antimicrobial drug therapy (see Chapter 16) should be used in horses with suspected or confirmed aspiration pneumonia . The prognosis for horses with gastric impaction is variable and dependent on the underlying cause. Some horses have an apparent gastric motility disturbance and the stomach can become enormous. The prognosis for these cases is poor. Recently, the survival for horses diagnosed with a gastric impaction was reported to be 5 out of 12, with the main causes of non-survival being gastric rupture, recurrent gastric impaction, or euthanasia for another primary intestinal disease.[29a]

Gastric neoplasia
Key points
- Gastric neoplasia should be considered in horses presenting for colic with severe and rapid weight loss with or without signs referable to the esophagus or stomach.
- Diagnosis can be made using gastroscopy, ultrasonography, and peritoneal fluid analysis.
- The prognosis is grave and euthanasia is recommended.

Definition
The most common gastric neoplasia in horses is squamous cell carcinoma (SCC).[36–38] SCC is associated with the cardia and fundus. Other neoplastic diseases include lymphoma, leiomyoma, leiomyosarcoma, adenocarcinoma, and mesothelioma.[29,38,39] Gastric neoplasia is rare in horses.

Etiology/pathogenesis
The etiology and pathogenesis of gastric neoplasia in horses is unknown.

Clinical features

Clinical signs most often associated with gastric SCC as well as other gastric neoplasias are anorexia or inappetence, weight loss, lethargy, and fever.[36–40] Abdominal distension, colic, tachypnea, dysphagia, ptyalism, and ventral edema are also clinical features. Abdominal masses were palpable per rectum in some horses.[36–38] Anemia, neutrophilia, hypoalbuminemia, hyperglobulinemia, hyperfibrinogenemia, and hypercalcemia have been observed.[36–40] Recurrent esophageal obstruction (Choke, p. 47) and pyloric obstruction can occur. Metastasis throughout the peritoneal and, in some cases, the pleural cavities is common.[36–38,40]

Differential diagnosis

Esophageal obstruction; gastric impaction; equine gastric ulcer syndrome; other causes of anorexia and weight loss.[41]

Diagnosis

Peritoneal fluid cytology is diagnostic for neoplasia in approximately 50% of horses with gastric SCC.[7,40] Exfoliation of neoplastic cells from the surface of the tumor is necessary for peritoneal fluid to be of diagnostic value. Gastroscopy and biopsy for gastric neoplasia[42,38] and thoracoscopy and biopsy for gastroesophageal neoplasia[43] has been used to make a definitive diagnosis. Abdominal ultrasonographic examination is also useful, particularly in horses with metastatic disease.[38] The diagnosis is often made during exploratory celiotomy[36] or at necropsy (**1.37**).[38]

Management/treatment

The prognosis for horses with gastric neoplasia is grave. Euthanasia is recommended following confirmation of the diagnosis, particularly if the disease is advanced. All horses with gastric neoplasia died or were euthanized and the median time from onset of clinical signs to death was 4 weeks.[38]

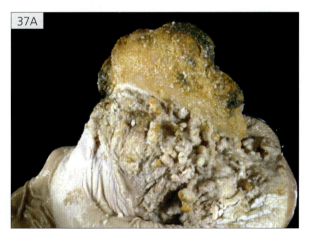
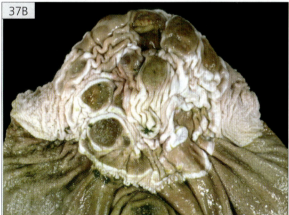

1.37A, B Gastric squamous cell carcinoma. (Courtesy Dr Perry Habecker)

Gastric rupture

Key points

- Horses with gastric rupture usually present with signs of shock and a diagnosis can be made with abdominal ultrasonographic examination and abdominocentesis/peritoneal fluid analysis.
- The prognosis for horses with gastric rupture is grave and euthanasia is indicated.
- Gastric rupture often occurs secondarily to a small intestinal obstruction and passage of a nasogastric tube is important in horses showing signs of colic to prevent gastric rupture.

Definition/overview

Full-thickness perforation of the stomach wall usually occurs along the greater curvature (**1.38A, B**) secondary to an increase in intraluminal pressure or a loss of gastric wall integrity. Gastric rupture was the reason for euthanasia in 11% of horses euthanized during abdominal surgery[44] and gastric rupture cases represented 3.0–5.4% of colic admissions.[44,45] Gastric rupture represented 20% of all GI tract ruptures.[46]

Etiology/pathogenesis

Small intestinal obstruction with secondary gastric accumulation of fluid and ingesta is the most common cause of gastric rupture, which emphasizes the importance of nasogastric tube passage in horses showing signs of colic. However, it is important to recognize that the presence of a nasogastric tube is not sufficient to prevent gastric rupture; 11% of horses that ruptured had an indwelling nasogastric tube.[44]

In 17–60% of cases, the cause for gastric rupture is unknown. There was no age, breed, or gender predisposition, or seasonal distribution in gastric rupture cases.[44,45] However, 50% of horses with gastric rupture were >15 years old.[47] Other proposed causes include grain overload, ulcerative gastritis, gastric impaction, nasogastric tube feeding, and trauma.[44]

Clinical features

The 'classic' presentation is a horse showing signs of severe colic that has progressed to dull demeanor. Horses generally present with signs of shock, including dull demeanor, sweating, muscle fasciculations, tachypnea, and reluctance to move. Tachycardia may initially be mild to moderate (60–70 bpm) and progresses to severe (80–120 bpm). Oral mucous membranes vary in color from bright pink to purple, are dry, and the CRT may be rapid initially followed by prolonged. Intestinal borborygmi are absent. Reflux was obtained following nasogastric tube passage in 40% of cases.[46] Abdominal

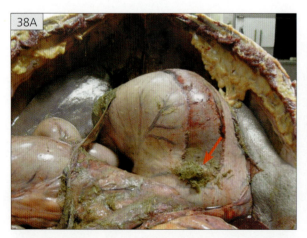
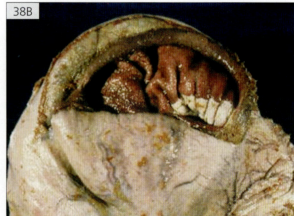

1.38A, B Gastric rupture along the greater curvature of the stomach. (A) Partial-thickness rupture with a focal full-thickness rupture (arrow) and abdominal contamination with ingesta. (B) Full-thickness gastric rupture. (Courtesy Dr Perry Habecker)

palpation per rectum may reveal a gritty serosal surface or free peritoneal gas; however, abnormal findings were more common in horses with colonic rupture than horses with gastric rupture.[46] Horses are usually leukopenic (leukocytes <4 × 10^9/l [4,000/µl]) and hemoconcentrated (PCV >0.5 l/l [50%]). Azotemia (creatinine >176 µmol/l [2 mg/dl]) and hyperlactatemia (lactate >2 mmol/l [18 mg/dl]) may be severe (see below).

Differential diagnosis

Cecal or colonic rupture; LCV; colitis (severe); enteritis (severe); small intestinal strangulating obstruction.

Diagnosis

A definitive diagnosis is made at surgery or necropsy. A tentative diagnosis can be made based on a history of moderate to severe pain followed by dull demea-nor with sweating, muscle fasciculations, tachypnea, reluctance to walk, severe tachycardia, and toxic mucous membranes. Horses are often febrile. Severe leukopenia (leukocytes <2 × 10^9/l [2,000/µl]), hemoconcentration (PCV >0.6 l/l [60%]), hypoproteinemia (total plasma protein [TPP] <55 g/l [5.5 g/dl]), and severe hyperlactatemia (lactate >8 mmol/l [72 mg/dl]) are typically observed.

Abdominal radiography can be used to diagnose pneumoperitoneum in cases of GI tract rupture in American Miniature Horses, ponies, and foals.[46] Ultrasonographic examination can be used to identify fluid and echogenic debris consistent with ingesta within the peritoneal cavity (**1.39A, B**) and can be used to identify an ideal site for abdominocentesis. Pneumoperitoneum can also be diagnosed using ultrasonographic examination.[46]

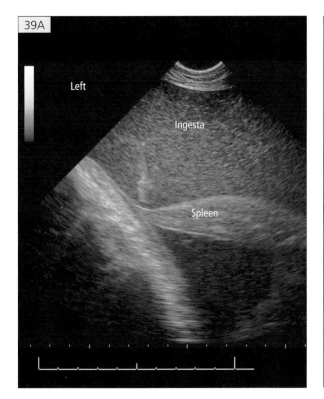
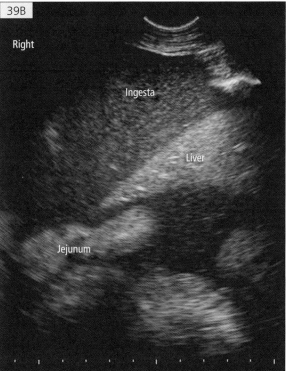

1.39A, B Ultrasonographic examination of the abdomen in a horse with a gastric rupture showing free fluid and ingesta within the peritoneal cavity. (Courtesy Dr JoAnn Slack)

Abdominocentesis can be performed to obtain peritoneal fluid. Gastric or other visceral rupture can be suspected based on the gross appearance of the peritoneal fluid obtained; however, cytology is necessary to distinguish intraperitoneal from intraluminal ingesta (i.e. from an enterocentesis) if abdominocentesis was not ultrasonographically guided. The appearance of intracellular bacteria on a Dif-Quik or Gram stain (**1.40**) can be used to make this distinction. Interestingly, peritoneal fluid nucleated cell counts were often erroneous because debris and bacterial clumps were counted and leukocytes were lysed.[45] Peritoneal fluid protein can also be within normal limits or low because of dilution.

Management/treatment

Euthanasia is indicated in almost all cases. Occasionally, an abdominal exploration is performed to obtain a definitive diagnosis. Rare cases with incomplete rupture or small perforation with no gross abdominal contamination have been managed with surgical repair of the tear.[48,49]

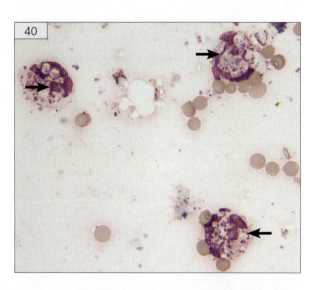

1.40 Intracellular bacteria identified in the peritoneal fluid of a horse with gastric rupture (arrows). (Courtesy Dr Raquel Walton)

Small intestine
Strangulating lesions

- Horses with strangulating small intestinal lesions usually have an initial period of moderate to severe pain that progress to more mild to moderate but persistent pain with dull demeanor and shock (tachycardia, injected or toxic oral membranes, poor jugular refill, and cool extremities) as the ischemia progresses.
- Tachycardia, tachypnea, and reduced to absent borborygmi are common physical examination findings. Rectal temperature is usually within normal limits.
- Abdominal palpation per rectum (p. 32) often reveals duodenal or jejunal distension.
- The presence of nasogastric reflux is highly suggestive of a small intestinal lesion, although not necessarily a strangulating small intestinal lesion (see Small intestine, Non-strangulating lesions). Nasogastric reflux is often not present initially, particularly with lesions affecting the distal jejunum and ileum.
- Abdominal ultrasonographic examination can be useful for identifying distended loops of small intestine and in some cases can be used to differentiate a strangulating from a non-strangulating obstruction. Horses with strangulating intestinal lesions often have an increase in the volume of peritoneal fluid identified ultrasonographically. There are usually markedly distended, amotile, and possibly thickened small intestinal loops in combination with more normal appearing and motile loops distal to the lesion (**1.41**).
- Peritoneal fluid is often serosanguineous (**1.42**) with a high protein and lactate concentration and a high nucleated cell count (p. 35). A peritoneal fluid:blood lactate ratio >1:1 is suggestive of intestinal ischemia (see Peritoneal fluid analysis).

- Surgery is always indicated for lesion correction. Jejunojejunostomy/jejunoileostomy or jejunocecostomy[8a] are generally indicated following resection of the affected bowel.[49a] Postoperative care following surgical correction includes IV fluid therapy, antimicrobial drugs (potassium penicillin and gentamicin) for 24 hours, flunixin meglumine for 4–5 days, antiendotoxin drugs, and motility modifying drugs (see Chapter 18).

- Common small intestinal strangulating lesions in alphabetical order include EFE (p. 64), gastrosplenic ligament entrapment (p. 66), intussusception (p. 66), strangulation through a mesenteric rent (p. 69), strangulating pedunculated lipoma (p. 71), and volvulus (p. 73). The small intestine can also become herniated with secondary strangulation including inguinal (p. 141), umbilical (p. 144), and diaphragmatic (p. 145) hernias.

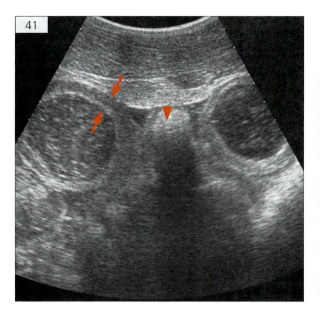

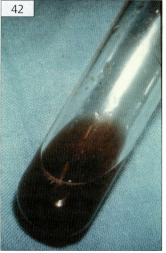

1.41 Ultrasonographic appearance of a thickened, amotile, and markedly distended loop of small intestine (arrows) adjacent to a more normal-appearing and motile loop (arrowhead) in a horse with a pedunculated lipoma causing intestinal strangulation. Note the mild increase in the amount of peritoneal fluid between the intestinal loops. (Courtesy Dr JoAnn Slack)

1.42 Serosanguineous peritoneal fluid from a horse with a small intestinal strangulating obstruction.

Epiploic foramen entrapment

Key points

- Crib-biting/aerophagia has recently been associated with EFE.
- Early referral and surgical intervention are critical for a favorable outcome.

Definition/overview

Entrapment of the jejunum or ileum through the epiploic foramen (**1.43, 1.44**). Jejunum or ileum passes through the foramen from left to right. The epiploic foramen (foramen of Winslow) is the opening into the vestibule of the omental bursa. It is found in the dorsal abdomen on the right side, cranial to the right kidney and adjacent to the caudate process of the liver. It is bordered by the caudal vena cava and caudate process of the liver dorsally and caudally, the portal vein cranioventrally, and the pancreas, right dorsal colon, and gastropancreatic fold ventrally.

Etiology/pathogenesis

While the exact etiology and pathogenesis have not been determined for EFE, risk factors have been identified. Crib-biting (cribbing, aerophagia, wind-sucking) is reportedly a predisposing factor for EFE. Horses undergoing an exploratory celiotomy that cribbed were at least 10 times more likely to have an EFE compared with horses that did not crib and >50% of horses with EFE cribbed compared with <10% of horses undergoing abdominal exploration for other causes of colic.[50] In a large controlled multicenter study, crib-biting/windsucking behavior was associated with an odds ratio for EFE of an approximately 70-times increase compared with horses that did not crib-bite/windsuck.[51,52] Other surgeons have questioned these findings, recognizing an association between this stereotypic behavior and colic, but not necessarily EFE.

Other identified risk factors for EFE were a history of colic in the previous 12 months, increased time in a stall in the previous 28 days, horses of greater height, and the daily care of the horse being provided by a non-owner.[51,52] Horses that were not fed at the same time as other horses and had access to a mineral or salt lick were at a decreased risk and horses that were easily frightened, excited, or inquisitive were at a lower risk compared with horses that were not.[51,52]

EFE usually occurs in mature horses, with a mean age of approximately 10 years.[53] It was previously thought that older horses were predisposed to EFE because of an enlargement of the epiploic foramen with age-related hepatic atrophy. It was recently shown, however, that horses with EFE are not older than

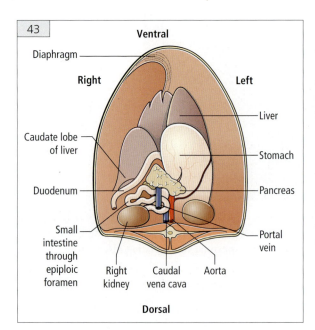

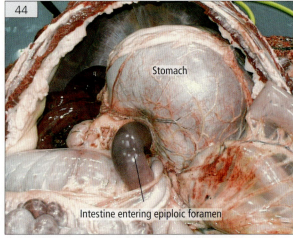

1.43, 1.44 Schematic illustration (1.43) and necropsy appearance (1.44) of small intestine entrapped in the epiploic foramen.

horses with other types of small intestinal lesions and the proportion of horses with EFE does not increase with increasing age.[53,53a]

EFE occurs most often in the winter months; 49% of cases occurred between November and February with most cases occurring in January.[51,52]

Clinical features

Horses with an EFE usually show signs of moderate and persistent abdominal pain (flank staring, pawing, and rolling). Abdominal distension is not a predominant finding. Heart rate may be within normal limits initially depending on previous analgesic administration, individual pain response, and extent of cardiovascular compromise. Horses become more tachycardic as intestinal ischemia progresses or as more intestine becomes entrapped. Respiratory rate is variable. Rectal temperature is usually within normal limits. Intestinal borborygmi may be ausculted initially but then rapidly become reduced or absent. Findings on palpation per rectum may reveal distended loops of small intestine. Reflux following passage of a nasogastric tube can be obtained in some cases; however, its absence does not rule out an EFE. An absence of distended small intestine on palpation per rectum and nasogastric reflux is often associated with a distal jejunum or ileal obstruction, which is common in horses with EFE.[54]

Peritoneal fluid is often serosanguineous; however, because the strangulated segment of intestine is sequestered in the craniodorsal aspect of the abdomen, peritoneal fluid analysis may also be within normal limits.

Differential diagnosis

Strangulating pedunculated lipoma (older horses); strangulation in a mesenteric rent; intussusception; segmental small intestinal volvulus; gastrosplenic ligament entrapment; proximal enteritis; ileal impaction.

Diagnosis

A definitive diagnosis is usually made during abdominal exploration or necropsy. Finding small intestine cranially on the right side of the abdomen between the liver and diaphragm during ultrasonographic examination is suggestive of an EFE (JoAnn Slack, personal communication, 2010).

Management/treatment

Abdominal surgery is necessary. The jejunum and ileum are most often affected and horses with EFE were more likely to have ileal involvement compared with horses with other types of strangulating obstructions.[53a] The entrapment is corrected by carefully manipulating either the proximal or distal aspect of the entrapped loop through the foramen. Particular care should be taken to avoid pulling up on the intestine as tearing of the portal vein may occur. Sodium carboxymethylcellulose can be used to lubricate the entrapped bowel to facilitate its manipulation through the foramen. If progress is not being made with simple manipulation: (1) the 'normal' distal aspect of the loop can be pushed further through the foramen from left to right and then the proximal part of the entrapped loop moved back through from right to left; (2) the contents of the intestine can be evacuated; or (3) the entrapped intestine can be transected and each part of the loop passed through the foramen independently. In some cases, the intestine is viable and decompression and replacement is all that is necessary. In many cases, a resection and anastomosis is necessary. Jejunojejunostomy or jejunoileostomy can be performed if the strangulation affects a more proximal segment of jejunum/ileum and a jejunocecostomy if a distal segment of ileum is affected.

Postoperative care includes IV fluid therapy, antimicrobial drugs, and flunixin meglumine. IV lidocaine, antiendotoxic and motility modifying drugs may be indicated. Feed should be reintroduced over 3–4 days if there is no postoperative reflux (see Chapter 18). Repeat celiotomy may be necessary in patients developing complications such as colic or postoperative reflux, which can be associated with ileus, obstruction at the anastomosis site, or adhesion formation.

While previous studies reported a less favorable prognosis compared with other causes of colic[55], more recently horses with EFE were more likely to be discharged compared with horses with strangulating lipoma or other small intestinal strangulating lesions.[54] The short-term survival for horses recovering from general anesthesia was 95%.[54] Recurrence is rare, possibly because of stenosis of the epiploic foramen (Dr Debbie Archer, personal communication).

Gastrosplenic ligament entrapment

Key points

- Incarceration of intestine through a rent in the gastrosplenic ligament is an uncommon cause of colic.
- The prognosis is excellent with early surgical treatment.

Definition/overview

The gastrosplenic ligament is confluent with the greater omentum and extends from the hilus of the spleen to the left part of the greater curvature of the stomach.[56] Jejunum or jejunum and ileum become entrapped most commonly and usually pass through the rent in a caudal to cranial direction.[56]

Etiology/pathogenesis

The cause of the rent in the gastrosplenic ligament is unknown and may be congenital or traumatic in origin.

Clinical features

Horses with intestinal incarceration through the gastrosplenic ligament were 8–23 years old.[56] Horses are often tachycardic and may be tachypneic. Distended small intestine is identified on palpation per rectum or abdominal ultrasonographic examination. Peritoneal fluid is usually serosanguineous with a mild to moderate increase in the TP concentration.[56]

Differential diagnosis

EFE; strangulating pedunculated lipoma (older horses); strangulation in a mesenteric rent; intussusception; segmental small intestinal volvulus; proximal enteritis; ileal impaction.

Diagnosis

A definitive diagnosis is usually made during exploratory abdominal surgery or necropsy.

Management/treatment

Abdominal surgery is necessary. Gentle traction is used to free the entrapped small intestine and enlargement of the rent may be indicated to facilitate atraumatic removal. Resection of the affected small intestine and jejunojejunostomy or jejunocecostomy was performed in all cases in one study.[56] The rent in the gastrosplenic ligament is inaccessible for closure and may be extended to the free margin of the ligament to prevent re-entrapment; however, this was not deemed necessary in a more recent report.[56]

(See Chapter 18 for postoperative management.) Reported complications included obstruction or stricture at the anastomosis site, postoperative reflux, incisional infection, diarrhea, laminitis, and postoperative intra-abdominal adhesions.[56] The prognosis was excellent with 13 out of 14 horses surviving to hospital discharge and 11 horses alive at long-term follow-up.[56]

Inguinal hernia

See Hernias, p. 141.

Intussusception

Key points

- A jejunal or ileocecal intussusception should be suspected in any young horse or foal presenting for acute colic.
- An ileocecal intussusception should be suspected in any horse <3 years old that has signs of recurrent colic with or without weight loss.

Definition/overview

An intussusception occurs when part of the small intestine invaginates or telescopes into an adjacent section of intestine (i.e. jejunum, ileum, or cecum). The part that invaginates into the other is called the intussusceptum, and the part that receives it is called the intussuscipiens. Jejunojejunal, jejunoileal, ileoileal, and ileocecal intussusceptions can occur (**1.45–1.49**). Ileocecal intussusceptions are most common, representing 74% of small intestinal intussusceptions.[57]

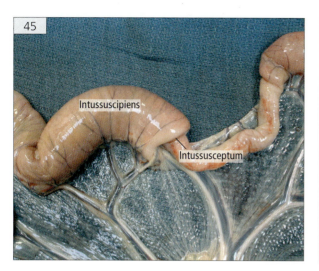

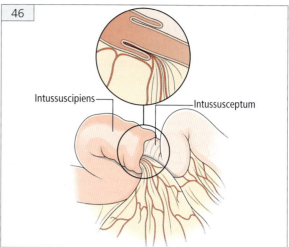

1.45, 1.46 Gross appearance (1.45) and schematic illustration (1.46) of a jejunojejunal intussusception showing the intussusceptum and the intussuscipiens. (Courtesy Dr Julie Engiles)

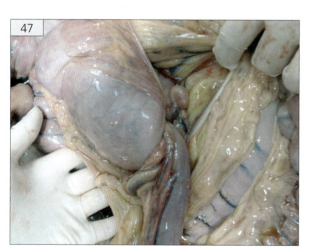

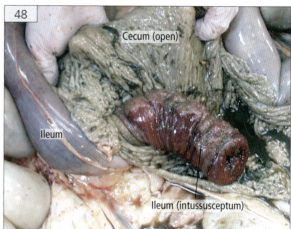

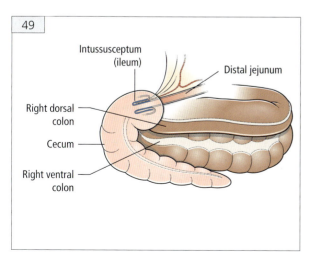

1.47–1.49 Gross appearance (1.47, 1.48) and schematic illustration (1.49) of an ileocecal intussusception.

Etiology/pathogenesis

An intussusception is thought to occur when there is a disparity in motility between adjacent intestinal segments. Intussusception has been associated with enteritis, diet changes particularly associated with weaning, ascariasis[58], cecal tapeworm infection (*Anaplocephala perfoliata*)[26,59], a pedunculated intraluminal mucosal mass (e.g. papilloma, granuloma) that pulls one segment of intestine into the adjacent segment, proliferative enteropathy with pseudodiverticula formation and jejunal muscular hypertrophy[60], transverse enterotomy in the small intestine[61], functional end-to-end anastomosis[62,63], end-to-end anastomosis[64], and the use of neostigmine.[65]

Clinical features

Young horses, <3 years old, are most frequently affected; however, a wide age range has been reported. Thoroughbreds and ponies are thought to be predisposed.[66] In 66 3–12-month-old foals, intussusception (ileocecal [n=5], cecocolic [4], jejunal [2]) and enteritis (11) were the most common cause of colic. Young foals (<3 months old) had only jejunal intussusceptions.[67]

Intussusception can be acute or chronic, with acute cases representing 73% of ileocecal intussusceptions.[57] Acute cases usually involve a long intestinal segment, whereas chronic or recurrent intussusceptions usually affect a short segment and do not cause a complete obstruction. Acute ileocecal intussusceptions were 6–457-cm long, whereas the chronic intussusceptions were less than 10-cm long.[57] Jejunojejunal intussusceptions usually present acutely and involve a long intestinal segment, whereas ileoileal intussusceptions are usually a very short dough-nut like segment.[66]

Acute cases present with signs of moderate to severe abdominal pain, tachycardia, tachypnea, and injected oral mucous membranes. A fever is often observed in horses with an ileocecal intussusception. Abdominal distension may be a feature in foals. Intestinal borborygmi are often absent.

Chronic cases usually have signs of recurrent mild to moderate colic, weight loss or failure to thrive, inappetence, insufficient fecal production, and low-grade fever.[66]

Reflux following nasogastric tube passage may be present in cases with a complete obstruction of sufficient duration to cause accumulation of fluid within the proximal small intestine and stomach.

Small intestinal distension can be identified on abdominal palpation per rectum. An ileocecal intussusception could be palpated in the right dorsal quadrant as a firm, tubular, painful structure in 30–50% of cases.[57,59,67] In chronic cases, the dilated thickened small intestine proximal to the ileocecal intussusception may be palpable.[67]

Differential diagnosis

- **Acute**: EFE; volvulus; proximal enteritis; primary ileus; ileal impaction; cecocecal or cecocolic intussusception.
- **Chronic**[41]: malnutrition; dental or oral disease; parasitism; infiltrative or inflammatory bowel disease; hepatic or renal disease; congenital GI tract anomaly.

Diagnosis

An ileocecal intussusception should be suspected in any horse <3 years old that has signs of recurrent colic with or without weight loss. An intussusception should be suspected in any young horse or foal presenting for acute colic. The final diagnosis is often made at surgery or necropsy.

Abdominocentesis and peritoneal fluid analysis can be performed (p. 35). Serosanguineous peritoneal fluid was obtained in 50% of horses with acute ileocecal intussusception; acute cases had a high peritoneal fluid nucleated cell count and TP, whereas chronic cases had high peritoneal fluid protein concentrations.[63,68]

Concentric intestinal rings (bull's-eye appearance) can be identified on abdominal ultrasonographic examination (**1.50**).

Management/treatment

Abdominal surgery is indicated for treatment of an intussusception. An attempt should be made to reduce the intussusception. Jejunal intussusceptions usually require resection of the ischemic segment and jejunojejunostomy.

Ileoileal and ileocecal intussusceptions can be managed by reduction only or reduction with bypass using an ileocecostomy if there are concerns about recurrence or obstruction postoperatively. Resection of any devitalized intestine is necessary. Reduction was not possible in 11 out of 16 ileoileal intussusceptions[69], 10 out of 19 acute ileocecal intussusceptions, and six out of seven chronic ileocecal intussusceptions. Resection of the intussusceptum through a typhlotomy[70] or bypass via a jejuno- or ileocecostomy can be used to manage cases that cannot be reduced.

In cases of acute ileocecal intussusception, bypass without reduction can cause hemorrhage and removal of the intussusceptum via a typhlotomy is reported to cause contamination.[68] Contamination can be minimized by suturing sterile plastic material (e.g. a sterile garbage bag) to the cecum as a drape. In chronic non-reducible cases, ileo- or jejunocecostomy can be performed as a bypass procedure, with a good prognosis. A hand-sewn technique is recommended because the proximal jejunum or ileum is usually thick. Long-term postoperative complications with this procedure include impaction at the stoma, ileal hypertrophy, and rupture distal to the stoma.

Tapeworms are often associated with intussusception and horses should be dewormed with pyrantel pamoate or praziquantel.

Strangulation through a mesenteric rent
Key points
- Small intestinal strangulation through a mesenteric rent should be considered as a cause of colic in broodmares and horses that have had a previous small intestinal surgery.
- Early referral is necessary for a favorable outcome.

Definition/overview
Mesenteric rents are defined as defects in the mesentery of the small or large intestine, with the small intestinal mesentery being affected most often (**1.51**).[71] Small intestine becomes entrapped in the rent and is often associated with a segmental volvulus of the entrapped intestine.

Etiology/pathogenesis
The etiology and pathogenesis is often unknown. Trauma, congenital malformations, and other primary lesions (e.g. ascarid impaction and ileal impaction) are likely etiologies.[71] Mesenteric defects can occur as a result of trauma associated with pregnancy and parturition. Interestingly, four out of 15 horses with mesenteric defects had a previous small intestinal resection procedure with either a jejunojejunostomy or jejunocecostomy.[71] However, the mesenteric defect was

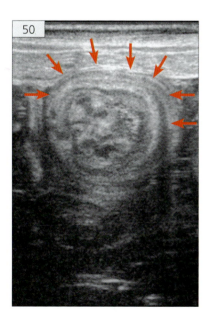

1.50 Ultrasonographic appearance of an intussusception. (Courtesy Dr JoAnn Slack)

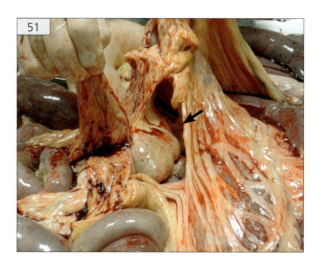

1.51 Mesenteric rent (arrow) through which a horse developed a segmental jejunal volvulus. Necrotic jejunum can be seen adjacent to the rent.

at a site remote from the original surgical site. This is likely to be related to a previous lesion or surgery, perhaps in association with mesenteric hemorrhage or focal necrosis. A mesenteric tear can occur adjacent to a mesodiverticular band (**1.52**) whereby the hernial sac formed by the band and the weight of the incarcerated intestine initiates a mesenteric tear.[71]

Clinical features

Mesenteric rents can occur in foals or horses of any age. Mares are likely affected more often.[71] Horses show moderate signs of abdominal pain, tachycardia, and tachypnea. Reflux following nasogastric tube passage is common, as is identification of distended loops of small intestine on palpation per rectum.[71] Peritoneal fluid is often serosanguineous with a high TP concentration.[71]

Differential diagnosis

EFE; intussusception; strangulating pedunculated lipoma (older horses); segmental small intestinal volvulus; enteritis; ileal impaction.

Diagnosis

Diagnosis is most often made during exploratory abdominal surgery or at necropsy.

Management/treatment

Surgical correction of the entrapment is necessary and resection and anastomosis of the affected intestine often required. Complications during surgery were common in one report and included an inability to reduce the obstruction and uncontrollable hemorrhage.[71] Other reasons for euthanasia during surgery were based on the length of the affected intestine, the presence of multiple rents, and an inability to close the mesenteric defect. Laparoscopic repair of a small intestinal mesenteric rent[72] has been described and should be considered in cases where the rent cannot be closed through a ventral midline celiotomy.

Postoperative complications were common in one report.[71] Long-term complications included adhesions and recurrence of the strangulating obstruction through a mesenteric rent. With early referral and careful surgical technique the outcome can be successful. (See also Chapter 18.)

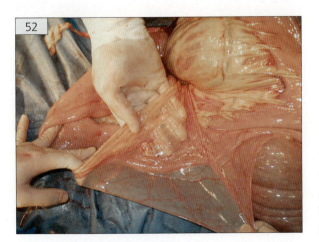

1.52 Mesodiverticula band (remnant of the vitelline artery) found in the distal jejunum. Intestine can become strangulated in a mesenteric rent that forms in the space.

Strangulating pedunculated lipoma
Key points

- A pedunculated lipoma causing small intestinal strangulation should be suspected in any older horse showing signs of abdominal pain.
- Older horses may not show as dramatic signs of colic as younger horses with a strangulating obstruction.
- Diagnosis can be further supported by identification of distended small intestinal loops on palpation per rectum, the presence of nasogastric reflux, and/or serosanguineous peritoneal fluid.
- Early referral and surgical intervention is critical for a favorable outcome.
- The prognosis for survival is good to excellent following surgery.

Definition/overview

A lipoma is an adipose (fat) tumor that is often associated with a pedicle (pedunculated lipoma). Lipomas are commonly found on the mesentery and mesocolon, as well as the intestinal serosal and peritoneal surfaces in the equine abdomen. Strangulating obstruction of the jejunum and/or ileum occurs most often (**1.53A, 1.53B**) and obstruction of the small colon (p. 135) occurs less frequently. The pedunculated lipoma can also strangulate a section of mesentery only, which may or may not affect bowel viability (**1.53C**). Strangulating obstruction associated with a pedunculated lipoma

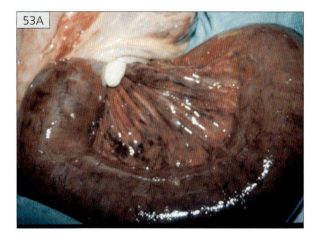

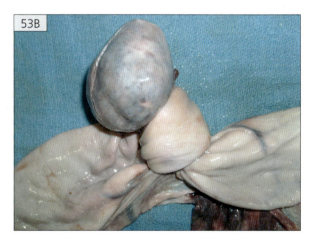

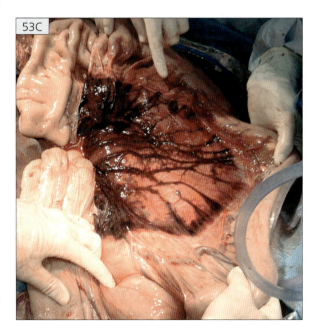

1.53A–C Pedunculated lipoma strangulating a jejunal segment (A) and a larger lipoma causing an obstruction of the jejunal lumen (B). (C) Strangulation of the mesentery only by a pedunculated lipoma. Note the line of demarcation. The bowel was viable and the mesentery hemorrhagic. Resection was not necessary.

occurs in adult horses and represented 10–15% of cases requiring abdominal surgery.[73,74] A large pedunculated lipoma weighing several kilograms was associated with recurrent colic in one horse[75] and another horse had spontaneous correction of a non-strangulating ileal obstruction caused by a pedunculated lipoma.[76]

Etiology/pathogenesis

The exact mechanism of intestinal strangulation is unknown. Pedunculated lipomas are commonly found incidentally at surgery, usually attached to the mesentery or mesocolon and occasionally to the omentum or the serosal surface of the intestine. In one study, lipomas that caused strangulation originated closer to the mesenteric route and weighed more compared with lipomas that did not cause strangulation.[73]

Clinical features

Old horses are affected more often than young horses.[77] The age of horses with pedunculated lipomas causing intestinal obstruction was older (16–19 years) than hospital- and colic-control populations.[53] Strangulating lipoma was one of the most frequent diagnoses made in geriatric horses at a tertiary care facility.[78] Pony breeds and Saddlebred and Arabian horses are reported to be at a higher risk compared with other breeds. Geldings were overrepresented compared with control hospital- and colic-control populations.[73,74] Pony breeds and Arabian horses as well as geldings are typically overrepresented in the geriatric horse populations, which may explain in part this predisposition.

Horses show signs of acute abdominal pain varying from mild (flank-staring and pawing) to severe (persistently rolling and thrashing). Some horses may be dull rather than show signs of abdominal pain. Geriatric horses may not demonstrate abdominal pain to the same extent as younger horses. Horses may be painful initially while the strangulated segment of intestine is viable; however, once the segment is non-viable or necrotic, signs of endotoxemia and shock (dull demeanor, mild abdominal pain, muscle fasciculations, cool extremities, tachycardia, injected oral membranes, reduced or absent borborygmi) may predominate. Respiratory rate is variable; however, geriatric horses may show nostril flare and tachypnea as a predominant sign of pain. Rectal temperature is usually within normal limits. Oral mucous membranes are pink initially but progress to injected or toxic and are usually dry. Intestinal borborygmi are usually reduced and are often absent.

Differential diagnosis

Proximal enteritis; primary ileus; EFE; intussusception strangulation through a mesenteric rent; gastrosplenic ligament entrapment; small intestinal volvulus.

Diagnosis

A strangulating lipoma should be suspected in any geriatric horse showing signs of abdominal pain. Distended small intestine on palpation per rectum (or abdominal ultrasonographic examination) is identified in most cases; however, its absence does not rule out a strangulating lipoma. Distended loops of small intestine could be palpated per rectum in most (13/17) cases.[79] Reflux following passage of a nasogastric tube is variable depending on the duration of clinical signs and the location of the obstruction (i.e. reflux may not be obtained early in the disease with strangulation of a distal jejunum or ileum). Horses with a strangulating lipoma were reported have 1–16 liters of reflux following passage of a nasogastric tube; however, half of the cases (9/17) did not have reflux.[79]

Abdominocentesis and peritoneal fluid analysis (p. 35) should be performed on any geriatric horses suspected of having a strangulating lipoma that is not particularly painful. Serosanguineous peritoneal fluid is strongly suggestive of a surgical lesion. In horses with a strangulating lipoma, peritoneal fluid was commonly serosanguineous (11/12 horses); however, this finding is dependent on the duration of intestinal strangulation. Peritoneal fluid TP, lactate concentration, and nucleated cell count are often high.

A definitive diagnosis is made during abdominal exploratory surgery or at necropsy.

Management/treatment

Early referral and surgical intervention is critical for a favorable outcome. Depending on the extent of intestinal damage, a resection of the strangulated intestine and anastomosis may be necessary. A jejunojejunostomy is performed if the jejunum is involved and a jejunocecostomy if the most distal aspect of the jejunum or ileum is involved. On rare occasions, the length of affected intestine is too extensive or inaccessible for resection and anastomosis and euthanasia may be necessary. Multiple non-strangulating pedunculated lipomas are often identified throughout a horse's abdomen and should be removed by pedicle ligation and transaction, if possible.

Postoperative care includes IV fluid therapy, antimicrobial drugs, and flunixin meglumine. IV lidocaine, antiendotoxic drugs, and motility stimulants may be indicated. Feed should be reintroduced over 3–4 days if there is no postoperative reflux (see Chapter 18). Repeat celiotomy may be necessary in patients developing complications such as colic or postoperative reflux, which can be associated with ileus, obstruction at the anastomosis site, or adhesion formation.

The most common postoperative complications are colic and postoperative reflux caused by ileus or obstruction at the anastomosis and, less commonly, intestinal obstruction associated with adhesion formation. The short-term prognosis is reported to be good with the most recently reported short-term survival rate being >80%.[53]

Small intestinal volvulus
Key points
- Small intestinal volvulus can affect the root of the mesentery or a segment of jejunum and/or ileum.
- Younger horses, particularly foals 2–4 months old, are more commonly affected.
- Horses with small intestinal volvulus are usually severely painful and rapidly begin to show signs of shock if not treated.
- Early surgical intervention is necessary for a favorable outcome.

Definition/overview

Rotation or twisting of more than 180 degrees of a segment of the small intestine around its mesentery.[66] Small intestinal volvulus can occur at the root of the mesentery or involve a jejunal segment (**1.54**).

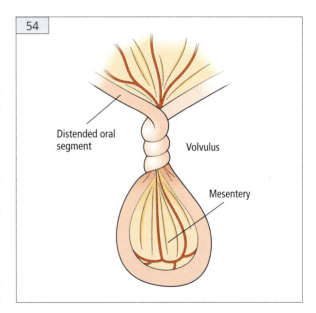

1.54 Schematic illustration of a segmental jejunal volvulus.

Etiology/pathogenesis

Small intestinal volvulus can be primary or secondary. Secondary volvulus has been associated with lipoma, acquired inguinal hernia, mesodiverticular band, Meckel's diverticulum, mesenteric rents, and adhesions (**1.55**).[77,80–82]

A volvulus is thought to occur as a result of hyperactive peristalsis adjacent to an intestinal segment, with cessation of peristalsis that may be temporary or permanent. Twisting of the intestine may occur at the junction of the hyperactive intestine with the amotile segment.[83]

Classically, small intestinal volvulus occurs most often in horses <3 years old[66] and in particular foals 2–4 months old.[84,85] It has been proposed that a change in diet from milk-based to solid feed can alter motility sufficiently to cause a volvulus. Thoroughbred horses appear to be most commonly affected.

Clinical features

Horses are usually acutely and severely painful and non-responsive to treatment with analgesia. Abrasions on the head and limbs are often seen because of the severity of the pain. In a recent study, 34% of horses had severe pain, 40% had moderate pain, and 27% had mild pain[85]; however, case selection for this study may have been quite liberal and included horses with a loose small intestinal volvulus secondary to another lesion. Abdominal distension is moderate to severe in horses with a volvulus involving the root of the mesentery; 13% of cases were reported to have abdominal distension at admission.[85] Horses are often tachycardic and tachypneic, and typically afebrile. Intestinal borborygmi are usually absent (61%) or markedly reduced (11%).[85] Reflux may be obtained following nasogastric tube passage; however, this depends on the duration of obstruction and lesion location (i.e. reflux is less likely if the obstruction is acute and the lesion is at the distal jejunum or ileum). Sixty-six percent of horses had reflux, with 4 liters being the median volume obtained (range 0.5–24 liters).[85] With a strangulation of longer duration and progression of ischemic necrosis, horses will begin to show signs of shock, with injected to toxic mucous membranes and marked tachycardia.

Differential diagnosis

EFE; intussusception; strangulation through a mesenteric rent; strangulating pedunculated lipoma (older horses); LCV.

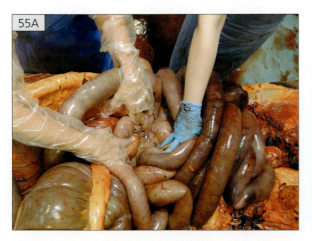
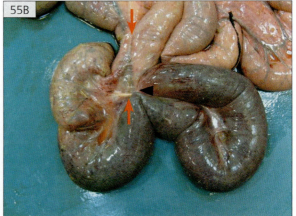

1.55A, B Jejunal volvulus involving most of the jejunum (1.55A). Ischemic necrosis of the affected jejunal segment is evident and resection and jejunojejunostomy would have been necessary. Segmental jejunal volvulus can also occur secondarily to an adhesion (1.55B). The red arrows demonstrate the adhesion and the black arrow the direction of the volvulus.

Diagnosis

Abdominal palpation per rectum (p. 32) can be performed in cases where the pain is responsive to analgesia. Distended loops of small intestine were palpated per rectum in 69% of horses.[85] Similarly, abdominal ultrasonographic examination (p. 39) can be performed to detect distended small intestinal loops if necessary. Peritoneal fluid analysis (p. 35) can be useful; however, in horses that are moderately to severely painful it is unlikely to alter case management. A tentative diagnosis can be made based on the horse's age, the severity of pain and/or signs of shock, and finding small intestinal distension on palpation per rectum (or ultrasonographic examination). A definitive diagnosis is made during abdominal exploratory surgery or at necropsy.

Management/treatment

Abdominal surgery is required to correct the lesion. If surgical intervention is early, a resection and anastomosis may be unnecessary. In horses with a segmental volvulus, resection and anastomosis is usually possible. If the jejunum is involved, then a jejunojejunostomy is performed and if the distal jejunum and ileum are affected, resection and a jejunoileostomy or jejunocecostomy is necessary. In horses with volvulus of the root of the mesentery involving >70% of the jejunum and ileum, resection and anastomosis is generally not possible because of the length of intestine affected. Therefore, the options are (1) to recover the horse and monitor it closely for signs of progressive intestinal necrosis (i.e. colic, reflux, tachycardia, fever, high PCV and hypoproteinemia, and leukopenia) or (2) euthanize the horse.

Postoperative care includes IV fluid therapy, antimicrobial drugs, and flunixin meglumine. IV lidocaine, antiendotoxic drugs, and motility stimulants may be necessary. Feed should be reintroduced over 3–4 days if there is no postoperative reflux (see Chapter 18). Repeat celiotomy may be necessary in patients developing complications such as colic or postoperative reflux, which can be associated with ileus, obstruction at the anastomosis site, or adhesion formation.

Recently, an overall survival rate of 58% was reported.[86] The survival rate was 80% for horses recovering from general anesthesia. The 20% of horses that did not survive following surgery had a higher heart rate, higher hematocrit or hemoglobin concentration, higher peritoneal fluid nucleated cell count, and higher pain score at admission compared with survivors.[86] Signs of colic after surgery and the necessity for a second surgery were associated with a poorer prognosis.

Non-strangulating lesions

- Horses with non-strangulating lesions of the small intestine can have a similar emergency presentation to horses with strangulating lesions, particularly on initial examination.
- Horses with non-strangulating small intestinal lesions that present with colic, however, are frequently less painful compared with horses with a strangulating obstruction, and often respond to medical treatment.
- Clinical features that may be used to differentiate a strangulating from a non-strangulating lesion include response to medical treatment (i.e. signs of colic and tachycardia abate with gastric decompression via a nasogastric tube and IV fluid therapy in horses with non-strangulating lesions); peritoneal fluid is typically not serosanguineous and has a lactate concentration equal to or less than that of the plasma in horses with a non-strangulating obstruction; and ultrasonographic examination may be used in some cases to differentiate strangulating from non-strangulating lesions.
- Some horses with inflammatory lesions may present with a chronic history of intermittent mild to moderate colic signs and weight loss.
- Abdominal exploration may be required in some cases to make the definitive diagnosis.
- Non-strangulating small intestinal lesions can be divided into: (1) functional obstruction including primary ileus and equine grass sickness; (2) mechanical obstructions including ileal impaction, ileal muscular hypertrophy, diverticula, ascarid impaction, adhesions, and neoplasia; and (3) inflammatory lesions including proximal enteritis (duodenitis–proximal jejunitis), inflammatory or infiltrative bowel disease, and proliferative enteropathy.

Functional obstruction
Primary ileus
Key points

- Primary ileus is generally used to describe cases of colic that have distended small intestine on palpation per rectum, with or without reflux following nasogastric tube passage, and that respond quickly to medical treatment, or cases with distended small intestinal at surgery with no other apparent lesion.
- Generally, horses with primary ileus have a good prognosis for survival; however, occasionally horses will not respond to medical or surgical management and euthanasia may become necessary.
- Ileus can occur secondary to many other problems (e.g. during the postoperative period and in horses with enteritis or peritonitis).

Definition/overview

Ileus or GI atony is a disruption of the normal propulsive GI motor activity due to non-mechanical causes. Ileus is generally used to describe horses showing colic signs who have distended small intestine on palpation per rectum and reflux following nasogastric tube passage and who respond rapidly to gastric decompression, analgesia, and IV fluid therapy, or horses with distended small intestinal at surgery with no other apparent lesion.

Etiology/pathogenesis

The etiology of primary ileus is often unknown. Electrolyte disturbances (i.e. hypocalcemia, hypokalemia, hyponatremia, or hypomagnesemia) causing alterations in neuromuscular function (see below), drugs (e.g. opiates), dietary changes causing alterations in digestion, and stress or pain causing alterations in the autonomic nervous system (see below) may contribute to primary ileus. Primary ileus is occasionally observed in the periparturient mare. It is also possible that these horses have very mild and self-limiting proximal enteritis (p. 90). Some horses may also have a primary enteric nervous system dysfunction.

Propulsion of ingesta along the GI tract is dependent on contraction of enteric smooth muscle in response to generation of an action potential (spiking activity). Each phase of activity moves along the intestinal tract.[87] Enteric smooth muscle generates slow waves (spontaneous oscillations of the membrane potential), which are inadequate to generate an action potential. Input from the enteric (intrinsic) and autonomic (extrinsic), namely sympathetic (adrenergic) and parasympathetic (cholinergic, vagus), nervous systems is required for sufficient depolarization to reach the threshold potential and generate an action potential.[87] The enteric nervous system consists of ganglia in the myenteric (Auerbach's) and submucosal (Meissner's) plexuses and uses neuropeptides and nitric oxide as neurotransmitters. Sympathetic hyperactivity results in splanchnic vasoconstriction and decreased propulsive motility; therefore, α-adrenergic agonists impair motility and α-adrenergic antagonists enhance intestinal motility. Parasympathetic hypoactivity causes a reduction in motility and a decrease in intestinal secretion. Cholinomimetics should, therefore, promote intestinal motility.[87] Any alteration in smooth muscle or enteric nervous system activity can cause ileus. (See also Equine grass sickness and Proximal enteritis).

Clinical features

Horses with primary ileus may have clinical signs consistent with a mild proximal enteritis (mild to moderate colic, reflux following nasogastric tube passage, distended small intestine on palpation per rectum, and dehydration); however, these horses usually respond to gastric decompression, analgesia, and IV fluid therapy within 6–24 hours of treatment. Horses with primary ileus do not show signs of shock and often do not have as marked clinical pathology abnormalities as horses with proximal enteritis, most likely because of the comparatively small reflux volume and lack of intestinal inflammation.

Differential diagnosis

Proximal enteritis; ileal impaction; equine grass sickness (non-US countries); EFE; strangulation through a mesenteric rent; strangulating pedunculated lipoma.

Diagnosis

No clinical signs or laboratory findings are pathognomonic for primary ileus and it can mimic other causes of colic including strangulating small intestinal lesions. The diagnosis is usually made by exclusion when horses with signs of colic, distended small intestinal loops on palpation per rectum, and reflux following nasogastric tube passage respond rapidly to medical treatment. Peritoneal fluid should be grossly normal and analysis should be within normal limits.

Abdominal ultrasonographic examination often reveals several loops of mild to moderately distended small intestine that is not thickened and usually has some motility (**1.56**).

Surgery is necessary in some horses with primary ileus that show persistent signs of abdominal pain. At surgery, small intestinal distension is the only abnormality. Intestinal biopsy should be considered in cases with recurrent intestinal problems or weight loss.

Management/treatment

Horses with primary ileus often respond to medical treatment with analgesia, IV fluid therapy, and gastric decompression. Occasionally, exploratory abdominal surgery is necessary to make a diagnosis and to decompress the small intestine. Motility modifying drugs, including IV lidocaine, metoclopramide, erythromycin, and neostigmine, may be necessary in some cases (see Chapter 18).

Most horses respond well to medical or surgical treatment. However, occasionally a horse will have signs of persistent colic, reflux, and small intestinal distension and euthanasia may be indicated. Biopsy should be considered in these cases at either exploratory abdominal surgery or necropsy to evaluate the histomorphologic appearance of the enteric nervous system as well as any evidence of inflammatory or infiltrative bowel disease (p. 93).

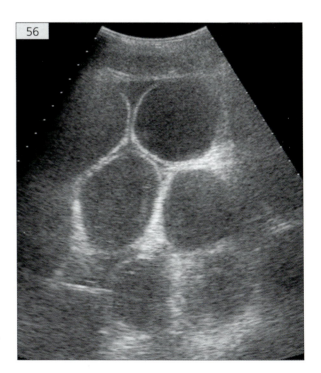

1.56 Abdominal ultrasonographic appearance of multiple loops of moderately distended small intestine of normal wall thickness consistent with ileus. (Courtesy Dr JoAnn Slack)

Equine grass sickness
Key points
- Equine grass sickness is reported to occur most commonly in Great Britain and Western Europe.
- Definitive diagnosis of equine grass sickness is made based on histologic examination of an ileal biopsy obtained during exploratory celiotomy or at necropsy. Histopathologic findings include chromatolytic changes of autonomic neurons.
- Acute grass sickness is fatal.

Definition/overview
Equine grass sickness is also known as equine dysautonomia because of the extensive autonomic dysfunction that occurs with the disease; however, it is actually a polyneuropathy because both central and peripheral nervous systems are affected.[88]

Etiology/pathogenesis
The specific cause of equine grass sickness is unknown.[88] However, based on the risk factors and pathologic findings (see below), ingestion of a potent neurotoxin-producing agent during grazing is the most likely etiology.[88] While various agents have been proposed, a toxicoinfectious form of botulism caused by *Clostridium botulinum* type C is currently thought to be the most likely etiology based on: reduction of mortality rates with vaccination; increase in *Clostridium* spp. in horses with grass sickness compared with controls; detection of C1 neurotoxin in the ileal contents and feces of horses with histologic evidence of grass sickness; and lower serum IgG concentrations to *Clostridium botulinum* type C and C1 neurotoxin in horses with grass sickness compared with controls.[88–91] BoNT/C and C2 binary toxin production and absorption occur mostly in the ileum, associated with overgrowth from normal large intestinal flora and/or spore germination associated with dietary trigger factors.[92]

The most important risk factor for equine grass sickness is access to grazing, particularly during the spring months and May (northern hemisphere). There is also a second peak in the autumn.[93–95] Young horses (2–7 years old) appear to be affected most often[93,95]; older horses are thought to have developed immunity or tolerance to the causative agent and younger horses ingest less grass and have maternal antibodies.[88] In addition to grazing, other reported risk factors include sand or loam soil type, grazing on previously affected pastures, increased horse numbers, pasture disturbance, dietary change, good to fat body condition, and frequent use of ivermectin-based anthelmintics.[88] Equine grass sickness has a strong geographic distribution with the most frequent occurrence in Great Britain and in Western European countries geographically close to Great Britain.[88]

Clinical features
Equine grass sickness can present as an acute/subacute or chronic disease. Horses with acute grass sickness show signs of colic with rapid development of clinical signs; cases of acute grass sickness are fatal within 7 days.[96] Acute grass sickness is characterized by gastric and small intestinal distension progressing to cecal and colonic obstruction with dehydrated ingesta.[88] Horses have a dull demeanor and signs of dehydration and hypovolemia. Intestinal borborygmi are often absent and fecal production is reduced to absent, with firm, small, mucus-covered fecal balls. Horses may have abdominal distension. Hypersalivation, dysphagia, inappetence, bilateral ptosis, and muscle fasciculations are also clinical features. A large volume of nasogastric reflux is obtained and horses may reflux spontaneously. Small intestinal distension and firm impacted ingesta in the cecum and large colon are identified on palpation per rectum.[88]

Chronic grass sickness is characterized by insidious onset of weight loss (**1.57**) or dysphagia.[88] Some other clinical features of chronic equine grass sickness include dull demeanor, rhinitis sicca, bilateral ptosis, patchy sweating, base-narrow stance, muscle fasciculations, and piloerection.[88]

Differential diagnosis
Proximal enteritis; primary ileus; ileal impaction; esophageal obstruction; botulism; peritonitis; small intestinal strangulating lesions.

Diagnosis
Diagnosis of equine grass sickness is made based on histologic examination of an ileal biopsy obtained during

exploratory celiotomy or at necropsy. Histologic evaluation of a 1-cm ileal sample had a 100% specificity and sensitivity for diagnosing equine grass sickness.[97] Histopathologic findings include chromatolytic changes of autonomic neurons (i.e. nerve cell bodies within the myenteric or submucosal plexus). At necropsy, samples from the peripheral sympathetic celiacomesenteric or cranial cervical ganglia can also be obtained.[88]

Abdominal exploration reveals distended small intestine without a mechanical obstruction, uncoordinated small intestinal spasms, and gastric distension. Severe or long-standing cases will have secondary impaction of the large colon with dehydrated ingesta and black coating of mucosa and ingesta.[98]

Management/treatment
Acute equine grass sickness is fatal. Management of chronic grass sickness cases involves supportive care including nutritional support, analgesia as necessary, and nursing care. Prevention includes (1) avoiding dietary changes during spring, (2) offering grazing animals supplementary forage, (3) avoiding disturbing pasture, and (4) tolerating low-level parasitism and avoiding overuse of anthelmintics.[88]

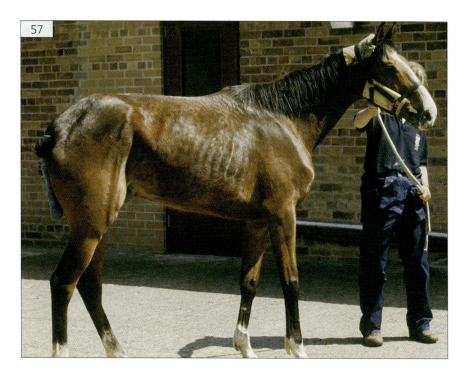

1.57 Horse with chronic equine grass sickness. (Courtesy Liverpool University)

Mechanical obstruction
Ileal impaction
Key points

- Ileal impaction occurs most commonly in the Southeastern USA, as well as in Germany and The Netherlands.
- Horses have a history of being fed Coastal Bermuda grass or poor-quality hay.
- There is a strong association with *Anaplocephala perfoliata* (tapeworm) infection.
- Medical management is successful if treated early.
- Prognosis is excellent with early treatment.

Definition/overview

Ileal impaction refers to obstruction of the ileum with dried ingesta forming a doughy-to-solid, tubular mass extending from the ileocecal orifice in a proximal direction for 90 cm.[99]

Etiology/pathogenesis

Ileal impaction is usually a primary disease; however, it can be secondary to a lesion at the ileocecal orifice or along the ileum. Ileal impaction has a high occurrence in the Southeastern USA, as well as in Germany and The Netherlands. It is associated with feeding Coastal Bermuda grass hay.[100] The odds ratio for a horse presenting with colic signs having an ileal impaction was 2.9-times higher for horses fed Coastal Bermuda grass hay compared with those not fed Coastal Bermuda grass hay.[100] Coastal Bermuda grass hay is a high-yield, warm-season perennial grass and stemmy, fine forage. The proportion of lignin and crude fiber increases and the dry matter, protein, and energy digestibility decrease with maturity.[101] These features make it a popular feed, but they predispose to impaction with maturity.

Weather changes, water intake, and the quality of hay are also thought to be important in the etiopathogenesis.[101] Ileal impactions are reported to occur most commonly in the autumn months.[102,103] Risk factors for ileal impaction have included (1) mares, (2) Arabian horses, and (3) recent introduction of poor-quality hay.

Feeding other hay with Coastal Bermuda grass hay did not lower the risk of ileal impaction; however, feeding a pelleted concentrate with hay did lower the risk.[100]

Ileal impaction has also been associated with *Anoplocephala perfoliata* (tapeworm) infection.[100,104,105] The risk of ileal impaction and gas colic increased with higher tapeworm burdens [105] The 'etiological fraction' for ileal impactions indicated that 81% of horses with ileal impactions were tapeworm associated.[104] For horses with colic, failure to administer a pyrantel salt within 3 months prior to admission resulted in an odds ratio of 3:1 for risk of ileal impaction.[100] Interestingly, orbatid mites, which are the intermediate host for *A. perfoliata*, prefer humid regions such as the Southeastern United States, which may also explain the regional case distribution.[99]

Occasionally, a diagnosis of ileal impaction will be made when the horse has another lesion proximal to the ileum, such as an EFE. In this case, the ileum is impacted with dried ingesta that has become dehydrated secondary to sequestration of fluid in the proximal jejunum, duodenum, and stomach.

Ileal impactions have also been associated with ileal muscular hypertrophy and thrombotic disease [101], as well as other lesions in the region of the ileum.

Clinical features

Horses initially present with intermittent, moderate to severe abdominal pain that is responsive to treatment with analgesics. The pain is thought to be associated with intestinal spasm in the region of the impaction.[101] The rectal temperature, pulse, and respiratory rate are within normal limits and borborygmi are present. There is usually no reflux following nasogastric tube passage at this point in the disease process.[101]

Small intestinal distension develops in cases that are not resolved with medical management within 8–10 hours of obstruction.[101] With the progression of small intestinal distension, abdominal pain becomes persistent, intestinal borborygmi decrease, and the horse becomes non-responsive to analgesia administration.

Nasogastric reflux develops in 15–20%[101] to 56%[106] of cases. The higher percentage of horses with reflux in the earlier study likely reflects a longer duration of obstruction. Horses that are not treated appropriately become dehydrated and develop signs of shock.

Differential diagnosis

Primary ileus; proximal enteritis; ileocecal intussusception; ileal muscular hypertrophy; EFE; strangulating pedunculated lipoma (older horses); small intestinal volvulus.

Diagnosis

A tentative diagnosis can be made based on the geographical location, history of feeding Coastal Bermuda grass hay, signs of abdominal pain, and the presence of reflux.

Findings on abdominal palpation per rectum are variable.[101] In 25–30% of cases, a firm, 5–8-cm diameter smooth-surfaced ileum could be palpated in the mid-abdominal region adjacent to the cecal base coursing in a cranioventral direction towards the left abdomen.[101,106,107] Palpation of the mass is more likely in cases without small intestinal distension. In one study, 96% of cases had palpably distended small intestine[106]; however, small intestinal distension is typically not palpated early in the course of the disease.[107]

Abdominal ultrasonographic examination can also be used to identify amotile, thin-walled, distended small intestine, which is more consistent with a mechanical obstruction than enteritis or ileus.[101] Peritoneal fluid analysis should be within normal limits (initially) and can be used to support diagnosis of an ileal impaction versus a small intestinal strangulating obstruction. A definitive diagnosis is often made at abdominal exploratory surgery.

Management/treatment

Medical treatment can be pursued initially when a diagnosis is made based on history and palpation per rectum findings and when the abdominal pain and small intestinal distension have not progressed, or in cases where economics preclude surgical management. IV fluids can be used to correct dehydration, provide maintenance water and electrolytes, and replace fluid and electrolyte loss from reflux.[101] Enteral fluids and mineral oil can be administered early in the course of the disease if reflux and small intestinal distension are not yet present or if reflux has ceased.[107] Analgesia can be provided with flunixin meglumine, firocoxib, xylazine and butorphanol, or detomidine. N-butylscopolammonium bromide (Buscopan®) can be given as a spasmolytic.[101] Horses managed medically should be checked frequently for reflux to avoid accumulation of fluid in the stomach and gastric rupture. The mean time for resolution of ileal impactions with medical management was 11.7 hours.[107]

Surgery is indicated in patients that are persistently or moderately to severely painful and have nasogastric reflux[107a], have small intestinal distension, and/or any signs of cardiovascular deterioration. Peritoneal fluid abnormalities are also an indication for surgery.[107a] Exploratory celiotomy is used to confirm the diagnosis. The impacted material can be massaged into the cecum. Sodium carboxymethylcellulose (1%) can be used on the serosal surface to minimize trauma and intraluminally (300–400 ml 1:1 ratio of sterile 0.9% saline and 1% sodium carboxymethylcellulose with or without 30 ml of 2% lidocaine hydrochloride) to help resolve the impaction.[101] If the intestinal wall is edematous and hemorrhagic, an enterotomy may be necessary[101]; however, this should be reserved for severe cases.[99] In cases with concurrent ileal muscular hypertrophy (p. 82), bypass via a jejunocecostomy is necessary. Resection of the affected intestine with jejunocecostomy is required in cases with thrombotic disease.[101]

Deworming with an anthelmintic against tapeworms (praziquantal or pyrantel pamoate) is recommended. It is also recommended to exclude Coastal Bermuda grass hay from the diet to avoid recurrence.[101]

The prognosis for survival for horses managed medically was 93% with 7% of horses being euthanized for economic reasons. The survival of horses managed surgically was 91%.[101,107a]

Ileal muscular hypertrophy

Key points

- Ileal muscular hypertrophy is uncommon.
- Horses with ileal muscular hypertrophy usually present with a chronic history of recurrent, mild colic.
- Side-to-side ileo- or jejunocecostomy with or without transection (or resection) of the affected ileum is reported to be successful.

Definition/overview

Ileal muscular hypertrophy refers to hypertrophy of the inner circular and outer longitudinal smooth muscle layers of the ileum (**1.58, 1.59**). The full length of the ileum is usually affected; however, on occasion the ileocecal junction and adjacent terminal ileum may be within normal limits.[66] Often there are acquired diverticula (p. 84) associated with the hypertrophied area. Full-thickness rupture can occur.[108–110] Compensatory hypertrophy of the distal jejunum, without luminal stenosis, can occur in chronic cases.[109] Similar lesions have been reported in the jejunum; however, this is less common.[109]

Etiology/pathogenesis

Ileal muscular hypertrophy is generally considered an idiopathic disease.[66,110] There are, however, several proposed pathogeneses including (1) chronic mucosal inflammation[111], (2) autonomic imbalance producing uncontrollable peristaltic activity or neurogenic ileocecal valve stenosis[112], and (3) infection with *Anaplocephala perfoliata* (tapeworms).[113] Ileal muscular hypertrophy was also reported in one case 3 years after an ileocecal intussusception that was managed with an incomplete ileal bypass via a jejunocecostomy.[110]

Clinical features

Horses most often present with chronic signs of recurrent, mild colic for up to 2.4 years.[109] Weight loss and inappetence may also be a feature of the clinical presentation. The clinical signs are a result of the marked but incomplete luminal constriction in the hypertrophied region.

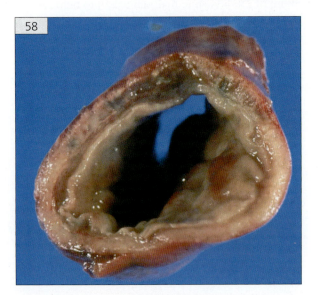

1.58 Gross appearance of ileal muscular hypertrophy.

An acute presentation has also been reported associated with ileal impaction[66] and full-thickness rupture of the affected ileum.[108–110] Horses with rupture develop septic peritonitis with associated signs of septic shock (tachycardia, tachypnea, fever, prolonged CRT, and injected or toxic mucous membranes).

No breed predisposition is reported. Mature horses are affected most often; however, the lesion has been reported in horses of all ages.[66]

Differential diagnosis

Ileocecal intussusception; ileal impaction; infiltrative or inflammatory bowel disease; neoplasia; gas or spasmodic colic; large colon or cecal impaction; perforation of other regions of the GI tract.

Diagnosis

A thickened, firm, tubular, ileum can occasionally be palpated per rectum.[109,110] Identification of small intestinal distension either on abdominal palpation per rectum or abdominal ultrasonographic examination is often possible; however, is not specific for ileal hypertrophy. In horses with rupture, septic peritonitis can be diagnosed with abdominocentesis and peritoneal fluid analysis. The diagnosis is usually made during abdominal exploratory surgery.

Management/treatment

Surgical treatment is necessary. Side-to-side ileo- or jejunocecostomy with (complete) or without (incomplete) transection (or resection) of the affected ileum is reported to be successful.[66] Euthanasia is indicated in cases with full-thickness rupture and septic peritonitis associated with leakage of intestinal contents. (See also Chapter 18.)

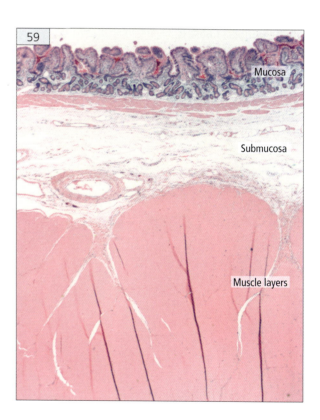

1.59 **Histologic appearance of ileal muscular hypertrophy showing hypertrophy of the inner circular and outer longitudinal smooth muscle layers of the ileum.**

Diverticula
Key points
- Diverticula formation is an uncommon cause of colic.
- Congenital Meckel's diverticulum is the most common diverticulum in humans and horses.

Definition/overview
A diverticulum (pleural diverticula) is a circumscribed pouch or sac. A true diverticulum comprises all layers of the intestinal wall and a pseudodiverticulum involves herniation of the submucosa and mucosa through a defect in the smooth muscle layer (**1.60A, B, 1.61**).[114]

Etiology/pathogenesis
Diverticula can be congenital or acquired and can occur along almost any part of the GI tract between the esophagus and the colon. Congenital diverticula are generally true diverticula, whereas acquired diverticula are usually pseudodiverticula. Congenital diverticula are usually solitary, whereas acquired diverticula are often multiple (**1.60A, B**).[60,114]

A Meckel's diverticulum is the most common congenital GI tract diverticulum in horses and humans. It occurs in the distal jejunum or ileum and is a remnant of structures within the fetal digestive tract (omphalomesenteric [vitelline] duct that provided communication between the yolk sac and embryonic gut) that were not fully reabsorbed prior to birth. Meckel's diverticula can become impacted and grow to an enormous size, become necrotic and perforate, or a small intestinal volvulus associated with persistence of a vitelloumbilical band between the diverticulum and umbilicus can occur.[66]

Acquired diverticula are uncommon. A traction diverticulum is formed by the pulling force of contracting bands of adhesion (true diverticulum) and is more commonly seen in the esophagus. A pulsion diverticulum is formed by pressure from within a hollow organ, often causing herniation of the mucous membrane through the muscular layer (pseudodiverticulum). Acquired diverticula of the small and large intestine are rare in horses and the exact etiopathogenesis is unknown. Possible causes include altered motility

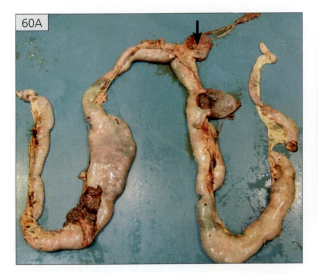

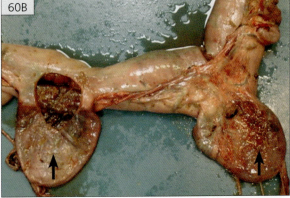

1.60A, B Multiple acquired jejunal pseudodiverticula (arrows).

leading to an increase in intraluminal pressure or visceral myopathy associated with smooth muscle function and structural abnormality (pulsion diverticulum[114]). Acquired diverticula formation has been associated with ileal muscular hypertrophy (p. 82). Diverticula formation can lead to impaction, inflammation and necrosis, rupture, and intussusception.[60]

Clinical features
While diverticula may be subclinical, a necropsy report found a Meckel's diverticulum in five horses and it was the cause of death in all five cases, suggesting that they are likely to become clinically important.[115] Clinical signs vary from acute colic associated with volvulus to chronic intermittent colic associated with an impaction. Horses with a ruptured diverticulum are likely to present with signs of shock similar to rupture of other parts of the GI tract (p. 60). Horses may also have a history of weight loss and inappetence.

Differential diagnosis
- **Acute colic**: strangulating small intestinal obstruction; other causes of non-strangulating small intestinal obstruction.
- **Shock**: GI tract rupture; colitis.

Diagnosis
Definitive diagnosis is generally going to be made during abdominal exploratory surgery or at necropsy.

Management/treatment
Surgical management is necessary. Diverticulectomy or complete resection of the affected intestine and anastomosis are necessary. Complete intestinal resection is recommended for patients with acquired diverticula because of the high incidence of intestinal surgical site dehiscence and septic peritonitis in human patients.[116]

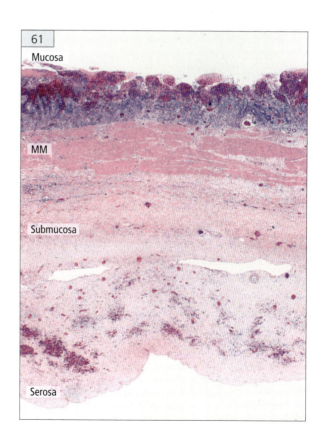

1.61 Histologic appearance of the acquired jejunal diverticula in 1.60A, B illustrating a lack of longitudinal and circular muscle layers. MM, muscularis mucosae.

Ascarid impaction

Key points

- Ascarid impaction is an uncommon cause of colic because of improvements in parasite management. However, with the emergence of anthelmintic resistance, ascarid impaction may become more common and fecal monitoring of anthelmintic efficacy is recommended.
- Ascarid impaction should be considered in a weanling foal with signs of acute colic and recent history of anthelmintic administration.
- Surgical management is necessary in many cases.
- The prognosis for survival is fair and prevention is important.

Definition/overview

Ascarid impaction refers to obstruction of the jejunum or ileum with *Parascaris equorum* (round worms) (**1.62**). Jejunal volvulus (p. 73) and intussusception (p. 66) are often associated with ascarid impaction. Abscessation, peritonitis, adhesion formation, and intestinal rupture can occur.[117]

Etiology/pathogenesis

P. equorum has a direct life-cycle with a free living and parasitic phase. The embryonated eggs are ingested and hatch in the small intestine; the larvae penetrate the intestinal mucosa and migrate to the liver and lungs. After traveling up the bronchial tree, they are swallowed and grow into 10–50-cm long adult ascarids in the duodenum and proximal jejunum.[118,119]

The pre-patent period of *P. equorum* is 72–110 days. The median age of affected foals is 5 months, with a range of 4–24 months.[58,117] Foals are, therefore, most likely affected at or soon after birth, with clinical signs of obstruction occurring when there are large numbers of mature ascarids. Foals >6 month old tend to develop immunity to infection with *P. equorum*[118] and most cases of ascarid impaction occur in horses <1 year.

Ascarid impactions occur most often in the autumn or fall months coinciding with the median age of the foal and pre-patent period of *P. equorum*.[58,117]

The association between recent anthelmintic administration and ascarid impaction is somewhat controversial. The most recent report was that 72% of foals presenting with ascarid impaction had been treated with an anthelmintic within 24 hours prior to the onset of colic signs.[58] Ivermectin, pyrantel pamoate, and trichlorfon were the anthelmintic drugs administered.[58,117] Rapid death of large numbers of *P. equorum* is thought to predispose to obstruction.

Heavy ascarid burdens can (1) cause a mechanical obstruction, (2) alter intestinal motility leading to volvulus or intussusception, (3) lead to GI rupture, and (4) penetration of the intestinal wall by the ascarid can lead to abscessation, peritonitis, and adhesion formation.

Clinical features

Classic signs of ascariasis are lethargy, inappetence, coughing, nasal discharge, and decreased weight gain. Ascarid impaction should be suspected in a weanling with signs of colic, particularly with a recent history of anthelmintic administration and concurrent signs of ascariasis. Physical examination findings can be variable. Foals are often tachycardiac and tachypneic and may also be febrile. Signs of dehydration are common. Reflux following nasogastric tube passage is a common feature and ascarids may be identified in the reflux. Abdominal palpation per rectum is often not possible because of the small size of the patient; however, it usually reveals distended small intestinal loops. Peritoneal fluid is often serosanguineous or consistent with peritonitis.[117] Foals with gastric or intestinal rupture present with signs of shock, tachycardia, tachypnea, injected or toxic mucous membranes, poor peripheral pulses, poor jugular refill, and cool extremities.

Differential diagnosis

Equine gastric ulcer syndrome; intussusception; small intestinal volvulus.

Diagnosis

Ascarid impaction is definitively diagnosed at surgery or necropsy. A tentative diagnosis can be made based on clinical signs and finding ascarids in the reflux or feces. Ultrasonographic and radiographic examination can be used to identify distended amotile small intestine; however, ascarids are not usually observed.

Management/treatment

Foals with ascarid impaction may be managed medically with analgesia, IV fluid therapy, and lubricants (i.e. mineral oil) administered via a nasogastric tube. Abdominal surgery is often necessary and involves manipulating the ascarids into the cecum for removal through a typhlotomy (preferred) or via a small intestinal enterotomy. Resection and anastomosis of the affected jejunum (and/or colon) may be necessary if it is discolored because necrosis of the bowel can occur postoperatively. Postoperative complications include colic, endotoxemia, fever, salmonellosis, diarrhea, septic peritonitis, pneumonia, incisional infection, and adhesions.[58,117] (See also Chapter 18.) With early surgical intervention and resection of severely affected bowel, these complications can be prevented.

Deworming of horses with heavy ascarid burdens is controversial.[119] Some parasitologists recommend deworming with a benzimidazole anthelmintic in foals suspected of having a heavy ascarid burden. Benzimidazoles starve ascarids by interfering with β-tubulin, whereas ivermectin and pyrantel pamoate interfere with neuromuscular transmission. Pasture management and monitoring of herd fecal egg counts are important to prevent the development of heavy ascarid burdens.

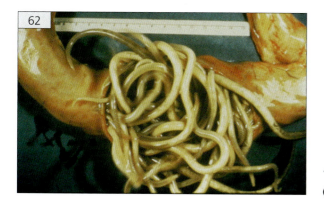

1.62 *Parascaris equorum* **causing intestinal obstruction. (Courtesy Dr Ted Stashak)**

Neoplasia
Key points

- Intestinal neoplasia is rare in horses.
- Horses with intestinal neoplasia may present on an emergency basis with a history of mild, intermittent colic signs associated with a partial intestinal obstruction.
- Horses with intestinal neoplasia usually have a history of weight loss, failure to thrive, or poor performance.
- Diagnosis can be made based on palpation of a mass(es) per rectum, ultrasonographic examination, peritoneal fluid analysis, rectal biopsy, and exploratory celiotomy.
- Prognosis for long-term survival is generally poor.

Definition/overview

The most common intestinal neoplasia is lymphoma followed by adenocarcinoma (**1.63**).[120] Leiomyosarcoma, leiomyoma[120], myxosarcoma, ganglioneuroma, nerve sheath tumor, carcinoid[120], and GI stromal tumor (**1.64A, B**) have also been reported. The small intestine is affected most commonly.[120]

Etiology/pathogenesis

The etiology and pathogenesis of intestinal neoplasia is unknown.

Clinical features

Horses with intestinal neoplasia typically have a history of weight loss and inappetence and present underweight. Signs of intermittent mild colic are also typical and are associated with a partial intestinal obstruction. Horses may also have a history of loose feces or diarrhea. Tachycardia, tachypnea, and fever are inconsistent clinical findings. Neutrophilia, lymphopenia, and hypoalbuminemia occur in about half of horses with intestinal neoplasia.[120] Other laboratory findings may include increased immature (band) neutrophils, hyperfibrinogenemia, hyperglobulinemia, anemia, and an increase in liver enzyme activity associated with hepatic metastases.[120] Hypercalcemia of malignancy is uncommon.[120]

Differential diagnosis

- **Colic**: inflammatory or infiltrative bowel disease; sand colic; enterolithiasis; right dorsal colitis; abdominal abscessation.
- **Weight loss**[41]: malnutrition; dental or oral disease; parasitism; hepatic or renal disease; non-intestinal intra-abdominal neoplasia; gastric neoplasia; gastric ulcers; proliferative enteropathy (young horses); right dorsal colitis; sand colic.

Diagnosis

Abdominal palpation per rectum may be useful for detecting intra-abdominal mass(es), small intestinal distension, and ascites.[120] An intra-abdominal mass(es) was diagnosed in 27% of horses on palpation per rectum.[120]

Peritoneal fluid analysis should be performed in horses suspected of having intestinal neoplasia. Approximately half of the horses with intestinal neoplasia in one study had a high nucleated cell count and/or TP concentration.[120] Neoplastic cells are typically identified in the peritoneal fluid of about 40–50% of horses with intestinal lymphoma; however, they are not found in horses with adenocarcinoma.[120]

Transabdominal and/or transrectal ultrasonographic examination is useful for detecting an increase in intestinal wall thickness and/or intramural masses; an increase in the amount of peritoneal fluid; cecal lymphadenopathy; hepatopathy or discrete hepatic metastases; and splenic abnormalities.[120] Intestinal wall thickening and enlarged cecal mesenteric lymph nodes are most consistently seen in horses with lymphoma, whereas an intramural mass with proximal intestinal distension and hypertrophy is more commonly seen with adenocarcinoma. Examination of the thorax ultrasonographically should be considered for identification of pulmonary metastases.

Rectal biopsy may be useful in some cases for diagnosis of lymphoma. Fecal occult blood, although non-specific for intestinal neoplasia, may be positive in horses with adenocarcinoma, particularly those with anemia as a result of luminal blood loss from the neoplasia.

Abdominal exploration through either a ventral midline celiotomy or laparoscopic approach, with biopsy of the affected intestine, can be used to make a definitive diagnosis.

Management/treatment

The prognosis for horses with intestinal neoplasia is generally poor and most are euthanized following diagnosis. Abdominal surgery with resection of the affected bowel may be possible in some cases, with anastomosis of adjacent normal segments. In three horses with intestinal adenocarcinoma that underwent resection and anastomosis, signs recurred 3–5 years following hospital discharge and the horses were euthanized without necropsy.[120] Two horses with intestinal lymphoma that were treated with corticosteroids survived to 5 and 12 months, respectively, following hospital discharge. Metastasis is common in horses with intestinal lymphoma and adenocarcinoma and less common in horses with smooth muscle tumors or GI stromal tumors.

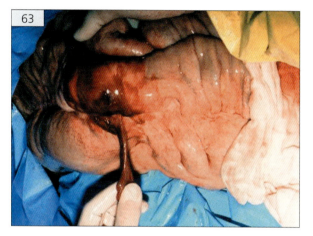

1.63 Intestinal adenocarcinoma (of the large colon). (Courtesy Dr Eric Parente)

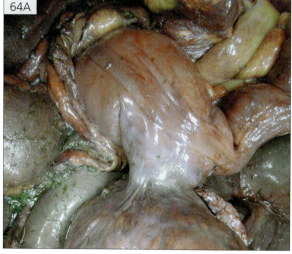

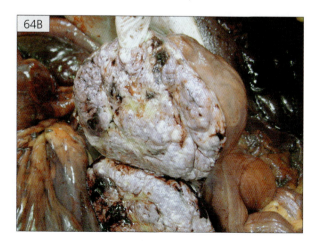

1.64 (A) GI stromal tumor (GIST) causing partial obstruction of the small colon in this case; (B) the same tumor transected to shown consistency of the mass.

Inflammatroy lesions
Proximal enteritis (duodenitis–proximal jejunitis)
Key points

- Proximal enteritis is relatively common in horses and has a geographic distribution.
- Classic clinical signs of proximal enteritis are mild colic, dull demeanor, and nasogastric reflux.
- It can be difficult to differentiate cases of proximal enteritis from strangulating lesions and in some cases surgery is necessary as a diagnostic tool.
- Large volumes of IV replacement and maintenance fluids are necessary to manage horses with proximal enteritis because of the large volume of nasogastric reflux.
- Persistent reflux and laminitis are the most common reasons for euthanasia of horses with proximal enteritis.

Definition/overviews

Proximal enteritis is acute inflammation of the small intestine and usually occurs in the duodenum and proximal jejunum (duodenitis–proximal jejunitis). Proximal enteritis is often managed medically and in these cases has been defined clinically as a horse with signs of colic that progresses to dull demeanor and a large volume of nasogastric reflux (>48 liters in 24 hours[121] or nasogastric reflux for >24 hours or at a rate >3 liters/hour for >8 hours[122]). Horses with proximal enteritis often have gastric ulceration and, therefore, it is possible that the disease is gastroenteritis rather than enteritis only.

Etiology/pathogenesis

In many cases, the etiology and pathogenesis of proximal enteritis is not determined. *Clostridium difficile* and *Salmonella* spp. have been isolated from the reflux of horses with proximal enteritis. Toxigenic strains of *C. difficile* were isolated from all 10 horses with proximal enteritis and only one out of 16 horses with other causes of reflux.[123] Histopathologically, intestinal injury in cases of proximal enteritis is similar to that created by *Clostridium* spp. exotoxins[124] and after experimental challenge with *C. difficile*.[125] *Salmonella* spp., particularly *Salmonella enterica* serovar *newport*, has been isolated from the reflux of horses with enteritis. Enteritis caused by *Salmonella* spp., however, is often not localized to the duodenum and proximal jejunum. *Fusarium moniliforme* has also been proposed as an etiological agent.[126,127]

Diet may also play a role in proximal enteritis. Horses with proximal enteritis were fed significantly more concentrate and were significantly more likely to have grazed pasture than colic and lameness control horses.[128]

Clinical features

Horses may initially present with signs of moderate colic; however, this often progresses to dull demeanor, fever, decreased intestinal borborygmi, reflux following nasogastric tube passage, small intestinal distension on palpation per rectum, dehydration, and leukocytosis.[124,129] Horses with salmonellosis are often leukopenic. Passage of a nasogastric tube generally reveals large volumes of reflux and signs of abdominal pain often resolve following gastric decompression via a nasogastric tube. Horses are usually tachycardic (60–120 bpm). Respiratory rate is variable. A mild fever is a notable feature of proximal enteritis; however, a lack of fever does not exclude a diagnosis of proximal enteritis. Horses with proximal enteritis may have hemorrhagic reflux and show signs of shock.[129] Hemoconcentration, hyponatremia, hypochloremia, hypokalemia, azotemia, and high hepatic enzyme activity are clinical pathology abnormalities consistent with proximal enteritis and mostly reflect small intestinal functional obstruction with loss of large volumes of water and electrolytes into the GI tract.

Differential diagnosis

Primary ileus; equine grass sickness; EFE; strangulation through a mesenteric rent; strangulating pedunculated lipoma; volvulus; ileal impaction.

Diagnosis

No clinical signs or laboratory findings are patho-gnomonic for proximal enteritis[129] and this disease can mimic other causes of colic including small intestinal strangulating lesions (p. 62). Horses with proximal enteritis had lower mean heart and respiratory rates, greater reflux volume, better intestinal borborygmi, lower mean plasma potassium and higher mean plasma bicarbonate concentrations, and lower mean perito-neal fluid nucleated cell count compared with horses with a mechanical intestinal obstruction.[130] Peritoneal fluid TP is typically high (>40 g/l [4 g/dl]) in horses with proximal enteritis.[129] Anion gap, abdominal fluid TP concentration, and the volume of reflux during the initial 24 hours were associated with outcome.[121]

Ultrasonographic examination can be used in some cases to differentiate proximal enteritis from a strangulating obstruction. Enteritis cases have dilated small intestinal loops that are often thickened and have poor motility (**1.65A, B**). Horses with a strangulating obstruction have normal small intestinal loops and markedly dilated amotile small intestinal loops with a normal wall thickness intermixed with thickened loops, as well as an increase in the amount of peritoneal fluid.

A tentative diagnosis of proximal enteritis can be made in a horse that was initially painful then became dull and ceased showing signs of colic; has a large volume of reflux following nasogastric tube passage; the signs of pain subside and heart rate decreases with gastric decompression; and the horse responds to rehy-dration with improved heart rate, oral mucous mem-brane color and moistness, and CRT. A high peritoneal fluid TP and normal total nucleated cell count is also indicative of proximal enteritis.

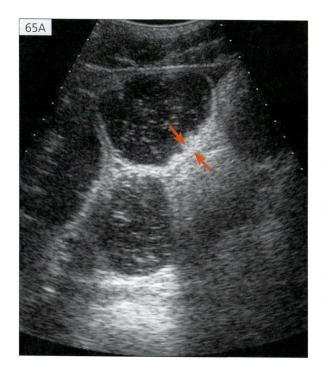 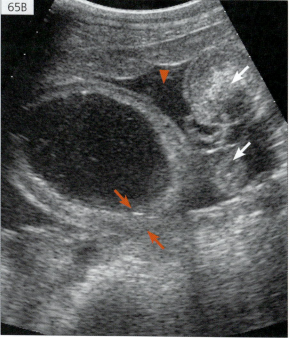

1.65 Ultrasonographic appearance of a horse with enteritis (A) and a horse with mechanical obstruction (B). Note the multiple loops of moderately distended small intestine with a mild increase in wall thickness in the horse with enteritis (arrows). The horse with a mechanical obstruction had a combination of markedly dilated and thickened small intestine (red arrows) as well as small intestine of normal thickness, which was contracting (white arrows), and an increase in the amount of anechoic peritoneal fluid (arrowhead). (Courtesy Dr JoAnn Slack)

The definitive diagnosis is often made during abdominal exploratory surgery. The gross appearance of the small intestine at surgery or necropsy in horses with proximal enteritis is distended, thickened, and hemorrhagic intestine with yellow discoloration (**1.66**).[124] The duodenum and proximal part of the jejunum are the only segments affected. The distal jejunum is usually not distended or thickened.

Management/treatment

Horses with proximal enteritis are generally treated medically with large volumes of crystalloid fluids (see Chapter 12). Maintenance fluids can be estimated at 2 ml/kg/hour and replacement fluids can be estimated based on the volume of reflux produced per hour. The horse should be monitored closely to determine if fluid therapy is adequate (see Chapter 11 and Chapter 18).

Flunixin meglumine is used as an anti-inflammatory and analgesic drug. Plasma and polymixin B can be given in cases with signs of endotoxemia. Metronidazole is given in some cases because of the possibility of *C. difficile* being the causative agent (see Chapter 12 and Chapter 16).

Promotility drugs can be used in horses with proximal enteritis or primary ileus. IV lidocaine has been shown to result in a more rapid resolution of reflux in horses with proximal enteritis or postoperative ileus compared with saline.[131] Of the IV lidocaine treated horses, 65% stopped producing reflux within 30 hours of starting treatment, including 8/13 with postoperative ileus and 3/4 with proximal enteritis. Only 27% of saline control horses stopped producing reflux within the same time period, including 4/11 with postoperative reflux and 0/4 with proximal enteritis.[131] The efficacy of IV lidocaine for treatment of proximal enteritis or ileus has not been investigated further and it is most likely that IV lidocaine has an anti-inflammatory rather than a promotility effect on the intestine. There was no clinical benefit observed during treatment with bethanechol or metoclopramide; however, horses that did not respond to treatment with these prokinetics within 24 hours did not survive.[132] (See also Chapter 18.)

Laminitis is a serious complication of proximal enteritis and was reported to occur in 28–31% of cases.[133,134] Factors associated with the development of laminitis were body weight >550 kg and hemorrhagic reflux.[133] Horses that were treated with heparin were less likely to develop laminitis (0/12) compared with horses that were not treated with heparin (31/104).[133] Currently, applying ice to the feet is the recommended treatment for preventing laminitis (see Chapter 2).

Exploratory abdominal surgery is necessary in some cases of proximal enteritis and is mostly used as a diagnostic tool to rule out a strangulating lesion and to decompress the small intestine. The small intestine contents are decompressed into the cecum. Bypass of the affected segment has been reported[124] and it is possible that some horses may benefit from gastrojejunostomy; however, this is not often performed in cases of proximal enteritis. Postoperative treatment involves continued treatment for primary ileus (p.76). Feed should be reintroduced over 3–5 days after reflux has ceased (see Chapter 18).

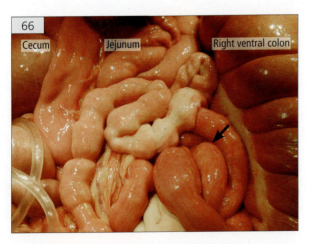

1.66 A horse with duodenitis-proximal jejunitis showing the thickened proximal jejunum with a hemorrhagic serosal surface (arrow). Normal jejunum is adjacent to the affected jejunum.

While it has been suggested that horses with proximal enteritis may benefit from surgical decompression of the affected small intestine, this was not demonstrated in a recent retrospective study.[122] Horses treated surgically had a greater total volume and a longer total duration of reflux compared with horses treated medically.[122] However, 28% of horses treated surgically produced ≤2 liters of reflux postoperatively, suggesting that there may be a benefit in some horses. Horses with proximal enteritis undergoing surgery were more painful and less likely to be febrile at admission compared with horses managed medically, suggesting that they were more critically ill than medically treated horses; however, other physical and laboratory findings were not different.[122] Exploratory abdominal surgery is still indicated as a diagnostic tool in horses that are refluxing and showing signs of colic.

The survival rate for horses with proximal enteritis is variable and is reported to range from 67%[121] to 77%[134] and, most recently, 87%, with 91% of horses managed medically and 75% of horses managed surgically surviving to hospital discharge.[122] Admission heart rate, PCV, plasma creatinine concentration, and peritoneal fluid TP and nucleated cell count were higher in horses that were euthanized compared with horses that survived.[122] The major life-threatening complications are persistent reflux, economic constraints imposed by the clients, and laminitis.[122]

Inflammatory or infiltrative bowel disease
Key points
- Inflammatory or infiltrative bowel disease is uncommon in horses.
- Horses with inflammatory or infiltrative bowel disease may present with chronic intermittent mild colic and weight loss or acutely with moderate signs of colic associated with a complete obstruction.
- Diagnosis can be made based on abdominal ultrasonographic examination, abdominocentesis, rectal biopsy, and/or exploratory celiotomy or laparoscopy with biopsy.
- Treatment predominantly consists of corticosteroids and dietary management unless the lesion is focal and a resection and anastomosis is possible.
- Long-term prognosis is unfavorable.

Definition/overview
Inflammatory or infiltrative bowel disease is defined as infiltration of the intestinal mucosa and submucosa with abnormal cells.[135] The diagnosis is based on the degree of inflammation and the type of cells.[136] The small intestine is affected primarily; however, the large intestine can be affected in severe cases. Types of inflammatory bowel disease are listed in *Table 1.3*.[137]

Table 1.3 **Inflammatory bowel diseases in horses**[137]

DISEASE	DEFINITION	PROPOSED CAUSES
Eosinophilic enteritis	Infiltration of the intestinal mucosa with eosinophils and lymphocytes	Type I hypersensitivity reaction to inhaled, dietary, or parasitic antigens
Granulomatous enteritis	Lymphoid and macrophage infiltration of the mucosal lamina propria with variable numbers of plasma cells and giant cells. Ileum most severely affected	Overactivation of mucosal T cells with the release of inflammatory cytokines leading to amplification and perpetuation of the disease process (similar to Crohn's disease in humans). Previously associated with *Mycobacterium* spp. infection and may be an abnormal inflammatory response to intestinal bacteria or diet
Lymphocytic/plasmacytic enteritis	Infiltration of the intestinal mucosal lamina propria with lymphocytes and plasma cells in the absence of granulomatous change	Possibly early stage of lymphoma
Lymphoma	Intestinal infiltration with malignant cells of lymphocyte origin	Unknown

Etiology/pathogenesis

The etiology and pathogenesis of inflammatory bowel disease in the horse is mostly unknown. It is thought to be an abnormal immune response to bacterial, viral, parasitic, or dietary antigens (*Table 1.3*).[138] Infectious causes include *Lawsonia intracellularis* and *Rhodococcus equi*.

Inflammatory or infiltrative bowel disease causes maldigestion (impaired breakdown of micronutrients) and malabsorption (defective nutrient uptake or transport by the intestinal mucosa), leading to clinical signs.[137]

Clinical features

Horses most commonly present with recurrent mild to moderate signs of colic and weight loss. They may have a history of inappetence and lethargy. Diarrhea may be a feature if the large intestine is also affected. Hypoproteinemia may also be a feature.

Horses with eosinophilic enteritis can present with acute signs of colic resulting from complete obstruction associated with circumferential mural bands (**1.67**).[139,140] Similarly, intestinal lymphoma can present as a discrete lesion causing obstruction and acute colic.[137]

Multisystemic disease is not uncommon. Clinical features may also be variable depending on other organs affected. Horses with eosinophilic enteritis may also have infiltration of skin, liver, pancreas, oral cavity, esophagus, lungs, and/or lymph nodes (multisystemic eosinophilic epitheliotrophic disease).[138] Even with multisystemic disease eosinophilia is rare. Granulomatous lesions can be observed in the lung and liver. Lymphoma can be primarily intestinal or secondary metastatic disease most commonly from the mediastinum.[137] Mesenteric lymph nodes are often affected. Horses with lymphoma often have anemia, thrombocytopenia, and hypoproteinemia. Lymphocytosis is rare.[137]

Horses of any age, breed, or gender are affected; however, eosinophilic and granulomatous enteritis is thought to affect young horses (1–5 years old) and Standardbreds and Thoroughbreds or Standardbreds, respectively.[138,141]

Differential diagnosis

- **Weight loss**[41]: malnutrition; dental or oral disease; parasitism; hepatic or renal disease; neoplasia; gastric ulcers; proliferative enteropathy; right dorsal colitis; sand colic.
- **Recurrent colic**: right dorsal colitis; sand colic; ileocecal intussusception; peritonitis.

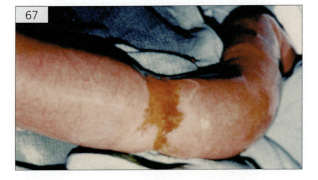

1.67 Focal eosinophic enteritis with mural fibrous bands causing stricture and leading to obstruction and acute signs of colic.

- **Acute colic**: primary ileus; proximal enteritis; ileal impaction; ileal muscular hypertrophy; ileocecal intussusception; strangulating small intestinal lesion.

Diagnosis

A thorough history should be obtained and physical examination completed to rule out other more common causes of weight loss. Fecal flotation for parasites should be performed.

Abdominal palpation per rectum (p. 32) may be used to identify thickened small intestine or any caudal masses associated with lymph node involvement. Abdominal ultrasonographic examination (p. 39) can be used to diagnose thickened small intestine and, on occasion, lymphadenopathy. A complete abdominal and thoracic ultrasonographic examination should be performed in horses suspected of having inflammatory or infiltrative bowel disease to identify multiorgan or multisystemic involvement or other diseases causing weight loss.

Abdominocentesis and peritoneal fluid analysis (p. 35) should be performed but is often non-diagnostic. Neoplastic lymphocytes may be identified in the peritoneal fluid in some horses with intestinal lymphoma and neutrophils or eosinophils in some horses with eosinophilic enteritis.

Rectal biopsy is diagnostic in approximately 30% of horses with inflammatory or infiltrative bowel disease when the disease involves the rectum.[137,142,143] Care should be taken with interpretation of a rectal biopsy.

Exploratory celiotomy or laparoscopy with intestinal biopsy using an 8-mm tissue biopsy punch is the best technique to obtain a definitive diagnosis. However, celiotomy and laparoscopy are invasive and expensive compared with other diagnostic methods.

Other diagnostic procedures include gastroduodenoscopy and biopsy and oral glucose or D-xylose absorption tests.[137] Skin or liver biopsy may also be diagnostic if these organs are affected.

Management/treatment

Dietary changes that have been recommended include (1) highly digestible and balanced feed, (2) frequent feeding of small amounts, (3) corn oil to increase caloric intake, and (4) simple high-fiber diets to minimize exposure to antigens and increase the proportion of feed digested in the large intestine (e.g. oats supplemented with corn oil and grass hay[137]).

Daily anthelmintic treatment with pyrantel tartrate to remove exposure to parasitic antigens and treatment with ivermectin and praziquantel in the spring and autumn to manage bots and tapeworms has been previously recommended.[137] However, because of the development of anthelmintic resistance, a targeted deworming regimen has recently gained more favor.[143a]

Corticosteroid treatment should be individually altered based on the horse's response and prolonged treatment is often necessary. One regimen[137] involves administering dexamethasone (2 mg/ml) at: 0.05 mg/kg IM q24h for 3 weeks; 0.03 mg/kg IM q24h for 3 weeks; re-evaluate patient; 0.03 mg/kg PO q24h for 3 weeks; and finally 0.03 mg/kg PO q48h for 3 weeks. HIgher doses (0.1 mg/kg) may be required for a short period of time.

Other treatments that have been used include: metronidazole for its anti-inflammatory and antimicrobial effects; hydroxyurea (antineoplastic drug) in horses with multisystemic epitheliotropic eosinophilic disease; and chemotherapy in horses with lymphoma.[137]

Some horses have focal lesions and resection of the affected bowel and anastomosis is possible and often curative. These horses have a good prognosis for survival.

The long-term prognosis for survival for horses with diffuse inflammatory or infiltrative bowel disease is guarded to poor. Early and appropriate treatment with corticosteroids was reported to be successful in about 50% of cases.[137] Prolonged treatment with corticosteroids may be necessary and can be associated with complications associated with infection, hyperadrenocorticism, and laminitis. The long-term prognosis for horses with lymphoma is poor.

Proliferative enteropathy
Key points

- Proliferative enteropathy should be suspected in a weanling with signs of colic, diarrhea, and weight loss or failure to thrive.
- Hypoproteinemia and markedly thickened small intestine identified on ultrasonographic examination support the tentative diagnosis of proliferative enteropathy.
- Diagnosis can be confirmed antemortem with fecal PCR and serum antibody titers and postmortem based on the gross and histologic appearance of the affected intestine.

Definition/overview

Proliferative enteropathy is an intestinal disease characterized grossly by segmental mucosal hypertrophy (**1.68**) and histologically by crypt hyperplasia, with a large number of small, curved, intracellular bacteria in the apical cytoplasm of proliferating enterocytes that are usually only visible when stained with silver stain (**1.69A, B**).[144] Proliferative enteropathy (also known as intestinal adenomatosis) is often endemic in swine populations, causing reduced growth rates and diarrhea in weanling pigs.[144]

Etiology/pathogenesis

The etiological agent for proliferative enteropathy is *Lawsonia intracellularis*. Proliferative enteropathy is a transmissible disease that occurs in foals and weanlings 3–9 months old.[145] In one study, most foals had been weaned prior to the onset of clinical signs.[146] Proliferative enteropathy has been reported in horses in the USA, Canada, Australia, and parts of Europe. Clinical signs are attributable to mucosal injury associated with the infection.

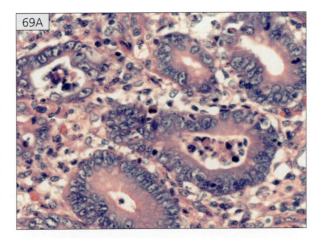

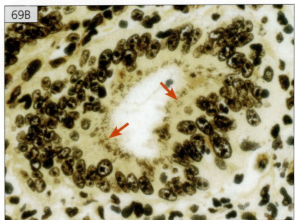

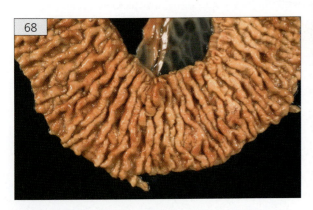

1.68 Gross appearance of a horse with proliferative enteropathy caused by *Lawsonia intracellularis*. (Courtesy Dr Perry Habecker)

1.69A, B Histologic appearance of a horse with proliferative enteropathy caused by *Lawsonia intracellularis*. (A) Hematoxylin and eosin stain showing a proliferative enteropathy and (B) Warthin-Starry silver stain showing curved intracellular bacteria in the apical cytoplasm of crypt cells (arrows). (Courtesy Dr Perry Habecker)

Clinical features

The characteristic clinical features of proliferative enteropathy are profound dull demeanor, lethargy, rough hair coat, inappetence or anorexia, rapid and marked weight loss and poor body condition, pot-bellied appearance, colic, mild to severe diarrhea, fever, intestinal hypermotility, dehydration, and hypoproteinemia causing ventral edema.[146–148] Affected horses often have a transient leukocytosis, mild anemia, mild to severe panhypoproteinemia, electrolyte abnormalities (hyponatremia, hypokalemia, hypocalcemia), and metabolic acidosis.[149] Occasionally, patients will have azotemia, hypoglycemia, hyperfibrinogenemia, and high serum creatine kinase concentration.[146,148] Peritoneal fluid analysis is usually within normal limits.[149]

Differential diagnosis

Malnutrition; parasitism; gastric ulceration; inflammatory or infiltrative bowel disease; ileocecal intussusception; colitis.

Diagnosis

Proliferative enteropathy should be suspected based on the patient's age and clinical signs. Ultrasonographic examination reveals markedly thickened small intestine (**1.70A, B**) and can be used to support the tentative diagnosis.

A definitive diagnosis can be obtained antemortem by detection of *L. intracellularis* in fecal samples with PCR and serum antibodies against *L. intracellularis*.[149]

While PCR is specific for *L. intracellularis*, it may lack sensitivity because of PCR-inhibitory factors that inactivate or interfere with the test and a lack of bacterial shedding.[149] Obtaining fecal samples prior to initiation of antimicrobial treatment and serial daily samples may improve the sensitivity. Refrigeration of fecal samples is recommended.[149]

Positive serum titers for naturally infected horses are often between 1:30 and 1:120[146], but can be up to 1:960.[147] Serum antibody titers are likely to be negative in acute infection because of inadequate time to mount an immune response[149] and serologically positive foals and horses have been detected on premises with a clinically affected foal.[149] Therefore, serial serum samples should be submitted.

In one case report, fecal PCR for *L. intracellularis* was negative and the serum antibody titer was positive.[147] Similarly, in a case series, only six out of 18 foals had a positive fecal PCR for *L. intracellularis* and in all cases tested the serum was positive for anti-*L. intracellularis* antibodies.[146]

Post-mortem diagnosis is based most often on the characteristic gross lesions of segmental mucosal hypertrophy involving the ileum and distal jejunum and, in severe cases, the entire jejunum.[144] Histologically, the lesions have mucosal hyperplasia and curved intracellular bacteria in the apical cytoplasm of crypt cells.[150] Staining with Warthin-Starry silver stain or immunohistochemistry can be used to confirm the presence of *L. intracellularis*.

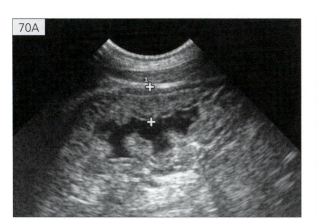 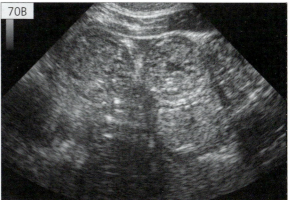

1.70A, B Ultrasonographic appearance of proliferative enteropathy showing single (A) and multiple (B) thickened loops of small intestine. (Courtesy Dr JoAnn Slack)

Management/treatment

Management is similar to that for enteritis and colitis and involves crystalloid and colloid IV fluid therapy and electrolytes, anti-inflammatory and analgesic drugs, antiulcer medication, and antidiarrheal treatment.[149] Parenteral nutrition may be necessary in patients not able to tolerate enteral feeding. Easily digestible complete pelleted feeds are recommended. *L. intracellularis* infection is treated with antimicrobial drugs:

- Erythromycin alone (15–25 mg/kg PO q6–8h for 21 days).
- Erythromycin (see above) and rifampin (5–10 mg/ kg PO q12h for 21 days).
- Azithromycin (10 mg/kg PO q24h for 5 days then 10 mg/kg PO q48h) and rifampin (5 mg/kg PO q12h).[149]
- Oxytetracycline (6.6 mg/kg IV q12h for 7 days) then doxycycline (10 mg/kg PO q12h for 8–17 days). Treatment with oxytetracycline and doxycycline may be as effective, less expensive, easier, and associated with fewer side-effects compared with treatment with erythromycin/ azithromycin.[148]
- Chloramphenicol (25–50 mg/kg PO q6–8h for 14 days).

Cecum

- Cecal disease is an uncommon cause of colic.
- Horses can present with variable clinical signs from very mild signs associated with a cecal impaction to severe signs with a cecal infarction.
- Palpation per rectum and abdominal ultrasonographic examination are useful diagnostic tools for evaluating horses with suspected cecal disease.
- Surgery is indicated in many horses with cecal disease. Procedures commonly performed include typhlotomy, partial typhlectomy, and jejuno- or ileocolostomy (cecal bypass).[8a,150a]
- Common lesions affecting the cecum include cecal impaction, cecocecal and cecocolic intussusception (p. 101), and less often, cecal infarction (p. 104).

Cecal impaction

Key points

- Horses with cecal impaction may not be particularly painful and the most notable features may be inappetence and insufficient fecal production. Pain is generally well managed with flunixin meglumine.
- Horses with cecal impactions are at risk of cecal rupture, which is rapidly fatal.

Definition/overview

Cecal impaction refers to the accumulation of solid ingesta or fluid within the cecum (**1.71**). The former is thought to be a primary impaction and the latter secondary to cecal dysfunction.[151] In many cases, however, the distinction between primary and secondary or solid and fluid contents is not as obvious as would be expected. Cecal impaction is the most common cecal disease in the horse. Cecal impaction can lead to cecal rupture, which is fatal in most cases (**1.72**) and has been reported to occur in 24–57% of horses with cecal impaction.[152,153]

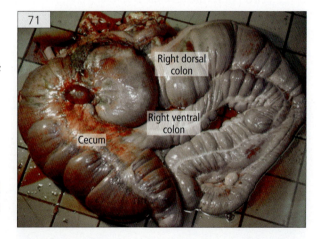

1.71 Gross appearance of a horse with a cecal impaction. (Courtesy Dr Michael Ross)

Etiology/pathogenesis

Cecal impaction is usually not associated with a mechanical obstruction and is thought, in most cases, to be functional.[154] Cecal impaction is commonly seen in horses receiving treatment for another, non-GI problem (e.g. post-arthroscopy, post-arytenoidectomy, horses with lacerations, fractures, or ocular lesions). While the exact etiology and pathogenesis of cecal impaction is unknown, many predisposing factors have been identified. Recent stall confinement or hospitalization, fasting, general anesthesia, surgery, and NSAIDs have been associated with cecal impaction.[154,155] General anesthesia, NSAIDs, and a lack of exercise have been shown to impair GI tract motility.[156–158]

Poor dentition, feeding poor-quality roughage, inadequate water intake, parturition, parasite-induced thromboembolism, and *Anaplocephala perfoliata* (tapeworms) are thought to be involved in the pathogenesis of cecal impactions.[154,159,160] Horses fed Coastal Bermuda grass hay may be predisposed.[160] Arabian, Appaloosa, and Morgan horses as well as horses >15 years old were more often affected than other horses in one study.[158]

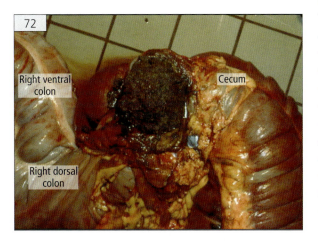

1.72 Cecal rupture. (Courtesy Dr Michael Ross)

Right ventral colon

Cecum

Right dorsal colon

Clinical features

Horses with cecal impaction are often only mildly painful. Signs may be as subtle as inappetence, dull demeanor, and reduced fecal output. Flank 'staring' and recumbency may be the predominant signs of colic. Colic signs can generally be controlled with analgesia, such as flunixin meglumine. Some horses with cecal impaction will be moderately painful. The heart rate, respiratory rate, and rectal temperature will often be within normal limits. Intestinal borborygmi are usually reduced compared with normal. Laboratory data are initially within normal limits.

Tachycardia and tachypnea and signs of shock will develop following cecal perforation and the oral mucous membranes will become injected to toxic with a prolonged CRT.

Differential diagnosis

Large colon impaction; right dorsal displacement of the large colon; NSLE; small colon impaction.

Diagnosis

Cecal impaction can be diagnosed based on abdominal palpation per rectum in most cases. A firm ingesta (or fluid and gas)-filled viscus with a tight band and sacculations can usually be palpated on the right side of the abdomen. The cecum is usually oriented more dorsoventrally; however, in some cases it may appear to be oriented transversely cranial to the pelvic inlet. The cecum can usually be distinguished from the large colon during palpation per rectum based on the location, orientation, and the inability to palpate dorsal to the cecum. In some cases, it can be difficult to distinguish the cecum from the large colon. Occasionally, a cecal impaction will not be palpable per rectum because only the cupula is involved.[161] Ultrasonographic examination can be used in these cases to diagnose a cecal impaction and to differentiate cecal from colonic disease. Ultrasonographic examination and abdominocentesis with peritoneal fluid analysis can be used to diagnose cecal rupture.

Abdominocentesis was not found to be useful in differentiating horses that would respond to medical treatment from those in which surgical treatment was necessary.[153]

Management/treatment

Some cases of cecal impaction can be managed medically. Medical management involves withholding feed, analgesia (flunixin meglumine and xylazine or butorphanol as needed), IV and/or enteral fluid and electrolyte therapy, laxatives, and cathartics (see Large colon impaction). Motility modifying drugs (see Chapter 18) can be used; however, anecdotally there is concern that these drugs may precipitate perforation. In a recent retrospective study, approximately half of the horses with cecal impaction were treated medically and 81% of horses with a cecal impaction managed medically survived to hospital discharge. The median duration of time to resolution of clinical signs was 2 days with a median hospitalization period of 11 days.[153] The 1-year survival rate was 95%.[153] However, in the latter study, several of these cases may have been a result of feeding Coastal Bermuda grass hay and cecal impactions with this etiology may be more likely to respond to medical treatment. More recently, in a population of horses with cecal impaction not associated with feeding Coastal Bermuda grass hay and with a high proportion of cases secondary to another non-GI problem, the success of medical management was lower (60%).[161a]

Because of the concern of cecal perforation or rupture, many clinicians will recommend surgical treatment of horses with a cecal impaction. Severity or persistence of colic signs, extent of cecal distension and tension on the cecal band, and a lack of response to medical treatment are used to make the decision for surgical treatment. The two major surgical procedures are typhlotomy alone (**1.73**) or typhlotomy plus complete or incomplete cecal bypass. Typhlotomy involves cecal exteriorization and a 10-cm incision at the cecal apex. It is important to empty the cupula as well as the body and apex of the cecum. This may necessitate placing an arm through the typhlotomy and into the cecal base. The typhlotomy can then be closed using 2-0 synthetic absorbable suture material in a simple continuous pattern oversewn with a Cushing pattern. If contamination is excessive, a partial typhlectomy of the cecal apex using stapling equipment (TA-90 or ILA-100, US Surgical Corporation) followed by oversewing the staple line can be performed.

Complete or incomplete cecal bypass via an ileo-/jejunocolostomy involves creating a side-to-side anastomosis between the ileum or jejunum and the right ventral colon. The anastomosis can be stapled or handsewn. Complete cecal bypass also involves transection of the ileum, which is usually performed using staples, and the two ends are oversewn. There was no improvement in survival or prevention of reimpaction in horses with a cecal impaction managed surgically by typhlotomy alone or typhlotomy with incomplete bypass.[161a] Complete cecal bypass is recommended in cases of recurrent or chronic cecal impaction (e.g. >5 days).

Postoperatively, horses are managed with perioperative antimicrobial drugs, IV fluids, and flunixin meglumine. Motility stimulants may be used in some cases. Slow refeeding over 7–10 days is thought to be important to prevent reimpaction. Feed should be withheld for 24–36 hours, followed by grazing, then small amounts of a pelleted low-residue feed, and then hay.

The most common postoperative complications are incisional infection (22%), diarrhea (19%), and postoperative ileus (19%). Recurrence of cecal impaction occurred in 13% of horses and 13% had undiagnosed colic episodes.[153] The short-term survival rate following surgery was ~80–95% and the long-term survival rate 65–89%.[153, 161a]

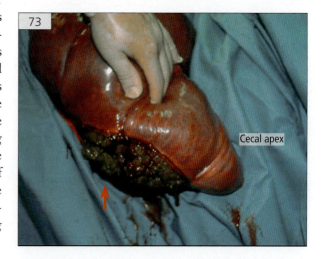

1.73 Typhlotomy (arrow). (Courtesy Dr Michael Ross)

Cecocecal and cecocolic intussusception

Key points

- Young horses and Standardbred horses are most often affected.
- Horses can present with acute to chronic signs.
- A good prognosis has been reported even in cases where manual reduction of the intussusception was not possible.
- Deworming with an anthelmintic against tapeworms is recommended.

Definition/overview

Cecocecal or cecocolic intussusception refers to the invagination of the cecal apex into the cecal body (cecocecal) or through the cecocolic orifice and into the right ventral colon (**1.74A–C**).[160]

Etiology/pathogenesis

Altered cecal motility is thought to be involved in the pathogenesis, although a specific etiology has not been determined.[160] Diet change, cecal wall abscess,

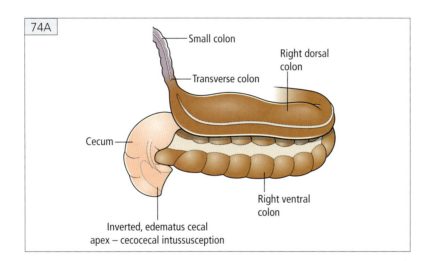

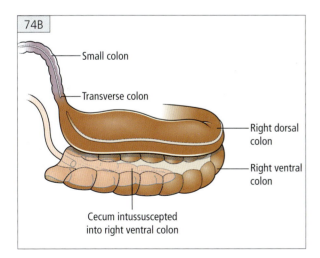

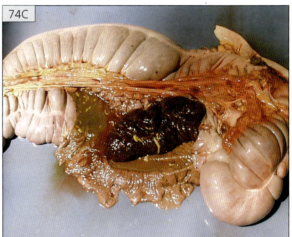

1.74A–C Schematic illustration of a cecocecal (A) and a cecocolic (B) intussusception. (C) Cecocolic intussusception diagnosed at necropsy. The right ventral colon has been opened and the hemorrhagic cecum is identified within the colonic lumen.

Salmonella spp., *Eimeria leuckarti*, *Strongylus vulgaris*, cyathostomes, organophosphates, parasympathomimetic drugs, and *Anaplocephala perfoliata* (tapeworms, **1.75A, B**) are thought to be risk factors.[162–166] Horses <3 years old and Standardbred horses appear to be at a high risk.[163,164]

Clinical features

Horse may present with acute or chronic signs depending on the extent of the mechanical obstruction and vascular compromise.[160] Most horses (55%) presented with acute, moderate to severe signs of colic (acute); 30% presented with intermittent mild to moderate colic signs with soft feces or diarrhea of 3–8 days duration; and 13% had chronic weight loss, scant soft feces, and mild colic signs for 6–180 days duration (chronic).[164] Cecocecal intussusception was more likely to result in chronic signs and cecocolic intussusception in acute signs, with complete obstruction to the passage of ingesta and vascular compromise to the cecal apex and part of the body.[164]

Differential diagnosis

Large colon impaction; cecal impaction; right dorsal displacement of the large colon; ileocecal intussusception

Diagnosis

In horses with cecocolic intussusception, abdominal examination per rectum may reveal a mass or edematous intestine in the right caudal abdomen, the cecum may feel malpositioned, or it may not be identified.[160] Cecocecal intussusceptions are usually not diagnosed on abdominal palpation per rectum.

Abdominal ultrasonographic examination can be used to identify the invaginated cecal apex within the cecum or the cecum within the colon (**1.76A–C**).

Peritoneal fluid analysis is often within normal limits initially because the abnormal intestine is sequestered; however, the TP and nucleated cell count will increase over time. Diagnosis is often made at surgery.

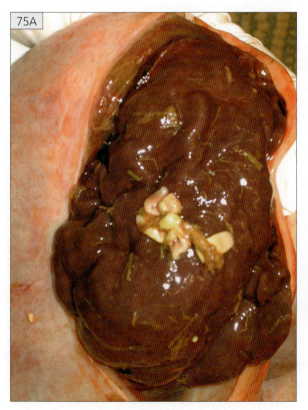

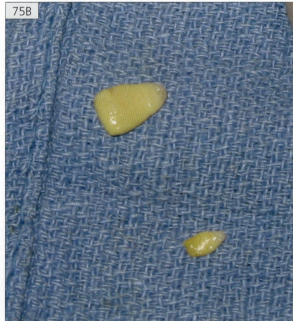

1.75A, B *Anaplocephala perfoliata in situ* **(A) and (B) isolated.**

Management/treatment

Exploratory celiotomy through a ventral midline approach is often necessary to make a diagnosis and correct the intussusception. Attempting to manually reduce the intussusception was reported to be successful in one-third of cases.[164] Typhlectomy is necessary if the intussusceptum (i.e. cecum) has vascular compromise.

If manual reduction is unsuccessful because of edema and adhesion formation, the cecal apex and part of the body can be amputated through a right ventral colon colotomy followed by reduction.[167] In cases where reduction is not possible following partial cecal amputation, a bypass via a jejuno- or ileocolostomy is necessary.

Postoperative treatment includes perioperative antimicrobial drugs, flunixin meglumine, and IV fluids (see Chapter 18).

Anthelmintic treatment with pyrantel pamoate or praziquantel is recommended because of the association between cecocecal or cecocolic intussusception and tapeworm infection.

The prognosis for horses with cecocecal intussusception is good.[59] A good prognosis for horses with irreducible cecocolic intussusception requiring partial typhlectomy through a colotomy has also been reported.[167] Additionally, 4/6[168] and 3/3[169] horses survived after bypass via a jejuno- or ileocolostomy of a cecocolic intussusception without partial typhlectomy.

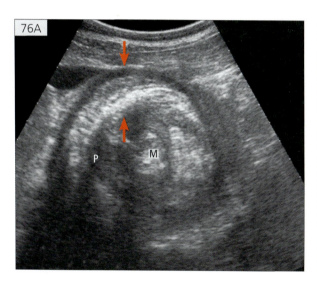

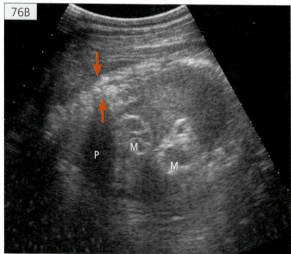

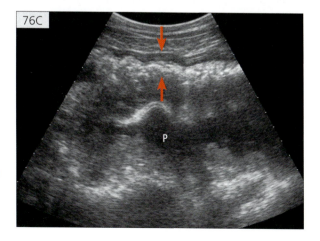

1.76A–C Ultrasonographic appearance of a cecocecal intussusception imaged through the right flank; cross-sectional (A, B) and longitudinal (C) views. The arrows show the outer (intussuscipiens) and inner (intussusceptum) walls of the cecum with gas in between (hyperechoic area). P, peritoneal fluid; M, mesenteric vessels. (Courtesy Drs Laura Johnstone and Rose Nolen-Walston)

Cecal infarction

See Colonic infarction.

Large colon
Strangulating or ischemic lesions

- Horses with large colon strangulating or ischemic lesions present with severe abdominal pain and distension.
- Signs of shock develop rapidly.
- Abdominal surgery is necessary for management (LCV).
- A favorable prognosis is dependent on early treatment.

Large colon volvulus
Key points

- A LCV should be suspected in any horse showing severe signs of colic particularly if there is marked or rapidly developing abdominal distension.
- LCV is a common cause of colic in postparturient mares.
- Early referral and surgical correction is critical for a favorable outcome.

Definition/overview

Abnormal twisting of the large colon causing obstruction of the intestinal lumen, arterial supply, and venous drainage. The twist occurs across the mesocolon and is usually at the colonic base with the ventral colon rotated medially and the dorsal colon rotated laterally (dorsolateral–ventromedial or counter-clockwise as viewed from the ventral abdominal wall) (**1.77A, B**). LCV represents 10–26% of surgical colic cases at referral hospitals.[5,170,171]

Etiology/pathogenesis

The exact etiology and pathogenesis of LCV is unknown. Broodmares appear to be predisposed and this may be because of alterations in intestinal motility or colonic positioning associated with pregnancy and parturition. Of 163 broodmares admitted on emergency within 30 days of parturition, 16.6% were diagnosed with a LCV; urogenital hemorrhage and LCV were the most common diagnoses in periparturient mares.[172] LCV occurred within 3 months of parturition in >80% of post-parturient mares presenting with an LCV.[171] While LCV appears to occur frequently in peri- and post-parturient mares, castrated and entire male horses represented 45% of the LCV cases and only 18% and 8% of 327 horses with a LCV had recently foaled or were pregnant, respectively.[171] LCV most commonly affects mature horses.

Interestingly, 33% of horses with a LCV had a history of at least one previous colic episode prior to the volvulus. Horses with a previous colic episode were significantly more likely to have an episode of colic following surgery for LCV compared with horses that did not have a previous colic episode (50% versus 17%) suggesting that some of these horses may be predisposed to colic and have alterations in intestinal function.[171]

Clinical features

Horses with a LCV are usually severely painful and have marked abdominal distension. The severe pain may have been acute in onset or may have been preceded by a period of mild to moderate pain. The pain is usually unresponsive to analgesia and the horse is often difficult to examine. Abdominal distension usually progresses rapidly and can be severe enough to inhibit adequate spontaneous ventilation. Heart rate, respiratory rate, and rectal temperature are variable depending on the use of alpha-2 agonists, duration of the LCV, as well as the degree of pain, endotoxemia, and cardiovascular and respiratory compromise. Oral mucous membranes vary in color from pink to purple, are usually dry, and the CRT may be short or prolonged depending on the stage of shock. Signs of shock (tachycardia, weak peripheral pulses, cool extremities, prolonged CRT, bright pink to purple mucous membranes, poor jugular refill) develop rapidly if the lesion is not corrected.

Differential diagnosis

Severe gas colic; small intestinal volvulus; large colon infarction; colitis; middle uterine artery hemorrhage (postpartum mare); uterine hemorrhage or tear (postpartum mare).

Diagnosis

A tentative diagnosis can be made based on the signalment (e.g. postpartum mare), severe pain, and marked abdominal distension. Abdominal palpation per rectum is often difficult and unsafe to perform because of the severity of the colic signs, and findings may be unremarkable despite obvious abdominal distension. Large colon distension can be palpated per rectum in many cases and is not specific for a LCV.

Ultrasonographic examination has been described to identify LCV. A colon wall thickness ≥9 mm had a sensitivity of 67% and a specificity of 100% for diagnosis of a LCV[4], and a finding of non-sacculated large colon ultrasonographically in the left ventral abdominal quadrant was consistently indicative of LCV in four horses.[173] Often one of the main differential diagnoses for LCV is severe colitis, and identification of thickened large colon is insufficient to differentiate ultrasonographically a LCV from a colitis. However, colitis should be considered if the horse has fever, leukopenia, hypoalbuminemia, and hyponatremia.

Ultrasonographic evaluation is usually unnecessary in horses with a LCV because surgery or euthanasia is indicated based on the severity of pain. Physical and laboratory data can provide prognostic information. A definitive diagnosis is usually made at surgery.

Management/treatment

Early referral and surgical correction is necessary for a favorable outcome. Horses should be resuscitated preoperatively with hypertonic saline (4 ml/kg) and polyionic isotonic fluids (>20 liters) (see Chapter 12). Antimicrobial drugs and flunixin meglumine are administered preoperatively. Analgesia (xylazine and butorphanol, or detomidine) is given as necessary to allow catheter placement and preparation for surgery. In some cases with severe abdominal distension, trocharization using either a 5-cm (2-in) 14-gauge needle or a 13.3-cm (5.25-in) 14-gauge IV catheter may be necessary to improve ventilation and venous return to the heart.

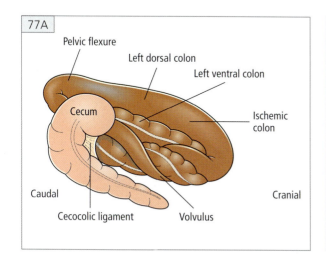
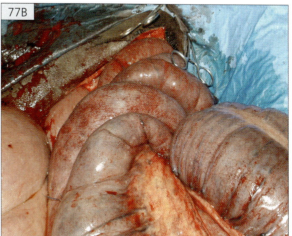

1.77A, B A large colon volvulus almost always occurs in a dorsolateral–ventromedial (counter-clockwise) direction at the colonic base. **(A)** Schematic illustration. **(B)** Experimentally created large colon volvulus with the colon exteriorized.

A ventral midline approach is made with the horse under general anesthesia and the LCV can usually be palpated in the right mid to cranial abdomen. The twist is usually in a dorsolateral–ventromedial (counter-clockwise direction) and is rotated dorsomedial–ventrolateral to correct the LCV. Key points for successfully correcting a LCV are to rotate the colon immediately adjacent to the twist, which is almost always deep within the abdomen at the base of the colon, create a large enough incision to allow for easy colonic manipulation, adequately decompress the gas from the colon prior to derotation, and empty the colon through a pelvic flexure enterotomy if the colon is markedly ingesta-filled and there is concern of colonic rupture. Use of sodium carboxymethylcellulose may be beneficial when manipulating the colon.

Assessment of intestinal viability is usually based on the serosal color, which is inherently unreliable. Mucosal color can be used if a pelvic flexure enterotomy is performed and is somewhat more reliable (i.e. a black or green mucosa and a lack of bleeding from the enterotomy indicate a poor prognosis for survival, **1.78**). Edema resolution, palpation of an arterial pulse, and motility are used as indications of adequate colonic viability. Other methods that can be used to assess intestinal viability include intraluminal pressure[174], IV fluorescein dye (11 mg/kg of a 25% solution), Doppler ultrasonography, laser Doppler velocimetry, surface and pulse oximetry, and histologic evaluation of morphological damage using frozen sections (**1.79A, B**)[175]; however, these methods all have inherent limitations and are rarely used in clinical cases. The author generally recommends recovering horses with a LCV, economics permitting, because often it is difficult to predict which horses will survive and which horses will not survive.

A pelvic flexure enterotomy may be performed to empty the contents of the damaged large colon and to administer intraluminal di-tri-octahedral-smectite for endotoxin absorption or psyllium mucilloid, which may help enterocyte healing. A large colon resection[8a] is performed by some surgeons in cases where there is uncertainty of colonic viability based on the appearance of the colon. Colonic resection and anastomosis may improve the prognosis for some horses with a LCV.[176,177] Interestingly, intraluminal pressure measurements were not useful for predicting survival in horses with a LCV undergoing colonic resection and anastomosis.[178]

Postoperative treatment includes analgesia and anti-inflammatory drugs (e.g. flunixin meglumine, IV lidocaine), antiendotoxin treatment (e.g. J-5 plasma, polymixin B), and carefully monitored fluid therapy (see Chapter 11 and Chapter 18). Additional treatments that may be used are anti-coagulants (e.g. heparin, aspirin), free radical scavengers (e.g. dimethylsulfoxide), and pentoxifylline.[179] However, the use of these drugs appears to have declined, likely based on apparent lack of clinical efficacy. Hay should be reintroduced over 2–3 days depending on fecal production, borborygmi, colonic distension, signs of pain, and appetite.

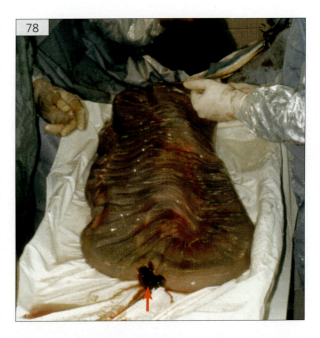

1.78 A pelvic flexure enterotomy can be performed to assess the mucosal color (arrow) and provide prognostic information. (Courtesy Dr Ted Stashak)

Postoperative complications include diarrhea, jugular vein thrombophlebitis, and ongoing colonic ischemia. Clinical signs associated with a non-viable colon include persistent tachycardia, tachypnea, fever, inappetence, abdominal distension, lack of fecal production, and colic. With non-viability, PCV tends to increase, TPP decreases, and blood lactate concentration remains high

The reported prognosis for horses with a LCV is variable and is mostly dependent of the duration of time between the onset of severe pain and surgery. Encouragingly, a recent study reported a short-term survival of 83%; however, horses in that practice are referred and operated on soon after the onset of clinical signs.[170] Importantly, survival rates did improve from the late 1980s (25%) to the late 1990s (70%).[171] The recurrence rate is between 10% and 20% and colonic resection and anastomosis or colopexy can be performed in recurrent cases.

Admission physical examination and laboratory data can be used to predict prognosis for survival. Admission heart rate, PCV, plasma glucose, and creatinine concentration have been associated with survival[171,179] and reflect the severity of colonic damage, endotoxemia, and systemic inflammatory response syndrome. More recently, plasma lactate concentration was significantly lower in horses with a viable colon compared with horses with a non-viable colon, and plasma lactate concentration <6 mmol/l [54 mg/dl] had a sensitivity of 84% and a specificity of 83% for predicting survival.[180] Importantly, except in the most extreme cases when there is obviously poor viability, it is recommended that horses are recovered from general anesthesia and monitored closely for colonic non-viability.

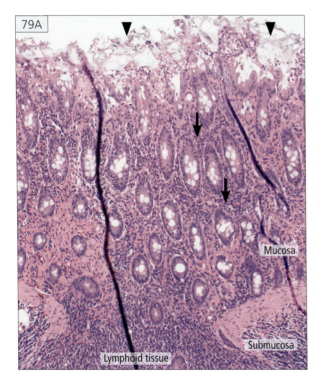
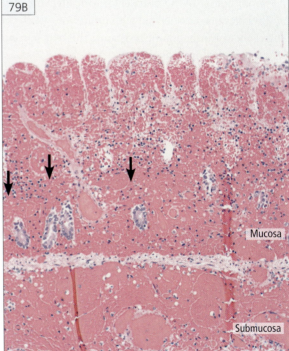

1.79A, B Histologic appearance of the colon from a horse that would survive (A) and one that would not survive (B). Note the loss of deep epithelium and crypt architecture (arrows) in the severely affected horse and loss of superficial epithelium only (arrowheads) in the horse that would have survived.

Infarction
Key points
- Colonic infarction is an uncommon cause of colic.
- Horses are initially in severe pain and rapidly develop signs of shock.
- Cecal infarction can occur concurrently or independently.
- Infarction is often associated with colitis or a postoperative complication following LCV.

Definition/overview
Infarction is defined as a localized area of necrosis resulting from obstruction of the blood supply (**1.80**).

Etiology/pathogenesis
The exact cause of infarction is often unknown. However, horses with severe colitis or postoperative LCV can develop an infarction as a complication of the primary disease. Damage to the intestinal vascular endothelium and a hypercoagulable state causing intravascular thrombosis are probably important in the pathophysiology of this disease. Historically, *Strongylus vulgaris* has been associated with infarction. With the emergence of anthelmintic resistance, this may become an important clinical disease.

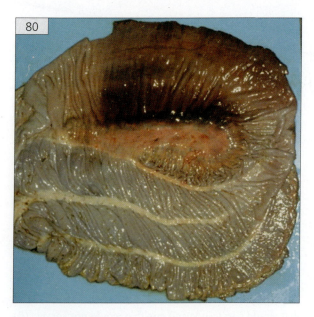

1.80 Infarct in the left dorsal colon adjacent to the pelvic flexure.

Clinical features
Horses with infarction are in severe pain during the initial ischemic phase. Clinical signs are variable depending on the extent of intestinal necrosis. Once necrosis has occurred, signs of shock including marked tachycardia, tachypnea, injected or toxic oral mucous membranes, prolonged CRT, cool extremities, and dull demeanor are observed. Horses may also present with signs of peritonitis (p. 148) if the infarction involves a segment of bowel only.

Differential diagnosis
LCV; colitis; peritonitis.

Diagnosis
Laboratory features include a high PCV and relative hypoproteinemia, leukopenia, and a markedly high plasma lactate concentration. Peritoneal fluid will frequently be serosanguineous or consistent with peritonitis depending on the duration of infarction.

Abdominal ultrasonographic examination may reveal an increase in the volume and possibly echogenicity of peritoneal fluid and the affected bowel will be thickened if it is observed. However, is unlikely to be useful for diagnosing an infarction. Diagnosis is frequently made at surgery or necropsy.

Management/treatment
Horses with extensive infarction are often euthanized because of severe systemic disease and a non-resectable lesion. Horses with local infarction in an area of the intestine that can be exteriorized (**1.80**) can be managed surgically with resection of the affected bowel. (See also Chapter 18.)

Non-strangulating lesions
- Horses with non-strangulating large colon lesions are in mild to moderate pain and responsive to treatment with analgesics, at least temporarily. Generally, horses do not shown signs of shock. Abdominal distension and colonic distension on palpation per rectum are typical features.
- Horses with non-strangulating colonic obstruction generally have an excellent prognosis.

- Non-strangulating lesions of the large colon include gas or spasmodic colic, intraluminal obstruction including impaction (p. 110), sand impaction (p. 113) and enterolithiasis (p. 115), displacements including nephrosplenic entrapment of the large colon (p. 118) and right dorsal displacement (p. 122), and inflammatory diseases including colitis (p. 124) and right dorsal colitis (p. 127). For neoplasia, see Small intestine.

Gas or spasmodic colic
Key points

- Gas or spasmodic colic is likely the most common cause of abdominal pain in horses.
- A diagnosis of gas or spasmodic colic is made when the horse responds to medical treatment without another cause for the colic being identified.

Definition/overview

Gas or spasmodic colic (also referred to as medical colic) is associated with signs of abdominal pain thought to be caused by dysmotility and/or intraluminal accumulation of gas in the cecum or large colon. Gas or spasmodic colic is likely the most common cause of abdominal pain in horses and is generally a diagnosis made by exclusion of other causes of acute colic.

Etiology/pathogenesis

While the cause of gas or spasmodic colic is unknown, predisposing factors have been identified in large epidemiologic studies. Predisposing factors for colic in general include: change in diet, type or batch of hay, and type of grain or concentrate fed; longer time in a stall and less time on pasture; feeding >2.7 kg of oats per day, hay from round bales, Coastal Bermuda grass hay; change in housing or weather; recent travel; Thoroughbred and Arabian breeds; horses >8–10 years old; previous colic or colic surgery; absence of or very recent anthelmintic treatment; infrequent dental care; and aerophagia.[181–184] These factors likely cause mild colic through alterations in hindgut fermentation, indigestion, mild inflammation, parasitic damage, or alterations in enteric or autonomic nervous system function.

Clinical features

Signs of abdominal pain are usually mild to moderate, but can be acute and severe. Occasionally, horses with colonic tympany can have severe abdominal distension. The most striking feature is that most horses respond rapidly to medical therapy with flunixin meglumine, xylazine, and butorphanol, and enteral fluids or mineral oil. Horses with gas or spasmodic colic do not show signs of shock (moderate to severe tachycardia, injected or toxic oral mucous membranes, sweating, cool extremities).

Differential diagnosis

Large colon impaction; right dorsal displacement of the large colon; entrapment of the large colon over the nephrosplenic ligament; small colon impaction; fecalith obstruction; enterolithiasis (depending on geographic location).

Diagnosis

A diagnosis of gas or spasmodic colic is made when a horse responds to medical therapy or when intraluminal accumulation of gas is the only abnormal finding at surgery.

Management/treatment

The vast majority of horses with gas or spasmodic colic recover with minimal or no treatment.[185] Analgesia with flunixin meglumine is often all that is necessary. In some cases, additional analgesia with xylazine and butorphanol or even detomidine may be necessary. N-butyl-scopolammonium bromide (Buscopan®), a parasympathomimetic or spasmolytic drug, is used by some veterinarians; however, its efficacy in a large randomized blinded clinical trial has not be evaluated.

Rarely, horses with severe colonic tympany undergo abdominal surgery because of the severity of pain and abdominal distension. Horses are decompressed using a 14-gauge needle and suction and the abdomen explored. Postoperative treatment involves flunixin meglumine for 2–3 days. Hay should be reintroduced over 36–48 hours. (See also Chapter 18.) The prognosis is excellent. Some horses may have recurrent gas or spasmodic colic.

Large colon impaction
Key points
- Large colon impaction is a very common cause of colic in adult horses.
- Most horses with large colon impaction respond to medical treatment.
- Large volumes of enteral fluids and electrolytes are necessary for hydration of the colonic impaction and successful medical management.
- Surgery is necessary in some cases not responding to medical treatment and care needs to be taken to avoid colonic rupture during surgery.
- The prognosis for survival is excellent.

Definition/overview
Obstruction of the large colon lumen with firm ingesta. Impactions occur most often in the right dorsal colon (**1.81A**) or pelvic flexure (left ventral colon, **1.81B**). Large colon impaction with ingesta is the second most common cause of colic after gas or spasmodic colic.

Etiology/pathogenesis
While the exact etiology and pathogenesis are unknown, identified risk factors, which are similar to those for gas or spasmodic colic, include increasing number of hours in a stall, residing at the present stable for <6 months, recent change in exercise regimen, infrequent dental care, absence of ivermectin or moxidectin anthelmintic treatment in the previous 12 months, travel within the preceding 24 hours, cribbiting and windsucking, recent lameness (<4 weeks), and having had a previous episode of colic.[184] In one study, 54% of horses with a large colon impaction had a change in routine within the previous 2 weeks and 12% developed an impaction while being hospitalized for a non-GI disease.[157] Alterations in intestinal motility associated with enteric or autonomic nervous system function, intestinal inflammation or injury from parasites, and inadequate digestion likely play a role with these predisposing factors.

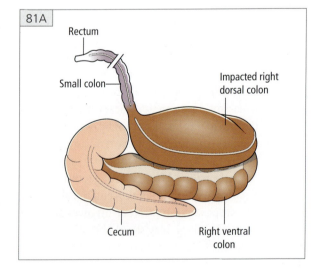

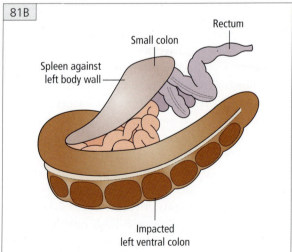

1.81A, B Schematic illustration of an impaction of the right dorsal colon (A) and left ventral colon/pelvic flexure (B).

Inadequate water intake is thought to be associated with large colon impaction. Water consumption was 40% greater in ponies offered warm drinking water compared with cold drinking water in cold weather.[186] This may explain the peak in large colon impaction colic observed in the autumn and winter months.[54]

Diets high in grain content resulted in a high right colon dry-matter content and feeding grain has been associated with an internal fluid flux and dehydration of ingesta, which may predispose to colonic impaction.[160]

Parasites may also play a role in the etiology and pathogenesis of colonic impaction, although currently there is little direct evidence supporting this proposition.[160] Poor-quality feed, old age, debilitation, overeating, and motility disorders have also been implicated.[187]

Amitraz, atropine, glycopyrrolate, and morphine have all been shown to prolong intestinal transit[188] and can predispose horses to impaction. Topical amitraz has caused impactions in horses.[189]

Clinical features

Horses usually show signs of mild abdominal pain including being quieter than normal, inappetence and decreased fecal output, stretching, lying down, and flank 'staring'.[157,190] Pain is usually responsive to treatment with analgesics (flunixin meglumine, xylazine, butorphanol). Heart rate is usually normal.[157,190] Rectal temperature should be within normal limits; however, it may be mildly increased during impaction resolution. Oral mucous membranes are usually pink, but may be tacky and the CRT may be prolonged if the horse is dehydrated or hypovolemic. Intestinal borborygmi are usually present. Abdominal distension is not typical of horses with large colon impaction and if present is usually mild to moderate. While reflux following passage of a nasogastric tube is not generally a feature of large colon impaction, horses can have reflux particularly if they have been treated with large volumes of enteral fluids, lubricants, and/or laxatives. Reflux (1–10 liters) was seen in 8% of horses at admission in one study.[157] Laboratory data should be within normal limits.[190] Horses can become moderately painful during resolution of the impaction with enteral fluids. Tachycardia, abdominal distension, and pain become progressively worse if the impaction is not resolved or becomes complicated.

Differential diagnosis

Right dorsal displacement of the large colon; entrapment of the large colon over the nephrosplenic ligament; enterolithiasis; fecalith obstruction; foreign body obstruction; cecal impaction.

Diagnosis

A large colon impaction should be high on the differential diagnosis list based on the time of year (autumn and winter) as well as historical and physical examination findings. A pelvic flexure/left ventral colon impaction can usually be diagnosed based on palpation per rectum. In one study, palpation per rectum was accurate for diagnois of a pelvic flexure/left ventral colon impaction in 90% of cases, but was useful for diagnosing a right dorsal colon impaction in only 10% of cases.[157]

Abdominocentesis should be performed with care because the impacted colon may be lying on the ventral abdominal wall and there is a risk for enterocentesis.

Management/treatment

Horses with a large colon impaction are usually treated medically. The duration of medical management necessary for impaction resolution is variable (1–4 days) depending on the size and firmness of the impaction, intestinal motility, and aggressiveness of fluid therapy. While IV fluids are important to ensure adequate hydration and intravascular volume, they are often unnecessary and are expensive. Enteral fluids delivered via a nasogastric tube are most important for hydration of the impaction. Enteral fluids and electrolytes (see below), lubricants (mineral oil, 2–4 l/500 kg horse via a nasogastric tube once), and magnesium sulfate (0.5–1.0 g/kg via a nasogastric tube once) have been used.

A balanced enteral electrolyte solution was shown to be good for hydrating the right dorsal colon contents and feces without causing electrolyte abnormalities.[191] The balanced electrolyte solution consisted of 5.27 g NaCl, 0.37 g KCl, and 3.78 g $NaHCO_3^-$ and was administered at a rate of 5 l/hour for 12 hours.[191] Impactions were resolved faster, horses had a shorter hospitalization period, and the cost of treatment was less following enteral administration compared with IV fluid administration.[190] Horses treated with 10–12 ml/kg (5–6 l/500 kg horse) of enteral isotonic fluids every 30 minutes for 2.5 hours or q1h for

5 hours, as well as magnesium sulfate (0.5 g/kg body weight in water), had the most rapid resolution of the impaction (12 and 24 hours, respectively).[190] Current recommendation is for enteral administration of 4–6 liters of water and electrolytes q2h. Horses should be checked for reflux prior to administration of water and electrolytes. If reflux is obtained, the horse should not be administered water and electrolytes until the next scheduled time.

Analgesia is often necessary during medical management (see Chapter 14). Flunixin meglumine, xylazine, butorphanol tartrate, and detomidine hydrochloride are most often used. COX-I- sparing NSAIDs such as firocoxib or meloxicam may be used as an alternative to flunixin meglumine. Some clinicians advocate the use of N-butylscopolammonium bromide (Buscopan®) and/or IV lidocaine.

Occasionally, abdominal surgery with a pelvic flexure enterotomy (**1.82**) is necessary in horses that do not respond to medical management. In one study at a referral hospital, 16% of horses with a large colon impaction required surgery.[157] The decision to undergo surgical treatment can be difficult and should be based on a lack of response to analgesics, abdominal distension, reflux, no resolution of the impaction based on palpation per rectum, and an absence of intestinal borborygmi and fecal production. A large ventral midline incision is often necessary to exteriorize the fluid- and ingesta-filled distended large colon. Sodium carboxymethylcellulose can be used to lubricate the colon and facilitate exteriorization from the abdomen. Care should be taken to avoid rupturing the colon during exteriorization or manipulation. The right dorsal colon was reported to rupture during exteriorization in approximately 20% of cases.[157]

Horses undergoing surgery are treated with perioperative antimicrobials (24 hours), flunixin meglumine, and IV fluids (see Chapter 18). Diarrhea (mild and short duration) is a common complication and was reported to occur in 16% of cases managed medically and 37% of cases managed surgically.[157] An incisional infection occurred in 16% of cases managed surgically.[157] The most frequent complication reported in another study was jugular vein thrombophlebitis, with 25% of horses developing this complication.[190]

The prognosis for horses with a large colon impaction is good to excellent with over 95% of horses surviving to discharge.[157,192] Non-survivors had a higher admission heart rate, respiratory rate, leukocyte count, blood lactate concentration, and peritoneal fluid TP concentration.[157]

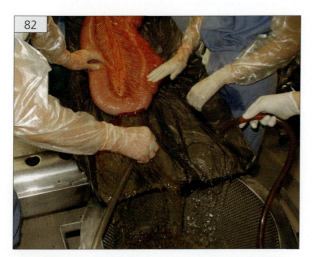

82

1.82 Pelvic flexure enterotomy.

Sand impaction

Key points

- Sand impaction should be suspected in a horse presenting with signs of colic or diarrhea living in a sandy geographic region.
- Surgical treatment is indicated in many cases.
- The prognosis is good with early and appropriate treatment.

Definition/overview

Sand impaction refers to the accumulation of sand in the large colon to the point where it causes a mechanical obstruction to the flow of ingesta. Obstruction usually occurs at the pelvic flexure (**1.83A, B**) or, more commonly, in the right dorsal colon (see Large colon impaction).

Etiology/pathogenesis

Sand impaction occurs as a result of horses ingesting sand, usually from the pasture. The amount of sand necessary to cause an obstruction is unknown. It is likely that horses accumulate sand over months to years and the ingested sand causes colonic mucosal irritation with impairment of intestinal motility and subsequent impaction.

Risk factors include access to sand, insufficient roughage in the diet, and the mineral content of the soil.[160] The occurrence of sand impaction is highest in coastal regions. Horses >1 year old are affected more commonly, although sand impaction can occur in foals. Miniature horses are thought to be predisposed because of environmental and management practices.[160]

Clinical features

Horses with sand impaction can present with signs similar to those for large colon impaction (p. 111), but pain and abdominal distension tend to be somewhat more severe and persistent. Signs include mild to moderate abdominal pain and distension, reduced to absent fecal output, and decreased intestinal borborygmi compared with normal. The sound of sand may be heard when the ventral abdomen is auscultated just caudal to the xiphoid.[160] Heart rate, respiratory rate, rectal temperature, and mucous membranes should be within normal limits; however, some horses will present with mild tachycardia, fever, and injected mucous membranes most likely associated with mucosal irritation and intestinal abrasion from the sand.

Other clinical signs associated with accumulation of sand within the GI tract include diarrhea, which may be chronic, weight loss, and poor performance.[160]

Differential diagnosis

Large colon impaction; right dorsal displacement of the large colon; entrapment of the large colon over the nephrosplenic ligament; fecalith obstruction; enterolithiasis; cecal impaction; small colon impaction.

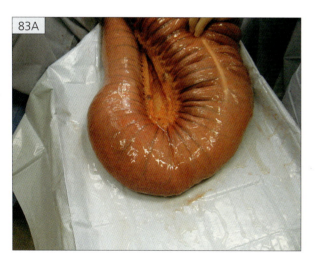
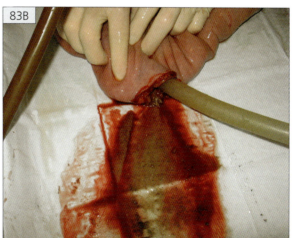

1.83A, B (A) Sand impaction at the pelvic flexure. (B) A pelvic flexure enterotomy removing the impacted sand.

Diagnosis

Observation of sand in the feces is an indication that there is sand within the GI tract. Fecal sedimentation can also be performed by adding water to six fecal balls in a rectal sleeve and allowing the sand to settle to the bottom; more than 1 teaspoon of sand is considered excessive.[160] Sedimentation of sand from feces is neither specific nor sensitive for diagnosing sand impaction because horses can have sand within their GI tract without showing clinical signs, and horses with sand impaction may not have sand in their feces. However, the appearance of sand in the feces during treatment is thought to be indicative of sand clearance.[193]

Auscultation of the ventral abdomen for sand (i.e. ocean sounds with water rushing over sand or the sound made by sand in a partially filled paper bag that is slowly rotated) may be diagnostic in some cases.[160] Abdominal examination per rectum usually reveals a gas-distended large colon and/or cecum and rarely is the sand impaction palpable.

Abdominal radiographic (**1.84**) and ultrasonographic examination can be used to diagnose sand accumulation as well as to monitor resolution. Radiographic examination of the cranioventral abdomen is the ideal projection. Horses can have some sand accumulation within the GI tract detected radiographically and show no clinical signs. There is no association between the presence of sand and sand colic[194], therefore a grading system based on the number of sand accumulations,

opacity and homogeneity of the accumulations, rib width to length of accumulation ratio, and the rib width to height of accumulation ratio was developed (*Table 1.4*).[195] Radiography is reported to be better than ultrasonography for evaluating sand accumulations.[196] Ultrasonographically, the ventral aspect of a sand accumulation is hyperechoic and causes varying acoustic shadowing, flattening of sacculations, and hypomotility.[196] The length but not the height of sand accumulations could be assessed ultrasonographically. The specificity and sensitivity of ultrasonography for detecting sand accumulations were both 87.5%, with small and dorsally located sand accumulations being more difficult to identify.[196]

Horses with severe colonic injury may be leukopenic and hypoproteinemic. Peritoneal fluid analysis is usually within normal limits; however, if there is compromise to the colonic wall, a high TP concentration may be observed. Peritoneal fluid analysis is not specific for sand impaction; however, in some cases sand can be palpated with the tip of the needle or teat cannula or even identified in the sample following enterocentesis. If sand impaction is suspected, the author does not recommend abdominocentesis unless it is performed with ultrasonographic guidance because of the potential complications associated with enterocentesis in a horse with colonic damage. A definitive diagnosis is often made at surgery.

Table 1.4 **Objective radiographic assessment scoring sheet for sand accumulation**					
LOCATION	**NUMBER OF ACCUMULATIONS**	**OPACITY***	**HOMOGENEITY**	**THICKNESS OF SAND: WIDTH OF RIB**	**LENGTH OF SAND: WIDTH OF RIB**
Other = 0	0 = 0	Much less opaque = 0	Heterogeneous = 0	1–3 × = 0	<10 × = 0
Cranioventral = 1	1–2 = 1	Mix = 1	Mix = 1	4–5 × = 1	10–20 × = 1
	3 or >3 = 3	More or as opaque = 2	Homogeneous = 2	>5 × = 2	>20 × = 2

*Relative opacity compared with a rib or vertebral body
A score of 7 out of 12 was found to have an 83% likelihood of being associated with a diagnosis of sand colic and a score less than 7 indicated that although there was sand present, it was unlikely to be associated with colic (Keppie *et al.*, 2007).[195]

Management/treatment

Medical management can be attempted in horses with none to mild signs of abdominal pain, that are passing feces, have no abdominal distension, and have a normal heart rate and intestinal borborygmi. Medical treatment includes psyllium mucilloid (at least 1 g/kg via nasogastric tube or PO), magnesium sulfate (0.5–1 g/kg in water via a nasogastric tube), or mineral oil (2–3 liters per day).[193] IV isotonic crystalloid fluids (2–4 ml/kg/hour) and analgesics (flunixin meglumine) can also be administered. While abdominal radiography can be used to monitor resolution of sand accumulations, this is unlikely to be practical in many cases because of the high exposures necessary.[193] Resolution of clinical signs occurred before the complete clearance of sand radiographically[193]; therefore, continuing treatment beyond the initial clinical improvement is recommended.

Surgery is indicated in horses with persistent or moderate to severe abdominal pain, a lack of fecal output, abdominal distension, persistently absent intestinal borborygmi, and tachycardia. Sand usually accumulates at the pelvic flexure or in the right dorsal colon. Sand is evacuated from the colon via a pelvic flexure enterotomy (**1.83B**). Concurrent large colon displacements or volvulus were found in 25% and 54% of horses with sand impactions, respectively.[197,198] Care needs to be taken during manipulation to avoid rupture of the damaged colon.

Postoperative management is similar to that for large colon impaction. (See also Chapter 18.) The prognosis for horses with sand impaction is good with 85% to 92% of horses recovering from surgery surviving to hospital discharge.[197,198] Prevention of sand ingestion can be challenging. Feeding the horse in a non-sandy area is recommended and routine use of psyllium mucilloid may be beneficial.

Enterolithiasis
Key points

- Enterolithiasis is a common cause of colic in certain geographic regions, such as California in the United States.
- Horses can have a chronic history of intermittent colic and/or can present acutely with signs consistent with a complete obstruction of the GI tract.
- Transmural necrosis and rupture can occur if the horse is not managed promptly with surgical removal of the enterolith.
- The prognosis for survival is excellent with early surgical treatment.

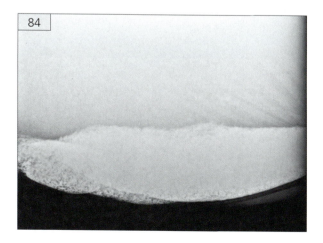

84

1.84 Radiographic image of the cranioventral abdomen revealing sand accumulation within the colon.

Definition/overview

Enteroliths ('stones') are composed of concentric layers of struvite (magnesium ammonium phosphate), usually surrounding a central foreign body nidus, and appear to form in the ampulla coli of the right dorsal colon (**1.85–1.87**).[199]

Etiology/pathogenesis

Based on the site of formation, obstruction is most common within the right dorsal, transverse, and small colon at sites where the intestine normally becomes narrow.

There is a strong geographical distribution with cases occurring most commonly in Southwestern regions of the United States, especially California.[160] Enteroliths also occur in other regions of the United States including Ohio, Texas, Florida, Missouri, and Minnesota. Internationally, enteroliths are common in Tahiti and also have been reported in France, the United Kingdom, and the Middle East. At the University of California, Davis, enteroliths were the cause of colic in 28% of horses undergoing celiotomy for treatment of colic. High concentration of magnesium in the water and feeding alfalfa hay are thought to be responsible for the high incidence; 99.3% of horses with enterolithiasis had a history of being fed alfalfa hay.[199] Horses with enterolithiasis had a higher colonic pH, lower colonic percentage dry matter, higher colonic mineral content, and were more likely to be fed alfalfa hay and spent less time on pasture compared with horses that did not have enterolithiasis.[199a] While the rate of enterolith formation is unknown, horses as young as 1 year of age have been affected.

A genetic predisposition has been proposed. Arabian and Arabian crosses, Morgans, American Saddlebreds, and donkeys were overrepresented and Thoroughbreds, Standardbreds, and Warmbloods were underrepresented compared with the hospital population.[199] Almost 10% of horses had a history of at least one sibling being affected.[199]

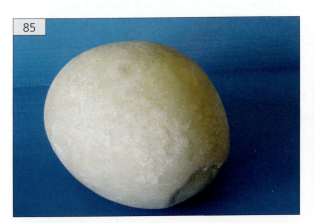

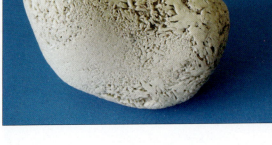

1.85 Spherical enterolith indicating a solitary enterolith.

1.86 Polytetrahedral enterolith indicating multiple enteroliths.

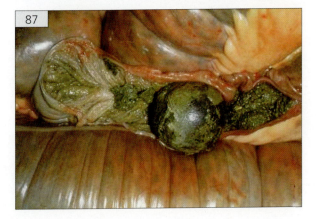

1.87 Enterolith in the small colon at necropsy.

Clinical features

Horses often have a history of recurrent colic. In one study, 33% of horses had a history of recent colic episodes and 14% had passed one or more enteroliths in their feces prior to admission for colic.[199] Horses can also have a history of lethargy and dull demeanor, agitation, weight loss, or loose feces.

Clinical findings are variable depending on the location of the enterolith(s) and degree of obstruction. Most horses show signs of mild to moderate abdominal pain. Horses with a small colon obstruction are more likely to have a complete obstruction and show signs of severe pain (65%) compared with horses with an obstruction(s) at another site(s) (29%).[199] Tachycardia is common and borborygmi are often reduced to absent, particularly if there is a complete obstruction. Complete obstruction also leads to abdominal distension.

Transmural necrosis and GI tract rupture can be caused by an enterolith and result in septic peritonitis with associated signs of shock (tachycardia, injected or toxic mucous membranes, prolonged CRT, cool extremities, fever). Rupture was seen in 15% of cases in one study and occurred most commonly in the small colon.[199]

Differential diagnosis

Gas or spasmodic colic; large colon impaction; sand impaction; small colon impaction; fecalith obstruction; foreign body obstruction; right dorsal displacement of the large colon; entrapment of the large colon over the nephrosplenic ligament.

Diagnosis

Abdominal palpation per rectum is usually non-specific with large colon distension being identified in the majority (58%) of cases; only 5% had a palpable enterolith.[199]

Abdominal radiographic examination can be used to diagnose enterolithiasis (**1.88**); however, the accuracy varies with the prevalence of enterolithiasis seen at the hospital and the location of the enterolith. In one study, radiographic evaluation had 84% sensitivity for enteroliths in the large colon but only a 50% sensitivity for identification of enteroliths in the small colon.[200] The use of computed radiography has slightly increased the sensitivity and specificity, particularly for detection of small colon enteroliths.[200a] Abdominal ultrasonographic examination can be used; however, the accuracy has not been evaluated. Abdominocentesis and peritoneal fluid analysis (p. 37) can be used to determine the extent of transmural necrosis and diagnose GI tract rupture. Horses with a complete small colon obstruction are more likely to have a high peritoneal fluid protein concentration.[199]

The diagnosis is often made at surgery, particularly in geographical regions where enterolithiasis is uncommon.

Management/treatment

Abdominal surgery is necessary to remove the enterolith(s). In one study, half of the horses had a solitary enterolith and half had multiple enteroliths. Solitary enteroliths are spherical (**1.85**) whereas the finding of a polytetrahedral enterolith is indicative of multiple enteroliths (**1.86**). Obstruction is usually at the right dorsal colon (32%), transverse colon (23%), or small colon (45%, **1.87**). Large enteroliths are always in the right dorsal colon. Enteroliths are removed via a single or multiple enterotomies at the pelvic flexure or in the small colon. Occasionally, resection of devitalized intestine is necessary.

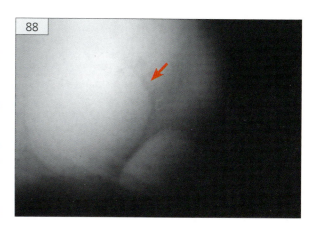

1.88 Radiographic image of an enterolith (arrow).

Horses are treated perioperatively with anti-microbial drugs (24 hours) as well as flunixin meglumine and IV fluids. Feed is gradually reintroduced over 48–72 hours or longer depending on the location of the lesion appearance of the intestine at surgery. (See also Chapter 18.)

Diarrhea was the most common postoperative complication (12%) followed by incisional infection (8%), incisional hernia (5%), salmonellosis (4%), laminitis (3%), septic peritonitis (3%), adhesions (2%), and impaction at the descending colon enterotomy site (2%).[199]

Of the horses successfully recovered from general anesthesia between 1991 and 1996, 99% survived until discharge and 97% were alive 1 year after surgery.[199] The confirmed recurrence rate was 8%; however, 14% of horses had colic episodes following hospital discharge. It is recommended to avoid feeding alfalfa hay and minimize feeding wheat bran to prevent recurrence.[160] Other recommendations include removing horses from dirt or gravel, which can act as a nidus, adding psyllium mucilloid to the diet, and supplementing with cider vinegar (1 cup twice daily).[160] Using an alternative water source in areas where the water supply has a high mineral content has also been recommended.[199]

Nephrosplenic ligament entrapment of the large colon

Key points
- NSLE can often be managed medically.
- The prognosis for survival is excellent.
- Horses with recurrent NSLE can be managed with laparoscopic ablation of the nephrosplenic space.

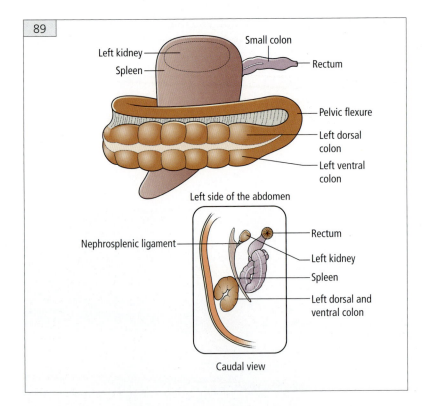

89

Left kidney
Spleen
Small colon
Rectum
Pelvic flexure
Left dorsal colon
Left ventral colon
Left side of the abdomen

Nephrosplenic ligament
Rectum
Left kidney
Spleen
Left dorsal and ventral colon
Caudal view

1.89 Left dorsal displacement of the large colon where the colon is positioned between the spleen and the left body wall.

Definition/overview

A left dorsal displacement of the large colon occurs when the left dorsal and ventral colons become displaced between the spleen and the left body wall (**1.89**); the colon can then rotate 180 degrees, moving dorsally to become entrapped in the nephrosplenic space (entrapment of the large colon over the nephrosplenic ligament, **1.90**). NSLEs represent 5–11% of horses admitted to referral hospitals.[65,201,202]

Etiology/pathogenesis

The exact etiology and pathogenesis is unknown. Entrapment of the colon in the nephrosplenic space has been found incidentally during laparoscopic abdominal exploration (**1.91**). It could, therefore, be concluded that horses often have their left colons in this location and that signs of abdominal pain are caused by colonic gas distension or positioning of the colon so that it creates tension on ligamentous structures. NSLE recurs in some horses.[202] Young-mature geldings and large-breed horses appear to be predisposed[74,203], suggesting that alterations in colonic motility or the individual anatomy of the nephrosplenic space may play a role. The depth of the nephrosplenic space appears to be important[204] and is defined by the dorsal extent of the dorsal border of the spleen in relation to the attachment of the nephrosplenic ligament. Splenic adhesions to a ventral midline incision scar can also predispose horses to NSLE.[205]

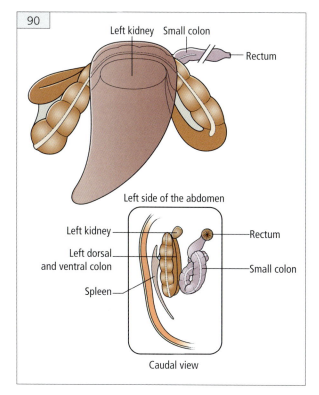

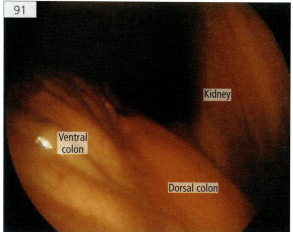

1.91 Laparoscopic appearance of the large colon entrapped over the nephrosplenic ligament.

1.90 Left dorsal displacement of the large colon where the colon is entrapped over the nephrosplenic ligament.

Clinical features

Horses with a NSLE are usually mildly to moderately painful. The level of abdominal pain varies with the amount of gas distension and the extent to which the left colons have been pulled through the nephrosplenic space. Abdominal distension can be absent and is often mild to moderate and may be appreciated more on the left side of the abdomen. The heart rate is usually within normal limits; however, horses showing signs of abdominal pain can be mildly tachycardic (heart rate 50–60 bpm). Respiratory rate is variable and rectal temperature should be within normal limits. Borborygmi are often present, but may be reduced compared with normal or absent on the left side of the abdomen. Horses with a simple NSLE do not have signs of shock (moderate to severe tachycardia, injected or toxic oral mucous membranes, sweating, cool extremities). About one-third of horses with NSLE had reflux following passage of a nasogastric tube.[206]

Differential diagnosis

Gas or spasmodic colic; large colon impaction; sand impaction; enterolithiasis; right dorsal displacement of the large colon; small colon impaction; fecalith obstruction; foreign body obstruction; cecal impaction.

Diagnosis

NSLE can be difficult to diagnose definitively because there are no diagnostic tests with 100% accuracy. Abdominal palpation per rectum is most commonly used. The caudal pole of the left kidney is identified and the left dorsal and ventral colon is palpated to the left of the kidney coursing over the nephrosplenic ligament. The dorsocaudal aspect of the spleen can then be palpated to the left of the entrapped colon. The spleen is often displaced ventral and axial to the normal position against the left body wall. Palpation of colonic bands or gas distended colon in the region of the nephrosplenic space can justify a tentative diagnosis of nephrosplenic entrapment, but not a definitive diagnosis. Occasionally, extensive colonic gas distension will be palpated and the nephrosplenic space is inaccessible for palpation per rectum.

Ultrasonographic examination through the upper part of the left flank can be used to assist with diagnosis of a NSLE (**1.92**). The left kidney and dorsal aspect of the spleen are no longer visible in the left paralumbar fossa because the gas-filled left colon lies between these structures and the left body wall.[207] The spleen may also be found to lie more ventral compared with normal. The accuracy of ultrasonographic examination for use in diagnosing a NSLE is reported to be high, with only five false-negative and no false-positive results reported in 82 horses.[207]

Many cases of NSLE are diagnosed at surgery and while surgery may be thought of as the 'gold standard' diagnostic tool, occasionally the NSLE may correct as the horse is moved into position for a ventral midline approach. Horses with a recently corrected NSLE often have petechiae on the colonic serosal surface and a presumptive diagnosis may be made if this is found and the clinical findings are consistent with a NSLE.

Laparoscopy has been used to diagnose NSLE and may be a more reliable diagnostic tool because the procedure is performed standing and the horse is not rolled into dorsal recumbency; however, reposition-

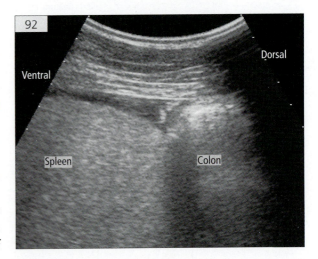

1.92 Ultrasonographic appearance of the nephrosplenic space through the left upper paralumbar fossa. (Courtesy Dr JoAnn Slack)

ing of the colon following abdominal insufflation has been reported.[202] The spleen often has fibrin deposition and a subtle indentation from the colon if recent entrapment has occurred. Horses in which NSLE is a problem generally have a deep and wide nephrosplenic space compared with horses in which NSLE is not a problem.

Management/treatment

NSLE can be corrected using phenylephrine, rolling the horse, or surgically. Phenylephrine (3 µg/kg/minute for 15 minutes) is an alpha-agonist that causes vasoconstriction and can be used to reduce the size of the spleen.[208] With gentle exercise (light jogging) for 5–10 minutes immediately following phenylephrine administration, the colon can fall back into its correct position. Excessive jogging is contraindicated because colonic rupture can occur. The spleen returns to its previous size within 35 minutes of phenylephrine administration;[208] therefore, the horse should be jogged immediately on completion of administration and jogging beyond 10–15 minutes is unlikely to be productive. Treatment with phenylephrine can be repeated several times. Recently, fatal hemorrhage was reported in five aged horses following phenylephrine administration for management of nephrosplenic entrapment.[209] The success rate for treatment of NSLE with phenylephrine is reported to be excellent (>90%)[202,206,210]; however, 'success' should be used cautiously because of the challenge with definitively diagnosing this type of displacement. Surgery is recommended for horses that are persistently or severely painful.

If phenylephrine treatment is unsuccessful, the horse can be rolled under general anesthesia. The horse is anesthetized with IV anesthetic drugs and positioned in right lateral recumbency. The hindlimbs are hoisted and the torso shaken vigorously. The horse is then positioned in left lateral recumbency. Phenylephrine did not appear to improve resolution of the entrapment with rolling under general anesthesia.[210a] Abdominal palpation per rectum or ultrasonographic examination can be performed at this time to assess the colon position. If the colon remains entrapped, rolling can be repeated

or surgery performed. Some clinicians also recommend allowing the horse to roll and self-correct the NSLE. The major limitation with medical management is that in some cases other lesions (e.g. LCV, right dorsal displacement) may be present.[206] Rolling under general anesthesia was used successfully to correct NSLE in 74% of cases.[206]

Abdominal surgery is indicated in cases that are severely painful, non-responsive to medical treatment, or when a diagnosis is not made preoperatively. Gastric reflux, pain, and abdominal distension were associated with the decision for surgical treatment in one study.[210b] The colon can be repositioned by manipulating the spleen axially over the colon beginning at the caudal aspect and moving cranially, using one or two arms, from the right or left side of the abdomen. The colon is then lifted to the incision. In some cases there will be a volvulus of the large colon at the sternal and diaphragmatic flexure or a right dorsal displacement. If colon exteriorization is difficult in a horse with a large colon displacement or volvulus, the nephrosplenic space should be checked for an NSLE. Postoperative management consists of flunixin meglumine for 1–2 days and feed should be introduced within 36–48 hours.

NSLE has also been corrected using a laparoscopic approach.[211] This may be indicated in cases that are not painful or when abdominal pain is easily controlled with analgesia and when there is minimal colonic distension.

Horses with the large colon displaced between the spleen and the left body wall can be successfully treated with hand walking, withholding feed, analgesia, and IV fluid therapy if necessary.

The prognosis for horses with a NSLE is excellent (>90%). The reported recurrence rate is 8–21%[202,206], and in some cases recurrence can occur on a regular basis. In recurrent cases, ablation of the nephrosplenic space can be performed using a laparoscopic approach with either suturing or mesh placement.[204,212,213] If laparoscopy is unavailable, colon resection or colopexy can be performed or the nephrosplenic space ablated through a left flank approach with resection of the 18th rib.

Right dorsal displacement of the large colon
Key point
- Horses with right dorsal displacement of the large colon have an excellent prognosis for survival following surgical correction.

Definition/overview
A right dorsal displacement of the large colon occurs when the left dorsal and ventral colon becomes displaced between the cecum and the right body wall (**1.93**). The pelvic flexure can move in a counterclockwise (more common) or clockwise (less common) direction as viewed from the ventral abdomen around the base of the cecum. Large colon displacement was one of the most common cause of colic overall (16.5% of cases) and the most common lesion found at surgery (24.5% of cases) in horses admitted to a referral hospital in western Canada.[5]

Etiology/pathogenesis
The etiology and pathogenesis of right dorsal displacement is unknown. Horses with a wide-body configuration are reported to be predisposed to right dorsal displacement[214], and in two retrospective studies Quarter Horses represented 40–45% of right dorsal displacement cases.[171,214] Of 167 horses with a right dorsal displacement, 22 were postparturient mares and 14 were in middle to late gestation.[171] Right dorsal displacement associated with late gestation and parturition is likely a consequence of colonic malpositioning and, possibly, alterations in intestinal motility. Factors such as change in diet, exercise, and housing may cause gas colic or a large colon impaction (p. 110) and predispose to a right dorsal displacement. Right dorsal displacement can occur as a complication of a pelvic flexure impaction. Forty-three percent of horses with a right dorsal displacement were reported to have had at least one previous colic episode[171], suggesting that some of these cases may have an underlying colonic dysmotility or inflammation.

Horses with right dorsal displacement were more likely to be 4–10 years old compared with a hospital- and colic-control population[214] and 75% of horses with right dorsal displacement were 5–15 years old.[171] This age distribution may be a consequence of colonic motility and management: young horses may still have good

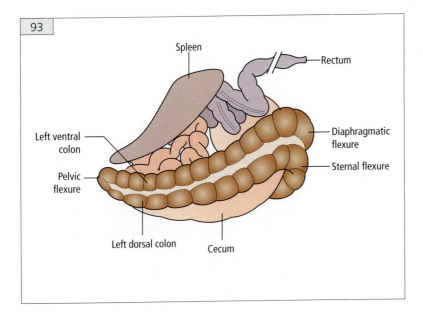

93

Spleen

Rectum

Left ventral colon

Diaphragmatic flexure

Sternal flexure

Pelvic flexure

Left dorsal colon   Cecum

1.93 A right dorsal displacement of the large colon occurs when the left colons become displaced between the cecum and the right body wall.

colonic motility; young and geriatric horses may live on pasture; and horses that are predisposed to right dorsal displacement may be euthanized prior to becoming geriatric.

Clinical features

Horses with a right dorsal displacement are in mild to moderate pain and have mild to moderate abdominal distension. The heart rate is usually within normal limits or there may be mild tachycardia (50–65 bpm). Respiratory rate is variable and rectal temperature should be within normal limits. Oral mucous membranes should be pink and may be slightly tacky. Reflux was obtained following passage of a nasogastric tube in 17% of cases.[171] Horses with a simple right dorsal displacement do not show signs of shock (severe tachycardia, injected or toxic oral mucous membranes, sweating, and cool extremities).

Differential diagnosis

Gas or spasmodic colic; large colon impaction; sand impaction; enterolithiasis; NSLE; small colon impaction; fecalith obstruction; foreign body obstruction; cecal impaction.

Diagnosis

A tentative diagnosis is made based on abdominal palpation per rectum; the ventral colon can be palpated coursing across the abdomen just cranial to the pelvic inlet. Colonic distension is often palpated per rectum and the ventral cecal band cannot be palpated.

Hematology and serum or plasma biochemistry is within normal limits in most cases.[171] Liver enzymes and bilirubin can be quite high in horses with a right dorsal displacement; however, there was no association between evidence of hepatobiliary injury or dysfunction or survival.[171,215]

Ultrasonographic examination can be used to diagnose right dorsal displacement. Ultrasonographic evidence supporting a diagnosis includes (1) medial displacement of the right liver lobe by a distended large colon or small intestine, (2) the right liver lobe may not be visible or displaced cranially, (3) markedly dilated colonic and/or cecal mesenteric vessels, and (4) the cecal mesentery and vessels cannot be followed from the right mid-paralumbar fossa region to the ventral midline.[216]

Management/treatment

Some horses with right dorsal displacement may respond to medical management by withholding feed and administering IV fluids and electrolytes and analgesia. Because of the difficulty with obtaining a definitive diagnosis preoperatively, it is generally unknown whether horses that respond to medical therapy truly had a right dorsal displacement. Surgical correction is necessary in the majority of cases. Indications for surgery include persistent or severe abdominal pain, absent borborygmi, and lack of defecation, as well as worsening abdominal distension and tachycardia.

Abdominal surgery is performed using a ventral midline approach. The pelvic flexure is identified, usually in the cranial abdomen, and exteriorized. Decompression of the cecum and colon using a 14-gauge needle and suction is almost always necessary. The colon and cecum are then repositioned by rotating them around the cecocolonic base. If there is a concurrent large colon impaction and pelvic flexure enterotomy may be necessary.

Postoperative treatment involves flunixin meglumine for 2–3 days. Hay should be reintroduced over 36–48 hours (see Chapter 18).

The prognosis for horses with a right dorsal displacement is excellent (>90%).[214] Clinical findings reported to be associated with survival were the duration of colic, heart rate, and peritoneal fluid TP concentration.[171] Recurrence of a right dorsal displacement can occur in approximately 10–15% of cases. Large colon resection or colopexy can be performed in these cases to prevent recurrence. Intestinal biopsy is recommended in horses with recurrence to document any underlying disease process.

Colitis

Key points

- Not all horses with colitis have diarrhea.
- Colitis should be suspected in any horse with fever, dull demeanor, or inappetence, particularly if exposed to predisposing factors.
- Early diagnosis and aggressive medical management is necessary for a favorable outcome.
- Causes of colitis may be infectious and horses should be isolated.

Definition/overview

Colitis refers to inflammatory disease of the large colon. The cecum is often involved (typhlocolitis). (See also Chapter 9.)

Etiology/pathogenesis

The major etiological agents for colitis that have been identified in horses and foals are *Salmonella* spp., *Clostridium difficile* or *Clostridium perfringens*, *Neorickettsia risticii* (Potomac horse fever or equine monocytic ehrlichiosis), and cyathostomiasis.[149] However, in the majority of cases the underlying etiology is not determined.

Salmonellosis: Horses can be latent subclinical carriers of *Salmonella* spp., acquire salmonellosis as a nosocomial infection (clinical or subclinical), or have primary clinical disease. Several risk factors have been identified for salmonellosis including transportation, high ambient temperature, withholding feed, gastrointestinal tract disease particularly foals, large colon impaction, nasogastric intubation, abdominal surgery, and antimicrobial therapy.[217–223] *Salmonella* spp. cause diarrhea by invading the intestinal epithelium via pinocytosis. Invasion induces an inflammatory response and stimulates cyclic AMP-induced secretion of water and electrolytes. The inflammatory response can result in intestinal injury. Cytotoxins and enterotoxins also cause intestinal injury and further secretion of water and electrolytes.

Clostridiosis: *C. difficile* is a spore-forming, obligatory anaerobic, gram-positive rod. Colitis caused by *C. difficile* is often associated with antimicrobial drug use. Other predisposing factors include hospitalization, transport, surgery, and dietary changes.[149] *C. difficile* is

not considered part of the normal flora of the equine adult GI tract[149]; however, up to 42% of horses with antimicrobial-associated colitis can have *C. difficile* isolated from the intestinal tract.[224,225] Clinically important disease associated with a *C. difficile* infection is dependent on toxin A (enterotoxin) and toxin B (cytotoxins) production that act synergistically to cause tissue damage and inflammation and subsequent clinical signs of colitis.

C. perfringens is widely distributed in the environment and has been isolated from normal horses. *C. perfringens* type C, less commonly type A, and β2-toxigenic strains have been associated with diarrhea in adult horses and foals. In neonates, type C is most often associated with infection. Infection and exotoxin production following colonization is thought to be associated with trypsin inhibitors in the mare's colostrum and other environmental (geographic and seasonal) factors.[226,227] Cytotoxic β toxin and α toxin are produced by *C. perfringens* type C and cause clinical signs. *C. perfringens* type A containing β2-toxin has been associated with typhlocolitis in adult horses[228]; however, this strain has also been isolated from normal horses, suggesting that other factors are involved in disease.[229]

Potomac horse fever: *N. risticii* (formerly *Ehrlichia risticii*) is the causative agent in Potomac horse fever or monocytic ehrlichiosis. *N. risticii* is a rickettsial organism. It is a gram-negative, obligate intracellular bacterium that infects mononuclear cells, specifically blood monocytes and tissue macrophages, with a preference for intestinal epithelial crypt cells and mast cells in the equine intestine, particularly the cecum and colon.[149] The organism multiplies in the cells, causing exfoliation. Potomac horse fever is an infectious but not a contagious disease. *N. risticii* infects horses via the oral route following ingestion of infected digenetic trematodes in the secretions of first (fresh water snails) and second (aquatic insects) intermediate hosts.[230] Peak incidence is between June and September (northern hemisphere) and generally occurs in horses grazing pastures bordered by creeks or rivers.

Cyathostomiasis: Cyathostomiasis (infection with small strongyles) has been identified as a major cause of acute and chronic colitis and colic.[149] While current anthelmintics are effective against large strongyles (e.g. *Strongylus vulgaris*), they are relatively ineffective at controlling cyathostomes.[231] Recent treatment with an adulticidal anthelmintic is a risk factor for the development of clinical cyathostomiasis. Disease is most common in young horses (1–6 years old) and occurs in association with emergence of larvae from a hypobiotic state in the large colon mucosa (i.e. late winter and spring in temperate regions and late fall and winter in subtropical regions).[149]

Clinical features

Horses with colitis have variable clinical signs. The most common clinical features include fever, dull demeanor, and diarrhea. It is important to recognize that not all horses with colitis have diarrhea. Horses with colitis may also show mild to moderate signs of colic, abdominal distension, and inappetence. Horses with moderate to severe disease will be tachycardic and tachypneic. Oral mucous membranes will be dry, injected or toxic, and with a prolonged CRT (see Chapter 17). Intestinal borborygmi are often hypermotile; however, in severe cases they will be reduced or absent. Horses are often leukopenic (neutropenic), at least transiently, and may subsequently develop a leukocytosis. The PCV may be high, associated with hemoconcentration and splenic contraction, and the TPP relatively low as a result of a protein-losing enteropathy and loss of albumin from the intravascular space. Hyponatremia and hypokalemia are common and severely affected horses may have a metabolic acidosis. Hyperlactatemia is associated with poor peripheral perfusion. A high creatinine concentration is also observed and is at least initially associated with poor renal perfusion (prerenal). Horses with severe colitis often have a coagulopathy. Severe laminitis, acute kidney injury, and colonic infarction are sequelae of severe colitis.

Differential diagnosis

Colonic or cecal infarction (severe disease); GI tract rupture (severe disease); LCV (severe disease); small colon impaction (mild to moderate disease and diarrhea); large colon impaction (mild to moderate disease and diarrhea); cecal impaction (mild to moderate disease and diarrhea); sand colic (mild to moderate disease and diarrhea); infiltrative or inflammatory bowel disease; peritonitis; right dorsal colitis.

Diagnosis

A tentative diagnosis of colitis is usually made based on the clinical features particularly fever, dull demeanor, diarrhea, leukopenia (neutropenia), hyponatremia, and hypoproteinemia. Other diagnostic tests that can be performed are palpation per rectum and abdominal ultrasonographic examination. Abdominal palpation per rectum should be performed to rule out another lesion such as a large or small colon impaction. Abdominal ultrasonographic examination reveals normal peritoneal fluid with a thickened and/or fluid-filled colon and/or cecum. Peritoneal fluid analysis can be performed to rule out GI tract rupture or peritonitis and to assess colonic injury.

Salmonellosis: *Salmonella* spp. can be isolated from the feces using bacterial culture.[232] Because *Salmonella* spp. are shed intermittently and cannot be consistently isolated from horses with salmonellosis, particularly horses with profuse watery diarrhea, five or more sequential daily fecal samples are recommended.[233] Because of the cost associated with performing bacterial culture and isolation on multiple samples and the 2–5 day delay with obtaining results, PCR techniques have been developed as a screening test for salmonellosis and are often used in conjunction with culture techniques.

Clostridiosis: A diagnosis of *C. difficile* colitis is dependent on fecal bacterial culture and toxin detection.[149] Because of the challenges with sample handling associated with bacterial culture and the lack of specificity and sensitivity for isolation of disease-causing *C. difficile*, toxin detection is most often used. Toxin (A and B) detection is performed using cell culture ('gold standard') or antigen and toxin immunoassays.[149,234]

C. perfringens typhlocolitis can be definitively diagnosed based on isolation of large numbers of the bacteria from the feces or GI tract and identification of the toxin gene (β2-toxin and enterotoxin) using PCR in a horse or foal showing classical clinical signs.[149] Necropsy findings in cases of clostridial enterocolitis include acute hemorrhagic enteritis, colitis, villi necrosis, mural emphysema, and large numbers of gram-positive rods in stained smears and histologic sections of affected intestine.

Potomac horse fever: Potomac horse fever can be definitively diagnosed based on isolation or detection of *N. risticii* in the blood or feces; however, this is time-consuming and often impractical.[149] Indirect fluorescent antibody tests have been used, but have false-positive results associated with recent exposure and vaccination.[149] PCR has been used to detect *N. risticii* in the blood or feces and is the most rapid, sensitive, and accurate method to definitively diagnose Potomac horse fever.[235,236] Necropsy findings include a lack of severe invasive lesions, foul odor, or inflammatory infiltration of the intestine and the presence of depleted inactive lymphoid tissue.[149] Histologically, *N. risticii* can be identified within the cytoplasm of host cells using immunoperoxidase or modified silver stains.[149]

Cyathostomiasis: Cyathostomiasis is difficult to diagnose. Cyathostome larvae can be seen with the naked eye in the feces and may be red or white and of variable size.[149] Fecal worm egg counts are not useful because it is the larval stages that cause disease. While rectal biopsy is non-diagnostic, cecal or colonic biopsy may show edema and eosinophilic inflammation with or without identification of mucosal larvae.[231] Research into immunodiagnostic techniques for detection of cyathostome larvae and molecular techniques for detection of anthelmintic resistance are in progress.[149]

Management/treatment

Medical management of colitis consists of IV fluid and electrolyte therapy for maintenance and to replace losses. Colloidal support is necessary in many cases to maintain colloid osmotic pressure (COP) (see Chapter 12). Enteral water and electrolytes can be provided in mild or resolving cases to maintain hydration (see Chapter 9).

Antiendotoxin therapy is necessary and includes J5 plasma, polymixin B, and flunixin meglumine (see Chapter 17). Analgesia can be provided with flunixin meglumine, IV lidocaine, or a butorphanol CRI. Antidiarrheal therapy (e.g. pepto bismol), di-tri-octahedral smectite (0.5 kg via nasogastric intubation q24h)[237,238], and probiotics (e.g. *Saccharomyces boulardii* 25–50 g PO q12h)[239] have been used to manage horses with colitis.

The use of antimicrobial drugs in managing horses with colitis is controversial. In general, their use is not recommended because antimicrobial drug use has been implicated as a cause of colitis and may contribute to the already documented emergence of multidrug-resistant *Salmonella* spp., for example. Antimicrobial drugs are recommended, however, in critically ill cases of colitis and cases with severe neutropenia. Care should be taken with the use of nephrotoxic antimicrobial drugs (e.g. aminoglycosides and oxytetracycline) in horses that are severely dehydrated or showing signs of renal failure. Metronidazole (15–25 mg/kg PO q6h) is recommended for treating horses with moderate to severe colitis associated with *Clostridium* spp. Metronidazole resistance has been documented in up to 43% of *C. difficile* isolates from horses.[240] Vancomycin could possibly be used in cases of resistant life-threatening *C. difficile* colitis; however its use is generally not recommended. Oxytetracycline (6.6 mg/kg IV q12h) is recommended for management of Potomac horse fever. Horses respond well to treatment.

Treatment of cyathostomiasis is challenging. Cyathostomes are generally resistant to benzimidazoles (e.g. fenbendazole). Resistance to ivermectin has not been recognized and repeat dosing is necessary to kill emerging larvae. Moxidectin is the only anthelmintic consistently effective against encysted larvae.

Laminitis is a common complication of colitis and the current recommendation for prevention is applying ice to the feet, correcting the underlying disease, and providing supportive therapy. Other complicating factors include colonic infarction (p. 108), renal failure (see Chapter 5), and hyperammonemic encephalopathy.

The mortality rate for colitis is variable. Tachycardia, high PCV, low TPP, and high plasma creatinine and blood lactate concentrations reflecting the severity of disease and the degree of shock are associated with non-survival.[241] Horses with antimicrobial-associated diarrhea had a less favorable outcome compared with horses that did not receive antimicrobial drugs prior to the onset of diarrhea.[241] Reasons for euthanasia include persistent signs of colic, unresponsive diarrhea, shock, and severe laminitis. The mortality rate for horses with Potomac horse fever was reported to be as high as 30%[149] and up to 60% with severe cases of cyathostomiasis.[231]

Right dorsal colitis
Key points

- Horses with right dorsal colitis typically present with a history of NSAID treatment, signs of colic or diarrhea, and hypoproteinemia/hypoalbuminemia.
- Diagnosis can be confirmed using abdominal ultrasonographic evaluation.
- Early recognition and treatment of horses with right dorsal colitis is important for a favorable outcome.
- TPP should be monitored in horses being treated with NSAIDs.
- Caution should be used when administering NSAIDs to dehydrated horses and high doses, prolonged treatment, or the concurrent use of multiple NSAIDs should be avoided.

Definition/overview

Right dorsal colitis refers to inflammation specifically of the right dorsal colon. Right dorsal colitis is characterized by mucosal ulceration and hemorrhage, submucosal edema, neutrophilic inflammation, and thickening of the right dorsal colon wall (**1.94**).

Etiology/pathogenesis

Right dorsal colitis usually occurs as a result of administration of NSAIDs, particularly phenylbutazone but also flunixin meglumine. Horses showing signs of dehydration or hypoperfusion at the time of NSAID administration, receiving high doses of NSAIDs for a long duration of time, and horses concurrently receiving multiple NSAIDs appear to be particularly susceptible to right dorsal colitis.[242,243] However, it is important to note that horses receiving phenylbutazone or flunixin meglumine dosages within the recommended range and for a brief period of time have developed right dorsal colitis.[244]

The exact pathogenesis is unknown. NSAIDs inhibit COX-1, which is constitutively produced, and COX-2, which is induced with inflammation, and, subsequently, prostaglandin production. Loss of the protective effects of prostaglandins on the mucosa likely plays an important role (see Gastric ulceration). Prostaglandin E is important for maintenance of mucosal blood flow and repair. Therefore, inhibition of prostaglandin E production results in hypoxic or ischemic mucosal damage and delayed mucosal healing.[244] Other mechanisms that may play a role include adherence of neutrophils to the vascular endothelium, with release of oxygen-derived free radicals and other enzymes from the activated neutrophils causing mucosal injury and attenuation of the synergy between prostaglandins and nitric oxide mediation of mucosal protection.[244] Infection, an immune-mediated response, behavioral traits, genetic factors, and stress may also contribute to the pathogenesis of right dorsal colitis.[245]

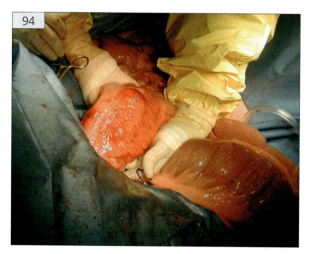

94

1.94 A thickened right dorsal colon identified at surgery.

While mucosal ulceration associated with NSAID use can occur at various locations along the GI tract, the right dorsal colon appears to be predisposed and the exact reasons for this predisposition are currently unknown.[244]

Clinical features

Horses with right dorsal colitis typically have signs of mild to moderate colic and/or diarrhea or soft feces. Other clinical signs include weight loss, inappetence, dull demeanor, and ventral edema.[242,243,245] Fever and tachycardia with signs of shock (prolonged CRT, poor pulse quality, poor jugular refill, cool extremities) can be seen in acute severe cases.[243,245] Ponies and young performance horses appear to be predisposed.[244]

A history of NSAID administration and moderate to marked hypoproteinemia (hypoalbuminemia) in a horse with signs of colic or diarrhea is highly suggestive of right dorsal colitis. Hypoalbuminemia was the first detectable clinical pathologic abnormality in a right dorsal colitis model and was detected as early as 3 days after beginning treatment with phenylbutazone.[246]

Hyperfibrinogenemia may or may not be seen.[242,243] Anemia (mild), hypocalcemia, leukocytosis, neutrophilia or neutropenia, and band neutrophilia have also been reported.[243,244,246] Horses with an acute onset of severe disease may have clinical pathologic abnormalities consistent with hypoperfusion (high PCV, azotemia, hyperlactatemia) and electrolyte disturbances.[245] Peritoneal fluid analysis is usually within normal limits.[244]

Rupture of the right dorsal colon[243] and stricture,[242,244] can occur.

Differential diagnosis

Colitis; inflammatory bowel disease or neoplasia; sand colic; large colon impaction; small colon impaction; gastric ulcers.

Diagnosis

Diagnosis of right dorsal colitis can be supported further by ultrasonographic examination of the abdomen (**1.95**). The right dorsal colon is imaged ultrasonographically on the right side between the 11th and 13th ICSs beginning at the ventral border of the lung. In some horses, the right dorsal colon should also be imaged in the 10th and 15th ICSs. The right dorsal colon can be identified by a lack of sacculations and its location axial and ventral to the liver, ventral to the duodenum, and dorsal to the right dorsal colon.[243] The thickness of the right dorsal colon relative to the right ventral colon can be measured. Horses with right dorsal colitis had a median right dorsal colon wall thickness that was 2.5-times thicker than the right ventral colon (range 2.0–3.3 times) and the median wall thickness of the right dorsal colon in affected horses ranged from 0.72–1.59 cm (normal horses 0.22–0.59 cm) between the 11th and 13th ICSs. The median right ventral colon thickness was no different between normal horses and horses with right dorsal colitis (0.36 and 0.43 cm, respectively).[243] A hypoechoic layer within the thickened wall of the right dorsal colon corresponding to submucosal edema, inflammatory cell infiltrates, and granulation tissue was observed in horses with right dorsal colitis.[243] False-negative results have been reported with ultrasonographic examination, most likely because only a portion of the right dorsal colon is imaged.[244]

Scintigraphy using technetium-99m hexamethylpropyleneamine oxime (HMPAO)-labeled white blood cells has also been used to diagnose right dorsal colitis.[247] A definitive diagnosis can be made during an exploratory celiotomy.

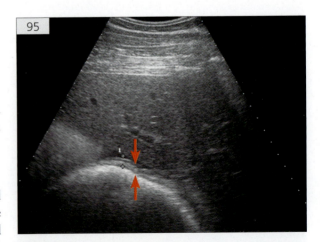

1.95 Ultrasonographic appearance of the right dorsal colon in a horse with right dorsal colitis.

Plasma creatinine concentration, urinalysis, and renal function should be assessed in horses with right dorsal colitis because of the potential for renal papillary necrosis in horses with NSAID toxicity (see Chapter 5). Gastroscopy should also be performed in order to diagnose concurrent gastric ulceration (p. 51).

Management/treatment

Medical: Most horses with right dorsal colitis are managed medically. Medical management includes discontinuing NSAID administration. A low-roughage pelleted complete feed with at least 25% dietary fiber should be fed instead of hay.[244] Feeding should be based on the manufacturer's recommendations and divided into several meals throughout the day. Fresh grass or alfalfa leaves can be given. Severely affected horses may require partial or total parenteral nutrition (see Chapter 15) for several days.

Corn oil or safflower oil (200–400 ml daily), psyllium mucilloid (50–100 g/horse daily), and sucralfate (20 mg/kg PO q6h) may be used to facilitate mucosal healing. Misoprostol is a synthetic prostaglandin that has also been used in the management of horses with right dorsal colitis (see Gastric ulceration). The recommended dosage for misoprostol is 2–3 µg/kg PO q6–12h.[244] Complications in human patients include colic and diarrhea and it may cause mild colic signs in equine patients.

A butorphanol CRI (13 µg/kg/hour) can be used to provide analgesia; however, horses should be monitored closely for signs of excitation associated with opiate use. Episodes of colic can also be managed with alpha-2 agonists (see Chapter 14).

IV lidocaine (1.3 mg/kg bolus over 15 minutes then 0.05 mg/kg/minute CRI) was recently shown to ameliorate the inhibitory effects of flunixin meglumine on recovery of the jejunal mucosal barrier from ischemic injury and may play a role in the management of horses with right dorsal colitis.[248]

Metronidazole is reported to inhibit leukocyte adherence to mesenteric vessel endothelial cells in laboratory animal models of NSAID-induced intestinal injury. The recommended dose is 10–15 mg/kg q8–12h.[244]

Stress should be minimized and horses with right dorsal colitis should be given a period of rest from exercise and performance during colonic healing. Access to fresh and palatable water is essential. Body weight should be monitored and caloric supplementation in the form of pellets or dietary oil provided if necessary.

Signs of colic and diarrhea should resolve, the TPP and albumin concentrations should increase, and the thickness of the right dorsal colon as viewed ultrasonographically should decrease towards normal with successful medical management. Horses often need to be managed for 3–6 months.[243]

Horses with acute and severe disease and showing signs of shock should be managed with IV fluid and electrolyte therapy. Hypoproteinemia can be managed with plasma or synthetic colloids (see Chapter 12). Antiendotoxin treatment includes polymixin B and J5 plasma (see Chapter 17).

Surgical: Horses that do not respond to medical management and horses that show persistent signs of colic can be managed surgically. In addition to obtaining a definitive diagnosis, the right dorsal colon can be bypassed via an anastomosis between the left dorsal colon and small colon, a resection and anastomosis of the right dorsal colon can be performed through a 16th rib resection, or a resection of the right dorsal colon with bypass can be performed also through a 16th rib resection or through a ventral midline approach.[249,250] There is limited experience with each of these techniques. Horses undergoing a bypass procedure only appear to have chronic intermittent signs of mild colic and persistent hypoproteinemia/hypoalbuminemia. Right dorsal colon resection and anastomosis or resection and bypass is associated with more rapid resolution of colic signs and hypoproteinemia; however, complications include deep surgical site infection, with thoracic abscess formation associated with penetration of the diaphragm during the surgical approach and leakage of the anastomosis.

Small colon

- Small colon lesions are uncommon relative to lesions of the small intestine and large colon.
- Non-strangulating obstructions (i.e. small colon impaction [p. 130], fecalith obstruction [p. 132], enterolithiasis [p. 115], concretions, and foreign body obstruction [p. 133]) are considerably more common than strangulating obstructions (e.g. strangulating lipoma [p. 135]). (See also Chapter 9.)

- Horses with small colon lesions are typically mild to moderately painful.
- Abdominal distension is common with complete obstruction
- Horses usually do not show signs of shock unless intestinal perforation or necrosis has occurred.
- Small colon impactions are usually diagnosed on palpation per rectum, whereas fecalith, enterolith or foreign body obstructions are typically in the proximal small colon and not palpable. Distended small colon on palpation is always abnormal and indicative of an obstruction.
- Horses with small colon lesions often require surgical correction. Surgical procedures routinely performed include enterotomy and small colon resection and anastomosis.[8a,49a]
- The prognosis for survival is good, particularly if resection and anastomosis is not necessary.[250a]

Small colon impaction

Key points

- Impaction is the most common problem affecting the small colon.
- Small colon impaction is more common during the winter months.
- Horses with small colon impaction may present with diarrhea.
- Small colon impaction is usually diagnosed on palpation per rectum.
- Aggressive medical management is necessary in horses with a small colon impaction and horses often require surgery.
- Salmonellosis, reimpaction, and adhesion formation are the most common complications following surgical correction of a small colon impaction.
- The prognosis is good to excellent.

Definition/overview

Diffuse obstruction of the descending or small colon with fecal material. Small colon impactions often involve the entire length of the small colon.

Etiology/pathogenesis

Poor-quality feed, inadequate water consumption, improper deworming, and infrequent dental care leading to improper mastication can be associated with small colon impaction. Seventy percent (20/28) of small colon impactions occurred during the winter months[251], supporting the notion that inadequate water consumption and poor-quality feed may play a role.

Alterations in small colon motility may also be contributing factors in some cases. Small colon impaction has been associated with salmonellosis.[251] Forty percent of horses requiring surgical management of a small colon impaction shed *Salmonella* spp. postoperatively; however, similar results have not been found in more recent reports.[252] Horses with a small colon impaction were 10.8-times more likely to have diarrhea at the time of initial examination compared with horses with a large colon impaction; it could not be determined whether the diarrhea was the cause of, or a result of, the small colon impaction.[253] However, 34% of these horses also had a fever at admission suggesting that colitis may have been the primary disease.[253] Small colon impactions may occur secondary to colonic inflammation, edema, and ileus in horses infected with *Salmonella* spp., or *Salmonella* spp. shedding may occur as a complication of the small colon impaction.

Horses <6 months of age were overrepresented among cases of small colon disease requiring surgery[254] and horses <1 year and >15 years old were most prevalent in cases of small colon obstruction, representing 29% and 57% of cases, respectively.[47] More recent studies, specifically of small colon impaction, have found no age, breed, or gender predisposition.[251,253,255]

Clinical features

Horses have a presenting complaint of mild to moderate colic with or without diarrhea. Heart and respiratory rates may be variable and 34% of horses were reported to have a fever at admission.[253] Oral mucous membranes are usually pink with a variable moistness and CRT. Borborygmi may be present initially, but may be reduced or absent in cases with a long duration. Horses with small colon obstructions develop abdominal distension over several hours to days depending on the degree of obstruction. Reflux following passage of a nasogastric tube is rare. There is usually an apparent lack of fecal production, except for a relatively small volume diarrhea consistent with passage of water around an obstruction.

Differential diagnosis
Intestinal concretions and foreign body obstruction; enterolithiasis; sand colic; colitis; gas or spasmodic colic; large colon impaction; small colon strangulating pedunculated lipoma.

Diagnosis
A tentative diagnosis of small colon impaction can be made based on the time of year (i.e. late autumn and winter) in a horse with mild to moderate signs of colic and abdominal distension with or without small volume diarrhea. In most cases a definitive diagnosis is made using abdominal palpation per rectum (p. 32).[251,253] The small colon is identified on palpation based on its small size, location in the caudal abdomen, and the prominent antimesenteric (and mesenteric) tenial bands. The rectal mucosa is often edematous and irritated.

Abdominocentesis and peritoneal fluid analysis (p. 37) can be performed in cases where there is concern regarding intestinal viability; a high TP (>25 g/l [2.5 g/dl]) or high nucleated cell count (>10 × 10^9/l [10,000 cells/μl]) may be an indication that the integrity of the small colon is compromised and surgical intervention is necessary.

Management/treatment
Horses with small colon impaction can be managed medically with IV fluid and electrolyte therapy to maintain hydration and electrolyte balance (see Chapter 12), enteral fluids and electrolytes to soften the impacted ingesta, and analgesia as needed (see Large colon impaction). Some clinicians use IV lidocaine (1.3 mg/kg IV bolus over 15 minutes then 0.05 mg/kg/minute CRI) or N-butylscopolammonium bromide (Buscopan®) as an analgesic, particularly if surgery is not an option. Lubricants, laxatives, and cathartics can also be used, including mineral oil and magnesium sulfate. The mean time from admission to impaction resolution with medical treatment was 55 hours (2–169 hours).[253]

Enemas are generally not recommended because the impaction is often quite proximal and the risk and consequences of rectal tear (p. 135) outweigh any benefit. However, if the impacted feces can be palpated in the distal small colon, surgery is not an option, and if the horse is not responding to other treatment, an enema can be performed using a small stomach tube and warm water. The client should be warned of the potential for causing a rectal tear with this procedure. Abdominal distension can be relieved using trocarization in cases where surgery is not an option.

Surgical correction of a small colon impaction is required in many cases[251]; however, some authors have reported a higher percentage of cases managed with medial therapy.[252] Indications for surgery are persistent or severe pain, lack of defecation, absent borborygmi, and abdominal distension.[251–253] Horses treated surgically were 5-times more likely to have abdominal distension at admission compared with horses treated medically.[253]

Surgery is performed through a ventral midline celiotomy; however, a small colon impaction can also be approached through a left flank incision in the standing horse. A small colon impaction is usually resolved surgically using a high enema with large volumes of warm water delivered via a small nasogastric tube attached to a hose. The use of sodium carboxymethylcellulose on the serosal surface may minimize injury to the bowel. Serosal tears can occur, particularly if the impaction is long standing, and these should be repaired using 2-0 synthetic absorbable suture in a continuous inverting (Cushing or Lembert) pattern. The decision to perform an enterotomy versus an enema is based on the ease with which the impacted ingesta is hydrated and broken down with manipulation, and surgeon preference. An enterotomy results in contamination and needs to be closed, but ultimately may be quicker and less traumatic compared with a high enema. The enterotomy is performed on the antimesenteric tenia[256] and closed using 2-0 synthetic absorbable suture material in a simple continuous pattern oversewn with a Cushing or Lembert pattern. Care should be taken to avoid lumen narrowing. Often with small colon impaction, the bowel is inflamed and edematous and prone to reimpaction. A pelvic flexure enterotomy (p. 44) can be performed to empty the intestinal tract proximal to the small colon to prevent reimpaction.

Perioperative antimicrobial drugs, flunixin meglumine, and IV fluids and electrolytes are the main postoperative treatments (see Chapter 18). Antiendotoxin therapy can be used in some cases. Other anti-inflammatory treatment includes low-dose dexamethasone (0.05–0.08 mg/kg IV), dimethylsulfoxide (20–100 mg/kg IV), and IV lidocaine. Hay should be slowly reintroduced over 5–7 days to prevent reimpaction and complete pelleted feed may be used as an alternative to hay. Hospitalization time is usually longer for horses treated surgically (7–14 days) compared with horses treated medically (3–7 days).[253]

The prognosis for horses with a small colon impaction is good. In the most recent report, 21/23 (91%) horses treated medically and 20/21 (95%) horses treated surgically survived to discharge.[253] The major complications following small colon impaction are reimpaction, salmonellosis, and adhesion formation (see Chapter 18).[251]

Fecalith obstruction

Key points
- A fecalith generally causes a complete obstruction of the proximal small colon.
- Horses with a fecalith obstruction usually require surgical management.
- Prolonged medical treatment can result in ischemic necrosis of the small colon at the site of the obstruction.
- The prognosis is good to excellent with early treatment.

Definition/overview
Focal obstruction of the small colon with a firm, large fecal ball (**1.96**)

Etiology/pathogenesis
Fecalith formation is infrequent and the etiology and pathogenesis are generally unknown but may be similar to that for small colon impaction (p. 130). American miniature horses, particularly foals, and ponies are predisposed to fecalith formation suggesting either a genetic or management component.[252,257] Of 15 American miniature horses referred for colic, nine had obstruction of the small colon.[258] In many cases, fec-

aliths in miniature horses have a large component of hair, which is thought to be from young horses eating tail hair.

Clinical features
Horses present with signs of mild to moderate colic. Because a fecalith generally causes a complete obstruction, signs of colic are usually persistent and abdominal distension tends to be a clinical feature. Intestinal sounds are usually reduced to absent, particularly if abdominal distension is marked. An absence of fecal production is apparent and horses may show signs of tenesmus. Horses usually do not show signs of shock except when bowel viability is affected.

Differential diagnosis
Large colon impaction; enterolithiasis; sand colic; intestinal concretions and foreign body obstruction; colitis; gas or spasmodic colic; strangulating pedunculated lipoma of the small colon (older horses).

Diagnosis
A tentative diagnosis is made based on breed and clinical signs. A definitive diagnosis of fecalith obstruction is usually made at surgery. The obstruction most often occurs at the proximal part of the small colon and is

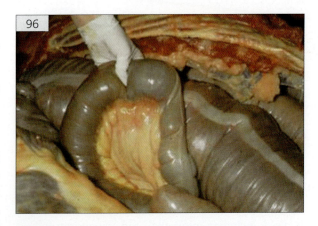

1.96 A fecalith causing small colon obstruction with a diffuse, long, and tubular impaction oral to the obstruction.

usually not palpable per rectum. In some horses, gas distension of the small or large colon may be identified on palpation per rectum.

Management/treatment

Some horses with fecalith obstruction may be managed medically (see Small colon impaction); however, most require abdominal surgery for diagnosis and treatment. The fecalith can be broken down by massage using tap water delivered intraluminally through a high enema or sterile fluid delivered through the intestinal wall using a 14-gauge 3.8-cm (1.5-inch) needle and fluid administration set. The use of carboxymethylcellulose on the serosal surface may minimize intestinal injury during massage. Fecaliths can also be removed via an enterotomy along the antimesenteric band of the small colon (see Small colon impaction). Transmural ischemic necrosis of the small colon (**1.97**) can occur in some horses, necessitating resection and anastomosis or careful inversion of the affected bowel if only a small focal area is affected.

Perioperative antimicrobial drugs, flunixin meglumine, and IV fluids and electrolytes are the main postoperative treatments (see Chapter 18). Hay should be slowly reintroduced over 5–7 days to prevent reimpaction and complete pelleted feed may be used as an alternative to hay. The prognosis for survival is good to excellent with early treatment.

Intestinal concretions and foreign body obstruction

Key points

- Foreign body obstruction should be considered in a young horse with mild signs of colic and scant or no feces.
- Horses may also have a history of recurrent colic.
- The prognosis is good to excellent with early surgical treatment.

Definition/overview

A phytoconglobate is a concretion of matted plant residue formed into a ball. A phytobezoar is plant material combined with struvite (magnesium, ammonium, phosphate) and a trichobezoar is hair combined with struvite. A phytotrichobezoar is composed of both plant material and hair in a struvite concretion (**1.98**).[160] (See also Fecalith obstruction and Enterolithiasis.) Ingested foreign material can also become mineralized and cause an obstruction.

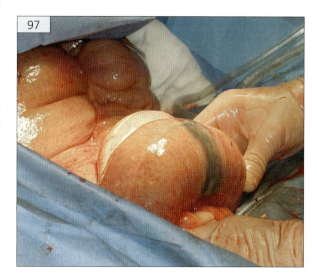

1.97 Ischemic necrosis of the small colon associated with a fecalith.

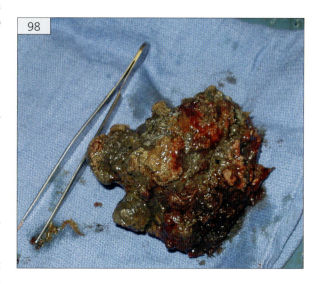

1.98 Rope that was covered with feces and struvite concretion and was removed from the proximal small colon in a young horse.

Etiology/pathogenesis

Ingested fibrous non-digestible (plant material or hair) or foreign material (e.g. rope, plastic, baling twine) becomes covered in ingesta and a concretion of magnesium ammonium phosphate (also called struvite) as it passes through the large colon. The concretion-covered foreign material is often irregularly shaped with a rough surface and becomes large and causes intestinal obstruction, which may be partial or complete. Obstruction most often occurs in the region of the right dorsal colon, transverse colon, and small colon. Young horses (<3 years old) are affected more often because of their indiscriminant eating habits. Poor-quality pasture may contribute to ingestion of inappropriate material.[259]

Clinical features

Horses may present with signs of mild to moderate colic and may have a history of recurrent signs. Horses have been seen to walk backwards and dog sit[259], and tenesmus may be observed in horses with a more distal obstruction.[260] Obstruction can be partial allowing gas and some soft or liquid ingesta to be passed through the intestinal tract. Horses with a partial obstruction show mild to moderate signs of pain, which may be intermittent, and pass small volumes of soft feces. Complete obstruction causes more severe signs of colic, abdominal distension, and a complete lack of fecal production. Heart rate will be within normal limits initially; however, horses will become tachycardic as abdominal distension progresses and in cases with associated intestinal wall necrosis. Intestinal borborygmi will be present initially, but will decrease or become absent with complete obstruction and progression of colonic distension. Reflux is usually not obtained following passage of a nasogastric tube. Abdominal palpation per rectum may reveal large colon (and on occasion small colon) distension and a lack of feces in the small colon and rectum. Rarely is the obstructing material palpable.

Differential diagnosis

Small colon impaction; fecalith obstruction; enterolithiasis; large colon impaction; large colon displacement; gas or spasmodic colic.

Diagnosis

GI tract obstruction with a foreign body is definitively diagnosed at surgery. A tentative diagnosis may be made in the case of a young horse showing signs of mild to moderate abdominal pain with abdominal distension and scant to no fecal production.

Hematology and biochemistry should be within normal limits unless perforation has occurred. Peritoneal fluid will be within normal limits initially; however, the TP concentration and nucleated cell count will increase and the fluid will change from yellow to serosanguineous as intestinal damage progresses.

Management/treatment

Abdominal surgery is necessary in most cases. The foreign material is most likely to cause an obstruction in the right dorsal colon/transverse colon/small colon region. The small colon will be relatively empty and the large colon distended with gas and impacted in the right dorsal colon. Because of the location of the obstruction it can be challenging to correct. An enterotomy is almost always necessary. This can be performed in the proximal aspect of the small colon using moistened laparotomy sponges to meticulously pack off the abdomen. A small colon enterotomy is performed in the antimesenteric band and should be made large enough to remove the foreign material. Sponge forceps may be necessary to retrieve the foreign body. A pelvic flexure enterotomy may be necessary to remove large concretions in the right dorsal colon. Necrotic intestine should be resected if possible. In some cases, inaccessible damaged areas can be inverted and oversewn. If the small colon is damaged or the large colon impacted, a pelvic flexure enterotomy may be necessary to empty the large colon proximal to the damaged intestine and allow the affected area to heal.

Antimicrobials, flunixin meglumine, and IV fluids are administered during the perioperative period. Reintroduction of feed will depend on the extent of intestinal damage (see Chapter 18). The prognosis for survival is good to excellent with early treatment.

Small colon strangulating pedunculated lipoma
Key points
- Strangulating pedunculated lipoma is a more common cause of small intestinal obstruction (p. 71), but it can cause obstruction of the small colon.[261,262]
- Strangulation of the small colon by a pedunculated lipoma should be considered in geriatric horses with signs of colic.
- Evidence of strangulation is usually identified on palpation per rectum.
- Prognosis is good to excellent with early surgical treatment.

Definition/overview
Strangulation of a small colon segment by a lipoma pedicle.

Etiology/pathogenesis
The etiology and pathogenesis are unknown. (See also Strangulating pedunculated lipoma.)

Clinical features
Strangulation of the small colon by a pedunculated lipoma usually occurs in older horses (>16 years). Horses show mild to moderate but persistent signs of colic. There is a lack of defecation and horses may appear to have a small colon impaction (p. 130) based on clinical signs and palpation per rectum.

Differential diagnosis
Small colon impaction; strangulating pedunculated lipoma of the small intestine; large colon impaction.

Diagnosis
In many cases a tentative diagnosis can be made based on the age of the horse and examination per rectum where the pedicle can often be palpated encircling the distal small colon/rectum. Small colon distension can also be palpated. Horses may also have an apparent small colon impaction. Definitive diagnosis is usually made during surgery. Peritoneal fluid can be serosanguineous with a high TP concentration and nucleated cell count.

Management/treatment
Abdominal surgery is necessary. Transection of the encircling pedicle is performed using Metzenbaum scissors. Tissue viability is assessed and a small colon resection and anastomosis performed if necessary.[49a,261] Often the distal small colon and rectum are involved; this precludes resection and anastomosis and emphasizes the importance of early surgical intervention.

Antimicrobials, flunixin meglumine, and fluid and electrolyte therapy are administered during the perioperative period. Reintroduction of feed should depend on the extent of intestinal damage (see Chapter 18). The prognosis for survival is good with early treatment.[261]

Rectum
- Rectal lesions are a rare cause of emergency admissions in horses.
- Clinical features, treatment, and prognosis are variable.
- Diagnosis is usually by rectal palpation.

Rectal tear
Key points
- Recognition that a rectal tear has occurred is critical and rapid appropriate first-aid treatment is important for patient care, as well as professional liability.
- Treatment of horses with grade 3 and 4 rectal tears involves either fecal diversion or repair.
- Horses with grade 3 tears have a fair to guarded prognosis and horses with grade 4 tears have a grave prognosis for survival.

Definition/overview

Tearing of the rectal mucosa and submucosa (grade 1); longitudinal and circular muscle layers only (grade 2); mucosa, submucosa, and muscle layers (grade 3A); mucosa, submucosa, muscle layers, and serosa with the mesorectum intact (grade 3B); or mucosa, submucosa, muscle layers, and serosa (full-thickness, grade 4) (**1.99A–E**).

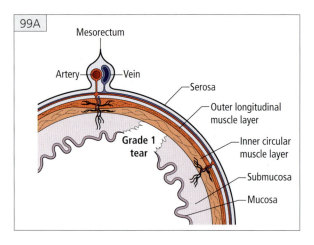

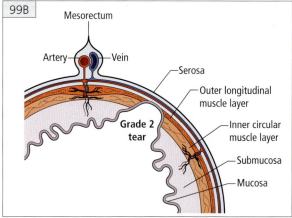

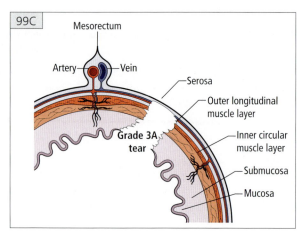

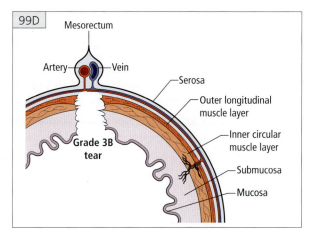

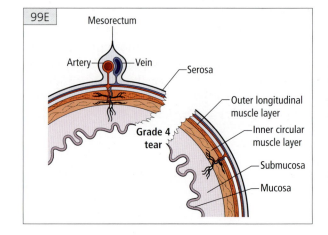

1.99A–E Schematic illustration of a grade 1 (A), grade 2 (B), grade 3A (C), grade 3B (D), and grade 4 (E) rectal tear.

Etiology/pathogenesis

Rectal tears are almost always secondary to trauma, the most common traumatic event being palpation per rectum of the reproductive or GI tract.[263,264] Aggressive palpation, failure to evacuate the rectum of feces prior to organ palpation, palpation while the horse is straining or against peristalsis, lack of lubrication, and inadequate restraint predispose to rectal tear. Other causes include parturition, dystocia, penetration of a stallion's penis into the mare's rectum, enemas, vertebral fracture, rectal prolapse, and trailer accidents.[264–267] Tears tend to occur on the mesorectal border (dorsally) where the vessels penetrate the rectal wall. Ischemic necrosis of the rectal wall caused by thrombosis or thromboembolism has been reported.[268,269] In some instances, rectal tears can occur spontaneously and the cause is not apparent.[267]

In one study, horses >9 years old, mares, and Arabian and American miniature horses were overrepresented compared with the hospital population.[267] Other studies, however, have reported that male horses and geldings are predisposed.[265,270]

Clinical features

When a rectal tear occurs during abdominal palpation per rectum, a loss of rectal tone can be appreciated. While blood on the rectal sleeve is the classic indication for a rectal tear, some veterinarians have reported no evidence of this in some cases of rectal tears. Rectal tears can be palpated as an irregularity or loss of integrity of the rectal wall. Most tears are located dorsally (51%) and occasionally ventrally (19%), laterally (16%), dorsolaterally (8%), and ventrolaterally (4%).[267] Tears are reported to range in size from 1 to 27 cm and occur approximately 35 cm (range 4–60 cm) cranial to the anus.[267]

Horses with grade 3 or 4 rectal tears rapidly develop signs of abdominal pain, septic peritonitis, and shock including dull demeanor, muscle fasciculations, sweating, reluctance to move, moderate to severe tachycardia, tachypnea, hyper-/hypothermia, and injected and dry oral mucous membranes.

Differential diagnosis

Rectal mucosal irritation (hemorrhage on rectal sleeve); anus tear (hemorrhage on rectal sleeve); perirectal abscess; GI tract obstruction (abdominal pain); GI or reproductive tract perforation (shock).

Diagnosis

Palpation per rectum is used to diagnose a rectal tear. When blood is identified on the rectal sleeve following routine palpation per rectum, the horse should be sedated (xylazine and butorphanol, or detomidine) and 2% lidocaine placed intrarectally either in the lubricant or using a 60 ml syringe and extension set. The rectum should be palpated gently using plenty of lubrication. Some clinicians recommend palpating the rectum using a bare arm because this increases stereognosis. Rectal tears are graded 1 to 4 (**1.99A–E**). Rectal endoscopy (proctoscopy) can also be used to evaluate the extent of the tear.

Management/treatment

Initial management involves parenteral administration of broad-spectrum antimicrobial drugs (e.g. penicillin and gentamicin, see Chapter 16), flunixin meglumine, and tetanus toxoid. Mineral oil may be given as a fecal softener (4 liters PO via a nasogastric tube). Epidural anesthesia should always be given at the sacrococcygeal space (xylazine 0.17 mg/kg diluted to 6 ml with sterile saline). Lidocaine (5–6 ml) can also be used in the epidural; however, it may make the horse ataxic, which may be undesirable for transportation.

The use of a rectal pack is controversial; if properly used with appropriate epidural analgesia/anesthesia, it can prevent fecal material from packing into the tear. However, feces are often passed around the rectal pack. If a rectal pack is to be used, once the epidural analgesia/anesthesia has taken effect, the recommended procedure is to place a povidone–iodine soaked and lubricated stockinet into the rectum and then begin to pack roll cotton into the stockinet.

Treatment for rectal tears involves a combination of one or more of the following: (1) repairing the tear (suturing the tear per rectum, via a ventral midline celiotomy, or laparoscopically) or (2) fecal diversion (rectal liner, pelvic flexure enterotomy, temporary colostomy, or repeated rectal evacuation).[271] Each technique has its advantages and limitations and success depends on the comfort of the surgeon with the particular technique.

In a recent report, the survival rate for horses with grade 1 and 2 rectal tears was 100%, grade 3 tears 38%, and grade 4 tears 2%. Loop colostomy and repair via a ventral midline celiotomy had the best success rate for horses with grade 3 tears (5/5) and only 2/5 horses with blind suture repair and 2/4 horses with repeated rectal evacuation survived.[267] The only horse with a grade 4 tear that survived had the tear suture repaired via a ventral midline celiotomy approach.[267] Other studies have reported a higher survival rate of 60–70% for horses with grade 3 tears[272,273], with 75% of horses with grade 3 tears surviving following direct suturing[273] and 60% of horses with grade 3 tears surviving following loop colostomy.[274]

Rectal prolapse

Key points

- Type I and II rectal prolapses respond well to treatment; identification and management of the underlying cause is important. Resection of the prolapsed tissue may be necessary.
- Type III and IV rectal prolapses usually occur in mares during parturition and can result in avulsion of the small colon vasculature, with subsequent small colon ischemic necrosis. The prognosis in these cases is grave.

Definition/overview

A rectal prolapse is defined as prolapse of the rectal mucosa and submucosa (type I) or full-thickness prolapse of the rectal ampulla (type II) through the anus. A type III prolapse is a type II prolapse with small colon intussuscepted into the rectum. A type IV prolapse is defined as the peritoneal rectum and a variable amount of small colon intussuscepted through the anus.[271]

Etiology/pathogenesis

Rectal prolapse is associated with straining. Type I and II prolapses are most common and occur in association with diarrhea, small colon impaction/obstruction, parasitism, colic, proctitis, and rectal foreign body or tumor. A type IV prolapse is most often seen in broodmares peripartum as a result of straining during parturition or dystocia. A type IV rectal prolapse almost invariably results in tearing of the mesocolon and detachment of the small colon vascular supply, with subsequent small colon necrosis (**1.100A, B**). Small colon necrosis causes small colon obstruction, signs of abdominal pain, septic peritonitis, and shock.

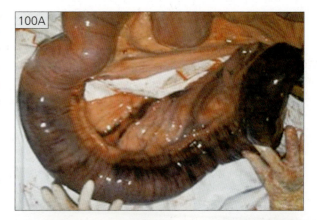

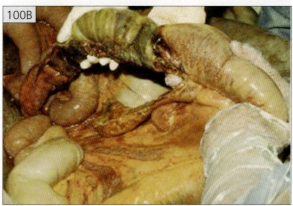

1.100A, B Small colon ischemic necrosis in a broodmare that had a type IV rectal prolapse postpartum. The prolapse was corrected and the mare developed signs of colic and shock.

Clinical features

Horses with a rectal prolapse have a rectal mass (type I, II, or III) or tube (type IV) protruding from the anus. The affected rectum and/or small colon is often edematous, hemorrhagic, cyanotic, and/or necrotic.[271] Horses with a type IV rectal prolapse with tearing of the mesocolon and small colon necrosis rapidly develop signs associated with small colon obstruction and intestinal necrosis including colic, lack of fecal production, septic peritonitis, and septic shock (tachycardia, tachypnea, fever, injected or toxic mucous membranes, cool extremities) after the prolapsed rectum has been replaced.

Differential diagnosis

Herniation of small colon/small intestine through a rectal or vaginal tear; other causes of postpartum shock.

Diagnosis

In horses with a type I or II rectal prolapse, diagnosis is made based on palpation of the mucosal mass. The cause of the prolapse should be determined by physical and laboratory examination, fecal examination for parasites, and, following correction of the prolapse, rectal examination and abdominal examination per rectum (see Colitis, Small colon impaction, Fecalith obstruction, Enterolithiasis, Intestinal concretions and foreign body obstruction).

Broodmares with a type III or IV rectal prolapse should be evaluated further for signs of mesocolon avulsion and ischemic necrosis of the small colon. Diagnosis of mesocolon avulsion is important because this is associated with a grave prognosis for survival. A presumptive diagnosis can be made based on a history of rectal prolapse and signs of colic, lack of defecation, and peritonitis (abdominocentesis and peritoneal fluid analysis). Laboratory data can include leukopenia, high PCV, hypoproteinemia, hyperfibrinogenemia or hypofibrinogenemia, prerenal azotemia, and hyperlactatemia.

A definitive diagnosis can be made using laparoscopy or abdominal exploration. It is important to recognize that even if the prolapse is corrected immediately, ischemic necrosis of the small colon can occur.

Management/treatment

Diagnosis and management of the underlying cause is important. Type I and II rectal prolapses can usually be managed by reducing the prolapsed rectum and maintaining reduction. Epidural anesthesia should be performed at the sacrococcygeal space using xylazine and/or lidocaine to reduce straining. Placement of an epidural catheter (see Chapter 14) should be considered in horses with recurrent rectal prolapse.

Edema of the prolapsed tissue can be reduced using topical hypertonic solutions (e.g. glycerine, sugar, magnesium sulfate). Lubrication and lidocaine can be used. The prolapsed rectum and/or small colon are reduced using massage and manipulation. Once the tissue is reduced, a purse-string suture can be placed in the anus using 1/4-inch umbilical tape. The anus can be left open enough for passage of feces or it can be loosened every few hours to allow manual or spontaneous rectal evacuation. The purse-string suture can be left in place for 48–72 hours, if tolerated. Mineral oil can be given via a nasogastric tube and a laxative diet fed to keep the feces soft. Diagnosis and management of the underlying cause is important.

In some cases the prolapsed tissue cannot be reduced or is necrotic or the prolapse is recurrent. Submucosal resection (types I and III) or resection and anastomosis (type IV) is necessary. Submucosal resection can be performed with epidural anesthesia (see Chapter 14). After surgical preparation, two 18-gauge 15-cm spinal needles (or 14 gauge 13-cm Teflon catheters with the stylet in place) are inserted at 90 degrees to each other through the external anal sphincter and healthy mucosa to maintain the position of the prolapsed tissue during resection and anastomosis. Beginning at the 12 o'clock position, the mucosa and submucosa are resected in increments of one-third of the circumference of the rectal prolapse. Alternating resection of necrotic tissue and anastomosis of healthy tissue is performed until the entire circumference of the necrotic tissue has been resected. The submucosa is apposed using #1 or #2 synthetic absorbable suture material in an interrupted horizontal mattress pattern. The mucosa is apposed using 2-0 synthetic absorbable suture material in a simple interrupted or simple continuous pattern interrupted at least three points around the circumference. Resection and anastomosis of the prolapsed rectum/small colon is performed similarly to a submucosal resection except that it is full thickness and care should be taken to ligate the mesenteric vessels. Postoperatively, horses should be treated with flunixin meglumine, perioperative antimicrobial drugs, and laxatives, and fed a laxative diet (e.g. fresh grass and alfalfa hay).[271]

Perirectal abscess

Key points

- Perirectal abscess should be suspected in a horse showing mild signs of colic, tenesmus, and reduced fecal production.
- Diagnosis is made via rectal palpation and ultrasonographic examination of the mass.
- The prognosis for uncomplicated perirectal abscesses is good to excellent.

Definition/overview

Abscess formation in the perirectal subcutaneous tissues or lymph nodes.

Etiology/pathogenesis

In most cases the cause of a perirectal abscess is unknown. Proposed etiologies include rectal tear, gravitation of a gluteal abscess post injection, and abscessation of anorectal lymph nodes.[275,276] *Streptococcus zooepidemicus* and *Escherichia coli* have been isolated from perirectal abscesses.[275,276]

Clinical features

Horses with perirectal abscesses usually present with signs of mild colic, tenesmus, and reduced fecal production. Dull demeanor, inappetence, and fever are also seen. Perirectal abscesses are identified on rectal palpation. A firm mass is palpable in the rectal wall, usually caudal to the peritoneal reflection. Often there is a soft area on the surface of the mass, which is usually an area of impending drainage. Fecal material is typically impacted cranial to the abscess. Urinary tract dysfunction (i.e. dysuria) can be seen in some cases associated with neuritis secondary to regional inflammation[276] or when the urinary tract is involved in the abscessation.

Differential diagnosis

Small colon impaction; rectal tear; lymphadenopathy; perirectal neoplasia; perirectal hematoma.

Diagnosis

Ultrasonographic examination of the mass can be performed to determine the consistency and provide some indication as to the whether the mass is an abscess, reactive lymph node, hematoma, or neoplasia (**1.101**), and if other pelvic structures are involved. A 14-gauge 1.5-inch (3.8-cm) needle with extension tubing can be used to obtain a sample from the mass per rectum for gross evaluation, cytology, and bacterial culture and sensitivity testing.

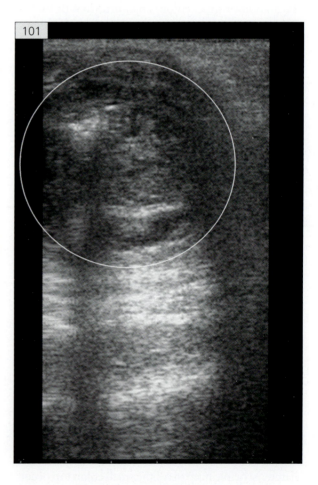

1.101 Ultrasonographic appearance of a perirectal abscess. The image was obtained with a linear probe per rectum. Note the circumscribed mass containing material with mixed echogenicity.

Rarely, the perirectal abscess involves the peritoneal cavity. In these cases, transrectal and transabdominal ultrasonographic examination can be performed to determine the extent of the abscess and the structures involved. Abdominocentesis and peritoneal fluid analysis (p. 37), including cytology and bacterial culture and sensitivity testing, should be performed.

Management/treatment
Epidural anesthesia is performed (see Chapter 14). Dorsal and lateral abscesses can be drained into the rectum. Once a sample is obtained, the mass can be distended with sterile saline to facilitate drainage. A #15 scalpel blade is guarded with the finger tips and taken into the rectum and used to create a 2–3-cm hole in the palpable soft area of the abscess. Ultrasonography can be used to guide drainage hole placement, but is usually not necessary. The abscess can be lavaged daily using saline until it heals. Ventral abscesses can be drained into the vagina in mares or ventral to the anus in males.[271] Perioperative management includes antimicrobial drugs, flunixin meglumine, laxatives, and a laxative diet (e.g. fresh grass and alfalfa hay).[271] Young horses and foals have also been managed with antimicrobials, analgesics, and laxatives without drainage.[276] The prognosis is good to excellent if other pelvic structures are not involved.

In cases where the abdominal cavity is involved, an exploratory celiotomy may be necessary to identify the extent of the abscess and for drainage. The prognosis is guarded to poor for these horses.

Hernias
- Hernia is a general term used to describe a bulge or protrusion of an organ through the structure or muscle that usually contains it.
- Herniation of intestine through either the inguinal canal, an umbilical defect (p. 144), or a diaphragmatic rent (p. 145) can result in signs of colic and necessitate emergency care.
- The small intestine tends to become herniated most commonly; however, herniation of various parts of the digestive system can occur.
- Horses with herniation of the digestive system typically present on an emergency basis with signs of colic. While inguinal and umbilical hernias can be readily diagnosed on physical examination,

diaphragmatic hernias require ultrasonographic or radiographic evaluation and are often diagnosed at surgery or necropsy.
- Surgery is indicated in most cases and involves repositioning the entrapped part of the digestive system, resection and anastomosis if intestinal viability is impaired, and repair of the abdominal cavity hernia site.

Inguinal and scrotal hernias
Key points
- Foals with inguinal hernias should be monitored closely for signs of colic and the herniated intestine becoming non-reducible and/or firm.
- The scrotum and testicle should be examined in any colt or stallion showing signs of colic.
- The prognosis for foals and horses with inguinal hernias is excellent with appropriate management.

Definition/overview
Inguinal hernias are defined as herniation of intestinal contents within the inguinal canal (**1.102**) and scrotal hernias as intestinal contents within the scrotum. Occasionally, a scrotal hernia can rupture (ruptured scrotal hernia). Distal jejunum and ileum are the most common parts of the GI tract that become herniated.

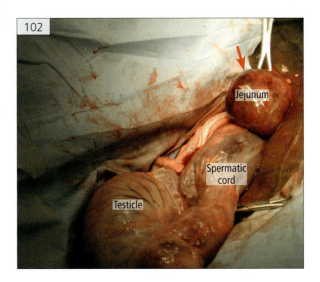

1.102 Inguinal hernia in a stallion at surgery. The jejunum (arrow) is identified in the inguinal area.

Indirect (true) inguinal hernias occur when the intestine passes through the vaginal ring and into the vaginal tunic (**1.103**). Direct (false) hernias occur when intestine passes through a defect in the peritoneum and transverse fascia adjacent to the vaginal ring and lies in the subcutaneous space of the scrotum and prepuce.[271,277] Indirect hernias are most common in horses.

Etiology/pathogenesis

The size of the inguinal ring is not thought to be a contributing factor to inguinal herniation because it is actually the vaginal ring through which the intestine initially herniates. Hernias in neonates are congenital. Inguinal hernias occur almost exclusively in intact males. A higher incidence of inguinal or scrotal hernias is reported in Standardbred horses, Tennessee Walking Horses, and American Saddlebreds.[278,279] Neonates and any age group over 1 year are at risk.[278] Reported predisposing factors include recent breeding or strenuous exercise and trauma.[278,279]

Clinical features

Neonates: Foals often present as neonates with a congenital indirect scrotal hernia. These hernias are easily reducible with the foal positioned on its back. Intestinal strangulation is uncommon because of the foal's shorter and wider inguinal ring[271]; however, foals with these hernias should be monitored closely for signs of colic and the hernia becoming non-reducible, larger, and firm.

Direct hernias or ruptured indirect scrotal hernias can occur in foals and are usually diagnosed within 4–48 hours of birth. Clinical signs include colic, dull demeanor, and marked scrotal and preputial swelling with skin abrasions and splitting.[271]

Colts and stallions: Adult male horses with an inguinal hernia usually present with moderate signs of colic. Scrotal swelling is observed (**1.104**). The testicle on the side of the herniation becomes cool and firm and the spermatic cord enlarged, firm, and painful to the touch because of obstruction of venous drainage from the testicle.[271,277]

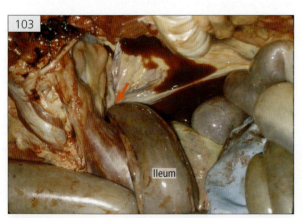

Ileum

1.103 Indirect inguinal hernia with the ileum (arrow) and distal jejunum herniated into the inguinal canal via the vaginal ring.

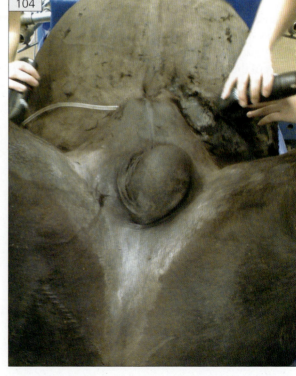

1.104 Swollen, cool, and firm left testicle in a horse with an inguinal hernia.

Differential diagnosis

Neonates: Ruptured bladder/uroabdomen with accumulation of urine in the subcutaneous tissue or scrotum; urethral tear with subcutaneous accumulation of urine.

Adults: Spermatic cord torsion (abnormal testicle); testicular thrombosis (abnormal testicle); scrotal seroma or hematoma (abnormal testicle); testicular neoplasia (abnormal testicle); gas or spasmodic colic (colic signs); large colon impaction (colic signs); EFE (colic signs); strangulating lipoma (colic signs); small intestinal volvulus (colic signs).

Diagnosis

Neonates: Diagnosis of a congenital indirect hernia is usually made in foals during a physical examination with identification of an enlarged scrotum. The swelling is typically soft, non-painful, and easily reducible. Ultrasonographic examination can be performed to determine the hernia contents. A direct hernia or ruptured scrotal hernia should be suspected in any neonate presenting with colic and extensive ventral swelling. Ultrasonography can be used to confirm the diagnosis; however, this is usually not necessary.

Colts and stallions: A tentative diagnosis of inguinal hernia can be made based on signs of colic, an enlarged scrotum, and a firm testicle in an intact male. Inguinal herniation in adult horses can be definitively diagnosed based on palpation per rectum of the inguinal ring. Small intestine, which is often dilated, can be palpated entering the internal inguinal ring. Ultrasonographic examination of the inguinal region and scrotum can be performed if the diagnosis is not confirmed based on palpation per rectum; however, this is unnecessary in most cases.

Management/treatment

Neonates: Congenital scrotal hernias usually resolve spontaneously within 3–6 months and surgical correction is recommended if the hernia does not resolve by this age.[271] Neonatal foals with a reducible hernia can be managed medically with repeated reduction of the herniated intestine. A closed castration with the horse under general anesthesia and closure of the inguinal area or vaginal tunic is recommended when and if the horse is castrated.

If a foal shows signs of colic or the herniated intestine is no longer reducible or becomes enlarged or edematous, surgery is recommended. Emergency surgery is necessary for direct hernias or ruptured scrotal hernias. An inguinal as well as a ventral midline celiotomy approach is usually made. The herniated intestine is reduced and the viability of the intestine assessed. In foals with non-viable intestine, resection and anastomosis is necessary. Castration or hemicastration is recommended through the previously created inguinal approach followed by closure of the inguinal rings. Laparoscopic inguinal ring closure has been described.[279a,279b]

Colts and stallions: Surgical management is necessary for correction of inguinal hernias in adult horses. Correction of an inguinal hernia and a non-surgical approach where the herniated intestine is massaged back through the inguinal ring with the horse in dorsal recumbency, with or without laparoscopic guidance, has been described.[271] However, a surgical approach is often necessary. An approach to the inguinal area and a ventral midline celiotomy is usually made. Castration or hemicastration is performed. Hemicastration should not affect fertility; however, an inguinal hernia can occur on the side where the testicle remains. Once the vaginal tunic is opened, the herniated intestine is identified. The herniated intestine is reduced, which often requires manipulation from the inguinal approach as well as gentle traction via the ventral midline celiotomy. Usually only a few centimeters of distal jejunum and ileum are affected. Resection and anastomosis of a short segment of affected intestine is often necessary and is performed following hernia reduction through a ventral midline celiotomy. Alternatively, resection and anastomosis can be performed through an inguinal approach. The vaginal tunic and the subcutaneous tissue in the inguinal area (and/or the inguinal ring) are closed. Absorbable sutures are placed in the skin if needed. Minimal postoperative care is necessary. (See also Chapter 18.) The prognosis for foals and horses with inguinal hernias is excellent with appropriate management.

Strangulating umbilical hernia
Key points
- Foals and weanlings with umbilical hernias should be monitored closely for signs of colic and the hernia palpated at least daily to ensure that it remains soft and reducible.
- Surgical repair of large umbilical hernias or hernias that have not resolved spontaneously by the time the foal is about 4 months old is recommended.
- The use of a hernia clamp should be avoided because of the potential for complications.

Definition/overview
Strangulating umbilical hernia refers to the incarceration of intestine in an umbilical hernia. A parietal hernia (also called Richter's or Littre's hernia) occurs when only the antimesenteric wall of the intestine becomes incarcerated. Necrosis of the intestinal wall associated with a parietal hernia can result in abscessation and enterocutaneous fistula formation.

Etiology/pathogenesis
Umbilical hernias are usually congenital and may be hereditary and occur when the body wall fails to close at the location of the umbilicus.[277] Trauma to the umbilical cord during birth, excessive straining, and omphalitis have been proposed as causes for umbilical hernia.[280] Thoroughbreds and females were at significantly higher risk for umbilical hernias compared with other breeds and males.[281] Umbilical hernias are reported to occur in 0.5–2% of foals and only on rare occasions does intestine become incarcerated in the hernia.

Complications associated with the use of a hernia clamp can also require emergency management and include intestinal obstruction, peritonitis, enterocutaneous fistula formation, and evisceration.[277]

Clinical features
Umbilical hernias are usually reducible, soft, and non-painful. The hernia should be dry. Careful monitoring of any umbilical hernia is important for early detection of intestinal incarceration. Foals and weanlings with strangulating umbilical hernias usually present with an acute onset of mild to moderate signs of colic.

Clinical examination of the umbilical hernia reveals an increase in hernia size, firmness, edema, and/or pain on palpation. Parietal hernias do not cause a complete intestinal obstruction and while signs of colic may be observed initially, following intestinal necrosis these signs may subside. An enterocutaneous fistula can be diagnosed on examination, with ingesta seen at the umbilicus and marked periumbilical edema and inflammation.

Differential diagnosis
Intestinal incarceration; parietal hernia; abscessation; omphalitis or omphalophlebitis (neonatal foals).

Diagnosis
Diagnosis is usually made based on the clinical features in patients presenting with acute signs of colic. Ultrasonographic examination of the hernia can be performed, particularly in neonatal foals, to distinguish infection of the umbilical structures from intestinal incarceration or in foals not showing signs of colic to distinguish abscessation from intestinal incarceration. In many cases, however, ultrasonographic examination is not necessary.

Management/treatment
Strangulating umbilical hernias are managed surgically. With the patient positioned in dorsal recumbency, the ventral midline is prepared and an elliptical incision made around the umbilical hernia through the skin and subcutaneous tissue. The external sheath of the rectus abdominis muscle and hernia ring is exposed using a combination of sharp and blunt dissection. A small incision is made cranial to the umbilical hernia to enable palpation of the umbilical region from within the abdominal cavity. The body wall incision is carefully extended in a caudal direction to the hernia ring and the entrapped intestine is removed. Small intestine, cecum, and large colon can be involved in a parietal hernia. Intestinal viability should be assessed and resection of devitalized intestine and anastomosis performed. Often, resection and anastomosis is unnecessary. The body wall is closed routinely. Minimal postoperative care is necessary. (See also Chapter 18.) The prognosis is excellent.

Diaphragmatic hernia

Key point
- A diaphragmatic hernia is uncommon, but should be considered as a differential diagnosis in a horse or foal showing signs of colic with a history of trauma (including birth) or a broodmare that has recently foaled, particularly post dystocia.

Definition/overview
Herniation of intestine and other abdominal structures through a defect in the diaphragm.

Etiology/pathogenesis
Diaphragmatic hernias can be congenital or acquired. Congenital diaphragmatic hernias occur as a result of fusion failure of the pleuroperitoneal folds or of one fold to the septum transversum.[282] The cause of acquired diaphragmatic hernias in neonatal foals is usually trauma associated with parturition, including rib fractures at the costochondral junction of ribs 3 to 8[283,284], and in adult horses trauma, parturition, and strenuous activity.[282,285] Many horses do not have a unique historical event to which the hernia can be ascribed.[285]

Clinical features
Horses with a diaphragmatic hernia commonly present with signs of acute colic, particularly cases with small defects and where the small intestine is involved.[285,286] Large defects, however, can cause signs of respiratory distress with a rapid and shallow respiratory pattern associated with herniation of the colon and other abdominal organs.[282,285] Occasionally, horses can present with a history of low-grade recurrent colic or other signs of trauma such as epistaxis or puncture wound; rarely, a diaphragmatic hernia is found incidentally at necropsy.[277,285]

Diaphragmatic defects vary in size and can be as small as 2.5 cm or large enough to involve the dorsal to ventral length of the hemidiaphragm (**1.105**). Congenital diaphragmatic hernias usually occur in the left dorsal crus and have smooth edges with an absence of hemorrhage or fibrosis.[277,282] Acquired hernias are often large, involving the dorsal aspect of the diaphragm, and have thin, irregular areas with evidence of trauma including hemorrhage and fibrosis.[277,282]

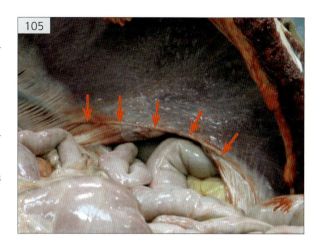

1.105 A large diaphragmatic hernia associated with trauma (arrows). (Courtesy Dr Fabio Del Piero)

Differential diagnosis
Small intestinal volvulus; EFE; pedunculated lipoma; proximal enteritis; mesenteric rent; large colon impaction; enterolithiasis; right dorsal displacement of the large colon; LCV; uterine tear (broodmare); uterine artery hemorrhage (broodmare); intestinal injury (broodmare); pneumonia (respiratory tract signs); pleuropneumonia (respiratory tract signs); heaves (respiratory tract signs).

Diagnosis
A diaphragmatic hernia should be considered as a differential diagnosis in a horse or foal showing signs of colic with a history of trauma or a broodmare that has recently foaled, particularly post dystocia. The diaphragm should be evaluated in foals with rib fractures involving the costochondral junction of ribs 3 to 8. Diaphragmatic hernia should also be ruled out either pre- or intraoperatively in horses showing signs of acute or recurrent colic with a history of exercise intolerance or a rapid and shallow respiratory pattern.

Rebreathing examination may exacerbate respiratory signs and horses may fail to take a deep breath. An absence of respiratory sounds may also be appreciated throughout the lung fields and intestinal borborygmi may be apparent within the cranioventral lung fields.[285]

Radiographic (**1.106**) and ultrasonographic examination can be used to identify the presence of abdominal viscera within the thoracic cavity and ultrasonography can be used to identify the actual diaphragmatic defect. Diagnosis, however, is often made at surgery.

Management/treatment

Diaphragmatic hernias associated with clinical signs are usually managed surgically with the horse under general anesthesia. Assisted ventilation is necessary. The diaphragm should be palpated in all horses undergoing abdominal exploration, particularly with a history of trauma or recent foaling or when a devitalized jejunal segment is identified with no obvious cause of strangulation.

Diaphragmatic hernias can be repaired via a ventral midline approach by suturing the defect primarily using a large-gauge suture material in a simple continuous pattern or by mesh herniorrhaphy. The incision should be made on the cranial ventral abdomen up to the xiphoid and the table tilted so that the head is elevated (reverse Trendelenberg) to gain access to the diaphragmatic defect. Lateral extension of the incision to the left or right in an L-shape may be necessary.[271] Following return of the intestine to the abdomen, its viability should be assessed. Resection and anastomosis of devitalized intestine is often necessary.[286] The pneumothorax should be corrected prior to recovery from general anesthesia and can be accomplished using a teat cannula or needle and suction.

Other reported approaches include repair in lateral recumbency through a rib resection that was made with guidance via a flank incision and thoracoscopy.[287] Inaccessible hernias can be left unrepaired; the stomach or other abdominal organs may adhere to the defect, leading to closure or partial closure.[287] However, if the horse reherniates and develops clinical signs associated with rehernation, reconsideration of repair or euthanasia may be necessary.

While the prognosis for horses with a diaphragmatic hernia, particularly a large or dorsally located hernia, is guarded, return to breeding or athletic activity, including racing and jumping, has been reported following hernia repair.[286,287]

In a recent retrospective study of 44 diaphragmatic hernia cases, the prognosis for survival was poor with 41% of horses dying or being euthanized prior to surgery and a further 39% being euthanized during surgery. Of the nine horses recovering from surgery, seven survived to hospital discharge and five were alive at least 1 year postoperatively.[285] Younger horses (≤2 years old) and horses with small and ventrally located diaphragmatic defects had a more favorable prognosis compared with older horses and horses with large and dorsally located defects.[285]

Liver
Acute hepatic disease
Key points

- Primary hepatobiliary disease is an uncommon cause of equine emergency admission.
- Liver enzyme activity is frequently high in horses with primary GI disease and is not typically clinically important.
- Clinical signs associated with liver disease include dull demeanor and anorexia, colic, icterus, and hepatic encephalopathy.
- Liver enzyme activity, liver function tests (blood ammonia and bile acid concentration), ultrasonography, and biopsy can be used to diagnose hepatic disease.
- Management of hepatobiliary disease is primarily supportive and the prognosis variable depending on the etiology.

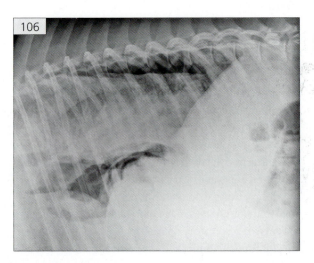

106

1.106 Radiographic appearance of abdominal contents within the thoracic cavity.

Definition/overview

Acute hepatobiliary disease refers to any disease of the liver or bile ducts. Hepatobiliary dysfunction refers to loss of a diverse group of physiologic functions and consequently has a variety of clinical features. Hepatic disease can occur without loss of hepatic function because most hepatic functions are not impaired until more than 80% of the hepatic mass is lost.[285]

Etiology/pathogenesis

The etiology of acute hepatic disease is variable (see Differential diagnosis). The pathogenesis also varies for the different etiological agents[288]; however, destruction of hepatic mass leads to loss of function including: protein, carbohydrate, and lipid metabolism; excretion of bile; detoxification; mononuclear phagocyte system; vitamin and mineral storage; and hematopoiesis. Loss of hepatic function is responsible for the clinical features observed.

Clinical features

Common clinical features include dull demeanor, anorexia, colic, hepatic encephalopathy, and icterus (hyperbilirubinemia). If there is chronic disease, weight loss is frequently observed. Less common clinical features include photosensitization, diarrhea, bilateral laryngeal paralysis, bleeding, ascites, and dependent edema.[288] Sudden death can occur with some causes of acute hepatic disease.

Specific clinical pathology indicators of liver disease in horses include increases in serum sorbitol dehydrogenase (SDH), gamma glutamyltransferase (GGT), bile acid concentration, direct (conjugated) bilirubin, ammonia, and urine bilirubin.[288] Non-specific tests include: increases in total or indirect (unconjugated) bilirubin, lactate dehydrogenase (LDH), aspartate aminotransferase (AST), alanine aminotransferase (ALT), alkaline phosphatase (ALP), blood urea nitrogen (BUN), globulin, and triglycerides; decreases in albumin and glucose; and prolongation of prothrombin and activated partial thromboplastin times.[288]

Differential diagnosis

Theiler's disease (serum-associated hepatitis, acute hepatic necrosis, serum sickness); Tyzzer's disease (*Clostridium piliforme*, acute necrotizing hepatitis in 7–42 day old foals); infectious necrotic hepatitis (*Clostridium novyi* type B, black disease); hyperlipemia; cholangiohepatitis; acute biliary obstruction (cholelithiasis, right dorsal displacement, liver lobe torsion); parasitic hepatitis; toxic hepatopathy (see Chapter 10); viral hepatitis (equine infectious anemia, equine herpes virus, equine viral arteritis).

Diagnosis

SDH, GGT, and serum bile acids are typically used to confirm a diagnosis of liver disease. Ultrasonographic examination and biopsy (histology and culture) are used to further evaluate the liver and potentially determine the etiology. Often, the disease is rapidly fatal (e.g. Theiler's disease, Tyzzer's disease, infectious necrotizing hepatitis) and diagnosis is made at necropsy.

Hyperlipemia describes the gross observation of lipid in the plasma and is typically associated with a plasma triglyceride concentration >5.65 mmol/l (500 mg/dl) and fatty infiltration of the liver and other organs. Hyperlipidemia is used to define a triglyceride concentration of 0.6–5.65 mmol/l (50–500 mg/dl), is not associated with lipemia or fatty infiltration of organs, and is a less severe form of the disease. Hypertriglyceridemia describes any increase in plasma triglyceride concentration above the reference limit (0.1–0.6 mmol/l [11–52 mg/dl]) and severe hypertriglyceridemia as serum triglyceride concentrations >5.65 mmol/l (500 mg/dl) and no signs of gross lipemia. If not treated, hypertriglyceridemia can progress to hepatic lipidosis, liver failure, multiple organ dysfunction, and death. (See also Chapter 10.)

Management/treatment

Management of acute hepatic disease is primarily supportive and aimed at supporting the patient until the liver can regain sufficient function. Hepatic encephalopathy can be managed with small doses of xylazine and detomidine. Note that most tranquilizers are metabolized by the liver and should be used with caution. Diazepam is contraindicated in hepatic encephalopathy because it enhances the effect of GABA on inhibitory neurons. IV polyionic isotonic fluids with 2.5–5.0% dextrose (see Chapter 12) is indicated. Hypokalemia and alkalosis increase renal production of ammonia and increase ammonia diffusion into the CNS; therefore, electrolyte and acid–base deficits need to be corrected.

Hyperammonemia associated with encephalopathy can be managed with oral lactulose/lactitol or oral antimicrobial drugs. Lactulose (0.3 ml/kg PO q6h) alters ammonia production from the GI tract through increased bacterial ammonia assimilation, decreased ammonia production, ammonia trapping, changes in microflora, and osmotic catharsis and can be used to decrease blood ammonia concentration.[288] Antimicrobial drugs (neomycin, metronidazole, rifaximin, vancomycin) can decrease blood ammonia concentration. Neomycin (10–100 mg/kg PO q6h) can cause diarrhea and salmonellosis and routine use of antimicrobial drugs such as vancomycin is not recommended. (See also Chapter 7.)

Anti-inflammatory drugs (e.g. flunixin meglumine; DMSO, 0.5–1.0 g/kg IV as a 10% solution for 3–5 days; and pentoxifylline, 10 mg/kg PO q12h) can be beneficial. Flunixin meglumine may help with hepatobiliary inflammation. DMSO may dissolve intrabiliary sludge and calcium bilirubinate stones. Pentoxifylline may decrease hepatic fibrosis. Avoid drugs that are dependent on hepatic metabolism. Long-term dietary modification is likely necessary in chronic liver disease.[288] Surgery may be necessary for hepatic lobe torsion or cholelithiasis causing biliary obstruction.

Tyzzer's disease and infectious necrotizing hepatitis are usually rapidly fatal, but they may be treated with high doses of penicillin, ampicillin, or trimethoprim/sulfa drugs and supportive care including parenteral nutrition. Cholangiohepatitis can be treated with trimethoprim/sulfa drugs, ceftiofur, penicillin and gentamicin, ampicillin, or chloramphenicol. (See Chapter 10 for management of intoxications causing liver disease.)

Resolution of hyperlipemia involves treatment of the underlying disease process, enteral nutrition, and/or dextrose administration with or without insulin. Enteral nutrition is the preferred form of calorie provision, particularly in patients with mild to moderate hypertriglyceridemia, and can be in the form of commercially prepared low-residue diets. If provision of enteral nutrition is not possible because of the underlying GI disease, calories can be provided with IV dextrose, typically administered as a 2.5–5.0% solution at a maintenance (plus losses) fluid rate. (**Note:** Lipids should be avoided.) Blood and urine glucose concentration should be monitored in patients receiving IV dextrose with or without insulin. Insulin inhibits fat mobilization by inhibiting hormone-sensitive lipase activity and promotes the uptake of triglycerides into peripheral tissues by stimulating lipoprotein lipase activity. Regular insulin can be administered as an IV CRI at 0.05 U/kg/hour or as a bolus at 0.2 U/kg IV q1–6h. Ultralente insulin can be given at 0.4 U/kg SC q24h. Insulin should be discontinued once the triglycerides are observed to decrease toward reference values. Exogenous insulin hastens the clearance of triglycerides from the blood, but does not necessarily impact survival. Heparin has been used as an adjunctive treatment because of its ability to act as a cofactor for endothelium-bound lipoprotein lipase; however, it is not commonly used.[288]

PERITONEAL CAVITY

- Peritonitis and hemoabdomen are the two most common problems affecting primarily the peritoneal cavity of horses presenting on an emergency basis. Peritonitis and hemoabdomen are often secondary to a primary lesion.
- Horses and foals with peritonitis or hemoabdomen can present with a variety of clinical signs including colic, fever, dull demeanor, inappetence, shock, weakness, muscle fasciculations, or recumbency.
- Peritonitis and hemoabdomen can be diagnosed with a combination of abdominal ultrasonographic examination (p. 39) and abdominocentesis (p. 35) and peritoneal fluid analysis (p. 37).
- Treatment and prognosis are variable and dependent on the underlying cause.

Peritonitis

Key points

- Peritonitis should be considered in horses showing signs of colic with an unexplained fever, hyperfibrinogenemia, and immature neutrophils in the peripheral blood.
- Peritonitis is diagnosed based on peritoneal fluid analysis with a white cell count >10 × 10^9/l (10,000 cells/μl).

- Bacterial culture and sensitivity testing is important in order to select an appropriate antimicrobial drug.
- Clinical findings can be used to decide whether or not exploratory abdominal surgery is necessary.
- The prognosis is dependent on the underlying cause and is excellent for horses with idiopathic or *Actinobacillus equuli*-associated peritonitis.

Definition/overview

Peritonitis is defined as inflammation of the peritoneal cavity with a peritoneal fluid white cell count >10 × 10^9/l (10,000 cells/µl).[289,290] Peritonitis can be considered aseptic, when there is no infection (e.g. following abdominal exploratory surgery), or septic, which is often associated with an abdominal abscess or following GI tract leakage.

Etiology/pathogenesis

Common causes of peritonitis include a primary GI tract lesion (e.g. small intestinal strangulating obstruction [p. 62]), GI tract rupture/perforation (e.g. stomach [p. 60], cecum, colon, or rectum), urogenital tract rupture/perforation (e.g. uterine tear [see Chapter 5]), omphalitis, and body wall or perirectal laceration. Peritonitis can also occur as a complication of castration and abdominal surgery. Neoplasia (p. 58), abscessation associated with *Streptococcus equi* or *Rhodococcus equi*, or any compromise to the GI tract (e.g. enteritis or colitis [p. 124]) can cause peritonitis.[291,292] Peritonitis has also been associated with *Actinobacillus equuli*.[292]

Idiopathic peritonitis is a diagnosis of exclusion where there is no other identifiable abnormality and the horse responds to medical therapy.[289,292] A small proportion of these horses can have underlying disease identified at a later time (e.g. gastric SCC [p. 58], infiltrative or inflammatory bowel disease [p. 93]); however, many horses have no further problems.[292]

Peritonitis occurs following abdominal surgery and is usually subclinical, aseptic, mild, and resolves without specific treatment. Peritonitis in this instance is attributed to the initial lesion, surgical trauma, and mild contamination. Septic peritonitis is a rare complication following abdominal surgery.

Clinical features

Horses with peritonitis most commonly have a presenting complaint of colic (65–85% of cases).[289,290,292] Fever, diarrhea, dull demeanor, inappetence, and weight loss are other common reasons for presentation.[289,290,292,293] Physical examination and laboratory findings are variable.[292]

GI tract rupture/perforation usually causes signs of severe shock including sweating, cool extremities, poor jugular refill, dull demeanor, reluctance to walk, tachycardia, tachypnea, fever, and injected or toxic mucous membranes. Horses with GI rupture are often severely hemoconcentrated (high PCV) with normoproteinemia or hypoproteinemia, leukopenia, and hyperlactatemia.[46]

Horses with peritonitis associated with *A. equuli* can present with signs of mild to severe abdominal pain, lethargy, inappetence, and occasionally weight loss. An important clinical feature of this disease is that horses respond to therapy within 24–48 hours of initiating treatment.[293]

Postoperative colic patients with clinically relevant septic peritonitis are febrile and are often dull and inappetent. Pain on abdominal palpation can be appreciated in some cases. Horses may show signs of colic and often begin to rapidly lose weight.

Differential diagnosis

GI tract lesion; urogenital tract lesion; abdominal or intestinal neoplasia; abdominal abscess (*S. equi* subsp. *equi*, *R. equi*); *A. equuli* infection; idiopathic peritonitis.

Diagnosis

Peritonitis should be considered in any horse presenting for signs of colic in conjunction with a fever and/or dull demeanor or with a history of weight loss. Unexplained fever, hyperfibrinogenemia, or immature (band) neutrophils on hematology are strong indications for performing an abdominal ultrasonographic examination (p. 39) and/or abdominocentesis (p. 35). Abdominal ultrasonographic examination may reveal an increase in the volume and echogenicity of the peritoneal fluid and the bowel wall may be thickened (**1.107**). An abdominocentesis site can be identified during the ultrasonographic examination. Depending on the underlying cause, the peritoneal fluid can vary in color from yellow–orange (**1.108**) to red to green–brown. Peritonitis is definitively diagnosed based on peritoneal fluid analysis with a white cell count >10 × 10^9/l (10,000 cells/µl).

The cause of peritonitis can be somewhat more difficult to diagnose. Historical information, such as recent foaling, trauma, or surgery, is critical for determining the most likely diagnosis and directing diagnostic tests.

The gross appearance of the peritoneal fluid can be an indication of the type of lesion (e.g. green–brown fluid with plant material is suggestive of GI tract perforation [or enterocentesis] and serosanguineous peritoneal fluid is most often associated with a lesion requiring surgery). Only 22% of horses diagnosed with peritonitis that had serosanguineous peritoneal fluid survived to discharge without surgery, whereas 74% of horses with yellow–orange peritoneal fluid survived to discharge without surgery.[292]

Cytology can be used to identify plant material and intracellular bacteria (GI tract rupture/perforation, p. 60) as well as neoplastic cells in some cases of abdominal neoplasia (p. 58). Cells are often lysed in horses with GI tract rupture, which may result in a falsely low peritoneal fluid nucleated cell count. Peritoneal fluid TP concentration is most often high in these cases.[46] Peritoneal fluid TP can be used to determine the need for surgery; horses with peritonitis that survived to discharge without surgery had a lower peritoneal fluid TP concentration (34 g/l [3.4 g/dl]) compared with horses that did not survive to discharge without surgery (46 g/l [4.6 g/dl]). (**Note:** The peritoneal fluid TP in horses with a GI rupture can be low as a result of dilution. The usefulness of peritoneal fluid lactate concentration for differentiating the need for surgery in horses with peritonitis is yet to be determined.) Bacterial culture and sensitivity testing of peritoneal fluid is important not only to identify the bacterial cause of the peritonitis, but also to select the optimal antimicrobial drug. Common bacteria isolated include *A. equuli*, *Escherichia coli*, *Streptococcus* spp., and *Bacteroides* spp.[292,293]

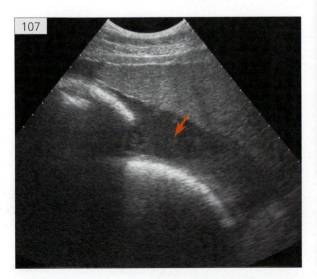

1.107 Ultrasonographic image of a horse with peritonitis. Note the increase in volume and echogenicity of the peritoneal fluid (arrow).

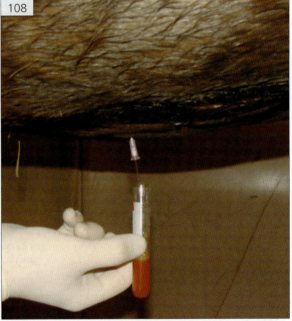

1.108 Peritoneal fluid from a postpartum mare with idiopathic peritonitis.

Abdominal palpation per rectum should be performed, but is often non-specific. Occasionally, a mass (e.g. abscess or tumor) or intestinal distension can be identified. Horses that were diagnosed with peritonitis that had small intestinal distension were more likely to have a primary GI tract lesion necessitating surgery compared with horses with no specific rectal findings or those with large intestinal distension.[292]

Abdominal ultrasonographic examination can be used in some cases to diagnose the cause of peritonitis including primary GI or urogenital lesions and abdominal masses. Ultrasonographic examination per rectum can also be performed in cases where a mass is palpated per rectum. Care should be taken to avoid rectal tear. Abdominal ultrasonographic examination is particularly useful to identify GI tract perforation with identification of free fluid and ingesta as well as pneumoperitoneum.

Exploratory abdominal surgery via laparoscopy or celiotomy may be the ultimate diagnostic tool for horses with peritonitis that do not respond to medical management and for which the cause cannot be diagnosed using other methods.

Management/treatment

The major decision once a diagnosis of peritonitis is made is whether to treat the horse medically or surgically. *Table 1.5* shows clinical findings that are associated with the presence of a concurrent lesion (e.g. GI tract lesion), survival to hospital discharge, and survival to hospital discharge without surgery.[292]

Medical management includes antimicrobial drugs, which should initially be broad spectrum (e.g. penicillin, gentamicin), and then selected based on bacterial culture and sensitivity testing. *A. equuli* is usually sensitive to penicillin, trimethoprim/sulfadiazine, and aminoglycoside antimicrobial drugs.[293] The duration of antimicrobial drug use is variable depending on the cause of the peritonitis and the response to treatment. Horses with *A. equuli*-associated peritonitis were treated with antimicrobial drugs for 5–21 days.[293]

Table 1.5 Clinical findings associated with outcome in horses diagnosed with peritonitis[292]

OUTCOME	PHYSICAL EXAMINATION OR LABORATORY FINDINGS
Concurrent abnormality diagnosed during hospitalization	• Moderate or severe abdominal pain at presentation or during hospitalization • Worsening or persistent fever during hospitalization • Absent intestinal borborygmi at presentation or during hospitalization • Distended small intestine on palpation per rectum
Survival to discharge	• No or mild signs of colic at presentation or during hospitalization • Normal or improved towards normal heart rate during hospitalization • Normal or improved towards normal rectal temperature during hospitalization • Normal intestinal borborygmi at presentation • Normal, soft, or less than normal feces during hospitalization • No nasogastric reflux • Yellow–orange peritoneal fluid
Survival to discharge without surgery	• No signs of abdominal pain • Normal intestinal borborygmi at presentation and normal or improved borborygmi during hospitalization • Normal feces during hospitalization • No nasogastric reflux • Yellow–orange peritoneal fluid

IV fluid therapy (see Chapter 12) and flunixin meglumine or firocoxib are also administered. Antiendotoxin therapy (e.g. polymixin B and J5 plasma) is indicated in some cases.

Peritoneal lavage may be necessary in cases that are not responding to medical management or in cases with a known etiology (e.g. uterine tear). Peritoneal lavage can be performed laparoscopically or using various catheters (e.g. Foley catheter) placed ventrally for ingress and egress, or in the flank region for ingress and ventrally for egress only. Exploratory celiotomy and lavage can also be performed in cases not responding to medical treatment.

The prognosis for horses with peritonitis is dependent on the underlying cause. Horses with idiopathic peritonitis or peritonitis associated with *A. equuli* have an excellent prognosis for survival and long-term complications are uncommon.[292–294] Horses with GI tract rupture/perforation have a grave prognosis and euthanasia is indicated.[290,291] None of the horses diagnosed with peritonitis associated with diarrhea survived and horses with bacteria identified on peritoneal fluid had only a 50% survival rate.[289] Septic peritonitis is an uncommon complication following abdominal surgery and is also associated with a poor prognosis for survival (44%).[289]

Hemoperitoneum
Key points
- Hemoperitoneum should be considered in any horse presenting with signs of colic with concurrent signs of hemorrhagic shock.
- Abdominal ultrasonographic examination reveals echogenic swirling fluid. A hemorrhagic effusion is seen with peritoneal fluid analysis.
- Cardiovascular stabilization is critical prior to pursuing further diagnostics and treatment.

Definition/overview
Hemoperitoneum is defined as an accumulation of blood within the peritoneal cavity caused by intraperitoneal hemorrhage.[295]

Etiology/pathogenesis
The etiology of hemoperitoneum is variable. In one study, the cause was diagnosed in 78% of cases. Causes included: trauma (25% of cases) causing splenic injury, pelvic injury or fracture, and diaphragmatic or peritoneal injury; neoplasia (18%); uterine artery rupture (13%); mesenteric injury (12%); and coagulopathy (6%).[295] Other causes include postoperative complications and penetrating abdominal wounds. Occasionally, the cause of hemoperitoneum is undetermined.[295]

Clinical features
Horses with hemoperitoneum can have variable clinical signs depending on the cause of the hemoperitoneum and the volume and rate of blood accumulation within the abdomen. The most common clinical features include signs of colic (79%) and shock (weakness, anxiety, muscle fasciculations, dull demeanor) (60%).[295] Horses can have a history of trauma, recent parturition or pregnancy (broodmares), or weight loss.

On physical examination, horses are often tachycardic, tachypneic, and have pale mucous membranes. A fever can be observed depending on the underlying cause. Abdominal distension may be apparent. PCV and TPP levels are variable depending on the volume of blood loss and the duration of time from hemorrhage to examination (see Chapter 4). TPP, however, is often at the lower limit of normal. Blood lactate and plasma creatinine concentrations are often high because of poor tissue perfusion and mean arterial blood pressure is low (see Chapter 11).

Abdominal ultrasonographic examination reveals swirling echogenic fluid and hemorrhagic fluid is obtained with abdominocentesis.

Differential diagnosis
Splenic injury; mesenteric injury; ruptured viscus; diaphragmatic tear; neoplasia (granulosa cell ovarian tumors, metastatic melanoma, multicentric hemangiosarcoma, metastatic SCC, lymphoma, pheochromocytoma); coagulopathy.

Diagnosis

Hemoperitoneum can be diagnosed based on abdominal ultrasonographic examination with the finding of a large volume of swirling fluid (**1.109**). Abdominocentesis and peritoneal fluid analysis (p. 37) can confirm the ultrasonographic findings.

Ultrasonographic examination can also help diagnose the cause of the hemoperitoneum. Ultrasonography was successfully used to obtain a diagnosis in 44% of horses with hemoperitoneum that were examined. Cytology should be performed on peritoneal fluid. A diagnosis of the cause of hemoperitoneum is often made at surgery or necropsy.

Management/treatment

IV catheterization and crystalloid fluid therapy (see Chapter 12) is necessary to stabilize patients with signs of shock. Overzealous fluid resuscitation should be avoided, particularly in patients that may have uncontrolled hemorrhage. Heart rate, extremity temperature, blood lactate concentration, and arterial blood pressure should be monitored in horses with signs of hemorrhagic shock during resuscitation. (See also Chapter 11 and Chapter 12.)

Fresh-frozen plasma can be administered to provide coagulation factors. Blood transfusion may be necessary based on the PCV and response to initial therapy. Flunixin meglumine is often necessary to control signs of abdominal pain. Prophylactic antimicrobial drugs (e.g. penicillin and gentamicin) are recommended. In cases where hemorrhage is ongoing, aminocaproic acid can be given.

Surgery is not recommended (if possible) until the patient is stabilized and a tentative diagnosis made based on ultrasonographic examination or historical and physical examination findings.

In a recent report, the survival rate to hospital discharge was 51% (34 out of 67); 25 horses were euthanized because of disease severity (shock or underlying disease) and eight horses died. Admission respiratory rate and cause of hemoperitoneum were associated with survival. The odds ratio for death was 18-times higher in horses with a respiratory rate ≥30 breaths/minute compared with horses with a respiratory rate <30 breaths/minute. Horses with neoplasia, uterine artery rupture, mesenteric injury, or a coagulopathy had a greater odds of death compared with horses with idiopathic hemoperitoneum.[295]

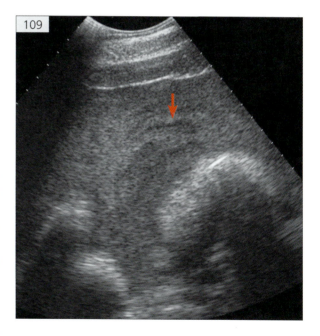

1.109 **Ultrasonographic image of hemoperitoneum. Note the echogenic (cellular) peritoneal fluid with a swirling appearance (arrow).**

CHAPTER 2

MUSCULOSKELETAL SYSTEM

Liberty M. Getman and
Troy N. Trumble

GENERAL APPROACH TO THE HORSE WITH A MUSCULOSKELETAL EMERGENCY

- Musculoskeletal conditions requiring emergency attention include fractures, septic synovial structures, myopathies, and laminitis. The majority of these types of problems require referral to a tertiary care or surgical facility for diagnostic tests and management. Identification of the potential problem and appropriate stabilization prior to referral is important.
- In general, horses and foals with a musculoskeletal problem requiring emergency care present with an acute onset of a readily apparent gait alteration (e.g. non-weight-bearing lameness, abnormal stance, reluctance to walk, recumbency).
- Early and appropriate diagnosis and treatment is essential for a favorable outcome. A detailed history and thorough physical examination is needed to differentiate between some of the less apparent causes of lameness or gait abnormality.
- One of the most common problems causing acute onset of non-weight-bearing lameness in horses is subsolar abscessation. Subsolar abscess should always be ruled out in horses with acute severe lameness where the diagnosis is not readily apparent.
- Drugs commonly used in the emergency management of horses with musculoskeletal problems are included in *Box 2.1*.

Box 2.1 **Dose rates of the most commonly used drugs in the emergency management of horses with musculoskeletal problems**

DRUG	DOSE RATE (AMOUNT FOR A 500 KG HORSE)
Non-steroidal anti-inflammatory drugs	
Phenylbutazone	2.2–4.4 mg/kg IV or PO q12–24h (5–10 ml or 1–2 tablets)
Flunixin meglumine	1.1 mg/kg IV q12h (500 mg or 10 ml)
	(also available as an oral paste)
Firocoxib	0.27 mg/kg IV (loading dose) (135 mg or 6.75 ml)
	0.09 mg/kg IV q24h (45 mg or 2.25 ml)
	(also available as an oral paste)
Meloxicam	0.6 mg/kg IV or IM q24h (300 mg)
Sedation	
Xyalzine HCl	0.3–0.4 mg/kg IV (150–200 mg or 1.5–2.0 ml)

(Continued overleaf)

Box 2.1 *(continued)*

DRUG	DOSE RATE (AMOUNT FOR A 500 KG HORSE)
Detomidine HCl	0.01–0.02 mg/kg IV or IM (5–10 mg or 0.5–1.0 ml)
Butorphanol	0.01–0.02 mg/kg IV (5–10 mg or 0.5–1.0 ml) (with xylazine or detomidine)
Antimicrobial drugs	
Procaine penicillin	22,000 U/kg IM q12h (11×10^6U or 37 ml)
Potassium penicillin	22,000 U/kg IV q6h (11×10^6U but volume depends on concentration following resuspension)
Gentamicin	6.6–8.8 mg/kg IV q24h (3.3–4.4 g or 33–44 ml)
Amikacin	500 mg (2 ml) intra-articularly q24–48h

- Horses with a fracture usually present with an acute onset of non-weight-bearing lameness:
  - Often, the site of fracture is readily apparent based on bony instability and/or marked swelling.
  - Radiographic or sonographic examination is necessary, depending on the fracture location, to determine the configuration.
  - Knowledge of the appropriate splint application for fractures (p. 170) can minimize further damage to the bone, soft tissue, and vasculature and can make the difference between a repairable fracture and a fracture that requires euthanasia of the horse or foal.
  - Owners and caregivers should have knowledge of the prognosis for survival and athletic performance and the expense associated with treatment before pursuing treatment of any musculoskeletal emergency, particularly an adult horse with a long bone fracture.

- Horses and foals with septic synovial structures usually present with moderate to severe lameness of varying duration. There is often an associated swollen joint with synovial effusion and periarticular edema or cellulitis:
  - In adult horses, there is usually a history of synoviocentesis or trauma. Lacerations or puncture wounds involving synovial structures should be immediately diagnosed and treated.
  - Foals often do not have such a history; however, bone involvement (e.g. septic physitis) is common and radiographic evaluation important.
  - Diagnostic tests include radiographic evaluation and synoviocentesis (p. 159). Sonographic evaluation can be helpful, particularly when there is a lot of periarticular edema or cellulitis.
  - Treatment involves local and/or systemic antimicrobial drugs, anti-inflammatory analgesic drugs (e.g. phenylbutazone, flunixin meglumine, firocoxib, meloxicam), synovial lavage with or without endoscopy, and wound care.

- Myopathy (i.e. exertional rhabdomyolysis) often occurs following a variable degree of exertion. There appears to be a breed and genetic predisposition. Horses have a stiff gait and affected muscles (usually epaxial and gluteal muscles) are firm:
  - Diagnosis is suspected based on history and physical examination and confirmed by measuring creatinine kinase and AST.
  - Treatment involves oral (mildly affected horses) or IV (moderately and severely affected horses) fluid therapy, anti-inflammatory analgesic drugs, acepromazine, and muscle relaxants.
  - Horses typically develop myoglobinuria and renal function needs to be monitored closely. Careful use of NSAIDs and other nephrotoxic drugs is recommended.
- Laminitis is a devastating disease affecting adult horses and ponies:
  - Horses and ponies present with a bilateral lameness, most commonly affecting the forelimbs but often affecting the fore- and hindlimbs. Occasionally, the hindlimbs only are involved. Affected animals may be recumbent.
  - A history of predisposing factor(s) is usually present (e.g. pony grazing spring pasture; non-weight-bearing lameness on contralateral limb; enterocolitis; retained fetal membranes).
  - Diagnosis is made based on the bilateral lameness, palpably increased or bounding digital pulses, and pain on hoof tester application. If the diagnosis is not readily apparent, abaxial sesamoid nerve blocks can be used for confirmation. Radiographic evaluation of the feet is recommended to determine the degree of rotation or sinking and the presence of gas between the hoof wall and distal phalanx.
  - Management involves early recognition with removal or treatment of any inciting causes, confinement to a well-bedded stall, administration of anti-inflammatory and analgesic drugs, and hoof care. Cooling the feet with ice is recommended in any horse with an identified predisposing factor.

COMMON PROCEDURES PERFORMED ON HORSES WITH MUSCULOSKELETAL EMERGENCIES

Diagnostic procedures
Physical examination
Indications

A thorough physical examination is indicated with any horse or foal presenting on an emergency basis with lameness or a gait abnormality.

Technique

Heart rate, mucous membrane color and moistness, CRT, jugular refill time, respiratory rate, and rectal temperature should be obtained. Intestinal borborygmi, extremity temperature, and digital pulses should be evaluated. The level of pain and cardiovascular status of the horse is determined based on this initial examination. Basic laboratory data including PCV, TPP, leukocyte count, fibrinogen or serum amyloid A (SAA), and creatinine concentrations is recommended.

If not readily apparent, the source of lameness or gait abnormality should be identified. In order to localize the affected area, the unsedated patient should be examined for:
- Stance abnormalities.
- Specifics of gait alteration at a walk and/or degree of lameness.
- Observed asymmetry between left and right limbs.
- Swelling (synovial effusion, edema, or cellulitis).
- Crepitus.
- Muscle firmness.
- Palpably increased or bounding digital pulses.
- Areas painful to palpation or manipulation.

For example, a septic synovial structure is associated with moderate to severe lameness, heat and pain on palpation of the affected structure, synovial effusion, and edema; horses with laminitis tend to stand with their forelimbs forward, shift weight from left to right, and have a bilateral increase in digital pulses; horses with a distal phalanx fracture or infection in the hoof have a unilateral increase in digital pulses on the affected limb; horses with rhabdomyolysis have painful, firm muscles; horses with fractures are typically non-weight bearing and have swelling, crepitus, and pain on palpation.

Auscultation for crepitis over the upper limb musculature during limb manipulation is recommended if a lower limb lesion is not diagnosed and a humerus, femur, or pelvic fracture suspected. Palpation per rectum may be necessary for pelvic injuries. Hoof testers should be applied to all horses where the source of lameness is not known. Neurologic deficits should always be considered in a horse presenting on an emergency basis with a presumed musculoskeletal injury or trauma.

Complications
None.

Diagnostic imaging
Indications
Several diagnostic tests are available including radiography (plain or contrast arthrography or fistulography), sonography, MRI, and CT. Once the affected site is identified, tests to confirm the tentative diagnosis and further evaluate the involved structures are necessary. Radiographic evaluation is indicated for horses with a suspected fracture, laceration or puncture wound, synovial sepsis, or laminitis. Sonography is particularly useful for evaluating synovial sepsis, periarticular swelling, wounds associated with synovial structures, clostridial myopathy, and fractures not easily amenable to radiographic evaluation (e.g. pelvic fracture).

Technique
Radiographic examination
- Sedation of the horse or foal is often necessary.
- The kVp, mAs, and anode-film distance are set according to those established for the particular X-ray machine.
- Multiple radiographic views; typically, four views (cranial–caudal or dorsal–palmer/plantar, medial–lateral, and oblique) are needed for full evaluation.
- Plain radiographs are used to evaluate the presence of a fracture as well as the fracture configuration, concurrent bony lesions or gas opacities within synovial spaces indicative of synovial involvement associated with wounds, and osteomyelitis associated with a penetrating wound or septic synovial structure.
- A malleable probe can also be inserted to the depths of the wound and the indicated radiographic views taken to evaluate the course of a wound.

- Contrast arthrography can be performed by aseptically preparing a site distant from a wound and injecting iodinated contrast material into the synovial space until the space is distended or contrast material is observed escaping from the wound. The necessary radiographic views are then taken to demonstrate any synovial communication with the wound.
- Alternatively, contrast fistulography can be performed by injecting contrast material directly into a puncture wound or wound tract, taking the indicated radiographic views, and evaluating nearby synovial structures for the presence of contrast material (**2.1**).
- Finally, for horses with metallic foreign bodies remaining in the wound (such as horses that have stepped on a nail), it is helpful to radiograph the area before removing the object to evaluate the proximity of the object to any synovial structures. This should only be done if radiographs can be taken immediately, because allowing a horse to continue to walk with a sharp foreign body in its limb can cause further tissue damage.

Sonographic examination
- Sedation is often necessary because the horse or foal may be painful in the area to be examined.
- The hair should be clipped and the skin cleaned prior to examination.
- Ample sonographic coupling gel should be used to obtain a good quality image.
- A thorough and systematic sonographic examination of the affected area should be performed. Details of superficial structures are obtained using a 7.5 MHz probe and deeper structures are evaluated using a 3–5 MHz probe.
- Sonography can be used to determine what tissue is affected (e.g. subcutaneous tissue, muscle, synovial structure) when there is severe swelling that prevents assessment by palpation. Identifying a pocket of fluid for sample collection for bacterial culture and sensitivity testing is also important. Large fluid pockets may warrant drainage, which can be performed using sonographic guidance.

- Sonography is used to determine the extent of damage to soft tissue structures such as tendons and ligaments.
- Careful evaluation of synovial structures, focusing on the volume and echogenicity of synovial fluid and thickness of synovial membrane, is particularly useful in at least determining the likelihood that a synovial structure is infected. Sonographic guidance for synoviocentesis is particularly useful if there is a great deal of subcutaneous tissue swelling or structures that are not readily accessible.
- Observation of fluid adjacent to bone and an irregular bony surface can be used to increase suspicion of osteomyelitis and loss of continuum of the bony surface can indicate a fracture.

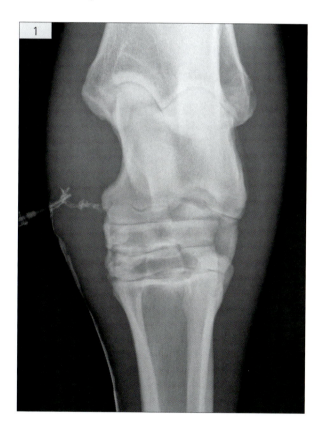

2.1 Dorsoplantar radiograph of the hock of a horse with a puncture wound to the medial aspect; contrast fistulography was performed through the wound and demonstrates communication of the wound with the proximal intertarsal joint.

- Sonographic examination is useful for delineating the course of wound tracts and determining their proximity to synovial structures. It may also provide additional information about the presence of foreign material that is not radiopaque, such as wood.

Other

Other advanced imaging modalities, such as CT and MRI, may be beneficial for interpreting complicated fractures or evaluating chronic wounds or obscure causes of lameness; however, these modalities are only available at large referral centers and often require general anesthesia.

Complications
None.

Synoviocentesis and synovial fluid analysis
Indications

Knowledge of the presence, location, and anatomy of synovial structures is critical for successful diagnosis and management of injuries to these structures. Synovial structures will be defined here as any structure that normally produces synovial fluid including joints, tendon sheaths, and bursae. Any time a synovial structure is involved in a traumatic wound in horses, the prognosis for return to athletic function is poor without prompt recognition of synovial involvement and adequate treatment. Therefore, it is of utmost importance to be able to diagnose accurately whether a synovial structure has been invaded. This may be as simple as identifying that a fracture extends into a joint or as complicated as determining whether a tendon sheath was punctured during a laceration. As a general rule, because of the environment that horses live in, all synovial structures that are punctured from an external wound should be assumed to be contaminated. These wounds are not necessarily infected, but they can become so if not managed properly. If diagnosed quickly and managed appropriately, many horses with traumatic wounds involving a synovial structure have a good prognosis for return to athletic function. Recent studies have shown a good prognosis for survival (90%) as well as return to athletic function (81%) with prompt, aggressive therapy including endoscopic surgery of the affected structure.[1] Negative prognostic indicators include marked fibrin accumulation in the synovial space, osteochondral lesions, and injuries involving the navicular bursa.[1] The importance of early recognition of synovial involvement and prompt, aggressive treatment cannot be overemphasized.

Understanding the anatomy of the distal limb is vital to the success of any equine practitioner. This includes understanding the location and anatomy of each joint, tendon sheath, and bursa in the limb. For example, when examining a laceration or a fracture, it is important to determine whether a synovial structure is involved, as this will determine the type of therapy that is indicated, the potential costs involved in treatment, and the overall prognosis. Indications for synoviocentesis and synovial fluid analysis include abnormal physical examination findings and changes identified using diagnostic imaging that may indicate the involvement of a synovial structure.

Technique

A simple approach, and usually one of the most revealing ways to identify involvement of synovial structures, is to perform synoviocentesis at a site distant to the wound (**2.2**). This requires extensive knowledge of the anatomy and location of all the synovial structures located in close proximity to the wound. When any doubt exists as to the involvement of an adjacent synovial structure, synoviocentesis should be performed because failure to identify such a communication can have disastrous consequences.

Synoviocentesis is performed by placing a needle into the synovial structure through healthy tissue distant from the site of injury in order to avoid contaminating the synovial cavity if it does not communicate with the wound. The goal is to obtain synovial fluid for analysis and to distend the synovial structure with sterile saline to evaluate if there is communication with the wound. If there is a communication, the fluid should exit through the wound. The limb can be flexed and extended while the synovial structure is distended to allow separation of fascial planes that may prevent fluid leaking while the horse is standing.

Synovial fluid analysis should be performed once a sample is obtained.[2] Fluid should be collected into a blood tube containing EDTA for cytologic analysis and, if possible, a separate sample collected and placed

into a tube containing culture medium for bacterial culture and antimicrobial sensitivity testing. In addition to submitting a sample of fluid for bacterial culture, it is often useful to perform a Gram stain on a sample of fluid to identify bacteria. This helps determine if bacteria are present and whether they are gram positive or gram negative, since false-negative culture results are common.

Gross evaluation of the fluid may give an indication as to whether the fluid is normal or abnormal (**2.3**):
- Normal synovial fluid is pale yellow and clear.
- The presence of opacity or flocculent material in the sample indicates synovitis.
- If the fluid is diffusely hemorrhagic, it is suggestive of acute trauma.
- Synovial fluid viscosity is directly related to the hyaluronan content, and this decreases with infection or inflammation. The string test is a crude test for viscosity and involves placing

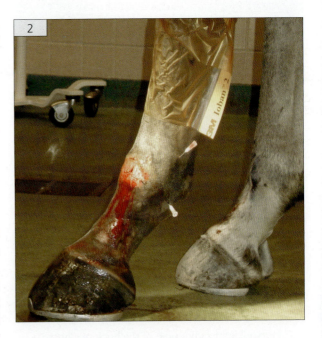

2.2 Locations for arthrocentesis and joint distension in the fetlock joint at a site distant to the laceration. Top needle, proximoplantar approach; bottom needle, distoplantar approach.

a drop of synovial fluid on the thumb. The thumb is touched to the index finger and then the fingers are separated; with normal synovial fluid a string of 2.5–5.0 cm should be produced before it breaks.

Cytologic examination of synovial fluid is useful for determining whether the fluid is inflamed or contaminated:

- Normal synovial fluid should have a TP of <25 g/l (2.5 g/dl), a white blood cell (WBC) count of <300 cells/μl, and contain <10% neutrophils.[2]
- In the presences of sepsis, fluid becomes grossly cloudy or turbid, with an average of 80–90% neutrophils, >75,000 WBCs/μl, and a TP of >50 g/l (5.0 g/dl).[3] However, WBC counts can be as low as 10,000 cells/μl in infected synovial structures due to sequestration of the cells within fibrin deposits. Therefore, the percentage of neutrophils present may be a more reliable indicator of sepsis.
- The normal pH of synovial fluid is 7.3, and this becomes acidic (as low as 6.2) when the joint is septic.

- The normal lactate concentration of equine synovial fluid is slightly greater than that of serum and ranges between 1.25 and 2.8 mmol/l (11.26–25.22 mg/dl). Intrasynovial lactate concentrations increase with inflammation and infection due to lactate production from anaerobic glycolysis of synoviocytes and neutrophils.

Distal interphalangeal joint

- Dorsal approach (**2.4**). The needle is placed 1.5 cm proximal to the coronary band and either on midline, through the common (or long) digital extensor tendon, or just off midline (medial or lateral). The needle should be directed distally and axially at approximately a 30–45 degree angle from the long axis of the second phalanx. Many horses are sensitive to this approach and will react when the needle is placed through the skin. An alternative dorsal approach is to insert the needle through the skin on the sagittal plane 1 cm proximal to the coronary band and direct it perpendicular to the skin surface.

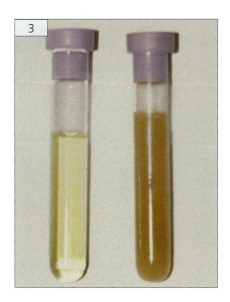

2.3 Visual inspection of synovial fluid. Normal synovial fluid is on the left and septic synovial fluid is on the right. (Courtesy Dr Murray Brown)

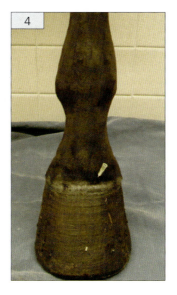

2.4 Needle placement for arthrocentesis of the distal interphalangeal joint using a dorsal approach.

- Palmar (plantar) approach (**2.5**). The landmarks for needle placement include the distal palmar (plantar) border of the middle phalanx dorsally and the proximal border of the lateral (or medial) collateral cartilage distally. The needle is inserted between these structures and directed in a dorsodistomedial (or dorsodistolateral) direction. With this approach, inadvertent entry into either the navicular bursa or digital flexor tendon sheath is common and radiographic guidance is recommended.

Navicular bursa

- With the limb placed slightly forward, an 18 gauge, 3½ inch spinal needle is placed through the deepest depression between the heel bulbs. The needle is then inserted parallel to the ground until bone is contacted (**2.6**). Lateral radiographs should be taken to confirm placement of the needle just palmar or plantar to the navicular bone (**2.7**). This is facilitated by first performing an abaxial sesamoid block.

Proximal interphalangeal joint

- Dorsal approach (**2.8**). The needle is placed just lateral or medial to the common (long) digital extensor tendon at the level of the distal palmar (plantar) process of the proximal phalanx. The needle is directed slightly distomedially (or distolaterally) until the joint is encountered.
- Medial or lateral palmar (plantar) approach (**2.9**). The joint can be identified by palpation of the proximal palmar (plantar) eminences of the second phalanx. Just proximal to these eminences is a V-shaped notch dorsal to the neurovascular bundle, between the distal palmar (plantar) process of the proximal phalanx and the insertion of the medial or lateral branch of the superficial digital flexor tendon. The limb is held off the ground with the digit flexed, and the needle is directed distomedially (or distolaterally) and slightly dorsally, at a 30 degree angle from the transverse plane.

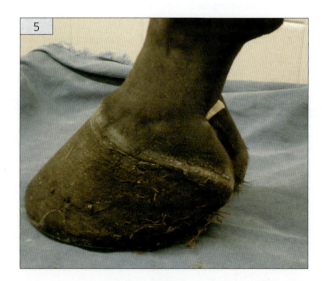

2.5 Needle placement for arthrocentesis of the distal interphalangeal joint using the palmar (plantar) approach.

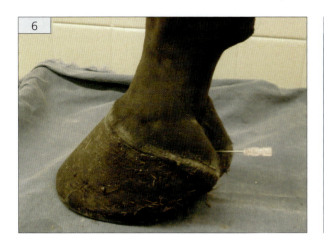

2.6 Photograph illustrating needle placement for synoviocentesis of the navicular bursa.

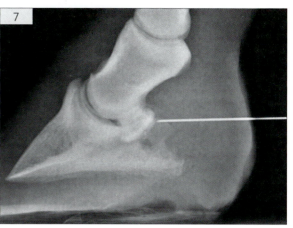

2.7 Lateral radiograph of a foot demonstrating correct needle placement for synoviocentesis of the navicular bursa.

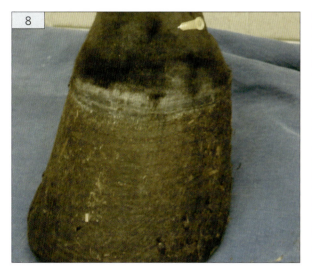

2.8 Needle placement for arthrocentesis of the proximal interphalangeal joint using the dorsal approach.

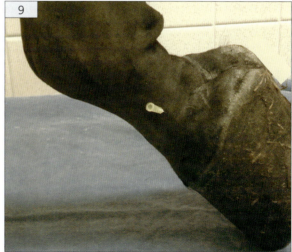

2.9 Photograph illustrating needle placement for arthrocentesis of the proximal interphalangeal joint using the lateral approach.

Metacarpo-/metatarsophalangeal joint
- Dorsal approach (**2.10**). The needle is placed either medial or lateral to the common (long) digital extensor tendon, angled parallel with the ground, axially and slightly palmar (plantar).
- Proximopalmar (plantar) approach (**2.2, 2.11**). The proximal palmar (plantar) pouch is identified just proximal to the collateral sesamoidean ligament, distal to the button of the splint bone, directly palmar (plantar) to the third metacarpus (metatarsus), and dorsal to the suspensory ligament branches. The needle is placed in the center of the pouch and directed slightly distally in the frontal plane (superficial insertion of the needle usually provides the best result). Large synovial villi can occlude the needle at this location, making it difficult to obtain fluid.
- Distopalmar (plantar) approach (**2.2, 2.12**). The needle is placed in a small, palpable depression just proximal to the proximal palmar (plantar) process

of the proximal phalanx. This site is just dorsal to the neurovascular bundle and most consistently results in the retrieval of fluid because it is located in the most distal aspect of the joint.
- Approach through the collateral sesamoidean ligament (**2.12**). The collateral sesamoidean ligament can be palpated between the third metacarpal (metatarsal) bone and the medial or lateral proximal sesamoid bone. The needle is placed into the distopalmar (plantar) pouch directly through this ligament with the horse standing or with the limb in slight flexion.

Digital flexor tendon sheath (2.13A, B)
- Proximal approach. A needle is placed between the superficial and deep digital flexor tendons, just proximal to the proximal sesamoid bones and palmar (plantar) to the fetlock joint. This approach is easier to perform when there is distension of the tendon sheath.

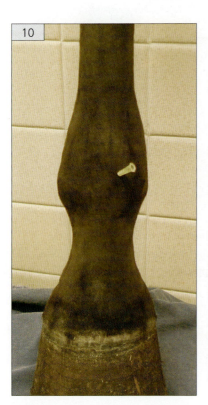

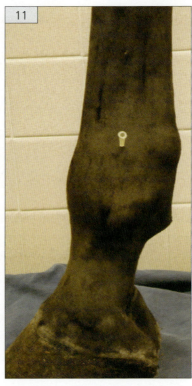

2.10 Needle placement for arthrocentesis of the metacarpophalangeal joint using the dorsal approach.

2.11 Needle placement for arthrocentesis of the metacarpophalangeal joint using the proximopalmar approach.

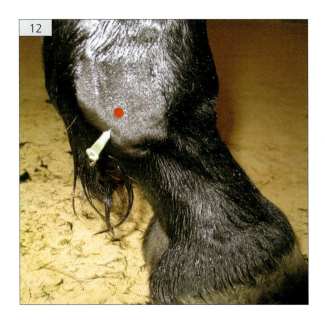

- Distal to the proximal sesamoid bones. The needle is placed in an out-pouching between the palmar annular ligament and the proximal digital annular ligament, at the base of the proximal sesamoid bones, just axial to the neurovascular bundle. This approach can be performed even if there is no obvious effusion.
- Distal approach. The needle is placed on the midline in an out-pouching of the sheath between the proximal and distal digital annular ligaments. This approach is easier to perform if effusion is present.

2.12 Needle placement for arthrocentesis of the metacarpophalangeal joint using the distopalmar approach (needle) and the site for the collateral sesamoidean ligament approach (red circle).

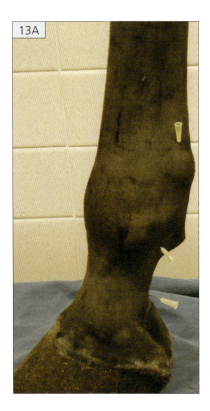

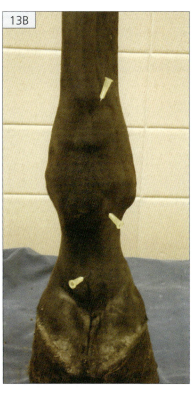

2.13A, B Lateral (A) and palmar (B) views showing needle placement for synoviocentesis of the digital flexor tendon sheath. Top needle, proximal approach; middle needle, distal to the proximal sesamoid bones; bottom needle, distal approach.

Middle carpal joint

- Dorsal approach (**2.14**). With the limb flexed, a needle is placed in a palpable depression between the proximal and distal row of carpal bones, either between the common digital extensor tendon and the extensor carpi radialis tendon, or medial to the extensor carpi radialis tendon. The needle should be directed axially to minimize iatrogenic damage to articular cartilage.
- Palmar lateral approach (**2.15**). This is performed with the horse standing by inserting a needle in the small depression between the distal aspect of the ulnar carpal bone and the proximal aspect of the fourth carpal bone (superficial insertion of the needle usually provides the best result). The synovial out-pouching is easier to identify if effusion is present. This approach is usually safest for use on a fractious horse.

Radiocarpal joint

- Dorsal approach (**2.14**). With the limb flexed, a needle is placed in a palpable depression between the proximal row of carpal bones and the distal radius, either between the common digital extensor tendon and the extensor carpi radialis tendon, or medial to the extensor carpi radialis tendon. The needle should be directed axially to minimize iatrogenic damage to articular cartilage.
- Proximal palmar lateral approach (**2.16**). This is performed with the horse standing. A needle is placed immediately palmar to the distal radius and proximal to the accessory carpal bone. The needle is inserted lateral to medial (superficial insertion of the needle usually provides best result). Care must be taken not to enter the carpal sheath with this approach. This approach is usually safest for use on a fractious horse.

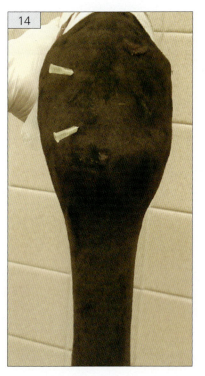

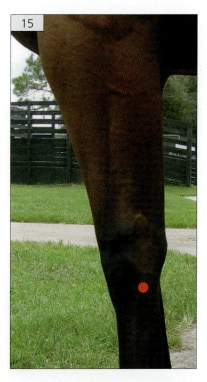

2.14 Dorsal aspect of the carpus with the carpus in flexion illustrating needle placement for arthrocentesis of the middle carpal joint (bottom needle) and radiocarpal joint (top needle) using the dorsal approach.

2.15 Lateral aspect of the carpus illustrating the site for needle placement for arthrocentesis of the middle carpal joint using the palmar lateral approach (circle).

- Distal palmar lateral approach (**2.16**). With the horse standing, a needle is inserted into the notch created by the distal radius, dorsal aspect of the accessory carpal bone, and the proximal ulnar carpal bone, in a lateral to medial direction.

Carpal sheath (2.17)

- The carpal sheath is approached laterally, just proximal to the accessory carpal bone, between the lateral digital extensor tendon and the ulnaris lateralis tendon. The needle is advanced in a lateral to medial direction, parallel to the ground.

Extensor carpi radialis or common digital extensor tendon sheaths

- These tendon sheaths closely surround their respective tendons at the level of the carpus. A needle can be inserted in either sheath by penetrating the sheath superficially and following an orientation parallel to the tendons.

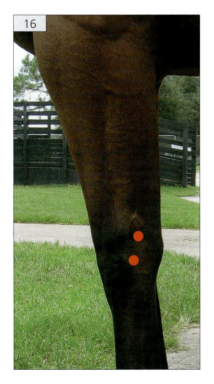

2.16 Lateral aspect of the carpus illustrating needle placement for arthrocentesis of the radiocarpal joint using the proximal palmar lateral approach (top circle) and the distal palmar lateral approach (bottom circle).

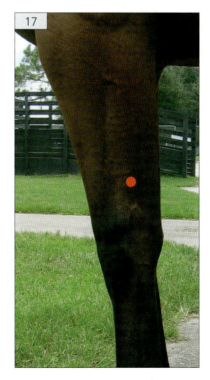

2.17 Lateral aspect of the carpus illustrating needle placement for synoviocentesis of the carpal sheath.

Tibiotarsal joint (2.18)

- Dorsal approach. The needle can be placed either lateral or medial to the extensor tendon bundle on the dorsal aspect of the hock. The dorsomedial pouch is the easiest area to obtain fluid from in horses without obvious effusion. It is entered distal to the medial malleolus, on either side of the saphenous vein. The needle is angled proximally and axially. The dorsolateral pouch can be entered similarly.
- Plantar approach. The plantar pouches can be entered between the medial or lateral aspect of the talus and calcaneus, with the needle directed slightly distally and dorsally. Care should be taken not to enter the tarsal sheath at this location.

Tarsometatarsal joint

- Lateral approach (**2.19A**). The needle is inserted just proximal to the fourth metatarsal bone. At this location, there is a slight depression through which the needle is inserted craniomedially and slightly distal.
- Medial approach (**2.19B**). This approach is more difficult and unreliable, but is located at the small depression at the articulation of the fused first and second tarsal bones and the third tarsal bone.

Distal intertarsal joint (2.20)

- The needle is placed medially, parallel with the ground, in a small depression formed at the junction of the fused first and second tarsal bones, the third tarsal bone, and the central tarsal bone. This is located at the distal aspect of the cunean tendon.

Tarsal sheath (2.21)

- The tarsal sheath surrounds the deep digital flexor tendon as it courses over the sustentaculum tali, medial to the calcaneus. It extends from 6–7 cm proximal to the medial malleolus of the tibia to the proximal quarter of the third metatarsal bone. It can be approached medially, 1–2 cm proximal to the sustentaculum tali at the level of the medial malleolus of the tibia, by identifying the tendon plantar to the tibiotarsal joint.[4] Care must be taken not to enter the plantar medial tibiotarsal joint with this approach.

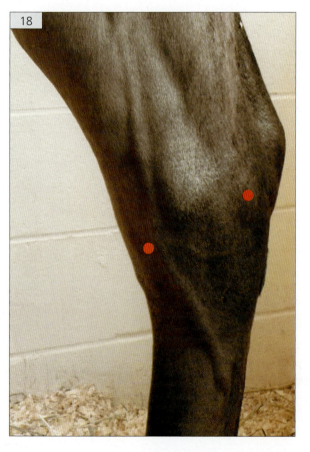

18

2.18 Medial aspect of the hock illustrating needle placement for arthrocentesis of the tibiotarsal joint; dorsal approach (bottom circle), plantar approach (top circle).

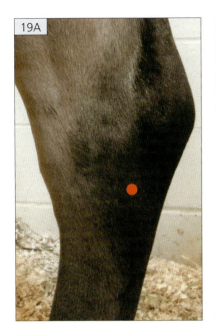

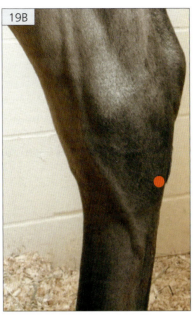

2.19A, B Lateral (A) and medial (B) aspects of the hock illustrating needle placements for arthrocentesis of the tarsometatarsal joint.

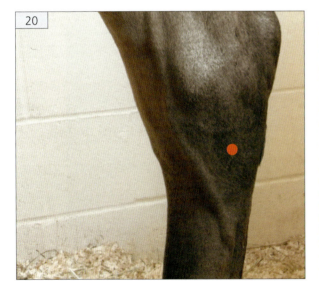

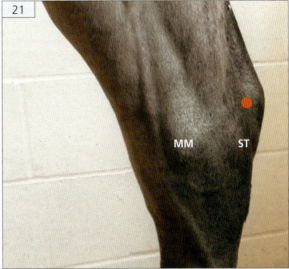

2.20 Medial aspect of the hock illustrating needle placement for arthrocentesis of the distal intertarsal joint.

2.21 Medial aspect of the hock illustrating the site for needle placement (star) for synoviocentesis of the tarsal sheath. MM, medial malleolus of the tibia; ST, sustentaculum tali of the calcaneus.

Complications

The main complication with synoviocentesis is infection. Infection is best prevented by using an aseptic technique and 500 mg of amikacin can be placed in the synovial structure at the completion of the procedure. (See also Septic arthritis and wounds involving joints.)

Therapeutic procedures
Splinting and casting
Indications

When evaluating horses with a fracture or complete disruption of a tendon or ligament, the first and most important step that must be taken is to stabilize the injured limb. If this is not done promptly, further injury to the limb will occur as the horse tries to bear weight on the limb. This occurs because bending forces are transferred through the fracture or laceration site instead of the joints as the horse continues to attempt to bear weight. This can have catastrophic consequences, such as causing a closed fracture to become open or compromising the blood supply to the fracture site. Either scenario can impede a successful surgical repair and can markedly lower the horse's prognosis for survival. Therefore, it is important to know how to correctly stabilize the limb and to have the materials available to do so quickly. Once the limb has been stabilized, the horse should be able to bear weight on the injured limb, which will decrease its anxiety and allow a more detailed examination to be performed.

Technique

Depending on the type of injury, stabilization can be accomplished using bandages, splints, or casts. A variety of splints or casts can be used in the distal limbs to accomplish these goals.[5–8]

Many different materials can be used as a splint. The splint must be rigid enough to provide the desired support, but it should ideally be lightweight and easy to apply over a bandage on the standing horse. A classic example of material that can be used as a splint for horses is polyvinyl chloride. This hard plastic can be cut into varying widths and lengths, which can be easily stored and transported in most veterinary vehicles. However, other common materials that are generally present in most barns can be used including wooden handles (e.g. broom, rake, axe), boards (5 × 10 cm or 2.5 × 15 cm [2 × 4 in or 1 × 6 in], **2.22**), or metal rods that can be bent (**2.23**). In addition, there are many commercially available splints, such as the Kimzey Leg Saver Splint, which can be applied quickly over a light bandage for first

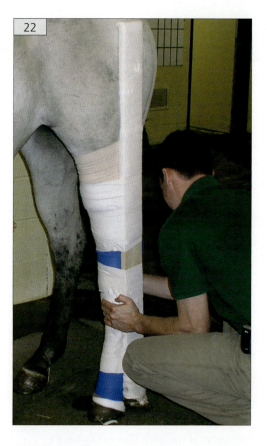

2.22 Use of a piece of wood as an extended lateral splint for the hindlimb.

and second phalangeal fractures and breakdown injuries (**2.24**). These splints are available in several sizes, with separate forelimb and hindlimb models available, and can be custom ordered to match specific measurements. Fiberglass casting material can be used circumferentially over bandage material to provide further rigidity, but is often hard to successfully apply because most horses with a fracture are anxious and will not stand completely still during application. However, large (10 cm [4 in]) casting material can be repetitively folded back and forth to create a splint of desired thickness and length, and this can be easily molded to the desired shape.

Note that an improperly placed splint or cast can do more harm than good. Specifically, the top of the splint or cast should never end at the same location as the fracture because it will act as a fulcrum, causing the fracture to displace and potentially become

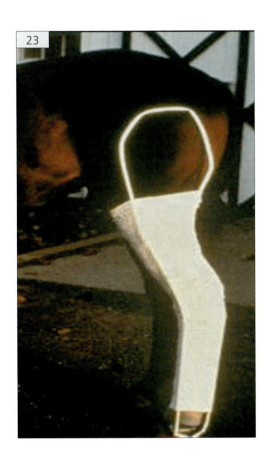

2.23 A horse with a splint constructed using a metal rod.

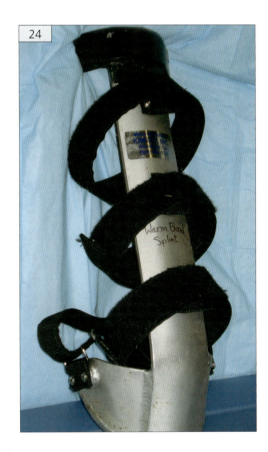

2.24 A Kimzey Leg Saver Splint.

open (**2.25**). Additionally, for most splints a light, compressive bandage should be applied before placing the splint. Excessive padding under the splint should be avoided because this will become compressed and loosen as the horse bears weight on the limb.

To determine the type of splint to apply, the horse's limb can be divided biomechanically into four regions. The proper location for splint application, depending on the type of injury present, is described in *Table 2.1*. The following are descriptions for application of each type of splint.

Dorsal or plantar splint: The goal of a dorsal splint is to place the dorsal cortices of the third metacarpal/metatarsal bone, first phalanx, second phalanx, and third phalanx in alignment in order to neutralize the bending forces that occur at the fracture site (**2.26**). In the forelimb, this is accomplished by placing a splint over a light bandage on the dorsal surface of the limb. The splint should extend from the toe to the proximal aspect of the metacarpus just distal to the carpus. The splint should be padded with cotton at the top to prevent the development of rub sores and then secured to the bandage with non-elastic tape. For the hindlimb, the splint is placed on the plantar surface of the limb. For both the forelimb and hindlimb, a heel wedge can be applied to help stabilize the limb (**2.27**). The strength of this coaptation can be increased by incorporating fiberglass cast material around the outside of the splint and bandage. Commercially available splints (e.g. the Kimzey Leg

Table 2.1 Splint required for stabilization of specific injuries

INJURY	DORSAL	90 DEGREE	CAUDAL	LATERAL	NO SPLINT
Middle phalanx fracture	✓*				
First phalanx fracture	✓*				
Traumatic disruption of the suspensory apparatus	✓*				
MC III/MT III condylar fracture					✓**
MC III/MT III diaphyseal fracture		✓			
Carpal fracture (unstable, comminuted)		✓			
Tarsal fracture (unstable, comminuted)		✓			
Olecranon fracture			✓		
Radial fracture				✓***	
Tibial fracture				✓	
Humeral fracture					✓
Femoral fracture					✓
Pelvic fracture					✓
Extensor tendon disruption			✓		
Flexor tendon disruption	✓				
Radial nerve paralysis			✓		
Articular luxation		✓			

*Kimzey Leg Saver Splint can also be used. If the fracture is in the hindlimb, use a plantar splint.

** If non- or minimally displaced. If displaced, instability will be medial to lateral requiring a lateral splint or circumferential splint, such as a bandage cast, or commercial braces such as the Fetlock Stabilizing Brace.

*** Distal radius fractures may benefit from the addition of a caudal splint that extends from the ground to the elbow. **WARNING:** The splint should not end at the fracture site.

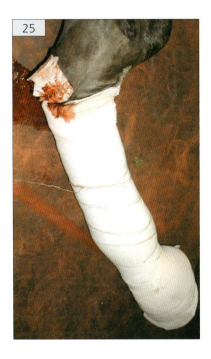

2.25 An inappropriately applied cast. The top of the cast ends at the same level as the proximal metatarsal fracture and has led to the development of an open fracture. (Courtesy Dr Curry Keoughan)

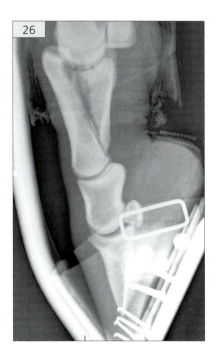

2.26 Lateral radiograph of the distal limb of a racehorse with a comminuted fracture of the first phalanx that was stabilized for transport with a Kimzey Leg Saver Splint. Note how the dorsal part of the splint is used to keep the dorsal cortices of the bones in alignment.

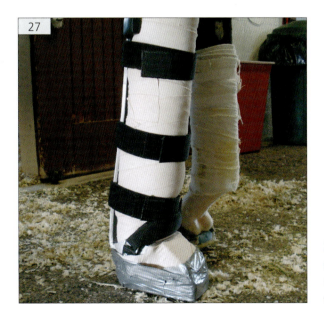

2.27 A horse with traumatic disruption of the suspensory apparatus (suspensory ligament rupture) wearing a Kimzey Leg Saver Splint on a hindlimb. Note the heel wedge, which is taped on to help stabilize the limb.

Saver Splint and the Straight to the Toe Brace) can also be used to achieve alignment of the dorsal cortices of the bones of the distal limb.

Double splints applied at 90 degrees to each other: Double splints placed at 90 degrees to each other are used to stabilize the limb in a dorsal to palmar/plantar direction and in a medial to lateral direction (**2.28**). A Robert Jones bandage should be placed on the limb extending from the ground to the elbow or stifle region. This is made of multiple layers of roll cotton, which is compressed to a thickness of about 2.5 cm (1 in) per layer with elastic bandage material. Ideally, the thickness of the bandage should be approximately 2–3 times the diameter of the limb at the site of the fracture. For the forelimb, splints should be placed caudally and laterally extending from the ground to the elbow. The foot can be maintained in a normal weight-bearing position. For the hindlimb, the caudal splint extends from the ground to the proximal aspect of the calcaneus, but the lateral splint should extend from the ground to the stifle. Fiberglass casting material can be added to the outside of the splints and bandage to increase the strength of the coaptation.

Caudal splint: A caudal splint should be placed on horses that are unable to place their limb in extension (**2.29**). Examples include horses that present with a 'dropped elbow' appearance due to a loss of function

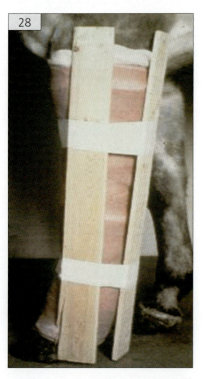

2.28 A horse with double (90°) splints applied caudally and laterally to stabilize an injury to the carpus. The splints are applied over a Robert Jones bandage.

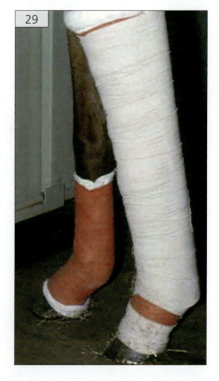

2.29 A horse with a caudal splint applied over a bandage to lock the carpus in extension.

of the triceps muscle caused by an olecranon fracture or radial nerve paralysis. Other horses requiring caudal splints are those that knuckle over at the fetlock joint due to disruption of an extensor tendon. Placing a caudal splint allows the horse to bear weight on the limb and also to advance the limb by utilizing upper limb muscles to abduct the limb slightly and swing it forward.

For horses unable to extend their carpus, a light bandage should be placed on the forelimb extending from the pastern to the elbow. The foot does not need to be incorporated into this bandage. The splint should be placed caudally, extending from the fetlock to the elbow to keep the carpus locked in extension.

For horses with an extensor tendon disruption, a slightly thicker bandage is placed extending from the ground to the carpus or tarsus. A splint is then placed on the palmar or plantar surface of the limb extending from the ground to the proximal metacarpus or metatarsus just distal to the carpus or tarsus. These caudal splints generally do not need to be reinforced with casting material.

Lateral splint: A lateral splint is used to prevent abduction of the limb in horses with radial (**2.30**) or tibial (**2.31**) fractures. When these fractures occur, the flexor and extensor muscles, which are located laterally, become abductors of the distal limb. This causes the fractured bone to displace medially, which often causes

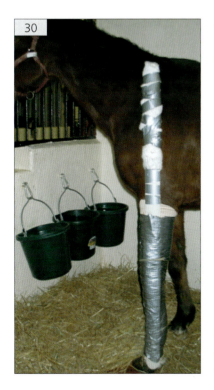

2.30 A horse with an extended lateral splint applied to a forelimb to stabilize a radius fracture.

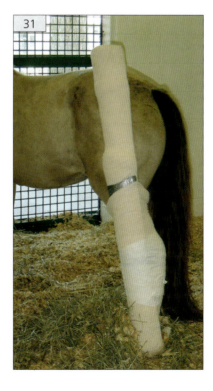

2.31 A horse with a Robert Jones bandage with an extended lateral and plantar splint for stabilization of a displaced tarsal fracture.

the fracture to become open due to the minimal amount of soft tissue that is present medially. A Robert Jones bandage should be placed on the limb extending from the ground to the elbow or stifle region. This is made of multiple layers of roll cotton, which is compressed to a thickness of about 2.5 cm (1 in) per layer with elastic bandage material. Ideally, the thickness of the bandage should be approximately 2–3 times the diameter of the limb at the location of the fracture. A splint is placed laterally extending from the ground up to the scapula on the forelimb and up to the hip on the hindlimb. Because of the angle of the hock, the hindlimb splint can be difficult to place and maintain. A wider board (15 cm [6 in]) or a metal rod contoured to match the angle of the hock works best (**2.22, 2.23**). These splints need to be well-incorporated into the bandage and, if possible, should be further secured around the axillary region or flank with tape to help prevent abduction (**2.32**).

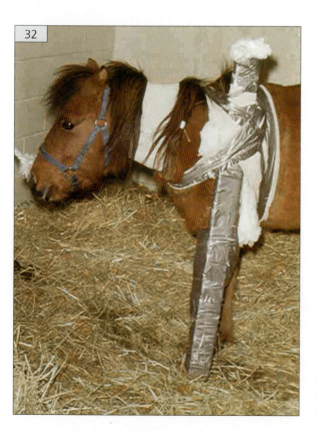

32

Regional limb perfusion
Indications
It is often difficult to achieve effective antimicrobial drug concentrations at the tissue level when treating orthopedic infections with systemic antimicrobial drugs alone. Adjunctive methods used to deliver high concentrations of antimicrobial drugs locally include intra-articular injections of antimicrobial drugs, regional limb perfusions with antimicrobial drugs, and the use of antimicrobial impregnated substances such as polymethylmethacrylate, plaster of Paris, or collagen sponges.[9–11]

Technique
Regional limb perfusion can be performed via the IV or IO route. Comparable antimicrobial drug concentrations are obtained in bone, synovial fluid, and soft tissue regardless of the chosen route. Because of the ease of performing IV regional limb perfusion, the rest of this section will focus on the IV route.[12] However, IO perfusions may be preferable if the vascular integrity of the limb has been compromised (**2.33**). IV regional limb perfusion maintains high concentrations of antimicrobial drugs in bone, synovial fluid, and soft tissues for approximately 24 hours after infusion depending on the drug and dose used.[13] Concentrations up to 50 times the MIC of susceptible organisms can be achieved with IV regional limb perfusion, which is greater than those achieved with systemic administration of antimicrobial drugs but less than concentrations obtained in synovial fluid following intra-articular injection. Bone concentrations of antimicrobial drugs are similar following IV regional limb perfusion and intra-articular administration.[14] Since the dose of antimicrobial drug used in IV regional limb perfusion is usually lower than the systemic dose, additional advantages of IV regional limb perfusion include minimizing systemic side-effects and lowering the cost of treatment.

2.32 Photograph of a pony with an extended lateral splint secured to the axillary region to help prevent abduction of the limb.

Ideally, the antimicrobial drug used for IV regional limb perfusion should be chosen based on the results of bacterial culture and antimicrobial sensitivity testing. However, since therapy is usually initiated prior to obtaining such results, the antimicrobial drug chosen should be effective against the most commonly isolated pathogens for a given type of infection. Traumatic injuries tend to result in polymicrobial infections containing gram-negative, gram-positive, and anaerobic bacteria. Iatrogenic infections are usually caused by *Staphylococcus* spp., most commonly *Staphylococcus aureus*.[3] Hematogenous infections in neonates are usually caused by gram-negative bacteria. Aminoglycosides are commonly used for IV regional limb perfusion because of their effectiveness against many of the common orthopedic pathogens and because of their concentration-dependent bactericidal effect. Amikacin is superior to gentamicin for resistant organisms and is often the drug of choice for IV

regional limb perfusion.[15] It has been suggested that time-dependent antimicrobial drugs can also be used effectively for IV regional limb perfusion because the MIC that is obtained at the tissue level is high enough to exert a therapeutic effect, despite the fact that the tourniquet is usually maintained for 30 minutes or less. Other antimicrobial drugs that have been used include ceftiofur, cefotaxime, timentin, potassium penicillin, enrofloxacin, imipenem-cilastin, and vancomycin.[9,16–18] Although enrofloxacin can be used, it may cause a local vasculitis that could interfere with future IV regional limb perfusion. Additionally, drugs such as imipenem-cilastin and vancomycin should only be used to treat infections caused by resistant organisms against which no other antimicrobial drugs are effective. The dose of antimicrobial drug used varies greatly between reports; however, it has been shown that higher doses are necessary to reach therapeutic concentrations in standing, awake horses than in horses under general anesthesia.[18] The authors routinely use one-third of the systemic dose for most antimicrobial drugs. This is diluted to a final volume of 60 ml with sterile saline. The volume can be adjusted depending on the size of the isolated region.

For IV regional limb perfusions performed with the horse under general anesthesia, a pneumatic tourniquet should be used. If performed standing, the horse should be heavily sedated and perineural anesthesia proximal to the region of interest should be considered to minimize movement during the procedure, because this reduces tissue concentrations of the antimicrobial drug (David Levine, unpublished data).

The region of interest is isolated using one or two tourniquets. In general, one tourniquet is placed proximal to the region of interest and another can be placed distal to the area if desired. The tourniquet should remain in place for 20–30 minutes following administration of the antimicrobial drug. The width of the

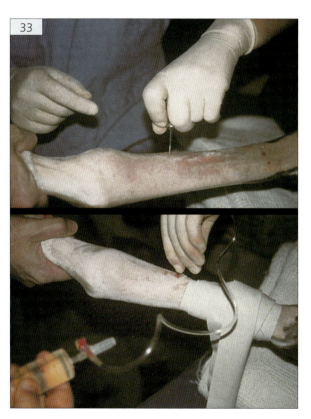

2.33 Placement of a cannulated screw (top) and administration of antimicrobials (bottom) via the intraosseous route. (Courtesy Dr Murray Brown)

tourniquet is important, with wide tourniquets (such as an esmarch bandage) providing higher tissue concentrations of antimicrobial drug than those obtained with smaller rubber tubing (David Levine, unpublished data) (**2.34**).

Superficial veins are isolated and aseptically prepared for venipuncture; this can be easily performed using a small (25–27 gauge) butterfly catheter. For the distal limb, the palmar or plantar digital arteries are commonly used. For the proximal limb, the cephalic vein (forelimb) or the saphenous vein (hindlimb) can be used (**2.35**). However, if these vessels are not easy to access, any superficial vessel can be used.

IV regional limb perfusion can be done as frequently as once daily to every other day for several weeks' duration.

Complications

The limiting factor in how long IV regional limb perfusion can be continued is the condition of the vessels, which varies between patients. It is beneficial to maintain a compressive bandage over the injection site and in some cases apply topical anti-inflammatory drugs (e.g. diclofenac or dimethylsulfoxide) to aid in resolution of mild vasculitis or cellulitis between perfusions.

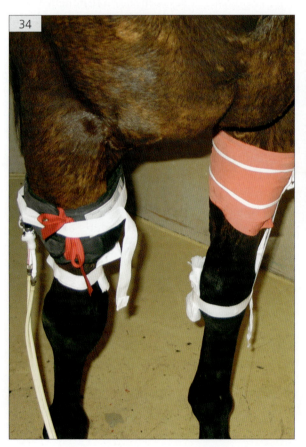

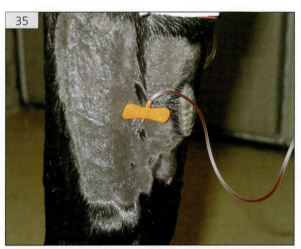

2.35 A 25-gauge butterfly catheter being used to perform an intravenous regional limb perfusion via the cephalic vein. (Courtesy Dr David Levine)

2.34 A pneumatic tourniquet (left) and esmarch tourniquet (right) used to perform intravenous regional limb perfusions in standing horses; the horse in this picture was heavily sedated, but no local analgesia was used. (Courtesy Dr David Levine)

Antimicrobial-impregnated polymethylmethacrylate

Indications

It is often difficult to achieve effective antimicrobial drug concentrations at the tissue level when treating orthopedic infections with systemic antimicrobial drugs alone. This is due to changes in the local environment that occur in response to infection such as alterations in blood supply, a decrease in pH, the accumulation of fibrin within synovial cavity, and the production of an impenetrable glycocalix or 'biofilm' by bacteria surrounding orthopedic implants. In addition, failure to achieve effective antimicrobial drug concentrations at the site of infection can favor the growth of resistant organisms. Therefore, delivery of high concentrations of antimicrobial drugs directly to the infected site is critical for resolution of orthopedic infections. Sustained high concentrations of antimicrobial drugs can be achieved by using antimicrobial-impregnated polymethylmethacrylate (AIPM).[10,11,19,20] Tissue concentrations of antimicrobial drugs up to 20 times those obtained with systemic therapy alone can be achieved with minimal risk of systemic toxicity.[21,22] Additionally, AIPM has been shown to aid in the resolution of equine orthopedic infections refractory to treatment with systemic antimicrobial drugs and surgical debridement.[20]

Technique

Elution of antimicrobial drugs from AIPM is influenced by several factors including the type and porosity of polymethylmethacrylate used, the surface area of the implant, the antimicrobial drug concentration and its diffusion characteristics, and the local tissue environment. The elution of antimicrobial drugs from AIPM occurs in a bimodal fashion, with the initial release occurring during the first 24 hours, followed by a sustained release that can result in therapeutic levels for weeks to months.

Ideally, the antimicrobial drug used in the AIPM should be based on the results of bacterial culture and antimicrobial sensitivity testing. However, since therapy is usually initiated prior to obtaining such results, the antimicrobial drug chosen should be effective against the most commonly isolated pathogens for a given type of infection. For example, traumatic injuries tend to result in polymicrobial infections with gram-negative, gram-positive, and anaerobic bacteria. In these cases, broad-spectrum coverage can be achieved by using AIPM beads made with a cephalosporin and an aminoglycoside in separate beads. Conversely, iatrogenic infections, such as those that occur postoperatively or after joint injections, are usually caused by *Staphylococcus* spp., most commonly *S. aureus*.[3] Many of these infections are susceptible to aminoglycosides, with amikacin being superior to gentamicin for resistant strains.[15] Hematogenous infections in neonates are usually caused by gram-negative bacteria, and AIPM beads made with an aminoglycoside are a good first choice for these infections.

Note that not all antimicrobial drugs can be incorporated into polymethylmethacrylate.[10,11] Antimicrobial drugs must be heat stable and must elute from the polymethylmethacrylate. Antimicrobial drugs that have been proven to elute effectively from polymethylmethacrylate include gentamicin, amikacin, cefazolin, tobramycin, and metronidazole.[9] It is generally recommended that only one antimicrobial drug is used in each AIPM bead, because studies have shown that combining some antimicrobial drugs (e.g. cefazolin and amikacin) within the same bead greatly increases the initial elution of the antimicrobial drugs from the bead and, therefore, significantly decreases the amount of time that affective antimicrobial drug concentrations will be achieved in tissues.[23]

AIPM is easy to prepare and can be made at the time of surgery, or it can be made in advance, gas sterilized, and stored for later use. There are many types of polymethacrylate that have demonstrated good elution rates (e.g. Surgical Simplex P, Palacos, Zimmer). The AIPM is prepared by mixing the liquid monomer with the powdered polymer and the crystalline form of the antimicrobial drug.

Reported doses of antimicrobials used are 1–2 grams of antimicrobial per 10 grams of polymethylmethacrylate powder.[9] The combination is mixed until it forms a paste, which can then be molded into the desired shape; examples include small beads connected to a single strand of suture or wire to expedite future removal, or larger individual beads or cigar shapes that can be placed directly into the tissues (**2.36**). The cement takes 5–10 minutes to harden, although AIPM made with metronidazole needs several hours to set up.[24] The AIPM will become warm as it sets because this is an exothermic reaction.

AIPM can also be used prophylactically in fracture repair at the time of surgery. (**Note:** Although the addition of antimicrobial drugs to polymethylmethacrylate weakens its biomechanical strength, this is not a concern if the AIPM is being used solely as an antimicrobial drug delivery device.)

Complications

AIPM beads are not biodegradable; however, they do not normally need to be removed. In rare instances, they can be the source of chronic inflammation and lead to the development of fistulous tracts; removal of the beads is usually curative. Because of the abrasive nature of the beads, they should not be used in synovial structures, especially joints. If they are placed in a synovial structure, they should be removed as soon as possible to minimize further damage.[25]

MUSCULOSKELETAL EMERGENCIES

Bone
Fractures
Distal phalanx fracture
Key points

- The distal interphalangeal bone often heals via a fibrous union, therefore when rechecking these horses, remember that a fracture line is often visible for many months after the fracture has clinically healed and the horse is sound.
- If clinical findings suggest a coffin bone fracture but radiographs are normal, scintigraphy and MRI are both more sensitive diagnostic tests. The horse can also be stall rested for 10 days and the foot re-radiographed after some bone resorption occurs at the fracture line.
- False-positive findings on radiographs are common when the foot is not properly packed. The fracture should be apparent on at least two views and the fracture line should not extend beyond the limits of the bone.

Definition/overview

Fractures of the distal phalanx are relatively rare and usually present as one of six previously classified configurations in adults (**2.37**).[26–28] Foals tend to have a different type of fracture than adults.[29]

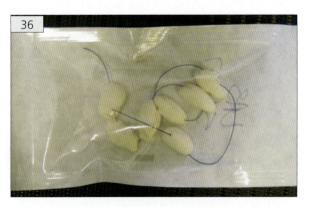

2.36 Antimicrobial-impregnated polymethylmethacrylate beads embedded around suture material that has been gas sterilized for future use.

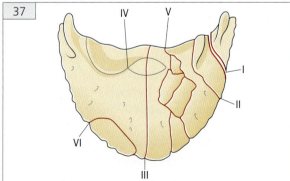

2.37 Classification of distal phalangeal fractures: type I (abaxial, non-articular), type II (abaxial, articular), type III (axial articular), type IV (extensor process), type V (comminuted, articular), type VI (solar margin).

Etiology/pathogenesis

Although high-speed work may predispose to fractures of the distal phalanx, the injury is seen in all breeds and all ages. Direct trauma, such as kicking an immovable object, is a common cause of fracture as well as lacerations sustained to the hoof capsule. Laminitic horses can sustain pathologic fractures of the distal phalanx.

Clinical features

Most horses present with an acute history of severe lameness (equal or greater than grade 3 out of 5), which is usually most evident when the horse turns. Minimal to no soft tissue swelling may be observed proximal to the coronary band. Prominent digital pulses are often palpable in the digital arteries. Most horses have obvious hoof tester sensitivity that can be focal or generalized.

Differential diagnosis

Subsolar abscess; septic osteitis; laminitis; navicular disease/fracture.

Diagnosis

Lameness examination can mostly be performed at a walk combined with hoof tester examination. Perineural anesthesia may be required to localize the lameness to the distal phalanx. A horse with an articular fracture should also improve with a distal interphalangeal joint block. Definitive diagnosis is made from radiographs (**2.38, 2.39A**). It is important to make sure that the foot

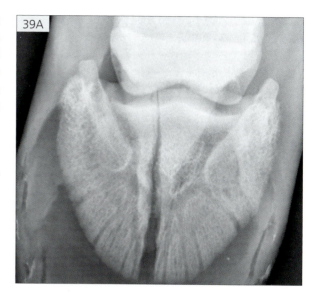

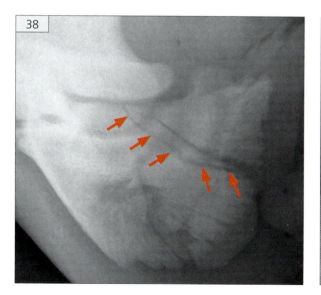

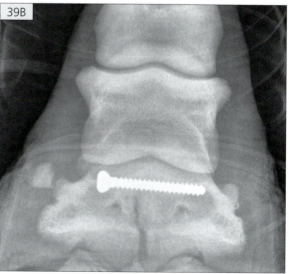

2.38 Oblique 60 degree dorsoproximal–palmarodistal radiograph of the foot highlighting a type II fracture of the distal phalanx (arrows).

2.39A, 2.39B Dorsoventral radiograph of a foot with a type III fracture of the distal phalanx (A) and a dorsopalmar radiograph of the same foot documenting subsequent surgical repair (B).

is adequately packed to minimize the superimposition that results from the sulci of the frog. Alternatively, the foot can be radiographed while it is submersed in water to eliminate gas pockets.

Management/treatment

Conservative treatment consists of stall rest for 6–8 weeks in combination with a shoe with clips or a full rim to prevent expansion of the foot. A foot cast can be applied as well. Surgical treatment should be considered in large mid-sagittal or parasagittal fractures and articular chip fractures (**2.39B**). The prognosis for all distal phalanx fractures is much better in young horses.

Middle phalanx facture
Key points

- It is important to take four radiographic views of middle phalanx fractures because many are comminuted.
- The prognosis for horses with middle phalanx fractures is based on whether an intact strut of bone is present between the proximal and distal interphalangeal joints, which can only be verified by obtaining a complete series of radiographic views.

Definition/overview

Fractures of the middle phalanx are often comminuted fractures of the forelimb or hind limb (**2.40**), but can also be palmar/plantar eminence fractures (medial, lateral, or both) (**2.41**).[30–32]

Etiology/pathogenesis

Fractures of the middle phalanx are common in Quarter Horses and performance horses that are required to make abrupt turns. The hoof may stay still while the rest of the limb rotates, leading to abnormal torsional forces being placed across the middle phalanx. These fractures can also occur as a result of severe trauma such as getting the limb trapped in a fence or cattle guard.

Clinical features

Horses with palmar/plantar eminence and comminuted fractures often present with a severe lameness (greater or equal to 4 out of 5). Soft tissue swelling distal to the fetlock and proximal to the coronary band is often present and crepitus can be palpated. Subluxation of the pastern joint may also be observed, especially in those horses with an eminence fracture. These fractures are rarely open.

Differential diagnosis

Proximal phalanx fracture; distal phalanx fracture; subsolar abscess.

Diagnosis

Diagnosis of middle phalanx fractures is made from the combination of history, palpation of the pastern area, and survey radiographs of the pastern region.

Management/treatment

For both palmar/plantar eminence and comminuted fractures, the limb should be stabilized by use of a dorsal splint (or a plantar splint in the hindlimb) that places the dorsal cortices of the digits in alignment so that the horse bears weight on its toe (see Splinting and casting). The digits are placed in extension in order to avoid motion at the fracture site in the frontal plane. Commercially available splints, such as the Kimzey Leg Saver Splint, can also be used to achieve alignment of the dorsal cortices of the bones of the distal limb. Palmar/plantar eminence fractures can rarely be satisfactorily reduced with lag screw fixation, therefore most horses should be treated early with an arthrodesis of the proximal interphalangeal joint.

The prognosis is worse for comminuted fractures and those with marked displacement at the distal interphalangeal joint. If there is an intact strut of bone extending the length of the middle phalanx, internal fixation (typically two bone plates and additional lag screws) can be performed to repair the fracture and fuse the pastern joint. This can be done with or without transfixation pin casting. Extremely comminuted fractures should be treated with a transfixation pin-cast or an external skeletal fixation device.[33,34]

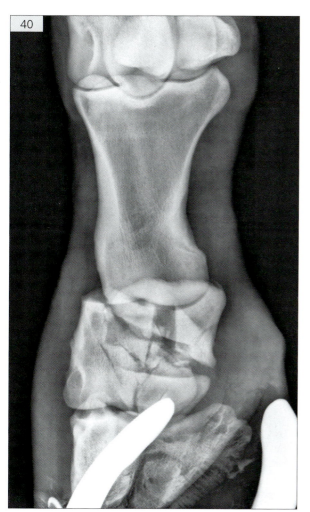

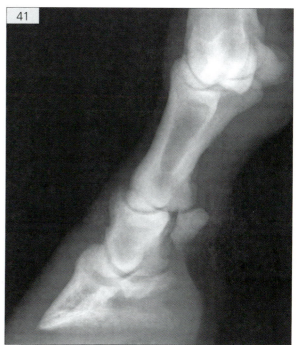

2.41 Dorsomedial plantarolateral oblique radiograph of the pastern demonstrating a plantar medial eminence fracture of the middle phalanx.

2.40 Dorsolateral plantaromedial oblique radiograph of the pastern demonstrating a severely comminuted fracture of the middle phalanx.

Proximal phalanx fracture
Key point

- If the signalment (racehorses) and history are even suggestive of a proximal phalanx fracture, the horse should undergo radiographs and/or nuclear scintigraphy prior to performing any perineural analgesia to minimize the risk of having further propagation of the fracture during the lameness examination.

Definition/overview

There are many configurations of proximal phalangeal fractures including dorsal frontal (**2.42**), collateral avulsions, palmar/plantar eminence, sagittal (**2.43**), and comminuted fractures (**2.44**).[32,35] Comminuted fractures are always displaced, but all other forms can be non- or minimally displaced.

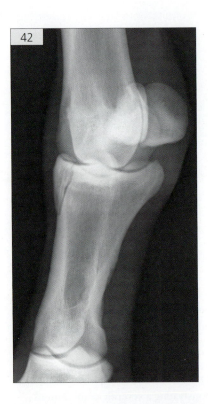

2.42 Dorsolateral palmaromedial oblique radiograph of a dorsal frontal fracture of the first phalanx.

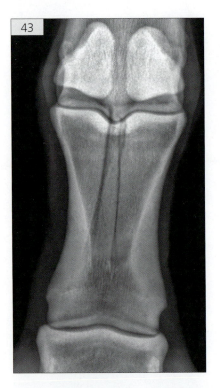

2.43 Dorsopalmar radiograph of an incomplete midsagittal fracture of the first phalanx.

Etiology/pathogenesis

The anatomy of the metacarpo-/metatarsophalan-geal joint articulation ensures proper alignment and mobility of the joint, but also predisposes the proximal phalanx to injury. The mid-sagittal ridge of the distal third metacarpus/metatarsus sits in a concave area in the middle of the proximal aspect of the proximal phalanx. Because of this anatomy, when the horse places longitudinal compression with rotational torque across the joint, a 'screwdriver fracture' can occur where the fracture originates and propagates from the concavity in the proximal aspect of the bone.

Clinical features

Clinical signs will vary depending on the severity of the fracture. Horses with minimally displaced fractures may present with a mild to moderate lameness at a trot (2 to 3 out of 5), but horses with complete fractures usually have a lameness observable at a walk (4 out of 5). Minimal soft tissue swelling is usually present with incomplete and complete non-displaced fractures. Pain may be elicited on direct palpation over the fracture or manipulation, but this is relatively unreliable. Comminuted fractures present with severe lameness (5 out of 5), pain on palpation/manipulation, crepitus, and obvious soft tissue swelling.

Differential diagnosis

Middle phalanx fracture; condylar fracture of the distal third metacarpus/metatarsus; subsolar abscess.

Diagnosis

History, physical examination and lameness examination combined with radiographs and/or nuclear scintigraphy can be used to diagnose comminuted fractures and most complete non-displaced fractures. However, many incomplete and some complete non-displaced fractures will be difficult to discern from the history, palpation, and even a complete lameness examination.

Management/treatment

For incomplete or complete non-displaced fractures, the horses can be placed in a support bandage for transport. However, if the fracture is displaced or comminuted, the limb should be stabilized by use of a dorsal splint or prefabricated splint so that the horse bears weight on its toe (see Splinting and casting). Repair of the fracture depends on the configuration.[36–38]

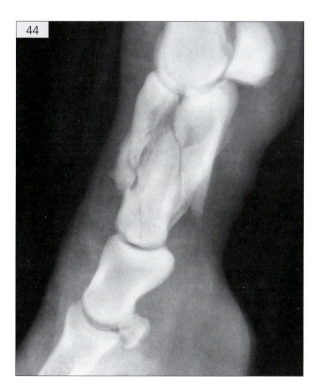

2.44 Lateromedial radiograph of a comminuted fracture of the first phalanx.

Incomplete or non-displaced complete fractures can be repaired via lag screw fixation or cast application (**2.45**). For comminuted fractures, lag screw fixation can be attempted to reduce the fracture and realign joint surfaces. Transfixation pin casts or an external skeletal fixation device may also be used to transfer weight to the metacarpus/metatarsus.[34] A later arthrodesis of the fetlock is often necessary in horses with severely comminuted fractures.

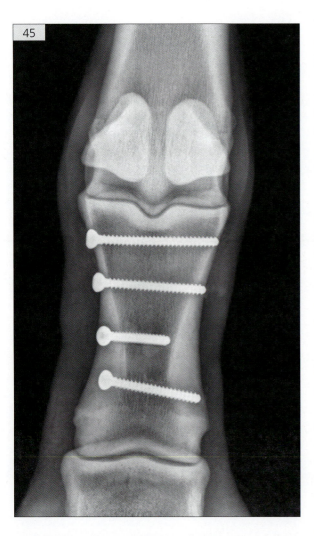

2.45 Surgical repair of the horse in 2.43.

Third metacarpus/metatarsus fracture
Key points
- If a condylar fracture is suspected during a lameness examination, a minimal lameness examination should be performed to reduce the potential for fracture propagation. Do NOT perform nerve blocks or intra-articular anesthesia or else the fracture could propagate.
- Aggressive first aid measures are very important for third metacarpal and metatarsal fractures because the minimal overlying soft tissues are so vulnerable to injury. If a fracture is open, the expense of treatment increases considerably and the prognosis conversely declines.

Definition/overview
Fractures of the third metacarpal or metatarsal bones occur in multiple configurations. The most commonly seen are those that occur in racehorses, which are either lateral condylar fractures that exit the lateral cortex (**2.46**) or medial condylar fractures that propagate from the medial condyle into the diaphysis. Less commonly, other variations of metacarpal/metatarsal fractures are seen with equally variable prognoses (**2.47A, B**).[39–42]

Etiology/pathogenesis
Most fractures of the metacarpus/metatarsus in non-racehorses are due to external trauma. In racehorses, repetitive stresses in the distal palmar condyle, experienced during racing and training, lead to the development of microcracks or osteonecrosis, which predisposes the area to developing condylar fractures.[43]

Clinical features
Horses and foals with diaphyseal fractures have obvious instability, swelling, and pain, which can be used to localize the problem. Racehorses with condylar fractures have a wider range of presenting signs. Although the effusion and periarticular swelling associated with displaced condylar fractures are generally greater than that seen in non-displaced fractures, many horses with non-displaced fractures are lamer than those with displaced fractures.

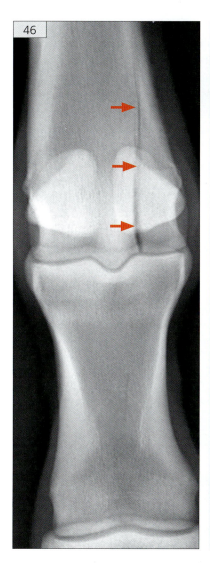

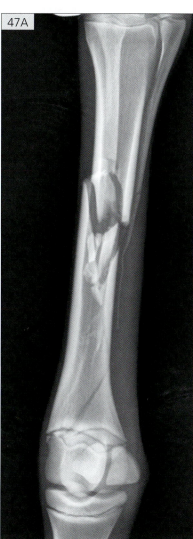

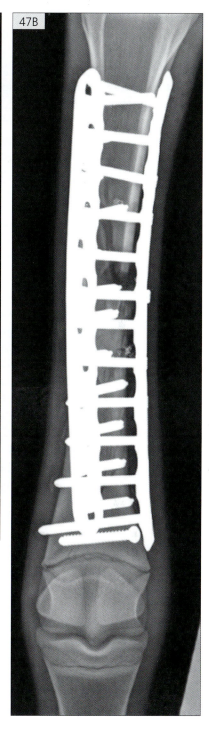

2.46 Dorsopalmar radiograph highlighting (arrows) a complete, minimally displaced lateral condylar fracture of the third metacarpus.

2.47A, B Dorsolateral plantaromedial oblique radiograph of a comminuted diaphyseal fracture of the third metatarsus in a 6-week-old foal (A) and dorsoplantar radiograph of the subsequent successful surgical repair (B).

Differential diagnosis

Sesamoid fracture; proximal phalanx fracture.

Diagnosis

For those fractures that are sustained from external trauma or for displaced condylar fractures, diagnosis is made from a thorough history, physical examination, and radiographic examination. For some condylar fractures, a lameness examination may need to be performed in combination with nuclear scintigraphy. A special 125 degree dorsopalmar metacarpal skyline view of the metacarpophalangeal joint is indicated to identify pathology of the distal palmar joint surface (**2.48**).

Management/treatment

If the fracture involves the diaphysis of the forelimb, a Robert Jones bandage extending from the ground to the elbow with at least two splints incorporated on the caudal and lateral sides of the limb should be applied (see Splinting and casting). It is NOT advisable to place an extremely thick bandage because this lessens the mechanical benefit of splints. If available, medial and dorsal/cranial splints can also be used. Overlapping staves of polyvinyl chloride pipe are particularly useful for third metacarpal fractures because the padded bandage can be made almost perfectly cylindrical. The splints should always be secured to the bandage with a non-elastic tape. Radiator hose clamps can be used to secure splints if overlapping staves are used. The splints should extend completely to ground level.

It is much more difficult to splint a third metatarsal bone injury because of the hock angle. The best temporary splinting is to use a plantar splint extending from the top of the calcaneus down to the ground, combined with a lateral splint extending up over the stifle and thigh. For either to be effective, the bandage should NOT be excessively padded.

For typical lateral condylar fractures, a simple well-padded bandage is usually adequate. Splints, including Kimzey splints, are not recommended.

Medial condylar fractures, especially those in the hindlimb, are extremely prone to catastrophic dehiscence so they should be handled with much more caution than other condylar fractures. This essentially means treating them more like a diaphyseal fracture. The method of repair depends on the configuration of the fracture.[39,41,42] Most diaphyseal fractures are treated with two plates, although severely comminuted injuries may require external skeletal fixation, usually a pin-cast. Lateral condylar fractures are best repaired by a combination of arthroscopy and lag screw fixation. Medial condylar fractures tend to spiral or 'Y' in the mid-diaphysis and are treated with lag screws in the condyle and a single plate spanning the length of the

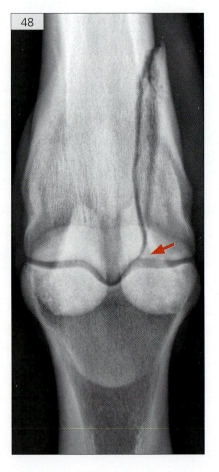

2.48 125 degree dorsopalmar metacarpal skyline view of the metacarpophalangeal joint. Note the osteochondral fragment (arrow) at the distal palmar joint surface, which was only identified on this radiographic view.

metacarpal or metatarsal bone. Any fracture other than a simple lateral third metacarpal condylar fracture is at considerable risk of catastrophic failure during anesthetic recovery, so maximal measures for protection during recovery should be considered. This includes pool recoveries or sling recoveries when available and full-limb casts when they are not available.

In small foals, it is best to sedate the foal and quickly bandage and splint the limb before physically restraining the foal in recumbency while it is being transported to a surgical facility.

Carpal fractures and luxations
Key points
- Nearly all acute injuries of the carpus that are not grossly unstable can be managed successfully and many horses can return to athletic function.
- Overtly unstable carpal injuries are extremely difficult to manage long term without internal fixation. Any carpal injury that results in gross deviation of the limb should be considered a very serious problem and surgical arthrodesis strongly suggested.

Definition/overview
Fracture sustained to one or a combination of the bones that make up the carpus including the accessory, ulnar, intermediate, radial, second, third and fourth carpal bones.[44,45] Luxations of the carpal joints are rare.

Etiology/pathogenesis
The most common type of carpal injury is a chip fracture involving the dorsal rim of the middle carpal or radiocarpal joints, but this injury is seen almost exclusively in racehorses and almost never presents as an emergency. The continuum of racehorse fractures due to high impact loading of the carpus includes more serious injuries such as slab fractures of the major carpal bones (**2.49, 2.50**). It is likely that the combination of

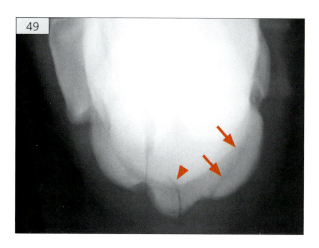

2.49 Skyline radiograph of the distal row of carpal bones highlighting a frontal slab fracture of the radial facet of the third carpal bone (arrows) and a sagittal slab fracture of the intermediate facet of the third carpal bone (arrowhead).

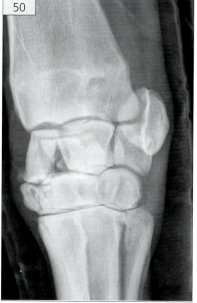

2.50 Dorsolateral palmaromedial oblique radiograph of the carpus of a racehorse with slab fractures of the radial carpal bone and third carpal bone (with comminution).

speed and fatigue of the carpal and digital flexors results in excessive dorsiflexion (hyperextension) of the carpus and overload, resulting in failure. Fractures involving the palmar aspect of the carpus occur primarily in horses that fall with their carpus flexed (**2.51**). This is seen most commonly in event horses, steeplechase horses, and horses recovering from general anesthesia. All the major types of carpal injuries can be seen in non-racehorses as a single event trauma. Multiple slab fractures and luxations occur most often as unwitnessed pasture accidents or due to direct blows in non-racehorses.

Clinical features

Racehorses with typical chip fractures are rarely very lame and most will not present as an emergency. Displaced slab fractures and other major injuries of the carpus may cause sufficient pain to warrant emergency attention. Diagnosis is rarely difficult because the middle carpal and/or radiocarpal joints will have prominent effusion and the horse will be reactive to carpal manipulation. The most important feature to recognize is medial to lateral instability because that is an accurate sign of marked displacement of fracture fragments. If the limb deviates laterally, the fourth carpal and ulna carpal bone are often fractured. If the limb deviates medially, the third carpal (most common) and/or radial carpal bone may be fractured. Comminuted fractures usually have palpable crepitus.

Fractures of the palmar carpus do not have medial to lateral instability and these horses often stand comfortably on their affected limb at rest. Horses with palmar carpal fractures are usually markedly sensitive to flexion and may have carpal sheath effusion.

Horses with accessory carpal bone (**2.51**) injuries (usually in frontal plane) are usually very lame initially (greater than or equal to grade 4 out of 5) and typically have pain on carpal flexion. Effusion may be present in the carpal canal of horses with accessory carpal bone fractures.

Differential diagnosis

Ligamentous injury; luxation/subluxation; septic arthritis.

Diagnosis

Thorough history, physical examination and lameness examinations, combined with radiographs, are usually diagnostic. As part of a thorough radiographic examination, a skyline of the distal row of carpal bones must be taken to diagnose slab fractures of the third carpal bone. If there is suspicion of a slab or comminuted fracture, the horse should be radiographed before performing intra-articular anesthesia.

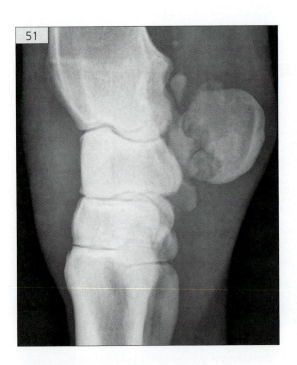

51

2.51 Lateromedial radiograph of the carpus of a steeplechase horse with a comminuted accessory carpal bone fracture sustained while falling over a jump.

Ultrasonography, CT (**2.52**), MRI, or nuclear scintigraphy can all be performed to diagnose complicated fractures or ligamentous tears.[46] Arthroscopic examination can also be used as a diagnostic tool.

Management/treatment

Although the treatment for carpal fractures depends on the severity of the injury and the intended use of the horse, nearly all are best treated with arthroscopic surgery. Smaller fragments are generally removed[44,47] and slab fractures repaired using lag screw fixation.[48] Although some complex multiple slab fractures can be repaired with individual screws, more serious comminuted fractures of the carpal bones are best treated with partial carpal (middle carpal and carpometacarpal) arthrodesis (**2.53**) or pancarpal arthrodesis if the proximal row is badly damaged.

Horses with chip fractures or typical slab fractures do not require extensive bandaging because the carpi are stable. Horses with unstable carpi should be placed in a heavily padded bandage, with caudal and lateral splints that extend from the foot to the elbow, until definitive surgical treatment can be performed (see Splinting and casting). Long-term casting is not a good option for unstable carpal injuries because these horses can rarely be managed in a cast long term, as the instability nearly always results in serious cast sores. Non-surgical treatment of unstable carpal fractures often results in an angular deformity that worsens over time. For example, combined third carpal and radial carpal fractures nearly always result in a severe carpus varus deformity. Accessory carpal bone fractures are treated with rest and have a good prognosis.

Tarsal fractures and luxations
Key points
- There is a broad range of tarsal bone fractures and the treatment of these injuries is equally diverse.
- Unstable fractures or luxations are difficult to stabilize and need urgent surgical attention.

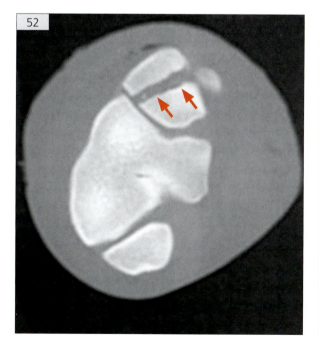

2.52 Computed tomograpic image of a transverse section through the distal row of carpal bones highlighting (arrows) a fracture of the fourth carpal bone.

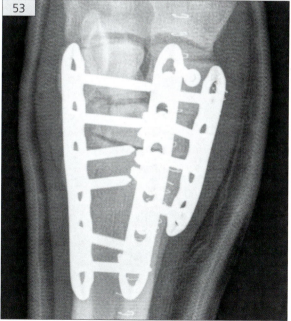

2.53 Dorsopalmar view of the repair via a partial carpal arthrodesis of the fracture shown in the horse in 2.50.

Definition/overview

Fractures can involve any of the tarsal bones, but calcaneal (fibular tarsal bone) fractures are probably most common. Fractures of the trochlear ridges or the body of the talus and frontal plane slab fractures of the central or third tarsal bone also occur. Luxations most commonly occur at the proximal intertarsal joint.[49–51]

Etiology/pathogenesis

Fractures of the tarsus are uncommon except for those secondary to external trauma from kicks or striking fixed objects. Trauma to the plantar aspect of the hock can lead to fracture of the calcaneal tuberosity or the sustentaculum tali (**2.54**). Slab fractures of the central or third tarsal bone occur almost exclusively in racehorses and are due to a combination of repetitive stress injury and focal overload (**2.55**). Direct kicks to the medial aspect of the hock can result in chip fractures of the dorsal or plantar medial trochlear ridge of the talus. Fractures of the lateral trochlear ridge are usually larger and not always associated with external trauma.

Clinical features

Most horses with calcaneal fractures will have obvious and localized swelling, but sustentacular fractures may be less obvious and may have tarsal sheath effusion.

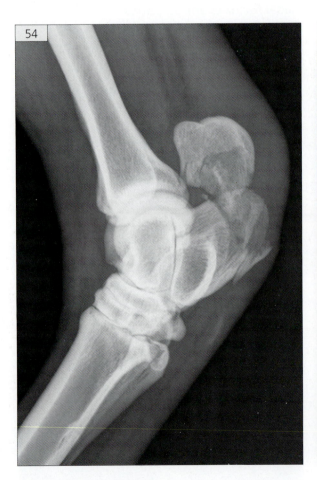

2.54 Lateromedial radiograph of the tarsus of a miniature horse with a communicated calcaneal fracture.

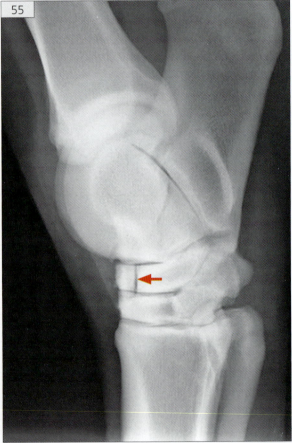

2.55 Lateromedial radiograph of the tarsus highlighting a frontal slab fracture of the central tarsal bone (arrow).

Fractures of the talus typically have marked tarsocrural effusion. The degree of lameness depends on the bone that is fractured and the fracture configuration. Most horses are moderately to severely lame (greater than or equal to grade 3 out of 5). If the horse has clinical signs referable to the tarsus and remains very lame for more than 3 days, one should be suspicious of a slab fracture (frontal or sagittal) or joint sepsis. Horses that sustain multiple tarsal fractures are severely lame (greater than or equal to grade 4 out of 5) and can have crepitus and a marked tarsal instability.

Differential diagnosis

Ligamentous injury; septic arthritis.

Diagnosis

A thorough history, physical examination, and lameness examination, combined with radiographs, are usually diagnostic. As part of the radiographic examination, a flexed lateromedial and a skyline view of the sustentaculum tali (**2.56**) should be performed. If there is suspicion of slab or comminuted fractures, the horse should be radiographed before performing intra-articular anesthesia. Depending on the size of the horse, CT, MRI, or nuclear scintigraphy (**2.57**) can

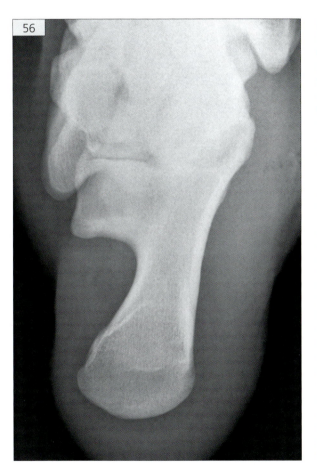

2.56 Skyline radiograph of the sustentaculum tali.

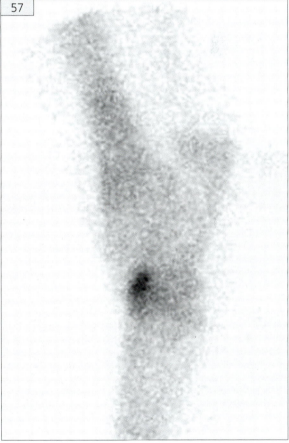

2.57 Lateral scintigraphic image (bone phase) of the horse with the slab fracture of the central tarsal bone shown in 2.55. There is focal increased radiopharmaceutical uptake in the cranial aspect of the central tarsal bone.

be performed to help diagnose occult or complicated fractures or ligamentous injuries.

Management/treatment

Horses should initially be placed in a Robert Jones bandage with a lateral splint that extends from the hoof to the thigh (see Splinting and casting). A second plantar splint from the hoof to the proximal tuber calcis should be placed (**2.58**). If materials are available (i.e. aluminum rods or heated and bent polyvinyl chloride staves), a cranial splint from the hoof to the proximal tibia will provide additional stability. Any type of bandaging and splinting of an unstable hock fracture in an adult horse rarely provides much comfort, only protection from further injury.

The type of treatment for tarsal bone fractures depends on the bone that is injured, the configuration of the fracture, and the intended use of the horse. Slab fractures can be repaired with lag screw fixation. Tarsal luxations without fractures, which can be successfully reduced, can be managed with external coaptation. Major fractures with gross instability are difficult to manage long term without internal fixation (**2.59**).

Olecranon fractures

Key point

- A caudal splint that holds the carpus in extension will make horses with olecranon fractures much more comfortable.

Definition/overview

Fractures of the olecranon have been categorized into one of five fracture types based on location (**2.60**) and configuration.[52,53]

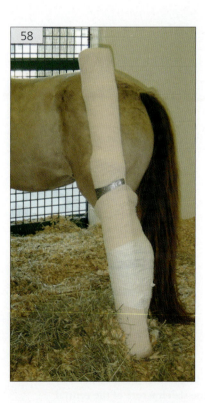

2.58 A horse with a Robert Jones bandage and lateral and plantar splints placed for stabilization of a displaced tarsal fracture.

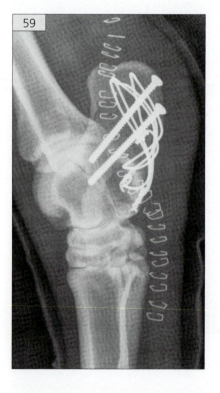

2.59 Surgical repair of the miniature horse with a calcaneal fracture in 2.54.

Etiology/pathogenesis

Direct trauma is the most common etiology for sustaining an olecranon fracture; most horses have history of a kick or a fall. The pull of the triceps inserting on the olecranon process can result in marked proximal displacement of complete fractures (**2.61**).

Clinical features

Horses with a displaced fracture of the olecranon process usually present with a dropped elbow stance and flexed carpus (**2.62**). They are severely lame (greater than or equal to grade 4 out of 5), have difficulty advancing the limb forward, and are unable to bear weight on the limb. Many horses with an ulnar fracture, including a mildly displaced olecranon fracture, can stand squarely

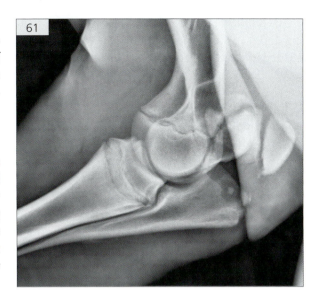

2.61 Medial to lateral radiograph of a horse with an olecranon fracture demonstrating marked proximal displacement of the fracture fragment due to the pull of the triceps apparatus.

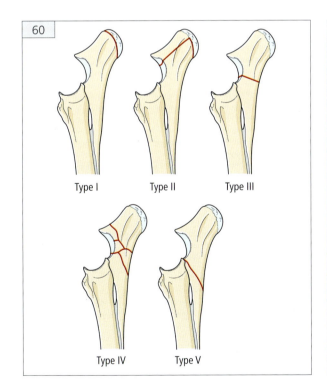

Type I   Type II   Type III

Type IV   Type V

2.60 Categorization of olecranon fractures as they would be identified on a lateral radiograph.

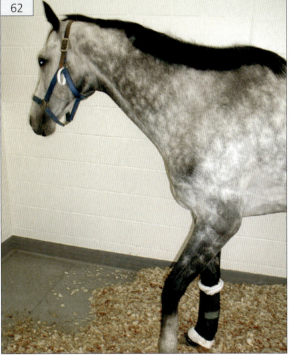

2.62 A horse with a dropped elbow stance and flexed carpus due to an olecranon fracture. (Courtesy Dr Murray Brown)

on the limb and bear weight. Moderate to severe swelling and occasionally crepitus may be noted. Pain is elicited by direct palpation and/or manipulation of the elbow joint.

Differential diagnosis
Radial nerve injury; humeral fracture; scapular fracture; proximal radius fracture.

Diagnosis
A thorough history and physical examination, combined with radiographs of the elbow, are required to make an accurate diagnosis. Diagnosis is nearly always possible with a single radiographic projection. The limb should be extended by an assistant and the radiograph taken in a medial to lateral direction with a second assistant holding the cassette. In young foals, there can be confusion about the appearance of proximal physis of the olecranon process. If possible, the radiographic appearance of the affected olecranon process should be compared with that of the contralateral olecranon process. In foals without an obvious fracture, the possibility of joint infection must always be considered.

Management/treatment
Horses with loss of triceps function will not be able to fix their limb in extension. In these horses, considerable relief is provided by applying a lightly padded bandage with a caudal splint extending from the ground to the proximal aspect of the olecranon (see Splinting and casting). With this splint, the horse can keep the carpus in extension and bear weight quite well (**2.63**). The splint gives the horse a 'post' to stand on, allowing it to use the limb for balance.

A displaced fracture is best treated with internal fixation. It is essential to recommend surgery for management of all displaced fractures that are proximal to the radial joint surface. Many of these horses become fairly comfortable quickly without surgery, but most will develop a painful non-union. Minimally displaced fractures distal to the joint can sometimes be treated conservatively in adult horses. In foals, minimally displaced fractures at or below the joint can usually be managed without surgery.[52–55] Horses have a good prognosis for soundness following internal fixation of an ulnar fracture.

Radial fractures
Key point
- Always have a high index of suspicion for radial fractures in any lame horse coming off a pasture with any wound in the antebrachial region.
- Superficial wounds should never be dismissed.
- The horse's lameness can improve quickly even though there remains enormous risk for catastrophic failure of the bone.

Definition/overview
Fractures of the radius can occur in any configuration, but usually affect the mid- or distal diaphyseal region (**2.64**). The most common fractures are non-displaced, minimally displaced, or comminuted.[53,56]

Etiology/pathogenesis
Radius fractures usually occur secondary to external trauma, most notably a kick from another horse. Often horses will sustain a kick to the medial aspect of the distal radius when fighting or playing with other horses.

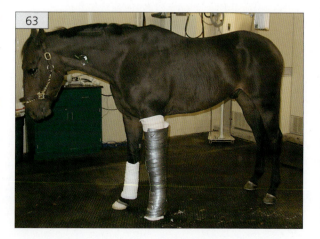

2.63 A horse with an olecranon fracture stabilized preoperatively by a full limb bandage and caudal splint in order to lock the carpus in extension.

Clinical features

Non-displaced fractures are one of the most important differentials to consider in a horse developing an acute, severe lameness while out at pasture. If a horse has any type of abrasion or laceration over the distal antebrachium, radiographs should be taken, especially if the horse seems disproportionately lame for the type of wound that is evident. It is quite common for owners to treat what appears to be a minor wound and turn the horse back out in a day or two when the lameness improves; this can be catastrophic. When in doubt, always recommend radiography of horses with wounds over the radius (**2.65**). Although some horses will have local pain, the presence of a superficial wound can make such an assessment difficult. Radiographs are essential.

Complete displaced fractures of the radius can occur in numerous configurations and many can be open.

Differential diagnosis

Septic carpal canal; subsolar abscess; cellulitis of the antebrachium; other fractures.

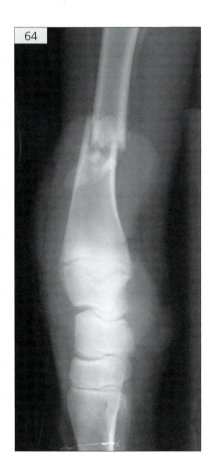

2.64 Lateromedial radiograph of a transverse, mildly comminuted fracture of the mid-diaphysis of the radius.

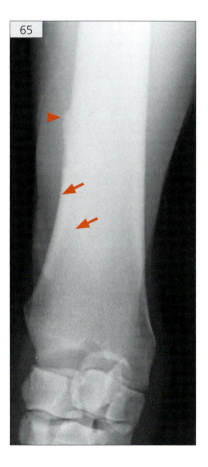

2.65 Craniocaudal radiograph highlighting a non-displaced fracture of the distal medial radius (arrows). Note the periosteal reaction (arrowhead).

Diagnosis

Diagnosis can be based on a thorough history, physical examination, and radiographic examination in most horses. If a non-displaced radial fracture is suspected, lameness examination, including perineural anesthesia, should not be performed. Nuclear scintigraphy can be performed to determine whether there is increased uptake present in the radius, which would be suggestive of a fracture.

Management/treatment

A simple Robert Jones bandage with splints extending from the ground to the elbow provides inadequate stabilization of a radial fracture because it fails to prevent abduction of the distal limb. This type of splint may actually make the injury worse by applying a heavy weight to the limb with a fulcrum (i.e. the top of the bandage) at the fracture site. The reason for this is that the extensor and flexor muscle groups lie on the lateral aspect of radius and when the radius is no longer intact, these muscles act as abductors of the distal limb, leading to penetration of the skin on the medial aspect of the limb with the fractured bone. Therefore, to prevent abduction, a lateral splint should be extended from the ground to the triceps/thorax (**2.66**) (see Splinting and casting).

The only treatment option for displaced radial fractures is open reduction and internal fixation[53,56] with two plates, but results in adult horses with this type of fracture are not good. In foals, radius fractures can be treated successfully. Neonates (<30 days old) with simple mid-diaphyseal fractures can be successfully managed with a single cranial plate.

Non-displaced radial fractures should be treated with strict stall confinement for at least 3–4 months with serial radiographs to evaluate fracture healing.[57] There is a great deal of variation in the radiographic appearance of non-displaced radial fractures. Some appear to be long, incomplete, spiral or oblique fractures and these probably have more risk of catastrophic dehiscence even when the horse is confined to a stall. In such cases, consideration should be given to maintaining long lateral and caudal splints in combination with a means of preventing the horse from lying down. The most common technique is to use a breakable tether attached to cross ties or a rope or wire running across the stall well above the horse's head.

Tibial fractures
Key point

- If a Thoroughbred racehorse presents off the track with severe hindlimb lameness and no palpable effusion or noticeable swelling, a lameness examination and perineural anesthesia should NOT be performed. A thorough examination of the foot, as well as radiographs of the tibia and/or nuclear scintigraphy, should be completed first.

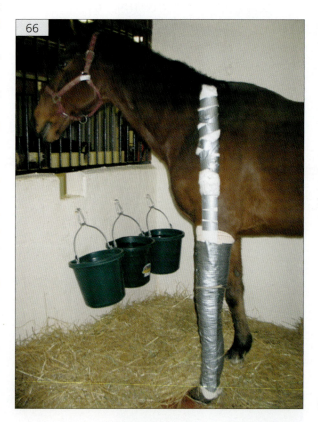

2.66 A horse demonstrating lateral splint application to stabilize the forelimb after fracture of the radius (in this case an incomplete, non-displaced fracture). The lateral splint prevents abaxial displacement and extends from the ground to the scapula.

Definition/overview

Fractures of the tibia can occur in any configuration including comminuted (**2.67**), proximal or distal physeal fractures (**2.68**), non-displaced fractures, and stress fractures.[58–61]

Etiology/pathogenesis

Tibial fractures usually occur secondary to external trauma. In addition to kicks, catastrophic missteps at speed and falls can also result in tibial fractures.

A common configuration of tibial fractures in foals is the proximal Salter–Harris II fracture in which the fracture breaks transversely across the physis from the medial side and then down the lateral metaphysis (**2.68**). This occurs when the foal is kicked on the lateral side of the stifle while bearing weight on the limb. Stress fractures of the tibia in racehorses are due to cyclic fatigue and can occur anywhere along the length of the bone.

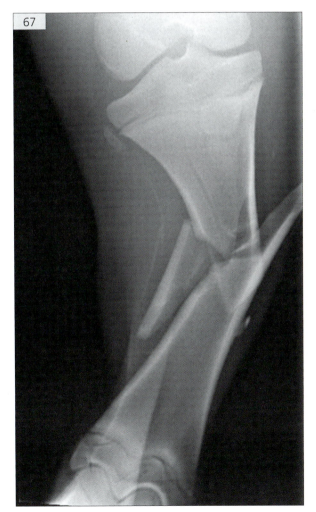

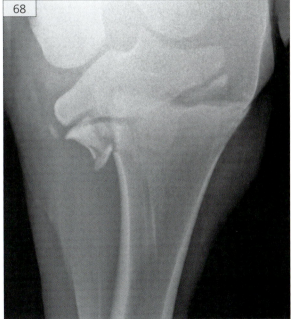

2.68 Caudocranial radiograph of a Salter–Harris type II fracture of the proximal physis of the tibia. Note the lateral metaphyseal spike.

2.67 Caudocranial radiograph of a comminuted, displaced fracture of the mid-diaphysis of the tibia.

Clinical features

Many tibial fractures are comminuted, especially in adults, but others will be oblique or transverse in configuration. Most are closed, but some may be open, especially on the medial side. Horses present with a severe lameness (greater than or equal to grade 4 out of 5) and pronounced swelling around the tibia. Instability and crepitus are often present as well. Horses with tibial stress fractures may be lame at a walk or trot (greater than or equal to grade 3 out of 5), but many will improve rapidly and are returned to work too quickly. Occasionally, direct palpation of the tibia directly over the stress fracture will elicit pain.

Differential diagnosis

Stifle/hock injury/sepsis; cellulitis of the gaskin region; subsolar abscess.

Diagnosis

Diagnosis in most horses can be made using the combination of a thorough history, physical examination, and radiographic examination. If a non-displaced tibial stress fracture is suspected, lameness examination, including perineural anesthesia, should NOT be performed. Nuclear scintigraphy is both sensitive and specific for tibial stress fractures and should be performed if a definitive diagnosis is desired (**2.69**).[62]

Management/treatment

A simple Robert Jones bandage with splints ending at the stifle is inadequate to stabilize a tibial fracture because it prevents abduction of the distal limb. This type of splint may, in fact, make matters worse by applying additional weight to the distal limb. The digital extensors and tarsal flexors on the lateral aspect of tibia tend to direct the fracture ends medially, where there is little protective soft tissue. This can result in an open fracture. To limit abduction, a straight lateral splint should be applied from the ground to the thigh/pelvis over a moderately padded bandage (**2.70**). If available, molded cranial or caudal splints (bent conduit or thick-walled polyvinyl chloride pipe staves) can also be placed (see Splinting and casting).

The only treatment option for horses with a displaced tibial fracture is open reduction and internal fixation.[58,61] Success is largely dependent on the horse's age and the fracture configuration. Tibial fractures are much easier to manage in smaller and younger patients (**2.71**). Comminuted fractures carry a worse prognosis than simple oblique or transverse fractures.

Horses with tibial stress fractures should be taken out of work for at least 3–4 months with serial radiographs/scintigrams used to evaluate fracture healing.

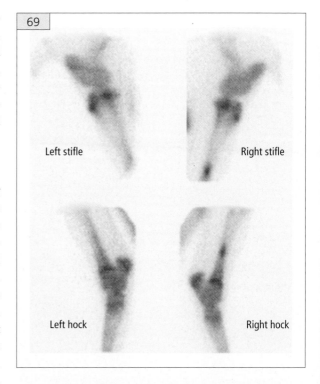

2.69 Lateral scintigraphic views (bone phase) of the left and right tibias demonstrating an area of focal, intense, increased radiopharmaceutical uptake in the mid-diaphysis of the right tibia due to a tibial stress fracture.

Humeral fractures

Key point

- The radial nerve courses across the distal diaphysis of the humerus and it can be injured by the fracture ends. Because the clinical appearance of the fracture is similar to that of a radial nerve injury, it is difficult to determine this prior to surgery.

Definition/overview

Fractures of the humerus can occur in any configuration, but oblique or spiral fractures of the mid- and distal diaphysis are most common (**2.72**). Non-catastrophic fractures of the greater tubercle are also common.[59,63,64] Stress fractures of the humerus are an important injury in racehorses.

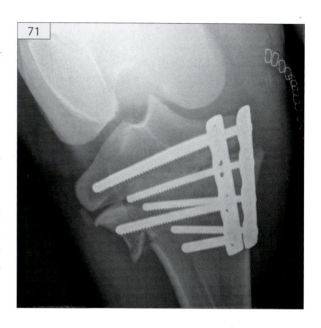

2.71 Surgical repair of the Salter-Harris type II fracture of the proximal physis of the tibia shown in 2.68. (Courtesy Dr Evita Busschers)

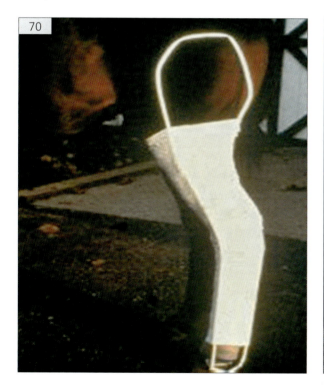

2.70 A horse with a lateral splint over a moderately padded bandage to stabilize a tibial fracture.

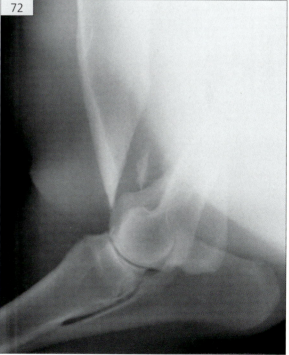

2.72 Medial to lateral radiograph of a horse with an oblique fracture of the distal diaphysis of the humerus.

Etiology/pathogenesis

In adult horses, humeral fractures occur most commonly as a result of a fall or working/racing on a pre-existing stress fracture. Fractures due to kicks can also occur, especially in foals.

Clinical features

Horses with diaphyseal fractures will present with a severe lameness (greater than or equal to grade 4 out of 5) and swelling present around the humerus and elbow (**2.73**). Crepitus may be palpable with limb manipulation, but it can be surprisingly difficult to appreciate in some cases. Most affected horses will present with a dropped elbow and flexed carpus. This may look similar to a radial nerve injury or an olecranon fracture, but the pain and location of the swelling help discriminate between these different types of injury. Most humeral fractures are long oblique or spiral fractures and they often have comminution along the fracture margins. Because of the forces exerted on the fractured bone by the extensive overlying muscles, there is usually considerable overriding of fracture ends.

Differential diagnosis

Radial nerve paralysis; olecranon fracture; radial fracture; scapular fracture; brachial plexus avulsion.

Diagnosis

Diagnosis is based on a thorough history, physical examination, and radiographic examination. Good-quality radiographs can be difficult to obtain under field conditions, but diagnostic images can almost always be obtained because the fractures are displaced. Nuclear scintigraphy is both sensitive and specific for humeral stress fractures and should be considered the most important diagnostic tool (**2.74**).

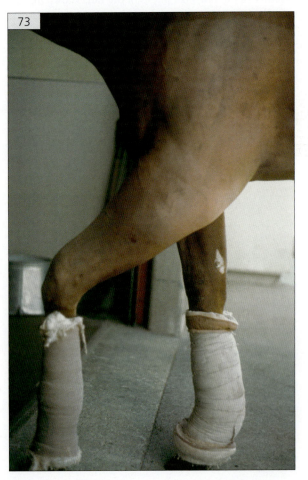

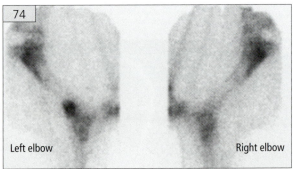

Left elbow   Right elbow

2.74 Lateral scintigraphic views (bone phase) of the left and right humerus demonstrating an area of focal, intense, increased radiopharmaceutical uptake in the distal diaphysis of the left humerus because of a humeral stress fracture.

2.73 Severe soft tissue swelling surrounding the elbow, a dropped elbow stance, and flexed carpus in a horse with a humeral fracture. (Courtesy Dr Murray Brown)

Management/treatment

There is no useful form of external coaptation to stabilize a humeral fracture. Because of the heavy musculature surrounding the humerus, minimal medial to lateral displacement will occur and very few will become open fractures.

Successful internal fixation of displaced humeral fractures in any animal older than a yearling has not been achieved to date, so euthanasia is a reasonable choice. However, some humeral fractures are adequately stabilized by the surrounding musculature and will heal with extended stall rest.[65] Humeral fractures in foals and yearlings can be successfully repaired with internal fixation using either bone plates and cortical screws, interlocking nails, or intramedullary pins.[63]

Racehorses with stress fractures respond well to being removed from hard exercise for at least 3–4 months.

Femoral fractures
Key points

- Femoral fractures are repairable in smaller horses, but there is still no successful technique for stabilization of displaced fractures in adult horses.
- Because of the massive musculature and an inability to apply a pressure bandage, hemorrhage and surgical site infections are major postoperative complications.

Definition/overview

Fractures of the femur can occur in any configuration. Diaphyseal fractures, often comminuted, occur in horses of all ages (**2.75**). Foals may sustain proximal physeal fractures (Salter–Harris I or II). Salter–Harris II fractures of the distal femur can occur in older horses because that particular physis is late to close (**2.76**). The metaphyseal spike of the Salter–Harris II fracture can be either cranial or caudal.[66,67]

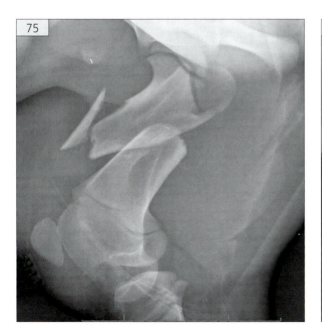

2.75 Medial to lateral radiograph of a foal with a mid-diaphyseal femoral fracture.

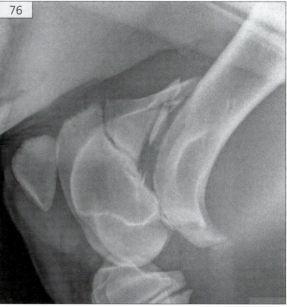

2.76 Medial to lateral radiograph of a foal with a distal diaphyseal Salter–Harris type II femoral fracture.

Etiology/pathogenesis

Femoral fractures in foals often are caused by kicks from mares. In horses of all ages, femoral fractures may occur during falls or other trauma. Stress fractures occur but are relatively uncommon compared with humeral or pelvic stress fractures. Fractures of the third trochanter are one of the few non-catastrophic fractures involving this bone.

Clinical features

Most horses with a femoral fracture will present with a severe lameness (greater than or equal to grade 4 out of 5) and massive swelling of the thigh (**2.77**). Crepitus may be palpated when the distal limb is manipulated, but the hemorrhage and muscle mass of the thigh may make it difficult to touch the bone ends together. Because of the extensive hemorrhage and pain, adult horses with femoral fractures may present in shock. Because of the forces exerted by the overlying muscle on the bone, there is usually considerable overriding of the fracture ends. Fractures of the femoral head or neck can also occur in young horses (**2.78**). These horses usually present with a severe lameness (greater than or equal to grade 4 out of 5), but the swelling is subtle. The typical appearance of a displaced proximal femoral fracture is that the entire limb is externally rotated and the point of the hock is clearly higher in the fractured limb. Pain and crepitus may be elicited when pressure over the greater trochanter of the femur is combined with manipulation.

Differential diagnosis

Severe soft tissue injury to the stifle; luxation of the coxofemoral joint; severe myositis; coxofemoral or stifle joint sepsis (foals).

Diagnosis

Diagnosis is based on a thorough history and a physical examination. Radiographs of the femur are difficult to obtain in an adult horse because of the amount of musculature as well as the degree of soft tissue trauma that is usually present. Radiographs of the distal diaphysis and epiphyseal region can be obtained standing to determine if the femur is fractured, but detailed

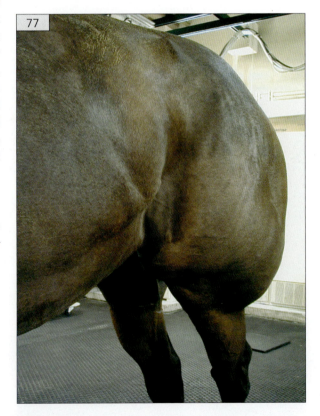

2.77 A horse with a right femoral fracture demonstrating severe soft tissue swelling of the thigh.

information of a proximal or mid-diaphyseal fracture is impossible without the horse being under general anesthesia (**2.79**). In cases of femoral head or neck fracture, the horse must be anesthetized to obtain diagnostic radiographs. Ultrasonographic examination can also be diagnostic of injuries in the proximal femur or coxofemoral region and, unlike radiographic examination, can readily be performed in the unanesthetized patient.

Management/treatment

There is no adequate form of external coaptation that can be applied to the limb to help stabilize a femoral fracture. Because of the amount of muscle surrounding the femur, minimal medial to lateral displacement will occur and very few will be open. Displaced femoral fractures in adult horses cannot be repaired with current techniques, so euthanasia is justified.

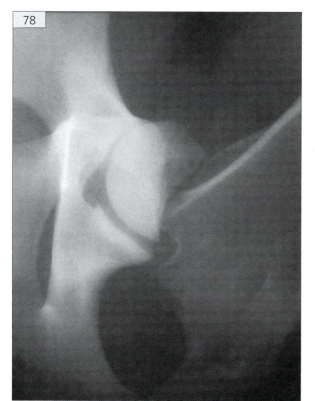

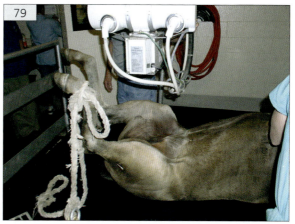

2.79 A horse under general anesthesia in dorsal recumbency to obtain radiographs of the proximal femur and pelvis.

2.78 Ventrodorsal radiograph of the coxofemoral joint of a foal with a femoral head fracture.

The prognosis for foals with internal fixation (double plating or a locking intramedullary nail) is reasonably good and success is possible in yearlings and smaller horses (**2.80, 2.81**).[67–70] Severe hemorrhage and incisional problems are major complications following femoral fracture repair. Proximal physeal fractures can be repaired using lag screw fixation, but the repair is difficult and osteoarthritis of the coxofemoral joint may develop.[71] Unlike the humerus, conservative management of femoral fractures is not usually successful. Fatal hemorrhage may occur. Adult horses usually develop contralateral laminitis or severe decubital sores. Foals will rapidly develop severe tarsal varus deformities in the contralateral limb.

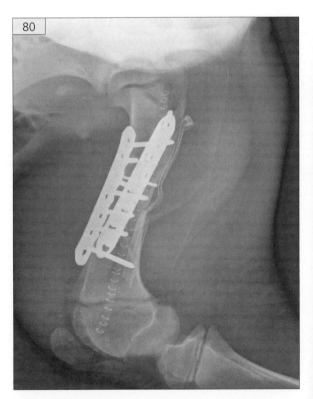

2.80 Surgical repair of the mid-diaphyseal femoral fracture in the foal in 2.75.

2.81 Caudal to cranial radiographic view of the surgical repair of the distal diaphyseal Salter–Harris type II femoral fracture in the foal in 2.76.

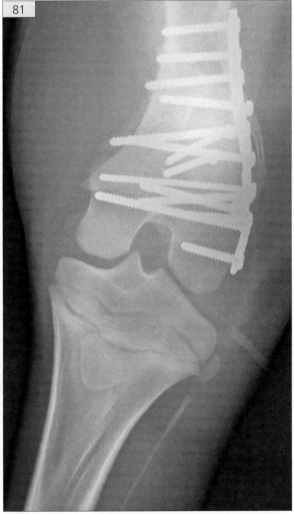

Pelvic fractures
Key point

- Horses with pelvic fractures are often severely lame initially; however, most of these horses will become acceptably comfortable within a few days. Therefore, any decision to euthanize the horse should not be made in haste. In one study 77% of horses with pelvic fractures that were not euthanized immediately had a successful outcome.[72]

Definition/overview
Fractures of any of the bones in the pelvis, including the ilium, ischium, pubic symphysis, and acetabulum.[60,67,72,73]

Etiology/pathogenesis
Most fractures of the pelvis are traumatically induced and can occur as the result of a fall, getting kicked, or running into a stationary object. These types of injuries can occur in horses of any age, but are most common in weanlings and yearlings (**2.82**). Stress fractures of the pelvis, typically involving the ilium, can also occur and are relatively common in racehorses (especially young fillies) (**2.83**). Although not technically a pelvic fracture, horses with coxofemoral luxations can have similar

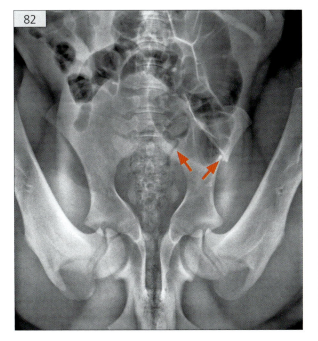

2.82 Ventrodorsal radiograph of the pelvis of a foal with a fracture of the left ilium (arrows).

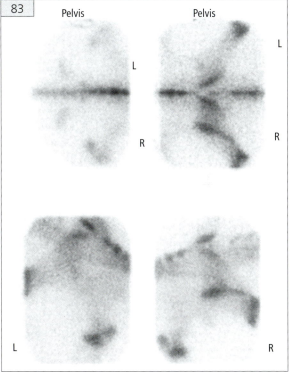

2.83 Dorsal (top) and dorsal oblique (bottom) scintigraphic views (bone phase) demonstrating an area of focal increased radiopharmaceutical uptake in the right ilium due to an ilial stress fracture.

presentations as those with pelvic fractures (**2.84**). However, these injuries are rare in horses and are seen more commonly in ponies and miniature horses. They can occur due to falls, attacks by other horses, or as the horse is struggling to free a trapped limb or upward-fixated patella. Horses and foals have also been reported to sustain coxofemoral luxations while wearing full-limb hindlimb casts.

Clinical features

The most common sites for pelvic fractures include the shaft of the ilium, the acetabulum, the pubic symphysis, and the tuber coxae ('knocked-down hip'). The degree of lameness varies depending on the location, the severity of fracture displacement, and the chronicity of the injury. In the acute stages, most horses are severely lame (greater or equal to grade 4 out of 5). In the more chronic stages, the degree of lameness tends to improve unless the acetabulum is involved in the fracture.

There may be asymmetry of external landmarks such as the tuber coxae, tuber ischii, tuber sacrale, and greater trochanter. In the acute stages, this asymmetry may be obscured due to the presence of soft tissue swelling or hematoma formation, but there may be palpable crepitus in the area when the limb is manipulated or the horse is walked. Externally, the swelling is often located in the region of the ventral medial thigh. In the chronic stages, atrophy of the gluteal musculature on the affected side occurs (**2.85**).

Occasionally, the fracture fragment may lacerate a major artery in the pelvic area (usually the internal iliac artery); these horses may present in hypovolemic shock, which can progress to death due to acute blood loss.

Horses with coxofemoral luxations tend to carry the affected limb externally rotated. The point of the hock is higher on the affected side than the normal side because most coxofemoral luxations are in the cranio-dorsal direction.

Differential diagnosis

Femoral head and/or neck fracture; coxofemoral joint arthritis; coxofemoral joint sepsis; greater trochanter fracture.

Diagnosis

A thorough history and physical examination can be used to localize the injury to the pelvis. Careful evaluation for any external swelling or pelvic area asymmetry should be performed. A pelvic examination per rectum should be performed with the horse standing; it is also helpful to have an assistant manipulate the limb on the affected side and to move the horse forward a few steps during the examination if possible. Pelvic examination per rectum is performed to identify any asymmetry, hematoma formation, or crepitus that can be palpated in the region of the pubic symphysis, ischium, or acetabulum. Ultrasonographic examination is useful for detecting displaced fractures and has the benefit of not requiring general anesthesia.[74] Limited radiographic views can be obtained with the horse standing[75], but the absence of a fracture on these views does not rule one out. A more thorough radiographic examination can be performed with the horse in dorsal recumbency under general anesthesia (**2.79**). However, because of the large size of the adult horse, radiographic examination even with the horse under general anesthesia is still an insensitive modality for diagnosis of pelvic fractures. If the horse does have a pelvic fracture, there is also the risk of

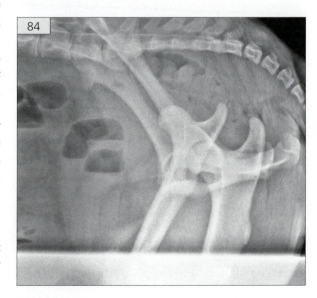

2.84 Lateral radiograph of the pelvis of a miniature horse with dorsal luxation of the left coxofemoral joint.

further injury at the fracture site during recovery from general anesthesia. Due to these limitations, nuclear scintigraphy may be the preferred method to diagnose pelvic fractures because the general location and presence of a fracture can be identified without having to anesthetize the horse (**2.83**).

Management/treatment

Because of the amount of musculature surrounding the pelvis, open reduction and internal fixation is not possible in the adult horse. Internal fixation has been reported for the repair of pelvic fractures of foals (**2.86**) and for reduction of coxofemoral luxations in ponies and miniature horses. The treatment for most adult horses with pelvic fractures is box stall rest for 3–4 months combined with analgesic therapy and support of the contralateral limb and foot. Some horses are severely painful in the acute period and may require judicious use of epidural analgesia or continuous rate infusions of analgesics such as butorphanol, lidocaine, or ketamine (see Chapter 14).

In general, the prognosis for horses with pelvic fractures depends on the degree of displacement. Horses with non-displaced fractures of any area of the pelvis (even the acetabulum) have the potential to successfully heal the fracture and resume athletic careers with rest alone. However, horses with displaced fractures do not heal as well and have a poor prognosis for survival due to the development of osteoarthritis of the coxofemoral joint and the potential for the development of contralateral limb laminitis. Mares with pelvic fractures, especially those that are displaced, are at risk of experiencing dystocia due to resultant narrowing of the birth canal.

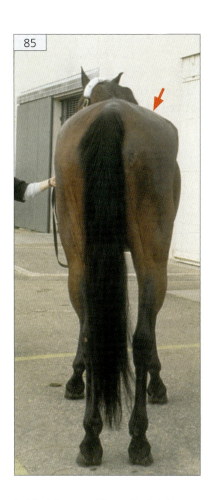

2.85 A horse with marked right gluteal muscle atrophy.

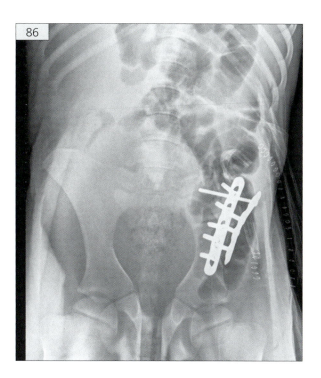

2.86 Surgical repair of the fracture of the left ilium in the foal in 2.82.

Skull fractures
Key points
- The prognosis for horses with skull fractures varies greatly depending on the location of the fracture.
- Horses with rostral mandibular and maxillary fractures have a good prognosis for survival and bone healing and surgical repair of these fractures is generally straightforward.
- Horses with skull fractures not involving the cranial vault or eye have a good prognosis; however, a sunken appearance in the area of the fracture may result (**2.87**).
- The prognosis for horses with neurologic involvement is less favorable, and these horses are often left with residual neurologic deficits.

Definition/overview
Fractures sustained to any area of the skull, including the maxilla and mandible.[76–78]

Etiology/pathogenesis
Most skull fractures are traumatic in origin. They can occur as the result of a kick, running into a stationary object, being startled while chewing on an object, or rearing up and falling over backwards.

Clinical features
Horses can present with a wide range of clinical signs depending on the type of trauma that has occurred and which bone(s) is/are fractured. Horses that flip over backwards often fracture areas of the poll such as the nuchal crest, paramastoid processes, and occipital condyles.

Cerebral injury can occur in any horse that sustains head trauma (see Chapter 7). These horses may be lethargic (**2.88**) or they may show obvious neurologic signs such as a head tilt. Horses with head trauma can also sustain more serious skull fractures of the basisphenoid or basioccipital bone due to the pull of the rectus capitis ventralis and the longus capitis muscles on these bones. Horses with these injuries often have signs of cranial nerve (CN) damage, specifically CNs V, VII, VIII, IX, and X. This can manifest as dyspnea, dysphagia, loss of facial sensation, and signs of vestibular disease. Horses with these fractures may also suffer from acute fatal hemorrhage.

Horses that sustain fractures to the maxilla or mandible may have malaligned incisors and can be dysphagic or anorexic. These horses may also drool excessively and are sometimes unable to keep their tongue in their mouth. Occasionally, the fracture initially goes unnoticed; these horses can develop dehydration and electrolyte abnormalities because of salivary loss.

Horses that sustain direct trauma to the head, such as a kick, often have fractures of the nasal, frontal, and maxillary bones. These fractures are often depression fractures and can cause damage to the eye, brain, nasal passages, and sinuses. There is often a laceration associated with these fractures (**2.89**). It can be difficult to palpate the fracture acutely due to extensive soft tissue swelling. If the fracture communicates with the nasal passages or sinuses, subcutaneous emphysema is usually palpable and epistaxis may be evident.

Differential diagnosis
Primary neurologic disease; ethmoid hematoma; guttural pouch mycoses; nasal passage or sinus neoplasia.

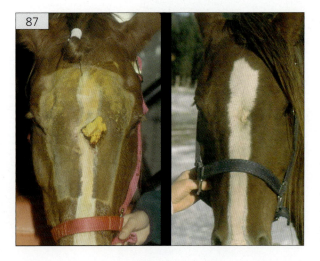

2.87 A horse with a wood foreign body that was impaled through the nasal bone (left). The same horse 3 months after foreign body removal and wound debridement (right).

Diagnosis

A thorough history and physical examination (including a complete neurologic and ophthalmologic examination) should be performed on these horses. Careful palpation of the affected area can be used to identify some fractures, although soft tissue swelling may prevent diagnosis in acute cases. Care must be taken to thoroughly assess the neurologic status of the horse prior to administering sedation. Radiographic examination, including multiple oblique views, should be performed to identify the location and extent of the fracture(s). Intraoral views should be taken of fractures of the rostral maxilla or mandible (**2.90**). Depending on the location of the fracture, skull radiographs can be difficult to interpret. CT or MRI may be beneficial in defining the exact location and extent of injury

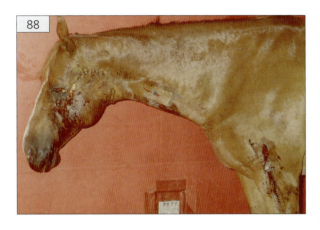

2.88 A horse that sustained severe head trauma after being hit by a truck. No sedatives were administered to this horse; note its lethargic state.

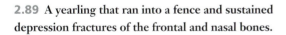

2.89 A yearling that ran into a fence and sustained depression fractures of the frontal and nasal bones.

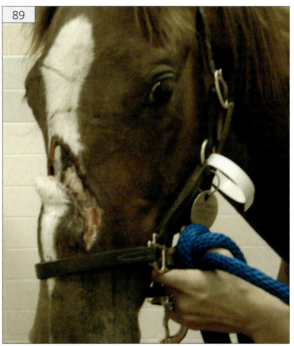

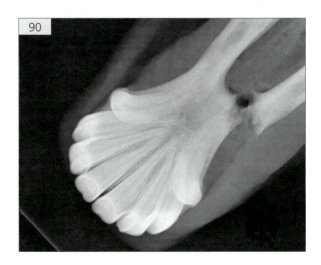

2.90 Intraoral ventrodorsal radiograph of the mandible demonstrating a rostral mandibular fracture of the left interdental space.

and can be performed immediately prior to surgery (**2.91**); however, the benefits of these modalities must be weighed against the risks of general anesthesia, especially if the horse has neurologic deficits. If the sinuses are involved in the fracture, or if a head tilt is present, endoscopy of the upper airway and guttural pouches should be performed. If the fracture is suspected to involve the cranial vault, cerebrospinal fluid (CSF) should be obtained for cytologic evaluation and bacterial culture and sensitivity testing.

Management/treatment

The management of these cases varies depending on the location of the fracture. Initial therapy should consist of stabilizing the patient systemically and addressing any neurologic abnormalities. Horses with neurologic signs should be treated for potential brain injury (see Chapter 7). Emergency treatment for these horses should include anti-inflammatory therapy (phenylbutazone, or flunixin meglumine) and administration of neuroprotective agents such as hypertonic saline (7.5%, 4 ml/kg) or magnesium sulfate (100 mg/kg).[79]

Horses with hemorrhage should receive isotonic crystalloid fluids IV, and in some cases colloid therapy (i.e. plasma) and/or hypertonic saline if the hemorrhage has ceased and the horse is showing signs of shock. If the blood loss is estimated to be >25% of the horse's blood volume, or if the horse's PCV is <0.2 l/l (20%), a blood transfusion should be considered (see Chapter 4).

Horses with significant CN deficits, fractures into the nasal passages, or severe hemorrhage obstructing the nasal passages may require a tracheostomy if they are in acute respiratory distress (see Chapter 3).

All external lacerations should be thoroughly cleaned and debrided and tetanus prophylaxis administered. Systemic antimicrobial treatment is also recommended, as skull fractures are often open and can communicate with the oral cavity, cranial vault, or nasal passages.

Although skull fracture patients do require emergency treatment and stabilization, the fracture itself does not usually require immediate surgical repair. Fractures of the rostral mandible and maxilla can be repaired with the horse standing or under general anesthesia once the horse is stable.

With other types of skull fracture, the size and location of the fractured bone and the degree of instability present will often determine whether the fracture requires surgical repair or if the fragments of bone will be removed. If fragments of bone are too small to repair, the periosteum can be sutured over the defect to provide a more rigid support and provide cells for bone defect healing.

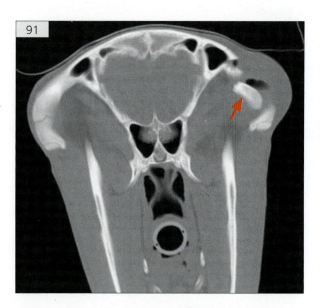

2.91 Computed tomographic frontal image of the caudal aspect of the skull highlighting a depression fracture of the zygomatic process of the temporal bone (arrow).

Infection
Septic physitis and epiphysitis
Key points

- Septic osteomyelitis should be considered in any foal with an acute onset of lameness with or without septic arthritis.
- Radiographic examination is typically used to make the diagnosis; however, it may need to be repeated because of the lack of sensitivity in identifying early bone lysis.
- Early and aggressive treatment with appropriate antimicrobial drugs, as well as joint lavage and bone debridement (if indicated), is important.

Definition/overview

Septic arthritis and osteomyelitis are more common musculoskeletal emergencies in foals. These infections are classified as:[80]

- S-type involving septic synovial membrane and fluid and typically affecting foals <1 week old.
- E-type involving the bone subjacent to the articular cartilage (articular epiphyseal complex). The distal femur, talus, radius (proximal and distal), and tibia (proximal and distal) are affected most commonly. Foals are often several weeks old, may have multiple joints involved, and frequently have a history of failure of passive transfer of immunity, pneumonia, or diarrhea.
- P-type involving a long bone physis, with the distal physis of the third metacarpal/metatarsal bone, radius, and tibia being most commonly involved, although any physis can be infected including the vertebrae and ribs. Affected foals can be weeks to months old and without a previous history of illness. P-type infections can occur with or without joint involvement.

Etiology/pathogenesis

Septic arthritis and osteomyelitis in foals are often associated with a history of failure of passive transfer of maternal antibodies, diarrhea, pneumonia, or umbilical remnant infection. Infection is thought to occur from hematogenous spread following a period of bacteremia. Common infecting organisms include *Streptococcus* spp., *Rhodococcus* spp., *Actinobacillus* spp., *Escherichia coli*, and *Salmonella* spp.[80]

Clinical features

Foals with septic arthritis or osteomyelitis are typically lame and have swelling (periarticular edema and/or synovial effusion) associated with the infection site. Heat and pain on palpation is common. Foals with S- and E-type lesions have lameness, effusion, and fever. Foals with P-type infections often have a history of mild lameness, which acutely becomes more severe and associated with swelling. These foals may not have synovial effusion, but there is periarticular edema and they are sensitive to palpation of the affected area.[80]

Differential diagnosis

Fracture; subsolar abscess.

Diagnosis

Radiographic examination of the affected areas is important to identify and monitor bone lysis. Foals with E-type infections have subcondral lysis and with P-type infections have lysis in the physeal region. Sonographic examination is useful for evaluating the volume and echogeneticity of the synovial fluid, the thickness of the synovial membrane, and bone irregularity. Diagnosis of S- and E-type infections is confirmed using synovial fluid analysis (p. 159). A sample should be collected for bacterial culture and sensitivity testing. Foals with osteomyelitis typically have an extremely high fibrinogen concentration.

Management/treatment

Early treatment is important for a favorable outcome. Management consists of initial broad-spectrum antimicrobials delivered systemically (e.g. potassium penicillin or ampicillin) and locally (e.g. intra-articular injection and/or regional limb perfusion [p. 176] with amikacin). Antimicrobial drugs should ultimately be selected based on results of culture and sensitivity testing as well as response to treatment. Aminoglycoside plasma peak and trough concentrations should be monitored to ensure that therapeutic drug levels are being achieved when these drugs are given systemically (peak) and that the drug is being cleared adequately by the kidneys (trough). Aminoglycoside dose rate and frequency of administration should be altered based on the plasma peak and trough concentrations, respectively.

Joint lavage using a large volume of polyionic isotonic fluid is recommended early during the course of disease. Joint lavage should be performed with the foal under short-acting general anesthesia. Arthroscopy can facilitate joint lavage particularly if there is a great deal of fibrin. Bone debridement is indicated in some cases.

Analgesia is usually provided with NSAIDs (e.g. phenylbutazone, flunixin meglumine, or firocoxib). NSAIDs should be used in low doses and for only 2–3 days to avoid complications with toxicity and to monitor response of the foal to treatment. Butorphanol can be used if NSAIDs alone are insufficient. Renal function (plasma creatinine concentration) should be monitored in foals administered nephrotoxic drugs.

The prognosis is generally good for athletic performance with early and appropriate management.

Septic osteomyelitis of the third phalanx
Key point

- Horses with draining tracts of the sole or coronary band should have foot radiographs taken to determine if septic osteitis of the distal phalanx (or any other condition such as a fracture of the third phalanx) is present that may complicate treatment and affect prognosis.

Definition/overview

Inflammation of the distal phalanx caused by an infectious agent.[81]

Etiology/pathogenesis

Penetrating wounds of the sole, subsolar abscesses, hoof wall avulsions (**2.92**), soft tissue infections (**2.93**), third phalanx fractures, and chronic laminitis (**2.94**) can all lead to the development of septic osteitis of the third phalanx.[82,83] In foals, the condition is often hematogenous in origin.[84] Any condition that compromises the vascular supply to the third phalanx can lead to ischemic necrosis, abscessation, and eventual sequestration of the avascular bone fragment (**2.95**). Secondary sepsis of the distal interphalangeal joint can also develop.

Clinical features

Horses with septic osteitis usually have a moderate to severe, intermittent but recurrent lameness. They typically have palpably increased digital pulses compared with normal, heat in the affected hoof, and soft tissue swelling proximal to the coronary band. Most horses have a positive response to hoof testers. A draining tract may be present (**2.93, 2.94**), but is not always identified at the time of examination.

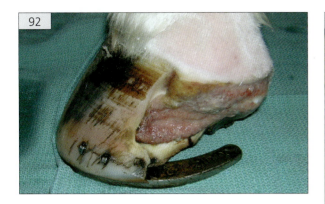

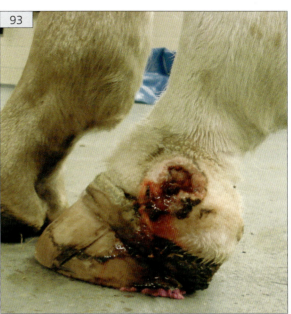

2.92 Hoof wall avulsion resulting in trauma to the wing of the third phalanx. (Courtesy Dr Patrick Colahan)

2.93 A horse with a chronic wound to the lateral coronary band that resulted in septic osteitis of the third phalanx.

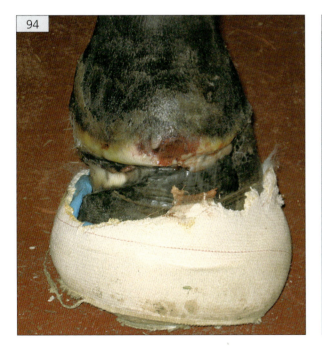

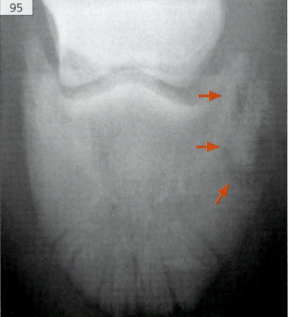

2.94 The foot of a horse with chronic laminitis and secondary septic osteitis of the third phalanx.

2.95 Dorsoventral radiograph of the foot of a horse with septic osteitis of the lateral wing of the third phalanx that resulted in the formation of a sequestrum (arrows).

Differential diagnosis

Subsolar abscess; third phalanx fracture; synovial sepsis (distal interphalangeal joint, navicular bursa, or digital flexor tendon sheath); navicular bone fracture; laminitis.

Diagnosis

The foot should be cleaned and carefully inspected to identify any defects caused by a penetrating wound. Gentle paring of the hoof wall or sole can be performed to identify a draining tract. Radiographs, especially dorsal proximopalmar/plantar distal oblique views at 60–65 degrees, are usually required to identify the presence of a lytic area or sequestered portion of the third phalanx (**2.95**). If a tract is found, contrast radiography or insertion of a malleable probe through the tract and then taking a radiograph may demonstrate the course of the penetrating object.

Management/treatment

The treatment of choice is surgical debridement and curettage of all the infected soft tissue and necrotic bone (**2.96**). This is performed through the sole or hoof wall and can be done standing under local anesthesia or with the horse under general anesthesia (**2.97**). Samples for bacterial culture and sensitivity testing should be obtained to direct future antimicrobial therapy; however, most infections are polymicrobial so initial antimicrobial therapy should be broad spectrum. Anaerobic infections are especially common in the foot so the regimen should include antimicrobials with good anaerobic coverage (e.g. metronidazole or high doses of penicillin). Regional limb perfusion with antimicrobial drugs may be performed in addition to, or in place of, systemic therapy (see Regionial limb perfusion). Polymethylmethacrylate beads (p. 179) or collagen sponges impregnated with antimicrobial drugs can also be placed into the surgically created defect.

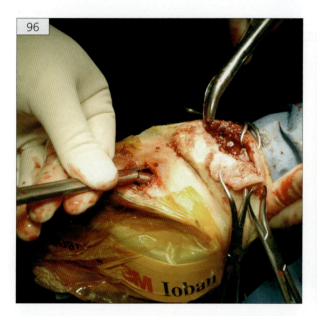

2.96 Surgical debridement of septic osteitis of the third phalanx caused by a chronic wound to the coronary band (same horse as in 2.93).

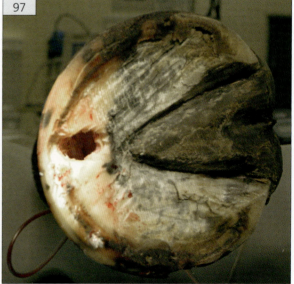

2.97 Debridement of a sequestrum of the third phalanx through the sole.

Tendons and ligaments
Traumatic disruption of the suspensory apparatus
Key point

- Some horses that sustain this injury stretch the digital vessels due to the distal displacement of the fetlock and lose perfusion to the distal limb.
- Horses with distal sesamoidean ligament injury are extremely difficult to manage conservatively.

Definition/overview
Displaced fractures of both proximal sesamoid bones, disruption of the suspensory ligament, or avulsion of the distal sesamoidean ligaments can result in loss of fetlock stability.[32,85]

Etiology/pathogenesis
This injury is almost exclusively seen in racehorses and predominantly in Thoroughbreds. Disruption of the suspensory apparatus may occur more often when the horse's digital flexors are fatigued, resulting in a greater load on the suspensory apparatus. The injury is career ending and life-threatening.[86,87] The forelimbs are much more commonly affected than the hindlimbs.

Clinical features
Horses with disruption of the suspensory apparatus present with severe lameness and the fetlock drops as the horse places weight on the limb (**2.98**). There is obvious local swelling and pain immediately after the injury.

Differential diagnosis
Condylar fracture of the third metacarpus/metatarsus (especially with an axial sesamoid fracture); comminuted fracture of the proximal phalanx; disruption of the superficial digital flexor tendon.

Diagnosis
A physical examination and radiographs can be used to diagnose this injury. In cases of biaxial proximal sesamoid bone fractures, the diagnosis is obvious radiographically (**2.99**). Horses with either disruption

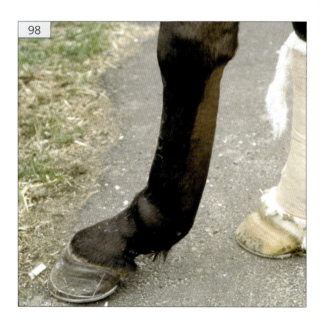

2.98 Horse with a 'dropped fetlock' stance due to a traumatic disruption of the suspensory apparatus.

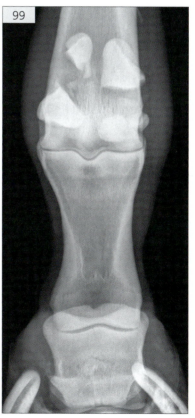

2.99 Dorsopalmar radiograph (non-weight bearing) showing traumatic disruption of the suspensory apparatus due to biaxial proximal sesamoid bone fractures.

of the suspensory ligament or the distal sesamoidean ligaments can be differentiated by the position of the proximal sesamoid bones on the radiographs; with disruption of the suspensory ligament, the sesamoid bones will be displaced distally (**2.100**), and with disruption of the distal sesamoidean ligaments, the sesamoid bones will be displaced proximally (**2.101**). Although it is not a sensitive indicator of vascular injury, the temperature and pulses in the foot should be assessed to see if damage is severe. If damage to the neurovascular structures of the distal limb is suspected, Doppler ultrasonography should be performed prior to any surgical repair to evaluate the blood supply to the distal limb.

Management/treatment

The digits are placed in extension by use of a dorsal splint or prefabricated splint so that the horse stands on its toe and bears weight through an aligned column of the phalanges and metacarpus/metatarsus (see Splinting and casting). Surgical arthrodesis of the fetlock joint is the optimal treatment. These horses no longer have an athletic career, but most are serviceable for breeding. Although some horses can be managed with long-term splinting, most horses so treated either develop laminitis in the contralateral limb or fail to become comfortable long term.

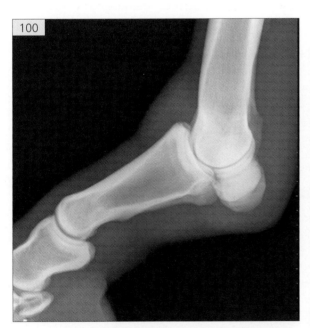

2.100 Lateromedial radiograph showing traumatic disruption of the suspensory apparatus due to disruption of the suspensory ligament. Note the distal position of the proximal sesamoid bones.

2.101 Lateromedial radiograph showing traumatic disruption of the suspensory apparatus due to disruption of the distal sesamoidean ligaments. Note the proximal displacement of the proximal sesamoid bones and the cortical screws placed in a previously repaired condylar fracture.

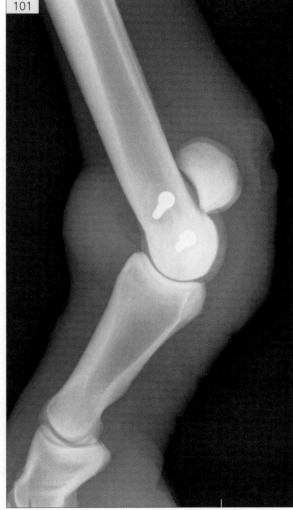

Flexor tendon disruption
Key points
- When trying to determine the amount of tendon damage present by palpation, the severity of the damage is often underrepresented.
- In general, horses with complete tendon disruption have a guarded prognosis for resuming an athletic career, with 45% returning to work.
- Complications after flexor tendon disruption are common and include necrotic tendonitis, synovial sepsis, cast complications, adhesions, and reinjury.

Definition/overview
Disruption of the superficial digital flexor tendon, deep digital flexor tendon, or both, causing misuse of the limb.[88–91]

Etiology/pathogenesis
Flexor tendon disruption is usually caused by external trauma to the distal limb, including lacerations, over-reaching injuries, kicks, and jumping injuries. Flexor tendon disruption can also occur secondary to proteolysis of the tendon due to sepsis or overuse injuries.

Clinical features
Horses with complete rupture of the flexor tendons are moderately to severely lame and show a characteristic change in their fetlock angle or foot position depending on the structure(s) involved (**2.102**). Horses that have completely ruptured their superficial digital flexor tendon will exhibit fetlock hyperextension (i.e. a 'dropped fetlock') (**2.103**). This may only be evident during the weight-bearing phase of the stride or when

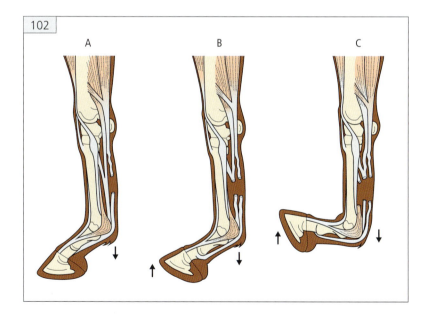

2.102 Changes in limb position due to flexor tendon disruption with respect to structure involved. A: superficial digital flexor tendon disruption causing a dropped fetlock; B: superficial and deep digital flexor tendon disruption causing a dropped fetlock and elevation of the toe off of the ground; C: superficial and deep digital flexor tendon disruption and suspensory ligament disruption causing the fetlock to drop to the ground.

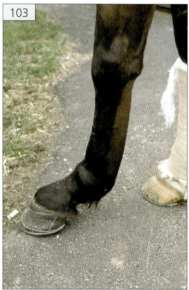

2.103 A horse with a 'dropped fetlock'.

the contralateral limb is picked up. When the deep digital flexor tendon is completely ruptured, the horse will exhibit hyperextension of the distal interphalangeal joint, evidenced by the toe being elevated off the ground during the weight-bearing phase of the stride (**2.104**). When both flexor tendons are ruptured, the horse will present with its toe flipped up in the air and a dropped fetlock. If the laceration continues through these structures and through the suspensory ligament as well, there is a complete loss of support to the fetlock joint and the fetlock will drop to the ground when the horse bears weight. Many horses with flexor tendon disruption appear to be anxious and in pain when bearing weight on the limb. It should be noted that up to 50% of a tendon can be disrupted without affecting the horse's gait at a walk.[92] The ends of the flexor tendons can usually be palpated through the wound if the disruption is incomplete. With complete tendon disruption there will be a large gap (at least 3 cm) present between the severed ends, making them difficult to palpate. Generalized limb swelling is usually present. Wounds into the digital flexor tendon sheath will often have synovial fluid leaking from the wound.

Differential diagnosis

Suspensory ligament rupture; sesamoid fractures; suspensory desmitis.

Diagnosis

A thorough history, lameness examination, and physical examination, including palpation of the severed ends of the flexor tendon through the laceration, are usually diagnostic for complete flexor tendon ruptures.

Ultrasonographic examination of the involved flexor tendon is recommended for incomplete disruptions to identify the amount of tendon that is involved because this will influence the method of treatment selected and the horse's prognosis. It may be difficult to definitively determine the extent of the tendon damage ultrasonographically if a laceration is present because of the resultant gas accumulation within the soft tissues.

Management/treatment

Emergency therapy should be aimed at stabilizing the limb so that no further soft tissue or neurovascular damage occurs before the horse is transported for further evaluation. In horses with rupture of the superficial flexor tendon, or both the superficial and the deep digital flexor tendons, the limb should be stabilized with a splint (either a dorsal, palmar/plantar, or a commercial splint (e.g. Kimsey Splint, **2.105**; see Splinting and casting). If only the deep digital flexor tendon is ruptured, the horse can be place in a shoe with a heel extension to prevent the toe from flipping up (**2.106**).

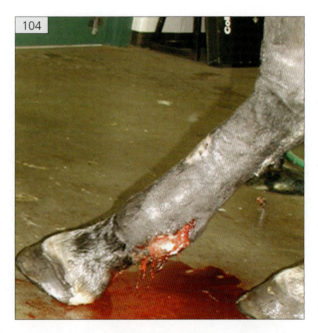

2.104 A horse with a laceration of the deep digital flexor tendon causing the toe to 'flip up' while weight bearing. (Courtesy Dr Curry Keoughan)

Laceration repair and, potentially, tenorrhaphy is best accomplished with the horse under general anesthesia. This also allows the full extent of the tendon damage to be assessed. Lacerations of <50% of the tendon do not require suture repair, but those of >50% should have tenorrhaphy performed whenever possible.

If the digital flexor tendon sheath is involved, appropriate treatment should be performed to prevent the development of septic tenosynovitis (see Septic tenosynovitis and wounds involving tendon sheaths).

Horses with forelimb flexor tendon disruption need to be maintained in a half-limb cast for at least 6–8 weeks and those with hindlimb tendon disruption require a full-limb cast to counteract the forces exerted by the reciprocal apparatus. After cast removal, an additional 3 months of stall rest is recommended and up to 8–12 months may be required before the horse can resume full athletic activity.

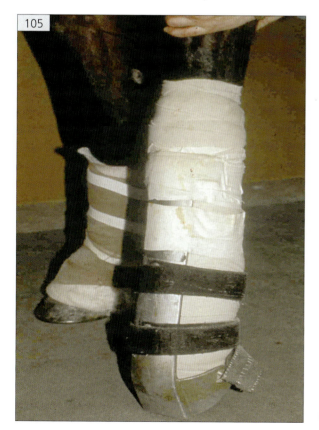

2.105 A horse with a dropped fetlock maintained in a Kimzey Splint in order to stabilize the fetlock joint.

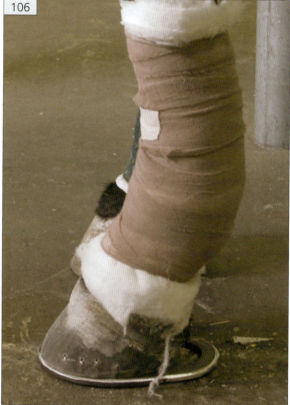

2.106 A horse with an extended heel shoe applied to prevent hyperextension of the distal interphalangeal joint following rupture of the deep digital flexor tendon. (Courtesy Dr Aloisio Bueno)

Extensor tendon disruption

Key points

- Horses with extensor tendon disruption have a good prognosis for returning to athletic activity (approximately 80%) if they are treated appropriately.[88]
- Tenorrhaphy is generally unnecessary, but horses should receive appropriate wound care, external coaptation, and stall rest to ensure a good outcome.
- Foals with rupture of the common digital extensor tendon also have a good prognosis unless they experience carpal or tarsal bone collapse secondary to incomplete ossification of these bones.

Definition/overview

Disruption of the common or long digital extensor tendon resulting in a gait abnormality where the horse cannot extend its foot when trying to advance the limb.[88,89,91,93]

Etiology/pathogenesis

Extensor tendon disruption in adults is almost always caused by external trauma such as running into stationary objects or sustaining a laceration to the dorsal (or cranial) surface of the limb (**2.107**). Congenital rupture of the common digital extensor tendon is common in foals and is not due to external trauma. The etiology of this condition is unknown, but it has been postulated to be due to contracture of the flexor tendons, which places excessive tension on the common digital extensor tendon, causing it to rupture. Rarely, extensor tendon disruption can occur by proteolysis of the tendon secondary to sepsis.

Clinical features

Horses with disruption of an extensor tendon demonstrate a characteristic mechanical lameness; they drag their toe when attempting to place their foot in extension and have trouble placing the foot squarely on the ground. Generally, once the horse has placed its foot squarely on the ground it is able to bear full weight on the limb. Most horses do not exhibit signs of pain associated with the gait abnormality, although they may have pain originating from a laceration and associated trauma. Focal swelling is usually present at the site of disruption and often the severed ends of the tendon can be palpated through the wound. Foals with congenital rupture of the common digital extensor tendon have swelling within the tendon sheath at the dorsolateral aspect of the carpus and tend to have a bow-legged or 'over at the knees' stance. These foals may knuckle over at the fetlock or buckle at the carpus when walking. Incomplete ossification of the carpal or tarsal bones is often present in these foals.

Differential diagnosis

Radial nerve paralysis; brachial plexus avulsion.

Diagnosis

A thorough history, physical examination, and lameness examination, combined with sonographic examination of the extensor tendon and its sheath, are usually diagnostic for extensor tendon rupture.

Management/treatment

Emergency management should consist of cleaning the wound, bandaging the limb, and placing a caudal splint to keep the fetlock (and carpus in the front limb) in extension if the horse is having difficulty protracting the limb. If the rupture is acute and the severed tendon edges are clean, the tendon can be sutured primarily. However, most extensor tendon injuries have some degree of contamination present and will heal well without primary apposition, therefore tenorrhaphy is not recommended for contaminated wounds. After appropriate treatment for the laceration, horses should be stall confined and kept in a bandage (and splint if needed) for 4–6 weeks. Some horses may benefit from the application of a shoe with a toe extension in order to prevent knuckling over once they are out of a splint; however, this can also exacerbate the problem in some horses (**2.108**).

Foals with common digital extensor tendon rupture respond well to treatment with splints over well-padded bandages and stall confinement. However, they should be evaluated radiographically for incomplete ossification of the carpal or tarsal bones and treated appropriately if present.

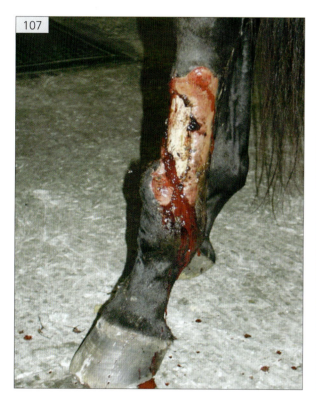

2.107 A laceration over the left metatarsal bone that extends through the long digital extensor tendon. (Courtesy Dr Ted Broome)

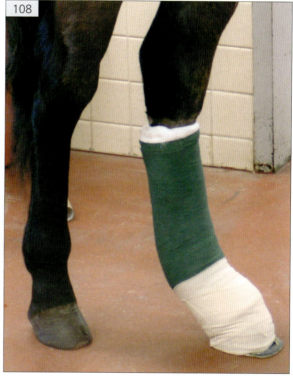

2.108 A horse wearing a shoe with a toe extension to prevent knuckling over due to long digital extensor tendon disruption.

Synovial structures
Articular luxations
Key points

- If the subluxation/luxation can be reduced and the joint is adequately stabilized, most horses will be able to bear weight on the limb if the surrounding soft tissue injury is not too severe.
- If the horse is going to be managed in a cast, the initial cast may need to be replaced in 2–3 days once the surrounding soft tissue swelling has resolved in order to prevent loosening of the cast and development of cast sores.
- Long-term prognosis is dependent on many factors including the joint involved, whether or not a septic arthritis develops, the nature of the surrounding soft tissue injury, and the degree of osteoarthritis that subsequently develops.

Definition/overview

A complete dislocation (luxation) or partial dislocation (subluxation) of a joint from its normal configuration such that normal forces can no longer be transmitted across the joint.

Etiology/pathogenesis

Most articular luxations/subluxations are traumatic in origin. Often they are a result of the horse getting its leg getting caught in fence, being kicked, or taking an awkward step. In order for the joint to become dislocated, at least one collateral or intra-articular ligament is usually disrupted. In horses, luxations/subluxations occur rarely, but have been reported to occur in the scapulohumeral[94], coxofemoral[72], carpal[95], tarsal (**2.109**)[49,96,97], metacarpophalangeal/metatarsophalangeal[98], proximal interphalangeal (**2.110**)[99], and distal interphalangeal joints.[100]

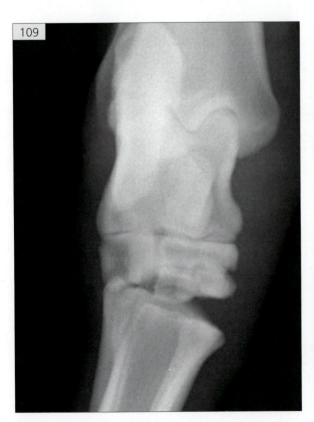

2.109 Dorsoplantar radiograph of the hock of a horse with a traumatic subluxation of the tarsometatarsal joint.

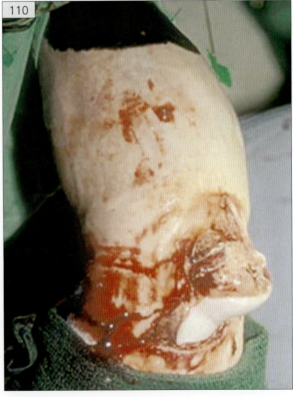

2.110 A complete, open luxation of the proximal interphalangeal joint.

Clinical features

Clinical signs are variable depending on the joint that is injured and the type of injury sustained to create the luxation/subluxation. With subluxations, the horse may exhibit a mild lameness when the joint is in its appropriate anatomic location, but it can become severely lame when the joint becomes dislocated. Often, these horses will have moderate soft tissue swelling surrounding the affected joint. These injuries may be open or closed. Subluxation of the distal joints in some horses will not be easily identifiable or palpable unless the horse is heavily sedated or anesthetized because the surrounding intact musculature, tendons, and ligaments will function to stabilize the joint.

Horses with complete luxation are non-weight-bearing lame and typically have a visibly abnormal joint angle or abnormal position of the affected limb. There is severe soft tissue swelling surrounding the affected joint and the luxation may be open or closed. Luxations of the scapulohumeral or coxofemoral joints are not as apparent as those involving the distal limb, but they will often present with a noticeably shorter leg on the affected side (**2.111A, B**). The affected limb of horses with a coxofemoral luxation is usually externally rotated with the point of the hock being higher on the affected side than the normal limb.

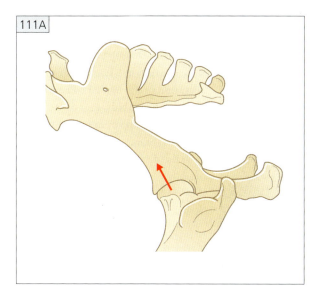

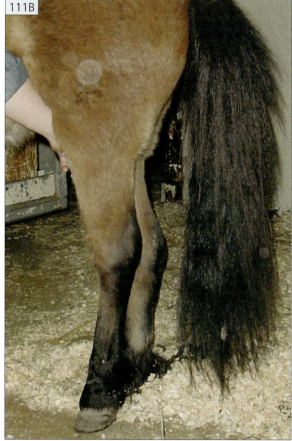

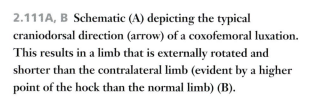

2.111A, B Schematic (A) depicting the typical craniodorsal direction (arrow) of a coxofemoral luxation. This results in a limb that is externally rotated and shorter than the contralateral limb (evident by a higher point of the hock than the normal limb) (B).

Differential diagnosis
Fracture; neuromuscular disease.

Diagnosis
The combination of a thorough history, physical examination, and radiographic examination can be used to diagnose most luxations/subluxations. In order to definitively diagnose subluxations in some horses, stress radiographs are needed to demonstrate disruption of a collateral ligament (**2.112A, B**). Stress radiographs are performed by actively manipulating the joint (usually medial or lateral) while the radiograph is being taken to identify whether there is an increase or decrease in joint space present on one side of the joint. This can be performed manually or by having the horse stand on a wood block placed under the medial or lateral side of the foot. Ultrasonographic examination may be useful in cases with a subluxation to identify injuries to the surrounding tendons or ligaments.

Management/treatment
If the injury is open, then the wound should be debrided and the joint stabilized with a Robert Jones bandage and a splint that will maintain the joint in normal anatomic alignment. These horses should be treated aggressively in order to prevent the development of septic arthritis (see Septic tenosynovitis and wounds involving joints). Horses with subluxation can be maintained in a splint, placed in a cast, or undergo surgical arthrodesis of the affected joint (**2.113**). For horses with luxation, the

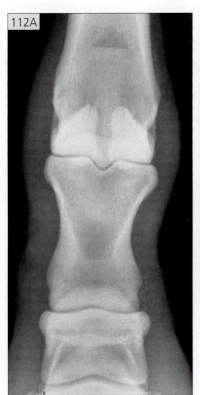

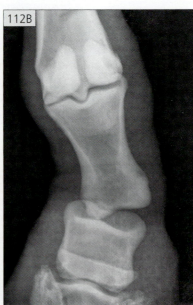

2.112A, B Dorsoplantar radiographs of the pastern of a horse with a laceration of the medial collateral ligament and subluxation of the joint that was only apparent on stressed views. (A) Standard view; (B) stressed view: the distal limb was pulled laterally.

initial goal of therapy should be to clean the wound, lavage and debride the joint if it is open, and attempt to reduce the luxation into normal anatomic alignment. This may require heavy sedation or general anesthesia since contraction of the muscles surrounding the joint may preclude reduction in the awake horse. Luxation of the coxofemoral or scapulohumeral joint always requires general anesthesia for correction and may need open reduction due to the large amount of musculature present at these locations. Once the joint is realigned, it can be stabilized by performing an arthrodesis or the horse can be placed in a cast if the injury is in the distal limb. Subluxation of the distal interphalangeal joint can often be addressed by placing the horse in a shoe with a heel extension; however, the integrity of the deep digital flexor tendon should be carefully evaluated in order to give an accurate prognosis.

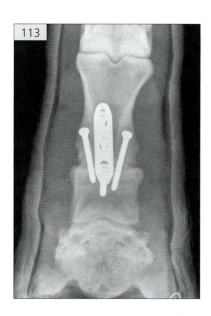

2.113 The horse in 2.112 after pastern joint arthrodesis to treat the subluxation.

Septic arthritis and wounds involving joints
Key points

- Early diagnosis and aggressive treatment via lavage and debridement is the most important component of obtaining a successful outcome for horses with synovial sepsis.
- Previously reported results with open surgical treatment indicated that approximately 73% of horses with a septic joint survived and 56% returned to athletic activity, while only 45% of foals survived.[101] However, more recent results indicate that the prognosis is improved by using arthroscopic surgery along with local antimicrobial drug therapy, with approximately 90% of horses surviving, approximately 80% of horses returning to athletic activity, and approximately 87% of foals surviving.[1,4,102]
- Owners should be aware that foals treated for septic arthritis are less likely to race than their peers, and those with more than one septic joint have only a 40% chance of survival.[102]

Definition/overview

Joints can become contaminated with bacteria or fungal organisms following lacerations or puncture wounds that communicate with the joint, hematogenous spread, extension of periarticular infection into the joint, or iatrogenic introduction into the joint. Septic arthritis occurs if these organisms replicate and then colonize the joint.

Etiology/pathogenesis

Once contamination of the joint occurs, a marked inflammatory response is initiated within the joint. Joints are lined by synovial membrane that produces and maintains a selective physical, cellular, and biochemical environment that responds to the presence of the con- taminating organisms in order to prevent their prolif- eration and colonization.[103,104] Septic arthritis occurs when the joint is inoculated with microorganisms that overcome these defense mechanisms, replicate, and colonize the synovial cavity. The number of microor- ganisms required to overcome the synovial defenses is determined by the number of organisms inoculated, the individual organism's virulence and pathogenicity, the presence of devitalized tissue or foreign material, and the host's immune status.[105] Following colonization, there is a release of a variety of inflammatory mediators that initiate a marked synovial inflammatory response, causing the influx of neutrophils. These neutrophils, along with the synoviocytes, release inflammatory enzymes and free radicals. Although this inflammatory response is initiated by the presence of the microorganism, it can lead to the degradation of normal intrasynovial structures. Proteoglycan synthesis is also inhibited in response to the inflammation. The inflammatory response causes synovial fluid to accumulate, increasing the intrasynovial pressure and causing pain. The inflammatory response also causes an excessive amount of fibrin to be produced, resulting in the formation of fibrinocellular conglomerates that trap devitalized tissue, foreign material, and bacteria (**2.114**). If the fibrin remains in the joint, it can act as a nidus for continued infection.[103–105]

Clinical features

In adult horses, septic arthritis is usually the result of a laceration or puncture wound (**2.115, 2.116**), although iatrogenic infections are not uncommon. In foals, the joint can become septic secondary to a laceration or puncture wound, but more commonly the sepsis is due to hematogenous spread (**2.117**). This is especially common in immunocompromised foals or foals with a primary site of sepsis (i.e. the umbilicus, lower respiratory tract [LRT], or GI tract).

With sepsis that is secondary to a laceration, horses are often comfortable and do not show any clinical signs of sepsis initially; joint effusion may not be present if synovial fluid is leaking from the open wound (**2.116**). However, once the wound heals and the synovial cavity is sealed, horses develop a rapidly progressive, severe lameness (greater than or equal to grade 4 out of 5), with moderate to severe joint effusion, and periarticular cellulitis, heat, and swelling. These horses are often anxious, inappetent, and febrile.

Horses with iatrogenic septic arthritis secondary to joint injections typically begin to show clinical signs of sepsis within 10 days after the injection; horses injected

with corticosteroids may have a delay in clinical signs because these drugs lessen the initial inflammatory response.

Differential diagnosis

Fracture; cellulitis; septic tenosynovitis; osteomyelitis; subsolar abscess.

Diagnosis

A complete history and physical examination should be performed on every horse suspected of having a laceration or puncture wound to a joint. The importance of determining whether the wound communicates with a joint cannot be overemphasized, as failure to promptly recognize and treat joint contamination markedly decreases the horse's prognosis for survival.

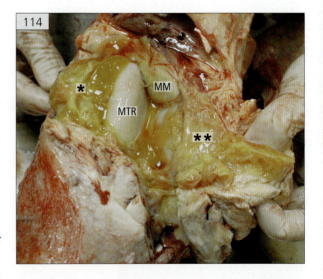

2.114 A post-mortem specimen demonstrating the production of an extensive fibrinocellular conglomerate in the tarsocrural joint of a foal due to hematogenous septic arthritis. MTR, medial trochlear ridge of the talus; MM, medial malleolus of the tibia; * fibrinocellular conglomerate between the medial and lateral trochlear ridges of the talus; ** fibrinocellular conglomerate adhered to the dorsomedial joint capsule.

Communication of a wound with a joint may be obvious because of the presence of synovial fluid. If it is not obvious, or if sepsis is suspected to be hematogenous or iatrogenic in origin, synovial fluid should be collected for analysis (**2.117**) (see Synoviocentesis and synovial fluid analysis). If there is question about communication of a wound with the joint, the joint should be distended with sterile fluids by placing a needle at a site

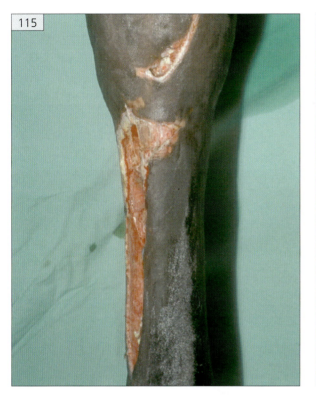

2.115 Lacerations near the tibiotarsal joint and the distal tarsal joints.

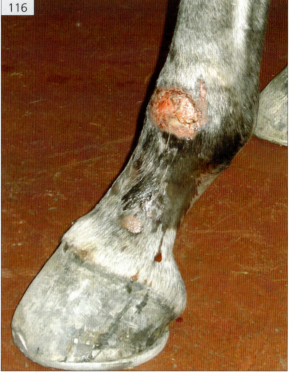

2.116 A laceration over the fetlock joint that communicated with the joint. Note the leakage of synovial fluid from the wound.

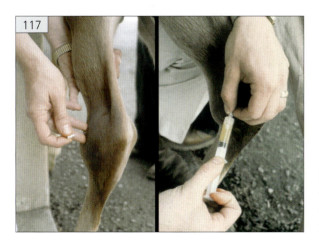

2.117 Severe distension of a tibiotarsal joint in a foal with septic arthritis (left) and arthrocentesis performed to obtain fluid samples for analysis (right). (Courtesy Dr Murray Brown)

distant from the wound and the limb should be taken through a range of motion to see if the fluid comes out of the wound (**2.118**).

Radiographs of the affected joint should be obtained to determine the presence and extent of bone involvement or identify any foreign material. Contrast radiographic examination can be used to help determine communication of a wound with an adjacent joint. This can be performed by either placing iodinated contrast material into the wound or by placing it into the joint aseptically at a site distant from the wound (**2.119**).

Ultrasonographic examination can be performed to determine the volume and echogenicity of the synovial effusion, assess the articular cartilage, identify the presence of foreign material or fibrin, and assess thickening of the synovium. CT and MRI may be useful to provide superior detail of bone and soft tissues, but these modalities are not widely available and are not needed to diagnose most cases of septic arthritis.

Blood should be collected for a CBC and biochemical profile, but the results are usually unremarkable in acute cases. As the time from the introduction of sepsis to sampling lengthens, hyperfibrinogenemia and neutrophilia may be seen.[101] Since many horses with septic arthritis will be treated with potentially nephrotoxic drugs, such as aminoglycosides and NSAIDs, special attention should be paid to renal function (i.e. BUN and creatinine concentrations) and hydration status.

Synovial fluid collection is paramount in establishing a diagnosis and properly directing therapy via cytologic analysis and microbial culture and sensitivity testing. Synovial fluid should be collected into blood culture bottles for culture and sensitivity testing because they contain ideal media for growth of most microorganisms.[106] Samples for cytology should be collected into an EDTA tube. Septic synovial fluid is generally cloudy or turbid. A synovial fluid TP of >40 g/l (4 g/dl) is indicative of severe inflammation and when this is seen in conjunction with a synovial fluid WBC count >3 × 10⁹/l (30,000 cells/μl), a diagnosis of septic arthritis can be made. A synovial fluid WBC count >10 × 10⁹/l (100,000 cells/μl) is pathognomonic for infection. However, not all infected synovial cavities

will have a high TP concentration or WBC count due to sequestration of cells and protein within fibrin clots. Therefore, cytologic evaluation may be a more sensitive indicator to detect sepsis, with one of the most consistent findings in synovial sepsis being an increase in the proportion of neutrophils to greater than or equal to 80–90% of the nucleated cells. In addition, septic synovial fluid is usually acidic, with a pH as low as 6.2, and has a high lactate concentration (6.9–11.9 mmol/l [62.2–107.2 mg/dl]).

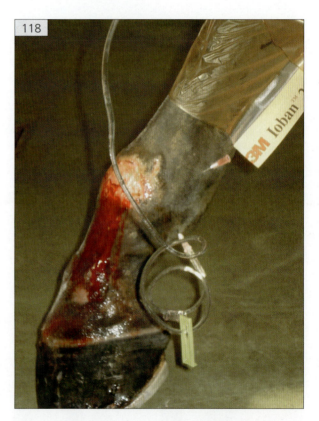

2.118 The joint of the horse in 2.116 is being distended at a site distant from the wound and joint communication is verified by fluid exiting the wound.

Management/treatment

Treatment for septic arthritis following lacerations or puncture wounds can be difficult. Successful outcomes are associated with early diagnosis and aggressive treatment.[101,107] Negative prognostic indicators include the presence of large conglomerates of fibrin, osteochondral lesions, navicular bursa sepsis, and concurrent septic osteitis/osteomyelitis.[1,4] Treatment for any infected synovial cavity should include lavage and debridement to remove any foreign material, necrotic debris, bacteria, and destructive enzymes, as well as systemic and local antimicrobial and anti-inflammatory therapy.[108]

Debridement and lavage can be accomplished using many different techniques. For horses with acute iatrogenic sepsis or many foals with septic joints, needle lavage of the joint using large (i.e. 16–14 gauge) needles can often be done standing with local analgesia and sedation in adults (2.120) or under short-acting IV anesthetics in foals. This procedure may need to be repeated every 48 hours depending on the horse's clinical signs. Needle lavage is most likely to be effective in acute cases only, because as the duration of sepsis increases so will the amount of fibrin within the joint. Fibrin accumulation results in the necessity of a more aggressive approach to thoroughly clear the joint of

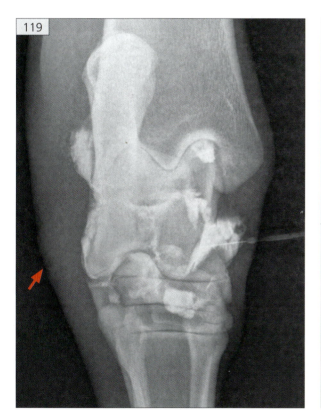

2.119 Dorsoplantar radiograph of the tarsus of a horse with a wound to the lateral aspect of the hock (arrow); contrast arthrography of the tarsocrural joint is used to rule out synovial communication with the wound.

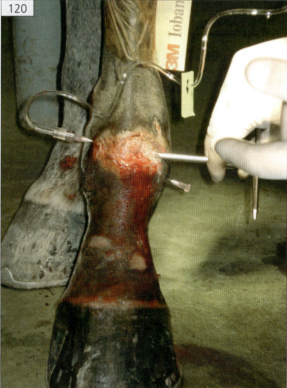

2.120 The horse in 2.116 illustrating standing fetlock joint lavage for treatment of synovial sepsis. Local and intra-articular analgesia was used. Ingress and egress needles are shown, as well as an arthroscopic lavage cannula (being held) that can be used to lavage large volumes of fluid through the joint.

all infected and necrotic debris. In these cases, or in horses with sepsis secondary to lacerations or puncture wounds, debridement and lavage via an arthrotomy or using arthroscopy with the horse under general anesthesia is the preferred approach (**2.121**).[101]

If there is a laceration, it should be thoroughly debrided and closed primarily if adequate debridement of the joint is possible; otherwise the wound can be left open to provide a portal for drainage. Other options for continued drainage include leaving the arthrotomy sites open or placing active (**2.122**) or passive drains at the time of surgery (see Drains). However, if thorough debridement of the joint is performed, open drainage is not necessary and all surgical incisions or traumatic wounds can be closed.

Arthroscopic debridement of septic or contaminated joints has several advantages including the ability to see the joint surface. This facilitates recognizing and removing debris and foreign material and identifying concurrent osteochondral damage.[1]

With an arthroscopic approach, almost all the areas of the joint can be accessed for debridement and lavage and, because all contaminated tissues and foreign material can be removed, the incisions can be closed. Arthroscopy is a minimally invasive surgical procedure associated with low postoperative morbidity. Finally, the information gained from performing arthroscopy can be used to estimate the prognosis for survival and future athletic activity.[4] Arthroscopic treatment of septic joints has been associated with shorter hospital times, a shorter duration of IV antimicrobial drug administration, higher survival rates, and a greater percentage of horses returning to athletic activity when compared with studies that used conventional open surgical techniques.[1]

Broad-spectrum systemic antimicrobial drugs should be started as soon as possible after a septic joint is suspected; however, it is important to obtain samples of synovial fluid for bacterial culture and antimicrobial sensitivity testing prior to initiating antimicrobial

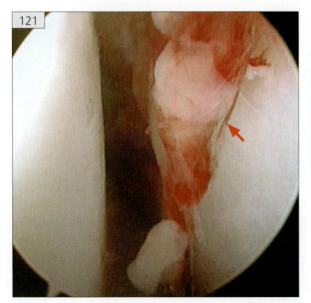

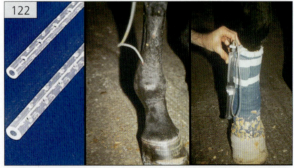

2.122 A Jackson–Pratt drain (a closed-suction drain) and its application in a metacarpophalangeal joint with chronic septic arthritis. (Courtesy Dr Murray Brown)

2.121 Arthroscopic image demonstrating the presence of fibrin within the joint (arrow).

therapy.[101,109,110] In cases of foals with septic joints or horses that show signs of systemic sepsis, it is useful to obtain a blood culture. The initial antimicrobial drugs will need to be chosen prior to obtaining culture and sensitivity results and should be based on the knowledge of common equine bacterial isolates. For horses with traumatically-induced synovial sepsis, the most common isolates are *Enterobacter* spp., *Staphylococcus* spp., *Streptococcus* spp., and *Pseudomonas* spp.; these types of infection are often mixed bacterial infections and can also involve anaerobic bacteria.[111] Horses with iatrogenic sepsis are often infected with *Staphylococcus aureus*.[101] Septic arthritis in foals is often hematogenous in origin; common bacterial isolates include *Escherichia coli*, *Klebsiella* spp., *Actinobacillus equuli*, *Streptococcus* spp., *Salmonella* spp., and *Rhodococcus equi*.[112] A good initial choice for antimicrobial drug therapy is a penicillin or cephalosporin in combination with an aminoglycoside. This combination provides broad-spectrum coverage that will be effective for most of the common infecting microorganisms.

Techniques to improve local concentrations of antimicrobial drugs should also be performed, such as intra-articular administration (via injection or continuous infusion, **2.123**), IV regional limb perfusion (p. 176), and placing antimicrobial impregnated material (e.g. Plaster of Paris or collagen sponges) into the joint. These local techniques increase the concentration of the antimicrobial drug within the synovial fluid, surrounding soft tissues, and bone compared with systemic therapy alone. Amikacin is the initial drug of choice for local therapy at the authors' hospitals, because most common equine bacterial isolates that cause joint sepsis are sensitive to amikacin and it is less susceptible to bacterial resistance than gentamicin. The antimicrobial drug used should be modified as needed based on bacterial culture and sensitivity testing results. For sepsis that is completely contained within the joint, intra-articular therapy (either by injection or continuous infusion) is preferred because higher concentrations of the antimicrobial drug (greater than or equal to 100 times the MIC of many organisms) are achieved in the synovial fluid compared with concentrations after performing IV regional limb perfusions (up to 50 times the MIC of many organisms). If the infection is

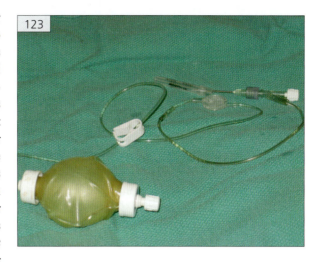

2.123 A Joint Infusion Kit that can be used for continuous antimicrobial infusions in cases with septic arthritis.

more diffuse or extends further into the surrounding soft tissues and bones, then IV regional limb perfusion should be performed; this can be done alone or in conjunction with intra-articular treatment. In general, either of these techniques (intra-articular injection or IV regional limb perfusion) will maintain levels of the chosen antimicrobial drug above the MIC for most organisms for 24–48 hours. Therefore, local antimicrobial drug therapy should be repeated daily or every other day until the horse's clinical signs resolve.

Anti-inflammatory therapy is also indicated for the treatment of joint sepsis, although some clinicians prefer to use systemic NSAIDs sparingly in these cases. In the authors' opinion, horses with septic joints should receive systemic anti-inflammatory drugs at moderate doses in order to reduce the inflammation within the joint and decrease the damage caused to the joint and periarticular structures by the inflammatory response. Additionally, topical therapy with anti-inflammatory substances (e.g. diclofenac or dimethylsulfoxide) can also be used to help prevent the development of capsulitis and periarticular fibrosis.

Septic tenosynovitis and wounds involving tendon sheaths

Key points

- Owners should be aware that treatment of horses with septic tenosynovitis can be protracted; however, early recognition and treatment can improve the outcome and lower the costs associated with treatment.
- Negative prognostic indicators include a prolonged time from injury to treatment (>24–36 hours), concurrent tendon laceration, and sepsis of an adjacent joint.
- With prompt treatment 80–90% of horses will survive, and 60–70% will return to their previous athletic use.[90,113,114]

Definition/overview

Lacerations or puncture wounds involving the digital flexor tendon sheath, tarsal sheath, carpal sheath, or calcaneal bursa, causing microbial contamination of the structure that can progress to septic tenosynovitis if left untreated. Less commonly, septic tenosynovitis can be iatrogenic in origin due to an injection into, or surgical procedure involving, the structure.

Etiology/pathogenesis

Contamination of a tendon sheath or bursa can occur with lacerations or small puncture wounds. These structures are lined by a synovial membrane and, therefore, respond similarly to a joint when contaminated. The synovial membrane produces and maintains a selective physical, cellular, and biochemical environment in order to prevent microbial proliferation and colonization.[103,104] Septic tenosynovitis occurs when the synovial membrane or synovial fluid is inoculated with microorganisms that overcome these defense mechanisms and proliferate, colonize, and establish an infection. The number of microorganisms required to overcome the synovial defenses and establish an infection is determined by the individual microorganism's virulence and pathogenicity, the number of organisms inoculated, the presence of any foreign material within

the synovial cavity, and the host's immune status.[105] Following colonization, there is a release of immune mediators that initiate a marked synovial inflammatory response leading to the release of multiple enzymes and free radicals. Although this inflammatory response is initiated by the presence of the microorganism, it can lead to the degradation of normal intrasynovial structures. The inflammatory response causes synovial fluid to accumulate, increasing the intrasynovial pressure. The increased synovial pressure causes pain and can lead to a compartment syndrome or compression of the soft tissue structures within the tendon sheath. The inflammatory response also causes an excessive amount of fibrin production, resulting in the formation of fibrinocellular conglomerates that trap devitalized tissue, foreign material, and bacteria. If the fibrin remains in the tendon sheath or bursa, it can act as a nidus for continued infection.[103–105] The end result of the inflammatory response and increased fibrin production is often the formation of adhesions between tendons or between tendons and the tendon sheath.

Clinical features

Septic tenosynovitis is usually caused by a laceration or puncture wound that communicates with the structure (**2.124**). Horses may remain comfortable as long as the affected structure is open and draining, but once the wound has sealed they develop an acute, severe lameness (grade 4 to 5 out of 5), with moderate to severe effusion in the tendon sheath or bursa (**2.125**). This is often accompanied by a surrounding cellulitis, and many horses are febrile. The affected region is usually painful on palpation. Some horses may have a partial or complete disruption of a tendon within the sheath or bursa, which can cause a mechanical lameness (**2.126**). Tendon disruption can be due to the primary injury or to the development of a septic tendonitis.[90] Other secondary complications include fibrosis and adhesion formation within the tendon sheath or bursa, osteomyelitis of the underlying bone, and contralateral limb laminitis.

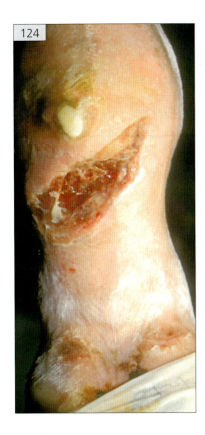

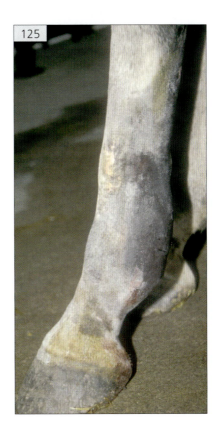

2.124 A laceration to the plantar aspect of the fetlock and pastern region that extends into the digital flexor tendon sheath and transects part of the superficial and deep digital flexor tendons.

2.125 Hindlimb with marked distension of the digital flexor tendon sheath.

2.126 A laceration of the proximal aspect of the digital flexor tendon sheath in a hindlimb that also transects the deep digital flexor tendon. Note that the horse's toe flips up during weight bearing due to this injury. (Courtesy Dr Curry Keoughan)

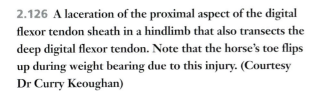

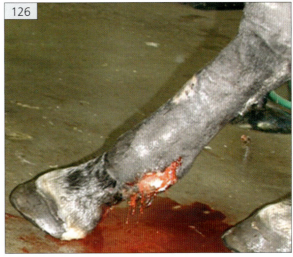

Differential diagnosis

Fracture; cellulitis; septic arthritis; osteomyelitis; tendon or ligament disruption; subsolar abscess.

Diagnosis

A complete history and physical examination should be performed on every horse suspected of having a laceration or puncture wound near a tendon sheath or bursa. The importance of determining whether the wound communicates with the structure cannot be overemphasized, as failure to promptly recognize and treat a communication markedly decreases the horse's prognosis for survival.[90,113,114] In order to diagnose a communication between the wound and an underlying synovial structure, it is imperative that the anatomy of each sheath and bursa is completely understood. If there is any question that such a communication exists, synovial fluid should be collected for analysis via aspiration at a site distant from the wound and from an area free of cellulitis, if possible. Following synovial fluid aspiration, the synovial structure should be distended with sterile fluid or iodinated contrast material if contrast radiography is to be performed.

Radiographs of the affected region should be obtained to identify the presence of gas within the area of the tendon sheath or bursa, the presence and extent of bone involvement, or the presence of foreign material. Contrast radiography can also be used to help determine communication of a wound with an adjacent tendon sheath or bursa. This can be performed by injecting the wound itself with an iodinated contrast material or by injecting the tendon sheath or bursa in question with contrast material at a site distant from the wound (**2.127**).

Sonographic examination can be very useful for determining the trajectory of the wound tract, the location, volume, and echogenicity of effusion, the presence of foreign material or fibrin, and to assess the degree of injury to the tendons enclosed in the sheath.

CT and MRI may be useful to provide detail of bone and soft tissues, but these imaging modalities are not readily available at many hospitals and are generally not required to determine if synovial contamination exists.

Blood should be collected for a CBC and biochemical profile, but the results are usually unremarkable in acute cases. Hyperfibrinogenemia and neutrophilia may be seen as the time from the initial injury to evaluation lengthens.[101]

Synovial fluid collection is paramount in establishing a diagnosis and properly directing antimicrobial therapy via cytologic analysis and microbial culture and sensitivity testing. Synovial fluid should be collected into blood culture bottles because they contain ideal media for growth of most microorganisms.[106] In chronic cases, synovial fluid may be difficult to obtain. Septic synovial fluid is generally cloudy or turbid. A synovial fluid TP concentration of >40 g/l (4 g/dl) is indicative of severe inflammation, and when this is seen in conjunction with a synovial fluid WBC count

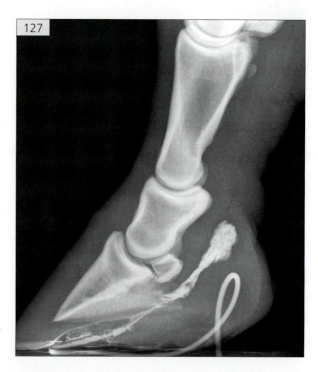

2.127 Lateral radiograph of the foot of a horse that stepped on a nail. Contrast fistulography was performed through the wound tract and demonstrated communication of the wound with the digital flexor tendon sheath.

of >3 × 10^9/l (30,000 cells/µl), infection should be suspected. A synovial fluid WBC count of >10 × 10^9/l (100,000 cells/µl) is pathogneumonic for infection. Not all infected synovial cavities will have high TP concentrations or WBC counts due to sequestration of cells and protein within fibrin clots. Therefore, cytologic evaluation may be a more sensitive method to diagnose sepsis, with one of the most consistent findings in synovial sepsis being an increase in the percentage of neutrophils to greater than or equal to 80–90% of the WBCs. In addition, septic synovial fluid is usually acidic, with a pH as low as 6.2, and it has a high lactate concentration, ranging from 6.9 to 11.9 mmol/l (62.2–107.2 mg/dl).

Management/treatment

Treatment of septic tenosynovitis can be difficult, and a successful outcome is significantly associated with early diagnosis and aggressive treatment.[90,101,107,109,110,113,114] Tendon involvement negatively influences the prognosis and necessitates more aggressive surgical debridement and treatment. The hallmarks of therapy for any infected synovial structure are surgical debridement, drainage and lavage, systemic and local antimicrobial drug therapy, and anti-inflammatory therapy. For horses with septic tenosynovitis it has also been shown that initiating early movement (i.e. hand walking) is

important to prevent the formation of adhesions within the tendon sheath.[115] Although lavage and drainage can be accomplished by needle lavage (**2.128**) or via incisions into the tendon sheath or bursa and blind removal of debris, tenoscopic debridement and lavage offers several advantages over these techniques and has been shown to improve outcome.[90,115] These advantages include the ability to lavage with a larger volume of fluid, direct visibility and capability to remove foreign material and fibrin, evaluation of damage to soft tissue structures within the sheath or bursa, and the ability to perform adhesiolysis (**2.129**). Additionally, as the procedure is minimally invasive and all gross contamination can be removed, the incisions made are small and can usually be closed, allowing for early postoperative hand walking.

Broad-spectrum systemic antimicrobial drugs should be administered as soon as possible after the diagnosis is confirmed or suspected.[101,109,110] The initial antimicrobial drug selection will need to be chosen prior to obtaining the results of microbial culture and sensitivity testing and should be based on the knowledge of common equine bacterial isolates. For horses with traumatically induced synovial sepsis, the most common isolates are *Enterobacter* spp., *Staphylococcus* spp., *Streptococcus* spp., and *Pseudomonas* spp.; these

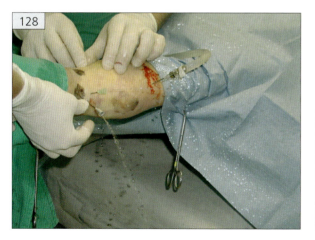

2.128 Needle lavage of the digital flexor tendon sheath under general anesthesia. (Courtesy Dr Murray Brown)

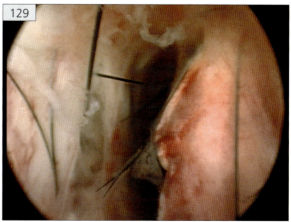

2.129 Tenoscopic image of the presence of hair in the digital flexor tendon sheath causing synovitis.

types of infections are often mixed and can also include anaerobic bacteria.[111] Horses with iatrogenic sepsis are often infected with *Staphylococcus aureus*.[101] A good initial choice for antimicrobial drug therapy is a penicillin or cephalosporin in combination with an aminoglycoside. This combination provides broad-spectrum coverage that will be effective for most of the organisms that are commonly isolated. Techniques to improve local concentrations of antimicrobials, such as intrathecal administration via injection or continuous infusion (**2.130**), IV regional limb perfusion (p. 176), and placing antimicrobial impregnated substances (e.g. Plaster of Paris or collagen sponges) into the sheath or bursa should also be performed.

Septic navicular bursitis
Key points
- It is imperative that synovial contamination is ruled out in any horse with a deep penetrating injury to the foot, because without prompt diagnosis and treatment these horses have a poor to grave prognosis for survival.
- With early recognition and aggressive surgical therapy the prognosis for horses with septic navicular bursitis is fair to good for athletic activity and survival.

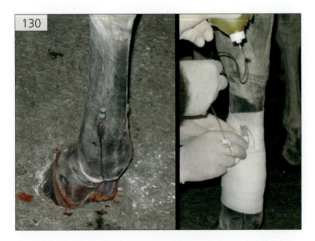

2.130 Photograph of the utilization of a Joint Infusion Kit (Mila International, Inc.) to treat sepsis in the digital flexor tendon sheath.

Definition/overview
Infection of the navicular bursa caused by a penetrating wound to the solar surface of the foot.[116,117]

Etiology/pathogenesis
Any deep puncture wound that occurs on the palmar/plantar half of the solar region of the foot (including the frog) has the potential to introduce bacteria into the synovial structures in the region, including the navicular bursa, digital flexor tendon sheath, and distal interphalangeal joint (**2.131**). The classic example of this type of injury is a horse that steps on a nail, but penetration by any foreign object can lead to the development of synovial sepsis. Because of the anatomy of the third phalanx and the navicular bone, the penetrating object usually extends through the deep digital flexor tendon, into the navicular bursa, and up towards the navicular bone (**2.131**). This introduces bacteria into the navicular bursa and deep digital flexor tendon. Without appropriate treatment an established synovial infection can develop.

Clinical features
Clinical signs are variable depending on the duration of the injury. Lameness is often mild at the time of the initial injury but worsens over the next 48–72 hours as the infection becomes established. Once septic navicular bursitis develops, horses are often toe-touching to non-weight-bearing lame and may be reluctant to put their heel completely down on the ground. Most horses do not have focal pain surrounding the tract, but do have generalized pain of the entire sole. There may be palpably increased digital pulses compared with normal, increased heat in the affected hoof, and soft tissue swelling proximal to the coronary band. Often, the penetrating object is no longer in place or has been removed by the horse's owner. If the object has been removed, carefully examining the solar surface of the foot and gently paring out the sole may reveal the puncture site.

Differential diagnosis
Subsolar abscess; septic distal interphalangeal joint; septic digital flexor tenosynovitis; third phalanx septic osteitis; third phalanx fracture; navicular bone fracture.

Diagnosis

If the penetrating object is present, radiographs should be obtained before removing it to determine its course and location with respect to the surrounding synovial structures. At least two views should be taken to definitively determine the trajectory of the object. If the penetrating object has already been removed but a tract can be identified, radiographic assessment of the wound can be performed after inserting a sterile malleable metal probe through the tract (**2.132A, B**) or after

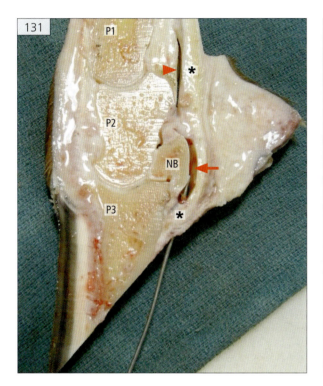

2.131 Post-mortem specimen (sagittal section) of the foot of a horse that stepped on a nail that penetrated the deep digital flexor tendon (*) and navicular bursa (long arrow). The metallic probe is inserted through the wound tract. P3, third phalanx; P2, second phalanx; P1, first phalanx; NB, navicular bone; arrow head, digital flexor tendon sheath.

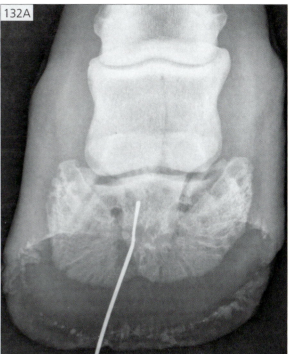

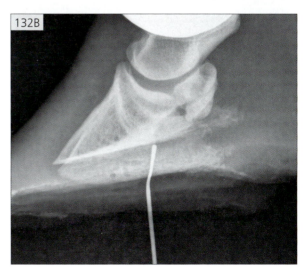

2.132A, B Dorsoventral (A) and lateromedial (B) radiographs of the foot of the horse in 2.131; a metallic probe is being used to delineate the wound tract.

injection of iodinated contrast material into the tract (**2.133**). Distension of the navicular bursa, digital flexor tendon sheath, or the distal interphalangeal joint with contrast medium aseptically at a distant site and then performing a radiographic examination can be used to determine if these structures are affected. If possible, synovial fluid should be obtained from the navicular bursa and submitted for cytologic evaluation and bacterial culture and sensitivity.

Management/treatment

Surgical management combined with systemic and local antimicrobial therapy is the treatment of choice for horses with septic navicular bursitis. An open surgical technique (i.e. 'street-nail procedure') in which a large hole is made in the sole and deep digital flexor tendon in order to debride the navicular bursa can be performed (**2.134**). However, the outcome after endoscopic surgery is significantly better, with more horses

2.134 A complete street nail procedure creating a window in the deep digital flexor tendon to provide drainage for the navicular bursa.

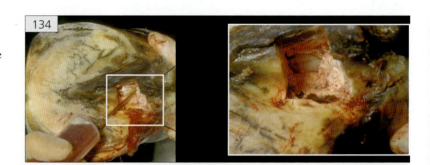

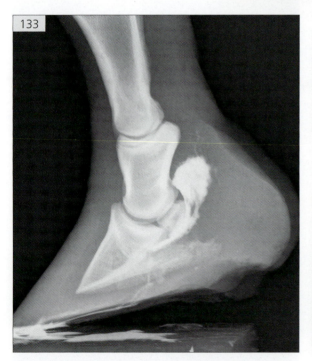

2.133 Lateromedial radiograph of the horse in 2.131. Iodinated contrast material was injected into the wound tract and is seen in the navicular bursa, demonstrating communication of the wound with the bursa.

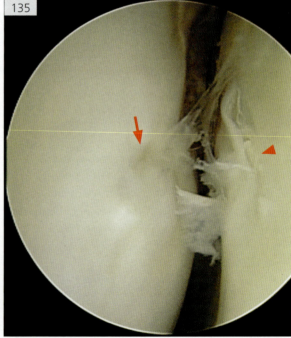

2.135 Arthroscopic image of the navicular bursa highlighting penetration of the bursa through the deep digital flexor tendon (large arrow) and cartilage damage on the flexor surface of the navicular bone (small arrow).

becoming sound and returning to their previous use (55–63%) than with an open approach.[118,119] (**2.135**). All of the necrotic debris and foreign material should be debrided regardless of the approach used.

Local antimicrobial therapy, such as performing IV regional limb perfusion (p. 176) or placing poly-methylmethacrylate beads (p. 179) or collagen sponges impregnated with antimicrobials into the solar defect is also indicated. It is often necessary to keep the horse in a shoe with a removable hospital plate in order to treat the solar defect locally and keep it clean until it has healed. In some cases there is enough damage to the deep digital flexor tendon to cause subluxation of the distal interphalangeal joint (**2.136A, 2.136B**). These horses should be placed in a shoe with a heel extension to prevent this from happening (**2.136C, 2.136D**).

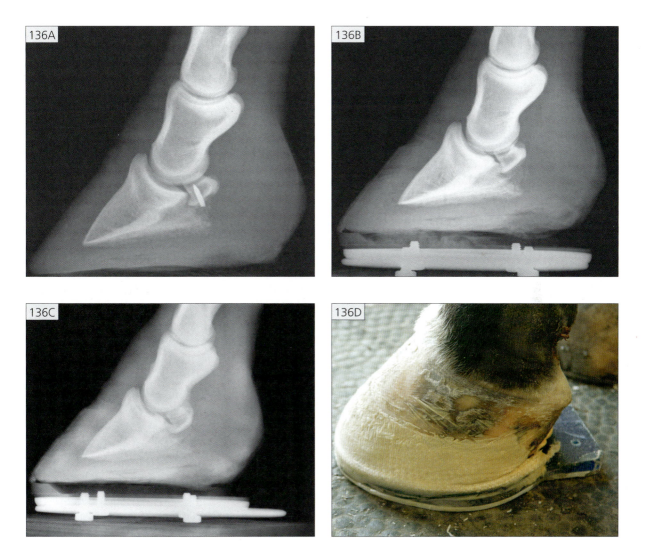

2.136A–D Lateral radiograph of the foot of a horse with a nail that penetrated the navicular bone (A) and resultant subluxation of the deep digital flexor tendon postoperatively due to damage to the deep digital flexor tendon (B). This was corrected after placement of a glue-on shoe with a heel extension and hospital plate (C, D)

Hoof
Subsolar abscess
Key points

- Subsolar abscessation is a very common problem, causing acute onset of non-weight-bearing lameness in horses.
- Subsolar abscess should always be ruled out in any horses with acute severe lameness where the diagnosis is not readily apparent.

Definition/overview
Infection of the subsolar tissue of the hoof.

Etiology/pathogenesis
Subsolar abscesses often occur as a consequence of small hoof cracks resulting in inoculation of the subsolar tissue with bacteria. Subsolar abscesses commonly occur in horses kept in areas with a great deal of dirt, particularly after rain.

Clinical features
Horses with a subsolar abscess have an acute onset of a unilateral moderate to severe lameness, an increase in digital pulses on the affected hoof, warm hoof surface, mild swelling of the distal limb, and focal or diffuse sensitivity to hoof testers.

Differential diagnosis
Fracture; hoof puncture wound; osteomyelitis of the distal phalanx.

Diagnosis
Diagnosis is typically based on the history, clinical features, and response to treatment. Radiographic examination can be performed if deeper structures are thought to be involved.

Management/treatment
Treatment involves drainage of the abscess through the sole of the hoof. Soaking the hoof in magnesium sulfate and application of poultices is often required to soften the hoof sole and encourage drainage. Horses should become markedly more comfortable following drainage of the abscess. Occasionally, the abscess will drain at the coronary band. Conservative use of NSAIDs (e.g. phenylbutazone) is often necessary. Antimicrobial drug therapy is not usually recommended unless involvement of deeper structures is suspected. The prognosis is excellent.

Hoof puncture wounds
Key points

- It is imperative that synovial contamination is ruled out in horses with penetrating injuries to the foot, because this greatly affects their prognosis for survival and athletic activity.
- Without synovial involvement and with prompt medical treatment, the prognosis for athletic soundness is good to excellent.
- Horses with synovial involvement that undergo prompt (i.e. <48 hours) surgical treatment have a fair to good prognosis for athletic soundness.
- Horses with prolonged synovial involvement (i.e. >7 days) without prompt surgical treatment have a poor to grave prognosis for survival and athletic soundness.

Definition/overview
Puncture of the solar surface of the foot with a nail, wire, or other sharp object causing acute, severe lameness in the horse.[116,117]

Etiology/pathogenesis
Puncture wounds commonly occur after a horse steps on a penetrating object; however, horse shoe nails placed close to the sensitive laminae can also cause the horse to become acutely lame. Because the hoof exists in a contaminated environment, the penetrating object often carries fecal material, soil, and rust deep into the underlying structures of the foot. Depending on the depth of penetration and the trajectory of the object, these injuries can result in subsolar abscessation, septic osteitis of the third phalanx or navicular bone, septic deep digital flexor tendonitis, or synovial sepsis of the navicular bursa, digital flexor tendon sheath, or distal interphalangeal joint.

Clinical features

Horses usually present with an acute, severe lameness (grade 4 or 5 out of 5). The penetrating object may still be in the foot, but the absence of a foreign body does not rule out a penetrating solar wound. The foot should be pared out and carefully examined for a wound tract in any horse that is acutely lame with clinical signs referable to the foot. Once the penetrating object is removed, the horse may initially become more comfortable as long as the wound is open and draining. Once the wound has sealed, the horse will again become acutely lame if sepsis of any of the underlying structures develops. In these cases, horses are usually toe-touching to non-weight-bearing lame. Digital pulses will often be palpably increased compared with normal and there may be excess heat in the affected hoof wall. Soft tissue swelling may extend proximal to the coronary band and into the palmar/plantar aspect of the fetlock region in cases of septic digital flexor tenosynovitis. With severe infections or the development of cellulitis secondary to the puncture wound, horses can demonstrate systemic signs of sepsis such as a fever, inappetence, and lethargy.

Differential diagnosis

Fracture (navicular bone or third phalanx); subsolar abscess; cellulitis.

Diagnosis

A thorough history and physical examination, combined with hoof tester application, can be used to localize the cause of lameness to the foot in most cases. Selective perineural anesthesia (medial or lateral palmar/plantar digital nerve branch) can be used to confirm that the pain is isolated to a specific area of the foot. The foot should be carefully evaluated by paring and trimming the sole to identify any puncture wounds or draining tracts. If a penetrating object is present, radiographs should be obtained before removing it to determine its course and location with respect to the surrounding synovial structures (**2.137A, B**). At least two views should be taken to definitively determine the trajectory of the object. If the penetrating object has already been removed but a tract can be identified, radiographic assessment can be performed after inserting a sterile malleable metal probe through the tract

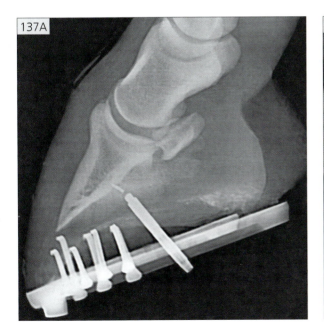
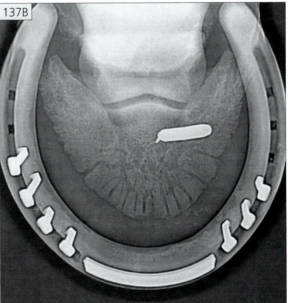

2.137A, B Lateral (A) and dorsoventral (B) non-weight-bearing radiographs of the foot of a horse that stepped on an eyeglass screwdriver. The object did not penetrate any synovial structures, but did go through the deep digital flexor tendon insertion and into the third phalanx.

(**2.138**) or after injection of iodinated contrast material into the tract. If there is any doubt as to whether there has been synovial contamination, synovial fluid should be obtained from the structure in question and contrast arthrography, bursography, or tenography performed to definitively determine the structure's involvement (see Septic navicular bursitis). The fluid should be submitted for cytologic evaluation and bacterial culture and sensitivity testing if there is communication with the wound. Foot baths or poultices may need to be used to soften the foot to allow localization of the abscess.

Management/treatment

In cases of wounds without synovial involvement, removal of the penetrating object, surgical debridement of the tract, and systemic and local antimicrobial therapy are recommended. This may be performed standing under perineural anesthesia or with the horse under general anesthesia if the wound is deep or if the horse is difficult to treat standing.

In cases of wounds with synovial involvement, both the wound tract and the synovial cavity must be debrided and lavaged. This is best performed with the horse under general anesthesia. Lavage can be performed by ingress and egress needles, stab incisions, or arthroscopy, tenoscopy, or burscoscopy. All of the necrotic debris and foreign material should be removed regardless of the approach used. Local antimicrobial therapy delivery by IV regional limb perfusion (p. 176) or placing polymethylmethacrylate beads (p. 179) or collagen sponges impregnated with antimicrobial drugs into the solar defect is also indicated. It is often necessary to keep the horse in a shoe with a removable hospital plate in order to treat the solar defect locally and keep it clean until it has healed (**2.139**). In rare instances, there may be damage to the deep digital flexor tendon, in which case a shoe with a heel extension may be required to prevent subluxation of the distal interphalangeal joint.

Other complications that can develop after penetrating injuries to the foot include septic osteitis of the third phalanx (p. 214), sequestra formation of the third phalanx, septic deep digital flexor tendonitis, and the development of adhesions within the digital flexor tendon sheath or the navicular bursa.

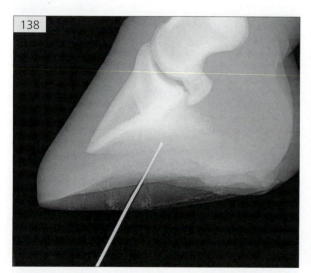

2.138 Lateromedial radiograph of the foot of a horse with a penetrating wound to the foot. The object had been removed prior to admission, so the trajectory of the object was evaluated by inserting a metallic malleable probe into the wound tract.

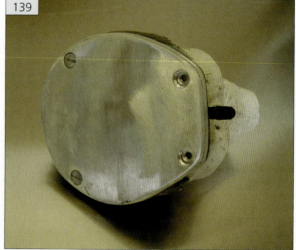

2.139 The bottom of a shoe with a hospital plate. The plate screws onto the shoe itself to help keep the sole clean.

Laminitis

Key points

- Laminitis can occur acutely, and affected horses may show clinical signs similar to those with a third phalanx fracture or hoof abscess. However, laminitis is the most common cause of severe bilateral lameness.
- Although many horses can become quite comfortable after an acute episode, owners should be warned that this is a chronic, incurable disease and relapses can occur.

Definition/overview

Inflammation of the digital laminae leading to separation of the sensitive and insensitive laminae of the hoof wall, which results in detachment of the third phalanx from the hoof wall.[117,120]

Etiology/pathogenesis

Although the pathophysiology of laminitis is not completely understood, there are several conditions that are known to be risk factors for development of the disease. Horses with any severe systemic illness that results in sepsis or endotoxemia, such as peritonitis, pneumonia, or metritis, are at risk of developing laminitis. Nutritional causes have also been implicated, such as horses with acute grain overload or those recently turned out on lush, rapidly growing pasture. Horses that are severely lame on one limb and, therefore, bear excessive weight on the contralateral limb are at risk for developing laminitis in the contralateral limb (i.e. support limb laminitis). Horses and ponies with metabolic derangements, such as equine metabolic or Cushing's disease, are also predisposed to developing laminitis. Horses with hyperthermia (heat exhaustion) are also at risk for developing laminitis.

Regardless of the cause, the acute stage of the disease results in separation of the sensitive laminae from the insensitive laminae of the hoof wall.[121,122] This leads to either rotation of the dorsal aspect of distal phalanx away from the hoof wall due to the pull of the deep digital flexor tendon (**2.140**) or sinking of the entire distal phalanx towards the sole if the laminar attachment is disrupted circumferentially (**2.141**). Laminitic horses that show the most severe clinical signs are

those in the acute and peracute stages of the disease, whereas those in the chronic stage are generally more comfortable.[123,124]

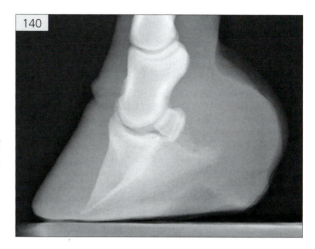

2.140 Lateral radiograph of the foot of a horse with laminitis demonstrating rotation of the third phalanx away from the dorsal hoof wall.

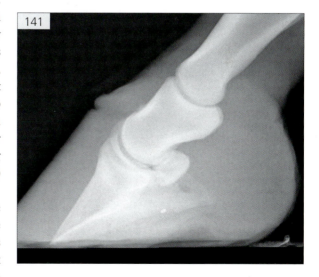

2.141 Lateral radiograph of the foot of a horse with laminitis demonstrating rotation and sinking of the third phalanx. Note the protrusion of the tip of the third phalanx through the sole of the foot.

Clinical features

Horses usually present on emergency with an acute onset of severe lameness (greater than grade 4 out of 5). Laminitis occurs most commonly in the forelimbs bilaterally, but it can affect any combination of limbs depending on the cause. Horses that are affected in their forelimbs exhibit a classic stance; they lean back and shift their weight to their heels while placing their hind feet forward underneath their body (**2.142**). Horses with bilateral hindlimb laminitis put their forelimbs further underneath their body and they bring their hindlimbs forward to try to shift weight to their heels, making it appear as if they have all four feet together. Horses with laminitis are usually reluctant to move and will continuously shift their weight from the left to right limb if they are bilaterally affected. In severe cases, the horse may be recumbent and reluctant or, rarely, unable to rise. The clinical signs of hindlimb laminitis are often confused with rhabdomyolysis or neurologic disease because of the abnormal stance and gait. Most horses with acute laminitis are tachycardic and tachypneic.

Digital pulses are normally elevated and may be bounding, and heat is usually present in the affected hoof wall. For horses that are sinking as well as rotating, a depression can be palpated along the coronary band (**2.143**).

Differential diagnosis

Subsolar abscess; third phalanx fracture; rhabdomyolysis; colic; neurologic disease.

Diagnosis

A thorough history and physical examination, combined with lateral radiographs of the feet, are usually diagnostic. Hoof tester examination can be attempted; however, many bilaterally affected horses will not stand on one limb long enough to allow this to be performed. Lateral radiographs should be taken to evaluate the degree of rotation and/or sinking of the third phalanx. **Note:** In many peracute causes, the initial radiographs may not show any rotation or sinking of the third phalanx, but will often have a radiolucent line present between the dorsal hoof wall and the third phalanx indicative of laminar separation. In these cases, radiographs should be repeated in 2–3 days and will often show evidence of sinking or rotation at that time. Most horses will need to have perineural anesthesia performed to allow radiographs to be taken and subsequent hoof care to be performed. If a diagnosis of laminitis is still in question following the initial examination, an abaxial sesamoid nerve block can be performed to localize the lameness to the foot region.

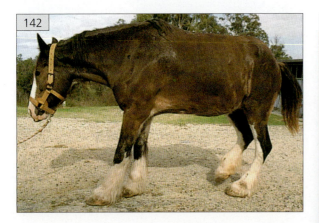

2.142 Typical stance of a horse with bilateral forelimb laminitis. (Courtesy Dr Patrick Colahan)

2.143 A cleft at the coronary band in a horse that has the combination of rotation and sinking of the third phalanx. (Courtesy Dr Patrick Colahan)

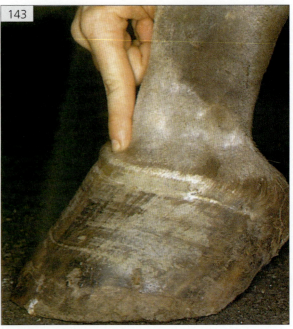

Management/treatment

Laminitis is an incurable disease; therefore, therapeutic strategies should be aimed at preventing at-risk horses from developing laminitis. This includes early and aggressive management of infection or endotoxemia, early treatment of and adequate analgesia for horses with non-weight-bearing lameness, and provision of contralateral limb support. Recent studies have also shown that icing the feet of at-risk horses may provide some protection from the development of laminitis.[125]

Once a horse develops laminitis, therapy is aimed at improving the comfort of the horse and attempting to bring the third phalanx and the hoof wall into a more normal alignment. Most horses respond well to treatment with phenylbutazone for analgesia; however, horses with more severe pain may require additional analgesics such as continuous infusions of ketamine, butorphanol, or lidocaine. Transdermal fentanyl patches may also be used. Horses with chronic laminitis receiving long-term NSAID therapy should be monitored closely for the development of renal or GI side-effects from these drugs (see Chapter 14).

Diligent foot care is of utmost importance in managing laminitic horses, and owners should be aware that these horses will require frequent trimming and consistent hoof care for the rest of their lives. The foot should be trimmed appropriately, and sole support (e.g. foam pads, commercially available boots, or special shoes) should be provided.

Surgical management, such as partial hoof wall resection or deep digital flexor tenotomy, may be indicated in cases that do not respond quickly to medical management (e.g. those with chronic abscessation and significant hoof wall separation, those where a venogram has indicated vascular compression, or those with severe rotation or sinking of the third phalanx).

Horses with chronic laminitis are predisposed to developing foot abscesses and this may cause a stable laminitic horse to become acutely lame. In these cases, therapy is aimed at debriding any abscess material and providing drainage of the area.

Muscle disorders
Clostridial myositis
Key points

- Once clostridial myositis is suspected, it is important to aggressively treat the horse with both medical and surgical therapy to achieve the best possible outcome.
- The prognosis for horses with clostridial myositis is generally poor, although recent studies have shown survival rates as high as 73% if early aggressive therapy is instituted.[126]
- Infections caused by *Clostridium perfringens* carry the best prognosis, while those caused by *C. septicum* have the worst prognosis.[127]

Definition/overview

Rapidly progressive soft tissue necrosis caused by infection with clostridial organisms[126,128–130]

Etiology/pathogenesis

In horses, clostridial myositis occurs most commonly as the result of IM injection with various types of non-antimicrobial agents, although infection through open wounds can occur.[127] Infection is typically caused by *C. perfringens*, although infection with other clostridial organisms (*C. septicum*, *C. chauvoei*, *C. fallax*, *C. sordelli*, or *C. novyi*) has been reported. Clostridial organisms are anaerobic gram-positive, gas-producing, spore-forming rods that are ubiquitous in the environment and are also commensal organisms of the skin and GI tract.

The clostridial infection results in local tissue inflammation that ultimately results in fulminant soft tissue necrosis, serosanguineous exudate, and free gas accumulation subcutaneously. The bacteria release potent exotoxins (e.g. alpha toxin) and enzymes capable of inducing systemic inflammation. The local response rapidly progresses into a severe systemic inflammatory response, after which horses begin to display signs of fever, dull demeanor, tachycardia, shock, disseminated intravascular coagulation, and multiple organ dysfunction. At this stage of the disease, death can occur even with aggressive therapy.

Clinical features

Focal painful swelling, often with palpable crepitus, is usually identified in the affected muscle within 6–72 hours following an IM injection (**2.144**). Many horses have a recent history of receiving IM drugs to treat signs of colic. The cervical musculature is most commonly affected, followed by the muscles of the hindquarters.[126] The overlying skin may initially be hot and inflamed, but later becomes cool with the progression of tissue necrosis. Large areas of edema may be present, which can eventually cause pressure necrosis, loss of vascular supply to the skin, and skin sloughing (**2.145**). Horses will generally demonstrate pain and reluctance to move. If the site of infection is in the neck, horses may carry their heads low and develop generalized edema of the head and neck, causing dypsnea that may progress to respiratory distress, necessitating a temporary tracheostomy. Signs associated with systemic inflammatory response include tachycardia, tachypnea, and fever (see Chapter 17). Most horses initially develop leukopenia with a left shift and hyperfibrinogenemia, but later may develop a leukocytosis. Muscle enzymes are often only moderately increased compared with normal and do not correlate well with the degree of myonecrosis. As signs of shock develop, horses become hemoconcentrated, azotemic, and can develop thrombocytopenia and disseminated intravascular coagulopathy (DIC).

Differential diagnosis

Focal rhabdomyolysis; cellulitis; foreign body; focal abscessation; colic.

Diagnosis

A history of previous injections or deep penetrating injuries, combined with palpation of subcutaneous emphysema in the affected muscle group, is highly suggestive of clostridial myositis.

Ultrasonographic examination can be used to rule out focal abscessation or the presence of a foreign body. In cases of clostridial myositis, severe edema and gas within the affected muscles is seen. Ultrasound-guided needle aspiration of the affected muscle should be performed to obtain a sample of fluid for cytology and bacterial culture and sensitivity testing. This fluid should be submitted for both anaerobic and aerobic culture,

but a presumptive diagnosis of clostridial myositis can be made quickly by performing a Gram's stain on the fluid and observing large gram-positive rods.

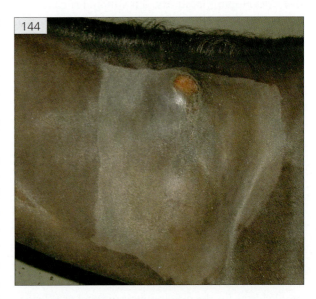

2.144 Focal swelling in the cervical musculature (head to the left) due to acute clostridial myositis following intramuscular injection. (Courtesy Dr Aloisio Bueno)

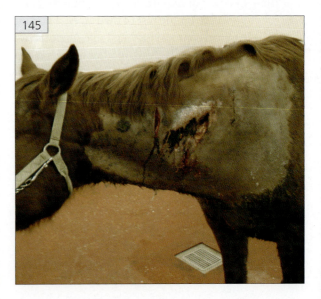

2.145 A horse with clostridial myositis secondary to an intramuscular injection in the more chronic stages. Note the large area of necrotic tissue at the injection site.

Management/treatment

Treatment for clostridial myositis needs to begin as soon as possible and should be aggressive. Treatment consists of antimicrobial therapy, surgical fenestration and debridement of necrotic tissue, and supportive care. High doses of penicillin-G (44,000–88,000 IU/kg IV q2–4h) are recommended; alternatively, the horse can be placed on a continuous infusion of potassium penicillin using the above dosages. The major disadvantage with the use of penicillin is the continued alpha toxin production by the bacteria; however, penicillin is an appropriate choice for treatment of clostridial myositis as long as high doses are used. Other antimicrobial drugs, such as tetracycline, rifampin, chloramphenicol, and metronidazole, are capable of causing complete suppression of the alpha toxin production.[131] A recent combination of antimicrobial drugs that has been used successfully is oxytetracycline (6.6 mg/kg IV q12–24h in 500 ml 0.9% NaCl) and metronidazole (20 mg/kg PO q6h).[130] No matter which treatment protocol is chosen, horses will require long-term therapy for 2–3 weeks.

Myofascial fenestration should also be performed as soon as a diagnosis is made to allow oxygen to penetrate the deeply affected tissues where an anaerobic environment is present (**2.146**). This also allows for debridement of necrotic tissue and provides drainage of exudate. Caution is indicated in horses with clinical evidence of a coagulopathy and these horses may benefit from treatment with fresh frozen plasma. If a hyperbaric oxygen chamber is available, it may be beneficial to expose the affected tissue to high oxygen concentrations under pressure. Wound care is an integral part of treatment and can become very intensive, especially if a large area of muscle is involved. Owners should be aware that deep necrosis (e.g. to the level of bone and joints) will require prolonged care and can lead to life-threatening complications (**2.147**). Horses with signs of shock may benefit from treatment with IV fluids, plasma, and flunixin meglumine.

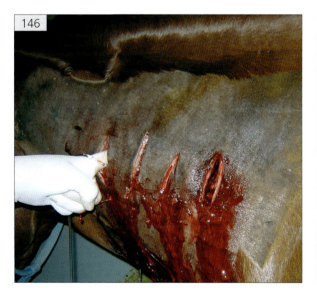

2.146 Myofascial fenestration of the cervical region to allow oxygenation of deep tissues and removal of necrotic material.

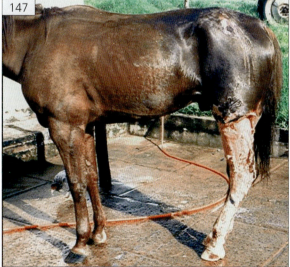

2.147 Complete skin sloughing on the left hindlimb secondary to clostridial myonecrosis from intramuscular injections. (Courtesy Dr Aloisio Bueno)

Rhabdomyolysis ('tying-up')

Key points

- Most horses with a single episode of rhabdomyolysis recover without further complications.
- In addition to providing sedation and analgesia, prevention of renal failure with diuresis and avoiding nephrotoxic drugs in horses with myoglobinuria is important.
- For horses with the recurrent form of rhabdomyolysis, there is no currently available treatment and several preventive strategies may need to be tried in order to control the clinical signs.

Definition/overview

Widespread muscle cell damage that results in clinical signs of muscle cramping, reluctance to move, a stiff gait, and sweating.[132–136]

Etiology/pathogenesis

There are several different forms of rhabdomyolysis that occur in the horse, many of which are known to be heritable within certain breeds. Exertional rhabdomyolysis is one of the most common types, where the horse experiences profound muscle pain and cramping after exercise. This is thought to be due to a genetic defect in the regulation of muscle contraction. Horses can become symptomatic due to the following triggers: overexertion (the most common cause), electrolyte depletion, or a deficiency in selenium or vitamin E. Horses on high-grain diets are also more commonly affected than horses eating low-grain/low-fat diets. This disease can become recurrent (i.e. recurrent exertional rhabdomyolysis) and is especially prevalent in Thoroughbreds, with up to 10% of Thoroughbred racehorses experiencing an episode while in training.[132,133] It is especially common in 2-year-old fillies with a nervous predisposition.[137] This genetic defect is postulated to have an autosomal dominant mode of inheritance.[136] Other racing breeds, including Quarter Horses and Standardbreds, have been reported to be affected by exertional rhabdomyolysis, and the syndrome can affect non-racing horses as well. Quarter Horses and draught horses are prone to developing a separate form of rhabdomyolysis called polysaccharide storage myopathy.[134] Rhabdomyolysis may also occur in horses that have undergone general anesthesia, with risk factors including prolonged hypotension, prolonged surgery time, inadequate padding of the surgery table, or improper positioning of the horse on the table.

Clinical features

Clinical signs can vary greatly, ranging from mild lameness or a stiff gait, to severe forms where the horse becomes recumbent. Most episodes occur shortly after the onset of exercise or recovery from general anesthesia. Affected horses are usually tachycardic and tachypneic and sweat excessively (**2.148**). Muscle fasciculations may be present and palpation of the lumbar and gluteal area reveals firm and painful muscles. In severe cases, the horse will be reluctant to move. Endurance horses with exertional rhabdomyolysis may show other signs of exhaustion, including dehydration, fever, synchronous diaphragmatic flutter, and collapse. If there is marked muscle cell damage, the horse may develop myoglobinuria due to the release of myoglobin from the damaged cells. Myoglobinuria can lead to the development of acute renal failure if proper treatment is not initiated.

Differential diagnosis

Colic; lameness; laminitis; tetanus; neurologic disease.

Diagnosis

A thorough history and physical examination is usually suggestive of exertional rhabdomyolysis, but the diagnosis is confirmed by demonstrating that serum CK and AST activity are markedly increased compared with normal. Serum CK is often in the 10,000–100,000 U/l range or higher, and AST is usually in the 1,000–10,000 U/l range.[138] If the horse has experienced recurrent episodes of rhabdomyolysis, or if a heritable form of the disease is suspected, then obtaining a muscle biopsy of the middle gluteal muscle for a definitive diagnosis of the specific form of rhabdomyolysis should be considered.

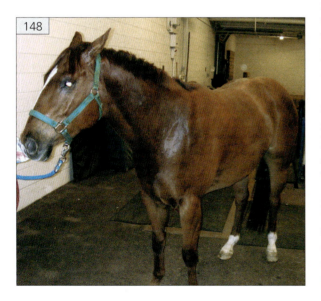

2.148 A horse with exertional rhabdomyolysis. Note the profuse sweating in the cervical region. (Courtesy Dr Stephanie Valberg)

Serum electrolytes, creatinine, and BUN concentration should be measured. Urinalysis should be performed to diagnose myoglobinuria and assess renal damage.

Management/treatment

The goals of treatment are to (1) correct any fluid, electrolyte, and acid–base deficits, (2) relieve the horse's pain and anxiety, and (3) prevent renal damage. Exercise should be stopped to prevent further muscle damage. Oral and/or IV fluid therapy with appropriate electrolyte concentrations should be instituted if the horse is dehydrated. If myoglobinuria is present, fluids should be given at a rate that will induce diuresis. This should be continued until the myoglobinuria has resolved. In severely affected horses, serial BUN and creatinine concentrations should be monitored.

Pain and anxiety can be minimized via the use of tranquilizers such as acepromazine, xylazine, or diazepam (see Chapter 14). Acepromazine does not provide analgesia, but may help improve blood flow to the injured muscles. NSAIDs, such as phenylbutazone or flunixin meglumine, can be of benefit in relieving pain, but should be used with caution in severely dehydrated horses or horses with myoglobinuria to prevent renal damage.

Prevention strategies for horses with the recurrent form include adjusting the diet so that the horse is fed a balanced vitamin and mineral supplement, high-quality grass hay, and minimal soluble carbohydrates such as sweet feed. Commercial diets high in fat but low in soluble carbohydrates are recommended if grain supplementation is necessary. Horses should also be exercised daily or kept turned out as much as possible. Some horses may benefit from the administration of acepromazine or dantrolene given as a preventive treatment approximately 30 minutes prior to exercise. Daily administration of phenytoin may also be used as a preventive treatment. None of these pharmacologic treatments are effective in every case and the expense of treatment with dantroline or phenytoin may prohibit their use.

Hyperkalemic periodic paralysis

Key point

- Hyperkalemic periodic paralysis (HYPP) can often be managed with careful feeding and exercise regimens.

Definition/overview

HYPP is a disorder caused by an abnormality in membrane permeability or a defective cation pump. This abnormality results in an altered electrochemical gradient across the sarcolemma and a change in the resting and threshold membrane potential, leading to a muscle fiber that is more or less excitable.[139]

Etiology/pathogenesis

HYPP is inherited as an autosomal dominant trait and is due to a mutation that causes an abnormal sodium channel in muscle cells. HYPP is an inherited disease in Quarter Horses, Paint Horses, Appaloosas, and Quarter Horse-crosses descending from the sire Impressive.

Horses have an increase in membrane sodium conductance because of the defective subpopulation of the voltage-dependent sodium channels failing to inactivate and remaining open or repeatedly opening. A small increase in plasma potassium concentration (e.g. diet, muscle activity) triggers a further increase in membrane sodium conductance, depolarization of the muscle cell membrane, and movement of potassium out of the cell. Initially, the membrane is hyperexcitable and myotonic behavior is observed. With continued depolarization, the muscle cell membrane becomes unexcitable and paralysis occurs.[139]

Clinical features

HYPP is characterized by intermittent attacks of weakness or paralysis often precipitated by potassium intake, fasting, cold, heavy sedation or general anesthesia, and rest after exercise. Affected horses tend to be well muscled. Horses are clinically normal between episodes, which may be mild to severe. Signs are usually first observed prior to 3 years of age. Prolapse of the membrana nictitans with or without facial muscle spasm and generalized muscle tension may be the first sign. Persistent contraction of the muzzle muscles and drooling, whole body sweating, and myotonia may be observed. Muscle fasciculations (especially shoulder, neck, and flanks) are common and may be all that is observed with a mild episode. Horses may remain standing but have an inability to raise their head and may buckle at the knees or hocks. Recumbency may occur; however, horses have normal demeanor. Some horses have altered vocalization and respiratory stridor associated with pharyngeal collapse, laryngeal spasm or paralysis, pharyngeal edema, or a displaced soft palate.[140] Homozygous horses are often exercise intolerant. Heart and respiratory rate are often within normal limits. An episode can last for 20 minutes to 4 hours, but typically between 30 and 60 minutes. Death may occur from cardiac arrest, respiratory failure, or asphyxiation from upper respiratory tract (URT) obstruction (associated with pharyngeal muscle flaccidity).[139]

Potassium is often normal in between attacks but high (5.0–11.7 mmol/l) during an attack.[140]

Differential diagnosis

Rhabdomyolysis; seizures; cardiac problems; syncopy; narcolepsy.

Diagnosis

Diagnosis is made by genetic testing using DNA extracted from hair or whole blood samples.[137]

Management/treatment

Mild episodes of HYPP can often be managed by owners, but moderate to severe attacks require emergency veterinary treatment. Management of mild cases involves light exercise and feeding a readily absorbed source of carbohydrate (e.g. oats or Karo syrup) to promote insulin-induced cellular uptake of potassium.[139] Acetazolamide (3 mg/kg PO) can be administered. Severe episodes require administration of 5% dextrose with sodium bicarbonate (1–2 mEq/kg), with or without insulin, to decrease plasma potassium concentration. Slow IV administration of 23% calcium gluconate (0.2–0.4 ml/kg) diluted in 1–2 liters of 5% dextrose is recommended to lower the depolarization threshold.[139] Use of glucocorticoids should be avoided.

Horses should be managed with acetazolamide (2–3 mg/kg PO q8–12h), feeding a low potassium diet (e.g. grass hay, oats, corn, rice bran, fats and oils, beet pulp), mild exercise, a regular feeding and exercise regimen, free access to clean water, and pasture turnout.[139]

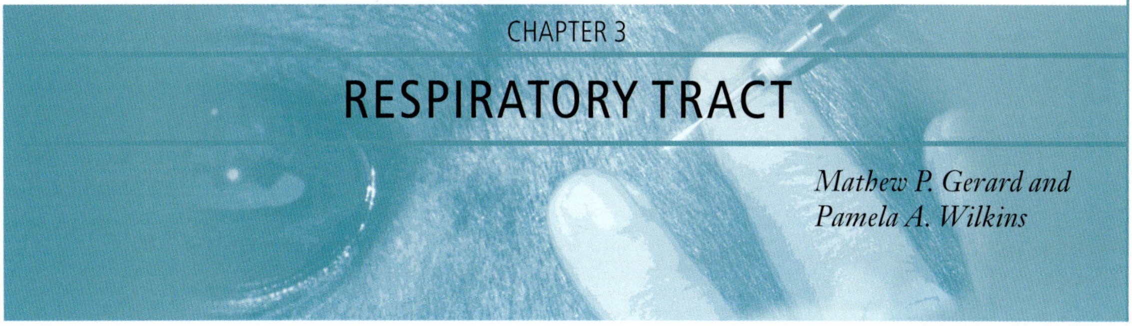

RESPIRATORY TRACT

Mathew P. Gerard and
Pamela A. Wilkins

GENERAL CONSIDERATIONS

- Horses can present on an emergency basis with upper (URT) or lower respiratory tract (LRT) disease. Care should be taken to differentiate between the two anatomic regions of respiratory tract disease because emergency treatment is different.
- The common presenting signs for horses with respiratory emergencies are shown in *Box 3.1*.
- The primary differential diagnoses for respiratory emergencies are listed in *Box 3.2*.
- The most useful diagnostic tests for horses with respiratory emergencies are listed in *Box 3.3*.

Box 3.2 **Primary differential diagnoses for respiratory emergencies**

Upper airway:
- The most common causes of URT obstruction are severe arytenoid chondritis, bilateral arytenoid cartilage dysfunction, cicatrix formation, and strangles (*Streptococcus equi* subsp. *equi* lymphadenopathy).
- The most common causes of epistaxis are guttural pouch mycosis, longus capitis/rectus capitis muscle rupture, ethmoid hematoma, trauma, and neoplasia.

Lower airway:
- Pleuropneumonia and acute exacerbation of heaves are the most common reasons for horses presenting on emergency with LRT disease.

Box 3.1 **Common presenting signs of horses with respiratory emergencies**

Upper airway:
- Respiratory distress with noticeable loud inspiratory noise and exaggerated respiratory effort.
- Air movement through the nostrils less than normal.
- Epistaxis.

Lower airway:
- Horses with LRT disease may also present in respiratory distress with exaggerated respiratory effort; however, these horses do not make a loud inspiratory noise characteristic of an URT obstruction.
- Pleuropneumonia and acute exacerbation of heaves are the most common reasons for horses presenting on emergency with LRT disease.

Box 3.3 **Useful diagnostic tests for horses with respiratory emergencies**

Upper airway:
- URT endoscopy is the most useful diagnostic test.

Lower airway:
- Thorough history, meticulous physical examination, particularly thoracic auscultation with and without a rebreathing bag, percussion, and palpation, in combination with ultrasonography, radiography, and cytology, should result in an accurate diagnosis.
- Bacterial culture and sensitivity testing from samples collected via a transtracheal wash (p. 262) should always be performed in horses suspected of having an infectious disease.

- Establishing a patent airway, facilitating ventilation, and providing oxygen are the key features of emergency resuscitation of horses with respiratory tract disease. Basic procedures are described below.
- Indications for immediate referral of horses with respiratory emergencies are presented in *Box 3.4.*

COMMON PROCEDURES PERFORMED ON HORSES WITH RESPIRATORY TRACT DISEASE

Intranasal oxygen administration

Indications

Intranasal oxygen insufflation is indicated in any horse or foal showing signs of respiratory distress associated with the LRT or following acute upper airway occlusive events. Administering humidified nasal oxygen at flow rates between 5 and 30 liters/minute improves arterial oxygen tension in horses with severe respiratory compromise.[1-3] Flow rates of 30 liters/minute (delivered by two nasal cannulae at 15 liters/minute) are associated with coughing and gagging in the horse. Transtracheal catheters have been used in both foals and adults to further increase FIO_2.[4] Nasal oxygen supplementation does not necessarily reduce breathing frequency, suggesting that stimulation of vagally-mediated afferents (perhaps responding to inflammatory mediators) is responsible for tachypnea.

Technique

- Intranasal oxygen insufflation tubes are relatively easy to place. Materials needed include:
  - An oxygen source. Most hospitals will have 'in wall' sources, but oxygen tanks may be used if necessary. Even large tanks will empty rapidly, so a good supply of these will need to be maintained under safe storage conditions.
  - An oxygen regulator. These are required to 'step down' the oxygen flow from the tank and set the flow (in liters/minute) that is desired.
  - An oxygen/gas humidifier. This attaches directly to the regulator and is filled with sterile water (NOT saline) in order to humidify the oxygen as it passes through the tubing to reach the patient. Dry air is very irritating to the mucous membranes of the upper airway.
  - Appropriate tubing to connect the humidifier to the intranasal cannula being used. An assortment of 'Christmas trees' will be helpful.

> **Box 3.4 Indications for immediate referral of horses with respiratory emergencies**
>
> - Any horse with clinically important airway compromise should be considered a candidate for referral. An emergency temporary tracheostomy (p. 258) or nasotracheal intubation (p. 257) may be necessary to stabilize the patient prior to completing a physical examination and diagnostic tests.
> - Chest tube placement (p. 265) and intranasal oxygen administration may be necessary to allow adequate ventilation and oxygenation, respectively.
> - Horses and foals with thoracic trauma and/or severe pulmonary parenchymal disease should be considered for referral for advanced imaging, diagnostic testing, and treatment.

- The intranasal cannula of choice. Many hospitals simply use variously sized soft stallion catheters.
- A variety of types of adhesive tapes such as Elasticon® and white tape.
- A popsicle or craft stick with rounded ends.
- Connect the regulator and the humidifier to the oxygen source, in addition to the initial tubing that will be used to reach the intranasal cannula:
  - Measure the distance from the medial canthus of the eye to the nostril using the intranasal cannula. At this point, place the cannula around the popsicle stick, making a bend in the cannula so it curves around the rounded end of the popsicle stick. Use white tape to secure the cannula to the popsicle stick in this position.
  - With the horse's mouth fully opened, make a circle of Elasticon® around its face above the nostril and below the medial canthus of the eye; two full wraps around the face should suffice.
- Place the end of the nasal cannula through the nostril such that the open end, which will deliver the oxygen, is within the nasal passage and approximately at the level of the medial canthus. The 'bend' created by using the popsicle stick should be snug against the nostril.
- Secure the popsicle stick and cannula (taped together now) to the previously placed Elasticon® by making wraps around the face with white tape (**3.1**).
- The cannula can then be easily removed from the nasal passage for cleaning and replacement without undue discomfort to the patient, as only the white tape needs to be removed.
- Attach the oxygen administration tubing to the nasal cannula and turn on the oxygen source, using the regulator to set the desired flow. A second cannula can be placed in the opposite nostril, if needed (**3.2**).

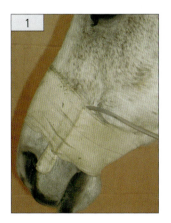

3.1 Adult horse with intra-nasal oxygen insufflation tube in place.

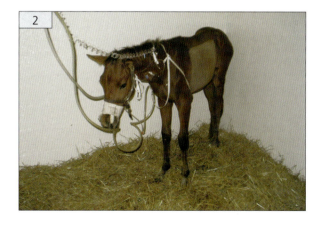

3.2 Foal with dual intranasal cannulas for oxygen insufflation in place. (Courtesy Dr Bettina Dunkel)

Endotracheal intubation
Indications

Endotracheal intubation is indicated in cases with severe URT obstruction and can be used as an alternative to a tracheostomy, depending on clinician experience. Endotracheal intubation can be performed more quickly than a tracheostomy if an endotracheal tube is available; however, intubation may not be possible with some causes of upper airway obstruction.

Establishment of a patent upper airway is achieved by successful intubation of the trachea via the nasal passage (**3.3**) or the oral cavity (**3.4**). The horse may be awake (typically sedated) or under general anesthesia for nasotracheal intubation. Usually, the horse is under general anesthesia if orotracheal intubation is being performed. Rarely, a heavily sedated horse will tolerate the procedure. Trauma to the tube from teeth is very likely in the non-anesthetized horse.

Intubation should be as atraumatic as possible. Excessive manipulation of the endotracheal tube at the larynx can result in soft tissue trauma, edema, and inflammation. Development of significant airway obstruction as a result of this tissue trauma may not be apparent until after the tube is removed, resulting in further rapid onset of respiratory distress.

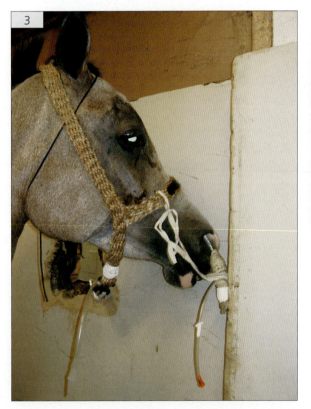

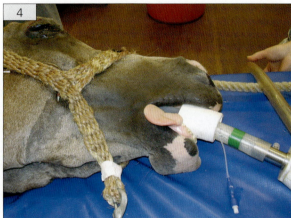

3.4 **Orotracheal tube in an anesthetized horse. Note the polyvinyl chloride mouth speculum.**

3.3 **Nasotracheal tube in a standing horse.**

Technique

Nasotracheal intubation

- Select a cuffed or non-cuffed nasotracheal tube or similar tubing of appropriate size (internal diameter 18 mm [range 14–22 mm] for an average adult horse). If possible, check the cuff if using a cuffed tube.
- Lubricate with a gel to reduce friction and abrasion trauma when passing the tube through the upper airway.
- The tube is passed along the ventral nasal meatus (similar to passing a nasogastric tube) by directing the tube ventrally and medially when inserted at the nostril.
- Extension of the head will facilitate the tube passing into the trachea rather than into the esophagus.
- Occasionally, a half twist of the tube if resistance is felt at the level of the larynx will help direct the tip of the tube dorsally over the epiglottis and on into the laryngeal lumen. Once in the laryngeal lumen the tube is rotated back to its original orientation so that the arch of the tube correlates with the curvature of the URT. Do not force the tube and if resistance is considerable, use a smaller tube.
- Correct placement is indicated by a strong flow of air through the tube.
- Inflate the cuff with air if needed; stop at the first sign of insufflation resistance.
- The tube is secured by taping the protruding end to the halter with white tape or similar material.

Orotracheal intubation

- The procedure is usually performed with the horse under general anesthesia.
- Thoroughly washing the mouth out with water to remove feed debris prior to intubation reduces contamination of the trachea.

- The horse is positioned in lateral or sternal recumbency.
- Select a cuffed, endotracheal tube appropriate for the size of the horse (internal diameter 26 mm [range 20–30 mm] for an average adult horse; 7–12 mm for a foal).
- The mouth is wedged open with a polyvinyl chloride pipe or other type gag placed longitudinally between the incisor arcades (5 cm diameter for adult, 2.5 cm diameter for a foal; 7.5–10 cm long for an adult, 5 cm long for a foal – pipe wrapped with elastic adhesive or white tape to make it less slippery on the teeth).
- The tongue is grasped with a gauze sponge and gently protruded out of one side of the mouth through the interdental space.
- The horse's head and neck are placed in mild extension.
- The endotracheal tube may be lubricated with a gel to facilitate passage over the tongue and through the oropharynx.
- The tube is passed through the polyvinyl chloride gag lumen and then directly through the center of the mouth, over the tongue to avoid trauma from dental structures, and directed towards the larynx.
- The tube can be used to displace the soft palate dorsally to allow passage over the epiglottis, through the larynx, and into the trachea.
- Minimal resistance to passage and obvious airflow back through the tube are indicative of correct placement (an assistant can compress the chest to allow airflow detection from the tube). If resistance is encountered at the larynx, the tube can be rotated and advanced gently.
- The cuff is inflated if present. Stop cuff inflation when resistance to insufflation is felt.

Temporary tracheostomy

Indications

A temporary tracheostomy is performed in any case with moderate to severe URT obstruction, ideally prior to the horse developing severe respiratory distress. There are several guidelines regarding when to perform a tracheostomy: (1) 'if you think about performing a tracheostomy, the horse probably needs one' and (2) if the horse is still in respiratory distress or has respiratory stridor when standing quietly, a tracheostomy is indicated.

Technique

- Temporary tracheostomy is typically performed at the junction of the upper and mid-cervical trachea, where the tracheal cartilages are readily palpable on the ventral midline of the neck. It is most frequently performed in the standing horse, with sedation as indicated (**3.5**). If a permanent tracheostomy is planned, the temporary incision should be made approximately 5–10 cm lower in the neck.
- Note that if there is a need for emergency airway establishment, little preparation of the surgery site is necessary.

- If time permits, the tracheostomy site should be clipped and prepared for sterile surgery.
- A subcutaneous line or inverted U-block of local anesthetic is placed if time allows.
- A 6 cm longitudinal skin incision is made on the ventral midline with a scalpel blade (**3.6A, B**).
- The incision is extended sharply through the subcutaneous tissues and the paired sternothyrohyoideus muscles are bluntly separated to expose the ventral surface of 2–3 tracheal cartilage rings.

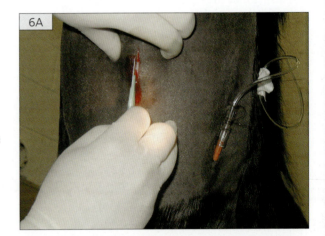

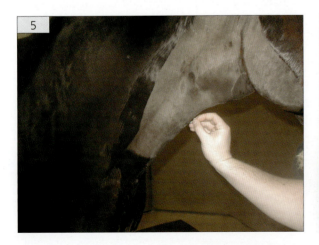

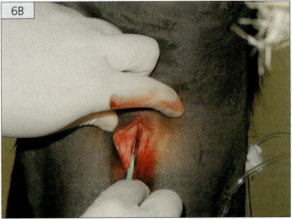

3.5 Site for temporary tracheostomy at the junction of the upper and middle third of the neck. (Courtesy Dr Eric Parente)

3.6A, B Incision on the ventral midline of the neck through the skin (A) and between the sternothyrohyoideus muscles (B). (Courtesy Dr Eric Parente)

- The annular ligament between two adjacent cartilage rings is sharply incised on the ventral midline by stabbing the scalpel blade horizontally (i.e. parallel to the cartilages) through the ligament and into the lumen of the trachea (**3.7**). Air will be heard rushing in and out of the incision once the tracheal lumen is entered.
- The incision in the annular ligament is then extended about 1–2 cm in each direction from the midline so that no more than one-third of the circumference of the trachea is cut. This is to avoid tracheal collapse, a complication due to incomplete tracheal rings.
- A tracheostomy tube (or any practical tube in a life-threatening emergency situation; e.g. section of stomach tube or garden hose or large syringe case) is inserted into the tracheal lumen to maintain patency of air flow and secured to the skin (**3.8A, B**). Placing the end of the tube against the 'upper' cartilage and forcing it in (dorsally) to collapse this cartilage helps to open up a gap between the two cartilage rings and allow insertion of the tube into the lumen of the trachea. In foals, miniature horses, and ponies, insertion

of the tracheostomy tube is facilitated by placing a length of suture around the dorsal and ventral tracheal rings to facilitate retraction. Care should be taken not to force the tube peritracheally into subcutaneous tissues.

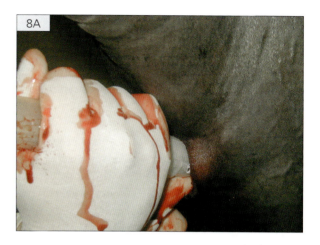

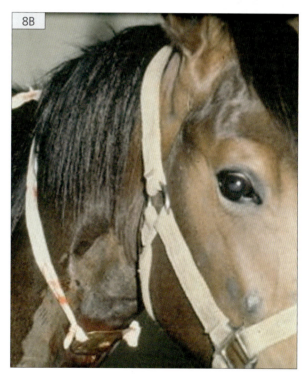

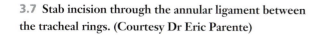

3.7 Stab incision through the annular ligament between the tracheal rings. (Courtesy Dr Eric Parente)

3.8A, B (A) Placing a silicone J-tube between the tracheal rings into the tracheal lumen. (B) Metallic J-tube in place. (Courtesy Dr Eric Parente)

- The tube and surrounding skin should be cleaned at least daily and more frequently in the first 2 days when wound exudate may be substantial.
- Alternating use of tubes allows adequate cleaning of the dirty tube.
- Once the tube is removed permanently, the surgical site is cleaned daily with moistened sterile gauze sponges and Vaseline® or a similar material is applied to the skin below the incision to prevent serum scald.
- Normally, wounds heal in 2–3 weeks by second intention. A firm knot of tissue, palpable and visible, may remain at the tracheostomy site.

Complications

The most common complications related to tracheostomy are often associated with unappreciated misalignment of the tracheostomy with the soft tissue and skin leading to localized subcutaneous emphysema (common) and/or localized cellulitis and edema (common). Misalignment is typically associated with a change in head and neck position during the procedure. Subcutaneous emphysema can develop into pneumomediastinum and, rarely, pneumothorax. In addition to ensuring an alignment of the tracheostomy with the skin, frequent changing and cleaning of the tracheostomy tube (at least daily) can minimize these complications. Tracheal collapse may occur if the tracheal rings are significantly damaged. Noticeable scarring at the tracheostomy site is rare. Tracheal chondroma formation with respiratory compromise (if large) may occur on rare occasions.

Arterial blood gas collection and analysis

Indications

Patients with respiratory disease are at risk for inadequate lung ventilation and inadequate tissue oxygenation.[5,6] Arterial blood gas sampling will provide information about lung ventilation through interpretation of the PCO_2 and tissue oxygenation through interpretation of the PO_2 and O_2% saturation.[7] Patients with certain metabolic diseases and selected toxicities are also at risk for acid–base abnormalities.

Arterial puncture sites

Readily accessible sites include:

- Decubital artery as it crosses the medial elbow (neonate only).
- Transverse facial artery lateral to the lateral canthus of the eye (adult).
- Facial artery as it crosses the ramus of the mandible.
- Dorsal metatarsal artery, located on the lateral metatarsus just distal to the hock.

Prior to performing an arterial puncture, all the necessary equipment should be ready at the stallside. Equipment includes:

- Gloves.
- Heparinized arterial blood gas syringe kit: these are readily available commercially.
- Alcohol for cleansing the area locally.
- 2 × 2 gauze.
- Patient label (put on syringe prior to submitting to laboratory).
- Sufficient restraint.

Technique

- Place the patient in an appropriate position to obtain adequate access to the desired artery.
- Put on clean, but not necessarily sterile, gloves.
- Identify the artery to be punctured by palpation using the non-dominant hand.
- Clean area with alcohol.
- Repalpate the artery gently to landmark for puncture. The index and middle fingers of the non-dominant hand can be used to 'bridge' the site for puncture by palpation of the arterial pulse with the tips of both fingers, allowing the space between the fingers to provide the landmark puncture area.
- Hold syringe in dominant hand like a pencil, with the plunger set to collect a 1 ml sample. The syringe is 'vented' at the plunger to allow the sample to enter under the pressure of the artery. Rest the dominant hand on the patient to steady the syringe.

- Holding the syringe at about 45 degrees (90 degrees for the transverse facial and decubital arteries), puncture the skin just distal to where the index finger is palpating the pulsation.
- Slowly advance the needle until there is a 'flash' of blood in the hub of the needle, then steadily hold the needle and syringe in that position.
- Allow the syringe to fill with blood to approximately 1 ml. The vented syringe will fill on its own. It is not necessary to draw the sample up into the syringe. The syringe should fill readily.
- Remove needle and immediately apply pressure to the area with a 2 × 2 gauze. Pressure should be maintained on the site for at least 5 minutes following puncture.
- Place a gauze sponge over the needle and expel any air in the syringe. Air in the syringe can affect the results.
- Puncture the rubber cube that comes with the syringe with the attached needle and then remove the needle from syringe, keeping the cube in place.
- Seal the syringe with the cap provided (usually a black rubber cap).
- Put patient label on the syringe (most laboratories will tell you 'no label, no results', so this is a good habit).

The dorsal metatarsal artery in the foal and the transverse facial artery in the adult are very superficial and this is the reason they are so frequently used for arterial blood gas sampling (**3.9, 3.10**).[8] One of the most common reasons for a puncture failure is missing the artery on the way through. This is often followed by attempts to find the artery even deeper by 'poking around'. This will be unsuccessful and much to the displeasure of the patient. If the artery is not encountered in the superficial subcutaneous tissue, pull the needle back and slowly redirect it towards the landmarked artery. It occasionally helps to place a 1 ml lidocaine (without epinephrine) 'bleb' over the artery prior to puncture. This helps with patient compliance and decreases arterial constriction following a failed attempt, allowing for another attempt. A 'trick' in foals with poorly palpable metatarsal arteries is to heat moistened gauzes in a microwave for a few seconds and place them over the artery for a minute or so prior to puncture. This will often help the artery 'pop'.

Complications

The most common complication from an arterial puncture is hematoma at the site. Less common but important complications are thrombus in the artery and infection at the site.

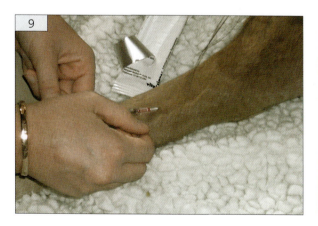

3.9 Successful arterial puncture of the metatarsal artery in a neonatal foal.

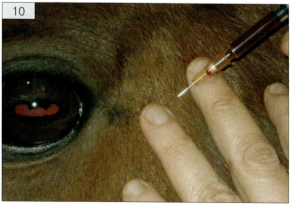

3.10 Successful arterial puncture of the transverse facial artery in an adult horse. (Courtesy Dr Ric Birks)

Transtracheal wash/tracheal fluid analysis
Indications
This technique is used for obtaining samples for cytologic evaluation and microbiologic culture from the lower airways of horses with lower airway disease.[8,9]

Technique
- The following materials are needed (**3.11**):
  - Transtracheal wash 'kit'. These kits are commercially available. Alternatively, human central venous pressure (CVP) catheters may be used. The kits will include a needle or a trochar and sterile flexible tubing that will fit through the needle or trochar and is of sufficient length to reach into the trachea for aspiration of the administered fluid.
  - Three sterile 60-ml syringes filled using sterile technique with ~20 ml sterile 0.9% saline.
  - Sterile gauze and surgical gloves.
  - Sterile tubes for samples. This includes an EDTA tube for cytology and culture media tubes for microbiologic samples. Sterile tubes not containing anticoagulant may be used for samples intended for virus isolation.
  - Materials for surgical scrub.
  - Clippers.
  - 3 ml local anesthetic.
  - Various sized needles and syringes.
  - #15 blade for stab incision.
- The area for puncture is identified by palpation of the ventral cervical trachea and strap muscles. Commonly, the best site is just cranial to the bifurcation of the strap muscles where the ventral trachea becomes readily palpable just under the skin, usually in the mid-third of the neck (**3.12**). A small area (1 cm × 1 cm) is clipped and aseptically scrubbed. Sedation is generally necessary in foals and is commonly used in adult

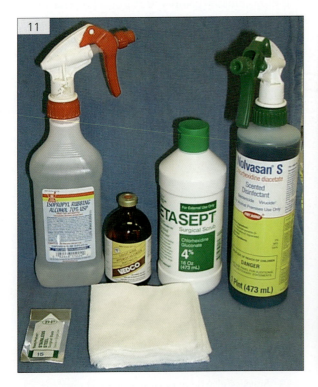

3.11 Transtracheal wash skin preparation 'kit'.

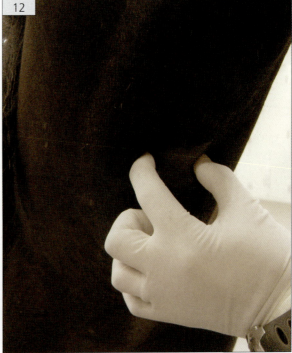

3.12 Area for performing transtracheal aspirate.

horses. All fluids used must be drawn up using sterile technique. Restraint in the form of a lip twitch can facilitate the procedure in many adult horses. Use of butorphanol (2 mg for a 50 kg foal; 5–10 mg for an adult horse) may decrease the possibility of initiating the cough response during the procedure.

- Once the area has been cleansed and surgically prepared, a small (2–3 ml) bleb of local anesthetic is placed at the predetermined site of puncture. Placement of the needle or trocar is facilitated by performing a small stab incision using a #15 blade (**3.13**). The trachea is stabilized with one hand while the needle or trochar is placed within the stab incision and advanced between the

tracheal rings on the middle of the ventral trachea. The needle or trocar is advanced down the trachea towards the bifurcation and held in place. At this point, the solid sharp portion of the trocar can be removed. If a needle is used, it is important that the bevel of the needle is oriented ventrally so that the sharp tip of the needle does not contact the catheter when it is placed through the needle. The catheter or tubing used for collection is then advanced through the needle or trocar down the trachea, approximately 30 cm (**3.14**). A syringe containing approximately 20 ml of 0.9% sterile saline is attached and the fluid injected slowly, followed by relatively rapid aspiration of the administered saline (**3.15**).

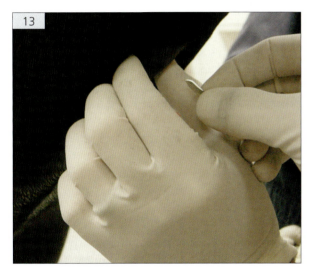

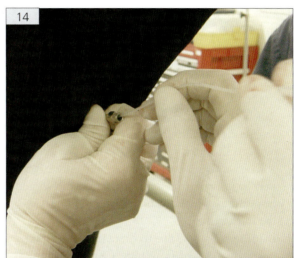

3.13 Making a 'stab' incision through the skin over the site prepared for transtracheal aspirate using a #15 blade. Note that the trachea is kept stabilized throughout the procedure.

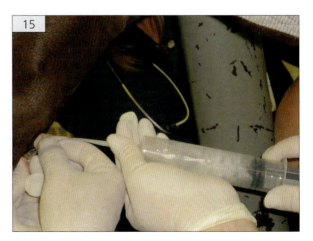

3.14 Tracheal trochar in place with sterile polyethylene tubing passed into the trachea and used for introducing sterile 0.9% saline for tracheal fluid wash.

3.15 Successful aspiration of transtracheal wash fluid.

- If no fluid is obtained, disconnect the syringe and expel accumulated air. Attempt aspiration again by slowly backing the catheter/tubing out while aspirating. Do not fully remove the tubing, and keep aspirating.
- If an inadequate sample is obtained, the flushing and aspiration can be repeated. After obtaining a sample, remove the catheter before removing the needle or trocar from the trachea to prevent inadvertent contamination of the puncture site.
- There is no need to close the stab incision or inject antimicrobials into the site if good technique has been used and the procedure has been performed without complication. This site should be closely monitored for evidence of local infection for several days, although some minor local inflammation is to be expected.
- Fluid is obtained for both cytologic and microbiologic examination. It is important to know in advance how the laboratory wants samples handled and submitted.

Complications

- Tracheal mucosal laceration. This occurs if the needle or sharp interior core of the trocar contacts the dorsal tracheal mucosa. The sample will be contaminated with blood and epistaxis may be present. Endoscopy of the trachea should be performed to evaluate the extent of injury to the trachea.
- Inadequate sample due to contamination by the pharynx or lack of an aspirate. Contamination occurs if a horse coughs the tubing retrograde so that the aspirated sample contains pharyngeal elements (identified by the presence of squamous cell epithelium and numerous mixed population bacteria on cytologic examination). Inadequate

sample volume occurs if there is insufficient tracheal fluid or if the end of the tubing in the trachea is not positioned properly.
- Subcutaneous emphysema. This is uncommon as the stab incision generally closes immediately. However, if the trachea has been injured during the procedure, air can leak subcutaneously.
- Subcutaneous infection at the site of the puncture due to leakage of infectious exudate from the trachea, contamination during catheter/tubing withdrawal, or other external contamination. This usually presents as local swelling or cellulitis within 24–36 hours following the procedure. Treatment is symptomatic, using hot packing and either systemic or local antimicrobials.
- Breaking off of tubing in the trachea can occur with use of a needle as opposed to a trocar and is usually due to malpositioning of the needle bevel. Horses generally cough up the severed end of the tubing, but it can be retrieved endoscopically if not coughed up.

Thoracocentesis/pleural fluid analysis
Indications
Thoracocentesis is an important diagnostic procedure performed when pleural fluid accumulation is evident, and it is desirable to sample that fluid in order to perform cytologic and microbiologic testing.[8,10]

Technique
The technique for thoracocentesis is fairly similar to that for indwelling chest tube placement. Similar materials are required except that thoracocentesis can be a one-time event performed for diagnostic purposes only using either an over-the-needle short catheter or a teat cannula.

Chest tube placement
Indications
An important decision in the management of horses with pleuropneumonia, pneumothorax, or hemothorax is determining whether pleural drainage is indicated. These include respiratory distress, poor response to conservative therapy, and/or pleural fluid or air with one or more of the following characteristics: sufficient volume to cause respiratory distress, empyematous fluid, putrid odor, cytologically visible bacteria and/or positive microbiologic cultures. When indicated, pleural drainage should be initiated as early in the disease process as possible, because if delayed, fibrin loculation can hinder adequate drainage.[11]

Technique
- Materials used for placement of an indwelling chest tube include:
  - Sterile gloves.
  - Clippers.
  - Sterile scrub materials.
  - Various sized syringes and needles.
  - 20 ml local anesthetic.
  - Fenestrated chest tubes of various sizes (16–32 French) with a blunt trocar (**3.16**).
  - #15 scalpel blade.
  - Non-absorbable suture material (e.g. O Nylon on a straight needle works well).
  - Non-lubricated condom or a Heimlich valve.[10,12]

- Manual restraint of the horse is usually adequate, but in some cases mild sedation may be required. The size of the chest tube to be used is determined by the character of the pleural fluid. Thick, tenacious pleural exudate necessitates a large bore (32 French) tube, whereas less tenacious pleural fluid may allow for a smaller bore tube (16 or 24 French).[13,14]
- The location for insertion of the chest tube is determined based on ultrasonographic assessment of the thorax (**3.17**). Place the tube at the most ventral extent of the pleural fluid, avoiding contact of the tube with the heart or diaphragm.[13,14]
- The site should be clipped and surgically prepared. Five to 20 ml of local anesthetic is deposited from the parietal pleura (3–6 cm deep) to the subcutaneous tissue at the selected site. A stab incision is made through the skin and subcutaneous tissue with a #15 scalpel at the center of the intercostal space.
- Prior to placing the tube, remove the trocar from the tube and then replace it; this allows for ease of tube separation from the trocar following placement. The chest tube with its blunt trocar is then inserted through the incision and forced bluntly through the intercostal muscles. Avoid the caudal aspect of the cranial rib as this is where blood vessels course down the ribs. Some prefer to 'slide' the trochar and tube over the cranial aspect of the caudal rib to prevent inadvertent damage to

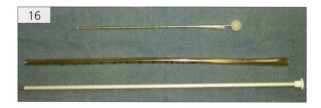

3.16 Fenestrated chest tubes of various sizes.

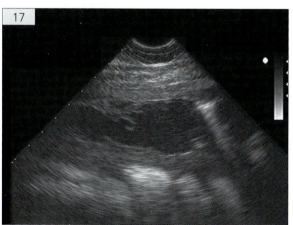

3.17 Ultrasonographic appearance of an appropriate location for chest tube placement. Note the depth of fluid within the pleural space and fibrin-coated pleurae.

those vessels. The tube should be advanced, with the hands 'choked up' at the end of the trocar to maintain control, and advanced gradually. It is helpful to estimate the distance the trocar needs to be advanced by measuring the depth during the ultrasonographic examination performed to identify the location. Do not 'tunnel' the tube subcutaneously. A sudden release of resistance occurs once the end of the tube enters the pleural cavity, but a surprising amount of force may be required to reach this point. The trocar is slowly removed, taking care to avoid allowing air to enter the pleural cavity.

- In cases of pleuropneumonia or hemothorax, fluid will usually start to drain immediately but if not, the tube should be clamped immediately to prevent inadvertent admission of air into the pleural space (**3.18**).
- At this point, fluid may be collected under sterile conditions for submission for cytologic and microbiologic testing (p. 262).
- If drainage does not commence, fibrin or lung may be overlying the fenestrations of the tube, the tube may incompletely passed through the parietal pleura, or the tube has been placed at an improper site.[13]

- With pleuropneumonia and hemothorax, a Heimlich valve, or non-lubricated condom with the tip snipped off, is attached to the end of the chest tube to facilitate unidirectional drainage.[13,14] In cases of pneumothorax, unidirectional valves may be used, and suction devices may be attached or air aspirated by hand through a 3-way stopcock valve.
- The unidirectional valve must be attached securely to the chest tube with white bandage tape. The chest tube is then secured to the body wall with a purse-string suture and a Chinese lock-stitch suture to prevent it from inadvertently sliding out (**3.19**).[13,14]
- When necessary, the thorax can be lightly bandaged with the drainage portal of the tube turned slightly caudal, so as to prevent drainage fluid from scalding the forelimb.
- Pleural fluid is allowed to drain by gravity flow (**3.20**).
- Indwelling chest tubes may be required unilaterally or bilaterally, depending on the patency of the mediastinal fenestrations. Place a chest tube in the hemithorax that appears to contain the most fluid first; following initial drainage the opposite hemithorax should be

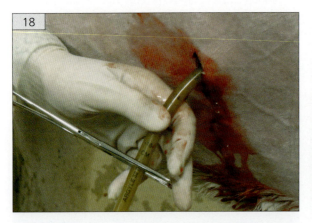

3.18 Chest tube in place with fluid draining. Note the clamp ready to occlude the tube to prevent possible air aspiration into the pleural space. (Courtesy Dr Kate McGovern)

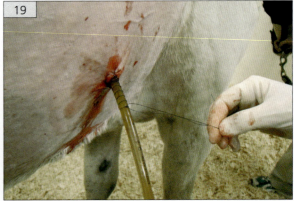

3.19 Chinese finger-trap suture used to hold the chest tube in place when the tube is used as an indwelling drain. (Courtesy Dr Kate McGovern)

re-evaluated with ultrasound to determine whether bilateral chest tubes are needed.[12] In many horses with bilateral effusion, both hemithoraces will drain from one side, indicating that the mediastinum remains fenestrated.

- In some horses with loculated pockets of pleural fluid, multiple drains may be necessary to effectively drain the pleural fluid.[13]
- Ultrasonography is used to determine the presence of loculations and to dictate the appropriate site for placement of multiple tubes.
- Chest tube sites should be evaluated daily. Evidence of local inflammation is expected, but signs of spreading or more generalized infection may prompt tube removal. In some cases, light bandaging may be desired, but generally this is not necessary. Chest tubes can be readily replaced through the same site using the same technique if they become irreparably clogged.
- Tubes should be removed once drainage has stopped for 12–24 hours and there is no ultrasonographic evidence of further fluid or air accumulation. There is generally no need to close the insertion sites following tube removal, as local inflammation quickly results in healing by second intention.

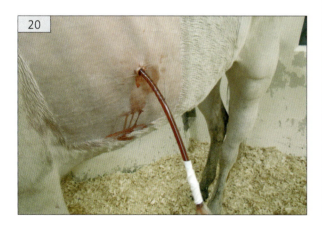

3.20 Horse with a chest tube drain in place allowing drainage by gravity flow. In this case a condom with the tip removed is used as the one-way valve device and is secured to the tube using white tape. (Courtesy Dr Kate McGovern)

UPPER RESPIRATORY TRACT DISEASES ASSOCIATED WITH OBSTRUCTION AND RESPIRATORY DISTRESS

Severe arytenoid chondritis
Key points
- Severe arytenoid chondritis is a common cause of acute URT obstruction in horses.
- Emergency temporary tracheostomy is necessary in some cases to stabilize the patient prior to further evaluation.
- Diagnosis is made using URT endoscopy.

Definition/overview
Chondritis refers to an inflammatory, often infectious, condition of cartilage. The paired arytenoid cartilages form the dorsal boundary of the narrowest part of the equine larynx and have a body and three processes: corniculate, muscular, and vocal. They are lined by respiratory mucosa (**3.21**).

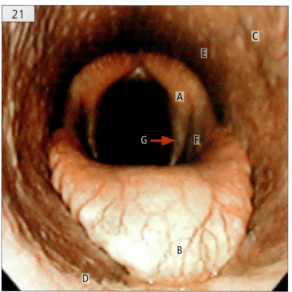

3.21 Normal laryngeal anatomy as viewed endoscopically. A, corniculate process of the arytenoid cartilage (left side); B, apex of the epiglottis; C, dorsal pharyngeal wall; D, soft palate; E, palatopharyngeal arch (not visible); F, aryepiglottic fold; G, vocal fold. (Courtesy Dr Eric Parente)

Etiology/pathogenesis

Trauma associated with severe coughing episodes (where the corniculate processes repeatedly contact and form a contact ulcer) or iatrogenic damage from nasogastric or nasotracheal intubation, endoscopy, or coarse feed material allow for bacterial invasion of the arytenoids cartilage.[15] Concurrent respiratory mucosa inflammation secondary to laryngitis may also contribute. Racehorses are most commonly afflicted by arytenoid chondritis.

In the acute stage there is often remarkable laryngeal and perilaryngeal inflammation and edema, causing sudden-onset airway obstruction.[16] Microbial infection of the cartilage leads to superficial chondritis and associated development of inflammatory granulation tissue and a fistulous tract.[15] Deep cartilage infection results in abscessation, enlargement, deformation, and loss of movement of the corniculate process.

Clinical features

Severe acute arytenoid chondritis, particularly if bilateral, can cause significant, rapidly developing respiratory distress. These horses may also have coughing, dysphagia, and nasal discharge of feed material.

Three clinical presentations are described affecting one or both cartilages: (1) mucosal ulceration, (2) intralaryngeal granulation tissue, and (3) arytenoid cartilage abscessation, deformation, and dysfunction.[15]

Exercise intolerance and abnormal respiratory noise are associated with granulation tissue formation and deformed cartilage, whereas mucosal ulceration is often asymptomatic at rest and during exercise.

Differential diagnosis

Laryngeal hemiplegia; laryngeal edema (anaphylactic reaction or purpura hemorrhagica); laryngeal neoplasia; fungal infection; epiglottitis; foreign body; retropharyngeal space-occupying mass; bilateral nasal passage obstruction; guttural pouch disease; pharyngeal paralysis.

Diagnosis

Diagnosis is made on endoscopy; careful assessment of the morphology and function of the arytenoid cartilage is required. With severe acute arytenoid chondritis, there will be marked obstruction of the laryngeal entrance by swollen, inflamed arytenoid cartilage mucosa and accurate assessment of cartilage conformation is not possible (**3.22**).

In chronic disease there will be a varying presence of protruding granulation tissue and deformity of the corniculate processes (**3.23**). To distinguish chondritic arytenoid cartilage from a grade IV laryngeal hemiplegia, look for the presence of a space lateral to the abnormal corniculate process and easy visualization of the palatopharyngeal arch. Normally, no space exists between an immobile grade IV hemiplegic arytenoid and the palatopharyngeal arch, making the rim of the arch difficult to see.[16] Abscessed cartilage may have draining tracts visible. Radiographs are useful to assess cartilage mineralization. Ultrasonographic examination of the larynx is very helpful for examining perilaryngeal and laryngeal structures that are not seen endoscopically.[17]

Management/treatment

A horse with marked respiratory distress should have a temporary tracheostomy performed (p. 258) to facilitate further patient evaluation. Minimizing stress on the horse, and thus its respiratory demand, may mitigate the need for a tracheostomy.

Systemic and topical (throat spray) anti-inflammatory and antimicrobial drugs (penicillin, gentamicin, trimethoprim sulfamethoxazole, doxycycline, chloramphenicol) are indicated for medical treatment of acute arytenoid chondritis. Typically, there is a dramatic improvement within several days of aggressive medical management (i.e. corticosteroids and antimicrobial drugs). If not, there is likely to be a secondary perilaryngeal infection, which may require drainage through an arytenoidectomy.

Granulation tissue on otherwise normally functioning cartilages is removed by laser excision and treated medically as for mucosal ulceration.[18]

Follow-up endoscopy to assess healing should be performed 2–3 weeks following initiation of treatment and then 2–3 months later to check for recurrence or cartilage involvement. About 30% of cases with granulation tissue will require a second surgery to remove the granulation tissue or will develop deeper chondritis despite treatment.[18]

Abscessed cartilage may be drained in the standing, sedated horse using endoscopic-guided instruments passed through a wide bore cannula inserted through the cricothyroid membrane.[19] Curettage of the abscessed cavity along with medical treatment can lead to complete healing of the cartilage and return to function.

Infected, deformed cartilage unresponsive to medical treatments is best managed by partial or subtotal arytenoidectomy. However, bilateral arytenoidectomy is not recommended due to the high risk of aspiration pneumonia. Horses with severe bilateral disease are unlikely to return to any athletic function.

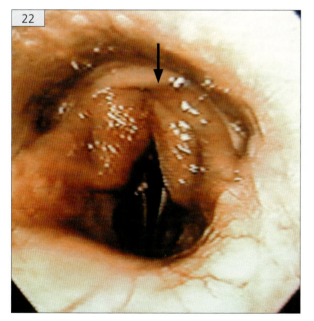

3.22 Endoscopic appearance of a horse with severe acute arytenoid chondritis. Arrow shows visible palatopharyngeal arch. (Courtesy Dr Eric Parente)

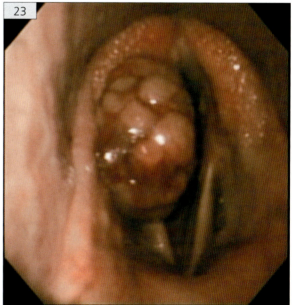

3.23 Endoscopic appearance of intralaryngeal granulation tissue.

Cicatrix

Key points

- Cicatrix is a regional disease, mainly restricted to the Texas panhandle region, but may be seen elsewhere in the southwestern US.
- Cicatrix may not be the primary cause of the airway obstruction.
- Immediate relief may require tracheostomy in severely affected horses.

Definition/overview

A cicatrix is a transverse circumferential scar within the nasopharynx. Affected horses frequently have lesions of the arytenoids cartilages, the epiglottis, and/or the opening to the guttural pouches.

Etiology/pathogenesis

This disease is most commonly recognized in the southwestern area of the US, in particular the Texas panhandle region. The age range is from 6–20 years with a mean age of ~12 years. The etiopathogenesis is unknown but is presumed to be a sequela of ulcerative laryngitis and pharyngitis. Lesions of the arytenoid cartilages or the epiglottis are the most frequent cause of airway obstruction in horses with cicatrix, although the cicatrix can, rarely, be the primary source of upper airway obstruction.

Clinical features

Respiratory stridor at rest or during exercise, exercise intolerance, abnormal vocalization (rare), and acute respiratory distress secondary to airway obstruction.

Differential diagnosis

Any other cause of upper airway obstruction

Diagnosis

Endoscopy of the upper airway is the diagnostic test of choice (**3.24**).

Management/treatment

Horses may acutely require temporary (p. 258) or eventual permanent tracheostomy if the problem is severe. Lesions of other portions of the airway are managed as described for those problems. The cicatrix can be relieved by dissection. Electrosurgery or laser surgery can be used to cut the wall of the cicatrix. A stent of the area might be used after surgery to help hold the cicatrix open, as recurrence is the major problem. The most common complication is coughing during exercise, most likely associated with irritation from dust particles. While surgical treatment will help acutely, definitive treatment involves removing the horse from pasture (Dr B. Buchanan, pers. comm., 2010). More significant complications have been reported associated with nasopharyngeal stomas that were too small.[20–22]

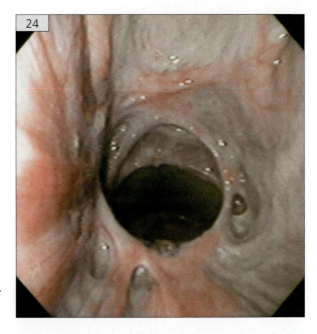

3.24 Endoscopic appearance of a pharyngeal cicatrix. (Courtesy Dr Ben Buchanan)

Bilateral laryngeal paresis

Key points

- Bilateral laryngeal paresis should be considered in any horse with neurologic disease or neck injury, and during recovery from general anesthesia in patients with untreated (or undiagnosed) laryngeal hemiplegia. It may also occur in horses with no underlying laryngeal disease.
- Severe URT obstruction often occurs following vocalization, excitement, or exertion.
- Bilateral laryngeal paresis can cause severe and acute URT obstruction necessitating emergency temporary tracheostomy (p. 258).

Definition/overview

Bilateral laryngeal paresis refers to loss of movement of the left and right arytenoid cartilage corniculate processes, resulting in a marked decrease in airway diameter at the glottic cleft (rima glottidis) (**3.25**).

Etiology/pathogenesis

The cricoarytenoideus dorsalis muscle (abductor of the arytenoid cartilage) is innervated by the recurrent laryngeal nerve (**3.26**). Recurrent laryngeal nerve dysfunction, trauma to the tissues of the larynx, or a combination of both mechanisms can result in laryngeal dysfunction. Any inflammatory, infectious,

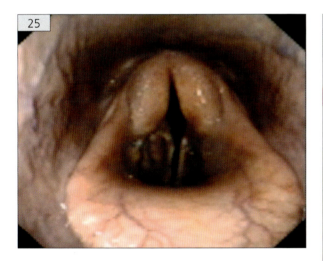

3.25 Endoscopic appearance of a horse with bilateral laryngeal hemiplegia. (Courtesy Dr Eric Parente)

3.26 Necropsy specimen showing normal and atrophied (arrow) cricoarytenoideus dorsalis muscles. (Courtesy Dr Eric Parente)

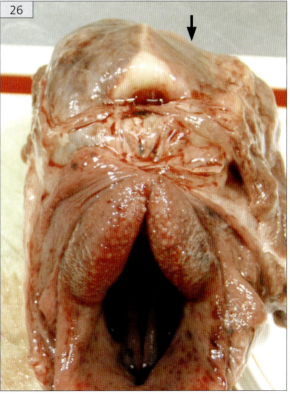

or traumatic event along the path of the recurrent laryngeal nerve has the potential to cause permanent or temporary laryngeal dysfunction. Laryngeal dysfunction may be secondary to perivascular jugular injection of caustic substances or trauma to the jugular furrow. In these cases, Horner's syndrome may also be present because the recurrent laryngeal nerve and the sympathetic trunk run in close association (**3.27**). Guttural pouch inflammation and infection may cause dysfunction of closely associated nerves including the recurrent laryngeal nerve.

Acute bilateral laryngeal paresis secondary to general anesthesia may be a consequence of laryngeal inflammation and edema (from endotracheal intubation and venous congestion from a dependent head position) or neuromuscular failure.[23,24] Trauma may cause swelling of the laryngeal tissues. Dysfunction of the recurrent laryngeal nerve may be a result of trauma in the cervical neck region; compression of the nerve between the endotracheal tube and neck structures; intraoperative tissue hypoxia and ischemia; and hyperextension of the neck when a horse is in dorsal recumbency causing compression of the blood supply to the nerve.

Horses with hemiplegia (recurrent laryngeal neuropathy) are at high risk for acute severe obstruction because of bilateral paresis if damage to the other recurrent laryngeal nerve occurs (e.g. from a perivascular injection). Horses with acute severe obstruction following general anesthesia are likely to have an underlying undiagnosed or untreated recurrent laryngeal neuropathy.

Bilateral laryngeal paresis has been associated with hepatic encephalopathy[23,25], organophosphate poisoning[26], *Hypochaeris radicata* toxicity (Australian stringhalt)[27], laryngeal edema secondary to anaphylactic reaction or purpura hemorrhagica, heavy metal poisoning, and botulism.[28]

Clinical features

Horses that develop acute bilateral laryngeal paresis will experience sudden severe dyspnea, stridor, and sometimes cyanosis usually following vocalization, excitement, or any type of even mild exertion. A loud, high-pitched, inspiratory stridor is observed with excessive inspiratory effort. Death is imminent secondary to severe negative pressure pulmonary edema if an airway is not rapidly established. Postanesthetic cases may not show signs for 24–72 hours after surgery.[24]

Evidence of injury or inflammation along the jugular furrows may be present. Ptosis, miosis, and sweating near the base of the ears are signs of Horner's syndrome. In addition, vascular dilation in the nasal passages can exacerbate reduced airflow, which may be detected. Hepatic encephalopathy cases demonstrate a range of clinical signs including CNS dysfunction (ataxia, circling, head pressing), colic, and inappetence.

Differential diagnosis

Arytenoid chondritis; laryngeal edema (anaphylaxis or purpura hemorrhagica); laryngitis; epiglottitis; cicatrix; laryngeal granuloma or neoplasia; cricopharyngeal–laryngeal dysplasia (rostral displacement of the palatopharyngeal arch); hepatoencephalopathy; botulism; heavy metal poisoning.

Diagnosis

Definitive diagnosis requires endoscopic examination, which can be difficult because there is no normal side for comparison. Endoscopy after the horse has been heavily sedated may be unreliable. Tissues will be swollen and collapsed within the larynx in the case of laryngeal edema and inflammation.

Palpation of the dorsal laryngeal structures to detect atrophy of the cricoarytenoideus dorsalis muscle can help increase the suspicion of laryngeal paresis in cases that are secondary to idiopathic recurrent laryngeal neuropathy or other gradual onset distal axonopathies.

Blood chemistry panels will help identify hepatic disease. Careful attention to the history of the horse will help determine likely causes of the laryngeal paresis.

Management/treatment

An emergency temporary tracheostomy (p. 258) is required in patients with marked respiratory distress. Alternatively, immediate passage of a nasotracheal tube (p. 257) may be possible and could prevent the need for a tracheostomy. Intranasal or intratracheal oxygen (10–15 liters/minute) is recommended. If pulmonary edema has occurred, furosemide (1 mg/kg IV) should be given. Dexamethasone (10 mg IV) and DMSO (0.1–1.0 g/kg diluted to a 10–20% solution in isotonic crystalloid fluids IV slowly) can also be administered.

IV fluids may counteract the hypotensive effects of systemic anaphylaxis, but should be administered with extreme caution if vascular leak is suspected.

If laryngeal edema is caused by an anaphylactic reaction, epinephrine (0.3–0.5 mg [0.3–0.5 ml of 1:1,000 or 3–5 ml of 1:10,000]) should be administered slowly IV.

If long-term dysfunction persists, definitive treatment is aimed at restoring an adequate, non-collapsing diameter to the rima glottidis to improve air flow. A unilateral laryngoplasty or arytenoidectomy may be sufficient to restore comfortable breathing in the retired pasture pet, even though this predisposes the horse to aspiration. Bilateral laryngoplasty or arytenoidectomy is not recommended because of the risk of aspiration and dysphagia. Certain horses may benefit from permanent tracheostomy (**3.28**).

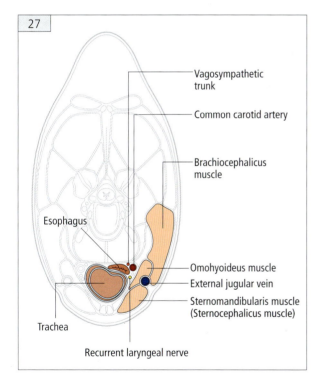

3.27 Schematic illustration of the jugular groove anatomy showing the relationship between the jugular vein and the recurrent laryngeal nerve.

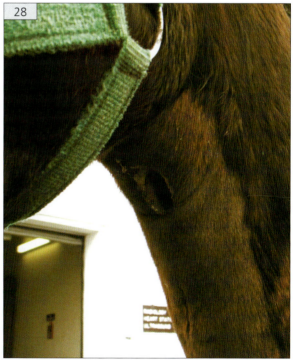

3.28 Horse with a permanent tracheostomy.

Strangles (*Streptococcus equi* subsp. *equi* lymphadenopathy)

Definition/overview

Strangles is a highly contagious bacterial infection principally affecting the URT. The term 'strangles' describes the compressive nature of retropharyngeal lymphadenopathy on the upper airway.

Etiology/pathogenesis

The infectious agent of strangles is *Streptococcus equi* subsp. *equi*. Following exposure of a naïve horse via mouth or nasal inoculation, *S. equi* subsp. *equi* penetrates lingual and palatine tonsils and after a few hours translocates by lymphatic drainage to local lymph nodes. The organism has numerous defense mechanisms (e.g. hyaluronic acid capsule, antiphagocytic SeM protein, and Mac protein) that protect it from neutrophil phagocytosis. There is typically an incubation period of 3–14 days before the first clinical signs of infection are observed. Nasal shedding of the organism begins 2–3 days after the onset of fever and may persist for 2–3 weeks.[29]

Metastasis of the organism via hematogenous or lymphatic routes results in abscess development in distant locations (i.e. 'bastard strangles'), which may affect the abdominal organs, lung parenchyma, and the CNS.[29,30]

After 2–3 weeks, systemic and mucosal immune responses are established and clearance of the organism is apparent; however, a proportion of horses can shed the organism for at least 6 weeks after apparently making a full recovery.

A strong, long-lasting immunity to strangles develops in about 75% of horses that experience the disease.[29] Horses that develop a less effective immune response can become clinically healthy, long-term carriers of the organism, with the usual site of persistent infection being the guttural pouch.[31] Persistent purulent exudate in the guttural pouch may become inspissated and form ovoid concretions called 'chondroids'.

Transmission of infection occurs through transfer of *S. equi* subsp *equi* in purulent discharges. This can be by direct horse to horse contact or indirectly through sharing contaminated housing, water, feed, tack, or twitches, and via personnel working with affected and susceptible horses.

Clinical features

The typical presentation is abrupt onset of fever followed by a mucopurulent nasal discharge. About 1 week after infection, retropharyngeal and submandibular lymphadenopathy and abscessation develops and is noted by unilateral or bilateral swelling of the throat latch (Viborg's triangle) and intermandibular region (**3.29**). The swollen regions are hot, edematous, and painful to the horse when manipulated. Lymph nodes may rupture spontaneously and drain a purulent discharge that does not have a foul odor. Dysphagia, inappetence or anorexia, signs of dullness, and listlessness are common findings and the horse may stand with its neck extended.[29,32]

Dyspnea and respiratory stridor will be present when severe lymphadenopathy and abscessation cause compressive obstruction of the airway and possibly temporary laryngeal hemiparesis. Nasal reflux of food and water may be seen during attempts to swallow. A moist, low-grade cough may be present, but is not a feature in many cases. Purulent ocular discharge can also develop.

Severity of clinical signs and disease depends on the immune status of the horse with older horses often exhibiting a milder form of disease compared to naïve, younger horses.

Differential diagnosis

Retropharyngeal foreign body; neoplasia; laryngitis; pharyngeal trauma; hematoma; cellulitis; lymphadenitis; esophageal obstruction.

Diagnosis

Known exposure to horses infected with *S. equi* subsp. *equi* strongly supports the clinical examination findings and presumptive diagnosis. Definitive diagnosis requires culturing of the organism from nasal or nasopharyngeal swabs/washes, guttural pouch swabs/washes, or fluid aspirated from abscesses. Nasal washes are more effective than swabs in detecting small numbers of organisms because a greater mucosal surface area is sampled. A Gram stain of aspirated fluid will show typical gram-positive cocci organisms linked in chains. Hematology may reveal leukocytosis and hyperfibrinogenemia to support pyogenic infection.

Rhinopharyngoscopy allows identification of the source of airway compression and examination of the guttural pouches for evidence of swollen lymph nodes bulging up from the ventral floor of the pouch (**3.30**). Rupture of lymph nodes into the pouch and guttural pouch empyema can be diagnosed.

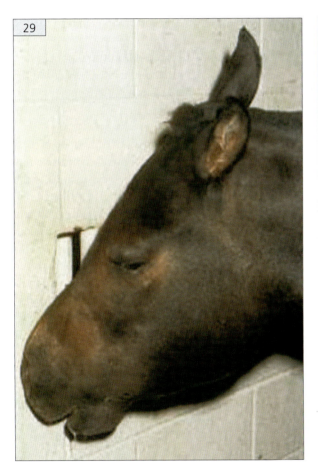

3.29 Horse with *Streptococcus equi* subsp. *equi* lymphadenopathy. (Courtesy Dr Josie Traub-Dargatz)

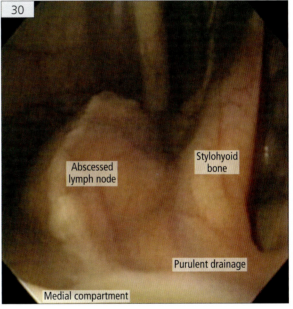

3.30 Endoscopic appearance of the medial compartment of the left guttural pouch illustrating a retropharyngeal lymph node protruding into the ventral aspect.

Radiographs reveal a soft tissue density in the retropharyngeal area, dorsoventral compression of the nasopharynx, and/or an irregular ventral border of the guttural pouches.

Ultrasonographic examination allows accurate assessment of the size and location of any abscesses and facilitates percutaneous needle aspiration of material.

PCR is a relatively sensitive and quick method compared with culturing to detect *S. equi* subsp *equi* DNA sequences and can be used to screen horses for potential carrier states where low bacterial numbers are shed.[29] Serologic assay for SeM protein is useful for diagnosing recent infection and the possibility of a metastatic abscess or purpura hemorrhagica.[33]

Management/treatment

Horses suspected of having strangles should be isolated and appropriate measures taken to control further bacterial transmission.[29] An emergency temporary tracheostomy (p. 258) may be required in horses that already have marked respiratory distress or that do not respond quickly to therapy and develop signs of airway obstruction.

Medical management with systemic antimicrobial drugs (penicillin is the drug of choice) and NSAIDs is effective in many cases of early disease. However, use of antimicrobials is controversial as they may inhibit an effective immune response, with treated horses remaining susceptible to reinfection.[29] Antimicrobial drug therapy is probably contraindicated in horses with palpable external lymphadenopathy that are otherwise healthy and alert.[29,33] Thick-walled abscesses respond less effectively to systemic antimicrobial drugs and surgical drainage of matured abscesses using ultrasonographic guidance in the standing, sedated, and locally anesthetized horse is often required. A technique of percutaneous needle lavage and antimicrobial drug infusion into abscessed cavities has also been described.[34]

Complications of strangles include chronic guttural pouch empyema, purpura hemorrhagica, myositis, agalactia, and infections at distant anatomic sites (metastatic or bastard strangles).

Any new horse with an unknown medical history introduced to other herd animals should ideally be isolated for 3 weeks and screened for *S. equi* subsp *equi* by PCR and culture of weekly nasopharyngeal samples.[29] Swabs of the guttural pouch or guttural pouch lavage fluid should be obtained and cultured for any suspect carrier animals.[35]

Guttural pouch tympany
Key points
- Foals with guttural pouch tympany present with a large soft swelling in the throat latch region.
- An emergency temporary tracheostomy is necessary in some cases.
- Treatment involves creating an outflow tract for the air to pass from the guttural pouch into the nasopharynx.
- An attempt to decompress the guttural pouches percutaneously is not recommended because of the risk of iatrogenic nerve and vascular damage.

Definition/overview

Excessive accumulation of air within the guttural pouch is referred to as guttural pouch tympany. The guttural pouches are large, sac-like expansions of the eustachian tubes lined by pseudostratified ciliated respiratory epithelium containing goblet cells. Left and right pouches are separated by a median septum and the dorsally located rectus capitis ventralis and longus capitis muscles. The pouches communicate with the nasopharynx through dorsolaterally located funnel-shaped openings, which have a cartilaginous medial flap binding their entrance (plica salpingopharyngea). Normally, guttural pouch air influx and efflux is regulated.

Etiology/pathogenesis

A definitive cause is not determined for most cases. Redundant or excessive mucosa on the ventral aspect of the plica salpingopharyngea may create a one-way valve allowing air to enter but not exit the pouch.[36] Malformed pharyngeal openings have been rarely implicated in the condition.

Foals are most commonly affected from birth to 1 year of age and fillies are more often affected than colts.[37] Congenital and acquired tympany can occur. Acquired tympany may be due to upper airway inflammation causing edema of the plica salpingopharyngea; this is more common than congenital disease with excessive mucosa development. Lateral expansion of the pouch is limited, therefore expansion is greatest in the medial compartment (**3.31**).[38] As the pouch inflates, there is collapse of the dorsal pharyngeal wall (and then the dorsolateral walls) into the nasopharynx, causing worsening respiratory obstruction. Most commonly, the condition is unilateral; however, severe unilateral distension can appear to be a bilateral disease.

Clinical features

The foal may present in severe respiratory distress with a grossly swollen throat latch region (**3.32**), or show little airway breathing difficulties at rest and have moderate swelling present at the throat latch. The owner may report hearing an inspiratory stridor that worsens when the foal is excited. Foals can have a white nasal discharge, which is usually a combination of milk and purulent exudate, and dysphagia is common. Signs of LRT infection (due to aspiration pneumonia) may also be present including dullness, coughing, inappetence, presence of a fever, and increased lower airway sounds and effort.

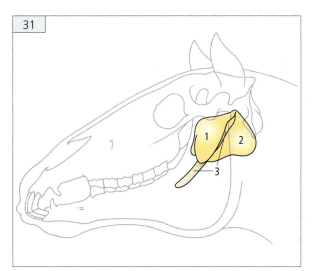

3.31 Schematic illustration of the anatomy of the guttural pouches. 1, lateral compartment; 2, medial compartment; 3, stylohyoid.

3.32 Foal with unilateral guttural pouch tympany. (Courtesy Dr Jock Tate)

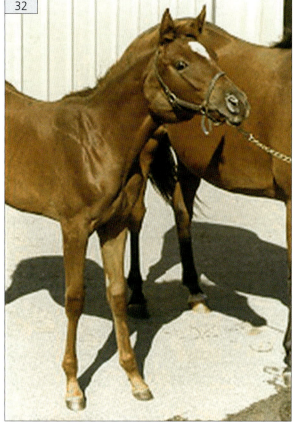

Differential diagnosis

Guttural pouch empyema; guttural pouch neoplasia; retropharyngeal lymph node hyperplasia/abscessation; salivary duct obstruction (sialocele); cellulitis; esophageal obstruction or perforation.

Diagnosis

Physical, endoscopic, and radiographic examination are used to obtain a definitive diagnosis. External palpation of non-painful swellings in the throat latch is consistent with guttural pouch tympany and sometimes manual compression will reduce the size of the pouch, indicating it was full of air.

Endoscopic examination of the upper airway may reveal dorsal collapse of the nasopharynx to varying degrees, with significant narrowing of the nasopharynx (**3.33**). When the endoscope or a catheter is passed into the affected pouch, there will be an immediate deflating of the pouch as air escapes. White, fluid material may be present in the guttural pouch.

Radiographic examination reveals an enlarged gas-filled pouch that can extend beyond the level of the second cervical vertebra (**3.34**). Determining the affected side is critical for treatment success when choosing a side-specific treatment option.

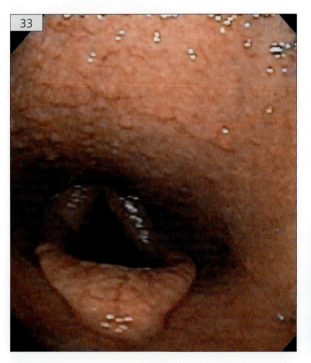

3.33 Endoscopic appearance of guttural pouch tympany illustrating dorsal collapse of the nasopharynx. (Courtesy Dr Eric Parente)

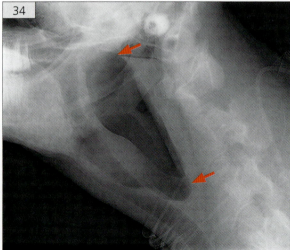

3.34 Radiographic image of a foal with guttural pouch tympany illustrating air-filled guttural pouches (arrows).

Percutaneous needle puncture of the pouch through Viborg's triangle can be performed under aseptic conditions to confirm an air-filled cavity, but is not recommended as a routine procedure because of the risk of iatrogenic neurologic or vascular damage.

Management/treatment

Some foals require an emergency temporary tracheostomy (p. 258) because of the severe dorsoventral compression of the caudal nasopharynx. Rarely, a case will be self-limiting. Most foals benefit from establishing an effective outflow tract for air accumulating in the affected pouch.

If upper airway inflammation and edema are considered the cause of the outflow obstruction, temporary catheterization of the affected pouch(es) with an indwelling Foley catheter or similar and treatment of the upper airway condition may be curative.

Surgical intervention is usually required and includes fenestration of the median septum so that air can flow from the abnormal side to the normal side and into the nasopharynx. Fenestration can be performed via a Viborg's triangle approach or via transendoscopic laser surgery. Plica salpingopharyngea opening enlargement by resecting the mucosal fold or the cartilaginous flap, or both, or by passing forceps into the opening and expanding them can be performed. If bilaterally affected, both plica salpingopharyngea openings need to be enlarged. An alternative minimally invasive transendoscopic laser surgery technique is to create a permanent fistula between the affected guttural pouch and the nasopharynx dorsocaudal to the existing opening (**3.35**).[39] This procedure is usually performed in the standing, sedated foal. Recently, salpingoscopy has been described as a minimally invasive approach to the guttural pouches that facilitates resection of tissue at the plica salpingopharyngea openings.[40]

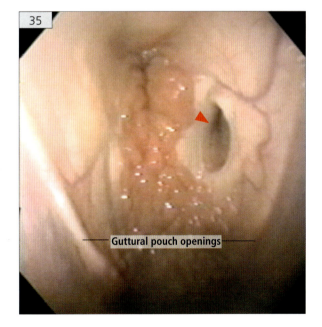

3.35 Endoscopic appearance of the pharynx 3 weeks following creation of a permanent fistula (arrow head) between the affected guttural pouch and the nasopharynx dorsocaudal to the existing opening. (Courtesy Dr Jock Tate)

Long-term prognosis after surgical intervention is good provided there is no iatrogenic neurologic damage. Fenestrations and fistulas may close with the subsequent recurrence of tympany requiring a second surgery.

Snake bite

Key points

- Snake bite is common in many geographic areas. It is important to be aware of problematic snakes in specific regions of the world.
- Horses are most commonly bitten on the muzzle and severe swelling in association with tissue damage from toxins in the venom can cause URT obstruction.
- Important aspects of treatment are maintaining a patent airway and managing the systemic effects of the venom toxins.

Definition/overview

Horses in certain geographic areas are commonly bitten on the nose by snakes, usually rattlesnakes. Swelling from the toxins in the venom causes URT obstruction, which is often severe.

Etiology/pathogenesis

Depending on the geographic region, there are a variety of snakes whose venom can cause local and systemic pathology. Rattlesnakes, cottonmouths (water moccasins), copperheads, and coral snakes are the four common species of venomous snake in the US. Rattlesnakes are widely dispersed and, therefore, are likely the most common species to cause snake bite injury. Copperheads are particularly prevalent in the eastern US. Different snake species are problematic in other regions of the world and local familiarity is important. Horses are susceptible to snake bite injury given their habitat and grazing practices. The face and distal limbs are most commonly bitten.[41]

Snake venom contains many enzymes and toxins and can be broadly classified as primarily neurotoxic, cytotoxic, or hematoxic. Viperids, also known as 'pit vipers' and found worldwide, typically contain an abundance of proteases in their venom (cytotoxic and hematoxic actions) that produce localized severe pain, swelling, tissue necrosis, and DIC. Many of the enzymes have a digestive function serving to 'predigest' the prey before it is consumed by the snake. These snakes are capable of giving a 'dry bite'. In this instance, there is no injection of venom into the animal and possibly only localized puncture wound reaction may be identified. Death from envenomation is usually the result of cardiovascular collapse.

Elapids (coral snakes) have venom that is mostly neurotoxic and causes paralysis that may result in death due to asphyxiation. Some snakes will produce a mixture of signs consistent with cytotoxicity and neurotoxicity.

The outcome following a snake bite is dependent on factors such as the species and size of the snake involved, location of the bite, how much venom was injected (if any), and the victim's body mass, age, and health.

Clinical features

Following viperid envenomation, the most common physical examination findings are progressive swelling at the bite location (usually on the muzzle, **3.36**), fever, tachycardia, dyspnea, epistaxis, and tachypnea.[41] Cardiac dysrhythmias, clotting abnormalities, diarrhea, colic, CN deficits, and laminitis may also be noted. Airway obstruction develops secondary to facial swelling. Warm swelling becomes cool as the skin necroses and severe cellulitis may occur with secondary *Clostridium* spp. infection.[42] Anemia and thrombocytopenia may be noted on CBC. High concentrations of muscle enzymes (i.e. CK and AST) on biochemical analysis are consistent with myonecrosis. Severe systemic affects are not common in adult horses; foals may be more susceptible to cardiovascular dysfunction and shock.[42] Unexpected death is possible, particularly in foals at pasture.

Differential diagnosis

Bee sting; spider bite (black widow); fire ant bites; penetrating foreign body or trauma to the head or limb; lymphangitis; cellulitis; clostridial myositis; anaphylaxis; acute obstruction of the jugular vein with concurrent low head carriage.

Diagnosis

The bite incident is rarely witnessed and diagnosis may be reached by ruling out other causes of swelling and tissue necrosis. The known presence of venomous snakes and time of year are important factors in considering the likelihood of snake bite injury. Shaving a suspected area may reveal fang marks. Upper airway endoscopy, radiography, and ultrasonography are useful for detecting the cause of acute airway distress and assessing swollen soft tissues. Hematology testing revealing hematologic dysfunction is supportive.

Management/treatment

The definitive treatment for confirmed snake envenomation is prompt IV administration of the specific antivenin for that species of snake. This appears to be rarely performed in the horse probably because of cost, lack of convenient access to treatment, inexperience with appropriate treatment, and time delay between the bite and clinical recognition of the problem.[41,43] In the US, an equine-derived IgG-based polyvalent antivenin is licensed for use in animals, as is an equine-origin elapid (coral snake) antivenin.[43] Antivenin (equine origin) is not recommended unless administered within the first 8 hours following the bite.[43] Antivenin administration may be useful in foals bitten by coral snakes. An Australian study revealed that the use of antivenin significantly improved the chances of survival of domestic animals bitten by snakes.[44]

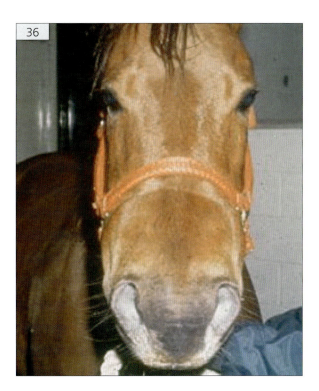

3.36 Horse with a swollen muzzle as a result of a rattlesnake bite. (Courtesy Dr Josie Traub-Dargatz)

Following suspected snake bite horses should be kept as calm and inactive as possible. The inclination to apply a tourniquet, ligature, or compression bandage should be strongly discouraged; these procedures increase local tissue damage because of ischemia. The historical practice of incising open identified fang puncture marks is of inconsequential value.[43] Likewise, surgical fasciotomy has very limited application in emergency management of snake bites. Tissue spread of venom may be promoted by the vasodilatory effects of alcohol, so its use to clean the wound is contraindicated.

It is critical to ensure maintenance of a patent upper airway and to monitor cardiovascular and pulmonary function closely. Passage of a stomach tube, a nasotracheal tube, or a 20–35 ml syringe case that has the end cut off, inserted into the ventral nasal meatus will help maintain an airway in the face of progressive muzzle swelling.[42] Elevation of the head will help reduce severe swelling associated with facial bites and may reduce the risk of airway obstruction. A temporary tracheostomy (see Temporary tracheostomy) is indicated if airway obstruction becomes severe.

NSAID and broad-spectrum antimicrobial drug administration and tetanus prophylaxis are routine supportive treatments. The use of corticosteroids is controversial and may not be beneficial.[41] Hypotensive patients showing signs of shock should be managed with IV fluids and inotropic or vasopressor drugs as indicated (see Chapter 13). Whole blood transfusion may be required in an acutely anemic patient. Monitoring coagulation parameters may be useful; plasma or heparin or low molecular weight heparin administration may be beneficial in patients with abnormal coagulation parameters.

Bite wound management includes cleansing, lavage, debridement of necrotic tissues, pressure bandaging of limbs, and hydrotherapy. Chronic complications include laminitis, pneumonia, colitis, and cardiac dysfunction.[41]

Mortality rates may reach 20–30%. Foals and miniature breeds are more likely to die from a snake bite than 450 kg mature animals or larger because of their smaller body size relative to the volume of venom injected.

Clostridial myositis
(See also Chapter 2)
Key points
- Clostridial myositis affecting the head and upper neck can cause severe URT obstruction.
- In addition to treatment of the clostridial myositis, providing a patent airway is necessary in some cases.

Definition/overview
This condition is also referred to as malignant edema, gas gangrene, or clostridial myonecrosis and is an acute-onset, fulminating, and necrotizing infection of the subcutaneous and deeper muscle tissues. Clostridial myositis can occur in the head and neck region, causing severe URT obstruction as a result of marked swelling around the airway. Quarter Horses and stallions may be at increased risk of developing the disease compared with other horses.[45,46] A typical preceding event is IM (or inadvertent perivascular) administration of a NSAID for treatment of colic or soft tissue wounds.

Etiology/pathogenesis
The infectious agent is a *Clostridium* spp. *C. perfringens* and *C. septicum* are most commonly isolated; however, other *Clostridium* spp. have been reported associated with the syndrome and multiple *Clostridium* spp. may be isolated from a single site.[45,46] Flunixin meglumine is the most common IM administered drug associated with clostridial myositis, perhaps because it is used IM more frequently than other drugs. B vitamins, dipyrone, phenylbutazone, dexamethasone, furosemide, vaccines, and perivascular leakage of 50% dextrose, selenium, epinephrine, and tripelennamine hydrochloride (antihistamine) have all been associated with the development of clostridial myositis.[45,46]

The source of the vegetative or spore form of the clostridial organisms remains unknown. The microorganisms may remain dormant in muscle tissue until a traumatic event leads to local necrotic and anaerobic conditions favoring spore germination, growth of vegetative organisms, and production of toxins. Variations in IM injection technique (e.g. the degree of skin preparation, swabbing the top of a multidose vial) do not appear to influence the incidence of clostridial myositis in horses.[47]

Clinical features

The rapid development (as soon as 6 hours in peracute cases) of painful, hot, soft tissue swelling at the site of IM or intended IV injection is the typical presentation. A traumatic wound may be associated with some cases. Subcutaneous emphysema (crepitus) is often palpable, but may be absent early in the disease course.[46] A stiff neck after cervical muscle or jugular vein injection and an inability or reluctance to lower or raise the head and neck may be observed. Horses with clostridial myositis affecting the upper neck region and head may also present with signs of respiratory distress (3.37). The soft tissue swelling will become cool and firm as tissue necrosis occurs. Horses may be toxemic, febrile, obtunded, and in cardiovascular shock.[48] Sudden death is possible.

Differential diagnosis

Abscesses caused by other bacteria; cellulitis; acute impact trauma; hematoma; esophageal or tracheal perforation.

Diagnosis

A history of recent IM, SC, or IV injection supports the presumptive diagnosis established by physical examination. Definitive diagnosis is by demonstration of large gram-positive rods in needle aspirates of the swelling and anaerobic culture of clostridial organisms. Fluorescent antibody analysis is also available. Ultrasonographic examination is useful to assess deeper necrotic tissues and identify the presence of gas in the soft tissues, supportive of a diagnosis of an anaerobic infection. URT endoscopy can be used to determine the extent of airway compromise as well as the extent of tissue damage.

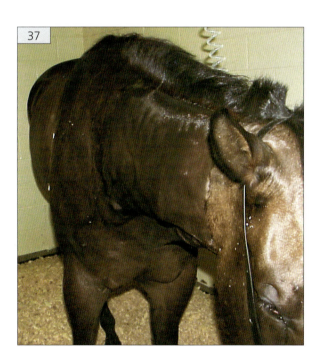

3.37 Head and neck swelling in a horse with clostridial myositis.

Management/treatment

Emergency treatment includes initiation of IV antimicrobial treatment and providing oxygenation and drainage of the infected tissues. Infrequently, tracheostomy (p. 258) or nasotracheal intubation (p. 257) is required in horses with severe facial swelling/edema. High-dose crystalline penicillin (44,000 IU/kg [20,000 IU/lb]) is commonly recommended and administered for at least 7 days. Anecdotal evidence suggests a combination of oxytetracycline and metronidazole may be a more efficacious antimicrobial treatment protocol and these drugs are less expensive than crystalline penicillin.[49] Clostridial toxins may cause erythrocyte, leukocyte, and platelet destruction, and this may be anticipated in the early treatment period. Treatment-associated penicillin-mediated hematologic abnormalities (e.g. anemia) usually occur a few days into treatment in an otherwise clinically responding patient.[46]

Early fasciotomy/myotomy is considered extremely important for successful outcome. The increased oxygenation of the infected area and access for lavage help reduce the spread of the disease. The procedure is performed under standing sedation with minimal need for local anesthetic infiltration in the necrotic tissues to be incised. Parallel incisions in a dorsoventral direction are made about 2.5 cm (1 in) apart extending into well-vascularized healthy tissue slightly beyond the perimeter of the necrotic tissue (**3.38**). Debridement of necrotic tissue is also performed. Wound lavage with penicillin solutions may be performed, but is not considered critical for resolution of the infection.[46] The use of hyperbaric oxygen therapy to improve oxygen delivery to tissues is a consideration and custom designed equine units are becoming more available.[45]

Other supportive medical care includes IV fluids as indicated and NSAID administration. Continued careful monitoring of wounds (pre-existing or created) is required to ensure infection is not spreading and further tissue debridement and incisions may be necessary. Appropriate antimicrobial therapy is continued for 2–4 weeks.

The overall survival rate of horses with clostridial myositis is approximately 75% with aggressive, early emergency treatment. The survival rate of horses with clostridial myositis affecting the URT is unknown.

Tracheal trauma
Key points
- Horses with tracheal perforation can have considerable subcutaneous emphysema.
- Many cases are managed medically with success.
- If tracheal collapse occurs, a temporary tracheostomy should be performed below the site of the tracheal perforation.

Definition/overview
Blunt or sharp impact injury to the trachea can result in disruption of the normal tracheal anatomy.

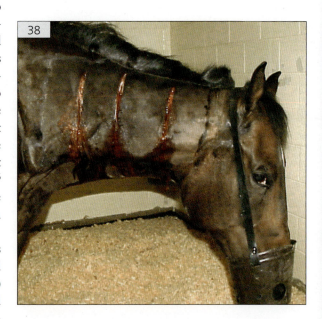

3.38 **Fasciotomy incisions in a horse with clostridial myositis.**

Etiology/pathogenesis

Kick injuries from other horses or collision injuries with fixed objects are common causes of tracheal trauma. The rostral two-thirds of the cervical trachea lies on the ventral midline, protected by a relatively thin layer of soft tissue, and is susceptible to blunt or penetrating trauma. Blunt trauma, with no associated open wound, may cause a tear in the wall of the trachea and subsequent development of spreading subcutaneous emphysema and local cellulitis. Sharp, penetrating trauma results in an open wound communicating between the tracheal lumen and the skin surface. Injuries can be fatal or complicated by trauma to the adjacent neurovascular and soft tissue structures (common carotids, jugular veins, vagosympathetic trunks, recurrent laryngeal nerves, and esophagus) in the neck (see **3.27**).

Clinical features

Horses may be in respiratory distress (dyspnea) if the trachea has been compressed to any degree, but this is uncommon. A history of observed trauma may be available at presentation. Open wounds are readily identified. Subcutaneous emphysema will develop with a closed laceration of the trachea and may also occur with open wounds. Regional swelling that is warm and painful to palpation is indicative of cellulitis. Coughing may be present if blood or other foreign materials have been aspirated. Frothy fluid may be present at the nares or open wound site. Disruption of adjacent vital neurovascular structures may be evident in the form of Horner's syndrome or rapid exsanguination.

Differential diagnosis

Esophageal perforation; esophageal obstruction; axillary wound; upper airway obstruction (laryngeal hemiplegia, arytenoid chondritis, neoplasia); cellulitis.

Diagnosis

History and physical examination will lead to a suspicion of tracheal perforation in most cases. Tracheoscopy is necessary to confirm the presence of a tear in the tracheal wall unless examination of an open wound reveals an open tracheal lumen. Tracheoscopy should be performed in all cases to fully assess the trauma to the trachea. Ultrasonographic examination can reveal subcutaneous air and foreign bodies. Radiographs are useful for evaluation of tracheal lumen diameter and the presence of intraluminal masses or peritracheal gas.[50]

Management/treatment

Acute respiratory distress caused by a compressed trachea can only be managed by a temporary tracheostomy (p. 258) placed distal to the compressed site; this is difficult in cases with caudal tracheal injuries. Many tracheal perforations can be managed medically with stall confinement to limit movement and progression of subcutaneous emphysema.[50,51] NSAIDs and antimicrobial medications are routinely administered. Surgical closure of a perforated trachea is performed where there is a large defect that might take months to heal by second intention.[50,52,53] The prognosis is favorable provided there are no aspiration pneumonia complications. Some horses develop an alarming degree of subcutaneous emphysema, which will eventually be resorbed. Rarely, increased pressure around the larynx from subcutaneous emphysema will necessitate a temporary tracheostomy distally to allow comfortable breathing and healing of the tracheal wound.[54] A large tracheal perforation with intact skin can be converted to an open wound at the injury site to prevent air being forced subcutaneously and the possible subsequent need for a tracheostomy.[50] On occasion, subcutaneous emphysema can lead to pneumomediastinum and pneumothorax.

UPPER AIRWAY DISEASES ASSOCIATED WITH EPISTAXIS

Longus capitis and rectus capitis muscle rupture/basi-sphenoid/occipital fracture
Key points (see also Chapter 7)

- Horses with longus capitis and rectus capitis muscle rupture usually present with epistaxis originating from the guttural pouch and the main differential diagnosis is guttural pouch mycosis.
- Horses with longus capitis and rectus capitis muscle rupture often have a history of falling over backwards.
- Treatment is supportive, although horses with severe accompanying neurologic signs will require immediate intervention.

Definition/overview
The longus capitis muscle is the largest flexor muscle of the head (**3.39**). The rectus capitis ventralis and the rectus capitis lateralis are the other two flexor muscles. The longus capitus and rectus capitus ventralis muscles are located in the dorsal aspect of the median septum of the guttural pouches. The longus capitis arises from the transverse processes of C3 to C5/6 and inserts on the basioccipital basisphenoid bone junction. The rectus capitis ventralis arises from the ventral arch of the atlas and inserts on the occipital bone.

Etiology/pathogenesis
Rupture of the muscles or fracture of the basisphenoid/basioccipital bones is traumatic in origin. Typically, the horse is reported to have fallen over backwards, hitting its poll on the ground in a hyperflexed position, which causes sudden violent hyperextension of the head and neck, although this may not be witnessed.[55] This causes acute rupture of the flexor muscles and possibly fracture of the basisphenoid/basioccipital bones due to a sudden pull on the insertion points of the muscles.

Clinical features
Horses present with acute epistaxis.[36,55] The neurologic status may vary from normal to severe dullness with or without CN signs or recumbency due to traumatic brain injury.

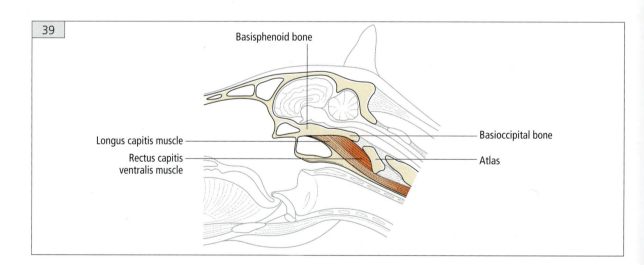

3.39 Schematic illustration of the anatomy of the longus capitis muscle.

Differential diagnosis

Guttural pouch mycosis (see Chapter 4); ethmoid hematoma; head trauma; foreign body; temporohyoid osteoarthropathy; guttural pouch empyema; guttural pouch neoplasia.

Diagnosis

Endoscopic examination and a history of falling over backwards support a definitive diagnosis. Endoscopic examination reveals dorsolateral pharyngeal wall collapse and blood exiting one or both guttural pouch openings. Within the guttural pouch, there will be accumulated blood clots and submucosal hematoma formation in the median septum. Blood clots and fresh hemorrhage may obscure the view and prevent a complete examination.

Radiographic evaluation will show a soft tissue opacification of the guttural pouch with nasopharyngeal narrowing due to collapse of the dorsal pharyngeal wall. Basisphenoid/basioccipital fracture may be evident by the presence of bone fragments ventral to the bone or an apparent displacement (**3.40**).[55,56]

Management/treatment

Treatment is supportive. Emergency care may include fluid therapy and/or a blood transfusion if blood loss is determined to be severe (see Chapter 12). Stall rest and anti-inflammatory drugs are indicated in combination with any necessary treatment for brain injury (see Chapter 7). The hematoma will usually resolve without complication over a few weeks. Treatment with antimicrobial drugs is indicated to reduce the risk of secondary bacterial infection. Mild neurologic deficits may persist in cases with neurologic disease at presentation. Severe neurologic signs warrant immediate intervention (see Chapter 7).

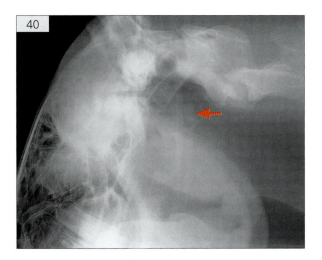

3.40 **Radiographic illustration of a basisphenoid fracture (arrow).**

Head trauma (sinus and nasal passage)

Key points
- The prognosis for horses with sinus and nasal passage head trauma is good.
- Conservative management usually results in a satisfactory outcome if the cosmetic appearance of the horse is not a concern.
- Maintenance of a patent airway and providing the necessary medical stabilization are the most important emergency treatments.

Definition/overview
The paranasal sinuses (caudal and rostral maxillary sinuses laterally; frontal and dorsal conchal sinuses dorsally) and nasal passages are protected by relatively thin plates of bone and minimal soft tissue in most areas. The ventral conchal and sphenopalatine sinuses are more medial and not typically affected by trauma.

Etiology/pathogenesis
Most facial injuries are the result of a kick from another horse or impact with a fixed object. The horse's natural flight response predisposes them to high impact trauma. Foal facial bones are more easily crushed compared with mature horses.

Open or closed fractures of the paranasal sinuses or nasal passages can occur. Typically, facial bones are depressed into the sinus cavity with or without skin disruption (**3.41**). When there is no skin disruption, a fracture may go unnoticed as the surface contour looks normal when the skin is detached from the bone during the impact.[57] Hemorrhage into the sinus or nasal passage space occurs with trauma. Significant nasal passage injury may lead to partial or complete air flow obstruction of the affected side. Severe impact trauma may cause ocular and CNS dysfunction. Healing or healed fracture sites will often appear as a concavity in the facial bone, with firm swelling along the fracture line where callous is present.[57]

Clinical features
Unilateral or bilateral epistaxis with obvious external facial injury is the common clinical presentation. Palpation will reveal subcutaneous emphysema when the paranasal sinus or nasal passage is breached.

Crepitus will also be felt when loose bone fragments are present. Air will flow in and out of a full-thickness defect as the horse breathes. Bubbles of blood may be apparent through smaller openings. Upper airway respiratory sounds will be increased in the case of partial obstruction of the nasal passage and airflow at the nares will be absent on the affected side if obstruction is complete. Nasolacrimal duct disruption can result in epiphora. Dullness or apparent visual impairment may be present with severe trauma. Injury involving the facial nerve branches will lead to muzzle asymmetry, with the lips being pulled to the unaffected side.

Differential diagnosis
Ethmoid hematoma; guttural pouch mycosis; nasal foreign body; neoplasia; fungal rhinitis; idiopathic epistaxis.

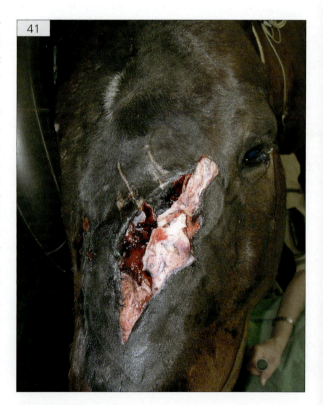

3.41 A horse with head trauma illustrating skin laceration with compression fracture of the facial bones.

Diagnosis

Observed trauma may be reported. Physical examination will provide the most specific evidence of facial trauma involving the paranasal sinuses and/or nasal passages. Rhinoscopy can be used to confirm the source of epistaxis and allow assessment of nasal passage integrity. Head radiographs will reveal fluid accumulation (blood) in the paranasal sinuses and subcutaneous air, and help with assessment of fractured bones (**3.42**). Multiple oblique views are required to definitively image the fractured area. Superimposition of head structures will limit the ability of radiographs to accurately determine the extent and configuration of a facial fracture(s). Fractures around the orbit need close evaluation to determine if there is any ocular damage. Careful assessment is also needed to rule out injury to tooth roots.

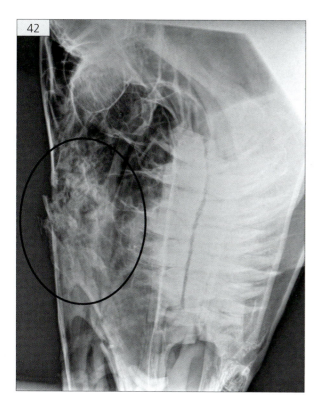

3.42 Radiographic image of a horse with a compression fracture of the facial bones (circled).

Management/treatment

Infrequently, a horse may need a temporary tracheostomy (p. 258) if injury results in bilateral nasal passage obstruction. Many fractures may be managed conservatively, particularly if cosmetic outcome is not a major concern.

Trephination at a stable site and lavage of sinus cavities to remove accumulated blood is recommended to reduce the risk of secondary sinusitis. Similarly, antimicrobial treatment should be administered for at least 7–10 days.

The most cosmetic outcome is usually achieved with surgical reduction and stabilization of the fracture.[50,58] Surgical repair of fractures often involves exposure of the site through a large curvilinear skin incision and flap elevation. Fragments are elevated to adjacent normal bone contours and stabilized with orthopedic wire or small bone plates if necessary.[50,58,59] Small bone fragments with no periosteal attachments are removed. A head bandage is applied if feasible.

Complications of conservative or surgical management include sinusitis, sequestra formation, facial deformity, abnormal bone growth in young horses, and nasal obstruction.

Foreign body obstruction

Key points
- Foreign body obstruction is uncommon in horses.
- Epistaxis, purulent nasal discharge, and, occasionally, acute respiratory tract obstruction are the most common clinical signs.
- Endoscopic or surgical removal is often necessary.

Definition/overview

Complete intraluminal obstruction of the upper airway by a foreign body is uncommon in the horse. Masses are generally not large enough to cause a reduction in airflow that becomes life threatening. However, inhaling or aspirating a foreign body into the nasal passages, nasopharynx, trachea, or primary bronchi, although rare, can lead to acute respiratory distress.

Etiology/pathogenesis

Inhaled or aspirated debris (e.g. small sticks or twigs) may become lodged in the upper or lower airway.[60,61] A mass of adequate size can cause respiratory distress if it is caught in the nasopharynx, larynx, or trachea, and impedes airflow. Foreign body lodgment in the trachea or primary bronchus results in severe, acute irritation of the respiratory tract. Chronic irritation and secondary bacterial infection may then develop.

Clinical features

An acute onset of coughing is noted with variable respiratory distress. Chronic, occasionally spasmodic coughing develops in the chronic case. Nasal discharge will occur, occasionally with evidence of fresh blood (epistaxis), in the acute or chronic case and progress to mucopurulent discharge if secondary infection develops. A foul odor may also be detected if local tissue necrosis accompanies foreign body lodgment. Relative to a normal horse, increased sensitivity to external tracheal palpation will often be present (i.e. induced coughing). Fluid 'rattles' may be auscultated over the cervical trachea. Increased lung sounds, compared with a normal horse, may be detected with a foreign body lodged in a bronchus. Signs of pleuropneumonia can develop in a chronic case where the foreign body has migrated into the lung parenchyma and then penetrated the pleural space (**3.43**).

Differential diagnosis

Pharyngitis; tracheitis; bronchitis/bronchiolitis; pulmonary abscess; dust inhalation; pharyngeal lymphoid hyperplasia; ethmoid hematoma; neoplasia; dorsoventral tracheal flattening.

Diagnosis

Careful endoscopic examination of the respiratory tract will allow detection of most foreign bodies.[60,61] A complete assessment of the respiratory tract accessible by the endoscope should be performed. The horse will typically require sedation with an alpha-2 agonist (xylazine or detomidine) and butorphanol, and perhaps instillation of local anesthetic solution into the airway to reduce airway sensitivity. Rarely, a small twig will lodge in a bronchus that is too narrow to pass the endoscope in to visualize it. If pulmonary signs are present, radio-graphic evaluation is indicated to visualize dorsoventral narrowing of the trachea as a possible cause of coughing and respiratory distress.[62] Ultrasonographic examination of the thorax is also indicated when pulmonary signs are noted.

Management/treatment

Removal of the foreign body by skilled endoscopic manipulations to grasp the object and gently withdraw it is required. This can be difficult to achieve, particularly for large diameter structures. A mid- to distal cervical tracheotomy may be considered for closer access to deeply lodged foreign bodies and allow introduction of a larger grasping forceps than can be passed transendoscopically. Most foreign bodies will be removed in the standing, sedated patient. Antimicrobial and NSAIDs are routinely administered. The prognosis is excellent for full recovery once all the foreign body is removed, assuming there are no secondary complications such as pleuropneumonia or severe hemorrhage, which can be fatal.

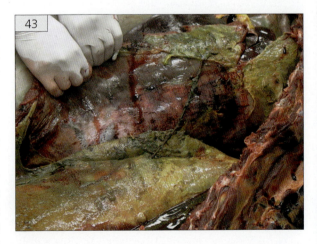

3.43 Pleuropneumonia associated with a foreign body. Note the stick that has migrated from the pulmonary parenchyma into the pleural space.

LOWER AIRWAY DISEASES

Pulmonary edema
Key points
- Acute onset pulmonary edema can frequently be successfully treated.
- Rapid establishment of an adequate airway is required in cases of negative pressure pulmonary edema (NPPE) to prevent death.
- Severe cardiogenic pulmonary edema associated with left heart failure carries a poor to grave long-term prognosis, although treatment of the edema may increase the comfort of the horse.

Definition/overview
Pulmonary edema rarely occurs as a primary event in the horse and, when present, is usually secondary to some other pathologic process. Extravascular fluid accumulates within the lung following events that alter hydrostatic and colloid osmotic interstitial and vascular forces, change the surface area and pore size of the blood–gas barrier, or diminish lymphatic drainage.[63]

Etiology/pathogenesis
Pulmonary edema can be classified as cardiogenic or non-cardiogenic (see Chapter 4). Pulmonary capillary pressure can be increased by any increase in left atrial or pulmonary artery pressure. Increases in microvascular permeability may occur with sepsis, DIC, hypoxic acidosis, or primary pulmonary pathology resulting in the release of mediators of inflammation that increase vascular endothelial or alveolar epithelial permeability. Pulmonary edema associated with even transient airway obstruction has been termed NPPE and has been reported in horses.[64–66] NPPE occurs secondary to inspiratory efforts against a closed glottis, which results in a precipitous fall in intrathoracic pressure. The large decrease in intrathoracic pressure increases the transmural pressure gradient for all intrathoracic vascular structures, favoring movement of water into the extravascular space. Neurogenic pulmonary edema, pulmonary edema associated with traumatic brain injury or seizure activity, may in fact be a form of NPPE.

Clinical features
Horses have a shallow rapid respiratory pattern and may be dyspneic. Fine crackles or wheezes may be audible on auscultation. Cases with volume overload (associated with renal failure or, rarely, too rapid fluid administration) or primary cardiac problems may have an increased CVP with pronounced venous distension. Fluid (clear or slightly yellow or pink-tinged) may drip from the nostrils and can increase in volume without necessarily becoming frothy (**3.44A, B**). Progression to this stage warrants a very grave prognosis.

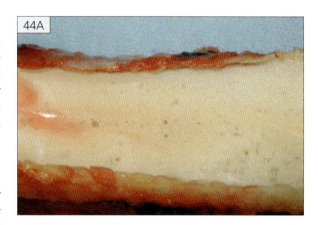

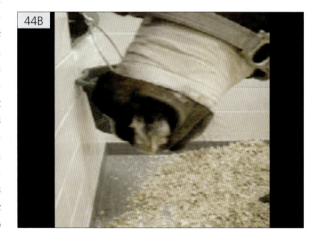

3.44A, B (A) Frothy tracheal contents in a horse with fatal pulmonary edema. (B) Froth at the nostril of an affected horse. This horse had severe acute-onset cardiac disease. (Courtesy Dr Steve Giguere)

Differential diagnosis

Any other cause of respiratory distress originating from the lungs or cardiovascular system.

Diagnosis

Diagnosis is based on clinical examination, a history of predisposing causes, and radiographs. Arterial blood gas analysis may reveal hypoxemia and hypercapnia. Radiographic findings are non-specific but include peribronchial and perivascular cuffing, increased prominence of vessels, and a hazy reticular interstitial pattern. Underlying pulmonary disease may obscure signs of edema and radiographs of sufficiently high quality to show relatively subtle changes may not be obtainable in mature horses. Radiography may not be as abnormal as lung pathology might suggest and in neonatal foals, CT might be the best imaging modality. Non-cardiogenic pulmonary edema (capillary leak) is a component of the definition for acute lung injury (ALI) and acute respiratory distress syndrome (ARDS).[67–69]

Management/treatment

Treatment consists of correcting the cause, reversing hypoxemia, decreasing plasma volume and left atrial pressure, and increasing plasma colloid osmotic pressure (COP).[69] Intranasal or intratracheal oxygen insufflation may be needed in severe cases (p. 254). Improvement in oxygenation can be monitored by sequential arterial blood gas analysis (p. 260) or by using transcutaneous oxygen saturation monitoring equipment applied to the nasal mucosa, tongue, or other available non-pigmented mucous membrane. In cases of NPPE, maintaining an adequate, low-resistance airway is very important to prevent further damage, and tracheostomy may be necessary. IV fluid therapy should be guided by the patient's needs and monitored by serial measurement of CVP if necessary. Furosemide may be given IV or IM (1–2 mg/kg, repeated in 1 hour). If helpful, the dosage can be titrated for each patient. At a dose of 1 mg/kg, approximately 8 liters of urine is produced in about 1 hour.[70] The effects of furosemide in horses with pulmonary edema have not been reported. Antiprostaglandin drugs (flunixin meglumine, phenylbutazone) and antihistamines may help. The use of corticosteroids (dexamethasone 10–20 mg IV or methylprednisolone 1 mg/kg IV q12h) remains controversial; if used, antimicrobial coverage is advisable, because pulmonary edema has been shown to impair pulmonary bacterial defense mechanisms.

Smoke inhalation

(See also Chapter 6)

Key points
- The diagnosis of smoke inhalation is straightforward.
- Clinical signs of pulmonary injury may progress for several weeks after the insult.
- Other organ systems are also generally compromised and should be evaluated and treated appropriately.

Definition/overview

Smoke inhalation injury is typically associated with exposure to fires and there are often concurrent problems in other body systems from thermal injury. Extensive or severe burns can magnify the severity of the injuries. Thermal injury along with smoke inhalation leads to both local and diffuse lesions.

Etiology/pathogenesis

Lesions are initiated by three mechanisms. The first is direct thermal injury, which can be limited to the URT. Toxic chemicals in the smoke can cause damage. Combustion consumes oxygen and the resulting low environmental and alveolar oxygen tensions can lead to pulmonary vasoconstriction as well as generalized hypoxia. Three phases of pulmonary dysfunction have been described in the horse:[71–74]

- The first is acute pulmonary insufficiency. Carbon monoxide may be present in sufficiently high concentration to cause toxicity within a short time after exposure. The acute phase includes progressive edema and necrosis in the upper airway, contributing to airway obstruction, while bronchoconstriction occurs in the LRT secondary to exposure to noxious products, and altered pulmonary blood flow.[75]

- The second phase is characterized by formation of pulmonary edema, lower airway obstruction, and pulmonary parenchymal lesions. Debris from the inflammatory cascade, along with fibrin and material deposited from smoke inhalation, may obstruct the small airways.[75]
- Bronchopneumonia, the last phase, may occur up to 1–2 weeks after the initial injury, and is a result of an impaired host immune system, both locally and systemically.

Clinical features

Horses exposed to fire with smoke will have a variety of clinical signs depending on the duration and type of exposure and the length of time from the insult.[74] Acutely, signs of carbon monoxide toxicity and shock may occur with the horse being dull, disoriented, irritable, ataxic, or moribund and comatosed. Dyspnea and stridor may develop due to injury to the upper airway. Auscultation of the thorax may be unremarkable initially, but reveal decreased air movement, crackles, or wheezes within 12–24 hours. Airflow may be severely restricted by edema of both the upper and lower airways.

Differential diagnosis

Given the history of exposure to fire and smoke, there are no significant differential diagnoses.

Diagnosis

Diagnosis is based on history and physical examination. A normal initial examination does not rule out exposure as clinical signs may require several days to manifest. A carboxyhemoglobin concentration >10% is consistent with carbon monoxide toxicity.[71] Other diagnostic tests include endoscopy of the URT and LRT (**3.45A–D**), thoracic radiography, blood gas analysis (see Chapter 11), hematology, and cytologic evaluation of tracheal aspirates.[74]

Management/treatment

Oxygen insufflation is used to overcome carbon monoxide toxicity and reduce hypoxemia (p. 254).[73] Upper airway obstruction may require temporary tracheostomy (p. 258). Sterile 0.9% saline nebulization may be beneficial, especially when pseudomembranous casts are present. Bronchodilators, diuretics, and NSAIDs are all potentially of benefit in treating airway inflammation and 'leakage' pulmonary edema. Corticosteroid use is controversial but may be beneficial.

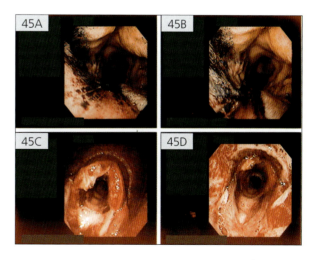

3.45A–D Effects of heat and smoke inhalation on the upper airway. A, B: Soot deposition and charring burn injury in nasal passages. C, D: Burn injury and soot deposition in laryngeal and tracheal regions. (Courtesy Dr Peggy Marsh)

Pneumonia/pleuropneumonia

Key points

- Pneumonia and pleuropneumonia are most commonly associated with stress and transport in adult horses.
- Although modern veterinary medicine and surgery have significantly reduced the death rate from pleuropneumonia, horses that develop the disease may not return to their prior use, particularly if significant complications have occurred.[76]
- Early recognition of the problem results in better outcome and a greater likelihood of returning to prior performance levels.
- Any horse being transported a long distance should be monitored closely at arrival for several days and should not undergo significant exertion until the health of its respiratory tract is known.

Definition/overview

Infection of the lung parenchyma by bacterial, viral, or fungal pathogens. Pleuropneumonia is used to describe the disease when the pleura space is also affected; typically, there is accumulation of fluid within the pleural space.

Etiology/pathogenesis

Equine pneumonia/pleuropneumonia results from contamination of the LRT with bacteria similar to the normal oropharyngeal inhabitants. Transportation of any mode, especially over long distances with no or short rest periods, is the single most important predisposing factor for this disease.[77–79] Strenuous exercise also results in LRT contamination combined with decreased immune function, therefore exercise, particularly shortly after transport, increases the risk of pleuropneumonia.[79,80] Pleuropneumonia can also occur secondary to aspiration of foreign materials, such as seen in horses with dysphagia from multiple causes, horses with choke, and horses receiving inadvertent tracheal intubation with nasogastric tubes.[81] Aspiration of mineral oil carries a particularly guarded prognosis.[82]

Pneumonia in foals is most commonly associated with equine herpesvirus (EHV) 1, 2, or 4 infection (viral pneumonia) or *Streptococcus equi* var *zooepidemicus* and *Rhodococcus equi* (bacterial pneumonia).

Pulmonary thromboembolism (PTE, also known as pulmonary infarction) can be associated with pleuropneumonia.[83] It is most commonly seen in racehorses, although it has been observed in horses with other uses. Acute or peracute onset of severe respiratory distress, with serosanguineous nasal discharge, ultrasonographic and radiographic evidence of severe pulmonary consolidation, and serosanguineous suppurative pleural effusion are all strongly suggestive of pulmonary infarction. These cases respond poorly to conventional treatment and have a poor prognosis for recovery.

Clinical features

A horse with pleuropneumonia will have fever, lethargy, and exercise intolerance. Nasal discharge is a variable finding, as is cough. Thoracic auscultation may initially be unremarkable, but as the disease progresses, abnormal lung sounds will become apparent, particularly during an examination performed using a rebreathing bag. Horses with significant lung pathology will not tolerate the bag well, may cough when the bag is removed, and may require more time to return to baseline respiratory patterns when the bag is removed.

Common abnormalities found during auscultation include ventral areas of dullness if pleural effusion is significant and dorsal harsh lung sounds. Crackles and wheezes may be variably present. Some horses with severe pleural involvement will have pleural friction rubs. The parenchyma of the right lung is commonly more severely affected, but pleural effusion is usually bilateral owing to the incomplete mediastinum present in most horses. Percussion of the thorax can reveal hyporesonance ventrally when pleural effusion is present and some horses will exhibit pleurodynia during this examination.

Differential diagnosis

Bacterial pneumonia; viral pneumonia; fungal pneumonia; heaves; pulmonary neoplasia; cardiac disease.

Diagnosis

Horses with pleuropneumonia of any duration will inevitably have hyperfibrinogenemia unless the disease has been severe enough to produce DIC, consuming fibrinogen, or they have severe concurrent liver disease resulting in decreased fibrinogen concentrations. Leukocytosis is variable, as is neutrophilia. Some horses with severe infection may have leukopenia and neutropenia.

Additional diagnostic tests include:
- Thoracic radiographic and ultrasonographic examinations. If significant pleural effusion is suspected, ultrasonography should be performed first (**3.46**). Thoracic radiographs should then be delayed until after drainage of the pleural space has been performed, as large volume pleural fluid accumulation can obscure ventral radiographic abnormalities (**3.47**).

- Samples for bacterial and fungal culture, virus isolation, and cytology should be obtained by tracheal aspirate (p. 262) early in the course of the disease, prior to initiation of treatment, in order to more appropriately direct antimicrobial therapy (**3.48**).

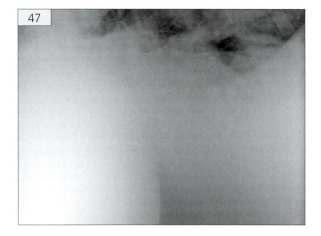

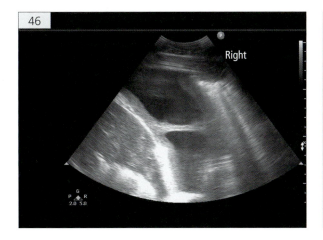

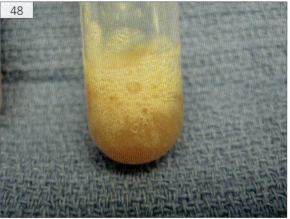

3.46 Ultrasongraphic appearance of lung affected by pleuropneumonia. There is fluid within the pleural space with fibrin adhering to the pleural surfaces and tethering the lung to the diaphragm. The lung shows variable echogenicity, demonstrating consolidation and variable aeration. (Courtesy Dr Kim Sprayberry)

3.47 Radiograph of middle and cranioventral lung following pleural drainage showing severe consolidation of cranioventral and caudoventral lung consistent with aspiration pneumonia.

3.48 Fluid obtained from transtracheal aspirate of a horse with severe pleuropneumonia. Note the yellow–orange color and purulent character of the fluid.

- Pleural fluid samples should be obtained when possible for the same purpose (p. 264). Primary pleuritis in the absence of pulmonary parenchymal infection is rare. If pleural fluid accumulation is small, samples may be obtained by ultrasound-guided thoracocentesis, performed with a teat cannula or spinal needle. If pleural fluid accumulation is significant, samples may be obtained at the time pleural drains are placed (**3.49**).

Management/treatment

Until culture and sensitivity results become available, broad-spectrum antimicrobial therapy directed against common aerobic and anaerobic organisms should be instituted. A combination of gentamicin, penicillin, and metronidazole is a good choice until microbiology testing is complete. Intranasal insufflation of oxygen may be required in severe cases (p. 254). Some cases benefit from nebulization of antimicrobial drugs such as gentamicin or ceftiofur sodium.

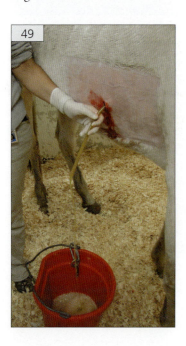

3.49 Fluid draining from a chest tube. Note the color (yellow–orange) and the froth in the bucket due to the high protein content of the fluid. (Courtesy Dr Kate McGovern)

No affordable specific treatment beyond rest and anti-inflammatory therapy exists for viral pneumonia in adult horses at present. Foals with herpes viral pneumonia may benefit from treatment with acyclovir (16–20 mg/kg PO 3–5 times daily)[84], while foals with influenza may benefit from oseltamivir phosphate (Tamiflu®) treatment.[85]

Treatment for fungal pneumonia is generally prolonged and may have a poorer prognosis. Local knowledge of common fungal pathogens and their responses to various fungicides will aid therapy.

Horses with pleuropneumonia frequently benefit from administration of NSAIDs, both for their analgesia and their anti-pyretic and anti-inflammatory properties. The use of corticosteroids (methylprednisolone, 1 mg/kg IV q12h) in the treatment of severe pneumonia is gaining acceptance, but remains controversial.

Antimicrobial treatment may be required for weeks to months in some patients. Some severe cases may require transthoracic abscess drainage, thoracoscopy, thoracic lavage, or removal of areas of necrotic lung/ large abscesses via rib resection.[86,87]

Pneumothorax/hemothorax
Key points

- Pneumothorax and hemothorax should be suspected in horses with subcutaneous emphysema and/or a history of thoracic trauma.
- Removal of air or blood is not always necessary, but should be performed if respiratory compromise is evident or progressive.

Definition/overview
Pneumothorax and hemothorax refer to the presence of air and blood, respectively, within the pleural space.

Etiology/pathogenesis
Pneumothorax and hemothorax have been reported secondary to trauma and pneumonia and also as a spontaneous occurrence in horses at maximal exertion.[88–94] Hemothorax has been reported as a complication of lung biopsy and associated with neoplasia.[89,95] Pneumothorax may be bilateral due to an incomplete mediastinum in some horses; hemothorax generally is bilateral. Pneumothorax can be closed, where air is trapped in the pleural space, or open, where there is free communication between the pleural space and the

external environment. Tension pneumothorax occurs when air accumulates in the thorax until intrapleural pressure exceeds atmospheric pressure; this can lead to cardiovascular compromise as compression of the vena cava decreases venous return to the heart and cardiac output.[96] Increased thoracic pressure is generally present with hemothorax.

Clinical features

Clinical signs include dyspnea, tachypnea, and cyanosis. In cases secondary to trauma, wounds may be present or a history of trauma elicited. Auscultation reveals absence of normal breath sounds in the dorsal thorax with pneumothorax and ventrally with hemothorax. Percussion reveals hyperresonance over the area of pneumothorax and hyporesonance ventrally over the area of hemothorax. Subcutaneous emphysema is frequently present in cases of pneumothorax and can make interpretation of auscultation and percussion findings difficult.

Differential diagnosis

Horses presenting with subcutaneous emphysema, and that are also dyspneic or in respiratory distress, should be fully evaluated for the presence of pneumothorax/hemothorax; in these cases the primary differential diagnosis is clostridial myositis. Other differentials, in the absence of trauma, are pleuropneumonia and cardiac disease.

Diagnosis

Radiographs of the thorax should be obtained and are usually diagnostic. The typical radiographic findings include the presence of pleural surfaces and lack of pulmonary vasculature in the dorsal aspect of the caudal lung fields (**3.50**). Hemothorax is revealed as a ventral 'white-out'.

Ultrasonography reveals an absence of lung excursions and 'comet tail' artifacts during breathing; however, subcutaneous emphysema may prevent accurate ultrasonographic evaluation. Fluid with an echogenicity consistent with blood may be seen ventrally in cases with concurrent hemothorax.

Aspiration of air and/or blood from the thorax is also diagnostic (see Thoracocentesis/pleural fluid analysis).

Management/treatment

Pneumothorax: The treatment for uncomplicated pneumothorax is rest and frequent monitoring for respiratory distress as the air is gradually reabsorbed. If hypoxemia (PaO_2 <80 mmHg, %O_2 sat <90%) or dyspnea are present, nasal insufflation of oxygen (10–15 liters/minute) should be administered (see Intranasal oxygen administration).

Any open wounds should be occluded. Wounds should be explored for any residual foreign material and the extent of the wounds determined, as extension to the abdomen is possible.

Air or blood can be removed from the pleural space by inserting a teat cannula or thoracostomy tube within the dorsal or ventral pleural space (see Thoracocentesis/pleural fluid analysis). Attaching a suction device aids air removal. If pneumothorax reoccurs or continues, chest tubes should be left in place to allow constant air removal. Gradual re-expansion of the lungs is recommended to avoid re-expansion pulmonary edema.[97] Broad-spectrum antimicrobial therapy is recommended as long as the tubes are in place.

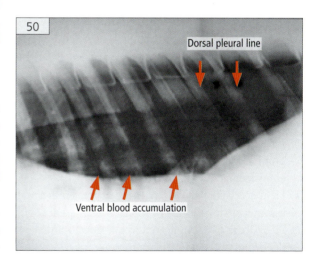

3.50 Lateral standing thoracic radiograph of a horse with both significant pneumothorax and hemothorax. Ventral arrows outline blood accumulation at its most dorsal extent; dorsally located arrows outline the most dorsal aspect of the lung collapsed secondary to pneumothorax.

If the cause of the pneumothorax requires surgical correction, the horse must first be stabilized and chest tubes inserted to remove air, correct atelectasis, and improve ventilation prior to induction of anesthesia.

Hemothorax: Hemothorax may be managed conservatively once the horse is hemodynamically stabilized and volume deficits are corrected. If the amount of blood in the thorax is not producing hypoxemia or respiratory distress, rest only can be attempted.[89]

The thorax may be drained, if necessary, by placing chest tubes ventrally in the thorax, using sonographic guidance (p. 264). Hemothorax may result in blood loss anemia and transfusion of whole blood from a cross-matched donor may be indicated (see Chapter 4). Techniques for autologous blood transfusion have been described but are not indicated if bacterial contamination is suspected or possible.

In general, horses with pneumothorax or hemothorax should be monitored closely for signs of shock during pleural drainage of either blood or air. With hemothorax, the thorax should not be drained until the clinician is satisfied that no active hemorrhage is occurring. NSAIDs (flunixin meglumine, phenylbutazone) may be administered for pain relief.

The prognosis for pneumothorax and hemothorax is good provided that air is removed and leaks are sealed, and infections are treated successfully. Major parenchymal lesions and esophageal rupture carry a poor prognosis.

Heaves/recurrent airway obstruction

Key points
- Heaves is also known as chronic obstructive pulmonary disease (COPD), equine asthma or emphysema, or broken wind.
- Heaves is a chronic disease that can present as acute respiratory distress due to severe exacerbation.
- Heaves can be complicated by the development of cor pulmonale secondary to pulmonary arterial hypertension (see Chapter 4).
- The mainstay of heaves management is control of airway inflammation by environmental control and administration of corticosteroids. Bronchodilators such as clenbuterol should be reserved for treatment of exacerbation and not used daily.

Definition/overview
Heaves is an obstructive airway disease of horses resulting from airway inflammation and bronchoconstriction characterized by difficult breathing and abnormal airway sounds. It is casually referred to as being similar to asthma in people.

Etiology/pathogenesis
Heaves, or recurrent airway obstruction (RAO)[98], is an inflammatory, obstructive airway disease of middle-aged horses that is most prevalent in the northern hemisphere where horses are stabled and fed hay. A similar syndrome, summer pasture-associated obstructive pulmonary disease (SPAOD) occurs in the southeastern US, the UK, and California in horses kept on pasture when the weather is warm and humid.[99] Evidence suggests that the two syndromes are the same disease with different initiating factors.[100]

When a horse with a history of heaves is moved from pasture to a stable (and fed hay), airway inflammation develops and neutrophils accumulate in the lung and invade the airway lumen within 6–8 hours. Concurrently, airway obstruction develops as a result of bronchospasm, mucus accumulation, and inflammatory changes in the wall of the airway.

Clinical features
A horse with severe heaves/RAO or SPAOD is easily recognized by its signs of respiratory distress. On physical examination the clinical signs are restricted to the respiratory system:[100]
- Nostril flare (**3.51**).
- Increased respiratory rate and effort; the horse uses its abdomen to assist expiration. Abdominal effort can be so marked that the horse may rock to and fro during breathing.
- If respiratory distress is very severe, the horse may be unable to eat adequately and therefore loses weight.
- Nasal discharge.
- Coughing associated with activity or feeding.
- Reduced exercise tolerance.
- Delayed recovery from exercise.
- A heave line due to hypertrophy of the external abdominal oblique muscle.

Abnormal lung sounds are heard to varying degrees depending on the severity of airway obstruction. Breath sounds are increased at all levels of the airways, but particularly over the peripheral lung fields. Wheezing can be intermittent and wheezes referred from deeper in the lung may be heard over the trachea and sometimes simply by listening at the nostrils. Percussion will reveal an increased size of the lung field in severely affected animals. In some severely affected animals, the lungs can be silent despite very strong inspiratory and expiratory efforts.

Differential diagnosis
Chronic interstitial lung disease; chronic pneumonia or chronic pleuritis/pleuropneumonia; equine multinodular pulmonary fibrosis; cardiac failure; pulmonary edema.

Diagnosis
CBC, fibrinogen concentration, and routine blood chemistry screen are within normal limits. Arterial blood gas analysis will reveal PaO_2 decreased to varying degrees but $PaCO_2$ normal or only slightly increased.

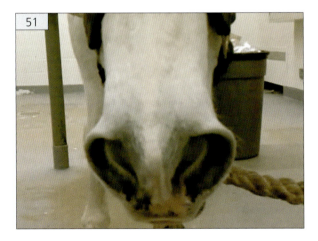

3.51 Nostril flare associated with heaves.

Bronchoalveolar lavage (BAL) is used to evaluate the severity of lung inflammation by cytologic evaluation of BAL fluid (BALF). In normal horses, lymphocytes and macrophages form the majority of cells in BALF and neutrophils comprise <10% of cells. In horses with heaves/RAO or SPAOD, there is an increase in the percentage of neutrophils and, in severely affected animals, non-degenerate neutrophils comprise over 50% of the cells. There is no evidence of bacterial infection. Some horses may have increased mast cells or eosinophils as their only cytologic abnormality. Increased mucus is also characteristic of the disease.

Transtracheal aspiration of tracheal mucus or a tracheal lavage can also be used to evaluate lung inflammation, but it is less reliable than BALF. Because there can be increased numbers of neutrophils in the tracheal wash, but not in BALF, peripheral lung inflammation should be evaluated based on BALF cytology. Mixed populations of bacteria are common in a tracheal wash and usually are of no significance.

Radiographs of the lung are useful to rule out other types of lung disease, but radiographic changes are not pathognomonic for RAO or SPAOD.

Reduction of respiratory distress after administration of a bronchodilator confirms the presence of bronchospasm, the major cause of airway obstruction in heaves. IV atropine (0.02 mg/kg) should relieve respiratory distress within 15 minutes in a horse with heaves/RAO or SPAOD. A single atropine dose is safe, but should not be repeated because of the risk of ileus.

Pulmonary function testing can be performed once the acute episode is resolved to confirm the diagnosis and monitor progression of treatment. This is beyond the scope and intent of this book.

Management/treatment
Management and prevention of RAO and SPAOD requires environmental control, use of corticosteroids to reduce inflammation, and administration of bronchodilator drugs to relieve respiratory distress.

NSAIDs (flunixin meglumine and phenylbutazone) are of no value and may be contraindicated as they decrease the production of prostaglandin E_2 (PGE_2), a prostanoid that inhibits inflammation and prevents bronchospasm.

The anti-inflammatory drugs of choice for treatment of RAO are corticosteroids. It is not helpful to initially use a topically active corticosteroid for the treatment of a horse with RAO because of severe airway constriction. IV or PO use of dexamethasone (0.1 mg/kg q24h for a maximum of 3–7 days) delivers the corticosteroid throughout the lung. Once there is a response to the initial corticosteroid treatment, topical treatment via the airway can be initiated.

Alternatively, the horse can be treated with a bronchodilator drug such as atropine (IV once only) or an inhaled β2-adrenergic agonist 15 minutes before administering the inhaled corticosteroid. Inhaled beclomethasone dipropionate (3,750 μg q12h) has been used with variable effect. Bronchodilators do not treat the airway inflammation, they are rescue medications. Once it is recognized that the horse has heaves, bronchodilators should be available at all times and horse owners need to be instructed to administer the bronchodilator whenever the horse is in respiratory distress. The prime example of a β2-adrenergic agonist used in horses is clenbuterol (0.8 μg/kg q12h). The side-effects of high doses of clenbuterol are those reported for all β2-agonists – sweating, trembling, tachycardia, and excitement. Large overdosing may result in death.

Equine multinodular pulmonary fibrosis
Key points
- Equine multinodular pulmonary fibrosis (EMPF) is a recently described severe pulmonary disease associated with infection by EHV-5.
- Definitive diagnosis requires lung biopsy, although the radiographic appearance is sufficiently suggestive to initiate treatment. PCR testing of BALF for EHV-5 is recommended.
- Treatment includes administration of corticosteroids and the antiviral medications acyclovir or valacyclovir (a prodrug of acyclovir) for a period of months. Intranasal oxygen supplementation is initially beneficial.
- Currently, the known survival rate in confirmed cases is approximately 50%.

Definition/overview
EMPF is a severe pulmonary disease of the horse characterized by the presence of multiple coalescing fibrotic nodules of the lung.[101]

Etiology/pathogenesis
The exact underlying pathophysiology is presently undetermined. There appears to be an association with EHV-5, an equine gammaherpes virus found much more commonly by PCR within pulmonary tissues and BALF in affected horses compared with controls.[101,102] It is thought that EHV-5 promotes a progressive profibrotic milieu within the pulmonary parenchyma, resulting in fibrosis of the lung and development of characteristic multinodular masses within the lung.

Clinical features
Clinical features of EMPF include high fever, lethargy, anorexia, cough, and acute respiratory distress (**3.52**).[102,103]

Differential diagnosis
All other causes of acute respiratory distress.

Diagnosis
Leukocytosis with neutrophilia and hyperfibrinogemia are typical and differentiate this disease from heaves.

Pulmonary radiographs reveal a multinodular pattern with an overlying interstitial pattern (**3.53**). The nodular pattern may be miliary or larger nodules may be distributed throughout the pulmonary parenchyma. The primary differential is fungal pneumonia as pulmonary neoplasia with this radiographic appearance is rare in horses (see Respiratory neoplasia).

Pulmonary ultrasonography will generally reveal discrete areas of pulmonary-altered echogenecity that are 2–5 cm in diameter and diffusely distributed (**3.54**).

Arterial blood gas analysis will reveal hypoxemia. BALF will show neutrophilia and PCR of BALF may be positive for EHV-5.

Lung biopsy using ultrasonographic guidance in the caudodorsal lung field will have characteristic histologic findings (**3.55**) and will also be PCR positive for EHV-5.)

Management/treatment[102]

Intranasal oxygen insufflation (see Intranasal oxygen administration) may need to be instituted immediately in cases presenting with respiratory distress.

Dexamethasone (0.037–0.4 mg/kg PO or IV q24h) and prednisolone (1.0–2.2 mg/kg PO q24h) have been used in the management of EMPF.

Treatment with the antiviral drug acyclovir, either as the parent compound acyclovir (10 mg/kg IV q12h diluted in 1 liter of isotonic crystalloid given over at least 1 hour, or orally at 20–30 mg/kg q8h) or as the prodrug valacyclovir (30 mg/kg PO q24h), has been used in most cases that have survived. The efficacy of these antiviral compounds against gammaherpes viruses such as EHV-5 has not been clearly demonstrated.

At this time the prognosis for EMPF remains guarded to poor.

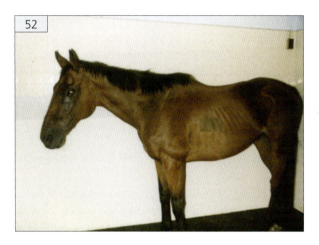

3.52 General appearance of a horse with chronic equine multinodular pulmonary fibrosis. The horse is thin, with a poor haircoat, and may have a 'heave' line.

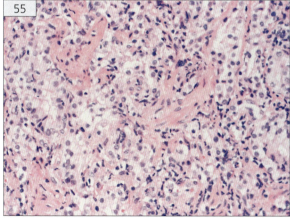

3.53 Radiographic appearance of a horse with equine multinodular pulmonary fibrosis. Note the multifocal distribution of radiodense 'nodules' in the caudal dorsal lung.

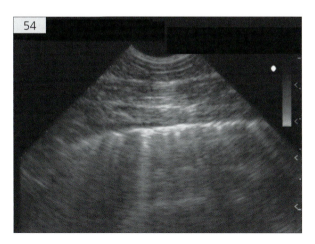

3.54 Ultrasonographic appearance of the pleural surface of caudal dorsal lung in a horse affected with equine multinodular pulmonary fibrosis.

3.55 Histologic appearance of lung from a horse with equine multinodular pulmonary fibrosis.

RESPIRATORY NEOPLASIA

Key points

- Horses with neoplasia can occasionally present on an emergency basis with signs of URT obstruction, epistaxis, and/or respiratory distress due to compression or loss of pulmonary parenchyma.
- Neoplasia should be differentiated from other respiratory tract diseases.
- Neoplasia of the lower airway is generally well advanced at diagnosis. Prognosis is grave and treatment is palliative.

Definition/overview

Upper respiratory tract: Neoplastic diseases that cause acute respiratory distress are uncommon. The astute owner will observe a gradually increasing respiratory noise and probable nasal discharge and will seek veterinary attention before significant airway obstruction occurs. However, because of the insidious nature of neoplastic growth it is not uncommon for the first noted sign of disease to be the development of a quickly progressing respiratory obstruction.

Lower respiratory tract: Primary pulmonary tumors are rare in the horse. The incidence of primary lung tumors of any type is reported to be less than 1% of all reported tumors in domestic animals.[104] Surveys of equine neoplasms indicate a low incidence of thoracic neoplasia in the horse.[105,106]

Etiology/pathogenesis

Upper respiratory tract: SCC is the most common sinonasal tumor in the horse; however, adenocarcinoma, osteoma, osteosarcoma, lymphoma, dental origin tumors, fibrosarcoma, and hemangiosarcoma have been reported.[107] SCC is also the most frequently reported tumor of the nasopharynx and larynx, with fibrosarcoma, lymphoma, and chondroma being recognized rarely. Guttural pouch tumors are frequently the result of metastatic disease (melanoma, hemangioma, adenocarcinoma, fibroma, and SCC).

In general, sinonasal tumors are locally destructive and rarely metastasize. Disease is typically advanced before clinical signs that prompt veterinary attention are noted. Once the tumor is of a size to cause significant airflow obstruction, respiratory distress can progress quickly as increased turbulence around the mass creates edema and swelling in local tissues, which contributes to airway obstruction.

Lower respiratory tract: Primary pulmonary tumors reported in the horse include granular cell tumor, bronchial myxoma, adenoma, adenocarcinoma, anaplastic bronchogenic carcinoma, pulmonary carcinoma, and, possibly, undifferentiated sarcoma. Other primary thoracic tumors reported in the horse include pulmonary chondrosarcoma, plural mesothelioma, thymoma, and malignant lymphoma. All these neoplasms generally occur in the mature or aged horse. The exception is malignant lymphoma, which may also be observed in young animals.

The lungs are susceptible to tumor emboli because of the filter action of the capillary bed associated with small capillary diameter and, perhaps, specific adhesion factors. It can sometimes be difficult or impossible to distinguish gross and microscopic patterns of metastatic disease from those of primary lung neoplasia, making exclusion of possible primary sites elsewhere in the body an important part of the diagnosis.

Clinical features

Upper respiratory tract: The main clinical signs of sinonasal tumors are facial swelling and unilateral mucopurulent nasal discharge. Increased respiratory effort with inspiratory and expiratory stridor and coughing may be present in advanced disease. Epistaxis may be a feature, particularly with an invasive tumor of the guttural pouch or pulmonary parenchyma. Ocular discharge, exophthalmos, enlarged regional lymph nodes, head shaking, and neurologic signs (blindness, dysphagia) are possible. Nasopharyngeal tumors will produce respiratory obstruction and clinical signs of dyspnea, stridor, and dysphagia. Malodorous breath may accompany respiratory tract neoplasia due to local tissue destruction and necrosis and secondary bacterial infection.

Lower respiratory tract: Clinical signs are generally related to the primary site of the neoplasm; thus the clinician often has no reason to suspect thoracic involvement. When respiratory signs such as dyspnea, tachypnea, hemoptysis, cough, cyanosis, nasal discharge, or epistaxis are present, relevant diagnostic tests are more likely to be performed. Ultrasonography and bronchoscopy, combined with transcutaneous lung biopsy, increase the frequency of antemortem diagnosis of thoracic neoplasia.

Differential diagnosis

Upper respiratory tract: Sinusitis; sinus cyst; ethmoid hematoma; guttural pouch mycosis; trauma; mycotic rhinitis; arytenoid chondritis; lymphoid hyperplasia; foreign body.

Lower respiratory tract: EMPF; fungal pneumonia; heaves; pleuropneumonia; viral pneumonia; thoracic trauma (pneumothorax, hemothorax).

Diagnosis

Upper respiratory tract: Diagnosis is dependent on biopsy and histopathology. Nasal passage invasion from paranasal sinus tumors is uncommon, therefore sinoscopy is required to directly see the mass and obtain a tissue sample. Rhinoscopy allows visibility of most respiratory tract masses (**3.56**). Head radiographs are useful for detecting masses inaccessible to rhinoscopic examination (**3.57**). CT or MRI of the head allows

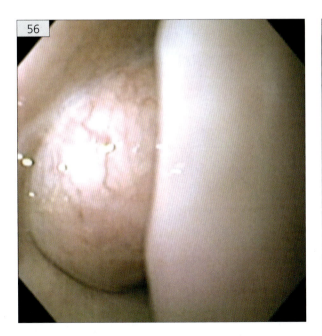

3.56 Endoscopic appearance of a nasal tumor.

3.57 Radiographic appearance of a nasal tumor (arrow).

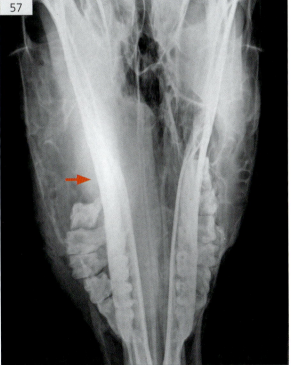

complete assessment of the extent of a tumor in that region and helps with treatment planning and prognostication (**3.58**).

Lower respiratory tract: Definitive diagnosis is based on biopsy. Certain pulmonary neoplasms may be visualized with bronchoscopy. In general, both thoracic radiography and ultrasonography are useful in aiding diagnosis and directing biopsy.

Management/treatment

Upper respiratory tract: A horse with significant respiratory distress due to upper airway obstruction can be managed with a temporary tracheostomy (see Temporary tracheostomy) to facilitate further diagnostic procedures. Complete surgical removal of carcinomas and sarcomas is often unsuccessful because of the advanced state of the disease when the diagnosis is made, and the long-term prognosis for survival is guarded to poor. Carcinomas and sarcomas are locally invasive and recur readily. Osteomas in the paranasal sinuses are benign, slow growing masses that are more easily removed and have a good prognosis.[108] Radiation therapy has been used successfully for treating lymphoma and SCC and should be a consideration in select cases.[109, 110]

Lower respiratory tract: Once clinical signs associated with pulmonary neoplasia are evident, and the diagnosis is confirmed by histopathology, the disease is generally well advanced. Palliative measures include drainage of thoracic fluid accumulation, administration of oxygen via nasal or tracheal insufflation, and pain control.

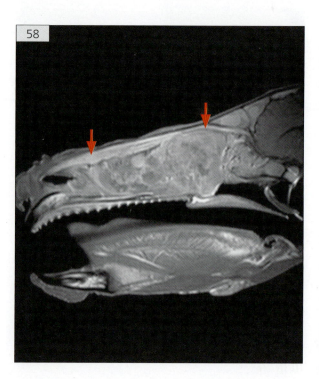

3.58 **Magnetic resonance image of a sinonasal tumor (arrows).**

CHAPTER 4

CARDIOVASCULAR SYSTEM

Melinda Frye,
Vanessa L. Cook,
Louise L. Southwood, and
Pamela A. Wilkins

GENERAL APPROACH TO THE HORSE WITH CARDIOVASCULAR DISEASE

- Cardiac disease is uncommon in horses, particularly cardiac disease requiring emergency care:
  - A thorough history including any previous or underlying disease, medication, or intoxications should be obtained.
  - Physical examination should include careful auscultation of the heart for rate, rhythm, and the presence of any murmurs; pulse quality; jugular refill; extremity temperature; edema formation; respiratory rate and auscultation of the lung fields for any indication of pulmonary edema or underlying LRT disease; and rectal temperature, which may indicate an infectious disease.
  - Cardiac disease is best evaluated using electrocardiography (p. 306) and echocardiography (p. 308).
  - Cardiac troponin I (cTnI) is a highly sensitive and specific biomarker of myocardial injury and is being used with increasing frequency to identify underlying cardiac muscle damage. cTnI measured by either the access immunoassay or the point-of-care analyzer i-STAT 1 is an accurate method of detecting cardiac disease in the horse.[1]
  - Laboratory data including CBC, fibrinogen or serum amyloid A concentration, and a biochemistry profile should be obtained.

- Hemorrhage is common and having a planned approach to the horse with substantial blood loss is critical for a favorable outcome:
  - A thorough history may indicate the source of hemorrhage.
  - Every attempt should be made to stop the hemorrhage.
  - Physical examination should be performed with a focus on heart rate, mucous membrane color, moistness, CRT (if visible), jugular refill time, demeanor, and extremity temperature. Laboratory data that can be useful in the acute phase include blood lactate concentration, base excess, and after 4–12 hours PCV and TPP. These findings can be used to determine the severity of hemorrhagic shock and monitor response to resuscitation.
  - If the source of hemorrhage is not readily apparent, abdominal (and thoracic) sonographic examination should be performed.
  - Conservative use of crystalloid fluids (p. 312), fresh frozen plasma (p. 312), and blood transfusion, if necessary, are components of the resuscitation regimen. (See Resuscitation following hemorrhage or hemolysis, p. 311.)

COMMON PROCEDURES PERFORMED ON HORSES WITH CARDIOVASCULAR DISEASE

Base-apex electrocardiography

Indications

Electrocardiography is indicated in any patient with a cardiac arrhythmia or unexplained tachycardia or bradycardia detected on physical examination, as well as in patients administered a drug or undergoing a procedure that may cause a cardiac arrhythmia.

Base-apex lead placement eliminates artifacts attributable to the panniculus reflex, which occurs when limb leads are used. Additionally, the vector of ventricular depolarization is directed dorsally and cranially, therefore the base-apex configuration displays the largest complexes. Because the wave of depolarization travels away from the positive electrode, the QRS complexes normally have a negative deflection. The electrocardiogram (ECG) cannot be used to approximate chamber size in equids and it is primarily used to characterize arrhythmias, usually making multiple lead configurations unnecessary.

Technique

- Shaving is unnecessary to record a diagnostic ECG. Saturating the area to which the alligator clip leads are applied with alcohol is recommended to maximize coupling when using such leads.
- When feasible, electrocardiography is best performed on an unsedated horse to avoid drug-induced arrhythmias and cardiac depression in an animal with potential hemodynamic instability. However, safety of the patient and caregivers, as well as humane considerations, should primarily dictate whether sedation is appropriate.
- To record a base-apex ECG (**4.1, 4.2**; *Table 4.1*):
  - The positive electrode should be placed on the right side of the horse in the area of the apex of the heart. Using external landmarks, this region lies at or slightly below, and caudal to, the olecranon.

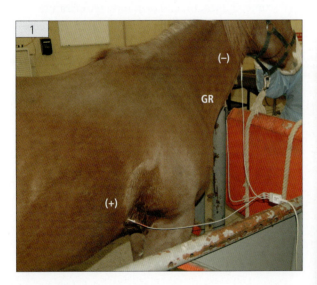

4.1 Lead placement for base-apex electrocardiography using a lead II configuration. (Courtesy Charlie Kerlee)

4.2 Negative and ground lead placement for base-apex electrocardiography in lead II. (Courtesy Charlie Kerlee)

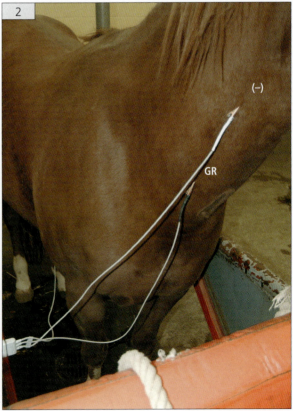

- The negative electrode is placed at the level of the heart base, either over the withers, along the right jugular furrow, or at the dorsal pectoral area cranial to the scapula.
- The ground electrode may be applied either at the withers or in the jugular furrow.
- All leads for recording the base-apex ECG can be placed from the right side of the animal, which is convenient if an echocardiogram is also being performed. However, the same lead configuration may also be placed from the left side of the horse, using identical landmarks on that side.
- The lead that is selected on the ECG machine (i.e. lead I, lead II) determines which electrodes are positive or negative. Standard ECG recorders are equipped with electrodes that are labeled for human use. In many countries, the black electrode is labeled LA (left arm), the white electrode RA (right arm), the red electrode LL (left leg), and the green electrode RL (right leg). In lead I, the RA electrode is negative and the LA electrode is positive; therefore, to record a base-apex ECG in the equine patient, the RA electrode (white) is placed over the area of the heart base and the LA electrode (black) is placed at the apex. In lead II (**4.1, 4.2**), the RA electrode is negative and the LL electrode is positive, therefore the RA electrode (white) is again placed over the heart base, while the LL electrode (red) is positioned at the apex. The green electrode is used as the ground in both leads I and II.

- When the base-apex lead configuration is employed:[2]
  - The P wave, representing atrial depolarization, normally has a positive deflection and is ≤0.16 seconds in duration.
  - The P-R interval is normally ≤0.5 seconds in duration.
  - The QRS complex, representing ventricular depolarization, is predominantly negative and is ≤0.14 seconds in duration.
  - The T wave reflects ventricular repolarization. Morphology is highly variable, although the deflection is usually positive.
  - The duration of the Q-T interval is normally ≤0.6 seconds.
  - At the standard paper speed of 25 mm/second, each small box on the electrocardiogram paper is equal to 0.04 seconds.
- Key factors to assess include heart rate and regularity of the P-P and R-R intervals. It is important to determine whether each QRS complex is preceded by a P wave and whether each P wave is followed by a QRS complex. The P-R interval should be measured to determine whether it is consistent or variable. Morphology of QRS complexes should be evaluated, as complexes with variable width, amplitude, deflection or shape are suggestive of multiple foci of impulse generation within the myocardium (*Table 4.2*).

Complications
None

Table 4.1 **Base-apex lead placement**

ELECTRODE	COLOR	PLACEMENT
Positive	Black in lead I Red in lead II	Just below and caudal to the olecranon
Negative	White	Jugular furrow, withers, or dorsal pectoral region
Ground	Green	Jugular furrow or withers

Table 4.2 **Electrocardiographic evaluation**

- Is the rate fast or slow?
- Does the ventricular rate equal the atrial rate?
- Is the P-P interval regular or irregular?
- Is the R-R interval regular or irregular?
- Is every P wave followed by a QRS complex?
- Is every QRS complex preceded by a P wave?
- Is the P-R interval regular, and is it normal?
- Are the amplitude, duration, deflection, and shape of the complexes similar or variable?

Echocardiography
Indications
Echocardiography is most often performed in emergency/critical care patients with a heart murmur or an arrhythmia. Additionally, a thorough cardiac examination including echocardiography should be considered in a patient with unexplained tachycardia or a fever of unknown origin.

Technique
- Echocardiography is best performed with the horse standing and restrained in stocks.
- When feasible, echocardiography should be performed on an unsedated horse to avoid drug-induced arrhythmias and cardiac depression in an animal with potential hemodynamic instability. (**Note:** The use of sedation is unlikely to alter echocardiographic interpretation in emergency conditions [i.e. the severity of the disorder is likely to be appreciated despite the effects of sedation]. The safety of the patient and caregivers, as well as humane considerations, should primarily dictate whether sedation is appropriate.)
- Ultrasonic coupling gel is required and should be applied liberally to the horse and probe. Saturating the area to which the probe is applied with alcohol is recommended in order to maximize coupling. If the hair coat is thick, the area for examination should be clipped. This region should extend cranially/caudally from the 3rd to 7th intercostal spaces, and dorsally/ventrally from 12.5 cm (5 in) above and below the olecranon. Horses with thin hair coats may require only coupling gel and rubbing alcohol.
- The critical views needed to diagnose cardiac conditions of an emergent nature can usually be obtained from the right side of the animal. It is helpful to remember that the 5th intercostal space is in the region of the caudal border of the triceps muscle. Because echocardiographic

images are interpreted in a standard manner, and the orientation of the probe dictates the image obtained, it is helpful to begin with the probe crystal in the 3rd to 5th intercostal space and the reference mark directed dorsally at 12 o'clock (**4.3**). Subsequent imaging will be accomplished by rotating the probe clockwise (i.e. directing the reference mark to the lower foreleg at 4 o'clock). The probe should be 5.0–7.5 cm (2–3 in) above

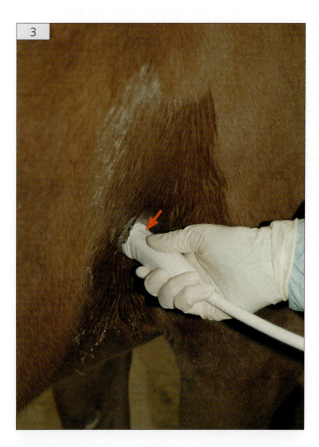

4.3 Because the echocardiographic image obtained is dependent on the probe orientation, it is helpful to orient the transducer initially so that the reference mark is in the 12 o'clock position, directed dorsally (arrow). Note that the head of the transducer is 5–7.5 cm (2–3 in) above the point of the olecranon, in the 3rd to 5th intercostal space. (Courtesy Charlie Kerlee)

the olecranon. To achieve and maintain a sufficiently cranial probe placement, some effort may be required (**4.4**) and it is helpful to have the patient's right forelimb extended cranially and slightly abducted.

- With the reference mark directed dorsally at 12 o'clock and the transducer held perpendicular to the thorax, long-axis 4-chamber views may be obtained (**4.5, 4.6**). These images may be used to evaluate mitral valve movement and to assess

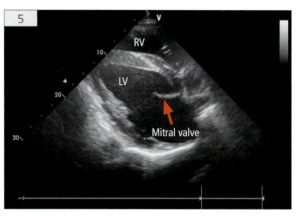

4.5 Right-sided long-axis 4-chamber view of the heart in diastole. Note that the open mitral valve is without thickening or irregularities. LV, left ventricle; RV, right ventricle. (Courtesy June Boon)

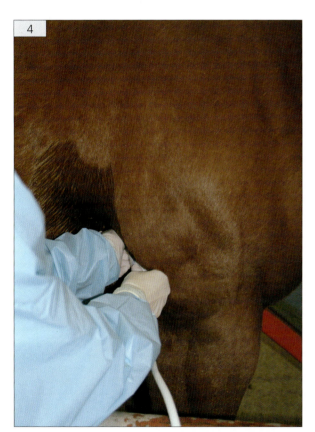

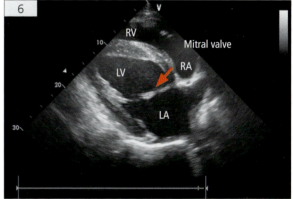

4.4 Because the 5th intercostal space is in the region of the caudal border of the triceps, it may be necessary to exert effort in order to achieve a sufficiently cranial probe placement. (Courtesy Charlie Kerlee)

4.6 Right-sided long-axis 4-chamber view of the heart in systole. Note the closed position of the mitral valve. LV, left ventricle; RV, right ventricle; LA, left atrium; RA, right atrium. (Courtesy June Boon)

for thickening or irregularity. This view allows better imaging of the right atrium and tricuspid valve (**4.7**) than does the long-axis left ventricular outflow view. Directing the crystal slightly cranial or caudal often allows imaging of the chordae tendinae (**4.7**).

- To obtain a long-axis left ventricular outflow view (**4.8**), it is necessary to rotate the probe clockwise to the 1 or 2 o'clock position. To better view the aorta, it may be helpful to rotate the transducer slightly clockwise (i.e. 2 o'clock).
- To view the maximal length of the left ventricle, it is often necessary to direct the crystal slightly caudal by pressing the cable into the right forelimb. Using this view, it may be possible to compare left and right chamber size and wall thickness. This view is best, however, for assessment of aortic valve movement and morphology. Myocardial contractility should be evaluated grossly for symmetry and appropriate thickening with systole.
- To obtain transverse views of the heart (**4.9, 4.10, 4.11**), it is necessary to rotate the transducer clockwise approximately 90 degrees from the

position used to obtain the left ventricular outflow images (i.e. 4 to 5 o'clock). Directing the crystal dorsal and slightly cranial will reveal a transverse image of the heart base (**4.9**), while directing the crystal ventrally and slightly caudal will provide images of the apex (**4.10, 4.11**). The transverse view of the heart base allows for observation of the aortic and pulmonic valves and subsequent assessment of movement and morphology. The size of the pulmonic artery should also be assessed using this view, by comparing the diameter with that of the aortic annulus. Unlike all other views, transverse images of the heart base will not reveal accumulation of pericardial fluid. Transverse imaging of the apex allows a comparison of left and right chamber size and wall thickness. As with the long-axis views, myocardial contractility may be roughly assessed.

The authors acknowledge June Boon for her assistance in obtaining these echocardiographic images.

Complications
None.

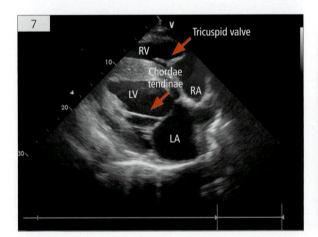

4.7 Right-sided long-axis 4-chamber view of the heart in systole, with closed mitral valve and visible chordae tendinae. The tricuspid valve is readily observed in this image. LV, left ventricle; RV, right ventricle; LA, left atrium; RA, right atrium. (Courtesy June Boon)

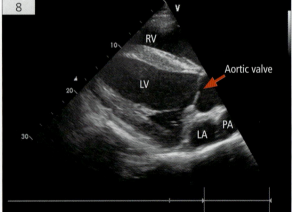

4.8 Right-sided long-axis left ventricular outflow image of the heart in diastole. Note that the closed aortic valve is thin and smooth. LV, left ventricle; RV, right ventricle; LA, left atrium; PA, pulmonary artery. (Courtesy June Boon)

Resuscitation following hemorrhage and hemolysis

Indications

The major indication for resuscitation is moderate to marked or ongoing hemorrhage or hemolysis. Blood volume is approximately 8% of the body weight (kg) (i.e. 40 liters in a 500 kg horse). Patients begin to show clinical signs of blood loss when 15–30% of the blood volume is lost (i.e. 6–12 liters of whole blood in a 500 kg horse) and become moribund and die when 40% of the blood volume is lost (i.e. 16 liters of whole blood in a 500 kg horse).

Any horse with moderate to marked blood loss will benefit from IV fluid therapy. Some specific measurements that can be used as 'blood transfusion triggers' for hemorrhage and/or hemolysis include:[3]

- Dullness and weakness.
- Tachycardia (heart rate >65 beats/minute).
- Poor pulse pressure (hemorrhage).
- Pale mucous membranes (hemorrhage).
- Hypotension (systolic arterial pressure <70 mmHg) (hemorrhage).
- Hyperlactatemia in euvolemic patients.
- Low $P_{cv}O_2$ and $S_{cv}O_2$ in euvolemic patients.
- Anemia:
  - PCV <0.2 l/l (20%) at 12 hours post hemorrhage or <0.12 l/l (12%) at 2 days post hemorrhage. Note that the PCV will not reflect the volume of blood loss for 4–12 hours post hemorrhage.
  - PCV <0.14 l/l (14%) (acute) or <0.12 l/l (12%) (chronic) in cases of hemolysis.
- Low hemoglobin concentration. A hemoglobin concentration <50 g/l (5 g/dl) results in inadequate tissue oxygen delivery.

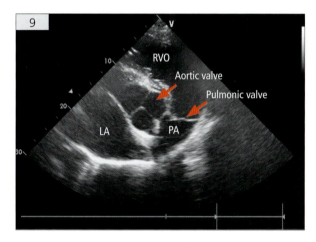

4.9 Right-sided transverse image of the heart base. LA, left atrium; PA, pulmonary artery; RVO, right ventricular outflow.

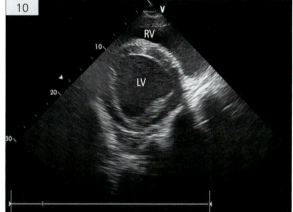

4.10 Right-sided transverse image of the apex of the heart in diastole (below the level of the mitral valve). LV, left ventricle; RV, right ventricle.

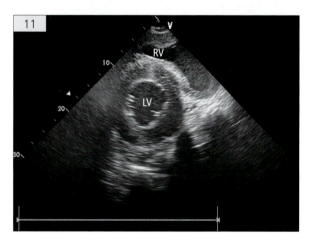

4.11 Right-sided transverse image of the apex of the heart in systole. Note that the interventricular septum and left ventricular free wall are uniformly thickened. LV, left ventricle; RV, right ventricle.

Technique
Hemorrhage
- Stop the hemorrhage using pressure (e.g. bandage) or vessel ligation, if possible.
- An IV catheter should be placed in any horse with hemorrhage (see Chapter 12).
- A cross-match should be performed if hemorrhage is not immediately life-threatening. If hemorrhage is severe and life-threatening, blood can be given without transfusion preferably from a Standardbred gelding. While this is often considered safe in horses that have not previously received a blood or plasma transfusion, complications associated with transfusion reaction are more likely if the patient is not cross-matched (see Chapter 12).
- IV isotonic crystalloids should be administered at 2–10 ml/kg/hour depending on the degree of shock, the source of hemorrhage, and whether or not hemorrhage has been controlled. Hypertonic saline can be administered if hemorrhage has stopped and the horse is showing signs of shock. Crystalloid fluids will help to improve tissue perfusion (see Chapter 12).
- Fresh frozen plasma (2–10 liters/500 kg horse) can be administered to replace clotting factors and protein.
- In cases of acute and severe hemorrhage, 15% of the patient's blood volume of whole blood can be given (i.e. 6–8 liters/500 kg horse). Another method to determine the volume of whole blood to administer is to estimate the volume of blood loss and initially replace 50% of the loss. Blood can be given at a rate of 10–20 ml/kg/hour using a blood administration set. The horse should be monitored for any signs of a transfusion reaction (see Chapter 12).
- Heart rate, arterial blood pressure, and lactate concentration should be monitored to assess tissue perfusion following resuscitation. (see Chapter 11)
- ε-aminocaproic acid (3.5 mg/kg/minute for 15 minutes then 0.25 mg/kg/minute, or 50 mg/kg loading dose then 25 mg/kg q6h for 24 hours) can be given if hemorrhage is ongoing.[4,5]

- 10% neutral buffered formalin (50 ml in 1 liter saline per 500 kg horse) has also been used to in cases of life-threatening and uncontrollable hemorrhage; its efficacy has not been demonstrated.

Hemolysis
- The amount of blood required for a transfusion of whole blood in an adult horse following hemolysis or blood loss can be calculated:[3]

$$\frac{desired\ PCV - current + PCV\ of\ recipient}{PCV\ of\ donor} \times$$

0.08 (body weight [kg]) = volume of blood to be transfused (liters)

- The cause of hemolysis should be determined and any underlying disease corrected and treated.[6]

Complications
The main complication following blood transfusion is transfusion reaction (see Chapter 12).

Cardiopulmonary resuscitation – foals
Indications
Most newborn foals make the transition to extrauterine life easily. However, for those in difficulty, it is of utmost importance to recognize the condition immediately and institute appropriate resuscitation.

A modified APGAR (Appearance, Pulse, Grimace, Activity, Respiration) scoring system has been developed as a guide for initiating resuscitation and probable level of fetal compromise (*Table 4.3*). It is also important that at least a cursory physical examination is performed prior to initiating resuscitation, as there are humane issues revolving around foals with serious problems such as severe limb contracture, microophthalmia, and hydrocephalus, amongst others.

Technique
Airway resuscitation
The first priority of neonatal resuscitation is establishing an airway and breathing pattern (**4.12, 4.13**). It should be assumed that foals not spontaneously breathing are in secondary apnea:
- Clear the airway of membranes as soon as the nose is presented.
- If the foal does not breathe or move spontaneously within seconds of birth, begin tactile stimulation.

Table 4.3 **APGAR score in the foal. Score at 1 and 5 minutes after birth. Scores of 7 to 8 generally indicate a normal foal; 4 to 6, mild to moderate asphyxia; and 0 to 3, severe asphyxia. A score of 4 to 6 should prompt stimulation, intranasal oxygen, or nasotracheal intubation and 'bagging'. For a score of 0 to 3, begin cardiopulmonary resuscitation.[6a]**

PARAMETER	ASSIGNED VALUE		
	0	1	2
Heart/pulse rate	Undetectable	<60 beats/minute; irregular	>60 beats/minute; regular
Respiratory rate/pattern	Undetectable	Slow; irregular	40–60 beats/minute; regular
Muscle tone	Limp	Lateral; some tone	Sternal
Nasal mucosal stimulation	Absent	Grimace; mild rejection	Cough or sneeze

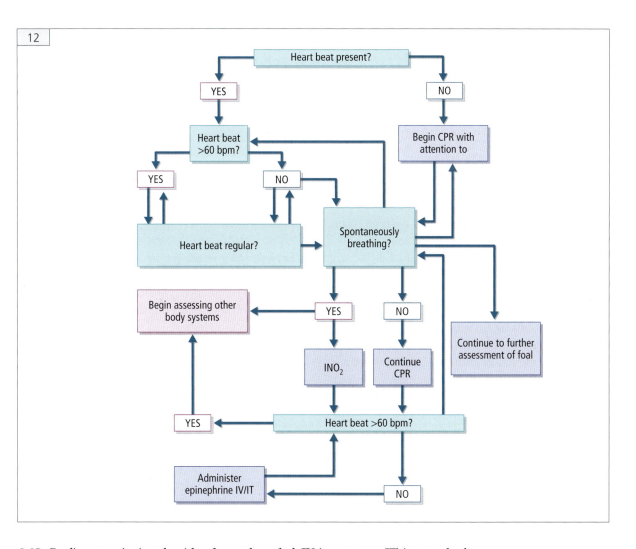

4.12 Cardiac resuscitation algorithm for newborn foal. IV, intravenous; IT, intratracheal.

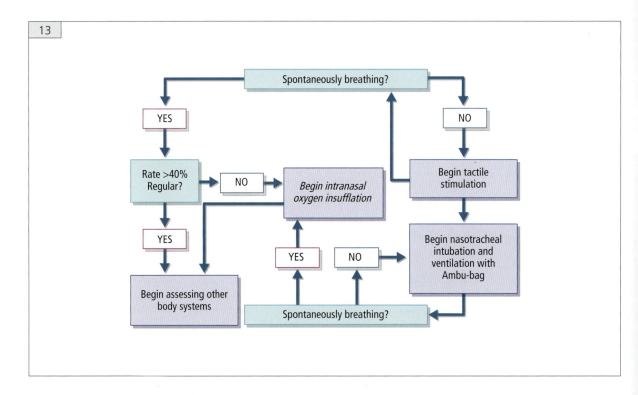

13

4.13 Decision tree for respiratory resuscitation of a foal at birth.

- If tactile stimulation fails to result in spontaneous breathing, the foal should be immediately intubated and manually ventilated using an Ambu-bag or equivalent.
- Mouth to nose ventilation can be used if nasotracheal tubes and an Ambu-bag are not available.
- The goal of this therapy is to reverse fetal circulation and hyperventilation with 100% oxygen is the best choice for this purpose. However, recent evidence suggests that there are no apparent clinical disadvantages in using room air for ventilation of asphyxiated human neonates rather than 100% oxygen.
- Almost 90% of foals requiring resuscitation respond to hyperventilation alone and require no additional therapy. Nasotracheal intubation can be initiated while the foal is in the birth canal if the foal will not be delivered rapidly, such as with a difficult dystocia. This is a 'blind' technique and will require some practice, but can be very beneficial and lifesaving.

- Once spontaneous breathing is present, provide humidified oxygen via nasal insufflation at 8–10 liters/minute.

Cardiovascular resuscitation
Cardiovascular support in the form of chest compression should be initiated if the foal remains bradycardic despite ventilation and a non-perfusing rhythm is present:
- Make sure the foal is on a hard surface, in right lateral recumbency with the top line against a wall or other support.
- Approximately 5% of foals are born with fractured ribs and an assessment for the presence of rib fractures is in order before initiating chest compressions. Palpation of the ribs will identify many of these fractures; they are usually multiple and consecutive on one side of the thorax, located in a relatively straight line along the part of the rib with the greatest curvature dorsal to the costochondral junction. Unfortunately, ribs 3–5 are frequently involved and their location over the

heart can make chest compression a potentially fatal exercise. Auscultation over the ribs during breathing will result in a recognizable 'click', identifying rib fractures that may have escaped detection by palpation.

- Initiate drug therapy if a non-perfusing rhythm persists for more than 30–60 seconds in the face of chest compression. Epinephrine (see p. 338) is the first drug of choice (**4.12, 4.13**).
- Do not use atropine in bradycardic newborn foals as the bradycardia is usually due to hypoxia and if the hypoxia is not corrected, atropine can increase myocardial oxygen debt.
- Do not use doxapram in resuscitation as its use wastes time and will not reverse secondary apnea, which is the most common apnea in newborns. Intubate and ventilate instead.

Complications

The most apparent complication is failure to resuscitate the foal and death. Epinephrine can induce arrhythmias. Rib fracture can occur with chest compressions.

Cardiopulmonary resuscitation – adults
Indications

The most common indication for cardiopulmonary resuscitation in adult horses is during anesthesia, typically associated with an overdose of an anesthetic drug. Attempts to resuscitate adult horses for other reasons (e.g. life-threatening hemorrhage, severe endotoxemia, or sepsis) are usually unsuccessful, primarily because of the underlying disease.

Technique

- Cardiac arrest should be verified by palpating peripheral pulses and ausculting the heart. Additionally, an ECG provides optimal assurance and further specifies whether the underlying rhythm is asystole (p. 337), ventricular fibrillation (p. 335) or, rarely, electromechanical dissociation. Appropriate pharmacologic treatment is then initiated after basic cardiopulmonary resuscitation (i.e. breathing, chest compression) is underway.

- If the cardiorespiratory arrest occurs during general anesthesia, administration of any inhalant or injectable anesthetic drugs should be stopped. Some injectable sedative and analgesic drugs can be reversed. (see Chapter 14).
- The 'ABC' of cardiopulmonary resuscitation applies. First, an Airway should be established by inserting an oro- or nasotracheal tube, or by performing a tracheostomy. The system is then connected to an anesthetic unit or demand valve (Breathing), and a flow of 100% oxygen established. Manual compression of a rebreathing bag may alternatively be used; moderate chest excursion, or compression to between 20 and 40 cm H_2O, indicates an adequate ventilatory effort.[7]
- To perform external compressions (Circulation) on an adult equine, the patient is placed in right lateral recumbency. A standing or crouching individual falls to a kneeling position, placing the knees on the cranial lateral thorax. While lower compression frequencies (40–60 beats/minute) achieve modest flow rates, higher rates (80 beats/minute) produce significantly greater flow and pressure.[8]
- A study of the hemodynamic effects of cardiopulmonary resuscitation in euthanized adult horses revealed that even with high compression rates (80 beats/minute), cardiac output was not adequate to sustain life.[8] The authors noted, however, that flow rates may be sufficient for resuscitative drug delivery to tissues, thus offering potential benefit to resuscitative efforts. Another study of cardiopulmonary resuscitation in anesthetized ponies experiencing unanticipated cardiac arrest demonstrated maintenance of >50% of baseline hemodynamic values with a thoracic compression rate of 20 beats/minute.[9] The ponies received ventilatory support and 6 out of 8 were successfully resuscitated.

Complications

The most apparent complication is failure to resuscitate the horse and death. Epinephrine can induce arrhythmias.

CARDIOVASCULAR DISEASE

Cardiac diseases
Congestive heart failure
Key points

- Signs of congestive heart failure (CHF) become evident when an acute onset of cardiac dysfunction precludes the development of compensatory mechanisms.
- A definitive diagnosis and, often, the underlying etiology can be identified with echocardiography.
- Goals of therapy are to improve cardiac output, reduce congestion, treat arrhythmias, reduce hypoxemia and anxiety, and manage the underlying cause.

Definition/overview

CHF occurs when reduced cardiac pumping results in inadequate provision of tissue oxygen and metabolic requirements, and in development of high arterial pressures proximal to the failing chamber(s). Signs of CHF become evident when an acute onset of cardiac dysfunction precludes the development of compensatory mechanisms. Alternatively, signs may manifest in cases of chronic, severe cardiac disease when adaptive mechanisms are exhausted. Fulminant CHF occurs rarely in horses[10], but it is a grave condition[11], with treatment aimed at reducing acute distress rather than permanently restoring functional myocardial contractility.

Etiology/pathogenesis

Equine CHF is most commonly attributed to valvular dysfunction[10] (i.e. due to degeneration or endocarditis) resulting in volume overload and dilative cardiomyopathy. Rupture of the chordae tendinae usually results in acute, uncompensated CHF due to valve incompetence. Myocardial disease may result from rattlesnake envenomation, ionophore or cantharidin toxicity, vitamin E or selenium deficiency, neoplasia (i.e. lymphoma), and exposure to viral, bacterial, or parasitic agents (see Myocarditis). Pericarditis attributable to trauma, infection, or neoplasia may inhibit myocardial relaxation, resulting in poor ventricular filling and reduced cardiac output (see Pericarditis). Systemic hypertension is rarely recognized in equids; pulmonary hypertension may occasionally occur in response to chronic hypoxic lung disease, contributing to cor pulmonale.[12] In foals, congenital heart disease may cause CHF.[13]

Decreased cardiac output from the compromised myocardium causes upregulation of the sympathetic nervous system. The resultant vasoconstriction and tachycardia initially serves to preserve cardiac output and blood pressure. Increased sympathetic activity and altered solute concentration at the kidneys activate the renin–angiotensin system. Subsequent vasoconstriction and sodium/water retention also act to preserve blood pressure.[14,15] Chronic activation of these mechanisms increases cardiac workload and contributes to myocardial remodeling.[15,16]

Clinical signs result from inadequate delivery of blood to tissues, as well as congestion and hypertension proximal to the failing heart chambers. Left- and right-sided CHF may occur concomitantly if primary left-sided disease results in secondary pulmonary hypertension sufficient to cause pressure overload in the right heart.[17] Valvular disease can be a primary contributor to CHF (i.e. degeneration, endocarditis, congenital malformation) or can result secondarily from progressively severe dilation of associated chambers.[18]

Clinical features

The non-specific sign of activity intolerance is often present in horses with heart failure.[19] The presence of a murmur and tachycardia are two of the most common cardiac findings.[11] The timing, character, and location of the murmur will vary depending on the valve(s) affected and degree of dysfunction. Heart sounds may be muffled if pericardial effusion is present.[11] An irregular heartbeat suggests the presence of an arrhythmia. Signs of right-sided CHF include edema of the ventrum, prepuce, and legs (**4.14, 4.15**) and jugular distension and/or pulsation.[19] Signs of left-sided

CHF include cough, dyspnea, white froth at the nares, tachypnea, and crackles on thoracic auscultation.[11] Reduced cardiac output may result in faint peripheral pulses, pallor, weakness, and syncope.[13] Cachexia may be present in chronic cases of CHF (**4.14**).

Differential diagnosis

Physiologic (innocent) murmur; arrhythmias attributable to underlying systemic disease or electrolyte imbalance; primary lung disease; hypoproteinemia; iatrogenic IV fluid overload.

Diagnosis

The CBC and biochemistry profile may be normal in a horse with CHF. Elevated liver enzyme activity may reflect hepatic congestion due to right-sided failure, and azotemia may be present with reduced renal perfusion. Evidence for consistent elevation of cTnI in horses with CHF is lacking. Elevated levels are observed in cats and dogs with cardiomyopathy[20,21]; in the latter population, plasma cTnI was correlated with left ventricle chamber size and wall thickness.[21] Increased circulating cTnI would suggest ongoing myocardial injury when echocardiographic confirmation is not feasible (refer to Myocarditis for reference ranges). Radiography may demonstrate cardiomegaly or pulmonary edema. The ECG cannot be used to estimate cardiac chamber size in horses, but should be used to characterize any arrhythmias. Catheterization of the jugular vein and use of a manometer or transducer can verify elevated CVP, while a Swan-Ganz catheter can measure pulmonary artery pressure. Sonography may reveal pleural or pericardial effusion, visceral edema, or excess peritoneal fluid.

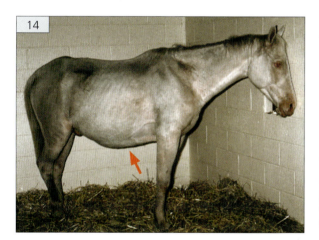

4.14 A horse with right-sided congestive heart failure. Note the ventral edema (arrow) and poor body condition (Courtesy Dr Josie Traub-Dargatz)

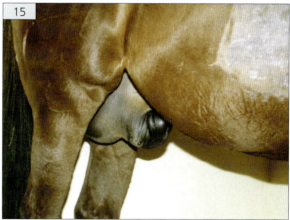

4.15 A horse with right-sided congestive heart failure. Scrotal, preputial, and ventral edema are present (Courtesy Dr Josie Traub-Dargatz)

A definitive diagnosis and underlying etiology can often be identified with echocardiography, making the aforementioned diagnostic tests unnecessary to perform. 2-D images may reveal enlarged chambers or great vessels (**4.16–4.18**), thickened valves, vegetative valvular growths (**4.16**), or abnormal valve motion. M-mode echocardiography may be used to assess myocardial contractility by calculating fractional shortening. Doppler imaging allows for gross quantitation of regurgitant volumes across valves and congenital defects.[13]

Management/treatment

Although treatment of horses with early or mid-stage CHF can improve hemodynamic parameters and myocardial contractility, management of the horse in

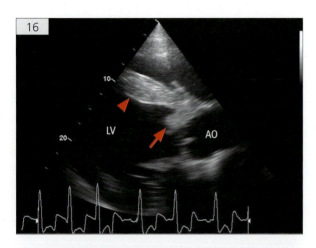

4.16 Right-sided long-axis left ventricular outflow image of an enlarged left ventricle. Note bowing of the interventricular septum (arrowhead). The left ventricular dilation was attributed to aortic regurgitation caused by aortic valvular endocarditis. Note the thickened, irregular aortic valve leaflet (arrow) compared with a more normal leaflet (see 4.8). AO, aorta; LV, left ventricle. (Courtesy June Boon)

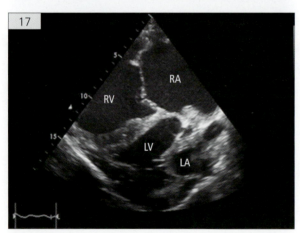

4.17 Right-sided four-chamber view of the heart of a foal with severe tricuspid regurgitation. Note the severe dilation of the right atrium and right ventricle. The tricuspid valve appears normal, but the leaflets do not approximate during systole. Whether the tricuspid failure is primary, or secondary due to severe right-sided dilation, cannot be determined from this view. LA, left atrium; LV, left ventricle; RA, right atrium; RV, right ventricle. (Courtesy June Boon and Dr Jan Bright)

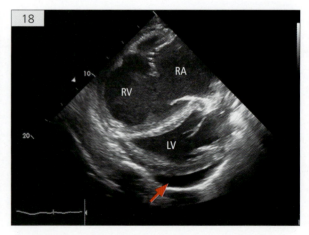

4.18 Right long-axis view of the heart imaged in 4.17. This image shows the heart in diastole. Note the pericardial effusion (arrow). RA, right atrium; RV, right ventricle; LV, left ventricle. (Courtesy June Boon and Dr Jan Bright)

fulminant heart failure is aimed at minimizing distress while accurately assessing the cause and severity of disease. Euthanasia is often the best option for these patients. Goals of emergency treatment are to (1) improve cardiac output, (2) reduce congestion, (3) treat arrhythmias, (4) reduce hypoxemia and anxiety, and (5) treat the underlying cause when possible.

Improve cardiac output: Cardiac output can be improved with the use of various drugs including digoxin, hydralazine, angiotensin converting enzyme (ACE) inhibitors (quinapril and enalapril), and dobutamine.

- Digoxin: loading dose 2.2 µg/kg IV slowly.[10] Maintenance dose 2.2 µg/kg IV q12h or 11 µg/kg PO q12h.[22] Signs of toxicity include somnolence, diarrhea, constipation, behavioral changes, sinus tachycardia, and ventricular arrhythmias.[23,24] Horses receiving quinidine or with hypoalbuminemia, renal disease, or electrolyte disturbances are more likely to develop digoxin toxicity.[23,25] If toxicity is suspected, digoxin treatment should be discontinued and blood submitted for measurement of albumin, electrolytes, creatinine, and serum digoxin. Correction of detected aberrancies should accompany treatment of arrhythmias.
- Hydralazine: 0.5–1.5 mg/kg PO q12h.[13] This drug also has positive inotropic effects.[10]
- The use of ACE inhibitors in horses has not been well characterized. However, the following agents and doses have been evaluated:
  - Quinapril: 120 mg PO q24h; when quinapril was administered over 8 weeks to horses with mitral valve insufficiency but without CHF, there was an increase in stroke volume and cardiac output while reducing severity of insufficiency in 5 out of 20 horses.[26]
  - Enalaprilat: 0.5 mg/kg IV once resulted in a reduction in ACE activity to <25% of baseline, without changes in exercise-induced cardiopulmonary hemodynamics or blood gas values.[27] In contrast, a single dose of enalapril (0.5 mg/kg PO) did not result in detectable serum concentrations or in significant ACE inhibition or hemodynamic effects in normal horses.[28] The same dose administered daily for

60 days also did not result in ACE inhibition, suggesting poor absorption and/or conversion to the active metabolite.[29]
- Dobutamine: 1–10 µg/kg/minute IV infusion may be used to promote positive inotropy and improve blood pressure in horses with acute heart failure.[30]

Reduce congestion
- Furosemide 1–2 mg/kg IV or IM q8h or q12h.[13,23] Administer with caution in horses with electrolyte disturbances, dehydration, or low cardiac output[31]; if indicated, pretreat or treat concomitantly with electrolytes, fluids, or positive inotropes. Hypokalemia may result from furosemide therapy[32] and can exacerbate digoxin toxicity[24], therefore routine electrolyte monitoring is warranted when the drugs are used concomitantly.

Treat arrhythmias: Arrhythmias should be identified and treated (p. 326).

Reduce hypoxemia and anxiety
- Oxygen at 5–10 liters/minute[7] administered via soft rubber tubing in the nares.
- Acepromazine 10–15 mg/450 kg (vasodilatory effect will also reduce afterload).[7]

Treat underlying cause when possible
- Antimicrobial drugs.
- Anti-inflammatory drugs.
- Removal of pericardial fluid.

Inflammatory diseases
- Inflammatory cardiac diseases are uncommon in the horse and should be suspected in any horse presenting with signs of CHF, exercise intolerance, lethargy, weight loss and inappetence, or fever of unknown origin when more common causes are not identified.
- Physical examination will often reveal tachycardia, arrhythmia, and/or abnormal heart sounds (e.g. murmur or friction rub).
- A diagnosis is made based on echocardiographic examination (p. 308) and elevated cTnI (myocardial disease).
- Treatment generally involves anti-inflammatory drugs and long-term antimicrobial drugs.

Endocarditis
Key points
- Emergency treatment of CHF or serious arrhythmias is the first priority.
- Echocardiography is necessary to confirm non-invasively the diagnosis of endocarditis.
- Once blood cultures are obtained, broad-spectrum antimicrobial drug treatment should be initiated immediately and continued if culture results are negative. Long-term treatment with antimicrobial drugs should be anticipated.

Definition/overview
Bacterial or fungal infection of the endocardium occurs by hematogenous dissemination and can affect the walls and septum of the heart (mural endocarditis) or the valves (valvular endocarditis).[33] Younger horses (i.e. 3 years of age) are more commonly affected.[34,35] Vegetative valvular endocarditis most commonly occurs on the mitral and aortic valves, though endocarditis of the tricuspid valve has been associated with septic jugular vein thrombophlebitis.[34] Pulmonic valvular endocarditis is rare in horses but has been reported.[36]

Etiology/pathogenesis
A primary nidus of infection is usually not identified in horses with endocarditis.[33,34] Bacterial endocarditis has been documented in horses with interstitial pneumonia, enterocolitis, ulcerative colitis, a visceral mast cell tumor[37], and jugular vein thrombophlebitis.[34] Common bacterial isolates include *Streptococcus* spp. and *Actinobacillus* spp.[34,38] Less commonly isolated organisms include *Serratia marcescens*[39], *Pseudomonas* spp.[40], *E. coli*, and *Candida parapsilosis*.[37] Fungal endocarditis has been attributed to *Candida* spp.[37] and *Aspergillus* spp.[41]

Hematogenous dissemination of microorganisms to the endocardium results in seeding of the underlying myocardium or valves with bacteria.[19,33] The invading organisms may be protected from host immune defenses by fibrin and platelets that converge at the site of infection.[33] Vegetative lesions develop when these factors, in addition to granulation tissue, form proliferative nodular lesions that prevent proper valve motion and/or approximation (**4.19**).[33] Myocardial, renal, and meningeal infarctions may occur when septic emboli break off from the primary vegetative lesion.[34,37]

Clinical features
Signs of endocarditis may include tachypnea, arrhythmias, recurring fever, anorexia, and weight loss.[19] If valvular incompetence is present, a murmur will be ausculted, the timing and location of which will be specific to the valve(s) affected.[19] Other signs may be present that reflect the original nidus of infection, such as jugular vein thrombophlebitis, cough, pyuria, swollen joints, or lameness.[19,35] Signs of heart failure may develop if valvular dysfunction contributes to volume overload and myocardial dysfunction.

Clinicopathologic findings usually include hyperfibrinogenemia, neutrophilia, hyperglobulinemia, hypoalbuminemia, and anemia (i.e. of chronic disease).[34,35] Renal compromise may be evident if renal infarction has occurred.[33]

Differential diagnosis
Myocarditis; pericarditis.

Diagnosis
Bacterial endocarditis affecting valvular function should be differentiated from myocarditis and pericarditis. Although the clinical signs may be similar, the treatment approach and prognosis may be quite different. It is necessary to perform an echocardiogram (p. 308) to confirm the diagnosis of endocarditis. The echocar-

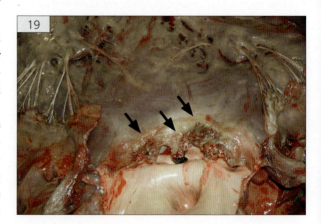

4.19 Thickened, nodular vegetative lesions on the aortic valve cusps (arrows). (Courtesy Dr Jan Bright)

diographic examination can be used to characterize any vegetative lesions (**4.20, 4.21**) in addition to quantitating the severity of subsequent valve or mural dysfunction.[33] This modality can also be used to identify chordate tendineae rupture and describe any existing chamber dilation, thus helping assess the prognosis.[34] Echocardiographic findings may rarely be normal in horses with endocarditis[42], such as in cases of acute endocarditis or those affecting only the septum or free wall (i.e. mural endocarditis). In a horse with fever of unknown origin, it is always prudent to perform an echocardiographic examination to determine whether valvular endocarditis is the focus of the persistent inflammatory response.

A positive blood culture strongly supports the diagnosis of bacterial endocarditis in the presence of appropriate clinical signs. A negative blood culture, however, does not rule out the diagnosis.[33] Three blood cultures should be obtained via sterile technique 1 hour apart and before antimicrobial treatment is administered.[33]

If arrhythmias are suspected based on auscultation, an ECG (p. 306) should be performed to characterize the arrhythmia and determine the need for treatment.

Management/treatment

Emergency treatment of CHF (p. 316) or serious arrhythmias (p. 326) is the first priority. Once blood cultures are obtained, broad-spectrum antimicrobial drug treatment should be initiated immediately and continued if culture results are negative.[19,33] Potassium penicillin (22,000–44,000 IU/kg IV q6h) combined with gentamicin sulfate (6.6 mg/kg IV q24h) is commonly used.[19] If a causative organism is identified with blood culture, appropriate antimicrobial drug treatment based on sensitivity results should replace initial broad-spectrum therapy. Long-term treatment (i.e. 4–8 weeks) with antimicrobial drugs should be anticipated, with resolution of neutrophilia, hyperfibrinogenemia, and fever, preferably for 2 weeks, being used to ultimately determine treatment duration.[19] It is also helpful to record the initial echocardiographic measurements and observations for comparison with future studies, because this can be used to assess treatment efficacy and guide decisions regarding length of therapy.[34] NSAIDs may be administered to relieve malaise and reduce fever.[19]

Vegetative valvular endocarditis affecting the aortic or mitral valve is associated with a grave prognosis despite treatment.[33,34] The prognosis for endocarditis affecting the tricuspid or pulmonic valves is slightly better, though still guarded.[33,34] Even with clearance of the bacterial infection with prolonged antimicrobial treatment, persistent vegetative lesions may prevent normal valve coaptation chronically, and CHF ensues.

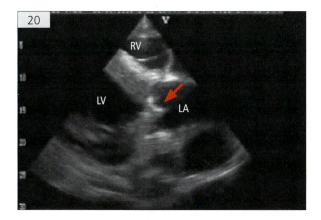

4.20 Echocardiographic image of a thickened, irregular aortic valve in closed position (arrow indicates abnormal valve). LA, left atrium; LV, left ventricle; RV, right ventricle. (Courtesy June Boon)

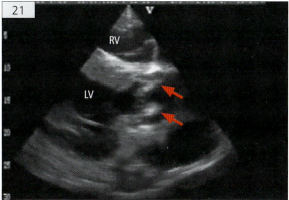

4.21 Echocardiographic image of the valve in 4.20 in open position (arrows indicate abnormal valve). LV, left ventricle; RV, right ventricle. (Courtesy June Boon)

Pericarditis
Key points
- Echocardiography is the most specific and sensitive non-invasive means for diagnosing pericarditis.
- For emergency treatment of excessive fluid accumulation and right heart failure, pericardiocentesis is indicated.

Definition/overview
Inflammation of the pericardium is uncommon in horses. The condition may result in pericardial thickening and fibrin formation, fluid accumulation between the visceral and parietal pericardium, or both.[19] It is now appreciated that early identification and aggressive therapy can often result in a positive clinical outcome.[43]

Etiology/pathogenesis
Pericarditis is most commonly idiopathic[43], but identified causes include hematogenous spread of infectious agents, local dissemination of infection from the lung and, less commonly, neoplasia or penetration by a foreign body.[44] Non-septic pericarditis can occur in the presence of viral or bacterial respiratory disease.[43]

Pericarditis may primarily manifest as pericardial effusion, accumulation of fibrin, or both.[33] Fibrin in the pericardial space can cause constrictive pericarditis[33] (**4.22**), and removal of pericardial fluid may not result in substantial clinical improvement due to persistently poor ventricular compliance. Horses with effusive pericarditis, or accumulation of pericardial fluid, have increased end-diastolic filling pressures, which cause reduced venous return.[33,43] Signs of right heart failure predominate initially, as the lower pressure system is more affected by forces exerted by the fluid.[7,33,43] In addition, the myocardium receives the majority of blood flow during diastole, so relative myocardial ischemia with reduced contractility contributes further to hemodynamic compromise.[33]

Clinical features
Most commonly, horses with pericarditis attributable to a known etiology have existing pleuritis or pleuropnuemonia, therefore predominant clinical signs may reflect respiratory disease.[43] Because of the chronic, inflammatory nature of pericarditis, horses often demonstrate non-specific signs of fever, anorexia, and lethargy.[43] Lung sounds may be reduced or absent ventrally when pleural effusion is present.[33,44] Muffled ventral lung sounds may be present with either pleuritis or pericarditis. In the former, however, heart sounds are more, rather than less, prominent and may be heard over a wider area of the thorax. Both fibrin and fluid can cause muffled heart sounds.[43] Tachycardia is often present.[44] A pericardial friction rub, likened to creaking leather, may be ausculted and is attributed to contact between inflamed pericardial surfaces.[33] If fluid accumulation is acute and/or severe, signs of right heart failure may be present.[33]

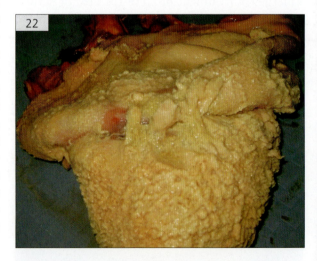

4.22 Postmortem image of the heart of a foal with severe fibrinous pericarditis and fluid accumulation. The pericardium is reflected back to reveal diffuse, severe fibrinous pericarditis. (Courtesy Dr Jan Bright)

Differential diagnosis

Pleuropneumonia/pleuritis; right-sided heart failure from primary valvular endocarditis or idiopathic dilative cardiomyopathy.

Diagnosis

Clinicopathologic testing is non-specific, often reflecting chronic anorexia, inflammation, infection, and/or heart failure.[33] Thoracic radiographic examination may reveal an enlarged and rounded cardiac silhouette[19], but this may also be present with global heart failure and cardiomyopathy.[7] Mild or constrictive pericarditis may not be evident radiographically and pericardial fluid may be difficult to differentiate from pleural fluid.

ECG examination may reveal decreased QRS amplitude compared with normal due to dampening of the electrical signal, but this finding may also be present with other conditions and is non-specific.[33] A regularly repeating change in P, QRS, and T morphology (electrical alternans) is pathognomonic for pericarditis and occurs due to regular movement of the heart within the pericardial fluid.[33]

Echocardiography is the most specific and sensitive non-invasive test for pericarditis.[33] Fluid is recognized as an anechoic or hypoechoic region between the visceral and parietal pericardium (**4.23**).[33] Fibrin may be hypoechoic to hyperechoic compared with the myocardium, and may be visualized on the visceral and parietal pericardial surfaces throughout the pericardial space.[33,43] Fibrin creates an irregular surface and longer tags may be seen floating or moving in the pericardial fluid (**4.24**). Signs of heart failure may include small chamber size, systolic right atrial collapse, and reduced fractional shortening.[43] With constrictive pericarditis, flattening of the left ventricular free wall during diastole may be seen.[33]

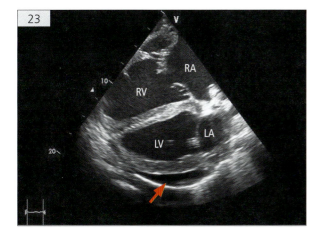

4.23 Right-sided four-chamber view of the heart of a foal with severe tricuspid regurgitation and right-sided heart failure (note dilation of right atrium and ventricle). Pericardial effusion is present (arrow). **RA**, right atrium; **RV**, right ventricle; **LA**, left atrium; **LV**, left ventricle. (Courtesy June Boon and Dr Jan Bright)

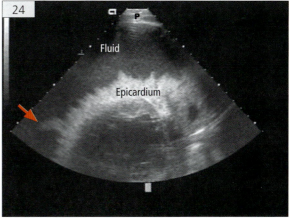

4.24 Two-dimensional echocardiographic image of the heart from the foal in 4.22. Note the irregular, proliferative epicardial surface with a large fibrinous tag (arrow). **P**, pericardium. (Courtesy Dr Jan Bright)

Analysis of pericardial fluid may assist in differentiating a septic from a non-septic process; however, non-septic pericardial fluid may be present with infectious respiratory disease[43] so does not preclude the need for antimicrobial therapy. Bacterial cultures of pericardial fluid are often negative for growth, even if there is cytologic evidence of sepsis.[43]

Management/treatment

For emergency treatment of excessive fluid accumulation and right heart failure, pericardiocentesis is indicated. This procedure is ideally performed with established IV access, ECG monitoring (p. 306), and under echocardiographic guidance (p. 308) using a large-bore (i.e. 28–32 French) Argyle flexible tube.[7,19,33,43] Local anesthesia of the intercostal muscles and pleura precedes catheter placement.[19] If ultrasonography is not available to guide catheter placement, the chest tube should be inserted in the left 5th intercostal space, 2.5–10 cm (1–4 in) dorsal to the olecranon or dorsal to the lateral thoracic vein.[19] The chest tube may be left indwelling for drainage and lavage 1–2 times daily until accumulated fluid is negligible (<1 liter over 12 hours) or until fluid drained after lavage is approximately equal to fluid instilled.[19,33,43] Suitable lavage fluids include normal saline and isotonic polyionic fluid, with or without the addition of antimicrobial drugs such as sodium penicillin G or gentamicin.[33,43] Volumes up to 1–2 liters may be infused, and smaller volumes (i.e. 1 liter) with antimicrobial drugs may be left in the pericardium until the next lavage treatment.[43]

Broad-spectrum antimicrobial drug treatment should be initiated if a bacterial cause is suspected, pending pericardial fluid analysis and bacterial culture and sensitivity testing. If respiratory disease is present and bacterial culture and sensitivity testing results are obtained from tracheal or pleural fluid samples, antimicrobial therapy should be adjusted appropriately. NSAIDs may be administered.[19,43] Corticosteroids may be used when immune-mediated or viral pericarditis is probable and there is no evidence of bacterial infection.[33]

Pericardiectomy, for cases of life-threatening restrictive pericarditis, should be undertaken only if the risk, expense, and relative lack of success in horses are fully understood by the owner.[45,46]

Myocarditis and myocardial degeneration
Key points
- Myocarditis presents a diagnostic challenge because it may be unaccompanied by cardiac signs or any specific signs that are present may be obscured by those attributable to the primary disease.
- Treatment of CHF and arrhythmias should be the first priority when accompanied by clinical signs.

Definition/overview

Myocarditis and/or myocardial degeneration occur with viral, bacterial, fungal, or parasitic infections, exposure to hypoxia or toxins, or nutritional deficiencies. These myopathies can be acute or chronic and may or may not cause myocardial dysfunction. The condition can be difficult to diagnose and the cause often remains unidentified.

Etiology/pathogenesis

Viral myocarditis has been diagnosed in association with equine infectious anemia, equine viral arteritis, equine influenza, and African horse sickness.[13,42] Myocarditis was identified in aborted fetuses infected by EHV-1.[47] Bacteria that most commonly contribute to myocarditis include *Staphylococcus* and *Streptococcus* spp.[13,42,48] Strongylosis[49] and onchocerciasis have been identified as parasitic causes of myocarditis. Fungal hyphae consistent with *Mucor* or *Rhizopus* spp. were seen histopathologically in the myocardium of a horse.[50] Less commonly, myopathy has also been attributed to ionophore[51] and cantharidin toxicity[52], rattlesnake envenomation[53,54] (see Chapter 9) (**4.25**), and to selenium and vitamin E deficiency.[55] Neoplastic infiltration of the myocardium has been described.[56,57]

Whether the underlying cause ultimately produces fibrotic, neoplastic, necrotic, or chronic inflammatory processes, there is degeneration or disruption of cardiac myocytes. If sufficiently widespread and/or in a critical focal area, myocardial contractile function or impulse conduction may be impaired.

Clinical features

Myopathies present a diagnostic challenge because they may be unaccompanied by cardiac signs. In addition, any specific signs that are present may be masked by those attributable to the primary disease (i.e. endotoxemia, acute viral syndromes). Acute myocarditis is more often accompanied by elevated fibrinogen, leukocytosis, fever, and malaise. Measurement of circulating cTnI, a contractile protein that serves as a highly sensitive and specific serum indicator of myocardial injury, may reveal elevated concentrations. Recently, use of a point-of-care analyzer was validated for measurement of plasma cTnI in horses.[1] Values for normal horses ranged from 0.0 to 0.06 ng/ml, while horses with monensin-induced myocardial necrosis had concentrations ranging from 0.08 to 3.68 ng/ml. Increased circulating cTnI was observed in cases of myocarditis attributed to sepsis[58] and experimental endotoxemia[59] and in a case of myocardial necrosis.[60] Elevated cTnI has also been measured in horses without primary cardiac disease in the presence of colic, renal failure, septicemia, skin disease, and mild leukocytosis.[61] Normal horses may have mildly elevated levels after racing or endurance activity.[62,63] The half-life of recombinant equine cTnI injected into ponies with normal renal function was determined to be short (0.47 hours)[64], therefore increased values represent acute or ongoing injury.

Otherwise, use of cTnI for monitoring or prognosticating has not been fully established in equids.

If dilated cardiomyopathy +/– valvular insufficiency is a sequela of myocarditis, signs of CHF may be present. Arrhythmias may occur if the conduction system is disrupted, and are likely to be specific to the region affected (i.e. multifocal premature ventricular contractions [PVCs] may be present with diffuse, active inflammation of the ventricular myocardium). Syncope or sudden death may occur[42], most often in association with stress or exercise.[65]

Differential diagnosis

Primary valvular disease with dilative cardiomyopathy; pericarditis; arrhythmias due to electrolyte abnormalities, general systemic disease, or dilative cardiomyopathy.

Diagnosis

A thorough history may reveal possible contributing factors (e.g. septicemia as a foal, rattlesnake envenomation), which can be used to form a presumptive diagnosis. If serum cTnI is elevated, a diagnosis of acute myocardial injury is strongly supported; however, if concentrations are within normal limits, the diagnosis cannot be ruled out, especially with chronic disease (see above). Electrocardiographic analysis may reveal arrhythmias, but this is non-specific. Echocardiographic findings may include decreased fractional shortening and dilative cardiomyopathy (i.e. increased LV camber size and decreased wall/septal thickness).[42]

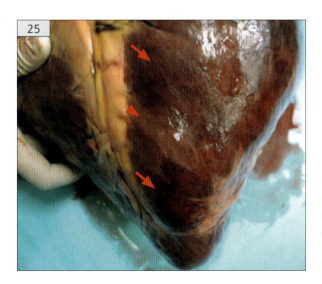

4.25 Postmortem heart from a horse with rattlesnake envenomation. Note the focal discoloration ranging from areas of darkened myocardium (arrows) to areas of pallor (arrowhead). This horse had a normal echocardiographic examination. (Courtesy Dr Jan Bright)

Rarely, focal areas of altered echogenicity within the myocardium may be identified (**4.26, 4.27**). If unaccompanied by cardiomyopathy, it is not unusual for a horse with myocarditis to have a normal echocardiographic examination (**4.25**).[60] Other signs attributable to the underlying pathology may be present (i.e. inflammatory leukogram, serologic evidence of viral infection, low blood selenium concentration).

Management/treatment

Treatment of CHF (p. 316) and arrhythmias should be the first priority when accompanied by clinical signs. In the absence of life-threatening arrhythmias or fulminant CHF, treatment of the primary disease, if defined, should be initiated and accompanied by rest.[19] Myocarditis may be treated with anti-inflammatory doses of corticosteroids in the absence of an active viral or bacterial infection.[19] If a bacterial etiology is suspected, broad-spectrum antimicrobial therapy is appropriate until a causative agent is identified by blood cultures or biopsy. In many cases, a causative agent is never identified, and broad-spectrum treatment with supportive care must continue for the duration of therapy.

Arrhythmias

- Arrhythmias are not uncommon in the horse.
- Horses can present with a range of clinical signs from mild exercise intolerance to collapse and sudden death.
- Arrhythmias are identified based on cardiac auscultation with identification of tachycardia or an irregular rhythm and are diagnosed using electrocardiography (p. 318).
- Treatment and prognosis is variable depending on the specific arrhythmia.

Atrial fibrillation
Key points
- Atrial fibrillation (AF) is the most common pathologic cardiac arrhythmia in the horse and is characterized by rapid, irregular atrial contractions that occur independently of ventricular contractions.
- AF can result from underlying heart disease, but most often occurs in the absence of identifiable cardiac pathology.

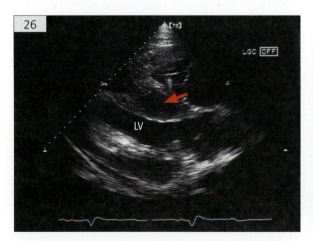

4.26 Right-sided long-axis view of the heart, with a focal lucency in the ventricular septum (arrow). A biopsy of this area revealed a mixed inflammatory infiltrate, with no organisms identified. LV, left ventricle.

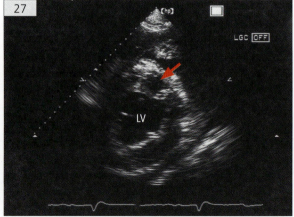

4.27 Right-sided transverse image of the heart shown in 4.26. The focal lucent area is again apparent in the ventricular septum (arrow). LV, left ventricle.

- An ECG allows definitive diagnosis of AF. Lack of P waves that are associated with each QRS, undulating baseline, irregular R-R intervals, and an irregularly irregular rhythm characterize this arrhythmia.
- If the AF is of short duration and associated with a causative event, the horse will likely convert to sinus rhythm with electrolyte replacement, fluids, and rest.
- Quinidine sulfate or quinidine gluconate is the treatment for AF that does not respond to electrolyte replacement, fluids, and rest.

Definition/overview

AF is widely appreciated as the most common pathologic cardiac arrhythmia in the horse, and is characterized by rapid, irregular atrial contraction that occurs independently of ventricular contraction. AF can result from underlying heart disease, but most often occurs in the absence of identifiable cardiac pathology.[66]

Etiology/pathogenesis

AF in the horse is most often attributed to hypokalemia induced by exercise or diuretics. Less frequently, it is caused by dilation of the atria secondary to valvular dysfunction. In many cases, the cause remains unknown.[66]

Horses have robust basal vagal tone and a large atrial mass, which renders this species more prone to development of re-entry phenomena and AF.[66] Myocardial fibrosis, atrial dilation, and electrolyte abnormalities further augment the risk for development of AF by disruption of normal electrical conduction and cellular depolarization.

Clinical features

Because the atrial 'kick' is not essential for maintenance of normal cardiac output at rest, the condition may be asymptomatic in non-athletes.[66] When a horse is asked to perform, however, even a minor decrement in hemodynamic function can contribute to inadequate provision of tissue oxygen and metabolic requirements.[19] Exercise intolerance is therefore the most common sign.[67] Indications of CHF may be present. An irregularly irregular rhythm with no S4 is heard on cardiac auscultation; the ventricular response rate may be normal or increased.[66,67] If tachycardia is present, underlying cardiac disease or increased sympathetic tone should be considered.[19]

Differential diagnosis

Arrhythmias: premature atrial contractions; PVCs; atrioventricular block. Exercise intolerance: upper airway obstruction; lower airway or pulmonary disease; neurologic disease; musculoskeletal disorders.

Diagnosis

An ECG allows definitive diagnosis of AF. Lack of P waves that are associated with each QRS, undulating baseline (fibrillation or 'f' waves), irregular R-R intervals, and an irregularly irregular rhythm characterize this arrhythmia (**4.28**).[19] The predominant QRS complex appears normal, although complexes with a ventricular derivation may occur and have an abnormal morphology.[66] It is critical to determine whether underlying heart disease is present (see Congestive heart failure), because this will greatly affect treatment recommendations.

4.28 ECG recording of a horse in atrial fibrillation. Note the irregular, multiform P waves (F) with irregularly irregular QRS complexes. Paper speed 25 mm/sec.

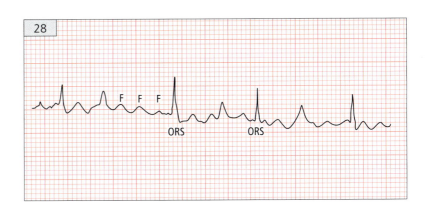

Whole body potassium depletion can be assessed by performance of a fractional excretion of potassium:

$$\text{fractional excretion K}^+ = (\text{urine } [K^+]/\text{serum } [K^+]) \times (\text{serum } [Cr]/\text{urine } [Cr]) \times 100$$

where $[K^+]$ and $[Cr]$ equal urine or serum concentrations

Normal values are between 15% and 65%. Because fluids and some medications can alter the fractional excretion of electrolytes, it is best to collect urine and serum samples prior to initiation of therapy.

Management/treatment

If the AF is of short duration and associated with a causative event (e.g. acute onset detected during competition), the horse will likely convert to sinus rhythm with electrolyte replacement, fluids and rest. It is therefore reasonable to withhold therapy for 72–96 hours after onset.[68] In horses with moderate to severe underlying heart disease, treatment of the AF is rarely successful long term. In these cases, treatment aimed at reducing cardiac workload and relieving congestion is more appropriate. Serum electrolytes should be supplemented as indicated prior to initiation of treatment.

Quinidine is available in two formulations: quinidine gluconate for IV administration and quinidine sulfate for oral administration:

- 12–24 hours prior to initiation of pharmacologic cardioversion, a test dose of quinidine sulfate in solution at 5 mg/kg may be administered by nasogastric tube to test for idiosyncratic effects or allergic reactions.[69]
- The dose rate for quinidine gluconate is 1.1–2.2 mg/kg IV every 10 minutes, not to exceed a cumulative dose of 12 mg/kg.[69]
- Quinidine sulfate is administered at a dose rate of 22 mg/kg PO q2h via a nasogastric tube, not to exceed 132 mg/kg. If AF persists and no adverse effects are present, administration may continue at a dose of 22 mg/kg PO q6h.[69] Alternatively, treatment may be withheld for 24 hours, and the protocol repeated with or without added digoxin (0.01 mg/kg PO q12h).[69]

Because quinidine decreases the renal excretion of digoxin[25], careful monitoring for digoxin toxicity (i.e. dull demeanor, diarrhea, prolonged P-R or QRS interval, atrioventricular block, sinus bradycardia, or ventricular arrhythmias) must be observed when the drugs are given concomitantly.

Adverse sequelae of quinidine include ataxia, behavioral changes, seizures, upper airway edema and obstruction, urticaria, laminitis, anorexia, colic, and diarrhea.[66,69–71] Mild depression and flatulence are frequent sequelae to quinidine administration and do not require treatment.[67] Ataxia, erratic behavior, and seizures suggest toxicity, therefore immediate discontinuation of quinidine is indicated, with subsequent environmental management and anticonvulsant treatment as needed.[66] Allergic responses may be treated with cessation of quinidine treatment and administration of corticosteroids and antihistamines depending on severity.[66] Patients with upper airway edema should additionally be monitored for development of dyspnea and obstruction, with emergency equipment readily available should nasal stenting, nasotracheal intubation, or tracheotomy be warranted.[66] Development of laminitis should preclude further quinidine dosing and warrants initiation of standard laminitis management.[66] GI signs often diminish with cessation of quinidine treatment; however, quinidine should be discontinued if colic or diarrhea is severe, and analgesics administered as required.[66]

Cardiac signs of quinidine toxicity include supraventricular or ventricular tachycardia, hypotension, and sudden death.[66,71] During treatment, the ECG should be monitored for >25% prolongation of the pretreatment QRS complex, which indicates toxicity and warrants immediate cessation of quinidine administration.[24,66] Signs of quinidine toxicity may be transiently reduced by administration of sodium bicarbonate (0.5–1.0 mEq/kg IV); relative alkalosis will promote protein binding of quinidine and therefore reduce active drug.[24,71] The first response to all cardiovascular sequelae should be discontinuation of quinidine; thereafter, treatment should be directed at restoring hemodynamic stability primarily with pressors and antiarrhythmics. Supraventricular tachycardia with a ventricular rate >100 bpm should be treated with digoxin (0.0022 mg/kg IV or 0.011 mg/kg PO).[66] Faint peripheral pulses, tachycardia, pallor, weakness, and syncope suggest inadequate cardiac output[13]; the β-adrenergic blocker propranolol may be administered to reduce heart rate and increase ventricular filling time (0.03 mg/kg IV) and the α-agonist phenylephrine may be used to promote vasoconstriction (0.1–0.2 µg/kg/min IV, up to 0.01 mg/kg total).[66] Ventricular tachycardia (p. 333) should be treated when signs of hypotension due to inadequate cardiac output are present, when the rate exceeds 120 bpm, or when multifocal complexes or R-on-T phenomenon are observed.[66] (See Ventricular tachycardia for pharmacologic management of this arrhythmia.)

Digoxin pretreatment of horses undergoing quinidine therapy has been described in cases of existing systolic dysfunction, resting tachycardia, or a history of tachycardia with previous quinidine administration.[67]

Successful pharmacologic cardioversion using amiodarone has been described in horses with a duration of AF ranging from 1 to 12 months and no contributing cardiac pathology.[72,73] Side-effects include transient hindlimb weakness and, more commonly, diarrhea. Amiodarone was administered at a dose of 5 mg/kg/hour IV for 1 hour, then 0.83 mg/kg/hour IV for 23 hours, then 1.9 mg/kg/hour IV for 30 hours.[72] Limited data regarding safety and efficacy of amiodarone use in horses are available.

To avoid the negative sequelae of quinidine in all patients, and to improve the chances for successful cardioversion in horses with chronic AF, electrical cardioversion may be attempted. This approach is very efficacious in patients with lone AF (i.e. without underlying cardiac disease).[74] Currently, this modality is available primarily in referral institutions, though a detailed description of the procedure has been published.[75]

While the prognosis for sustained cardioversion and return to function is fair to good in horses with lone AF[68], the presence of underlying heart disease or chronicity (>4 month's duration) is associated with persistent AF that is refractory to treatment.

Third-degree atrioventricular block
Key points
- Third-degree atrioventricular block (AVB) is never a normal finding.
- Horses have exercise intolerance and the 1st and 2nd heart sounds are slow and heard independently of the 4th heart sound, which occurs at a higher rate reflecting a normal sinoatrial or atrial origin.
- To characterize and verify the arrhythmia, ECG assessment is needed. Relatively frequent P waves are dissociated from the less common QRS complexes.
- Pharmacologic treatment includes corticosteroids unless an acute viral or bacterial myocarditis is suspected, atropine, isoproterenol, and/or dopamine.
- Pacemaker implantation is indicated in patients that do not respond to pharmacological treatment.

Definition/overview
Unlike 1st- and 2nd-degree AVB, 3rd-degree AVB is an uncommon arrhythmia in horses and is not a normal finding.[19] Contractile activity of the atria occurs independently from ventricular contraction, contributing to hemodynamic compromise at rest, syncope, and exercise intolerance.[66]

Etiology/pathogenesis
Third-degree AVB has occurred transiently immediately after electrical cardioversion of AF[76] and in association with duodenitis/proximal jejunitis[77], rattlesnake envenomation[54], and mediastinal lymphoma.[57] The arrhythmia was also present in four foals that underwent general anesthesia.[78] A congenital etiology was suspected in a young female Jerusalem donkey.[79]

The underlying cause of 3rd-degree AVB is presumed to be fibrosis, inflammation, ischemia, dilation, or neoplasia of the impulse generation or conduction pathway[78], although the cause often remains unknown. Third-degree AVB may be transient in young or middle-aged horses, suggesting that the underlying myocardial changes may be reversible in these cases.[68] Whether transient or permanent, interruption of the normal conduction pathway results in disrupted transmission of the electrical impulse generated in the sinoatrial node or atria, with subsequent development of an independent atrioventricular nodal or ventricular rhythm.

Clinical features

Because 3rd-degree AVB creates hemodynamic inefficiency and renders the ventricles insensitive to sinoatrial-mediated chronotropic influences, heart rate does not sufficiently increase with activity, and severe exercise intolerance exists.[66] Horses may become recumbent due to syncope.[66] The 1st and 2nd heart sounds are slow (<20 bpm), and heard independently of the 4th heart sound, which occurs at a higher rate reflective of normal sinoatrial or atrial origin.[66] Prominent heart sounds may occasionally be ausculted if the 4th heart sound occurs concomitantly with the 1st or 2nd heart sound.[66] If there are few ectopic beats, the rhythm is regular; if premature atrial or ventricular beats occur, the 4th or 1st/2nd heart sounds, respectively, may be irregular.[67]

Differential diagnosis

Second-degree AVB with a variable P-R interval; premature atrial or ventricular contractions; AF.

Diagnosis

Representative auscultation findings with appropriate clinical signs strongly support the diagnosis of 3rd-degree AVB. If ectopy is present, the irregular rhythm may make diagnosis based on auscultation and signs difficult. To characterize and verify the arrhythmia, ECG assessment is needed. Relatively frequent P waves are dissociated from the less common QRS complexes (**4.29**). Unless ectopy is present, both are regular. The QRS complexes may or may not be wider than established normal values, but are likely to be wider and of different morphology than those associated with the normally generated sinus complex (if available for comparison).[66]

Management/treatment

If the conduction aberrancy can be attributed to reversible inflammation, dexamethasone (0.05–0.22 mg/kg IV) is used.[66] If acute viral or bacterial myocarditis is suspected, the use of dexamethasone should be critically evaluated until appropriate antimicrobial drug therapy is initiated and/or active infection is likely to have resolved.

Emergency management includes use of the parasympatholytic drug atropine (0.005–0.01 mg/kg IV).[66]

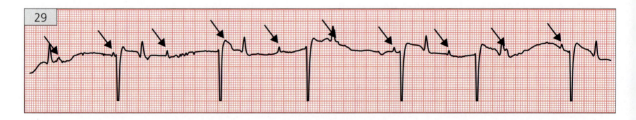

4.29 Third-degree atrioventricular block in a horse with rattlesnake envenomation. Arrows indicate P waves that occur regularly. Note that the P waves are often hidden in other complexes. QRS complexes occur independently of P waves, evidenced by prolonged and inconsistent PR intervals (paper speed 25 mm/sec). (Courtesy Dr Jan Bright)

If severe hemodynamic compromise results from a very slow ventricular rate, isoproterenol (0.05–0.2 µg/kg/minute IV infusion) may be administered.[66] This drug may initiate or exacerbate ventricular ectopic beats, in which case the isoproterenol should be discontinued and resultant arrhythmias treated appropriately.[54,66] Dopamine HCl (5–6 µg/kg/min) has been used to restore normal sinus rhythm in foals under general anesthesia with atropine-resistant 3rd-degree AVB.[78] A dopamine dose of 2.5–3.75 µg/kg/min IV was used to control 3rd-degree AVB in an adult horse without occurrence of ventricular arrhythmias and agitation observed at higher doses.[54]

If the horse is hemodynamically unstable or fails to respond to pharmacologic intervention, the optimal treatment is pacemaker implantation.[66,68] Successful implantation of permanent pacemakers in equids has been reported.[79] With profound hemodynamic compromise, a temporary transvenous pacemaker may be used. The temporary electrodes must make sufficient contact with the right atrial or right ventricular myocardium to ensure capture of pacemaker-generated impulses.[80]

Premature ventricular contractions

Key points

- PVCs are beats arising from ventricular foci that are independent of atrial and atrioventricular nodal activity.
- The presence of PVCs is best confirmed with electrocardiography.
- If the horse is hemodynamically stable and the rhythm is not characterized by frequent, polymorphic, or exercise-associated PVCs, or if the R-on-T phenomenon is not observed, initial treatment should be aimed at correcting the underlying disease and existing fluid or electrolyte imbalances.
- Lidocaine is the antiarrhythmic treatment of choice.

Definition/overview

PVCs are beats arising from ventricular foci that are independent of atrial and atrioventricular nodal activity. PVCs occur uncommonly in horses, and may be normal or associated with systemic or cardiac anomalies.

Etiology/pathogenesis

Sporadic monomorphic PVCs can occur in normal horses during rest or in the immediate post-exercise period, and are not considered to be clinically important.[66,68] When PVCs are polymorphic or occur frequently at rest or during exercise[66], or when the R-on-T phenomenon is observed[81], antiarrhythmic treatment should be initiated. Clinically relevant PVCs have been associated with ventricular remodeling secondary to dilative cardiomyopathy, as well as hypoxia, inflammation, and necrosis of the ventricular myocardium.[68,82] In addition to primary cardiac disease, electrolyte abnormalities, GI disease, systemic infection, and anesthesia have all been associated with the occurrence of PVCs.[66,81,82]

Little is known about the pathophysiology of ventricular dysrhythmias in equids, so information must be extrapolated from other species. The common disturbance is assumed to be ectopic foci, increased automaticity, and re-entry phenomena attributable to irritability[68], with disruption of normal conduction pathways within the ventricular myocardium.

Clinical features

Observed signs are more likely to reflect underlying disease (i.e. CHF, colic) rather than the PVCs, unless there is hemodynamic compromise attributable to frequent or paroxysmal PVCs (see Ventricular tachycardia). On auscultation, sounds associated with the PVC will be earlier and possibly louder than those of the normal sinus beats.[67] If the PVC occurs very soon after a normal contraction, there may be a pulse deficit appreciated on palpation of a peripheral artery.[66,68]

Differential diagnosis

Premature supraventricular (including atrial) complexes.

Diagnosis

The presence of PVCs is best confirmed with electrocardiography. Premature beats with a QRS that is wider and of different morphology than the sinus beats, and accompanied by a compensatory pause, strongly support a diagnosis of PVCs.[82] Additionally, ventricular complexes often have large T waves that are of opposite polarity to the QRS (**4.30**).[66,82] The frequency, number of foci (i.e. monomorphic versus polymorphic) (**4.31**), timing (i.e. exercise versus rest), and coupling interval (i.e. presence of R-on-T) should be characterized to determine whether treatment of the arrhythmia is indicated.[81,82]

Echocardiographic examination and serum cTnI measurements may assist in defining primary cardiac disease, although these may be normal even with existing cardiac pathology.

Management/treatment

If the horse is hemodynamically stable and the rhythm is not characterized by frequent or polymorphic PVCs, or if the R-on-T phenomenon is not observed, initial treatment should be aimed at correcting the underlying disease and existing fluid or electrolyte imbalances. In some cases, PVCs may be eliminated or greatly reduced after stall rest, with or without anti-inflammatory drug treatment.[81]

Lidocaine is the antiarrhythmic treatment of choice and should be given slowly and in small increments to avoid an excitatory response and seizures. The dose is 0.5 mg/kg IV slowly every 5 minutes, not to exceed 2–4 mg/kg total dose.[69] Alternatively, the drug can be administered as a continuous intravenous infusion at a rate of 20–50 µg/kg/minute.[69] If excitement or seizures occur, diazepam (0.05 mg/kg IV) should be administered.[7]

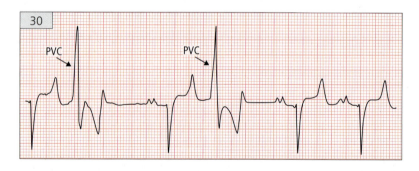

4.30 Bigeminal premature ventricular complexes (PVC). Note that normal sinus complexes precede the premature ventricular complexes. Paper speed 25 mm/sec.

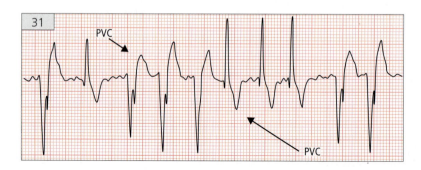

4.31 Two triplets of premature ventricular complexes (PVC) with different morphologies suggestive of distinct ventricular origins. Paper speed 25 mm/sec.

Another treatment option is phenytoin sodium (20 mg/kg PO q12h for 3–4 doses). If the arrhythmia persists, continue with 10–15 mg/kg PO q12h. Adverse sequelae associated with high serum phenytoin concentrations include sedation and recumbency.[83]

If lidocaine and phenytoin are ineffective, other treatment options include quinidine gluconate (1.1–2.2 mg/kg IV)[69] or procainamide (1 mg/kg/min IV, to a maximum cumulative dose of 20 mg/kg).[69] Both quinidine and procainamide can be negative inotropes at high doses[66], therefore care must be taken when treating patients with pre-existing heart failure or hemodynamic compromise.

Ventricular tachycardia

Key points

- Ventricular tachycardia is defined as five or more consecutive PVCs.
- Ventricular tachycardia can cause hemodynamic compromise at rest, can deteriorate into fatal arrhythmias, and is usually attributable to underlying systemic or cardiac disease.
- An ECG will best confirm and characterize ventricular tachycardia.
- Lidocaine is the antiarrhythmic treatment of choice.

Definition/overview

Ventricular tachycardia is defined as five or more consecutive PVCs.[68] Ventricular tachycardia can cause hemodynamic compromise at rest, can deteriorate into fatal arrhythmias, and is usually attributable to underlying systemic or cardiac disease.

Etiology/pathogenesis

Ventricular tachycardia has been documented to occur in a healthy young horse postoperatively[84], after strenuous exercise in an unconditioned horse[85], with electrolyte abnormalities and proarrhythmic drugs[66], and with renal tubular acidosis.[86] Cardiac etiologies include myocardial infarction secondary to endocarditis and septic embolization of the coronary arteries[33], as well as hypoxia, inflammation, necrosis[68], and fibrosis[87] of the myocardium.

Little is known about the pathophysiology of ventricular dysrhythmias in equids, so information must be extrapolated from other species. The common disturbance is assumed to be ectopic foci, increased automaticity, and re-entry phenomena attributable to irritability[68], with disruption of normal conduction pathways within the ventricular myocardium.

Clinical features

Signs may include lethargy[87], syncope, CHF[66], and tachycardia.[48] Signs may be related to underlying systemic disease (e.g. colic, anorexia). The severity of signs is often related to the ventricular rate, which determines filling time and cardiac output.

The ventricular response rate often exceeds 60 bpm.[7,66] An irregular rate may be appreciated if the ventricular tachycardia is multifocal. In most cases, however, the heart rate is regular due to a single ectopic focus (**4.32**).[7,66] Loud heart sounds may be appreciated if atrioventricular dissociation is present.[66]

Differential diagnosis

Supraventricular tachycardia; AF or 3rd-degree AVB with accelerated junctional or ventricular response.

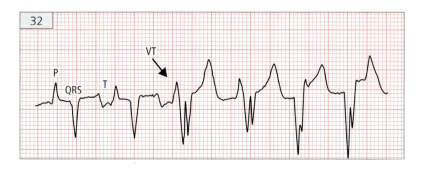

4.32 Normal sinus beat followed by ventricular tachycardia (VT). Paper speed 25 mm/sec.

Diagnosis

An ECG will best confirm and characterize ventricular tachycardia. In most cases, the heart rate is regular due to a single ectopic focus and this may aid in differentiating ventricular tachycardia from supraventricular tachycardia. Additionally, large T waves that are of opposite polarity to the QRS complex are observed. P waves are regular but dissociated from the QRS complexes and this may be difficult to appreciate if P waves are obscured in the QRS complexes (**4.33**). The presence of the following characteristics are associated with a greater chance of life-threatening hemodynamic compromise and progression into ventricular fibrillation:[7,66]

- Severe or progressive hemodynamic compromise.
- Multiform ventricular complexes.
- 'R-on-T' phenomenon, or QRS complexes occurring during myocardial repolarization (T wave).
- 'Torsades de pointes', a type of ventricular tachycardia characterized by QRS complexes that appear to be 'twisting' around the baseline; and/or
- Rapid ventricular rate (>120 bpm).

Echocardiographic examination (p. 318) and serum cTnI measurements may assist in defining primary cardiac disease, although these may be normal even with existing cardiac pathology.

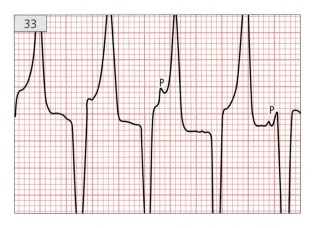

4.33 Ventricular tachycardia. Note that P waves (P) do not regularly precede the ventricular complexes. Paper speed 25 mm/sec.

Management/treatment

If the horse is hemodynamically stable and the rhythm is not characterized by any of the life-threatening characteristics listed under Diagnosis, initial treatment should be aimed at correcting underlying disease and existing fluid or electrolyte imbalances. If any of the aforementioned life-threatening characteristics are present, treatment of the arrhythmia should be initiated as an emergency.[66]

Lidocaine is the antiarrhythmic treatment of choice, given slowly and in small increments to avoid an excitatory response or seizures. If these effects occur, diazepam (0.05 mg/kg IV) should be administered.[7] The dose for lidocaine is 0.5 mg/kg IV slowly every 5 minutes, not to exceed 2–4 mg/kg total dose.[69] Thereafter, the drug can be administered as a continuous intravenous infusion at a rate of 20–50 µg/kg/minute.[69]

Although data in horses are minimal, the intratracheal (IT) route has been used to administer lidocaine in human[88] and small animal patients when IV access cannot be established. This is facilitated by tracheal intubation and extension of a soft catheter past the tip of the tube for drug deposition in the distal airways.[88] Subsequent ventilation, not necessarily mechanical, will further serve to distribute the drug in the airways. Commonly, the IV dose is doubled for IT administration, and diluted in a large volume of saline (e.g. up to 10 ml in humans[88]).

Other treatment options are:
- Quinidine gluconate (1.1–2.2 mg/kg IV[69]) or procainamide (1 mg/kg/min IV, to a maximum cumulative dose of 20 mg/kg[69]). **Note:** Both quinidine and procainamide can be negative inotropes at high doses[7,66], therefore care must be taken when treating patients with pre-existing heart failure or hemodynamic compromise.
- Propranolol (0.03 mg/kg IV[7]). Propranolol is a less desirable treatment option because of infrequent efficacy and negative inotropic effects. Its use should be reserved for persistent ventricular tachycardia that is refractory to conventional treatment.[7,66]
- Magnesium sulfate (slow IV bolus at a dose of 4 mg/kg every 2 minutes up to a maximal cumulative dose of 50 mg/kg[69]) can be given

to horses that have a low or normal serum magnesium concentration, quinidine-associated ventricular tachycardia, and to those with refractory ventricular tachycardia.[7,69]

- Amiodarone, an antiarrhythmic used commonly in humans, blocks potassium channels and prolongs repolarization.[30] Information regarding use of this drug in horses is limited, but successful conversion of two episodes of ventricular tachycardia in a horse with myocarditis has been described, each time using a dose of 5 mg/kg/hour IV for 1 hour, followed by 0.83 mg/kg/hour IV for 23 hours.[89] Tapering doses were used over 7 weeks to maintain sinus rhythm after the recurrence. Transient hindlimb weakness and diarrhea were observed in horses that received amiodarone for >36 hours.[72]
- Phenytoin sodium (20 mg/kg PO q12h for 3–4 doses) is another treatment option. If the arrhythmia persists, continue with 10–15 mg/kg PO q12h. Adverse sequelae associated with high serum phenytoin concentrations include sedation and recumbency.[83]

Ventricular fibrillation
Key points

- Ventricular fibrillation is a fatal arrhythmia characterized by uncoordinated and weak contractile activity of the ventricles that does not produce sufficient cardiac output to maintain the forward flow of blood.
- In an adult horse, thoracic compressions may be accomplished by a strike to the thorax just caudal to the elbow, delivered by a human dropping to his/her knees from a standing position onto the horse.
- Electrical defibrillation is the treatment of choice in foals and ponies.
- Lidocaine is the antiarrhythmic treatment of choice.

Definition/overview
Ventricular fibrillation is a fatal arrhythmia characterized by uncoordinated and weak contractile activity of the ventricles that does not produce sufficient cardiac output to maintain the forward flow of blood. Death

occurs if the arrhythmia is not immediately resolved. The occurrence of ventricular fibrillation is verified by an ECG, therefore the arrhythmia is primarily detected in anesthetized horses, since sudden death associated with ventricular fibrillation often precludes ECG recording.

Etiology/pathogenesis
In horses, ventricular fibrillation has been associated with intensive training in racehorses[90] and arrhythmogenic drugs.[90–93] Severe non-cardiac (e.g. GI tract, renal) disease and electrolyte abnormalities may also be causative. Ventricular tachycardia can also degenerate to ventricular fibrillation.

Little is known about the pathophysiology of ventricular dysrhythmias in Equidae, so information must be extrapolated from other species. Disturbances are likely to include ectopic foci, high automaticity, and re-entry phenomena attributable to irritability[68] and disruption of normal conduction pathways within the ventricular myocardium. Histopathologic lesions identified in five racehorses that experienced death from presumptive cardiac pathology included myocardial fibrosis of impulse generation and conduction regions and arterial sclerosis in the vessels supplying the sinoatrial and atrioventricular nodes.[90]

Clinical features
Because ventricular fibrillation causes acute, severe loss of cardiac output and death within minutes[90], the diagnosis of ventricular fibrillation outside the surgical suite is often a presumptive diagnosis made by ruling out other causes of sudden death. A study of five racehorses that died suddenly, one with confirmed ventricular fibrillation, revealed that all horses went down during or after intensive training.[90] Subsequent signs included dyspnea and tachypnea, severe sweating, and trembling.[90] There is loss of palpable pulses, auscultable heart sounds, and measurable blood pressure. Death occurs between 2 and 8 minutes after the onset of signs.[92]

Differential diagnosis
Asystole; any other cause of sudden death; technical problems with the ECG.

Diagnosis

A definitive diagnosis is made with electrocardiographic evidence of an undulating baseline with irregular, low-amplitude waves and absence of discernible QRS complexes (**4.34**).[66] If ECG monitoring is unavailable, the presence of clinical signs and concomitant absence of a heart beat, peripheral pulses, and blood pressure strongly support the diagnosis of ventricular fibrillation or asystole.

In the case of sudden death, ventricular fibrillation cannot be ruled out unless electrocardiographic confirmation is obtained ante-mortem. If the ECG reveals the characteristic waveform but the animal does not show the aforementioned signs, one should ensure that the gain is sufficiently augmented, all leads are adhered to the horse, and artifactual noise is minimized.

Management/treatment

In an adult horse, thoracic compressions may be accomplished by a strike to the thorax just caudal to the elbow, delivered by a human dropping to his/her knees from a standing position onto the horse.[94] While this technique does not create flow or pressure compatible with life, it may improve drug distribution and prolong the window for treatment. Cardiopulmonary cerebral resuscitation (p. 312) in foals can be effective in achieving functional blood flow and pressure.

Electrical defibrillation is the treatment of choice in foals and ponies, but should only be conducted by trained individuals as the risk for human injury is high with improper use. This modality may be impractical in adult horses due to large electrical impedance[7],

although newer biphasic cardioverter/defibrillator units may offer improved efficacy over older models.

Pharmocologic treatment includes:
- Bretylium tosylate (3–5 mg/kg IV; may repeat, not to exceed a total of 10 mg/kg).[7]
- Lidocaine (0.5 mg/kg IV slowly, not to exceed 2–4 mg/kg total dose[69]); if seizures occur, diazepam 0.05 mg/kg IV may be administered.[7]
- Magnesium sulfate can be given as a slow IV bolus at a dose of 4 mg/kg every 2 minutes, up to a maximal cumulative dose of 50 mg/kg[69], or 55.5 mg/kg diluted in saline over 20 minutes.[30]

Although data in horses are minimal, the IT route has been used to administer lidocaine in humans[88] and small animal patients when IV access cannot be established. This is facilitated by tracheal intubation and extension of a soft catheter past the tip of the tube for drug deposition in the distal airways.[88] Subsequent ventilation, not necessarily mechanical, will further serve to distribute the drug in the airways. Commonly, the IV dose is doubled for IT administration and diluted in a large volume of saline (up to 10 ml in human patients[88]). Direct installation of drugs into the left ventricle may be attempted when IV or IT access cannot be established.[7]

If bretylium and lidocaine, with or without magnesium, are ineffective, other treatment options include quinidine gluconate (1.1–2.2 mg/kg IV) and procainamide (1 mg/kg/min IV to a maximum cumulative dose of 20 mg/kg).[69]

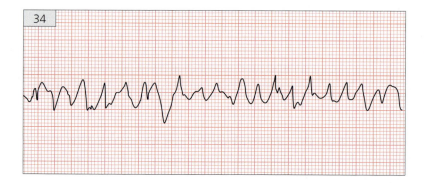

4.34 Ventricular fibrillation. Note the irregular baseline and complete lack of organized activity and recognizable complexes. Paper speed 25 mm/sec.

Asystole

Key points

- Cardiopulmonary cerebral resuscitation should be initiated immediately.
- Emergency pharmacologic treatment involves atropine and epinephrine/adrenaline.

Definition/overview

Asystole is the absence of electrical activity recorded on the ECG, with underlying absence of myocardial contractility and cardiac output. The conscious horse loses consciousness in seconds. Death can result within minutes.

Etiology/pathogenesis

Because of the acute and grave nature of this arrhythmia, it is most often verified in the anesthetized horse with continuous electrocardiographic monitoring.[95,96] No common etiology has been identified.

Asystole has been documented in association with low mixed venous oxygen tension, suggesting inadequate tissue perfusion may play a role.[96] Two horses developed asystole that had normal arterial oxygenation, presumably clinically insignificant hypercarbia, and normal serum electrolyte concentrations (venous oxygen tension not measured).[95] Although the arrhythmia has been identified in horses under halothane anesthesia[95,96], concomitant or preceding respiratory depression or hypotension were absent, suggesting that generalized depressant effects attributable to oversedation were not contributory.[95] Asystole can occur with manipulation of the bladder, reproductive organs, joints, or eyes and is presumed to be vagally mediated in these cases.[97]

Clinical features

Asystole is recognized on the ECG as a flat line representing a lack of electrical activity. Ventricular asystole may also occur, as evidenced by P waves in the absence of QRS complexes (**4.35**). During electrocardiographic monitoring of the anesthetized animal, asystole has been documented to occur both spontaneously and in association with preceding bradycardia or AVB.[95,96] Spontaneous breathing may be present.[95,96] There is a precipitous decrease in blood pressure and peripheral pulses are absent.

Differential diagnosis

Ventricular fibrillation; any cause of sudden death; technical problems with electrocardiographic monitoring.

Diagnosis

A definitive diagnosis is made with electrocardiographic evidence of a flat baseline accompanied by severe hypotension, absent peripheral pulses, and loss of consciousness (in the unanesthetized horse). If electrocardiographic monitoring is unavailable, the presence of clinical signs and concomitant absence of a heart beat, peripheral pulses, and blood pressure strongly support the diagnosis of asystole or ventricular fibrillation.

Other causes of sudden death in the unanesthetized horse cannot be ruled out ante-mortem unless electrocardiographic confirmation is immediately obtained. If the ECG reveals the characteristic waveform but the animal does not show the aforementioned signs, one should ensure that the gain is sufficiently augmented and that all leads are adhered to the horse.

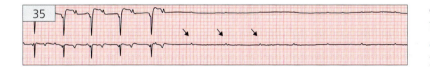

4.35 Normal sinus rhythm followed by ventricular asystole. Arrows denote non-conducted P waves. Paper speed 25 mm/sec.

Management/treatment

Cardiopulmonary cerebral resuscitation should be immediately initiated (p. 315). If asystole occurs during surgical manipulation, removal of the mechanical stimulation may restore sinus rhythm.[97] If the arrhythmia persists with reinitiation of the surgery, the horse can be premedicated with atropine or epinephrine prior to further manipulations.[97] Pharmacologic treatment of asystole is as follows:

- Epinephrine (0.03–0.05 mg/kg IV or 0.3–0.5 mg/kg in sterile saline IT, followed by robust ventilation).[7]
- Atropine (0.01–0.02 mg/kg).[7]
- Glycopyrrolate (0.001–0.005 mg/kg IV), as an alternative to atropine; and/or
- $NaHCO_3$ (0.5–1.0 mEq/kg IV if metabolic acidosis is present).[7]

Epinephrine/adrenaline can cause ventricular ectopy.[97] If hemodynamic compromise occurs as a result of this, the horse may be treated with lidocaine (0.5 mg/kg IV slowly every 5 minutes, not to exceed 2 to 4 mg/kg total dose).[69]

Although data in horses are minimal, the IT route has been used to administer atropine, lidocaine, and epinephrine in human patients[88] and small animals when IV access cannot be established.[7] (See Ventricular fibrillation.)

Congenital cardiac defects

- Congenital cardiac defects are uncommon in foals, with the Arabian breed being affected most frequently.[98]
- Foals present with poor growth, failure to thrive, exercise intolerance, respiratory distress, and death.[98]
- Ventricular septal defect (VSD) and tetralogy of Fallot (p. 340) are the most common.[98] Others include tricuspid and pulmonic valve atresia, truncus arteriosus, and aortic stenosis.
- Clinical signs include a loud murmur, tachycardia, tachypnea, and cyanotic membranes.[98]
- A diagnosis can be made with echocardiography (p. 308).
- Concurrent congenital defects are common.[98]
- Prognosis is generally grave except for foals with a VSD.

Ventricular septal defect

Key points

- VSD is the single most commonly diagnosed congenital anomaly of horses.
- Horses with a small VSD may continue to perform for some time, although generally not at the highest level.
- Horses with a VSD should have regular repeated echocardiographic evaluation to follow progress and evaluate for deterioration of cardiac function.

Definition/overview

A VSD is a defect, or communication, between the left and right ventricles of the heart present in the interventricular septum. It is the most common congenital cardiac lesion in the horse.

Etiology/pathogenesis

The defect is usually situated at the base of the interventricular septum in the membranous or semi-membranous portion, just below the aortic root, where the septum fuses with the endocardial cushion early in fetal development (**4.36**). Occasionally, defects are found in the septum just below the base of the pulmonary valve and are due to abnormal development of the bulbus cordis. Defects in the muscular portion of the septum have also been reported. A VSD can also be found as a component of more severe complex congenital cardiac disease such as tetralogy of Fallot, tricuspid atresia, and endocardial cushion defects.

Clinical features

The clinical signs seen in animals with a VSD depend on the hemodynamic effects of the defect. Large defects will result in volume overload early in life and CHF may be the presenting sign. Tachypnea and dyspnea may be noted and may be directly due to pulmonary edema. Some foals with less severe disease may have difficulty in keeping up with their dams at pasture, or reduced exercise tolerance compared with other foals. A murmur is detected in foals as an incidental finding when they are examined for other purposes. Some are only detected later in life when the horse shows signs of reduced exercise tolerance or is examined for another reason. VSDs have been detected well into adult life, particularly in horses that are not athletic. A characteristic loud plateau-type murmur may be ausculted with the point of maximal intensity on the right side of the chest, just above the sternum in the apex beat area. A palpable thrill may be present.

Differential diagnosis
Other cardiac anomalies.

Diagnosis
A definitive diagnosis of a VSD is best achieved using echocardiography (**4.37**). Contrast echocardiography is a useful technique to document the presence and location of a left-to-right shunt. Doppler echocardiography is a useful and sensitive technique for detecting the abnormal shunt flow. Pulsed-wave Doppler echocardiography is used to detect blood flow by placing the sample volume on the right ventricular side of the suspected defect.

Management/treatment
No specific treatment is available. Surgical repair is impracticable at present. CHF should be managed if it develops (p. 318). Small defects may allow for continued use of the horse, but follow-up evaluations should be regularly scheduled to follow any progression of cardiac dysfunction. Clinical and historical evidence is also pertinent in giving advice on the use of horses with VSDs for athletic work. A recent, normal performance record is supportive evidence for the presence of a relatively insignificant lesion.

Tetralogy or pentalogy of Fallot
Key points
- Tetralogy or pentalogy of Fallot is an uncommon complex cardiac defect with four elements: a VSD, an overriding aorta (the aortic root straddling the interventricular septum), right ventricular outflow obstruction, and right ventricle hypertrophy.
- One of the cardinal signs of tetrology or pentalogy of Fallot is central cyanosis.
- Euthanasia is usually warranted.

Definition/overview
Tetralogy or pentalogy of Fallot is an uncommon complex cardiac defect with four elements: a VSD, an overriding aorta (the aortic root straddling the interventricular septum), right ventricular outflow obstruction, and right ventricle hypertrophy. Sometimes the

aorta is termed 'dextraposed', which means that the root is entirely within the right ventricle. The cause

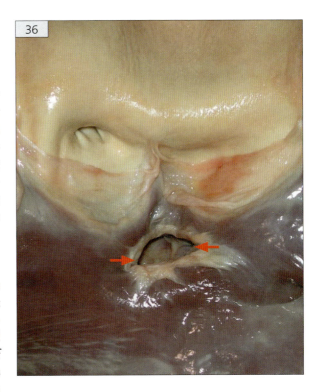

4.36 Ventricular septal defect located in the membranous portion of the interventricular septum (arrows). (Courtesy Dr Virginia Reef)

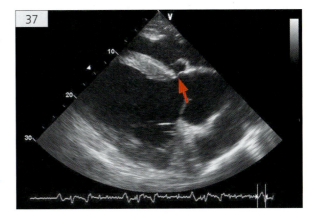

4.37 Echocardiographic image of a ventricular septal defect located in the membranous portion of the interventricular septum (arrow). (Courtesy Dr Virginia Reef)

of the right ventricle hypertrophy may be pulmonary valve stenosis or pulmonary artery hypoplasia. The latter is more common in the horse.

Etiology/pathogenesis

Embryology studies show that it is a result of anterior malalignment of the conal septum, resulting in the clinical combination of a VSD, pulmonary stenosis, and an overriding aorta. Right ventricular hypertrophy results from this combination, which causes resistance to blood flow from the right ventricle.

Clinical features

Owing to the presence of a right-to-left shunt, one of the cardinal signs of tetralogy or pentalogy of Fallot is central cyanosis, which may or may not be apparent on clinical examination, depending on the degree of shunting. Other signs include profound exercise intolerance, poor growth, and CHF. Auscultation reveals loud (grade 4 to 6 out of 6) murmurs on both sides of the chest, predominantly at the left base. A thrill is often present.

Differential diagnosis

Other cardiac anomalies.

Diagnosis

Diagnosis is based on clinical signs (particularly if cyanosis is present) and echocardiography. Echocardiography shows a VSD (usually quite large), an overriding aorta, and right ventricle hypertrophy, with thick walls and marked trabeculation. Pulmonary stenosis may be identified if present; pulmonary hypoplasia is more difficult to image due to interference from the lung. Doppler echocardiography and contrast studies are useful to demonstrate right-to-left flow. Injection of echo-contrast into the jugular vein results in opacification of the right atrium, right ventricle, and aorta.

Management/treatment

There are no surgical repair techniques described or attempted in the horse and the prognosis for life with tetralogy or pentalogy of Fallot is, at a minimum, poor. These horses will not become athletes. Euthanasia is usually warranted.

Patent ductus arteriosus
Key points

- Patent ductus arteriosus (PDA) is a congenital disease.
- Confirmation requires angiography and/or echocardiography.
- If combined with other significant cardiac defects the prognosis is grave.

Definition/overview

PDA (or persistent ductus arteriosus) is a congenital defect whereby the normal fetal vascular channel between the pulmonary artery and the aorta fails to close.

Etiology/pathogenesis

In utero, approximately two-thirds of fetal blood bypasses the pulmonary artery and is shunted by the ductus arteriosus directly to the aorta. In late gestation, the ductus arteriosus narrows and with expansion of the lungs at the first breath post parturition, pulmonary resistance falls and systemic arterial pressure rises, resulting in the reversal of blood flow within the duct until the duct begins to close. Although the mechanisms are not yet completely understood, initial closure of the duct is believed to be due to the reflex contraction of the muscular layer of the vessel, resulting in a stoppage of blood flow across the duct (functional closure). Gradually, the ductus arteriosus is replaced by a fibrous band called the ligamentum arteriosum (anatomic closure).

Clinical features

In normal foals, functional closure of the ductus arteriosus begins by 320 days of gestation and is generally complete at about 3 days of age; because of this a diagnosis of PDA is not usually made until 4–5 days of age. Clinical signs include a loud (grade 4 to 6 out of 6) continuous murmur with cyanosis.

Differential diagnosis

Transposition of the great vessels; persistent truncus arteriosus. Concurrent anomalies: persistent right aortic arch; interruption of the aortic arch; pseudotruncus arteriosus; tricuspid atresia; VSD; tetralogy of Fallot.

Diagnosis

Definitive diagnosis is made by angiography and/or echocardiography. Following diagnosis of a PDA at necropsy, the area must be very carefully evaluated to determine if it was patent, anatomically closed, or functionally closed.

Most equine congenital cardiac defects are diagnosed in foals that exhibit exercise intolerance and cardiovascular insufficiency; however, there are reports of 'aged' horses being diagnosed with a PDA.

Management/treatment

There are no reports of surgical correction of PDA in the foal. Marked shunting through the PDA that persists and results in continued cyanosis generally results in humane euthanasia, as does recognition of its association with other congenital cardiac defects.

Vascular diseases
Hemorrhage

(See p. 311)

Post-castration hemorrhage
Key points

- Post-castration hemorrhage is defined as hemorrhage that is more than that expected after castration.
- A thorough physical examination is necessary to assess the extent of hemorrhagic shock and the need for resuscitation (p. 315).
- Patient stabilization with crystalloid fluids and blood transfusion may be necessary.
- General anesthesia is usually necessary to identify and ligate the affected vessel.

Definition/overview

Post-castration hemorrhage is defined as hemorrhage that is more than that expected after castration. Although a slow drip of blood may be observed after the horse stands, a steady stream of blood or bleeding persisting for more than 30 minutes is an indication that additional investigation and intervention is required.

Etiology/pathogenesis

Severe hemorrhage is usually from the testicular artery and occurs because of improper use of the emasculator and failure to adequately crush the artery, or from a loose ligature in closed castrations. Good surgical technique can eliminate many of the potential causes of hemorrhage and these are outlined in *Table 4.4*.

Because the testicular artery is a branch of the aorta, hemorrhage from it can result in marked loss of blood. Bleeding is unlikely to resolve spontaneously and requires direct pressure or ligation to prevent serious hypovolemia and hemorrhagic shock.

Clinical features

Hemorrhage is usually not observed until the horse is standing after castration, when blood pressure rises and pooled blood drains from the incision. A slow drip

---

Table 4.4 Steps during castration to reduce the risk of post-castration hemorrhage

- Avoid large superficial vessels when creating the scrotal incision.
- Ensure the cutting blade of the emasculator is adjacent to the testicle and the crushing blade is adjacent to the inguinal canal.
- Apply the emasculator at 90 degrees to the spermatic cord.
- If the spermatic cord is large, separate emasculation of the vascular and muscular parts of the cord should be performed.
- Grasp the stump with forceps before the emasculator is removed and inspect the cord for hemorrhage without tension before it is released.
- If a closed castration is performed, ensure a transfixation ligature is placed and that the ligature is tight.
- Once hemorrhage has been corrected, the horse should be kept quiet in a stall for several days to allow a secure clot to form.

of blood from the castration site can be seen normally, but it should resolve within 30 minutes. However, if the rate of hemorrhage is more rapid, is persistent, or the horse shows signs of hypovolemia due to the hemorrhage, then immediate investigation to locate and ligate the source of the bleeding is essential. Signs of blood loss include dull demeanor, weakness, tachycardia, pale mucous membranes, and hypotension.

Differential diagnosis

A diagnosis of post-castration hemorrhage is inherently obvious. Other sources of hemorrhage should be considered in a horse showing signs of hemorrhagic shock without hemorrhage from the castration site.

Diagnosis

The diagnosis is usually made based on the history of recent castration and obvious bleeding from the surgery site. When the testicular artery recoils into the abdomen after surgery, hemorrhage can continue into the abdomen without overt exterior signs of a problem. Abdominal ultrasonography can be used to identify intra-abdominal hemorrhage.

Management/treatment

In order adequately to examine the castration site and locate the source of the hemorrhage, general anesthesia is necessary. A thorough physical examination of the horse should be performed first to determine if blood loss is clinically important. Hypovolemia should be corrected prior to anesthesia with crystalloid fluids (p. 312) and a blood transfusion (p. 312) if indicated. If intra-abdominal hemorrhage occurs, shed blood can be collected for autotransfusion.[99]

Initially, the skin and subcutaneous areas should be examined for hemorrhage from the external pudendal vein or artery or from subcutaneous vessels. If the source appears to be from the testicular artery, the testicular stump should be identified within the inguinal canal and a transfixation ligature applied.

Identification of the testicular stump within the inguinal ring is not always possible. The testicular stump may have retracted deep within the inguinal canal and swelling of the inguinal ring can make visibility difficult. In such situations, laparotomy sponges can be packed into the canal and the scrotum secured over the top to exert pressure on the artery for at least 24 hours. However, this is not always effective and may cover ongoing hemorrhage. Laparoscopy with the horse standing[99] or under general anesthesia can be used to identify the testicular stump and locate the testicular artery in such situations. The testicular stump should be identified and retracted through the internal inguinal ring into the abdomen and cauterized or re-ligated laparoscopically.[100]

Peripheral artery/vein hemorrhage
Key points
- Lacerations involving the distal limb can result in marked hemorrhage.
- The goals of treatment are to stop the hemorrhage and stabilize the patient.

Definition/overview

Hemorrhage from peripheral vessels is usually a result of a sharp traumatic injury that severs a vessel. Although these are peripheral vessels, ongoing hemorrhage can be marked and result in hemorrhagic shock.

Etiology/pathogenesis

Severance of a peripheral vessel is most likely to occur with lacerations to the lower limbs. Lower limb vessels are superficial and easily damaged as there is little soft tissue protection. Heel bulb lacerations are likely to result in marked hemorrhage, as the lateral or medial digital arteries are frequently involved. Ongoing blood loss from peripheral vessels can result in clinically important hypovolemia and shock if not addressed in a timely manner.

Clinical features

While the presence of a laceration may be obvious, the fact that a peripheral vessel has been involved is not always immediately apparent. Ongoing hemorrhage from the laceration or blood in the animal's environment may be obvious when the horse is first examined. Even if hemorrhage has resolved, it is possible for the clot to become dislodged with movement of the horse.

Lacerations that involve a peripheral vessel may have also compromised adjacent synovial structures or tendons, and careful evaluation of the entire area should be performed.

Differential diagnosis

Acute hemorrhage with no signs of a laceration: guttural pouch mycosis; ethmoid hematoma; rupture of the longus capitis muscle from trauma; URT neoplasia; URT trauma; LRT tract hemorrhage (e.g. exercise-induced pulmonary hemorrhage); hemoabdomen; hemothorax.

Diagnosis

In all horses with a laceration, a physical examination to detect signs of blood loss should be performed prior to repair of the laceration. Indicators of acute blood loss include pale mucous membranes, tachycardia, trembling, and weakness. (**Note:** The PCV does not change with acute hemorrhage and it may take up to 24 hours to fully reflect the degree of blood loss.)

Management/treatment

The aims are two-fold: (1) stop the hemorrhage and (2) assess the patient for signs of hypovolemia. If multiple competent personnel are available, it is advisable for one person to address the hemorrhage while another assesses the patient and provides supportive care if indicated.

A horse that has sustained a deep laceration is frequently agitated and may require sedation prior to wound exploration. Rapid assessment of the horse's cardiovascular status, particularly heart rate, pulse pressure, and CRT, is advisable prior to administration of any drugs. Acepromazine should be avoided as a sedative because its use can result in profound hypotension if the animal is already hypovolemic and it provides little sedation in an excited animal. Sedation is better achieved with one of the alpha-2 agonists, which result in adequate sedation for a defined period of time with fewer cardiovascular effects.

Application of direct pressure to the wound is the most rapid method of reducing hemorrhage. This can be performed by the owner with cotton padding and bandages in an emergency situation. The aim is for the external pressure applied to exceed the blood pressure in the vessel and thus prevent flow and allow platelet aggregation to occur. This is most effective for management of general capillary oozing and provides only temporary hemostasis for larger vessels.

If the vessel that is the source of the hemorrhage can be identified, it should be grasped with hemostats and a secure, circumferential ligature of absorbable suture material (most often size 2-0) placed to provide permanent occlusion of the vessel. If the vessel is particularly large, a second transfixation ligature should also be placed.[101]

Locating the severed end of the vessel can be challenging. Excellent visibility of the area is particularly important and can be improved by spot lighting and frequent blotting of the area with gauze sponges. It is possible for the proximal end of the vessel to retract due to the elastic recoil of the vessel wall as it is traumatized. In such situations, the skin may need to be incised proximally from the wound edge to locate and ligate the severed end.

If the source of hemorrhage cannot be identified and ligated, a topical hemostatic agent can be applied to the wound underneath a pressure bandage. Hemostatic agents are made of biodegradable gelatin or collagen, which promote platelet aggregation.[102] They are more effective against low pressure capillary ooze than hemorrhage from a specific vessel.

Once hemorrhage is controlled, the overall cardiovascular status of the patient should be evaluated to determine if fluid therapy (see Chapter 12) is required to correct hypovolemia and if a blood transfusion (p. 312) is necessary.

Guttural pouch mycosis
Key points

- Guttural pouch mycosis is associated with growth of fungal plaques on the major vessels and nerves associated with the medial and lateral compartments of the guttural pouches and can result in life-threatening hemorrhage or neurologic signs, or both.
- Occlusion of normograde and retrograde blood flow to the site of the plaque is necessary.
- The cardiovascular status of the patient should be assessed and crystalloid fluids, plasma, and/or blood transfusion given as necessary (p. 312).

Definition/overview

Fungal infection of the guttural pouch can result in either acute hemorrhage or dysphagia, depending on the location of the mycotic plaque. Frequently, there are no clinical signs or indication of disease prior to an episode of acute epistaxis.

Etiology/pathogenesis

The mycotic infection is caused predominantly by *Aspergillus* spp. *Aspergillus fumigatus* is the most commonly identified species.[103] The incidence of infection is relatively low and the reason why some horses are affected while others in the same herd are not is not understood. As these fungi are ubiquitous in the environment, predisposing factors, such as prior infection with an URT disease, may allow invasion of the respiratory epithelium in some individuals. However, there is no known breed, age, or sex predilection, and lesions have been found in foals and bilaterally.

The fungus usually colonizes the guttural pouch over one of the arteries that lie beneath the epithelial lining of the pouch (**4.38, 4.39A, 4.39B**). The artery most commonly affected is the internal carotid artery, followed by the external carotid and maxillary arteries. The fungal plaque can erode the wall of the artery, causing hemorrhage. Alternatively, local inflammation from the mycotic plaque can irritate the adjacent glossopharyngeal and hypoglossal nerves and cause dysphagia.

Clinical features

Prior to acute hemorrhage there is often no indication of the presence of mycosis. Occasionally, a slight nasal discharge or a few drops of blood at the nostrils is seen prior to a catastrophic bleed. The most common presentation is that the horse is found with epistaxis from one nostril. If the hemorrhage is severe, it is possible for

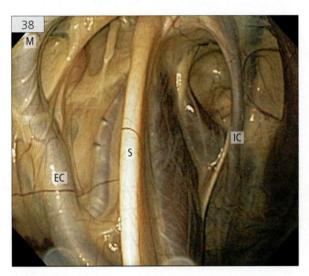

4.38 Anatomy of the normal right guttural pouch as seen endoscopically. S, stylohyoid bone; IC, internal carotid artery; EC, external carotid artery; M, maxillary artery. (Courtesy Dr Eric Parente)

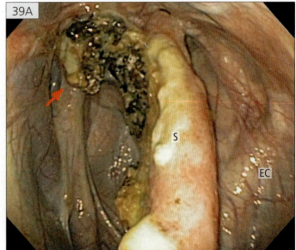

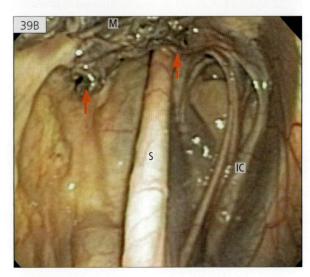

4.39A, 4.39B Endoscopic appearance of a guttural pouch mycosis in the left (A) and right compartment (B) (arrows). S, stylohyoid bone; IC, internal carotid artery; EC, external carotid artery; M, maxillary artery. (Courtesy Dr Eric Parente)

the epistaxis to occur bilaterally as the guttural pouch openings are caudal to the end of the nasal septum. Once a horse has had an episode of epistaxis from guttural pouch mycosis, it is highly probable that fatal epistaxis will occur at any time.

Dysphagia can also be seen in horses with guttural pouch mycosis, although this occurs less frequently than hemorrhage. Irritation and damage to the pharyngeal branches of the vagus and hypoglossal nerves causes difficulty swallowing. Additionally, damage to the recurrent laryngeal nerve by the mycotic plaque can cause laryngeal hemiplegia. In general, horses with dysphagia tend to respond less favorably to treatment than those with hemorrhage due to persistent nerve damage.

Differential diagnosis

Respiratory tract hemorrhage: ethmoid hematoma; LRT hemorrhage (e.g. exercise-induced pulmonary hemorrhage); rupture of the longus capitis muscle from trauma.[104] Dysphagia: stylohyoid osteoarthropathy; botulism.

Diagnosis

The use of endoscopy to identify the mycotic plaque in the guttural pouch provides definitive evidence of the disease. If hemorrhage has recently occurred, blood can usually be seen draining from one of the guttural pouch openings in the roof of the nasopharynx (**4.40**). Great care should be taken when entering the pouch with the endoscope as it is easy to dislodge a clot or the plaque, resulting in acute and severe hemorrhage. It is important to assess both guttural pouches endoscopically to confirm if the lesion is unilateral or bilateral, prior to making treatment decisions.

Management/treatment

Horses that have had an episode of hemorrhage from guttural pouch mycosis are at extreme risk for sudden fatal hemorrhage. Therefore, surgical management to occlude the blood supply to the affected artery should be performed as soon as possible. Even in cases with dysphagia and no history of hemorrhage, occlusion of the blood supply to the affected artery results in a more rapid and effective resolution of the lesion than topical antifungal treatment.

In a horse that has had an episode of severe epistaxis, expansion of the intravascular volume with crystalloids, colloids, and whole blood is advisable prior to general anesthesia. However, because these procedures increase the blood pressure, it is possible for the clot that has formed to become dislodged and epistaxis to recur. Therefore, hypotensive resuscitation is crucial in these cases to reduce the risks associated with general anesthesia while not initiating another episode of hemorrhage. In horses that are actively bleeding, delaying surgery to administer whole blood and fluids is not advisable and the horse should be taken to surgery immediately and medical therapy initiated during general anesthesia.

During an episode of acute hemorrhage, ligation of both common carotid arteries can be performed as an emergency measure to reduce the pressure in the internal carotid artery and slow the rate of bleeding.[105] Ligation of only the ipsilateral common carotid artery actually increases blood flow through the internal carotid artery and, therefore, is contraindicated.[105]

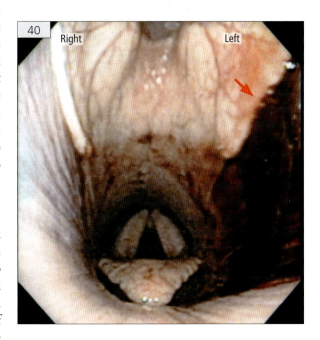

4.40 Hemorrhage from the left guttural pouch seen endoscopically (arrow). (Courtesy Dr Eric Parente)

Prior to surgery, it is vital to confirm which artery is affected (**4.41A**). Due to the abundant collateral blood supply to the head, both normograde and retrograde flow through the affected vessel must be prevented. In cases with hemorrhage from the internal carotid artery, it must be occluded distal to the fungal lesion at the sigmoid flexure and at its origin from the common carotid artery (**4.41B**). If the external carotid or maxillary artery is involved, retrograde flow must be occluded via the major palatine artery in addition to occluding the external carotid artery (**4.41C**).

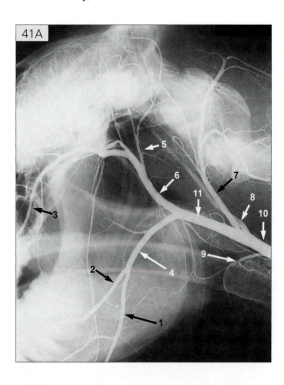

4.41A Normal arterial anatomy of the equine head. (Radiograph courtesy of Drs Tony Pease and J. Brett Woodie) 1; Facial artery, 2; Lingual artery, 3; Major palatine artery, 4; Linguofacial artery, 5; Caudal auricular artery, 6; Maxillary artery, 7; Occipital artery, 8; Internal carotid artery, 9; Cranial thyroid artery, 10; Common carotid artery, 11; External carotid artery.

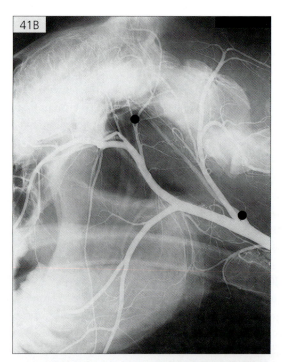

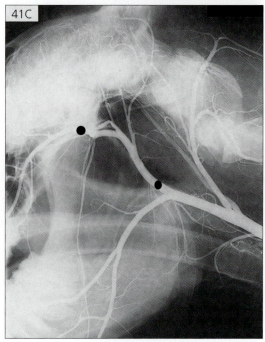

4.41B, C Vascular occlusion necessary for mycotic lesions associated with the internal carotid artery (medial compartment) (B) and the external carotid and/or maxillary artery (lateral compartment) (C).

Occlusion of the vessels can be achieved with a balloon thrombectomy catheter[106,107] and ligation of the proximal artery, or with detachable latex balloons[108] or coils.[109] Because transarterial coil embolization utilizes fluoroscopy to identify the vessels, there is less risk of complications from aberrant vasculature, which appears to be relatively common.[110,111] Two-year survival rates when this technique is used are reported at 84% with no recurrence of the mycotic lesion.[112]

Uterine artery rupture

Key points
- Rupture of the middle uterine, ovarian, or external iliac artery usually occurs shortly after parturition and results in severe hemorrhage that is often rapidly fatal unless the hemorrhage is contained within the broad ligament of the uterus.
- The most important aspect of management is to keep mares suspected of having a uterine artery rupture quiet to prevent clot dislodgement.

Definition/overview
Rupture of the middle uterine (4.42), ovarian, or external iliac artery usually occurs shortly after parturition. It results in severe hemorrhage, which is often rapidly fatal unless contained within the broad ligament of the uterus (4.43). The incidence is increased in older, pluriparous mares. Urogenital hemorrhage and large colon volvulus were the most common reasons for post-partum mares presenting to a university referral hospital on an emergency basis.[113]

Etiology/pathogenesis
The uterine artery runs in the broad ligament and is torn when the ligament stretches or is traumatized during pregnancy or parturition. In one study, approximately 14% of mares had prepartum hemorrhage with the remaining 86% occurring post partum.[114] The proximal uterine artery lying within 15 cm of the bifurcation of the iliac artery is reportedly the most frequent site for rupture, with lesions occurring preferentially at bifurcations, the lateral part of curvatures, and abrupt flexures of the artery.[115] If the middle uterine artery ruptures into the abdomen, the hemorrhage is not contained and rapid blood loss and death occurs. If the hemorrhage is contained within the broad ligament, a hematoma can form within the ligament, which may result in enough pressure on the artery to control the bleeding. Although the majority of cases are seen immediately following parturition, it is possible for hemorrhage to become clinically apparent several weeks later if a clot is dislodged from the site of hemorrhage. Although dystocia is likely to increase the risk of trauma to the artery, this problem is also seen in mares that have a normal delivery. Severe hemorrhage from the uterine arteries is also possible after correction of a

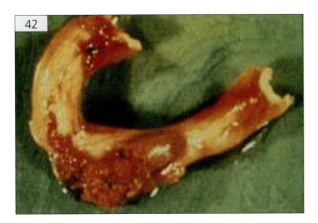

4.42 Middle uterine artery showing the site of rupture. (Courtesy Dr Patrick McCue)

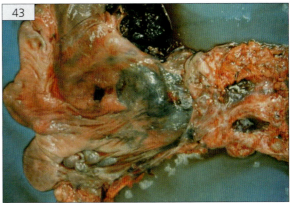

4.43 Broad ligament hematoma subsequent to middle uterine artery rupture. (Courtesy Dr Patricia Sertich)

uterine prolapse (see Chapter 5) due to stretching and damage to the vessels.

The risk of the artery rupturing increases with the number of previous pregnancies and age, probably because the artery becomes less elastic.[115] There is a 14% increase in risk of urogenital hemorrhage with each increase in year of age.[113] Most mares with periparturient hemorrhage (91%) are multiparous, with the majority having had more than four foals.[114] Histologically, the arterial wall adjacent to the rupture develops smooth muscle cell atrophy with fibrosis of the tunica media and disruption and/or calcification of the internal elastic lamina.[115] Low serum copper levels at the time of parturition may also reduce the elasticity of the artery wall.[116]

Clinical features

Clinical signs are those of pale mucous membranes, tachycardia, and shock. Therefore, all mares should be monitored closely for signs of shock after foaling, especially after a dystocia is resolved. Colic signs, trembling, and sweating are also seen, especially if there is a hematoma in the broad ligament. It is possible for the hemorrhage to be so rapid that sudden death occurs with little prior indication.

Differential diagnosis

Uterine wall or vaginal hemorrhage; uterine tear; large colon volvulus; hemorrhage from intestinal injury.

Diagnosis

Confirmation of the ruptured artery can be achieved by physical examination, abdominal sonography (**4.44A**, **B**), and abdominocentesis. However, great care should be taken to minimize stress and excitement to the mare, as this could disrupt a clot that has formed. Hemorrhage into the abdomen can be seen as swirling free fluid around the viscera. Abdominocentesis will confirm that the fluid is blood. It is also possible to confirm the presence of a hematoma in the broad ligament by palpation per rectum or transrectal ultrasonography (**4.44A**, **B**). Extreme care should be taken not to dislodge a clot that may have formed. These additional procedures are only indicated if the diagnosis is uncertain. A large firm swelling can be palpated in the broad ligament, which is seen as a hyperechoic mass with ultrasonography. Interestingly, abdominal palpation per rectum was diagnostic in 12 out of 16 cases of urogenital hemorrhage in post-partum mares.[113]

The PCV will not be low immediately following acute hemorrhage and so is not necessarily a useful indicator of acute hemorrhage. However, post-partum mares with urogenital hemorrhage are more likely to be anemic, hypoproteinemic, and hypofibrinogenemic compared with post-partum mares presenting as emergency for other reasons.[113]

Management/treatment

Treatment of mares with a uterine artery rupture is challenging. In many cases, blood loss is so rapid that the mare dies before therapy can be initiated. The best chance of success occurs if the hemorrhage is contained within the broad ligament. Surgical correction of the hemorrhage is not likely to be successful; it is usually impossible to identify and ligate the artery, anesthesia in a horse that is hypotensive is risky, and the stress of induction can elevate the mare's blood pressure and restart the hemorrhage.

Therefore, the goal of treatment is permissive hypotension in which blood pressure is maintained below normal to minimize hemorrhage, but at a sufficient pressure to supply vital organs. The first step is to avoid spikes in the mare's blood pressure by keeping her calm and avoiding unnecessary stress, such as transportation or removal of the foal. Mean arterial pressure should be monitored using an indirect blood pressure cuff on the tail. The aim is to keep the mean arterial pressure (MAP) between 70 and 90 mmHg. If the pressure is above this, or the mare is agitated, small doses of acepromazine can be given, with great care, to prevent severe hypotension. If the MAP is <70 mmHg, isotonic crystalloids can be given to expand the circulating volume. Fresh frozen plasma can also be given to provide clotting factors and for additional volume expansion (p. 312). Colloids that may reduce coagulation, such as hetastarch, should not be administered. Hypertonic saline is rarely indicated in situations of uncontrolled hemorrhage, as it can result in a rapid elevation in blood pressure, which can dislodge previously formed clots.

Blood transfusion may be necessary to improve tissue oxygen delivery. If there is hemorrhage into the abdomen, autotransfusion of the shed blood can be performed (p. 312). Alternatively, allogeneic transfusion can be used.

Some clinicians advocate the use of antifibrinolytic drugs to stabilize the clot. IV administration of formalin had been thought to enhance hemostasis. However, its administration to normal horses had no effect on bleeding time or activated clotting time[117] and, therefore, its use is not recommended. Aminocaproic acid (20–40 mg/kg slowly with IV fluids q6h for 24 hours) prevents the activation of plasminogen to plasmin and, therefore, prevents fibrinolysis of the clot.

Naloxone is an opioid antagonist that may be beneficial in hemorrhagic shock by attenuating the effect of opioids. A study of horses with endotoxic or hemorrhagic shock showed that administration of naloxone prevented some of the associated cardiovascular changes.[118] However, in the model of hemorrhagic shock, an extremely high dose of 0.2 mg/kg was used to achieve the beneficial effect. The dose that is more frequently used clinically is a single IV dose of 8 mg per 400–500 kg horse.

Administration of oxytocin will not reduce hemorrhage from a uterine artery. It should not be given if there is a hematoma in the broad ligament as the induced uterine contraction and associated pain may disrupt the clot.

The survival of mares presenting to a referral hospital with periparturient hemorrhage was recently reported to be good (84%) and 49% of mares for which follow up was available went on to produce a live foal at a subsequent pregnancy.[114] Mares that have had a uterine artery rupture and survived are at high risk for it to reoccur in subsequent pregnancies.

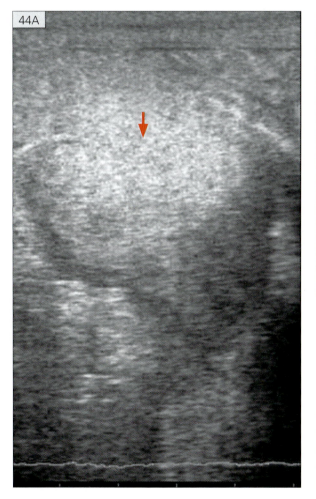

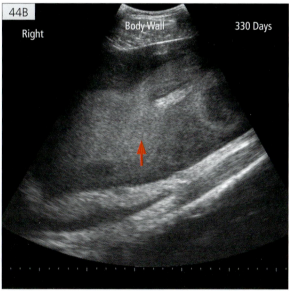

4.44A, B Ultrasonographic appearance of a hematoma in the broad ligament as viewed from a transrectal ultrasound examination (A, arrow) and hemoabdomen as viewed from a transabdominal ultrasound examination (B, arrow). (Courtesy Dr Audrey Kelleman)

Aortic aneurysm or rupture

Key points

- Aortic rupture is catastrophic and usually rapidly fatal.
- Cardiac arrhythmias and signs of right-sided heart failure may be observed if hemorrhage dissects into the interventricular septum or with rupture into the atrium/ventricle, respectively.
- There is currently no treatment; however, some horses may survive with supportive treatment for CHF.

Definition/overview

Aortic rupture most commonly involves the right aortic sinus (sinus of Valsalva).[119] The aortic root can rupture into the right atrium, right ventricle, interventricular septum, or pericardial space.[119–122] The extrapericardial aorta can also rupture, leading to rapidly fatal hemorrhage (**4.45**).

Etiology/pathogenesis

Aortic root rupture occurs most commonly in older horses, particularly older breeding stallions[120], but can occur in mares and young horses.[119] Dystrophic changes in the aortic media have been observed. Hypertension associated with breeding is thought to cause the abnormal aortic wall to rupture.[123] Aneurysms of the right sinus of Valsalva have been reported and are associated with congenital defects in the aortic media adjacent to the right coronary sinus.[123] Aorto-pulmonary fistulation in conjunction with aortic rupture has been reported to be common in Friesian horses and was associated with progressive pathology rather than sudden death.[124]

Clinical features

Most aortic ruptures are rapidly fatal. Horses can present with signs of distress and exercise intolerance associated with right-sided heart failure when aortic root rupture or rupture of a sinus of Valsalva aneurysm communicates with the right atrium or right ventricle (aorto-cardiac fistula, **4.46**). In horses with an aorto-cardiac fistula, a bounding pulse can be palpated and a right-sided continuous murmur loudest over the 4th intercostal space can be ausculted.[119,123] If dissection of blood occurs within the interventricular septum following rupture, cardiac arrhythmias, particularly ventricular tachycardia (p. 333), can occur.[119] Horses may also present with signs such as recurrent colic, peripheral edema and persistent tachycardia prior to cardiac failure.[124]

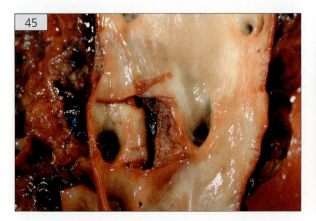

4.45 Abdominal aorta rupture. (Courtesy Julie Engiles)

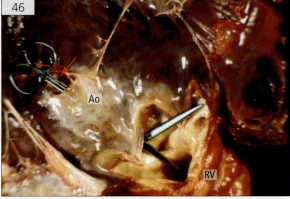

4.46 Aortocardiac fistula. RV, right ventricle; Ao, aorta. (Courtesy Dr Perry Habecker)

Differential diagnosis

Any other cause of sudden death.

Diagnosis

While ante-mortem diagnosis of an aortic sinus of Valsalva aneurysm or aorto-cardiac fistula can be made with echocardiography, most aortic ruptures are diagnosed at necropsy.

Management/treatment

There is currently no treatment; however, some horses may survive with supportive treatment for CHF (p. 318).[123] Owners should not use horses with aortic aneurysms or arterial-cardiac fistulae for any athletic activity. Horses may be used with caution for breeding.

Inflammatory
Thrombophlebitis and septic thrombophlebitis
Key points

- Intravenous catheter sites should be monitored closely for signs of redness, heat, pain, swelling, and drainage indicating thrombophlebitis.
- If there is any indication of thrombophlebitis, the catheter should be aseptically removed and bacterial culture and sensitivity testing performed on the catheter.
- Sonographic examination can be used to determine the extent of the thrombophlebitis.
- Antimicrobial drugs are indicated in cases of septic thrombophlebitis to treat the disease and prevent endocarditis.

Definition/overview

Thrombophlebitis and septic thrombophlebitis usually occur in the jugular vein (**4.47**) secondary to catheter placement or repeated blood draws. Damage to the vessel endothelium by the catheter allows a clot to form at the site. Infection of the thrombus with bacteria results in the more serious problem of septic thrombophlebitis.

4.47 Jugular vein thrombophlebitis.
(Courtesy Dr Perry Habecker)

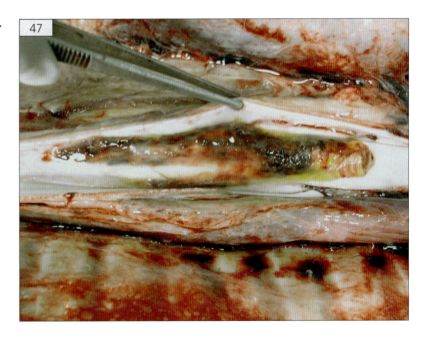

Etiology/pathogenesis

The factors that influence the development of thrombophlebitis are those of Virchow's triad (*Table 4.5*): (1) a hypercoagulable state, (2) venous stasis, and (3) damage to the vascular endothelium. These factors increase the coagulability of the blood and allow a clot to form within the vessel lumen. The presence of a catheter can result in bacteria entering the thrombus via three routes: (1) through the catheter line, (2) from skin bacteria migrating along the catheter tract, or (3) from systemic circulating bacteria seeding the catheter site.[125] In horses, the most common bacteria isolated are *Staphylococci* spp.[126], suggesting that it is bacteria from the skin that are the most frequent cause of infection. However, *Staphylococci* spp., especially *Staphylococcus epidermidis*, are frequently found in the intestinal flora of hospitalized patients, especially those receiving antimicrobial drugs.[125] Compromised intestinal mucosa is common in equine intensive care unit patients and allows translocation of bacteria from the lumen into the systemic circulation. Therefore, the systemic circulation may be an important source for infection of the thrombus in horses with GI disease. Once the thrombus is infected, bacteria can be seeded into the systemic circulation and result in septicemia and intermittent fever spikes.

Many disease processes found in hospitalized horses, including endotoxemia, hypoproteinemia, and colitis, result in the loss of antithrombin III and reduced fibrinolysis, ultimately resulting in a hypercoagulable state.[127] Reduced blood flow and blood stasis occur if there is reduced cardiac output, recumbency, or the horse is standing with its head down. Damage to the vascular endothelium occurs from IV catheters, irritant drugs, and due to underlying disease processes such as endotoxemia. Therefore, all three components of Virchow's triad are common in hospitalized horses, resulting in a dramatic increase in the risk of developing thrombophlebitis.

Clinical features

Diagnosis of thrombophlebitis is first made by visual inspection and palpation of the catheter site and jugular vein for thickening, heat, swelling, and pain. Redness and edema of the area, and drainage from the puncture

---

Table 4.5 Virchow's triad for thrombosis and methods to reduce their impact in the at-risk horse

VIRCHOW'S TRIAD	PREVENTION OF THROMBOPHLEBITIS IN AT-RISK HORSES
Hypercoagulability	Treat the underlying disease process.
	Monitor platelet count, activated partial thromboplastin time, prothrombin time, fibrinogen, and fibrin (ogen) degradation products.
	Administer fresh frozen plasma with 40 IU heparin/kg if antithrombin III concentrations are low.
Blood stasis	Correct hypovolemia to improve cardiac output.
	Cross tie and support the head of standing horses.
	Elevate the head of recumbent horses.
Endothelial damage	Use the smallest feasible gauge catheter.
	Use polyurethane or silastic catheters.
	Flush catheters with heparinized saline every 6 hours.
	Use commercially made sterile fluids.
	Avoid hypertonic solutions.

site are suggestive of septic thrombophlebitis. In severe cases, edema of the head is seen as venous drainage is impaired. Careful examination of the catheter site daily for signs of inflammation is critical for early identification of the problem. Horses with septic thrombophlebitis are often febrile and thrombophlebitis should always be considered in a horse with a fever of unknown origin with a catheter in place. Horses may also become inappetent because of the fever or neck pain.

Differential diagnosis
Jugular distension: right-sided heart failure. Head swelling: anaphylaxis; snake bite.

Diagnosis
Apart from clinical examination of the catheter site, sonographic examination of the vein can be used to determine the size of the thrombus and the degree of obstruction to blood flow (**4.48**). Additionally, the structure of the thrombus can be evaluated to determine if it is heterogeneous or contains hypoechoic areas consistent with fluid or necrosis, which may indicate septic thrombophlebitis.[128] If cavitations are found in the thrombus, ultrasound-guided aspiration of the area can be performed after sterile preparation to collect samples for aerobic and anaerobic bacterial culture and sensitivity testing. Blood culture with the sample collected at the peak of the fever and culture of the catheter can also help determine the causative organism.

Management/treatment
If thrombophlebitis is suspected, the catheter should be immediately removed. To avoid thrombosis of both jugular veins, it is advisable not to place a new catheter in the opposite jugular vein and to collect future blood samples from the transverse facial venous sinus. Therefore, a new catheter should be placed at an alternative location, such as the lateral thoracic or cephalic veins. Topical treatment such as hot packing and application of dimethylsulfoxide several times a day will reduce local inflammation. Diclofenac, a topical NSAID, can also be used. Frequently, a small abscess at the catheter puncture site will be found. This should be opened with a small stab incision to allow drainage. If septic thrombophlebitis is suspected, systemic antimicrobial drugs should be considered once the necessary cultures have been obtained. Antimicrobial drug therapy can be tailored to the individual once bacterial culture and sensitivity testing results are known.

In addition to treating the thrombophlebitis, steps should be taken to minimize the risk of further clot formation. This is best achieved by considering the three causal factors in Virchow's triad and minimizing the risk of each (*Table 4.5*).

4.48 Sonographic appearance of jugular vein thrombophlebitis: (A) cross-sectional and (B) longitudinal views. T, thrombus; J, jugular vein. (Courtesy Dr JoAnn Slack)

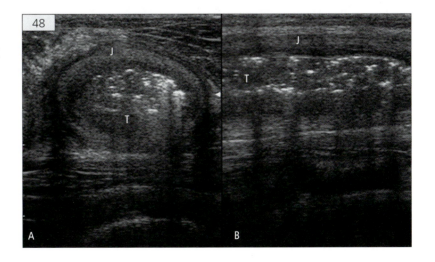

Thromboembolic disease
Key points
- Thromboembolic disease results in occlusion of a vessel by an embolus or thrombus leading to infarction to the area it supplies.
- Clinical signs are variable depending on the affected organ.
- The prognosis is generally hopeless and the animal should be euthanized.
- Patient management to avoid coagulopathy is critical to prevent thromboembolic disease.

Definition/overview
Thromboembolic disease results in occlusion of a vessel by an embolus or thrombus leading to infarction to the area it supplies. In general, smaller vessels are involved and multiple branches supplying the same organ are usually affected. In horses, organs that are commonly affected include the intestine, lungs (**4.49**), kidneys, liver, and distal limbs.

Etiology/pathogenesis
As in thrombophlebitis, the three factors in Virchow's triad that predispose to thrombus formation are prerequisites to this disease. Horses affected frequently

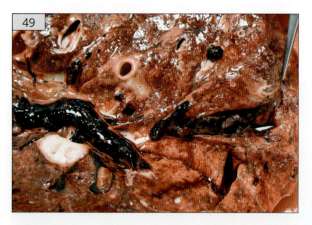

4.49 Pulmonary thromboembolus. (Courtesy Dr Julie Engiles)

have DIC, which results in fibrin forming in the circulation.[129] These fibrin deposits become lodged in the microcirculation and occlude the blood supply to the organ. This can ultimately result in ischemia and organ failure.

The key to development of thromboembolic disease is a hypercoagulable state. Endotoxin is known to induce shortened coagulation times in horses[130], therefore any disease process that results in endotoxemia will predispose the horse to developing abnormal coagulation profiles and ultimately DIC. This has been documented most frequently in horses with GI disease including large colon volvulus[131] and colitis.[132] Circulating fibrin deposits that form as a result of DIC were most frequently found in horses with severe GI disease, such as an ischemic intestine, or enteritis, and were not present in animals with simple intestinal obstruction.[129] Additionally, fibrin deposits were most frequently found in horses with an ischemic intestine (33%) compared with those with enteritis (19%) or peritonitis (11%).[129] These results suggest that absorption of endotoxin increases with the severity of the disease, resulting in coagulopathy and fibrin deposits in multiple tissues. In particular, the lungs appear to be the most severely affected organ, followed by the kidneys and liver.[129]

The pathophysiology of classic thromboembolic colic in horses is slightly different. In this disease, an underlying systemic coagulopathy is not usually present. Instead, local damage to the cranial mesenteric artery by migration of *Strongylus vulgaris* larvae results in a thrombus forming within the lumen. Occlusion of the vessel by the thrombus results in a non-strangulating infarction of the section of intestine supplied by the artery. Although this disease had become rare due to the use of ivermectin, drug resistance has recently resulted in an increased incidence.

Non-strangulating infarction of the intestine can also occur secondary to necrotizing enterocolitis.[133] Bacterial toxins from *Salmonella* spp. and *Clostridium* spp. are thought to damage the endothelium of the intestinal microvasculature, resulting in thrombosis and ischemia of focal areas.

Thrombosis of the limb arteries is also found is horses, usually foals, and can result in complete ischemia of the distal limb.[134] An underlying disease process such as bacteremia or enterocolitis, which results in thrombocytopenia and hypercoagulability, is usually present.

Clinical features

The presentation of this disease depends on the organs affected by the thromboembolism. With non-strangulating infarction of the intestine, colic is the predominant sign, which ranges from mild to severe depending on the amount of intestine affected. When the kidneys or liver are affected, a problem is not usually identified until abnormal values indicative of organ dysfunction are obtained on a blood chemistry panel.

In foals with distal limb thrombosis, occlusion of the vessels results in gangrene of the distal limb, which is cold with no evidence of pain, and focal areas of skin sloughing or even loss of the hoof.

Differential diagnosis

Depends on the specific organ involved.

Diagnosis

In all cases, the presence of a coagulopathy can be determined by a coagulation panel. Thrombocytopenia is frequently the first indication that a coagulopathy is present.[134] Other abnormalities seen are those associated with DIC, such as prolonged activated partial thromboplastin time (aPTT) and the presence of fibrin degradation products.[133]

An evaluation of the specific organ affected should also be performed. A full colic work-up, including abdominocentesis and transabdominal ultrasonography, are indicated for horses with abdominal pain. However, these diagnostic tests usually indicate that compromised bowel is present, but the cause of the ischemia is usually not confirmed until surgery or necropsy.

Likewise, diagnosis of limb thrombosis is not usually detected until clear clinical signs are apparent. Ultrasonography with Doppler flow of the digital vessels can be used to confirm a lack of blood flow to the distal limb. Pricking the coronary band with a needle can also be performed to check for fresh blood indicative of perfusion.

In horses with renal insufficiency, serum electrolyte measurements, ultrasonography, fractional excretion of electrolytes, and potentially renal biopsy are required to characterize the renal damage.

Management/treatment

In all types of thromboembolic disease, the prognosis is extremely guarded because infarction of the affected organ cannot be reversed. Therefore, every effort should be taken to prevent coagulopathies occurring rather than attempting to manage the consequences. Horses with GI disease appear to be particularly predisposed to this problem and should be monitored carefully.

Treatment of coagulopathy is a much debated topic, but the most effective treatment appears to be administration of heparin. Heparin is a cofactor for antithrombin, a serine protease inhibitor, which binds to, and inactivates, several of the activated clotting factors, including thrombin. In coagulopathy, antithrombin levels are often low due to decreased synthesis by the liver and increased consumption compared with normal. Therefore, if possible, antithrombin levels should be measured directly. If low, fresh frozen plasma can be given as a supplement. Traditionally, unfractionated heparin (40 IU/kg SC q8h) has been used. However, unfractionated heparin causes agglutination of red blood cells (RBCs), which is seen as a decrease in PCV. Therefore, low molecular weight heparin, such as dalteparin (50 IU/kg SC q24h) can be used instead.[135] Low molecular weight heparin does not have as many side-effects in horses as unfractionated heparin, but is more expensive. Horses with GI disease that were treated with dalteparin had significantly fewer fibrin deposits in the liver, kidneys, and lungs than untreated horses.[129]

The only instance in which management may be successful is when discreet ischemic sections of intestine can be surgically removed. However, multifocal areas, as are usually seen with enterocolitis, are impossible to resect and euthanasia at surgery is usually indicated. The prognosis is generally hopeless and the animal should be euthanized.

CHAPTER 5

UROGENITAL SYSTEM

Barbara L. Dallap Schaer and Dietrich H. Volkmann

GENERAL APPROACH TO MARES WITH UROGENITAL PROBLEMS

- Problems in the periparturient mare are common, with animals presenting with signs of colic and shock that may be GI (see Chapter 1) or urogenital in origin. Dystocia and traumatic injury associated with pregnancy and parturition are also common and require emergency care. Dystocia (p. 358) is one of the more important emergency conditions affecting the pregnant mare because it is life-threatening for the mare and fetus, and time, even minutes, can alter the outcome.

- While certain periparturient emergencies are readily apparent (e.g. dystocia [p. 358] and retained fetal membranes [RFMs] [p. 369]), others can be both diagnostically and therapeutically challenging.

- The clinician's attention needs to be focused on both the mare and the fetus or foal.

- Signalment and historical information pertaining to breeding, including gestational age of the fetus or time since parturition, previous complications during pregnancy and parturition, specific signs being shown by the mare, and any underlying disease, are particularly critical to obtaining an accurate diagnosis.

- Initial physical examination should focus on the cardiovascular status (heart rate, mucous membrane color, moistness and CRT, extremity temperature, pulse quality, and jugular refill time), respiratory rate and pattern, rectal temperature, and intestinal borborygmi. Examination of the body wall should be performed, looking for edema or any palpable abnormalities. Digital pulses should be closely monitored as laminitis is a common complication of many periparturient problems. Palpation per rectum is important for evaluation of both the GI and urogenital tracts, but can be somewhat unrewarding in the late pregnant mare.

- Transabdominal and transrectal ultrasonographic examination can be particularly useful for differentiating between the various causes of colic and shock in periparturient mares.

- Abdominocentesis and peritoneal fluid analysis (see Chapter 1) can be useful in the post-partum mare, but should be performed with ultrasonographic guidance in the late pregnant mare.

- The course of treatment varies dramatically depending on the different causes of periparturient emergencies. Cardiovascular stabilization is important (see Chapter 11 and Chapter 12). Obtaining an accurate diagnosis combined with early medical or surgical intervention and meticulous client communication are essential for a favorable outcome.

GENERAL APPROACH TO STALLIONS WITH UROGENITAL PROBLEMS

- Specific urogenital problems requiring emergency attention are uncommon in stallions.
- Emergency conditions affecting stallions include priapism and paraphimosis, inguinal hernia, testicular torsion, and testicular or penile trauma. While these problems are generally not immediately life-threatening, if not treated appropriately, they can lead to loss of breeding capabilities.

COMMON PROCEDURES PERFORMED IN MARES AND STALLIONS WITH UROGENITAL PROBLEMS

The procedures are discussed under individual diseases.

REPRODUCTIVE TRACT PROBLEMS

Mares
Dystocia
Key points

- Dystocia is a true emergency, in which minutes may determine fetal survival and mare prognosis.
- Foal survival is best when the response to a dystocia is rapid (i.e. delivery within <1 hour of the onset of second-stage labor) and conducted by a team that can provide all the options for delivery including obstetrical manipulation, general anesthesia, controlled vaginal delivery, and cesarean section.
- Implementation of a dystocia protocol to guide case management may optimize chances for a favorable outcome.
- If possible, a clear preconceived plan for the options available for dystocia resolution should be agreed on with the client prior to the onset of any treatment.

Definition/overview

Dystocia is the failure of a mare to give birth without assistance, resulting in a prolonged second-stage labor. Dystocia can be associated with maternal (e.g. uterine torsion, abdominal hernia) or fetal (presentation, position, posture, or rarely size) problems. Dystocia

occurs in approximately 10% of mare deliveries with malposture of the fetal head and limbs being the most common cause.[1,2]

During stage 1 of labor the fetus changes from a dorsopubic to a dorsosacral position, the cervix and pelvic ligaments soften, and uterine contractions begin but are not visible (usually 0.5–4 hours but may be interrupted and last for a few days). Stage 1 progresses to stage 2 when the chorioallantoic membrane ruptures at the cervix and the allantoic fluid passes. Stage 2 labor ends when the fetus is delivered (usually 20–30 minutes and if >20 minutes, should be treated as a dystocia). Stage 3 labor begins after delivery of the fetus and ends with passage of the fetal membranes (usually 0.25–4 hours and if >6 hours, treatment of RFMs is recommended [p. 369]).[3]

Equine dystocia is a true emergency where time to resolution will impact neonatal survival.[2,4-7] Given the rapid nature of equine parturition, a delay in stage 2 labor often results in fetal hypoxia and subsequent neonatal hypoxic/ischemic disease (see Chapter 9).

The definitions pertaining to the foal's orientation within the birth canal are:[7]

- Presentation: orientation of the fetal spinal axis to that of the mare; part of the fetus that enters vaginal canal first:
  - Cranial or caudal longitudinal.
  - Ventro- or dorsotransverse.
- Position: relationship between fetal dorsum (longitudinal presentation) or head (transverse presentation) and the quadrants of the mare's pelvis:
  - Dorsosacral.
  - Right/left dorso-ileal.
  - Dorsopubic.
  - Left cephaloilial.
- Posture: relationship between the fetal extremities (head, neck, limbs) and its body.

Etiology/pathogenesis

While most cases of equine dystocia are caused by postural deficits of the cranially presented foal (flexion of one or more joints of the front limbs or flexion of the head and/or neck, **5.1A–F**), some are caused by inappropriate presentation of the fetus (caudal or transverse) or by the faulty positioning of the foal (dorso-ileal or even dorsopubic).[7] Failure of

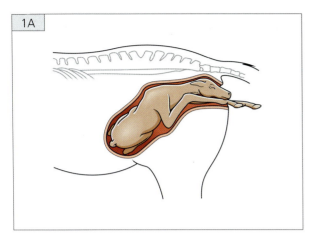

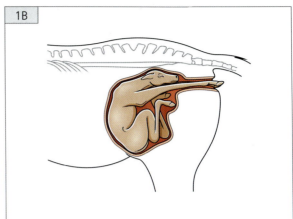

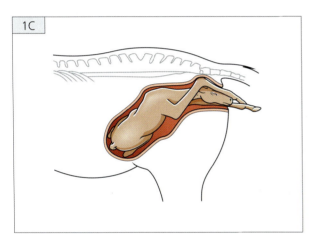

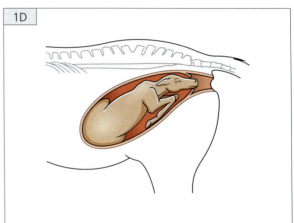

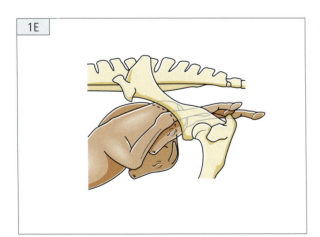

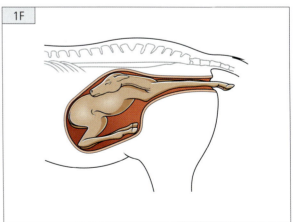

5.1A–F Schematic representation of common postural defects of the cranially presented foal: (A) elbow lock, (B) ventrovertical presentation with hip flexion, (C) foot-nape posture, (D) carpal flexion, (E) head/neck flexion with poll posture progressing to neck posture, and (F) lateral head/neck flexion. (Modified from Frazer G (2011) Dystocia management. In: *Equine Reproduction*, 2nd edn. (eds AO McKinnon, EL Squires, WE Vaala, DD Varner) Wiley-Blackwell, Ames, pp. 2479–2496.)

the allantochorion to rupture spontaneously (**5.2**) at the end of first-stage labor can also lead to the delay in the delivery of the foal, premature placental separation, fetal hypoxemia, and death. Twinning and fetal malformations, such as hydrocephalus, arthrogryposis, or schistosomus reflexus, account for rare cases of dystocia.

Clinical features

Most mares in dystocia present with forceful and unrelenting abdominal straining. The diagnosis is obvious when either fetal body parts or membranes protrude from the vulva without evidence of progression towards the delivery of the entire fetus. Stage 2 of labor should take no more than 20 minutes. Affected mares usually have a full udder and many have colostrum dripping or streaming from the teats. When no fetal parts or membranes can be seen at the vulvar opening, a vaginal examination is indicated in order to confirm that the mare is in labor. Dystocia is usually accompanied by tachycardia, tachypnea, and hyperthermia. Many mares sweat profusely and some roll excessively. Prolonged dystocia leads to dehydration and shock. Failure of the allantochorion to rupture (red bag delivery, **5.2**) is recognized by the appearance of the red, villous surface of the chorion at the vulvar opening.

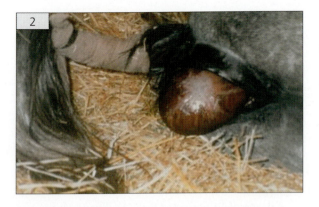

5.2 Failure of the allantochorion to rupture (red bag delivery). The cervical star can be seen. (Courtesy Dr Patrick McCue)

Differential diagnosis

Colic in late gestation (large colon volvulus; right dorsal displacement; mesenteric rent with entrapment of bowel; uterine torsion; uterine artery hemorrhage); false labor (passing episodes of Braxton–Higgs-like myometrial contractions during late gestation); abortion.

Diagnosis

Dystocia is confirmed by manual vaginal exploration revealing the presence of a fetus in the birth canal. If the cervix is not obviously effaced, manual exploration of the cervical canal is contraindicated as it may lead to ascending placentitis in mares that are not in labor.

Management/treatment

Swift intervention is required in order to optimize survival of the foal and a speedy recovery of the mare. Foal survival decreases dramatically as the duration of dystocia increases.[2,5-7] Following initial evaluation of the physiologic status of the mare, the examination then focuses on the reproductive tract. A red bag delivery should be relieved immediately by manual rupture of the allantochorion, followed by extraction of the fetus. It is critical with any dystocia to ascertain the cause for the dystocia prior to attempting any correction. The key steps to this examination are:

- Application of a tail bandage and a brief, but thorough, cleansing of the perineum should precede any vaginal examination.
- Vaginal examination (**5.3**) should be conducted with a clean obstetric glove and ample sterile lubricant.
- The birth canal should be evaluated for evidence of lacerations and the degree of cervical dilatation.
- Fetal presentation, posture, and position should then be accurately determined. Minor postural deficits (e.g. elbow flexion, poll presentation, or a front foot malpositioned dorsally across the head and neck) are corrected immediately by manipulation of the appropriate limb or the head and neck (see below), followed by prompt extraction of the foal (assisted vaginal delivery). With adequate lubrication only minimal traction is necessary to deliver a foal in normal orientation. One forelimb should be advanced about 10–15 cm

ahead of the other. Normal orientation entails a foal in cranial presentation with its forequarters in a dorsosacral position and with full extension of the head, neck, and forelimbs.[7]

- Clinicians may opt for caudal epidural anesthesia, particularly if a vaginal delivery without general anesthesia is deemed possible (e.g. carpal flexion, head flexion, neck flexion, foot-nape posture).

Traction without first correcting the malposition can worsen the problem. Care should be taken when repelling the fetus to avoid a uterine tear. Common, sometimes relatively easy fetal mutations include:[7]

- If there is apparently normal positioning but the foal is not being delivered, consider:
  - Incomplete extension of a forelimb (elbow lock, **5.1A**). The fetal muzzle lies at the same level as the fetlock rather than halfway down the metacarpus resulting from the partial flexion of the elbow, which is caught on the pubic brim of the mare. Gently repel the fetus and apply traction to the affected limb to lift the elbow over the pubis and fully extend the limb.
- Fetopelvic disproportion. Uncommon in mares. Apply copious lubrication prior to attempting delivery by forceful extraction. If two strong men cannot achieve delivery of the foal, cesarean section or fetotomy (if the foal is dead) is indicated.
- Ventrovertical presentation with hip flexion affecting one ('hurdling' posture, more common) or two ('dog sitting' posture) limbs (**5.1B**). Carefully repel the fetus sufficiently to allow the examiner to sweep the mare's pelvic inlet and push the hindlimb into the uterus. Rotating the fetus may help. General anesthesia is recommended if resistance is encountered with repositioning. Care needs to be taken to avoid trauma to the tissues of the mare's reproductive tract (cervix and especially the uterine body immediately cranial to the pelvic floor).
- Dorsopubic or dorsoileal presentation. Rotate the foal by crossing its forelimbs during extraction and by applying lateral pressure over the shoulder; allow the mare to roll and re-examine or apply torque with gentle traction on obstetrical chains.

- Foot-nape posture. One or two forelimbs are positioned over the fetus' head (**5.1C**). The fetus is carefully repelled into the uterus and the limbs lifted off the neck and placed in a lateral position; the head is elevated while ventromedial traction is applied to the limbs until they lie underneath the head. This malposture is often the cause of rectovestibular lacerations/fistulas, particularly in maiden mares.
- Carpal flexion (**5.1D**). When attempting correction of a flexed limb, the leg must be repelled as deeply as possible into the uterus and then extended by turning the flexed joint laterally (away from the fetus) and the foot

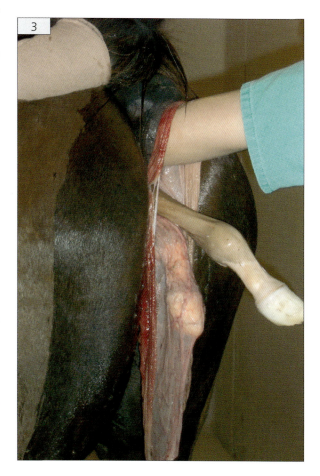

5.3 During obstetric intervention the obstetrician should always keep his/her arms inside the fetal membranes when working on the fetus.

medially (towards the fetus). Care must be taken to protect the reproductive tract by covering the fetus' hoof. Note that contracted tendons should be considered in any fetus with carpal flexion, particularly if it is bilateral. If carpal flexion and head and neck malposture occur concurrently, it is important to correct the latter first (see below).

- Head and neck malposture. Referral and controlled vaginal delivery should be considered for head and neck malposture because the long neck and head make it difficult to correct. Ventral deviation (**5.1E**) with the fetal nose just below the pelvic brim (poll posture) can be corrected by rotating the head laterally and then bringing the nose up over the pelvic brim. When the head is tucked down between the forelimbs (nape posture), a mandibular snare may be used to gently lift the nose while repelling the poll. However, if the flexure is extreme, the fetus may need to be repelled into the uterus and the forelimbs placed in carpal flexion to facilitate repositioning of the head and neck. Lateral flexion of the neck (**5.1F**) is difficult to correct, but can be achieved with gentle traction on a mandible snare (**5.4**). Note that excessive traction can result in mandibular fracture. Note also that a wry neck should be considered.

- Shoulder flexion. Controlled vaginal delivery by an experienced obstetrician or a cesarean section should be considered because of the difficulty with correcting this postural defect, particularly if bilateral. The obstetrician pulls on the skin overlying the shoulder until the radius can be reached and pulled into the birth canal. This results in the same posture as a carpal flexion and can then be corrected as described above.

- Caudal presentations. Presentation with the soles of the hooves facing upwards and palpation of the hocks (or tail) will confirm a caudal presentation. Caudal presentations have an increased risk of fetal hypoxia and death because of compression or rupture of the umbilical cord. With uncomplicated caudal presentations the fetus can usually be delivered by careful traction, using ample lubrication. Hock and hip flexions are difficult to correct because of the limb

length and difficulty with adequately repelling the fetus into the uterus. Uterine tear can be a complication of manipulating the hindlimbs within the uterus. Controlled vaginal delivery by an experienced obstetrician or cesarean section is recommended.

- Transverse presentations. Transverse presentations are extremely rare and require considerable obstetrical experience to correct. Cesarean section is generally recommended if the fetus is alive.

When more severe postural deficits are diagnosed, the mare should be brought to her feet and walked to limit the force of abdominal contractions while a plan for the resolution of the dystocia is formulated and discussed with the client. Questions that need to be answered as soon and as clearly as possible include:

- How important and how likely is foal survival?
- Is a cesarean section both desirable and logistically possible?
- Can the mare be transferred to a tertiary care facility, and how fast?

Outcome desired by the owner is a critical factor in determining treatment options available for dystocia resolution. Prioritizing mare or foal survival, as well as the possibility of a cesarean section or fetotomy, are options that should be discussed with the client, if possible, prior to referral.

Controlled vaginal delivery: Tertiary care facilities capable of accepting equine dystocia patients should have a protocol in place that focuses on timely resolution of the dystocia. The successful management of severe dystocia requires several clinicians and technicians working together on the execution of a well-rehearsed plan.

Controlled vaginal delivery involves placing the mare under general anesthesia and hoisting her hind end to approximately a 60 degree angle from the ground (**5.5, 5.6**). This facilitates repelling the fetus back into the abdomen and often permits manual correction of neck, carpal, elbow, or shoulder flexions that were impossible to resolve in the conscious, recumbent, or standing mare.

Ideally, preparation of the operating room, mare receiving area, and foal resuscitation area should be completed prior to the arrival of the mare. The following clinical procedures and treatments should happen simultaneously:

- Systemic support to the mare should begin immediately, including:
  - IV catheter placement.
  - Fluid administration (see Chapter 12).
  - Antimicrobial (see Chapter 16) and anti-inflammatory drugs.
  - Intranasal oxygen.
  - When available, administration of IV clenbuterol (0.3 mg total dose). Although its efficacy is unsubstantiated, oral clenbuterol can be given if the IV formulation is unavailable.

Clenbuterol will greatly reduce myometrial contractions and facilitate retropulsion and subsequent manipulation of the fetus.

- Sedation (see Chapter 14) may be given when necessary. Note that heavily sedated parturient mares are less likely to lie down than non-sedated ones.
- Blood collection for hematology, serum or plasma biochemistry, and blood gas analyses.
- The mare should be prepared, as previously described, for a vaginal examination and assessment of the size, presentation, position, and posture of the foal.
- When second-stage labor has been ongoing for more than 1 hour, the initial examination should include attempts to determine if the foal is

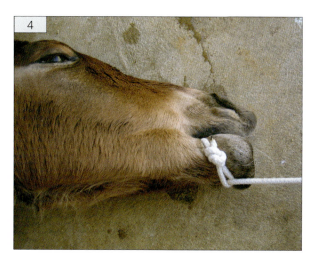

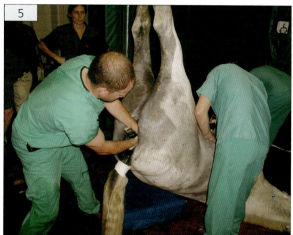

5.4 A thin rope is very useful when correcting a flexed head or neck, initially for the extension and then particularly when guiding the head nose-first into the birth canal. No forceful traction should be applied, because the mandible is relatively fragile.

5.5 Controlled vaginal delivery with the mare under general anesthesia and her hind end tilted to a 60 degree angle. Simultaneous preparation of the mare for a cesarean section is occurring while dystocia resolution is progressing. (Courtesy Dr Margot MacPherson)

5.6 Controlled vaginal delivery demonstrating the lowering of the mare once partial delivery of the foal has been achieved. (Courtesy Dr Rolf Embertson)

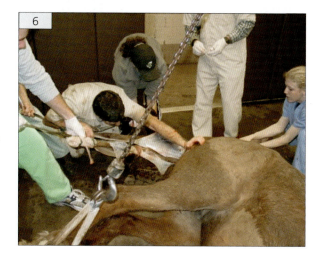

still alive. While gross motor movement of the foal provides immediate evidence that the foal is still alive, it may be necessary to use transabdominal ultrasonography, fetal heart rate monitoring, or intubation with capnography to determine with certainty that a foal is still alive or already dead. Nasotracheal intubation of the fetus can be performed to provide ventilation during delivery (EXIT procedure) if the nares are accessible. If the fetus is proven to be dead, delivery can proceed more slowly and more time can be devoted to attempts at vaginal delivery on the standing mare, possibly by fetotomy. As the erroneous use of dystocia equipment can result in very severe, non-reversible trauma to the mare's birth canal, fetotomy should be performed by a well-trained clinician (**5.7, 5.8**). Fetotomy can be performed either under caudal epidural anesthesia and heavy sedation (sedation usually prevents the mare from lying down) or under general anesthesia.

- Assign a non-essential person the task of time keeping during dystocia resolution. This person should notify attending clinicians of the duration of time elapsed from admission and for each portion of the process.

Once the mare is anesthetized, simultaneous preparations should be made for cesarean section in the event that controlled vaginal delivery is unsuccessful. Clipping of the ventral abdomen for a caudal ventral midline approach and aseptic preparation should begin immediately, while an experienced obstetrician works to resolve the dystocia. Simultaneous preparation for surgery during controlled vaginal delivery prevents wasting critical time under general anesthesia should controlled vaginal delivery fail.

Dystocia resolution requires ample warm lubricant; carboxymethyl cellulose-based lubricants are recommended. Resolution usually begins with careful retropulsion of the fetus from the pelvic inlet into the uterus to provide sufficient room for manipulation of the fetal extremities in order to correct postural defects (fetal mutation).[7]

A previously agreed time allotment for controlled vaginal delivery should be adhered to (typically 15–20 minutes) unless the owner has decided against a cesarean section. During the final 5 minutes of delivery, the surgeon(s) should be scrubbing for surgery. In order to justify this approach to the resolution of a dystocia, no more than 60 minutes should elapse between admission of the mare and surgical delivery of the foal. Once the decision for cesarean section has been made, the mare should be positioned in dorsal recumbency and final preparation for a ventral midline approach completed.

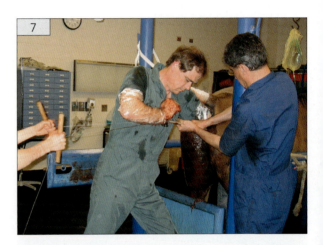

5.7 A fetotomy in progress. Systemic support (IV fluid therapy as well as antimicrobial and NSAIDs) should be provided prior to commencing the fetotomy. This mare was heavily sedated and under caudal epidural anesthesia. The head, followed by the neck, both distal forelimbs and then one shoulder were removed before the remainder of the fetus was delivered by traction. The mare required only standard aftercare and recovered uneventfully.

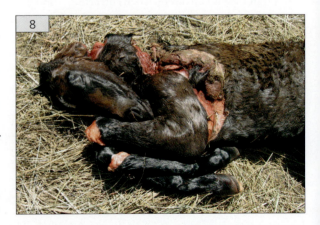

5.8 The fetus that was delivered in 5.7.

Cesarean section: Typically, the ventral midline incision is started 5–10 cm caudal to the umbilicus to facilitate exteriorization of the uterus. Using the hocks and fetlocks, typically present in the gravid horn, the uterus is elevated to the level of the incision. A combination of laparotomy sponges and additional impermeable drapes can be used to minimize contamination of the abdomen on hysterotomy. Stay sutures are commonly placed near the tip of the uterine horn and near the body of the uterus at the most cranial and caudal extent of the proposed uterine incision. The uterus and allantochorion are sharply incised between the stay sutures and the amnion opened (**5.9A**). The hindlimbs are grasped and the fetus is lifted through the hysterotomy incision (**5.9B**). Chains may be placed to assist in extracting the fetus, and can be handed to an assistant responsible for receiving the foal as the surgeon lifts the fetus up and out of the uterine body. The umbilical cord is clamped and transected (**5.9C**) and the foal is transferred to an area designated for foal resuscitation (see Chapter 9).

Following removal of the foal, 3–4 cm of the allantochorion is peeled from the uterine wall all along the edges of the hysterotomy incision.[8] A hemostatic suture line (simple continuous) is placed along the uterine edge to decrease the risk of postoperative hemorrhage using #2 polyglactin 910 (**5.9D**). Large vessels should be individually ligated using 0 synthetic absorbable suture material. The hysterotomy is closed using #2 polyglactin 910 in a double inverting pattern (Cushing or Lembert). The abdomen is thoroughly lavaged and closed routinely.

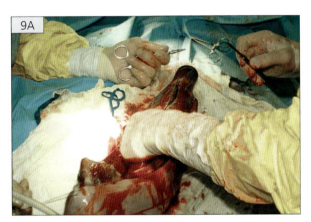

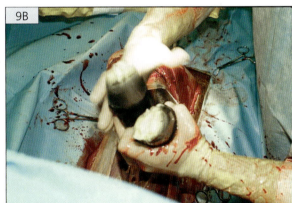

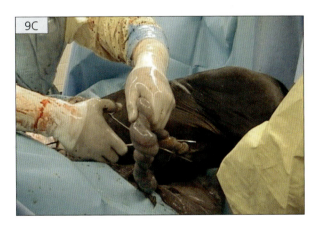

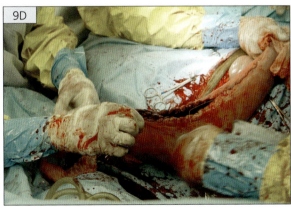

5.9A–D A cesarean section in progress. (A) A hysterotomy incision is performed. (B) The hindlimbs of the fetus are exteriorized and obstetric chains can be applied to facilitate extraction of the fetus. (C) The umbilical cord is clamped and transected. (D) After ligation of any large vessels, a hemostatic suture line is placed to prevent post-partum hemorrhage. (Courtesy Dr Rolf Embertson)

Complications associated with cesarean section may include any of those typically seen following abdominal surgery in the horse and include postoperative ileus or incisional infection, as well as hemorrhage. A common complication of dystocia is retention of the fetal membranes, regardless of the method of resolution (see Retention of fetal membranes and metritis).

Perioperative care often includes IV fluid therapy, antimicrobial and anti-inflammatory drugs. In addition, uterine lavage and appropriate anti-endotoxin therapy may also be helpful if RFM or metritis is suspected.

Prognosis for future breeding may be better than previously assumed, with 59% live foaling rates in mares bred in the year of the dystocia and 67% live foaling rates in subsequent years following dystocia.[1]

Partial fetotomy: Partial fetotomy can be used to resolve the dystocia if controlled vaginal delivery is unsuccessful and the fetus is dead. Partial fetotomy is performed with the mare under standing sedation or preferably under general anesthesia, positioned in dorsal recumbency and with the hindlimbs hoisted (see Controlled vaginal delivery). Fetotomy should be performed by an experienced obstetrician to minimize trauma to the mare's reproductive tract. The uterus is infused with copious volumes of lubricant. Partial fetotomy generally involves 1–3 cuts using a fetotome (e.g. Utrecht or Thygesen) and obstetrical wire. The fetotome is introduced into the birth canal and the wire passed over the extremity to be amputated. An obstetrical chain is attached to the fetus and then secured to the handle of the fetotome so that traction on the obstetrical wire during cutting does not result in movement of the fetotome relative to the fetus. The relative position of the fetotome is further accomplished by holding it firmly against the body of the fetus. Handles are applied to the wire and cutting is begun with slow, short to-and-fro movements. Once cutting has begun, the cutting strokes should be as long as possible so that the friction on the wire is distributed over the longest possible section of the wire, thus preventing it from overheating and snapping[7,9,10] Administration of anti-inflammatory and antimicrobial drugs is recommended before the fetotomy is begun and continued for several days after. The mare survival rate following partial fetotomy is excellent (>95%).[9] Complications include RFM, laminitis (see Chapter 2), vaginal and cervical lacerations (p. 279), and delayed uterine involution.[9] Short-term fertility for mares bred 2–3 months post fetotomy is good (>80%).[9,10] While comprehensive fetotomies, often involving 5, 6, or even 7 cuts, are not commonly performed, they can be executed efficiently and have resulted in both excellent survival and acceptable rebreeding rates.

Post-parturient shock
Key points
- A variety of conditions exist that can result in signs of post-parturient shock.
- Regardless of the cause of the shock, initial resuscitative efforts are relatively similar.
- Prognosis depends on diagnosis and the duration of post-partum shock, as well as the timeliness of intervention.

Definition/overview
Post-parturient shock is characterized by either acute or subacute physiologic deterioration of the mare with signs of dull demeanor and/or colic, tachycardia, tachypnea, and poor peripheral perfusion. A variety of conditions exist that could result in signs of post-parturient shock (**5.10, 5.11**).

Clinical features
Post-parturient shock could manifest itself clinically as tachycardia, tachypnea, abdominal discomfort, pale or toxic mucous membranes, weak peripheral pulses, fever, inappetence, or dull demeanor. Clinicopathologic findings may include anemia or hemoconcentration, hypoproteinemia, hyperlactatemia, leukopenia with or without left shift, hyperfibrinogenemia, azotemia, or other metabolic derangements. Many of the conditions are associated with secondary septic peritonitis or blood loss.

Differential diagnosis

- GI tract: large colon volvulus or displacement; cecal tympany, dysfunction, or perforation; small intestinal incarceration through a mesenteric rent; bowel trauma secondary to parturition, either vascular damage or direct trauma (i.e. small intestine, small colon, cecum, rectal prolapse).
- Urogenital tract: uterine tear/rupture; uterine hemorrhage; vaginal tear; puerperal metritis; bladder necrosis and rupture.

Diagnosis

Because a variety of conditions can cause post-parturient shock, a thorough work-up is necessary to identify the cause and develop an appropriate treatment plan. Careful evaluation of the medical history may provide important clues regarding the diagnosis. Early in the evaluation, it is important to determine if reproductive hemorrhage, either from the uterus or associated vasculature in the mesometrium, is the cause of the abdominal discomfort or the physiologic status of the mare. Because surgical intervention is rarely successful and typically contraindicated in mares with hemorrhage from a ruptured uterine artery, this is an important diagnostic rule-out. A complete physical examination and careful rectal palpation are necessary. Pale mucous membranes as opposed to bright pink to purple congested membranes may help distinguish between post-partum hemorrhage and other causes of shock. Identification of distended large or small bowel on abdominal examination per rectum should direct the veterinarian towards a GI cause of shock. Passing a nasogastric tube to determine the presence or absence of gastric reflux should be performed.

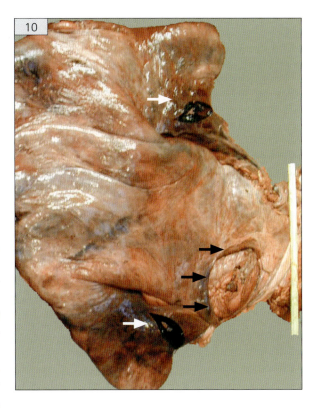

5.10 The reproductive tract of a mare that foaled 1 day prior to being euthanized. The uterus contains a large hole (black arrows) and a hematoma in each broad ligament (white arrows). Both hematomas were contained within the broad ligaments and were thus not life-threatening. The referring veterinarian had diagnosed a uterine torsion prior to assisting with the delivery of the foal. The torsion was corrected using a vaginal approach, which involved rolling the fetus with the uterus.

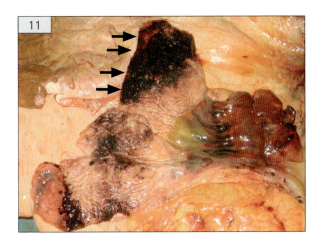

5.11 The bladder wall of this mare suffered a crushing injury with subsequent necrosis (arrows) and rupture. She had foaled 3 days prior to her death.

Routine hematology and serum chemistry may help determine if clinically important blood loss is a problem, although in acute hemorrhage PCV and TPP may not change initially.[11] PCV and TPP measurements should be repeated after initial fluid resuscitation to detect an appreciable decrease. High blood lactate concentration on initial evaluation, or persisting after resuscitation, could also be associated with marked blood loss. Profound leukopenia may be associated with puerperal metritis (with or without retention of all or part of the fetal membranes) or septic peritonitis. The latter can be caused by uterine or vaginal lacerations or by a GI lesion. Azotemia may be pre-renal or, rarely, due to bladder rupture during parturition.

Ultrasonographic evaluation of the abdomen and the reproductive tract is often useful in determining whether the cause of shock is of reproductive or GI origin. Transcutaneous imaging through a high flank position can be used to identify a uterine hematoma or hemorrhage into the broad ligament with relatively little risk of exacerbating any hemorrhage through disruption of a freshly formed blood clot (see Chapter 4). Such a risk is higher when affected mares are examined by transrectal palpation and ultrasonography.

Abdominocentesis, with or without ultrasonographic guidance, is indicated in most cases of postpartum shock. Confirmation of septic peritonitis and obtaining peritoneal fluid for bacterial culture and sensitivity testing is important regardless of the source of the peritonitis. Immediate cytologic evaluation to determine the presence or absence of bacteria and Gram stain characteristics, as well as the presence or absence of plant material, should be performed. A RBC count and PCV of the peritoneal fluid may also provide useful information in determining the likelihood of intra-abdominal hemorrhage.

Management/treatment

Regardless of the cause of the post-parturient shock, initial resuscitative efforts are relatively similar. Depending on the physical examination findings, most mares in this position warrant rapid fluid volume resuscitation with at least 40 ml/kg of polyionic isotonic pH balanced fluids (see Chapter 12). More severely affected mares may warrant placement of large-bore (9 French or 12 gauge) catheters to facilitate resuscitation or, alternatively, venous access through two separate sites (i.e. bilateral jugular catheterization).

Hypertonic saline (4 ml/kg) can also be given if rapid intravascular fluid volume expansion is needed and the likelihood of intra-abdominal hemorrhage is minimal (see Chapter 12). Some studies indicate a higher morbidity and mortality if hypertonic saline (7.2%) is used as a resuscitative fluid in the face of uncontrolled abdominal hemorrhage.

Depending on the results of the initial hematologic evaluation, colloidal therapy may be added to the resuscitative plan (see Chapter 12). Colloid options include hetastarch (10 ml/kg), dextran 70, or plasma. Plasma has a less immediate oncotic pressure contribution, but may be advantageous for its anti-endotoxic properties and prevention of hemostatic disorders.

Monitoring the success of resuscitative therapy can be achieved by observation of clinical progression with improvement or stabilization of cardiovascular parameters (i.e. heart and respiratory rates, mucous membrane color) or, more objectively, by measuring direct or indirect blood pressure or serial CVPs (see Chapter 11). Return of blood lactate concentration to within normal limits or a decrease in the lactate concentrations within the first 6 hours of resuscitation has been associated with improved clinical outcome in human patients.[12]

In cases of severe uterine hemorrhage (after cesarean section) or hemorrhage from the mesometrial arteries, blood transfusion may be necessary (see Chapter 12). The need for transfusion can be determined by hematologic measurements (PCV, total RBC counts) or on physiologic measurements such as persistent hyperlactatemia, unresponsive hypotension, metabolic acidosis, or sustained tachycardia. Depending on the urgency, cross-matching may or may not be feasible.

One of the most critical decisions to be made, following initial resuscitation, is whether or not surgical intervention is indicated. Mares with GI lesions, severe peritonitis, uterine tear, or bladder rupture are likely to need surgical intervention. Depending on the severity and source of the septic peritonitis, surgical exploration may or may not be warranted and, in some cases, treatment may be dictated by the client's financial constraints.

Prognosis depends on diagnosis and the duration of post-parturient shock, as well as the timeliness of intervention. In a study evaluating mares referred to a tertiary care facility for post-partum complications, overall survival was 68%, being highest in mares diagnosed with urogenital hemorrhage (88%).[13] That finding may be, in part, due to the fact that the hemorrhage did not result in immediate death prior to the opportunity to refer; these may be moderately and not severely affected mares in the referral population. Critical assessment of all available clinicopathologic data is important in obtaining an accurate diagnosis within 4 hours of the mare's presentation.

Uterus
Retention of fetal membranes and metritis
Key points
- RFM beyond 2–4 hours is a serious complication during the puerperal period of the mare.
- RFM requires prompt and comprehensive care in order to prevent or treat life-threatening complications such as metritis, endotoxemia and laminitis.

Definition/overview
RFM is failure of passage of part or all of the allanto-chorionic membrane with or without the amniotic membrane within a specific time limit (i.e. prolonged third-stage labor).[14] While the time limit varies from 0.5–6 hours, the fetal membranes of the horse are generally considered retained when they have not been passed completely within 2 hours of the foal's delivery. RFM can often lead to metritis, which is an acute bacterial infection of the uterine wall. Metritis is associated with signs of endotoxemia and shock, which can lead to laminitis.

Etiology/pathogenesis
The exact cause of fetal membrane retention is unknown, but the condition is more common after dystocia, induced parturition, abortion, or uncomplicated deliveries in certain breeds of horses (especially heavy breeds such as Friesians and other draft horses). Sporadic cases can occur in any breed after normal delivery of a foal. Mechanical interference and hormonal imbalance are thought to be important in the etiopathogenesis. Some cases are associated with inversion of the tip of a uterine horn (possibly after excessive treatment with oxytocin), resulting in entrapment of the membranes in the intussuscepted portion of the uterus. Among other reproductive problems, RFM are commonly encountered in cases of tall fescue poisoning.

Clinical features
Most mares with RFM show no signs of systemic disease unless metritis, an acute bacterial infection of the uterine wall, develops. Metritis may develop within 12 hours post partum and is characterized by signs of endotoxemia (pyrexia, tachycardia, dehydration, leukopenia, and a markedly dull demeanor). Laminitis, presumably as a consequence of endotoxemia, is more likely in heavy mares. Metritis is, therefore, a severe, potentially life-threatening condition.

Differential diagnosis
Uterine tear; septic peritonitis; damage to the GI tract during parturition (GI tract rupture, ischemic necrosis of intestine [e.g. small colon] associated with damage to the arterial blood supply); other GI disorders resulting in endotoxemia (enteritis, colitis, large colon volvulus, mesenteric rent with strangulation of entrapped bowel, ischemic necrosis of intestine [e.g. small colon] associated with damage to the arterial blood supply, GI tract rupture).

Diagnosis

Diagnosis of RFM is obvious when portions of the fetal membranes are hanging from the vulva (**5.12**), but can be challenging when only a small portion of the allantochorion has torn off and is retained after the bulk of the fetal membranes have been passed. Routine examination of the membranes for completeness (**5.13**) following passage will identify mares that have retained a small portion. Retention of a portion of the fetal membranes is more likely to occur in the tip of the non-gravid horn than in the gravid horn.[14]

Any mare with clinical signs of endotoxemia during the puerperal period should be examined by deep vaginal and even deep uterine exploration in order to rule out retention of a small piece of the allantochorion (usually in the tip of the non-gravid horn).

While transrectal ultrasonographic examination will often reveal accumulation of free fluid inside the involuting uterus, its use often fails to identify the presence of the retained part of the fetal membranes. When retained membranes are identified using ultrasonographic examination, they have a hyperechoic appearance (**5.14**). Many affected mares show no uterine fluid accumulation, while some mares present with a profuse, foul-smelling vaginal discharge.

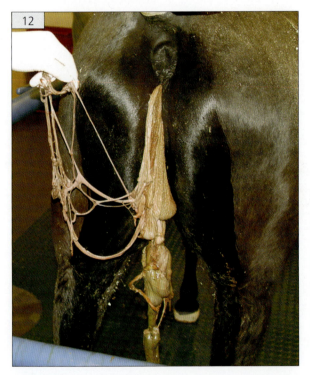

5.12 Retained fetal membranes 4 days after foaling. If the mare is treated with broad-spectrum antimicrobial drugs and the uterus is lavaged daily to remove toxic exudate, such mares should remain systemically healthy. This mare's membranes were finally released and removed 7 days after foaling and she recovered uneventfully.

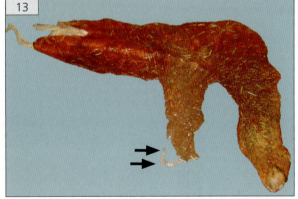

5.13 Routine examination of the freshly passed fetal membranes of a mare reveals that the tip of the non-fetal horn was torn off (arrows) and retained. Early identification of a retained portion of the fetal membranes allows for timely intervention and treatment.

Management/treatment

Any mare that retains all or part of her fetal membranes for more than 4 hours post partum should receive immediate veterinary care. Initial treatment consists of small doses of oxytocin (10–20 IU IV or IM every 30–120 minutes). Oxytocin can also be administered by CRI (60 IU oxytocin in 1 liter of fluid, administered over 1 hour). Transrectal massage of the uterus facilitates uterine contractility and often aids in the release of the retained portion of the chorion. Administration of broad-spectrum antimicrobial drugs will protect the mare from developing metritis.

Forceful removal of the fetal membranes by pulling on the released portion of the membrane or by 'peeling' the attached membrane from the endometrium are likely to result in tearing, leading to retention of one or more smaller pieces of the membrane (**5.15**). Forceful removal may also lead to uterine prolapse or cause endometrial damage, possibly compromising the mare's future breeding soundness. When the initial treatment fails to result in release of the membranes, inversion of the tip of one or both uterine horns should be ruled out by transrectal palpation or, preferably, by deep intrauterine palpation.

A large volume (10–20 liters) of fluid (saline, sterile water, or even tap water with a small amount of povidone–iodine solution) can be infused into the allantoic cavity by means of a stomach tube inserted through the

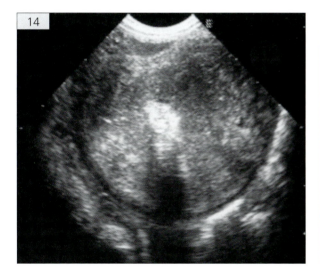

5.14 Ultrasonogram of a mare that retained only the tip of the non-fetal horn of the allantochorion. The retained membrane cannot always be depicted using ultrasonography, but when it is evident, it is characterized by its hyperechoic appearance.

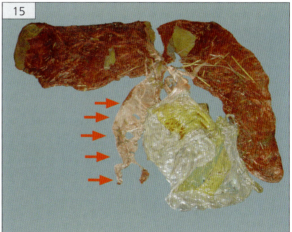

5.15 The fetal membranes from a mare that suffered a dystocia. After the foal had been delivered the attendant forcefully removed the membranes by traction, resulting in shredding of the non-fetal horn and the retention of a large portion of the same horn. Note the meconium staining on the inner surfaces of the amnion and allantois (arrows).

cervical star (**5.16**). The fluid must be prevented from escaping by holding the allantochorion closed around the stomach tube (it can also be tied in place with string or umbilical tape). The mare often strains in response to the expansion of the uterus. After 30 minutes the fluid is released, often resulting in the immediate passage of the membranes. Other clinicians prefer to 'cord' (twist up) the detached portion of the membranes inside the vagina, followed by very gentle traction with one hand inside or just outside the vulva, while the other hand is used to massage transrectally that portion of the uterus where the membranes can be felt to still be attached. Others prefer to make no attempt at all to remove the retained membranes, focusing rather on prevention of metritis by medical management including antimicrobial drugs, NSAIDs, polymyxin B, endotoxin hyperimmune plasma, IV balanced polyionic crystalloid fluids, and oxytocin (see above).

Uterine lavage is usually unrewarding while the bulk of the fetal membranes are still inside the uterus, but if only a small portion is retained, this procedure can serve to remove exudate and toxins from the uterus and should be performed at least once per day (**5.17**).

Once the membranes have been released, the uterus should be lavaged with liberal volumes of sterile saline to remove debris, exudate, and smaller fragments of autolyzed fetal membrane tissue. Medical treatment should continue for at least 24 hours or until signs of systemic disease (i.e. hyperemic mucous membranes, hyperthermia/fever, tachycardia, leukopenia, and pronounced digital pulses) have resolved.

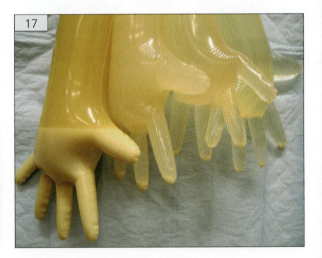

5.16 One method to facilitate release of retained fetal membranes involves filling the allantoic cavity with saline or clean water using a sterile nasogastric tube. Once filled, the fluid is held inside the distended membranes for 30 minutes and then drained. This method is not very useful when the allantochorion has holes in it.

5.17 Saline recovered during lavage of the uterus of a mare that suffered from acute puerperal metritis secondary to retention of a small portion of the fetal membranes. The vast bulk of the sediment in the first sleeve consisted of neutrophils, an indication of accumulation of waste, debris, and toxins within the uterus.

Some mares will develop endotoxemia (see Chapter 17) and/or laminitis (see Chapter 2) within as little as 12 hours of parturition. Preventive measures against laminitis should thus be part of the medical management of RFM and metritis (i.e. icing the feet, application of frog supports, deep bedding, withholding of grain or green grass; see Laminitis).

Retention of fetal membranes does not affect future fertility, except during the first estrus (foal heat) after foaling. Some clinicians recommend treatment with oxytocin immediately after foaling in mares with a history of RFM after previous deliveries.[14]

Uterine tear

Key points

- Uterine tear or laceration should be suspected in post-partum mares with fever, dull demeanor, tachycardia, inappetence, leukopenia, or mild colic.
- Uterine tears can be managed medically or surgically, although there is clinical evidence indicating an improved outcome with surgical intervention.
- The choice for medical or surgical management may be based on clinical progression, disease severity, or financial constraints.
- Early diagnosis of uterine tear and appropriate intervention improves outcome.

Definition/overview

Uterine tears are partial or full-thickness defects in the wall of the uterus. Uterine tear or laceration can occur during normal parturition or be secondary to complications such as dystocia, uterine torsion[15] or hydramnios.[16] Small tears are usually diagnosed 24–72 hours following parturition based on clinical progression and subsequent diagnostics. Large tears or uterine rupture secondary to uterine torsion may be discovered on abdominal exploration for cesarean section or torsion correction.

Etiology/pathogenesis

Uterine tears most commonly occur during the peripartum period. They may result from excessive force during fetal extraction, rough obstetric manipulations during dystocia, or the accidental penetration of the uterine wall by a fetotomy instrument or lavage tube (iatrogenic). Spontaneous uterine tear can also occur if the foal's foot (usually a hind foot) inadvertently traumatizes the uterus during labor, without human intervention. Such tears are usually small and located near the tip of the gravid uterine horn. Prepartum uterine tears may occur with uterine torsion or hydramnios. On rare occasions, the uterine wall may be penetrated by an endometrial biopsy punch, insemination pipette, endometrial swab or lavage tube, or during laser surgery for endometrial cyst removal.

Clinical features

Clinical signs can vary in severity depending on the presence or absence of peritonitis. During the immediate post-partum period mares may present initially with signs of mild colic. As peritonitis progresses, colic signs may be replaced by dull demeanor, fever, tachycardia, dehydration/hypovolemia, moderate to severe neutropenia, and shock. Some mares will progress very slowly or even recover spontaneously, provided the peritoneal cavity remains sterile or the mare is treated very aggressively with antimicrobial drugs. Abnormal fluid obtained on abdominocentesis may confirm peritonitis as a cause of the clinical signs, and diagnosis of uterine tear as the cause may be definitively confirmed on surgical exploration. Hemorrhage from the vulva is not a feature of a uterine tear.

Differential diagnosis

GI tract trauma (e.g. cecum, jejunum, small colon); large colon volvulus; enteritis; colitis; vaginal and cervical lacerations; uterine artery hemorrhage, other causes of peritonitis (GI tract perforation, urinary tract perforation).

Diagnosis

Many cases are diagnosed immediately during the manipulation of a malpostured fetus or during fetotomy. Tears immediately cranial to or involving the cervix are easily diagnosed by manual exploration of the vagina, cervix, and caudal uterus. Care should be taken during such explorations to avoid converting a partial-thickness tear into a full-thickness tear. Contamination of a potentially uncontaminated peritoneal cavity must be prevented by diligent hygiene during the examination. Many full-thickness tears are associated with extreme uterine contraction, which can be identified on transrectal uterine palpation. Uterine wall defects must be suspected in all cases where all or some of the fluid infused during a post-partum uterine lavage cannot be retrieved. The infused and retrieved volumes of fluid used in uterine lavage should always be measured.

On transrectal ultrasonographic examination (**5.18**), the uterus will usually contain no free fluid and be surprisingly small in size, while transabdominal ultrasonographic examination may reveal variable amounts of free peritoneal fluid. Abdominocentesis and peritoneal fluid analysis will reveal septic peritonitis. Depending on the time elapsed from parturition and the degree of uterine involution, abdominal ultrasonographic examination may be useful to determine involvement of the uterus versus compromise of GI viscus as a cause of the peritonitis. Abdominal ultrasonographic examination may also aid in determining the extent and the severity of the peritonitis (i.e. amount and echogenicity of peritoneal effusion, bowel wall thickening, and the amount of fibrin present).

In mares that fail to respond as expected to aggressive medical management, small uterine tears in the uterine horn are a possible differential diagnosis; exploratory celiotomy may be required for definitive diagnosis.

Management/treatment

Both conservative medical management and surgical intervention have been used to treat horses with uterine tears[17–19] as well as a combination of laparoscopic diagnosis and conservative therapy.[20] Therapeutic choices probably depend on disease progression and severity of illness; rapidly progressive clinical decline typically directs the veterinarian to more aggressive intervention.

Medical management consists of broad-spectrum parenteral antimicrobial therapy, including anaerobic coverage (see Chapter 16). Antimicrobial therapy can be adjusted based on bacterial culture and sensitivity testing of the peritoneal fluid. Flunixin meglumine used either at anti-inflammatory (1.1 mg/kg IV q12h) or anti-endotoxemic (0.25 mg/kg IV q8h) doses should be considered. Polymixin B may also be used as anti-endotoxic therapy (1,000–6,000 IU/kg IV q8–12h for

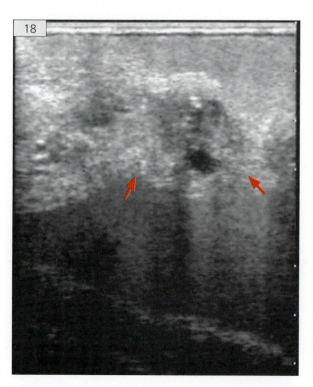

5.18 Transrectal ultrasonogram depicting a small hole in the uterine wall (margins marked by arrows). Note the large amount of free fluid in the peritoneal cavity. This mare presented with advanced peritonitis 2 days after foaling uneventfully. Correction and treatment were cost prohibitive and the mare was euthanized. The location and size of the hole were confirmed at necropsy.

no more than 6 total doses). IV fluid therapy may be necessary to help maintain appropriate perfusion and hydration in the face of the ongoing inflammatory process. Depending on the severity of the peritonitis, as reflected by either cytologic evaluation, abdominal ultrasonographic examination, or clinical progression, abdominal lavage using a large bore chest tube and 5–10 liters of sterile polyionic isotonic fluids q8–12h may be indicated. It was concluded in one case series that medical management was a reasonable alternative to surgical treatment of uterine tears in mares, with survival rates of 73% and 76%, respectively; however, the severity of tears that resolved with medical management was unknown and medical management was not less expensive than surgical correction.[17]

One report describes early surgical intervention in 33 mares suspected of having uterine tears, reporting survival in nearly 80% of cases, which was a marked improvement compared with previous reports.[8,19] The majority of the tears were near the tip of the uterine horn (**5.19**) and were repaired using #1 multifilament absorbable suture material in a two-layer closure (simple continuous followed by inverting pattern) from a caudal ventral midline incision. Aggressive abdominal lavage should be performed during the exploration, as well as assessment of other viscera. In a study evaluating 33 mares with uterine tear, drain placement was performed at the time of surgery and abdominal lavage performed for 3–4 days postoperatively. Caudal tears involving the body of the uterus can also be approached vaginally in the standing mare, closing the laceration with simple interrupted or continuous sutures, depending on the surgeon's preference and ease of access.[8] Some clinicians have reported good exposure to uterine tears by deliberately everting the uterus and repairing the defect outside the vulva before returning the prolapsed uterus into the peritoneal cavity. If this approach is to be tried, it is helpful to induce uterine relaxation by IV administration of a beta-2 agonist (clenbuterol, where available, or epinephrine as an alternative). Incisional infection in the body wall is a relatively common complication of the direct surgical approach, likely as a consequence of contamination of the incision with septic peritoneal fluid.

With delayed diagnosis or ineffective intervention, uterine tear or rupture can be fatal as a result of severe septic peritonitis leading to septic shock or a combination of septic peritonitis and hemorrhage causing septic and hemorrhagic shock. Early diagnosis and prompt intervention are critical in improving outcome in mares with uterine tears. Non-surviving mares with a uterine tear were reported to have a higher heart rate and anion gap, lower total CO_2 and leukocyte count, and nasogastric reflux compared with survivors.[17]

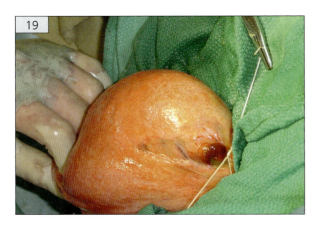

5.19 A small hole in the uterine wall near the tip of the fetal horn of a mare that had foaled 4 days earlier and was suffering from persistent pyrexia and mild peritonitis (as diagnosed by abdominocentesis), the cause of which could not be explained despite elaborate clinical tests and examinations. The hole was repaired. The mare recovered uneventfully and subsequently carried another pregnancy.

Uterine prolapse

Key points

- Uterine prolapse is a life-threatening condition that must be corrected immediately.
- Correction is usually easy and the prognosis for recovery is generally good.

Definition/overview

Uterine prolapse is eversion of the uterus through the cervix and vagina, and usually occurs immediately after foaling or abortion (**5.20, 5.21**).

Etiology/pathogenesis

Most cases occur for no particular reason. Some cases are associated with excessive straining by the mare while the partially detached fetal membranes add some traction on the inner surface of the uterus. Excessive traction by the attending veterinarian or owner on RFM can lead to uterine eversion. In rare cases of severe gas colic, pregnant mares were found dead with a prolapsed uterus and the fetus still inside the intact membranes lying next to her.

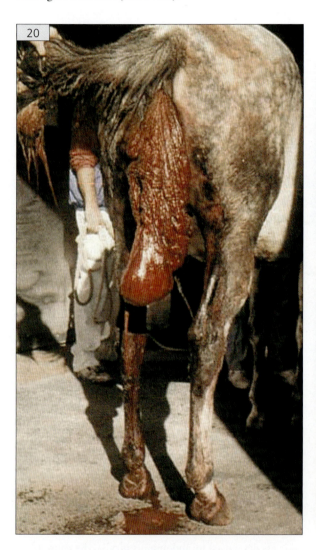

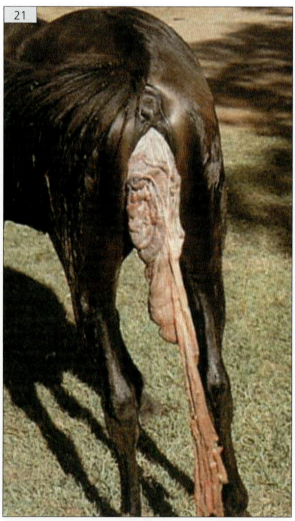

5.20 Uterine prolapse in a mare. The fetal membranes were expelled prior to prolapse of the uterus. The endometrial villi on the inner surface of the uterus resulted in the dark red color of the everted organ.

5.21 Uterine prolapse in a mare. The retained fetal membranes are still covering the inner surface of the uterus, resulting in the bluish color of the everted organ.

Clinical features

Most mares present during the early post-partum period or soon after prolapse and show relatively few systemic signs of disease or pain. Some mares, especially those foaling without supervision, may be found moribund or dead. Abdominal straining is consistently present. As the duration of the condition increases, signs of acute shock develop within hours, presumably due to circulatory compromise of the large, everted organ.

Differential diagnosis

RFM; eversion of the urinary bladder; rectal prolapse.

Diagnosis

Diagnosis is apparent on visual inspection in all cases. The inner surface of the uterus is characterized by its dark red, velvety endometrial villi (**5.20**). When the fetal membranes are still attached to the endometrium, the bluish-white allantoic surface of the allantochorion, with its many large blood vessels, will cover the endometrium (**5.21**).

Management/treatment

Caudal epidural anesthesia will suppress abdominal straining and improve patient compliance during the replacement procedure. Sedation will be helpful. A tail wrap is applied and the perineum is thoroughly washed with soap and water. The everted uterus is thoroughly cleansed with saline or clean water, inspected for lacerations, and then returned to its intra-abdominal position. A prolapsed equine uterus usually does not swell as much as that of a ruminant and the application of hygroscopic agents or pressure bandages is not necessary prior to replacement of the organ. Replacing the uterus is facilitated by placing the prolapsed portion on a tray, which is lifted to the level of the vulva by two assistants. The clinician then inverts the organ, starting with the cervix, followed by the uterine body, and finishing with the uterine horns. Once the organ has been returned to the abdomen, it should be filled with fluid to ensure that even the tips of the horns are completely extended. The fluid is then drained and the mare is given 10–20 IU oxytocin (IM or SC) to induce uterine contraction. Retention sutures in the vulva are not usually necessary. Systemic supportive therapy is the same as for RFM and metritis.

Uterine artery hemorrhage
See Chapter 4.

Uterine torsion
Key points
- Uterine torsion may be life-threatening for both mare and foal.
- Mares with uterine torsion often display signs of colic, although violent colic is not often noted.
- Rapid diagnosis via careful transrectal palpation and correction of the torsion is necessary to improve outcome.
- Uterine torsion occurring before 320 days of gestation may be associated with better survival of mare and foal. Correction through a standing flank laparotomy in these mares may result in better foal survival than correction through a ventral midline incision under general anesthesia.

Definition/overview

Uterine torsion is defined as rotation of the uterus through more than 90 degrees around its long axis. It usually occurs in mid to late gestation, with mares commonly presenting with signs of colic. The torsion may be 180 degress or 360 degrees. Uterine torsion places both mare and fetus at great risk of death and rapid diagnosis and intervention are critical to achieve the best outcome.

Etiology/pathogenesis

Uterine torsion is suspected to result from fetal activity during mid to late gestation, and may also occur at term.

Clinical features

Most mares with uterine torsion present with mild to severe signs of colic during the last 4 months of gestation. Other signs associated with GI causes of colic (i.e. poor intestinal borborygmi and lack of fecal production) are absent, and perineal edema may be present.

Differential diagnosis

Colic of GI origin; rupture of the uterine artery; transient prepartal myometrial contractions; abortion or impending parturition.

Diagnosis

Transrectal examination usually correctly identifies uterine torsion. Vaginal palpation often fails to detect uterine torsion in mares because most cases do not involve the reproductive tract caudal to the cervix. Carefully tracing the cranial edge of the uterine broad ligaments from their origins at the dorsolateral body wall to the insertion along the uterus during transrectal examination will reveal that one ligament is stretched horizontally from one side of the abdomen across the dorsal surface of the uterus towards the opposite side of the abdomen, while the other ligament is stretched in a ventral direction, passing the uterus on the same side as its origin. In cases of counterclockwise torsion as viewed from the rear (i.e. uterus twisting to the left), the left broad ligament is encountered first as it steeply descends on the left side of the uterus; the right broad ligament will lie more cranially and is stretched across the uterus.[21] A study involving 63 affected mares reported clockwise torsion (torsion to the right when the mare is viewed from behind) to be more common (59%).[22]

Management/treatment

Uterine torsion can be corrected surgically or by rolling the mare under general anesthesia (**5.22–5.25**). Rolling the mare is less expensive and can be performed relatively easily in the field, but is considered more risky as it may occasionally lead to uterine rupture. Rolling is accomplished by induction of general anesthesia and positioning the mare in lateral recumbency so that she lies on the same side as the direction of her uterine torsion (torsion to the right requires that the mare lies on her right side). A plank (approximately 20 cm wide and at least 3 m long) is then placed into her left (or right) paralumbar fossa. One person stands or sits on the plank, thus applying pressure to the pregnant uterus and preventing the fetus and uterus from rolling during the procedure. Using long ropes tied to the mare's legs, two other people then roll the mare over her spine, in the same direction as the torsion. This implies that the mare rotates around her immobilized uterus, thus correcting the torsion. Immediately after a transrectal palpation has confirmed that the torsion has been resolved, the mare is allowed to recover from general anesthesia.

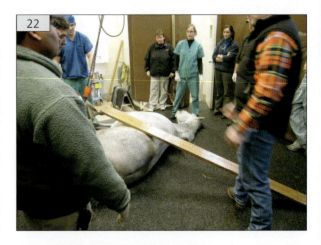

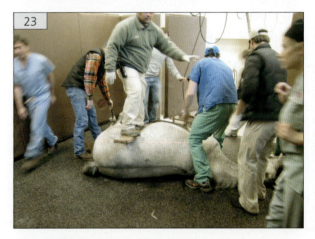

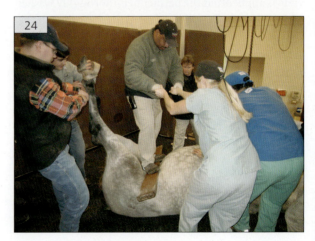

5.22–5.24 Mare with uterine torsion. The mare is placed under general anesthesia and a plank is placed in her flank (5.22) to hold the uterus in position while the mare is rolled in the same direction as the uterine torsion (5.23, 5.24). (Courtesy Dr Jacob Goodin)

Surgical management of uterine torsion involves either a flank approach in the standing mare or correction through a ventral midline approach with the mare under general anesthesia. Factors determining the choice of surgical approach are the disposition and clinical status of the mare, financial constraints, and the experience of the surgeon. Many surgeons correct all uterine torsions through standing flank laparotomy performed on the side of the direction of the torsion through a grid incision.[21,23] In order to maximize fetal oxygen delivery, it may be prudent to provide the mare with intranasal oxygen therapy during the standing procedure. Suspicion of a concurrent GI lesion may increase the motivation for exploration through a ventral midline incision with the mare under general anesthesia; 15–50% of mares have been reported to have concurrent GI lesions, most commonly involving the small or large colon.[22,24] Suspicion of uterine rupture could also be confirmed and potentially corrected through a ventral midline approach. Using either surgical approach allows for evaluation of the degree of vascular compromise of the uterus, an advantage over the general anesthesia with rolling technique.

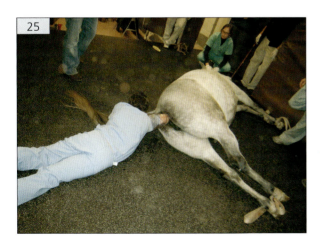

5.25 Abdominal palpation per rectum is performed with the mare under general anesthesia to confirm that the torsion is corrected. (Courtesy Dr Jacob Goodin)

Prognosis following uterine torsion may depend on the stage of gestation at which the torsion occurs and the method chosen for correction.[22] Previous studies sited mare survival of 60–70%, with foal survival ranging from 30 to 50%.[23] In a more recent retrospective study on a larger number of mares, overall mare survival was >80% and improved survival was associated with uterine torsion occurring before 320 days of gestation.[22,24] Foal survival ranged from 32% to 72% in one study and 87% in another[22,24], with highest survival rates in mares that developed the torsion before 320 days of gestation. Additionally, when the torsion occurred at <320 days of gestation and was corrected surgically, more foals survived after correction through a flank incision than after correction through a ventral midline incision.[22]

Cervix, vagina/vestibule region, and perineum
Vaginal and cervical lacerations
Key points

- Vaginal and/or cervical lacerations are rare presenting complaints, but are commonly associated with dystocia.
- Any bleeding seen at dismount or during the first hour after a natural breeding may indicate a breeding accident, leading to a potentially life-threatening, semen-induced peritonitis.
- Vaginal lacerations can be severe and life-threatening, depending on the location, degree of peritoneal involvement, and presence or absence of evisceration and hemorrhage.
- Rapid assessment of structures involved, followed by replacement of viscera into the abdominal cavity and aggressive medical or surgical management may result in a favorable outcome.

Definition/overview
Vaginal lacerations are defined as disruption of the vaginal floor or vault either during a breeding accident or at the time of parturition. During parturition, this can occur during propulsion of the foal or from interventions to facilitate delivery. Intestinal prolapse or bladder prolapse (p. 384) can result from vaginal lacerations, requiring rapid intervention.

Etiology/pathogenesis

Most lacerations occur during parturition, especially when the foal was forcefully extracted or when elaborate obstetrical manipulations were applied during a dystocia. Superficial erosions and abrasions are commonly seen in mares that underwent fetotomy or any other protracted obstetrical procedure.

Occasionally, vaginal and/or cervical lacerations occur in smaller or primiparous mares when they are naturally bred to stallions with disproportionately long penises (**5.26**). Ejaculation into the peritoneal cavity also results in severe, acute life-threatening peritonitis. The colpotomy procedure is an iatrogenic, intentional cause of vaginal laceration that will heal uneventfully in the overwhelming majority of mares.

Cervical tears may also result from dystocia or difficult parturition, but provided they do not extend vaginally or into the peritoneal cavity, are treated medically followed by delayed surgical treatment, if indicated.

Clinical features

Mares with retroperitoneal vaginal tears may present with mild dullness, reluctance to defecate, or possible vaginal abscessation. Dorsal vaginal tears may extend through the vagina into the rectum, resulting in a rectovaginal fistula. Vaginal tears located either in the rectogenital or urogenital pouches surrounding the cervix can result in penetration of the peritoneal cavity and possible herniation of intestinal viscera[25]; such a progression can prove fatal, even with rapid intervention. Mares with disruption of the peritoneal cavity due to a vaginal tear develop signs of septic peritonitis, including fever, dullness, mild colic, tachycardia, and anorexia.

A laceration in the ventral aspect of the vagina may result in bladder prolapse, subsequent occlusion of the urethra, and bladder protrusion through the vulva lips. Vaginal trauma or lacerations in the floor of the vagina secondary to aggressive attempts to relieve dystocia may make urethral obstruction secondary to inflammation more likely.

Differential diagnosis

Severe tears with peritoneal involvement: bladder prolapse; bladder eversion, with or without intestinal incarceration; rectal tear (grade 4) with intestinal herniation; peritonitis due to other causes (uterine tear, GI tract compromise). Vaginal tears/trauma without peritoneal involvement: vaginal hematoma or hemorrhage; vaginal bruising; urethral damage or trauma.

Diagnosis

Most lacerations are diagnosed only when they are specifically searched for by vaginal palpation or speculum examination. Such examinations are considered routine on many well-managed stud farms during the first 24 hours after foaling.

Cervical lacerations are difficult to diagnose by speculum examination immediately post partum when the cervical folds are usually bruised and swollen and the cervix is positioned so far cranially that it cannot be seen through a speculum. Careful direct palpation of the entire circumference of the cervix is the best way of detecting cervical lacerations and the depth and extent of such lesions.

With intestinal or bladder prolapse (**5.27**), it is obvious that a defect must be present in either the rectum or caudal reproductive tract. Extreme caution must be taken to evaluate carefully what structures are involved in the herniation to avoid further damage to the herniated viscera prior to reduction. Sedation of the mare, aseptic preparation of the perineal area, and cleansing of the involved viscera, followed by replacement into the abdominal cavity, will facilitate identifying the tear.

Ultrasonographic examination can be used to further characterize and evented organ (see Bladder eversion), if deemed necessary. Abdominocentesis should be performed to determine the degree of abdominal contamination and to obtain samples for bacterial culture and sensitivity testing.

Management/treatment

Vaginal tears with intestinal evisceration, or tears into the peritoneal cavity resulting from a breeding accident or parturition, can be evaluated with careful digital palpation or with the use of a Caslick's speculum.[26] If necessary, endoscopic examination may help determine the location and extent of the tear.

Eviscerated bowel can be lavaged with copious amounts of polyionic electrolyte solution, evaluated for vascular devitalization, and returned to the abdominal cavity.

The vaginal tear may be closed through a vaginal approach with the mare standing. Alternatively, the tear can be repaired with the mare anesthetized and placed in a position similar to that used for controlled vaginal delivery.[27] Care should be taken not to incorporate any intestine into the closure.[25] The tear may be left to heal by second intention, which should occur in 7–10 days.[26] A Caslick's procedure should be performed to decrease the likelihood of further contamination.[25,26]

Broad-spectrum antimicrobial drug therapy should be initiated immediately; this can be later modified based on the results of bacterial culture and sensitivity testing. Supportive care including anti-inflammatory drugs and fluid therapy should also be implemented and continued until the mare is hemodynamically stable. Depending on the severity of the peritonitis, abdominal lavage may be necessary. It has also been recommended to cross-tie the mare to reduce the likelihood of evisceration when the mare lies down.[28] Exploratory celiotomy is indicated if the mare develops signs of more severe abdominal discomfort, possibly indicative of vascular compromise to the involved intestine.

Prognosis depends on the severity of the vaginal tear, the degree of involvement of the peritoneal cavity, presence or absence of evisceration, and the extent of hemorrhage. Severe vaginal tears can obviously be life-threatening. Mares with vaginal tears in a retroperitoneal location should respond well to medical management, providing patency of the urethra is maintained. Fibrosis leading to adhesions and stricture can cause delayed reproductive or urinary tract complications.

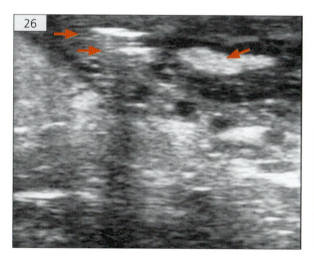

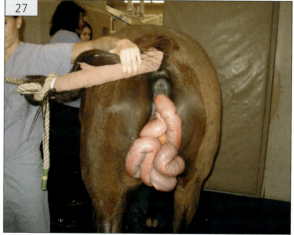

5.26 Transrectal ultrasonogram of the caudal uterine body of a mare that presented after developing a bloody vaginal discharge subsequent to having been bred naturally. The caudal uterine body contained air (small arrows) as well as a blood clot (large arrow). During a vaginal speculum examination, a tear was found, extending from the cranial vagina into the caudal half of the cervix. The mare was treated with systemic antimicrobials and NSAIDs and was cross-tied in a stall for 3 days. Recovery was uneventful.

5.27 Small colon prolapse through a vaginal tear following parturition.

Perineal lacerations
Key points

- Superficial lacerations of the vulva, vestibule, and perineal body should be repaired immediately after foaling.
- Wounds that are more than a few hours old, heavily soiled wounds, and all grade 3 lacerations should be left to heal before any reconstructive surgery is performed to restore the normal anatomy of the vulva, vestibule, and perineum.

Definition/overview

Perineal lacerations involve the dorsal commissure of the vulva, the ceiling of the vestibule, variable layers of the perineal body, and the floor of the rectum. Grade 1 lacerations involve the skin of the vulva and the mucosa of the vestibule (**5.28**), grade 2 lacerations extend deeper to involve the constrictor vulva muscle as well as the superficial portion of the perineal body (**5.29**), and grade 3 lacerations extend through the vestibular mucosa, the perineal body, and the rectal wall

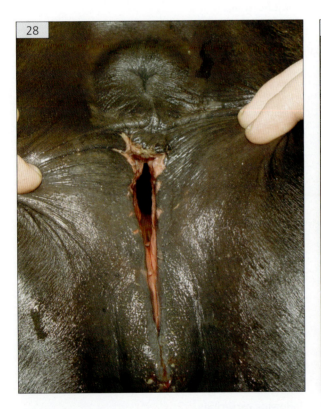

5.28 Superficial tear in the skin dorsal to the vulva of a mare that had foaled 1 day earlier. Usually such superficial tears require no repair, but this mare's vulvar conformation resulted in such severe pneumovagina that an immediate Caslick's procedure was indicated.

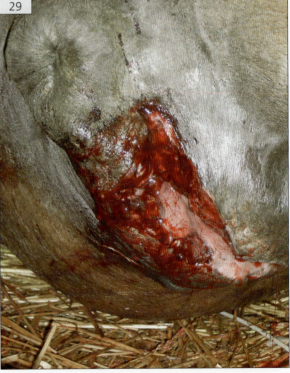

5.29 Grade 2 perineal laceration in a mare immediately after foaling. If performed within a few hours of foaling, such lacerations can be repaired successfully. Dead space in the deeper tissues is closed with buried sutures of absorbable material while the skin is apposed routinely. The vestibular mucosa can be left open for drainage.

(**5.30, 5.31**). The latter can be divided further into complete rectovaginal lacerations (anal sphincter torn, resulting in a common opening for the rectum and vestibule) and rectovaginal fistulas (anal sphincter intact).

Etiology/pathogenesis

Almost all perineal lacerations occur during foaling. Such trauma to the birth canal is more common in maiden mares, but can also occur in multiparous mares. Lacerations are also more common in mares that received obstetrical assistance during parturition. Occasionally, grade 1 lacerations occur in mares that were bred naturally without having had their Caslick's suture opened.

Clinical features

Lacerations vary from barely evident to gross disruption of the entire perineal area. Hemorrhage is usually not severe and minor tears often go unnoticed until the mare has her routine post-foaling examination. Even rectovaginal fistulas may go unnoticed until they are identified during a subsequent vaginal speculum examination that reveals the presence of fecal material inside the vestibular lumen. In some mares, a persistent purulent vaginal discharge is evidence of a chronic vaginitis that develops as a consequence to the persistent fecal contamination of the vaginal tract.

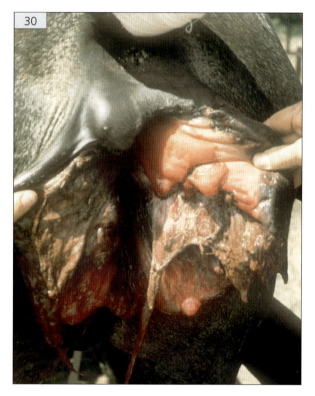

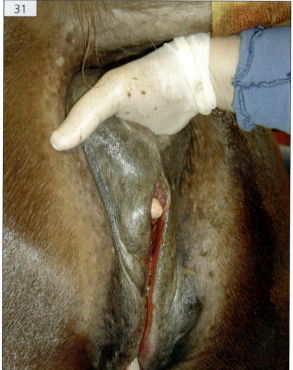

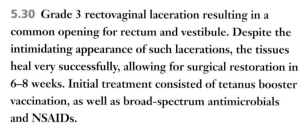

5.30 Grade 3 rectovaginal laceration resulting in a common opening for rectum and vestibule. Despite the intimidating appearance of such lacerations, the tissues heal very successfully, allowing for surgical restoration in 6–8 weeks. Initial treatment consisted of tetanus booster vaccination, as well as broad-spectrum antimicrobials and NSAIDs.

5.31 Grade 3 rectovaginal laceration resulting from a penetrating fetal foot during delivery. The foaling attendant saw the fetal foot coming through the anus and repelled it back into the birth canal, thus limiting the defect to a rectovaginal fistula.

Differential diagnosis
Vaginitis; cystitis; vaginal hematoma formation (**5.32**)

Diagnosis
Diagnosis is usually obvious, but may require a vaginal speculum examination in some cases.

Management/treatment
Grade 1 lacerations of the perineum usually require no therapy and heal quickly and with minimal scarring. Provided the laceration is attended to within the first few hours of foaling, grade 1 and 2 lesions can be sutured immediately after the exposed tissues have been thoroughly cleaned. When repairing such defects, the mucosal wound edges inside the vestibule can be left open to allow for drainage from the wound. Deeper

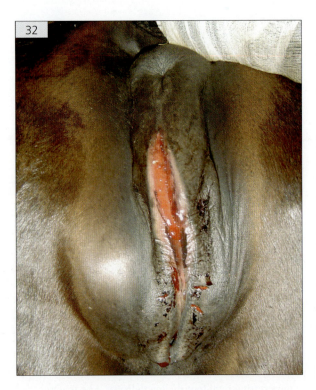

5.32 A large hematoma in the left vulvar lip of a mare immediately after foaling. After it had been confirmed that there was no vestibular laceration associated with the hematoma, it was allowed to resolve (uneventfully) without any treatment.

grade 2 lacerations may require a layer of buried sutures of absorbable material to close subcutaneous portions of the fibromuscular perineal body.

The repair of grade 3 defects should be postponed until the swelling and infection in the disrupted tissues have resolved completely. This process can take up to 6 weeks. The open wound should be cleaned once daily until it is covered by healthy rectal and vestibular mucosa. While most clinicians will treat the affected mare with NSAIDs and tetanus prophylaxis, others will also prescribe antimicrobial drug therapy for approximately 1 week. The vast majority of grade 3 lacerations can be repaired successfully and only a very small proportion of mares will suffer similar trauma during subsequent parturition.

Bladder eversion, prolapse, or rupture
Key points
- Bladder eversion, rupture, or prolapse can occur as a complication of difficult parturition.
- Proper identification of the prolapsed structure defines the plan of action and helps guide prognosis.
- Ruptured bladder should be considered in peripartum mares with signs of dullness and azotemia or, more critically, uroperitoneum.

Definition/overview
Bladder eversion results from the bladder protruding through the mare's urethra, with exposed mucosa evident (**5.33**). Bladder prolapse is characterized by identification of the serosal surface of the bladder on perineal examination of the mare, and must occur through a rent in the vaginal wall. Bladder rupture describes a tear or defect in the wall of the bladder, intra-abdominally or as a result of either of the above-mentioned conditions (**5.34**).

Etiology/pathogenesis
Bladder eversion occurs through the mare's relatively large urethra, with excessive straining, usually during parturition. Bladder mucosa may be evident either within the vaginal vault or protruding between the vulvar lips. Bladder prolapse occurs secondary to a vaginal tear, most often in the urogenital reflection, with the serosal surface of the distended bladder

protruding through the vulva. Bladder rupture or tear may result from trauma secondary to either condition in combination with parturition, or due to attempts to reposition or replace the bladder to its normal anatomic position.

Clinical features

Mares with bladder prolapse or eversion are identified by observing a protruding structure during perineal examination. Mares may also show signs of straining and or mild signs of colic and agitation. In cases of bladder rupture without either of the other two conditions, dullness, fever, and azotemia may be present, along with the absence of urination.

Differential diagnosis

Bladder prolapse; bladder eversion; in cases of bladder tear, other causes of uroperitoneum.

Diagnosis

Careful identification of the protruding structure at the vulva directs the veterinarian's plan for correction. Differentiation between mucosal and serosal surfaces

may be possible, depending on the duration of the condition. Identification of the ureteral openings would confirm bladder eversion. Songraphic evaluation of the viscus may help to determine if intestinal loops are also involved in the prolapse or eversion. Abdominocentesis should be performed to assess peritoneal involvement, degree of peritonitis, and to obtain samples for bacterial culture and sensitivity testing. Passage of a urinary catheter may help to locate the course of the urethra and relieve potential urinary obstruction in cases of bladder prolapse.

Management/treatment

The use of sedation and caudal epidural anesthesia (see Chapter 14) facilitates evaluation and treatment of traumatic bladder conditions in the mare. In cases of eversion, the mucosal surface should be closely evaluated for any defects and thoroughly lavaged prior to replacement. If no intestinal incarceration is associated with the eversion, the bladder can be gently massaged with sterile lubricant and reduced through the urethral opening. If intestine is confirmed to be involved in the eversion, exploratory celiotomy should be discussed

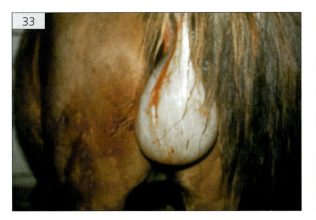

5.33 Bladder eversion. (Courtesy Dr Patrick McCue)

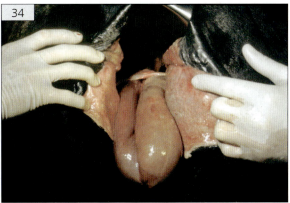

5.34 Small intestine has prolapsed through the urethral orifice in a mare with a ruptured bladder post foaling. The mare also has a rectovaginal fistula. (Courtesy Dr Dean Richardson)

with the owners, because vascular compromise of the involved intestine is likely. If reduction is difficult, it may be necessary to perform an urethrotomy to facilitate replacement.[25] Placement of a Foley catheter through the urethra and into the bladder helps to keep the bladder expressed and maintains the patency of the urethra. Broad-spectrum antimicrobial and anti-inflammatory drug therapy is indicated.

Bladder prolapse can be corrected by passing a urinary catheter (if possible) in order to evacuate the accumulated urine and facilitate bladder reduction. Again, the bladder should be carefully evaluated for defects, cleaned meticulously, and returned to the abdomen. If feasible, the vaginal tear can be repaired with the mare standing, still under the effects of the epidural anesthetic. Maintenance of a Foley urinary catheter during the immediate post-reduction phase will minimize straining and help to keep the bladder appropriately positioned. The mare should be treated aggressively for suspected peritonitis, including broad-spectrum antimicrobial drug therapy, which could be modified if and when indicated by the results of the bacterial culture and sensitivity testing of peritoneal fluid.

Bladder tears can occur as a result of the previously described bladder trauma, due to parturition alone, or to idiopathic causes. Surgical repair of the bladder can be approached through a caudal ventral midline approach[29,30], an incision through the vaginal floor, with prolapse of the bladder into the vagina[30], or after bladder eversion with or without[30] urethral sphincterotomy. The method chosen and suture pattern used may depend on the experience of the surgeon and the exact location and extent of the tear. Broad-spectrum antimicrobial drug therapy, anti-inflammatory drugs, and placement of a Foley urinary catheter are the mainstays of perioperative care. Only a small number of cases have been reported in the literature, but mares have been reported to have produced foals following bladder tear repair.[30]

Rupture of the abdominal wall during pregnancy

Key points

- Body wall ruptures are usually fatal if left untreated.
- Immediate delivery of the foal is indicated in most mares carrying twins and those with hydrops allantois or with advanced progressing disruption of the body wall.
- In cases identified early, initial management consists of supporting the body wall for sufficient time for the owner and veterinarian to define a management plan for the preferred outcome.
- It is possible to provide body wall support, nursing care, and medical therapy for long enough to allow the pregnancy to go to term and achieve delivery of a live foal.

Definition/overview

Life-threatening rupture of the abdominal wall in a late pregnant mare usually involves the prepubic tendon, but breakdown of the muscular portion of the caudoventral body wall can also occur.

Etiology/pathogenesis

Mares suffering from abdominal wall rupture usually suffer from excessive uterine weight during late gestation (e.g. twins, hydrops allantois, oversized foal), but some cases occur in aged, somewhat debilitated mares, or have no known predisposing cause.

In a recent retrospective study of 13 cases of body wall tears in pregnant mares, the median age of affected mares was 13 years with a range from 11 to 19 years and the median duration of gestation at the time of the tear was 323 days with a range from 312 to 334 days. Interestingly, this retrospective study did not include any draft horses or twin pregnancies.[31]

Clinical features

Mares commonly present with signs of colic and ventral abdominal edema.[31] Affected mares in which the condition is diagnosed in the early stage will present with misshapen abdominal walls (**5.35–5.38**). In the case of prepubic tendon rupture, the ventral body wall will be excessively edematous. The caudal abdomen will sink unusually low just cranial to the pubis; the udder will

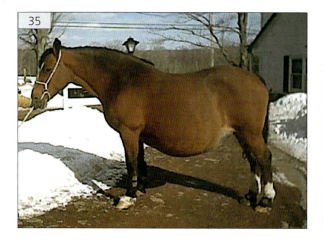

5.35 A Warmblood mare at 345 days of gestation. The mare was reluctant to move but was otherwise normal. The owner was advised not to move the mare and to apply a support wrap to the mare's abdomen; this she failed to do. Two days later the mare was found with intestines hanging through a complete rupture of the abdominal wall at the umbilicus. The mare was euthanized and the fetus did not survive.

5.36 The typical stance of a mare with partial abdominal wall rupture.

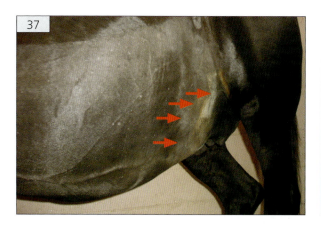

5.37 A mare with a partial body wall tear (arrows) 3 weeks prior to her anticipated foaling date. She was supported by a tight abdominal wrap and foaled uneventfully.

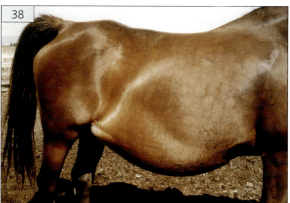

5.38 A mare with very severe edema of the ventral abdomen during late pregnancy. This mare did not show signs of discomfort or pain on abdominal wall palpation and her mammary secretion remained free of blood. She carried this pregnancy and at least one more pregnancy to term without requiring assistance or supportive care.

become severely edematous and break away from its pubic attachment, causing the teats to point caudally rather than hang vertically. In most cases bloody fluid can be expressed from the teats. Most affected mares are painful and reluctant to move and assume a stretched stance with their pelvis tilted more cranially than normal. When complete rupture is imminent, bloody serum may ooze through the overlying skin (**5.39, 5.40**). When the rupture involves a more muscular portion of the caudoventral body wall and the prepubic tendon remains intact, a striking asymmetry of the shape of the abdomen may be most noticeable. The distribution of the resulting subcutaneous swelling and edema will be equally asymmetric. If initially unnoticed or left untreated, the rupture may progress to herniation of viscera into the subcutis or complete dehiscence of even the skin, leading to fatal evisceration.

Differential diagnosis

Trauma to the body wall; snake bite or excessive reaction to insect sting or spider bite (edema).

Diagnosis

In most cases the diagnosis is obvious from the mare's misshapen abdomen and her classic stretched stance. Less advanced cases may require transcutaneous ultrasonographic examination (**5.41**) to demonstrate the rupture of one or more layers of the abdominal wall. Mares will show pain when the affected area is palpated or scanned. In addition to identification and characterization of the specific defect, ultrasonographic examination is useful for diagnosing underlying conditions such as hydrops allantois or amnion or twins.[31]

Abdominal palpation per rectum may reveal the rupture of the prepubic tendon from its insertion onto the pubic bone. Excessive udder edema, caudally directed teats, and the presence of blood in the fluid expressed from the teats are highly suggestive of an imminent prepubic tendon rupture. If the condition is associated with an excessively distended abdomen, the mare should be examined for hydrops allantois (a domed, excessively taut uterine wall will be palpable on palpation per rectum) or the presence of twins inside the uterus (usually requires very careful, systematic transabdominal ultrasonographic examination of the pregnant uterus).

Management/treatment

Disruption of the body wall is life-threatening in most cases. The immediate response should always be the application of a strong and tight abdominal support bandage. Mares should be moved only as much as is

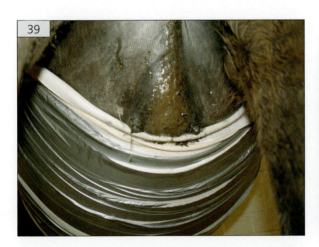

5.39 Oozing of serum form the pre-mammary area, the mammary glands, and escutcheon of a mare that was hospitalized for an impending abdominal rupture. One day later, the abdominal wall ruptured.

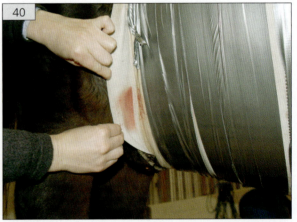

5.40 Bleeding from the skin of the abdominal wall is a sign of imminent body wall rupture. A terminal cesarean section was performed and the fetus was delivered alive.

absolutely necessary to transfer them to a facility where advanced care is available. Once informed of the seriousness of the problem, the likelihood of an abnormal pregnancy, the potentially rapid deterioration of the condition of the mare, and the poor prognosis for the mare to carry another pregnancy to term, owners must be urged to indicate their preference for the mare's or the foal's survival. They need to be informed that long-term hospitalization and nursing care will be required to support the mare to near full term.

Options for management include:

- Induction of fetal maturation by means of dexamethasone treatment, followed by the induction of labor with extensive obstetric assistance under caudal epidural anesthesia to limit abdominal straining during delivery.
- Immediate induction of labor (possibly preceded by cervical 'ripening' through the intracervical application of prostaglandin E_2) and delivery with obstetric assistance under caudal epidural anesthesia.
- Induction of fetal maturation, followed by terminal cesarean section.
- Immediate cesarean section with recovery, which is only possible when the body wall is in sufficiently good condition for a celiotomy. Further offspring from valuable surviving mares may be produced by embryo transfer.

- Support of the abdominal wall until term, when the foal will be delivered with extensive obstetric assistance. This approach may often be the preferred choice in cases that have been detected early. When this conservative approach is taken, an emergency response plan should be formulated for the eventuality of a sudden deterioration of the abdominal defect or the onset of labor.

When hydrops of the fetal membranes is diagnosed, the intra-abdominal pressure should be relieved as soon as possible by gradually draining the excessive fetal fluids through a large-bore tube inserted through the cervix into the expanded allantoic or amniotic fluid body. Drainage of the fluid will usually result in induction of labor.

Recently, a higher foal survival rate was reported with conservative management, which consisted of allowing parturition to occur naturally and avoiding induction of labor and/or cesarean section.[31] The conservative approach involved strict stall confinement, body wall support bandage, NSAIDs, and foal monitoring.

The prognosis for foal survival is less favorable in cases with an underlying disease, such as hydrops allantois or amnion, and is also less favorable if the body wall tears at an earlier gestational age.[31]

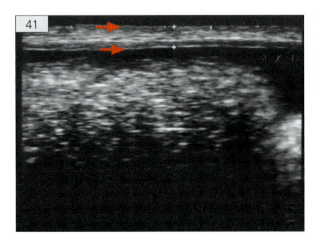

41

5.41 Ultrasonogram of a mare that had previously sustained a partial tear of the abdominal wall. The total thickness (arrows) of the body wall at the site of the defect was 4 mm. The mare was subsequently used as an embryo donor.

Stallion
Post-castration complications
Key points
- Post-castration complications occur with relative frequency and can be life-threatening if not treated promptly.
- Horse owners should be made aware of the potential complications and educated about how to monitor their horse following castration.

Definition/overview

Complications to castration commonly result in malpractice claims against veterinarians.[32] Common post-castration complications requiring emergency evaluation include hemorrhage, evisceration, iatrogenic penile injury, and severe infection. Because severe hemorrhage or evisceration subsequent to castration can be fatal, attention to detail while performing this routine procedure and postoperative vigilance are important.

Etiology/pathogenesis

Castration complications can occur for a variety of reasons, from improper surgical technique or inappropriate surgical equipment, to idiopathic causes in situations in which all accepted surgical recommendations were followed. Draft breeds, Standardbreds, and Arabian horses may be at higher risk for post-castration complications than other breeds.[33–35] Older stallions may also be more likely to develop post-castration complications than younger stallions or colts.

Clinical features

Hemorrhage described as rapidly dripping or streaming for longer than 15–30 minutes, particularly if the horse is standing quietly, should be considered excessive. Any tissue (e.g. omentum, mesentery, or loops of bowel) protruding through the surgery site necessitates emergency evaluation. Horses with herniated bowel usually present with signs of moderate to severe colic. Exposure of the corpus cavernosum or urethra during castration should alert the veterinarian that iatrogenic penile trauma has occurred, and immediate steps should be taken to prevent long-term complications. Horses that develop excessive edema, fever, reluctance to move, inappetence, or a dull demeanor may have a surgical site infection.

Differential diagnosis

Hemorrhage: testicular artery (most common); branches of the external pudendal artery (scrotal tissue); coagulopathy. Herniation or evisceration: omentum; mesentery; bowel (usually jejunum). Fever, dull demeanor: superficial surgical site infection; scirrhous cord; peritonitis; colitis; respiratory tract disease.

Diagnosis

In many cases, diagnosis of post-castration hemorrhage or evisceration is made on physical examination. Abdominal palpation per rectum may provide additional information regarding the amount of tissue herniating through the inguinal rings. Post-castration infection, either focal or extending into the peritoneal cavity, may be more difficult to diagnose and the work-up should include abdominocentesis, exploration of the surgical site, routine hematology and chemistry, and ultrasonographic evaluation. Rarely, severe anaerobic infections have been observed, including wound botulism or clostridial myonecrosis.

Management/treatment

Hemorrhage: The most severe cases of post-castration hemorrhage seem to occur with equipment failure, use of inappropriate equipment, or if castration is performed by an unqualified individual. Prolonged hemorrhage, either immediately following castration or during the postoperative period, necessitates careful scrutiny of the surgical site. If possible, the spermatic cord containing the testicular artery should be located and stretched slightly to facilitate clamp or hemostat placement.[36] Immediately following castration, it may be feasible to reapply the emasculators or ligate the cord, followed by re-emasculation. If the cord is not visible, or if bleeding is suspected to be coming from another source, packing with gauze and closure of the scrotum may decrease blood loss until the horse can be further evaluated at a surgical facility.

If the cord is not accessible, hemorrhage continues despite packing, or efforts to control hemorrhage seem ineffective, surgical intervention is indicated. Laparoscopic surgery can be performed with the horse standing or under general anesthesia positioned in dorsal recumbency.[36] Laparoscopic ligation of the testicular artery and vein has been described for post-castration hemorrhage[37] and is similar to techniques used for removal of intra-abdominal testicles via laparoscopy. If laparoscopy is not an option or is not preferred by the surgeon, exploration of the surgical site with the horse positioned in dorsal recumbency under general anesthesia should be considered. With appropriate inspection of the surgical site under optimal conditions, the source of hemorrhage can usually be located and either ligated or ligated and emasculated. Depending on the surgical findings, the surgeon may still elect to pack the site with sterile gauze and close the scrotum with large gauge, non-absorbable suture material, which can be removed 2–3 days postoperatively.

Broad-spectrum antimicrobial therapy is indicated in cases of post-castration hemorrhage. Administration of NSAIDs and modification of the original exercise program (i.e. stall confinement with hand walking after a few days) are also indicated. The most immediate concern on initial evaluation is the degree of blood loss, and determining the requirement for fluid volume resuscitation (see Chapter 12) or even the need for a blood transfusion (see Chapter 12). IV catheter placement and 20–40 ml/kg fluid resuscitation should be initiated in horses with persistent tachycardia, tachypnea, hyperlactatemia, or a low or decreasing PCV (see Chapter 4).

Evisceration and omental herniation: Evisceration (**5.42**) or omental herniation (**5.43**) are relatively uncommon yet life-threatening complications. In a study reporting commonly encountered complications after 23,229 castrations performed by equine practitioners, the incidence of evisceration (eventration) was 0.2%.[34] Draught breeds were more likely to suffer from these complications, with rates of 4.8% and 2.8% for evisceration or omental herniation, respectively.[35] It has been proposed that a pre-existing inguinal hernia might be a risk factor for postoperative herniation[36], but definitive data are lacking. Additional factors may

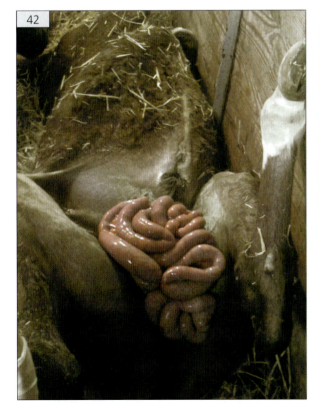

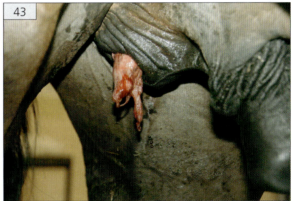

5.42 A 1.5-year-old colt castrated earlier in the morning on the day of presentation. The colt underwent a significant jejunostomy (approximately 6 meters [20 feet] of small intestine resected) and recovered uneventfully. (Courtesy Dr David Levine)

5.43 Herniated omentum leading to subsequent cord and surgical site infection following routine castration. Omentum had been surgically resected in this photo. (Courtesy Dr David Levine)

include difficult recovery from general anesthesia, large inguinal rings, or high intra-abdominal pressure.

Treatment of horses with post-castration evisceration is an emergency, with the initial steps depending on the type of castration performed (open versus closed) and the degree of herniation. If large amounts of bowel are protruding though an open castration site, the bowel should be suspended in a sling to prevent further trauma and damage to the mesentery (plastic garbage bag supported by a sheet or elastic cloth can work well), lavaged, and kept moist. Broad-spectrum antimicrobial drugs and flunixin meglumine (1.1 mg/kg IV or PO) should be administered.

Referral to a surgical facility is preferred, but if that is not an option, it is possible to treat evisceration in a field setting provided appropriate surgical equipment, lavage solutions, and the ability to induce anesthesia are available.[33] Smaller segments of small intestine herniating through an open castration site (or closed site that has opened) might be reducible, at least to within the scrotum, which could then be closed with suture or towel clamps.

If the horse is in shock, 20–40 ml/kg of crystalloid fluids can be administered IV. Fluid therapy can be started either before or during transportation to a surgical facility.

Young draught colts that eviscerated and received prompt surgical care on site have a relatively high survival rate of 72.2%.[35] This is better than might be expected at surgical referral practices that are situated some distance from their referral base. Surgical intervention consists of thorough lavage and evaluation of the exposed bowel with the horse anesthetized, followed by a decision to proceed to resection and anastomosis as opposed to manual reduction of the bowel. Depending on the amount of bowel involved and the degree of damage, ventral abdominal exploratory surgery may be necessary in order to further evaluate, reduce, and possibly resect the involved bowel segments. Severely devitalized or contaminated bowel should be resected and blind ends created at the sites of resection through an inguinal approach. Bowel resected via an inguinal approach also allows for less contaminated bowel to be returned to the abdomen, thus decreasing the magnitude of peritoneal contamination. Once the closed ends of the transected bowel have been returned to the abdomen, an anastomosis is performed through a ventral midline approach. If possible, the vaginal tunic should be ligated. Often, attempts to close the superficial inguinal rings with pre-placed, simple interrupted absorbable suture material are made, but the efficacy of this is unknown and it is left to the surgeon's discretion. It may help to pack the site and close the scrotum to decrease the likelihood of re-herniation.

Herniation of the omentum usually does not cause the horse discomfort, although it may increase the risk for infection and/or evisceration. In most cases the omentum can be emasculated and the horse confined to a stall for 2–3 days. If adhesion of the omentum to the inguinal ring is cause for concern for the client or the veterinarian, laparoscopic removal and subsequent ligation of the omentum can be performed on an elective basis. Small intestine can become incarcerated in this type of adhesion. Again, broad-spectrum antimicrobials and NSAIDs are indicated.

Iatrogenic penile trauma: Cases of iatrogenic penile trauma should be referred to a surgical facility. Repair of the urethra, if affected, is accomplished by use of 2-0 or 3-0 absorbable suture in a simple continuous pattern, followed by similar closure of the overlying tunic.[33] Possible long-term complications of iatrogenic penile laceration include surgical site infection, stricture formation, or paraphimosis (p. 394).

Other complications: Hematoma formation, surgical site infection, and peritonitis are treated by careful evaluation of the surgical site and judicious medical management. Broad-spectrum antimicrobials and NSAIDs are administered. Ultrasonographic evaluation may be indicated if peritonitis is suspected or to identify the exact location of the surgical site infection. On occasion, elective surgery may be needed to treat unresponsive infection of the cord (funiculitis [acute] or scirrhous cord [chronic]) or related structures associated with the castration site.

Post-castration edema or excessive swelling can occasionally result in paraphimosis. Typically, this is managed with penile support and topical emollients. Often, manual enlargement of the surgical site or removal of the median raphae (if left intact during an open castration) may facilitate drainage and reduce edema. Proper surgical technique and thorough education of the client prior to performing castration can decrease postoperative complications and improve client communications if complications do occur.

Priapism
Key points
- Priapism requires emergency attention, particularly if there is a desire to maintain breeding soundness.
- Priapism is almost always associated with phenothiazine treatment.
- Timely treatment with benztropine mesylate is the only documented medical therapy that has resolved the persistent erection.
- Lavage of the corpus cavernosum should be considered in cases that do not respond to treatment with benztropine mesylate.
- Surgery is necessary in cases that do not respond to medical therapy or corpus cavernosum lavage.

Definition/overview
Priapism is defined as a persistent penile erection without sexual stimulation. The persistence of engorgement is usually limited to the corpus cavernosum penis, leaving the glans penis and the remaining portion of the corpus spongiosum penis not engorged and small (**5.44**).

Etiology/pathogenesis
The etiology of priapism is essentially unknown; however, there is an association with phenothiazine tranquilizers (e.g. acepromazine). Phenothiazine tranquilizers are alpha-1 adrenergic antagonists and are thought to block the sympathetic pathway associated with detumescence. Priapism has also been reported as a complication of hemorrhagic colitis in a breeding stallion[38] as well as viral infection, spinal injuries, cachexia and starvation, strangles, and exhaustion.

Regardless of the etiology, there is neuromuscular and/or vascular dysfunction. Vascular stasis increases the CO_2 concentration, causing erythrocyte sickling and leading to occlusion of venous outflow. Trabecular edema, venous clotting, and arteriolar occlusion develop. If left untreated, sinusoidal trabecular fibrosis results in impotence despite a persistent erection.

Clinical features
Horses with priapism present with a history of recent phenothiazine (usually acepromazine) therapy for a variety of reasons. Affected horses show no signs of discomfort or systemic illness. The corpus cavernosum penis will be erect (firm, stiff, and unyielding to compression), while the corpus spongiosum (the glans and the erectile tissue surrounding the urethra) will usually not be engorged or enlarged. It is important to recognize that priapism can result in an inability of the horse to urinate.

Differential diagnosis
Paraphimosis.

Diagnosis
Diagnosing priapism is easy. An otherwise healthy male horse will present with a history of recent phenothiazine treatment (or underlying systemic disease) followed by a persistent erection. It will be impossible to force the blood out of the corpus cavernosum by compression of the penis.

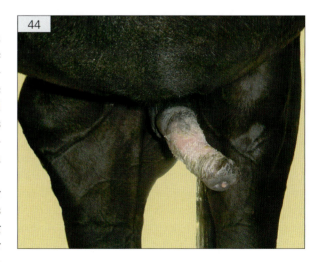

5.44 A gelding with acute priapism after administration of acepromazine. Note that the corpus cavernosum is erect, while the corpus spongiosum, including the glans penis, is not erect.

Management/treatment

Initial treatment includes administration of diuretic and anti-inflammatory drugs, penile massage and bandaging, hydrotherapy, and sling support. While this treatment does not usually resolve the priapism, it is important to prevent penile injury. If the horse appears to be unable to urinate, a urinary catheter should be passed to empty the bladder and prevent rupture.

The only published cure for priapism with return to full function has been achieved in a few horses where the condition was diagnosed correctly and treated with benztropine mesylate (8 mg total dose IV in 1 liter 0.9% sterile saline) within 2–4 hours of onset. Cases treated later, or treated repeatedly after initial treatment failed, did not resolve.

If treatment with benztropine mesylate is unsuccessful, the corpus cavernosum can be lavaged using sterile heparinized polyionic isotonic fluids with the horse under general anesthesia.[38] A 14 or 16 gauge needle is placed in the corpus cavernosum caudal to the glans penis (ingress) and one or two needles are placed 10–15 cm caudal to the scrotum (egress). The corpus cavernosum is then lavaged using several liters of sterile saline until the penis becomes flaccid and fresh blood is seen in the lavage fluid. If fresh blood is not observed, it is an indication that the arterial supply to the corpus cavernosum is occluded and the stallion is likely to become impotent. The penis is then replaced into prepuce and a purse-string suture placed in the opening to the prepuce. Care should be taken to leave the preputial opening large enough to allow for urination.

Paraphimosis is a relatively common sequela to priapism. Chemical induction of ejaculation with imipramine HCl and xylazine may provide a means of rescuing the stallion's breeding value.[38]

Unresponsive cases carry a poor prognosis and surgery is the only treatment option. Initially, the creation of a cavernosum-spongiosum venous shunt may be tried, but if this fails to resolve the erection, a penile amputation (phalectomy) is indicated. Return to breeding soundness after surgical intervention is unlikely.

Paraphimosis

Key points

- Persistent penile protrusion, regardless of its cause, must be considered a clinical emergency in geldings and stallions.
- Prompt decompression of the extended penis and its retention as close as possible to the body wall, preferably inside the preputial cavity, is the most important goal of initial therapy.
- Lack of progress towards spontaneous retention of the penis inside the preputial cavity is associated with a poor prognosis and is an indication for surgical intervention.
- Persistent paraphimosis will necessitate penile amputation.

Definition/overview

The inability to retract the penis into the prepuce is termed paraphimosis. The condition can be reversible if treated promptly, but may become permanent without appropriate treatment.

Etiology/pathogenesis

The most common cause of paraphimosis is trauma to the prepuce and/or penis (**5.45**). This is most commonly caused by a kick to the erect penis from a mare, but can also result from breeding attempts over a fence. Trauma is associated with penile enlargement (hematoma and edema formation) that renders the penis too heavy or large to be accommodated inside the preputial cavity, or reduced intrapreputial space (edema and hematoma formation) that pushes the penis cranially and out of the preputial cavity. Any other condition resulting in preputial swelling or limiting luminal space inside the preputial cavity (**5.46**) (e.g. tumors, insect stings, spider bites, dependent edema, and edema associated with balanoposthitis or swelling after castration) will also push the penis out of the prepuce.

Anesthesia and almost all tranquillizers can result in transient, reversible paralysis and relaxation of the retractor penis muscles, followed by protrusion of the penis (**5.47**). Occasionally, even after the systemic effects of the drugs have worn off, the penis will remain extended beyond the preputial orifice.

A particularly severe and devastating form of drug-induced penile paralysis and paraphimosis is seen infrequently, but regularly, after acepromazine administration to a male horse (**5.47**). While many consider this to be contraindicated, some use this drug deliberately to facilitate the passing of a urinary catheter, endoscope, or culture swab or for the cleansing of the penis and prepuce. A recent retrospective study and opinion poll on the use of acepromazine in horses undergoing general anesthesia reported that the complication rate for the development of penile prolapse, paraphimosis, or permanent penile dysfunction was low (0.2%, or less than 1 in 10,000, respectively[39]).

Penile paralysis, presumably caused by insufficient tone in the retractor penis muscles, is also frequently encountered in male horses suffering from neurologic conditions (e.g. equine protozoal myeloencephalitis, EHV (see Chapter 7), and spinal injury or disease), severe emaciation, or debilitating systemic diseases (**5.48**).

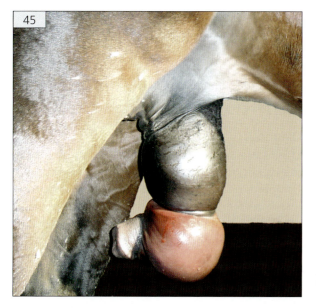

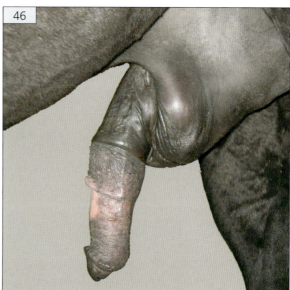

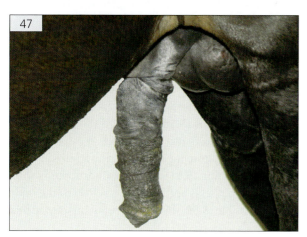

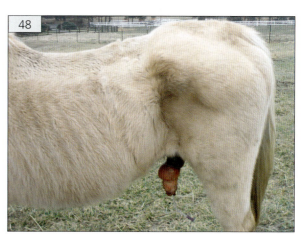

5.45–5.48 Causes of paraphimosis. (5.45) Preputial trauma, in this case caused by a kick to the prepuce during breeding. (5.46) Preputial swelling, presumably caused by an insect sting in this case. (5.47) Phenothiazine-derivative treatment. (5.48) Severe emaciation or debility.

Regardless of the initial cause, the course of the syndrome is rather uniform and predictable. Lack of venous and lymphatic drainage causes penile swelling and edema, further preventing the return of the penis into the preputial cavity (**5.49**). Lack of flow in the blood that accumulates inside the corpus cavernosum penis will result in coagulation, thrombus formation, firmness, fibrosis, and loss of elasticity. Chronic damage can result in desensitization of the penis, a critical impediment to the animal's use for breeding.

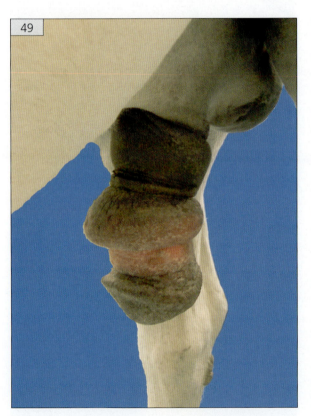

5.49 **If left unattended, the extended penis and surrounding soft tissues will start swelling, further reducing the likelihood of spontaneous recovery from paraphimosis.**

Clinical features

Unless associated with trauma, paraphimosis is not a painful condition. Most cases present with a history of recent trauma to the penis or prepuce. When associated with neurologic disease, emaciation, or general debility, the associated disease will be evident on presentation. When the urethra has been damaged, dysuria may be evident. In chronic cases, the penis may show variable degrees of desiccation, mucosal sloughing, and secondary trauma or ulceration. While the penis is extended, yet soft and flexible in most cases of paraphimosis, a much firmer, almost erect penis will be encountered once blood clots have formed inside the erectile tissues of the penis.

Differential diagnosis

Priapism.

Diagnosis

Diagnosis is self-evident in all cases, but many confuse the condition with priapism (a persistent erection). Paraphimosis is not associated with penile engorgement (erection), but it may lead to it in some cases. The cause of the paraphimosis can usually be determined on physical examination.

Management/treatment

Horses with paraphimosis should be attended to without delay with the primary goal of initial first aid being to prevent further edema formation and trauma. Once the cause of the paraphimosis has been identified, the protruding penis should be decompressed and returned into the prepuce whenever possible. The application of a pressure bandage applied from the glans towards the base will greatly facilitate reduction in size of the penis (**5.50**). Provided the penis can be completely reduced into the prepuce, it can be held in that location by placing a purse-string suture into the preputial opening (**5.51**), by the application of a sling that holds the penis and prepuce as close to the body wall as possible (**5.52**), by a penis retaining device that

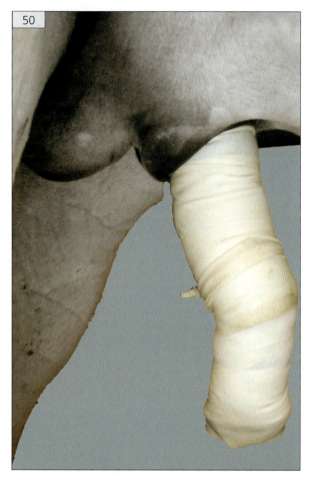

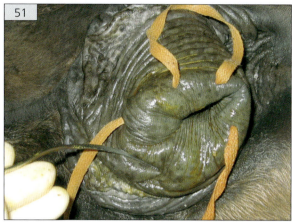

5.51 Placement of a purse-string suture in the outer preputial ring of a stallion. The umbilical tape is impregnated with iodine in order to limit the likelihood of infection tracking along its course. The suture is tied with a bow so that it can be loosened from time to time to allow for treatment of the penis.

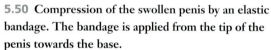

5.50 Compression of the swollen penis by an elastic bandage. The bandage is applied from the tip of the penis towards the base.

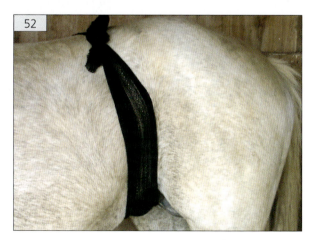

5.52 An inexpensive support strap for the retention and/or elevation of the penis of a stallion suffering from paraphimosis can be fashioned from lace material obtained from a sewing craft shop. The material is pervious enough to allow for urination, but it should be washed and dried at least once a day.

can be constructed from a plastic bottle and bandages (**5.53**), or by using a 'racing support' (**5.54**). Preputial purse-string suture placement may require brief general anesthesia or can be accomplished under local anesthesia in the compliant patient. When complete reduction is not immediately possible, elevation of the penis and prepuce as much as feasible is the most important initial therapy.

Swelling and edema of the affected tissues can be reduced by repeated application of a hygroscopic agent (e.g. glycerol) and regular hydrotherapy (20 minutes q8h, alternating hot and cold water). The penile skin should be kept moist by regular application of a topical emollient. Controlled exercise rather than forced stall confinement will also be beneficial. NSAIDs will help reduce swelling and antimicrobial drug therapy is indicated in cases associated with an infected wound. Sexual arousal must be prevented.

Paraphimosis secondary to preputial swelling and edema should resolve in 2–3 days. Segmental posthectomy (reefing) is indicated for treatment of preputial cicatrization causing paraphimosis. Cases that do not respond favorably to initial treatment have a poor prognosis for breeding. Chemical ejaculation (see Priapism)

may be indicated in stallions that remain impotent. Castration with phalopexy (Boltz procedure) or phalectomy is often recommended to prevent further penile injury.

Torsion of the spermatic cord
Key points
- Torsion of the spermatic cord is extremely uncommon, but should be considered in any intact male horse with signs of colic.
- Torsion of the spermatic cord up to 180 degrees is often clinically unimportant.
- Clinically important spermatic cord torsion usually results from a 270–360 degree rotation.
- Ultrasonographic evaluation of the scrotal contents and/or inguinal ring is often very useful in diagnosing spermatic cord torsion.

Definition/overview
Torsion of the spermatic cord occurs when the associated testicle rotates around the long axis of its spermatic cord. Torsions of 180 degrees are often encountered incidentally and usually are of no clinical importance. It has been hypothesized, however, that this condition may lead to low fertility due to poor blood flow to the

5.53 Retention device for the penis after it has been decompressed and returned to the prepuce. The bottom of a plastic bottle is cut off, the free edge rendered atraumatic by covering it with several layers of bandage tape, and four ties are fitted to the neck of the bottle to hold the device in place (tied above the horse's croup). The stallion can urinate through the open neck of the bottle.

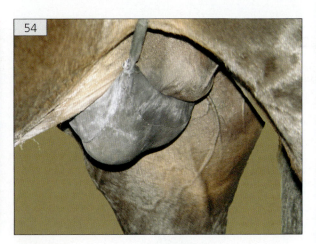

5.54 A 'racing support' for stallions is another useful device for the elevation and/or retention of the penis.

testicle.[36] Torsion of the spermatic cord of 270–360 degrees is clinically important, resulting in edema, limb or scrotal swelling, or signs of mild colic.[36,40]

Etiology/pathogenesis

The etiology of cord torsion is unknown, although a long ligament of the tail of the epididymis/proper ligament of the testis has been suggested to contribute to the condition.[40] Standardbreds may be more susceptible than other breeds.[36] Torsion of retained testicles may also occur.

Clinical features

Clinically important torsion of the spermatic cord requiring emergency evaluation is characterized by scrotal edema or swelling, mild or moderate colic signs, or even limb edema. The swelling may make it more difficult to determine the orientation of the tail of the epididymis. With 180 degree rotation of the spermatic cord, the tail of the epididymis will be oriented cranially instead of caudolaterally (**5.55**). If the torsion of the cord is approaching 360 degrees, the epididymal tail will lie close to its normal anatomic position, making diagnosis on palpation less definitive. Recurrent bouts of mild colic, responsive to NSAID therapy, have been associated with torsion of the spermatic cord.[40]

Differential diagnosis

Inguinal hernia; testicular or scrotal hematoma; neoplasia.

Diagnosis

Torsion of the spermatic cord, or other lesions affecting the reproductive tract, should be considered in the intact male showing signs of colic. Abdominal examination per rectum may be used to confirm thickening of the cord as it passes through the inguinal ring, and can be used to rule out inguinal herniation of abdominal contents. Transcutaneous ultrasonographic examination of the scrotum and its contents and transrectal ultrasonographic examination of the inguinal ring are useful in ruling out inguinal hernia, identifying the diameter and course of the spermatic cord, and providing information regarding testicular blood flow. Hydrocele (excessive fluid surrounding the testicle) may also be observed ultrasonographically in cases of spermatic cord torsion.

Management/treatment

Diagnosis is usually confirmed with surgical exploration through an inguinal incision made directly over the affected spermatic cord. The testicle and cord are evaluated, typically followed by a hemiorchidectomy (hemicastration). In horses not used for breeding, bilateral castration should be performed.[41] In breeding stallions, or horses intended for breeding, an orchipexy can be performed at the cranial and caudal poles of the remaining testis, using small diameter nonabsorbable suture.[40] Similarly, if the spermatic cord torsion was corrected rapidly and no vascular compromise was evident, an orchipexy can be performed on the affected testicle.[41] The extent of vascular compromise and reperfusion injury and its effect on future fertility may, however, be difficult to assess at the time of surgery. Although published reports are scarce, stallions on which this procedure had been performed were reported to have retained acceptable fertility.[40] The prognosis for survival after bilateral castration should be excellent, barring any post-castration complications.

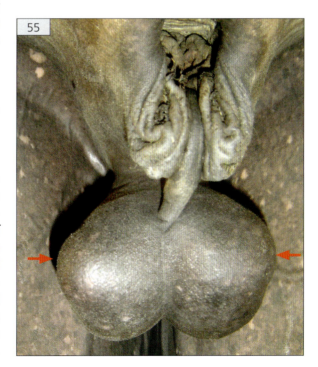

5.55 A stallion with bilateral spermatic cord torsion. Note that both epididymal tails are facing cranially (arrows). This horse was asymptomatic.

Penile and testicular trauma
Key points
- While the diagnosis may be readily apparent, determination of structures involved is important for penile/prepucial and testicular trauma.
- Penile and preputial lacerations are usually superficial.
- Penile hematoma formation should be controlled with compression bandages.
- Persistent hemorrhage warrants emergency surgical exploration because it is likely associated with disruption of the tunica albuginea. Preputial/penile lacerations should be debrided and sutured.
- Testicular trauma may require hemicastration.

Definition/overview
Injury to the penis/prepuce or testes including superficial and deep lacerations or blunt trauma.

Etiology/pathogenesis
Penile and testicular trauma often occurs as a result of a kick or the horse unsuccessfully attempting to jump a fixed structure.

Clinical features
Penile and preputial lacerations are usually superficial. Penile hematomas are often associated with injury to the dorsal superficial vessels. However, deep lacerations can involve the cavernous tissue and urethra. 'Fractured' penis is typically associated with disruption of the tunica albuginea surrounding the corpus cavernosum. Testicular trauma is often associated with scrotal swelling. Lacerations may also be evident.

Differential diagnosis
Penis: diagnosis is usually apparent. Testicle: inguinal hernia; testicular torsion; neoplasia.

Diagnosis
While the diagnosis may be readily apparent, exact determination of structures involved is important for the appropriate treatment of penile/preputial and testicular trauma. Specifically, the involvement of penile cavernous tissue and urethra should be evaluated using either ultrasonography or surgical exploration with urethral catheterization.

The affected testicle(s) should be evaluated ultrasonographically for the extent of damage including edema and hematoma formation and evidence of testicular rupture or rupture of the vaginal tunic. If the traumatic event was not observed, palpation per rectum should be used to rule out inguinal hernia and ultrasonography undertaken to rule out testicular torsion or neoplasia.

Management/treatment
Penile hematoma formation should be controlled with compression bandages and penile support. Hydrotherapy (cold initially) can also be used to slow down hemorrhage. Persistent hemorrhage warrants emergency surgical exploration because it is likely associated with disruption of the tunica albuginea. Preputial/penile lacerations should be debrided and sutured to prevent infection and associated cellulitis, swelling, and paraphimosis. Sexual and stall rest are recommended until swelling has resolved and wounds healed (3–14 days). Paraphimosis is a common sequela secondary to swelling. Preputial injury can lead to preputial cicatrix formation, resulting in paraphimosis (or phimosis). Segmental posthectomy (reefing) may be necessary. Urethral obstruction can occur secondary to penile trauma and hematoma formation and this can lead to bladder rupture (p. 384). Urethral lacerations often result in urethral stenosis. Penile lacerations can result in shunting with impotence (e.g. corpus cavernosum–superficial vasculature) or urination problems (e.g. cutaneous–urethral, cavernosum–urethral).

Minor testicular trauma can be managed with NSAIDs and hydrotherapy. Hemicastration is recommended for severe testicular trauma and delay can cause permanent dysfunction of the unaffected testis. Compensatory hypertrophy of the remaining testis occurs as a result of increased secretion of interstitial cell-stimulating hormone from the hypophysis.

URINARY TRACT

Urolithiasis

Key points

- Urolithiasis, particularly urethral calculi, may be the cause for emergency evaluation of a horse with hematuria, dysuria, or pollakiuria.
- Intermittent mild colic and weight loss are more commonly associated with renal or ureteral calculi, as opposed to bladder calculi.
- Surgical intervention, through perineal urethrotomy, routine cystotomy, or laparoscopic-assisted cystotomy, may be necessary to treat bladder calculi.

Definition/overview

Formation of calculi in the equine urinary tract can occur in the bladder, kidney, ureter, or urethra.[42] Calculi are most commonly observed in the bladder and are typically comprised of calcium carbonate, more specifically calcite, which is the mineralized form.[42] The majority of the cases are seen in males >8 years of age.[43] The size of the urethra in the mare facilitates passage of small calculi, lessening their clinical relevance.

Etiology/pathogenesis

The etiology and pathogenesis of urolithiasis in the horse remain unknown. Contributing factors may include incomplete emptying of the bladder during urination due to discomfort, neurogenic causes, pre-existing cystitis, or renal damage. Supersaturation of urine in the bladder and an environment promoting crystal precipitation have been implicated in other species.[42] Diet has not been shown to contribute to the formation of urinary calculi in the horse.

Clinical features

Most horses with bladder calculi show signs of hematuria and/or difficulty during micturition, including dysuria, stranguria, oliguria, or incontinence.[29,42] Because of the difficulty with urination and the sometimes chronic nature of the disease, urine scalding of the hindlimbs may be evident.[29] Weight loss can be a prominent feature, particularly in horses with renal calculi.[42] Urolithiasis should be considered in patients suffering from weight loss and intermittent mild colic. In cases of urethral obstruction, azotemia or uroperitoneum secondary to bladder rupture can occur, particularly if diagnosis and treatment are delayed. On occasion, urolithiasis can be the cause of inappropriate breeding behavior and should be considered in cases in which other more common diagnoses have been ruled out.[44]

Differential diagnosis

Urinary tract infection (e.g. cystitis, pyelonephritis); urinary incontinence due to other causes (e.g. neurogenic); urovagina; neoplasia or an abscess within the urinary tract.

Diagnosis

Presumptive diagnosis of urolithiasis may be based on history, signalment, and clinical signs. Confirmation is usually made by examination of the bladder per rectum, cystoscopy or ultrasonographic evaluation of the urinary system. The nature of the clinical signs might suggest the anatomic location of calculi. For example, signs of colic are more likely to be associated with renal, ureteral, or urethral calculi. Complete urethral obstruction, most commonly seen on an emergency basis, is characterized by complete failure to urinate or minimal micturition and is often associated with high serum creatinine concentrations. Calculi lodged in the extrapelvic urethra may be palpated or imaged via transcutaneous ultrasonographic examination. Calculi within the urinary bladder may be palpable per rectum or may be associated with a thickened bladder wall.[44]

Cystoscopy confirms urethral obstruction (if present), allows for visual inspection of the bladder and any calculi, and confirms urine flow from both ureters. Size and surface characteristics of the calculi may help in the formation of a treatment plan, guiding decisions with regard to the best surgical approach, or likelihood of success with medical management.[44] Ultrasonographic evaluation of the urinary system can aid in the identification of calculi inside the bladder and confirm the absence of nephrolithiasis. Approximately 10% of affected horses in one study developed calculi at more than one anatomic location.[42] In cases in which renal or ureteral calculi are suspected, ultrasonographic evaluation of both kidneys and ureters should be performed. Additional diagnostics include routine hematology and measurement of fibrinogen concentration, to assess the likelihood of ongoing cystitis, and serum creatinine concentration. Depending on the severity of the disease, biochemical analysis of serum electrolytes and further renal function tests are indicated.

Management/treatment

Calculi inside the bladder of mares can often be removed manually through the urethral opening with the mare under sedation and caudal epidural anesthesia. Particularly large calculi may require crushing or sphincterotomy or, rarely, alternative surgical approaches (see below).

In males, surgical options include cystotomy from a caudal midline incision, perineal urethrotomy in the standing horse under caudal epidural anesthesia, or laparoscopic-assisted cystotomy.[29,42,45] Choice of surgical approach is dependent on the clinical presentation of the case, surgeon experience, and equipment available. Urinary samples for bacterial culture and sensitivity testing should be collected aseptically prior to surgery or intraoperatively. Perioperative management should include antimicrobial drug administration in horses with suspected or documented cystitis, anti-inflammatory drugs (nephrotoxic NSAIDs must be used with caution in horses with suspected renal compromise), and possibly bladder lavage.

For many male patients, particularly with urethral calculi or smaller or fragmentable calculi, perineal urethrotomy under caudal epidural anesthesia may be sufficient for removal of calculi (**5.56–5.58**). Possible complications of this surgical approach include trauma to the pelvic urethra, rectum, or bladder, or postoperative urethritis.[42] Commonly, the urethrotomy incision is left to heal by second intention.

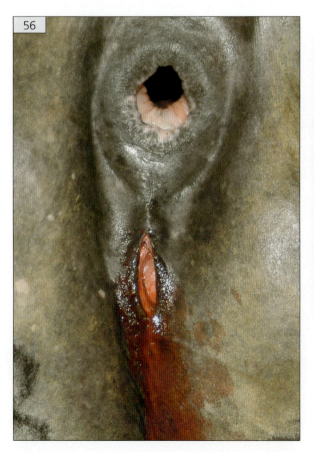

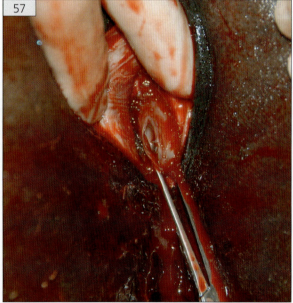

5.56, 5.57 Surgical approach to perineal urethrostomy (5.56), with entrance into the urethra visible at the end of the instrument (5.57). (Courtesy Dr Dean Richardson)

Removal of larger calculi from the bladder (**5.59, 5.60**) or urethral calculi that cannot be accomplished through a perineal urethrotomy can be achieved by routine cystotomy through a parainguinal or caudal midline approach.[29] Access can be difficult, depending on patient size and surgical exposure. Decisions regarding the surgical approach may relate to clinical features of a specific case (e.g. calculi size, patient disposition), surgeon preference, or equipment availability. Complications of the parainguinal or caudal midline approaches include incisional infection or dehiscence, difficult access, or problems with the cystotomy incision.

Laparoscopic-assisted cystotomy for the removal of cystic calculi has been described in a small number of geldings.[45] Reported advantages of this approach include relatively short surgery time, minimal postop-erative patient care, and no recurrence of urolithiasis at long-term follow-up.

Renal or ureteral calculi are challenging from a surgical standpoint and careful evaluation of both kidneys and renal function is indicated. Although nephrectomy is not common in the horse, it has been described for unilateral nephrolithiasis.[46]

Recurrence of urolithiasis can often occur regardless of the treatment method. Because the etiology of urolithiasis is still unclear, it is difficult to prescribe preventive measures or limit potential risk factors. Horses with urolithiasis may do well provided a diagnosis is made promptly and minimal complications are encountered during or after surgical intervention. Relatively few cases with long-term follow-up after surgical treatment for urolithiasis are reported.[42,45]

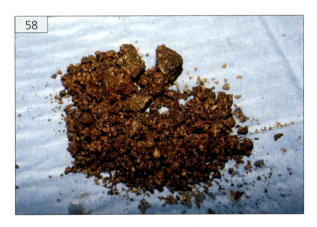

5.58 Crumbled calculi removed from the bladder following urethrostomy. (Courtesy Dr Dean Richardson)

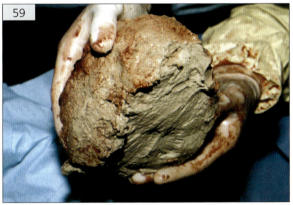

5.59 A large urolith removed from the bladder of a mare. (Courtesy Dr Dean Richardson)

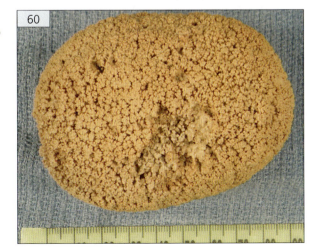

5.60 Large, speculated urolith. (Courtesy Dr Dean Richardson)

Acute kidney injury (previously known as acute renal failure)

Key points

- The best approach to acute kidney injury (AKI) is prevention by avoiding administration of nephrotoxic drugs in hemodynamically unstable patients.
- Aggressive medical management can result in the reversal of AKI, particularly if the disease is of short duration.
- Resolution of the primary disease and careful monitoring of hemodynamic status in the critically ill horse will lessen the likelihood of further renal damage.
- Therapeutic drug monitoring in relatively healthy patients receiving nephrotoxic drugs may help to avoid AKI.

Definition/overview

AKI in the critically ill equine patient is usually a component of other inflammatory disease processes that result in a decreased glomerular filtration rate (GFR) and impaired renal function. Renal function may be transiently affected or the process may persist, progressing to more significant renal damage. Decreased GFR allows nitrogenous wastes to accumulate in the body and, depending on the duration and severity, may result in electrolyte abnormalities and disturbed acid–base regulation.[47]

Etiology/pathogenesis

In the horse, renal failure is typically classified as having a pre-renal, renal, or post-renal/obstructive origin. AKI in the adult horse is usually of pre-renal or renal origin, and is often secondary to underlying disease or toxicity, or a combination of both. Post-renal or obstructive renal compromise can be seen in the adult horse, although rarely, and is usually related to urinary tract obstruction or bladder rupture (see Urolithiasis).

Decreased glomerular filtration rate due to pre-renal causes is primarily a result of poor cardiac output, leading to impaired renal perfusion without ongoing cellular damage.[47] Poor cardiac output in the horse can be due to a variety of primary clinical conditions, most commonly GI inflammation, septicemia, endotoxemia, acute hemorrhage, or severe dehydration. In many cases, pre-renal azotemia may progress to renal azotemia depending on the severity of the primary disease, associated inflammatory response, and clinical progression. If the inciting cause cannot be readily resolved, ischemic damage to the kidney becomes prolonged, and subsequent tubular damage may result.[48] The damage may be worsened by administration of nephrotoxic drugs (e.g. aminoglycoside antimicrobial drugs or NSAIDs) during a state of reduced renal perfusion, increasing the likelihood of renal tubular damage and subsequent renal failure.

The medullary portion of the kidney is particularly sensitive to ischemic damage because it only receives 10–20% of the renal blood flow in normal physiologic conditions, and rapidly becomes hypoxic in conditions of prolonged renal hypotension and endogenous catecholamine release.[47,48] As a result of the systemic inflammatory process, the intrinsic renal vasodilators may become overwhelmed by endogenous catecholamines, resulting in further reduction of renal blood flow and exacerbation of ischemia. Nephrotoxic drugs primarily affect the renal cortex, which receives the majority of renal blood flow.[49] The addition of nephrotoxic drugs to these patients' therapeutic regimen may add to the proximal tubular damage by reducing prostaglandin production (i.e. NSAIDs) or accumulation in the tubular epithelial cells (aminoglycoside antimicrobial drugs).[47,49]

AKI is also described by anatomic location, and in humans is identified as tubular, glomerular, or vascular. In horses, tubular necrosis is the most commonly observed clinical presentation, usually due to hemodynamic or nephrotoxic causes. Glomerulonephritis is diagnosed infrequently at necropsy or during histopathologic evaluation of a renal biopsy, while a vascular cause of AKI in the horse is not a clinically important entity.[47] Acute tubular necrosis is often the result of ischemia and microvascular coagulation[48], administration of nephrotoxic drugs (alone or in combination) to healthy patients, or in horses with an ongoing systemic inflammatory response syndrome (SIRS) (see Chapter 17).

As the primary disease progresses, the kidney attempts to respond to its state of poor perfusion by increasing renal vasoconstriction, signaling the renin–angiotensin system, and increasing vasopressin release.[47] Prolonged hypoperfusion may result in failure of the autoregulation system of the kidney and ischemic tubular damage may result.

In situations of nephrotoxicity related to drug administration in initially healthy animals, renal pathogenesis is slightly different. Nephrotoxic drugs are primarily taken up in the brush border of the proximal tubule in the renal cortex.[47] Prolonged administration or repeated daily dosing of these agents results in accumulation of the drug and cellular dysfunction and death. Proximal tubules become plugged with cellular debris, further decreasing glomerular filtration rate and exacerbating renal damage.

Glomerulonephritis is primarily an immune-mediated renal disease characterized by the accumulation of immune complexes in the glomeruli, activating the complement system, and resulting in local inflammation. In horses, this disease process has been associated with *Leptospira* spp. infection and group C streptococcal antigens.[50,51] It is infrequently diagnosed in horses perceived as suffering from AKI.

Clinical features

In many cases, horses with AKI present with a primary condition that results in hemodynamic instability or SIRS, and the majority of the clinical signs are typically associated with the primary disease. When developing a resuscitative and therapeutic plan, the veterinarian should consider low GFR, poor renal perfusion, and the potential for AKI or further renal damage in these patients. Horses may present with severe endotoxemia secondary to enterocolitis, severe acute GI disease, or sepsis. Acute hemorrhage can cause renal hypoperfusion and secondary AKI. Diseases that cause myoglobinuria (e.g. rhabdomyolysis) or hemoglobinuria (e.g. hemolysis) can also cause AKI. The initial management of these patients is critical, as developing AKI is commonly pre-renal and reversible. Avoidance of potential nephrotoxic drugs in this early stage is important, and ongoing attempts should be made to monitor renal function during the early phases of patient stabilization. Clinical signs might include a dull demeanor, azotemia (high creatinine and BUN concentrations) and low urine output. Oliguria is probably the most consistent clinical finding associated with AKI in the horse. Prolonged oliguria in the face of appropriate fluid resuscitation and failure of rapid resolution of azotemia are ominous signs that AKI may not be reversible.

Horses with AKI secondary to nephrotoxic drug administration only may present with clinical signs of dull demeanor, mild anorexia, and oliguria. Azotemia and associated metabolic disturbances, as well as hyponatremia and hypochloremia, may be present on biochemical analysis.[49] Mild colic and subcutaneous dependent edema may be observed. Horses with an obstructive or a post-renal cause of AKI often show signs of abdominal discomfort along with stranguria or dysuria.

Differential diagnosis

Severe SIRS may accompany AKI, resulting in a variety of organs similarly affected; pyelonephritis; nephrolithiasis; congenital renal disease (rare); other primary renal disease.

Diagnosis

High serum creatinine and BUN concentrations are salient biochemical features of AKI, but they are not predictive of outcome. Biochemical analysis should include evaluation of electrolytes to determine the degree of hyponatremia, hypochloremia, and hyperkalemia, if present, and to appropriately direct fluid administration.

Following initial evaluation, the veterinarian should attempt to rule out pre- and post-renal causes of AKI. Response to rapid fluid volume resuscitation and assessment of urine SG are indicated. SG of 1.025–1.055 has been associated with pre-renal acute renal failure.[47]

Urinalysis should be performed, paying particular attention to the degree of proteinuria and the presence or type of casts on cytological evaluation. Proteinuria and high red cell numbers may be more severe in cases of glomerulonephritis, and urine may be concentrated compared with horses with tubular disease.[47] Sodium fractional excretion may be useful to distinguish between pre-renal and renal azotemia in the horse[52] and should be performed once the horse is adequately volume resuscitated.

Post-renal obstruction can be ruled out based on history, clinical signs, passage of a urinary catheter, or cystoscopy, if necessary.

Management/treatment

Often, initial management is focused on fluid volume resuscitation and supportive therapy directed towards resolution of the primary disease. Again, it is preferable to prevent AKI in patients that are hemodynamically compromised by endotoxemia or severe dehydration, as opposed to attempting to treat established renal dysfunction. Isotonic, pH-balanced polyionic fluids can be used for initial fluid volume resuscitation, and can be adjusted if concerns regarding specific electrolyte abnormalities are evident on initial biochemical evaluation. If concerns regarding potassium excretion emerge, 0.9% sodium chloride solution may be used instead, bearing in mind the potential acidifying effect of the administration of this fluid. Fluid volume resuscitation can begin at 20–40 ml/kg, depending on the severity of the hypovolemia. Careful patient monitoring, including clinical observation, recording of urine output and SG, repeated venous blood lactate concentration determination, direct or indirect blood pressure measurements, or measurements of CVP (see Chapter 11), can be used to direct a resuscitation or maintenance fluid therapy plan.

If the horse remains oliguric following several hours of fluid therapy, critical patient reassessment and consideration of alternative therapy should follow. In patients suffering from severe volume depletion or endotoxemia, it must first be determined whether the patient has been appropriately fluid volume resuscitated or is still suffering from an overall lack of volume-limiting cardiac output. Other possibilities might include impaired cardiac output due to poor myocardial function or vascular tone resulting from endotoxemia or sepsis-mediated SIRS. Addition of a vasopressor or cardiac inotrope (see Chapter 13) may be indicated. The use of dopamine (3–5 µg/kg/minute) to increase renal perfusion has been advocated in the horse, but this is a much debated topic in human and veterinary critical care medicine and definitive evidence of its efficacy is lacking. If dopamine or other vasopressor/inotrope therapy is implemented, blood pressure and heart rate should be monitored. Electrolytes should be closely monitored in patients that remain oliguric, paying close attention to potassium and calcium concentrations, in addition to hyponatremia and hypochloremia. Placement of a urinary catheter will allow for the monitoring of daily urine output. Attempts to match IV sodium administration to the kidney's ability to handle sodium fractional excretion may be worthwhile.

Administration of 20% mannitol (0.25–1.0 g/kg), given over 20 minutes, may transiently increase renal blood flow due to the systemic osmotic activity of the drug.[47] Other potential benefits include enhanced prostaglandin E_2 synthesis and improved urine output due to an osmotic effect in the tubule. The use of furosemide or other loop diuretics is controversial, but has been applied frequently to promote urine output by natriuresis and possibly protect tubular cells from metabolism in a potentially hypoxic environment.

Providing a prognosis for an AKI patient can be difficult and is likely related to the severity of the underlying disease or initial nephrotoxic insult. Renal biopsy may be helpful in situations where a more definitive diagnosis, which might influence therapy, is needed.[53] Rate of response to initial therapy might provide some indication as to the likelihood of a full recovery or the possibility of progression to chronic renal dysfunction. Prolonged oliguria in the face of aggressive medical management can be considered indicative of a poorer prognosis for future renal function.[47]

CHAPTER 6

SKIN

*Troy N. Trumble and
Louise L. Southwood*

GENERAL APPROACH TO THE HORSE WITH LACERATIONS AND PUNCTURE WOUNDS

- Skin emergencies are most often lacerations or puncture wounds. Other problems such as burns, primary limb cellulitis, pruritus, photosensitization, and, rarely, pemphigus foliaceus or toxic epidermal necrosis (TEN) may require emergency attention.
- Referral to a tertiary hospital on an emergency basis should be considered in cases where the laceration potentially involves deeper structures, the horse does not appear to be cardiovascularly stable, further diagnostic tests are necessary, and surgical management with the horse under general anesthesia is warranted.
- A thorough history should be obtained from the caregiver. Pertinent historical information for a horse with a laceration or puncture wound is listed in *Box 6.1*.
- Hemorrhage should be stopped immediately and resuscitation performed if necessary. Hemorrhage from a distal limb laceration is rarely life-threatening and resuscitation not usually required. Hemorrhage from vessels associated with a laceration is usually controlled using digital pressure, pressure bandage, and vessel ligation (see Chapter 4).

Box 6.1 Pertinent history for horses with lacerations and puncture wounds

- Patient signalment.
- When the injury occurred or when the horse was last observed to be normal.
- How the injury occurred, including damage to fences, stalls, or feed bins, and whether the horse is pastured with other horses.
- Any medications that the horse is currently receiving and medications given by the owner or caregiver for the injury.
- Previous history of lameness or other illness.
- Vaccination history, particularly tetanus toxoid.
- Current use of the horse and expectations of the owner or caregiver for the horse following recovery from the injury.

- A rapid patient assessment (i.e. heart rate, respiratory rate, mucous membrane color, moistness, and CRT, rectal temperature, and borborygmi) should be performed on any injured horse because: (1) signs of shock may be associated with blood loss as well as thoracic or abdominal cavity injury; (2) there may be pre-existing or underlying disease (e.g. colic); and (3) involvement of other structures (e.g. joint, bone, trachea, esophagus) may not be initially apparent.
- The gait should be assessed, particularly for horses with limb lacerations, by walking the horse for a few steps to determine the degree of lameness and ability to weight bear. Any gait deficits (e.g. hyperextension of the distal interphalangeal joint) should be noted. Gait evaluation should be performed, preferably with the bandage removed and prior to sedation and desensitization with perineural anesthesia.
- Sedation (*Box 6.2*) is recommended prior to evaluating the laceration if the horse is cardiovascularly stable. Performing perineural anesthesia (local nerve block) (p. 409) or desensitizing the skin is also beneficial prior to any manipulation of the wound.
- When evaluating any laceration, sterile lubricant should be placed in the wound, the surrounding hair clipped, and the skin aseptically prepared (p. 412).
- The wound should be thoroughly evaluated using digital palpation and/or a probe to assess the involvement of deeper structures such as bone, joints, tendon sheaths, ligaments and tendons. The limb should also be examined for swelling, synovial effusion, crepitus, and instability. Comparison with the contralateral limb can be beneficial in some horses to differentiate normal from abnormal.
- Radiographic and sonographic examination may be used to assess bone damage and synovial structure involvement by observing air within the synovial structure. Sonography can also be used to determine direct communication between the wound and deeper structures and can be particularly useful if there is marked swelling, which prohibits palpation and synoviocentesis.
- If synovial structure involvement is suspected, a needle should be aseptically inserted into the structure and a sample aspirated for cytologic evaluation (p. 412). The structure should be distended with sterile isotonic fluid and communication with the wound determined by observing fluid exiting the wound. The limb often needs to be taken through a range of motion so that communication can be thoroughly evaluated.
- The wound should be carefully debrided and thoroughly lavaged (p. 412).
- The wound edges should be apposed, if possible (p. 412).
- Topical treatment of traumatic wounds is generally not recommended.
- Bandaging (p. 416) is important for managing swelling and wound protection. Cast application may be warranted in horses with lacerations in highly mobile areas.
- NSAIDs and antimicrobial drugs (*Box 6.2*) are often indicated in horses with wounds involving deep structures. Local delivery of antimicrobial drugs using regional limb perfusion (see Chapter 2) is indicated in horses with distal limb lacerations involving deeper structures.

Box 6.2 Dose rates of the most commonly used drugs in the emergency management of horses with skin problems

DRUG	DOSE RATE (AMOUNT FOR A 500 KG HORSE)
Non-steroidal anti-inflammatory drugs	
Phenylbutazone	2.2–4.4 mg/kg IV or PO q12–24h (5–10 ml or 1–2 tablets)
Flunixin meglumine	1.1 mg/kg IV q12h (500 mg or 10 ml) (also available as an oral paste)
Firocoxib	0.27 mg/kg IV (loading dose) (135 mg or 6.75 ml), then 0.09 mg/kg IV q24h (45 mg or 2.25 ml) (also available as an oral paste)
Meloxicam	0.6 mg/kg IV or IM q24h (300 mg)
Sedation	
Xyalzine HCl	0.3–0.4 mg/kg IV (150–200 mg or 1.5–2 ml)
Detomidine HCl	0.01–0.02 mg/kg IV or IM (5–10 mg or 0.5–1ml)
Butorphanol	0.01–0.02 mg/kg IV (5–10 mg or 0.5–1 ml) (with xylazine or detomidine)
Acepromazine	0.02–0.06 mg/kg IV (10–30 mg or 1–3 ml) 0.03–0.1 mg/kg IM (15–50 mg or 1.5–5 ml)
Antimicrobial drugs	
Procaine penicillin	22,000 U/kg IM q12h (11 x 10^6 U or 37 ml)
Potassium penicillin	22,000 U/kg IV q6h (11 x 10^6 U but volume depends on concentration following resuspension)
Gentamicin	6.6–8.8 mg/kg IV q24h (3.3–4.4 g or 33–44 ml)
Ceftiofur	2.2 mg/kg IV or IM q12h (1 g or 20 ml) (adult) 10 mg/kg slow IV q6h (neonate)
Trimethoprim sulfa	30 mg/kg PO q12h (15 g or 15–16 tablets)
Amikacin	500 mg (2 ml) intra-articularly q24–48h

COMMON PROCEDURES PERFORMED ON HORSES WITH LACERATIONS AND PUNCTURE WOUNDS

Abaxial sesamoid and low 4-point nerve blocks

Indications

Wound repair can be performed with the horse standing or under general anesthesia. Many lower limb lacerations can be thoroughly examined, lavaged, debrided, and reapposed with the horse standing and sedated. In general, if severe injury is suspected or additional therapies are proposed, such as arthroscopy, then it is best to have the horse under general anesthesia. Otherwise, perineural or local anesthesia can be utilized effectively. Local anesthesia is effective for mobilizing and suturing large flaps of skin, but is not very good at desensitizing enough area so that sufficient wound debridement can occur. Perineural anesthesia is generally better because it will facilitate the standing horse being able to tolerate debridement, multiple arthrocentesis, and distension of one or more synovial structures. Two of the most common sites for perineural anesthesia in horses with distal limb lacerations are the abaxial sesamoid and low 4-point nerve blocks.

An abaxial sesamoid nerve block can be utilized for lacerations involving the foot, including the coronary band, avulsion fractures, or deep puncture wounds to the navicular bursa. It will also desensitize the entire pastern region and the distal aspect of the digital flexor tendon sheath. It will not be effective for lacerations surrounding the fetlock.

A low 4-point nerve block can be utilized for any distal limb laceration that encompasses the fetlock or structures distal to the fetlock. The main difference between the low 4-point and the abaxial nerve block is desensitization of the entire fetlock and digital flexor tendon sheath with the low 4-point nerve block.

Technique
Abaxial sesamoid nerve block

- This block can be performed using 1–3 ml of local anesthetic per medial and/or lateral branch. In general, when performing this block for repair of lacerations, 3 ml is used because proximal migration of the anesthetic is not a concern.
- The name of this block identifies the location of where the nerve should be identified.
- The neurovascular bundle can be palpated as it courses over the abaxial surface of the proximal sesamoid bones (**6.1**). Often, a pulse can be palpated in this location. The nerve is located on the most palmar/plantar aspect of the neurovascular bundle.
- The block can be performed with the horse standing or with the limb held.
- The needle (25 gauge, 0.5 inch) is typically placed in the subcutaneous space directly parallel and superficial to the palpable nerve.

Low 4/6-point nerve block

- A low 4-point nerve block will desensitize the palmar nerves and the palmar metacarpal nerves (four injection sites) in the forelimb (**6.2**) and a low 6-point nerve block will densitize the plantar nerves, plantar metatarsal, and dorsal metatarsal nerves on the hindlimb (six injection sites) (**6.3**).
- It is preferable to place the needle in each location for this block.
- This block can be performed using 1–3 ml of local anesthetic per site.
- On both the forelimbs and hindlimbs, the palmar/plantar nerves can be palpated as the most palmar/plantar structure in the neurovascular bundle located next to the deep digital flexor tendon at the level of the button of the splint. The needle is placed in the subcutaneous space directly parallel and superficial to the palpable nerve.
- The palmar/plantar metacarpal/tarsal nerves are located directly beneath the button of the splint bones. One needle can be used to block both sides or each site can be blocked independently. The needle can be placed directly underneath the splint bone.

- The dorsal metatarsal nerves can be identified by placing the needle approximately 3 cm dorsal to the button of the splint bones. The nerve is difficult to palpate in this location, so the needle is placed in the subcutaneous space.
- These blocks can be performed with the horse standing or with the limb held.

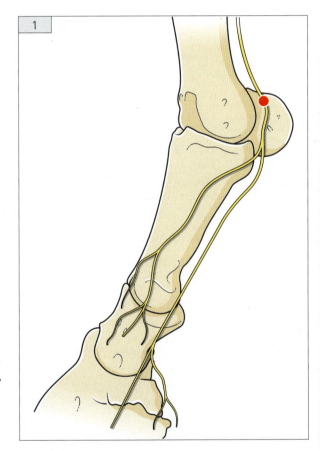

6.1 Schematic representing the lateral location of an abaxial sesamoid nerve block (red dot) to desensitize the lateral palmar/plantar nerves.

Complications

Complications with perineural analgesia are uncommon. The most common complication is failure of the block to be effective, in which case it can be repeated.

Rarely, a needle may break off and be retained in the subcutaneous tissue if the horse moves suddenly. If this occurs, the needle should be retrieved.

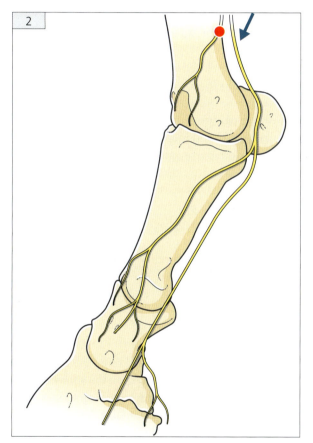

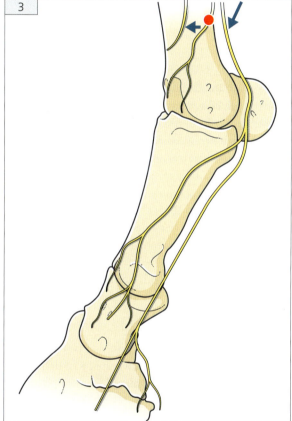

6.2 Schematic representing the lateral location of a 4-point nerve block. The arrow indicates the area to desensitize the lateral palmar nerve, which is located next to the deep digital flexor tendon. The red dot represents the location directly below the button of the splint to desensitize the lateral palmar metacarpal nerves. The procedure is also completed on the medial aspect of the limb.

6.3 Schematic representing the lateral location of a 6-point nerve block. The large arrow indicates the area to desensitize the lateral plantar nerve, which is located next to the deep digital flexor tendon. The red dot represents the location directly below the button of the splint to desensitize the lateral plantar metatarsal nerves, and the small arrow represents the location to desensitize the lateral dorsal metatarsal nerves. The procedure is also completed on the medial aspect of the limb.

Wound preparation
Indications
All wounds should be thoroughly cleaned and debrided.

Technique
- Sterile lubricant is placed in the wound to prevent contamination with hair and other debris during wound preparation.
- The skin in the region of the wound should be clipped and aseptically prepared. This includes the entire area of skin that will be covered by the bandage.
- The wound should be meticulously debrided with removal of all dirt, hair, and foreign material. A piecemeal approach is most commonly used for equine wound debridement. Gentle curettage can facilitate removal of debris from deep wounds. Necrotic appearing subcutaneous tissue can be debrided; however, **do not** remove any skin, particularly from distal limb wounds. It is often not possible to identify what portion of skin will live or die when treating a laceration. Therefore, try to use all of the skin present to close the wound; usually, even if some skin dies, it will serve as a bandage and allow development of a good granulation tissue bed underneath.
- The wound can be scrubbed with a chlorhexidine or povidone–iodine-based scrub and the scrub completely removed with sterile saline.
- The wound should be thoroughly lavaged, preferably with sterile saline.
- If the wound is extensive and severely contaminated, water and a hose can be used to lavage the wound and remove the gross debris.
- Alcohol should **never** be placed in a wound.

Complications
If hemorrhage was controlled with bandaging, it often recurs when the wound is cleaned and may necessitate vessel ligation with the horse standing, or re-bandaging and anesthetizing the horse for vessel ligation. Care needs to be taken during debridement to avoid further injury to vessels, synovial structures, and tendons or ligaments.

Synoviocentesis and synovial fluid analysis
(See also Chapter 2.)

Synoviocentesis and synovial fluid analysis is indicated as part of the management of any laceration potentially involving a synovial structure. The synovial structure should also be distended with 20–60 ml (depending on the size of the structure) of sterile isotonic fluid to determine if there is communication with the wound.

Suturing techniques
Indications
Wounds can be closed using primary, delayed-primary, or secondary closure or allowed to heal by second intention:
- Primary closure is defined as closing the wound following wound preparation and should be the goal of wound management.
- Delayed-primary closure is performed prior to granulation tissue formation and usually within 4–5 days post injury.[1] Delayed-primary closure is used to manage wounds with severe contamination, contusion, and swelling.
- Secondary closure is defined as wound closure following granulation tissue formation and is used in cases with chronic, severely contaminated, or infected wounds.[1]

Technique
- Equine wounds can be closed using 2-0 to #2 suture material depending on the animal's size, wound location, and type of laceration. Monofilament, synthetic non-absorbable suture material (e.g. polypropylene, nylon) is used most often to appose the skin. Use of bright colored suture material, if available, is recommended for use in the distal limb. Synthetic monofilament absorbable suture material (e.g. polydiaxanone, polyglyconate, poliglecaprone 25) can be used on

the distal limb, ventral abdomen, inguinal area, or in any horse that is difficult to handle to avoid the need for suture removal. Long tags should be left in these locations if non-absorbable suture material is used. If a cast is to be applied to the limb for longer than 2 weeks, use of absorbable suture material is recommended.

- Large vertical mattress (**6.4A, B**) or near-far–far-near (**6.5**) suture patterns can be used to bring the wound edges into close proximity if wound apposition results in tension at the wound edges. Stents or quills can be made using extension set tubing cut into 5–10 mm pieces (**6.4A**), Penrose drain, or gauze (**6.4B**) to increase the surface area over which the load is distributed and prevent the suture material from tearing through the skin.

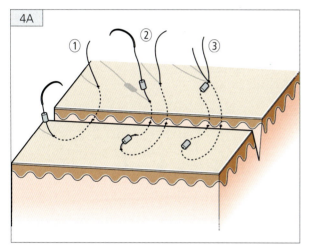

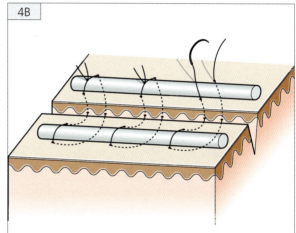

6.4A, B Large vertical mattress suture pattern with stents or quills made from extension tubing (A) or rolled gauze (B).

6.5 Near-far–far-near suture pattern.

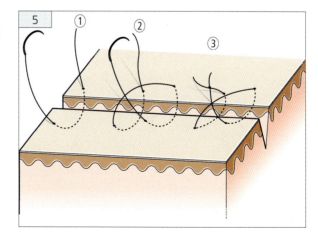

- Once the wound edges are in close proximity, simple interrupted (**6.6**), cruciate (**6.7**), or vertical mattress (**6.8**) suture patterns can be used to appose the wound edges.
- For example, the technique described can be used to repair partial degloving (**6.9**) and heel bulb (**6.10**) lacerations.

Complications

The most common complications following wound repair are infection and dehiscence. These complications can be avoided to some degree by meticulously preparing and debriding the wound, using tension-relieving suture patterns and appropriately sized suture material, providing adequate wound drainage, immobilizing the wound, and keeping the wound clean during the early healing phase. Judicious use of anti-inflammatory and antimicrobial drugs is also recommended. When a wound infection occurs, drainage should be provided by removing some of the skin sutures and the wound kept clean and dry. Bacterial culture and sensitivity testing is indicated if the infection is severe. In the case of a wound that continues to drain, a foreign body (e.g. piece of devitalized bone or tendon, or wood) should be considered.

Skin staples
Indications
Skin staples are indicated to appose small skin wounds where the wound edges are not under tension (e.g. head, back). Staples are easy to apply, but can be relatively expensive.

Technique
- Forceps are used to pull the skin edges together. The arrow on the staple instrument is aligned with the wound edge and the handle squeezed, releasing the staple.

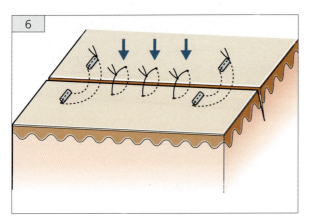

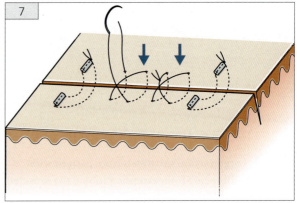

6.6 Simple interrupted suture pattern (arrows) used to appose the skin in between tension-relieving vertical mattress sutures.

6.7 Cruciate suture pattern (arrows) used to appose the skin in between tension-relieving vertical mattress sutures.

6.8 Vertical mattress or split thickness vertical mattress suture pattern (arrows) used to appose the skin between tension-relieving vertical mattress sutures.

- Staples should be placed about 5–10 mm apart depending on the wound configuration.
- Staples can be removed with commercially available staple removers or by placing a closed hemostat under the staple and then opening the hemostat.

Complications

Wound dehiscence is the most common complication. Staples may be of inadequate strength to hold the skin edges together, in which case they can be replaced with suture material.

Wound drains
Indications

Drains are used in traumatic wounds when there is a large volume of dead space that would delay wound healing and potentiate infection (**6.11**). Dead space results in accumulation of blood and serum, which inhibit healing by reducing the blood supply to the healing tissue, providing a medium for bacterial proliferation, and inhibiting bacterial killing by leukocytes. Drains facilitate the debridement phase of healing by providing a means of cellular debris removal; however, they should never be used in place of meticulous surgical debridement.

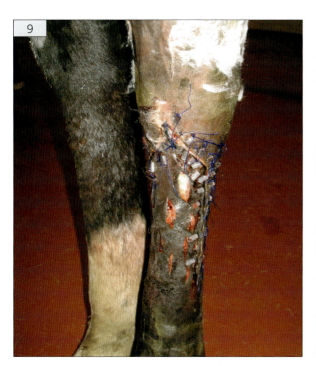

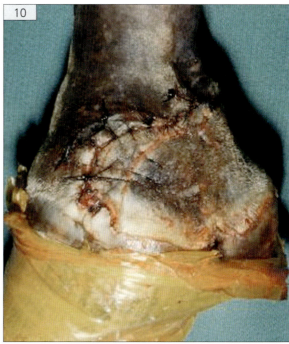

6.9 Large vertical mattress suture pattern with stents made from extension tubing used to appose a partial degloving wound of the metatarsal region. Note that stab incisions have been made in the skin to relieve tension on the wound edge as well as to provide drainage.

6.10 Large vertical mattress and near–far–far–near suture patterns used to appose a heal bulb laceration.

6.11 Penrose drains used in an extensive body laceration (arrows).

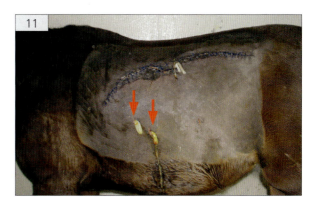

Technique

- Drains should always be placed and maintained aseptically and should be removed ideally within 48–72 hours (following the debridement phase of healing) or as soon as possible after drainage is minimal.
- Passive drains, such as Penrose drains, are generally used for traumatic wounds (**6.12**).
- Penrose drains are manufactured from soft latex, which does not cause discomfort, and drainage is driven by gravity and surface tension.
- Intraluminal drainage from Penrose drains is minimal and, therefore, fenestration is unnecessary and actually contraindicated because it decreases the surface tension and increases the risk of the drain breaking during removal.
- It is important to note that there is only an egress hole and not an ingress and an egress hole (**6.12**). The egress hole for drain placement is located at the most distal or most dependent area of the dead space.
- The drain should not be placed directly underneath the healing wound (**6.12**).
- If the dead space is particularly large, multiple drains may be used (**6.11**).
- The drain is sutured to the skin proximally and distally to prevent it becoming dislodged. It is recommended to use different colored suture material to that used to repair the wound because the sutures used to secure the drain will be removed prior to the sutures used to repair the wound.
- Patients are often treated with broad-spectrum antimicrobials (see Chapter 16 and *Box 6.2*) up to 24 hours after drain removal.
- Wounds with drains should be bandaged to reduce the risk of ascending infection.

Alternative methods for addressing dead space and drainage include: creating several small stab incisions in the skin (see Suturing techniques, **6.9**); leaving the most dependent part of the wound open to allow drainage through the wound; tacking the subcutaneous tissue together (this increases the amount of foreign material [suture] in the wound); or packing the wound with gauze soaked in dilute povidone–iodine solution. Packing should only be used during the debridement phase of healing (i.e. <48–72 hours) and should be replaced daily. Only material that does not fray should be used to avoid small pieces of packing material being left in the wound. All segments of the packing should be securely tied together (e.g. multiple rolls of gauze) to ensure that it is all is removed; it is not uncommon for wounds to drain chronically as a result of packing material being inadvertently left in a wound. Packing can be sutured to the skin at the point of wound exit using an interrupted suture.

Complications

Complications with drain placement include ascending infection, which can be prevented by keeping the site clean and avoiding leaving the drain in for a prolonged period of time. The drain can break if care is not taken during removal, resulting in a piece of the drain being left in the wound and necessitating removal. If the piece of drain is not removed, it will likely act as a foreign body potentiating infection, causing persistent drainage, and preventing wound healing. The drain may also become dislodged if it is not secured in place effectively. If a portion of a Penrose drain is left in the wound, a radiograph can be taken to identify its exact location.

Bandaging
Indications

Bandages are important for reducing edema formation and hemorrhage and protection of a laceration or injured skin from contamination and further trauma. They provide a favorable environment for wound healing and immobilization of wound edges to facilitate healing. Bandages with a wet-to-dry dressing can be used to enhance wound debridement. Stent bandages can be used at sites not conducive to conventional bandaging to protect small wounds from contamination and they can be used to reduce the tension at the wound edges.

Technique

- Conventional bandages consist of two major parts: (1) primary dressing that is applied directly over the wound and (2) secondary dressing that is applied over the primary dressing.

Primary dressing

- The primary dressing consists of a sterile, usually non-adherent semi-occlusive, dressing applied to the wound and secured in place using soft sterile conforming gauze (**6.13**). Non-adherent semi-occlusive dressings are typically applied to wounds where the skin edges have been apposed.
- Semi-occlusive non-adherent dressings allow movement of moisture away from the wound. Non-adherent dressings can be removed without disrupting cells and immature collagen on the wound surface. Semi-occlusive non-adherent dressings should be used when managing granulating or epithelializing wounds.

- Petrolatum-impregnated gauze can be used as an alternative to keep the wound moist.
- If the wound is open and still in the debridement phase of healing (days 1 to 3), a wet-to-dry dressing can be used. A wet-to-dry adherent dressing consists of fine mesh gauze that is saturated in sterile saline (+/- an antiseptic solution) and covered with a dry secondary bandage. When the primary adherent dressing is removed, the top layer of the wound is also removed and the wound gradually debrided.
- Occlusive dressings can be applied to open wounds during the early phase of healing prior to wound coverage with granulation tissue (days 2 to 6). While occlusive dressings are reported to provide a more suitable environment for migration and proliferation of fibroblasts and epithelial cells, wounds dressed with occlusive dressing have more exudate, exuberant granulation tissue, and delayed healing.

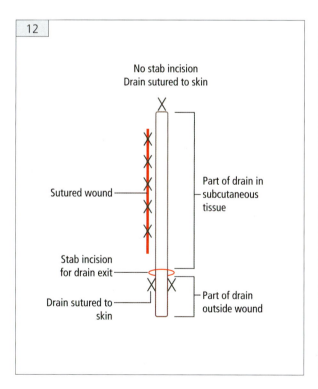

6.12 Schematic illustration of the principles of drain placement.

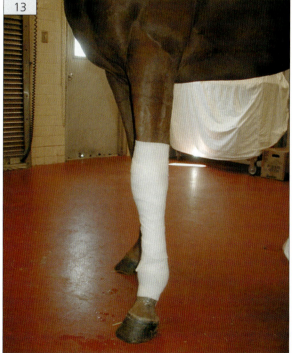

6.13 Primary dressing. A sterile non-adherent semi-occlusive dressing is applied over the wound and kept in place with soft sterile gauze dressing.

Secondary dressing

- Padding (secondary dressing) is applied over the primary dressing. This can consist of roll cotton, sheet cotton, or combine cotton (**6.14**). Roll cotton is less expensive compared with combine cotton and tends to slip less compared with sheet and combine cotton. Combine cotton, however, is easier to apply. Roll cotton is best when a heavy bandage with multiple layers is needed or under splints when immobilization is required. Roll cotton should be separated either longitudinally into two approximately 15-cm (6-in) full-thickness pieces or two half-thickness 30-cm (12-in) pieces to facilitate wrapping the limb. Padding should be at least 1 cm thick to ensure that boney prominences are protected. The amount of padding used will depend on the amount of wound drainage and the degree of immobilization needed. Padding should be applied evenly and snuggly.
- Non-sterile gauze is then applied to keep the cotton in place (**6.15**).
- An elastic bandage is then applied (**6.16**). An elastic adhesive bandage can be useful to secure the proximal and distal aspect of the bandage and prevent slipping, and to prevent dirt, straw, shavings, and fecal material getting under the bandage (**6.17**). Elastic adhesive bandage can also be used for the full length of the bandage.

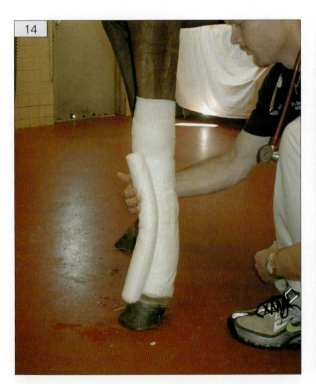

6.14 Secondary dressing. Combine cotton bandage padding.

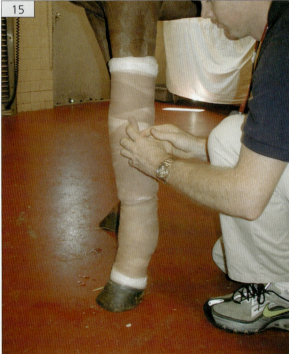

6.15 Secondary dressing. Non-sterile gauze used to keep the bandage padding in place.

Stent bandages

- A stent bandage can be made with rolled gauze sponges or gauze bandage material. An appropriate number of sponges or amount of bandage material should be used so that the stent bandage is not too large or too heavy for the wound.

- The stent bandage is sutured over the wound using #2 nylon interrupted sutures or by placing loops with #2 nylon on either side of the stent bandage and using umbilical tape threaded through the loops in a 'shoe lace' pattern to keep the bandage in place (**6.18**). The latter technique makes replacement of the stent bandage simple because the stent does not need to be sutured in place each time it is replaced.

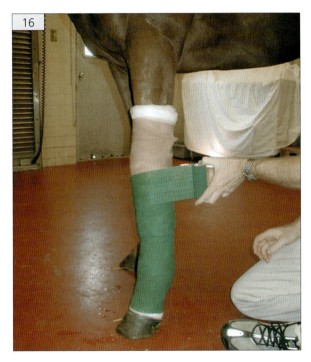

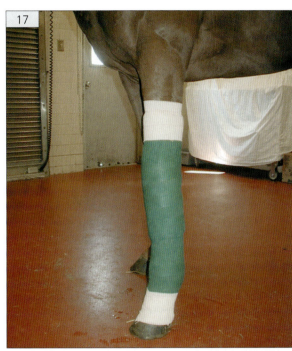

6.16 Secondary dressing. Elastic bandage material applied over the non-sterile gauze.

6.17 Secondary dressing. Elastic adhesive bandage applied to the proximal and distal aspect of the bandage.

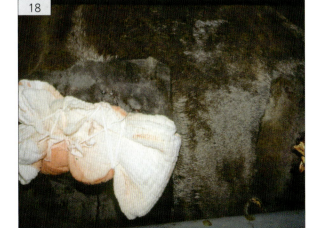

6.18 Stent bandage being used to cover a wound on the upper body.

Distal limb bandages

- Distal limb bandages extend from the coronary band to just below the carpus or tarsus.
- Bandaging is performed using a primary and secondary dressing.
- If the wound is very distal on the limb, the hoof should be cleaned and the hoof wall included in the bandage. The hoof should be covered with duct tape or other impermeable material to prevent wicking of urine and feces into the bandage.

Upper and full-limb bandages

- The carpus can be bandaged using padding either over the carpus alone or along the full length of the limb from the coronary band to just below the elbow.
- The padding component of the secondary bandage can be roll cotton or stacked combine cotton. When the latter is used, the distal limb is wrapped with combine cotton and then a second combine cotton is stacked proximally and slightly overlapping to cover the carpus.
- Following application of a padded carpus bandage, a release hole can be made in the elastic bandage over the accessory carpal bone to prevent pressure necrosis of the skin in this area. Some clinicians also recommend making a hole over the distal medial radius to prevent pressure necrosis of the skin overlying the bony prominence created by the distal radial physis.
- Tarsal bandages can be applied similarly to carpal bandages; however, the main difference is to avoid placing excessive pressure over the gastrocnemius tendon and the point of the hock. When applying a primary dressing to the hock region, the conforming gauze can be applied in a figure-of-eight pattern around the point of the hock, with the crossing of the eight over the cranial aspect of the hock and leaving the point of the hock out of the bandage.

Head bandages

- While bandaging of the head is often unnecessary, it is imperative that it is performed well to prevent complications associated with dislodgement as well as provide adequate wound protection. A poorly bandaged head can cause respiratory tract obstruction associated with slipping and occlusion of the nares, distress associated with the horse being unable to see because the bandage has moved and is covering the eyes, and wound complications such as hemorrhage, dehiscence, and infection.
- Types of bandages that can be used include:
  - Sterile primary dressing with secondary adhesive elastic bandaging material applied to create pressure at the wound site.
  - Stent bandages.
  - A light sterile primary dressing with a small piece of adhesive elastic bandage material applied with cyanoacrylate adhesive.
  - 15-cm (6-in) stockinet (with holes cut for eyes and ears).

Complications

Complications with bandages are uncommon *per se*; however, if the bandage becomes dislodged or is applied incorrectly, damage to deep structures such as tendons can occur and the wound will be inadequately protected, increasing the risk of infection and dehiscence. Lameness can be observed when the bandage is not placed correctly.

Cast application

(See also Chapter 2.)

Casts are primarily indicated for immobilization of distal limb lacerations in highly mobile areas (e.g. heel bulb lacerations and lacerations over the dorsal aspect of the fetlock joint).

Regional limb perfusion

(See also Chapter 2.)

Regional limb perfusion is indicated for local delivery of antimicrobial drugs to distal limb lacerations involving deeper structures.

Skin scraping

Indications

Skin scraping is rarely indicated on an emergency basis; however, when horses present on emergency with pruritus, (p. 446) a skin scraping may be indicated to definitively identify mites as the cause.

Technique
- Using a #10 scalpel blade, the superficial epidermis is scraped from the skin leaving a small area of irritation.
- The scraped material is transferred to a microscope slide to identify the presence and type of mites (p. 447).

Complications
None.

Skin biopsy
Indications
Skin biopsy is rarely indicated on an emergency basis; however, if a horse presents with pruritus (p. 446) or crusting and exfoliative dermatoses, such as dermatophilosis (p. 448), dermatophytosis (p. 448), or pemphigus foliaceus (p. 451), a biopsy can be performed.

Technique
- A skin biopsy is performed using an 8 mm biopsy punch. The skin is desensitized using 1 ml 2% lidocaine and aseptically prepared. Sterile gloves should be worn.
- The biopsy punch is used to cut a circular piece of skin. Care should be taken to ensure the dermis and epidermis is included in the sample (i.e. full thickness). A scalpel blade or scissors can be used to transect the subcutaneous tissue attached to the sample.
- The site can be closed using 2-0 nylon in an interrupted or cruciate pattern. Several samples should be obtained from areas with varying stages of disease. Samples at the junction of normal and abnormal skin can be particularly useful.

Complications
If the biopsy site is sutured, local infection or dehiscence may occur. Local infection can be managed by removing the suture and keeping the site clean. The wound will heal well by second intention.

SKIN PROBLEMS

Lacerations and puncture wounds
Distal limb
Key points
- Hemorrhage associated with a distal limb injury should be controlled immediately.
- Successful management of horses with distal limb lacerations and puncture wounds is dependent on early recognition and treatment of affected deep structures.
- The wound should be debrided and closed once deeper structures have been treated.

Definition/overview
Distal limb lacerations and puncture wounds refer to injuries occurring at or below the level of the carpus or tarsus associated with disruption of the skin and subcutaneous tissue.[2] A laceration may be superficial involving only the skin and subcutaneous tissues (**6.19**)[3,4] or deep involving neurovascular structures and/or structures such as bone, tendons, ligaments,

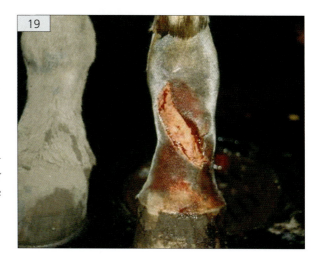

6.19 A superficial laceration involving the skin and subcutaneous tissue.

or synovial cavities (**6.20**).[5–8] A puncture wound refers to an injury that is penetrating and deep and often the skin wound is small relative to the wound depth (**6.21**). Lacerations and puncture wounds may occur concurrently with a single injury. Hoof puncture wounds are discussed in Chapter 2.

Etiology/pathogenesis

Lacerations or puncture wounds to the distal limbs in horses occur commonly. The 'fight or flight' response of horses predisposes them to injury. Horses live and work in an environment in which they can sustain lacerations or puncture wounds readily. Most lacerations heal successfully with minimal long-term

effect; however, this is largely dependent on the injured structures. Many horses sustain lower limb lacerations from jagged objects, such as barbed wire. These lacerations will cause a combination of uneven superficial and deep lacerations and puncture wounds (**6.22**). They may not lacerate all the way through a structure, but tend to infect deeper tissues more readily because most barbs will be contaminated with bacteria (gram-positive and gram-negative). When a horse sustains a laceration from a sharp object, such as metal, the laceration is usually sharp, dissecting, and deep (**6.23**). These type of injuries will often do more damage to deeper tissues such as ligaments and tendons.

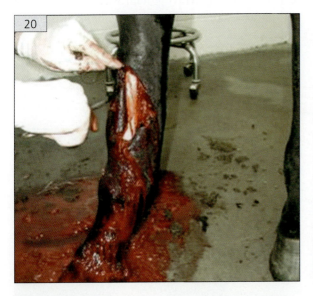

6.20 A partial degloving injury that extends through the common digital extensor tendon to the bone. (Courtesy Dr Ted Broome).

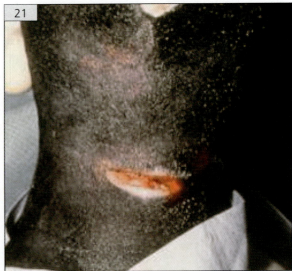

6.21 A puncture wound to the plantar aspect of the pastern region. The wound appears minor at the skin surface, but communicates with the digital flexor tendon sheath.

Horses may also sustain one or multiple lacerations secondary to limb entrapment in a solid structure. The depth and extent of the laceration and deeper injury depends on the type of structure in which the limb was entrapped (e.g. cattle guard, wire, or wood fence). Often, these horses will have a combination of lacerations and blunt trauma. The blunt trauma can often be worse because the ultimate effects (e.g. bone sequestrum) may not be visible for weeks after the trauma. The vascular supply to the distal limb can also be damaged as a result of this type of injury.

Clinical features

The clinical features will vary depending on the location, depth, and severity of injury. Two major clinical features are important with regard to emergency care of horses with distal limb lacerations: (1) hemorrhage and shock, and (2) injury to deep structures. Horses that have superficial lacerations involving the skin and subcutaneous tissue only usually have minimal hemorrhage or swelling; in addition, a painful or mechanical lameness is generally not a feature of these injuries. Physical examination of horses with superficial lacerations should be within normal limits.

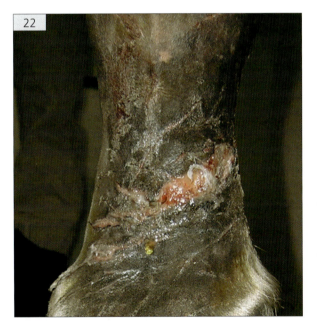

6.22 A laceration sustained to the palmar aspect of the pastern from a barbed wire fence.

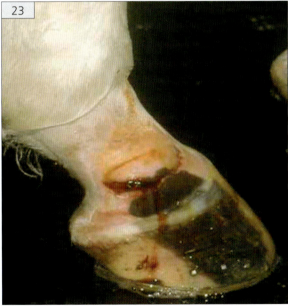

6.23 A laceration sustained to the lateral aspect of the pastern from kicking metal siding. The wound extends through part of the lateral collateral ligament and to the proximal interphalangeal (pastern) joint.

If the laceration extends through a vascular structure, severe hemorrhage may be present (**6.20**) (see Chapter 4). Horses with severe hemorrhage will often have signs of weakness, tachycardia, and pale oral mucous membranes. If the laceration is deeper, the horse usually has more swelling surrounding the laceration. Lacerations or puncture wounds that are infected will often have a local cellulitis or cellulitis of the entire limb. The horse's gait may be altered as a result of the laceration or puncture wound (**6.24**). This could be due to pain, instability, and/or infection.

Differential diagnosis

Fracture; cellulitis; myositis; septic synovial structure; abscess.

Diagnosis

A complete history should be obtained and physical examination performed on every horse with a distal limb laceration or puncture wound (*Box 6.1*).

A thorough physical examination should be performed to assess the horse's cardiovascular status, particularly heart rate, oral mucous membrane color and moistness, and CRT. Horses are often mildly tachycardic (50–68 bpm) after sustaining a laceration. Severe tachycardia (>70 bpm), particularly in combination with pale mucus membranes, should raise concern about blood loss or other underlying problems such as additional trauma. The oral mucous membranes should be pink; however, they may be tacky with a slightly prolonged CRT. The rectal temperature should be taken to obtain a baseline value and can be used to screen for infection associated with the injury if the duration of time since the injury is long or unknown or there is

another apparently subclinical disease (e.g. pneumonia, enterocolitis). The thorax should be ausculted and intestinal borborygmi assessed. Any signs of abdominal distension or colic should be noted because occasionally a horse will sustain a laceration during a colic episode.

It is necessary to examine the horse for lameness prior to administering sedation or performing local nerve blocks. Lameness examination should be performed with the horse at a walk only to avoid further damage to musculoskeletal structures. Lameness can be painful, mechanical, or both. The lameness can be classified as: none, if the horse walks normally; slight, if some asymmetry is observed; mild, if obvious asymmetry is observed; moderate, if the horse is able to bear some weight on the limb but has an obvious lameness; or severe, if the horse is non-weight bearing. A mechanical lameness indicates that deep structures are affected. For example, if the horse hyperextends its metacarpophalangeal joint, then it is highly likely that either the suspensory apparatus (including proximal sesamoid bones) or the superficial digital flexor tendon has been injured (**6.24**). If the distal interphalangeal joint is hyperextended (i.e. the toe flips up) then the deep digital flexor tendon function is affected (**6.24**).

The wound should be thoroughly examined. It is vital to determine what structures may be involved with the laceration since the more vital structures (i.e. synovial structures, tendons, ligaments, nerves, arteries, and bone) are involved in the wound, the worse the prognosis. This is where it is paramount for the practitioner to have a good working knowledge of the distal limb anatomy (**6.25**). Deeper structures that may be affected in horses with distal limb lacerations or puncture wounds include:

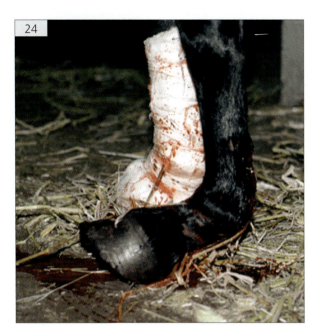

6.24 A laceration that has disrupted the superficial and deep digital flexor tendons. The horse demonstrates hyperextension of both the metacarpophalangeal and distal interphalangeal joints. Suspensory apparatus disruption would have a similar dropped fetlock appearance. (Courtesy Dr Ted Broome)

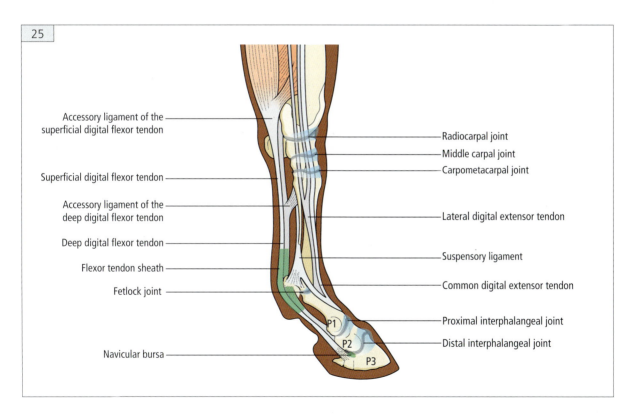

6.25 Distal limb anatomy showing the synovial structures (joints and sheaths), bones, tendons, and ligaments.

- Distal interphalangeal (coffin) joint (**6.26**).
- Proximal interphalangeal (pastern) joint (**6.23**).
- Metacarpophalangeal (fetlock) joint (**6.27, 6.28**).
- Tarsal or carpal joints (**6.29A, B**).
- Collateral ligaments (**6.23**).
- Ungulate cartilage (**6.26**).

- Digital sheath (**6.30, 6.31**).
- Superficial digital flexor tendon (**6.24, 6.32**).
- Deep digital flexor tendon (**6.24**).
- Suspensory ligament (body or branches) (**6.24**).
- Metacarpal (**6.20**), proximal/middle phalangeal (**6.33**), and carpal/tarsal bones.

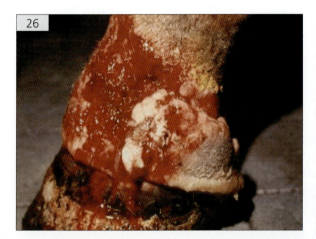

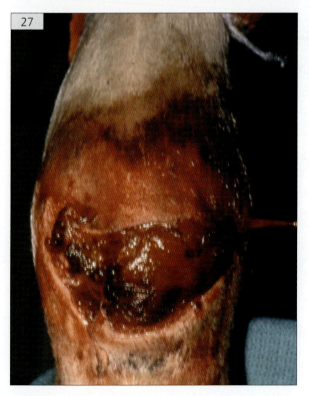

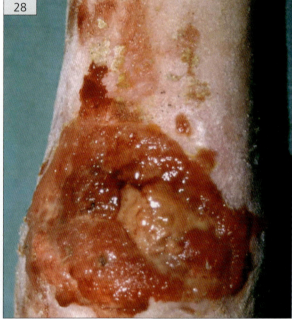

6.26 A heel bulb laceration that may affect the distal interphalangeal (coffin) joint depending on the depth and direction of the injury. The ungulate cartilage and pastern joint may also be involved in these types of lacerations.

6.27 A laceration associated with the dorsal aspect of the metacarpophalangeal (fetlock) joint.

6.28 A laceration associated with the palmarolateral aspect of the metacarpophalangeal (fetlock) joint and the proximal aspect of the digital flexor tendon sheath.

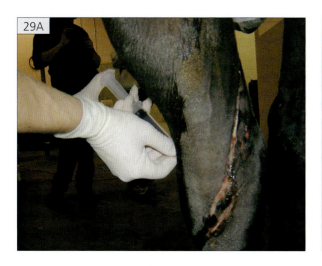
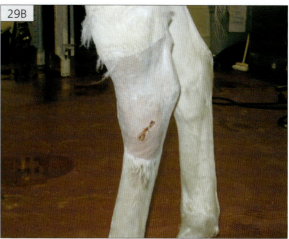

6.29A, B A laceration associated with the tibiotarsal (A, B) and possibly the proximal and distal intertarsal (B) joints. Arthrocentesis and distension of the tibiotarsal joint is being performed at a site distant to the wound to assess communication between the wound and the joint (A).

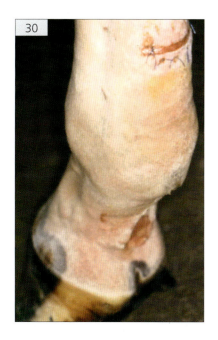

6.30 Lacerations associated with the digital sheath proximal and distal to the metacarpophalangeal joint.

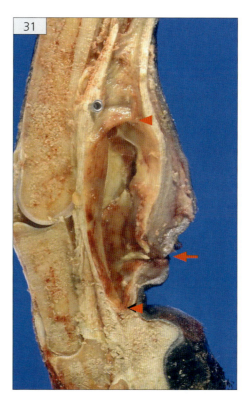

6.31 Necropsy specimen from a horse with a plantar pastern wound (arrow) that resulted in a digital sheath septic synovitis (arrowheads).

The wound should be protected with sterile lubricant. The hair around the wound should then be clipped and the wound and surrounding skin aseptically prepared. Digital palpation can provide basic information about the direction and depth of the wound as well as involvement of deeper structures (i.e. bone, joints, or tendons). The wound can also be examined using a blunt probe. The limb should be manipulated to assess damage to ligaments, such as the collateral ligaments stabilizing a joint, and different tracts that may become apparent with limb repositioning. Palpation of synovial structures can be used to assess joint involvement (i.e. if a synovial structure has effusion and associated subcutaneous edema, then it is likely involved); however, if there is no effusion, it does not rule out involvement but makes it less likely. Further diagnostics can then be performed based on the wound location and palpation findings.

Radiographs of the affected region should be performed to evaluate bone damage (**6.33**) or the presence of radiopaque foreign material. Radiographic examination using contrast material can be used to help determine the extent of the injury, communication with synovial structures (**6.34**), and the presence of foreign material by observing a space-occupying defect in the outline created by the contrast material. Radiography should be performed prior to synoviocentesis to assess the presence of air within synovial cavities, which indicates communication of the synovial cavity with the wound.

Sonographic examination can be used to determine the presence of foreign material and to subjectively assess the extent of structural damage to a tendon (**6.35A, B**), ligament, joint, or bone.

Assessment of synovial structures is necessary. The presence of synovial fluid or the palpation of articular

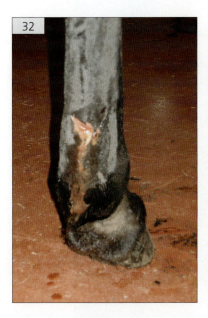

6.32 A laceration that completely transected the superficial digital flexor tendon. The laceration is proximal to the digital sheath.

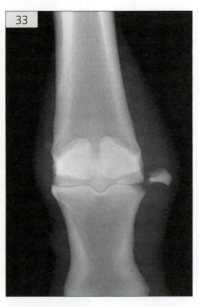

6.33 An avulsed fragment from the proximal lateral aspect of the first phalanx that is associated with a laceration.

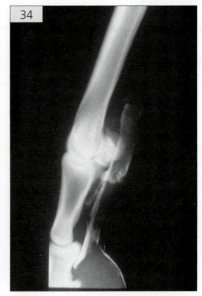

6.34 Contrast material injected into a wound illustrating involvement of the digital sheath.

cartilage or tendons within the digital sheath indicates synovial structure involvement. Occasionally, wounds can produce serum that is similar in appearance to synovial fluid. If synovial involvement is not obvious, a needle should be placed in the joint at a remote site from the wound and synovial fluid collected for analysis. The joint should then be distended and taken through a range of motion to see if the fluid exits the wound (**6.29A**). (See also Chapter 2: Septic arthritis and wounds involving joints, Septic tenosynovitis and wounds involving tendon sheaths, and Synoviocentesis and synovial fluid analysis.)

Hematology (leukocyte count and differential and PCV), TPP, fibrinogen concentration, and creatinine should be measured in horses with lacerations to obtain baseline values in cases where infection may develop,

monitor signs of blood loss, and to assess renal function prior to treatment with aminoglycosides and NSAIDs.

Management/treatment

Treatment of the laceration depends mostly on the location and the extent of deep structure injury. Hemorrhage should be controlled immediately using vessel ligation or bandaging. As a general rule, management of deep structures prior to addressing laceration repair is necessary. This may include lavage of a synovial structure (see Chapter 2: Septic arthritis and wounds involving joints and Septic tenosynovitis and wounds involving tendon sheaths) regional limb perfusion with antimicrobial drugs (see Regional limb perfusion), or repair of a tendinous injury (see Chapter 2: Flexor tendon disruption).

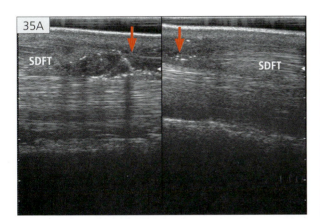

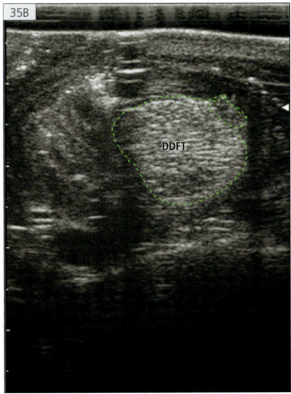

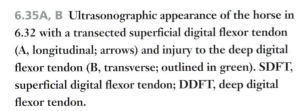

6.35A, B Ultrasonographic appearance of the horse in 6.32 with a transected superficial digital flexor tendon (A, longitudinal; arrows) and injury to the deep digital flexor tendon (B, transverse; outlined in green). SDFT, superficial digital flexor tendon; DDFT, deep digital flexor tendon.

It is best to attempt closure of almost all distal limb wounds (**6.36**) (see Wound preparation and Suturing techniques). Skin debridement should be avoided if possible. All available skin and soft tissue is incorporated into the repair and no decision is made with regard to the health of the skin flap. If the skin flap is unhealthy, a line of demarcation will become obvious within a few days and by this time healthy granulation tissue formation has usually occurred underneath the skin flap. Wound repair (primary closure) is recommended for many reasons: (1) repairing as much of the laceration as possible will provide a good soft tissue 'bandage' for deeper structures, such as exposed bone; (2) the more wound that is closed initially, the less area that needs to heal by second intention (second intention healing in the distal limb is complicated due to areas of high motion and the propensity for the exuberant granulation tissue formation); and (3) 'closing in infection' is rarely a concern since most wounds are contaminated at the time of closure, but not truly infected. If the site becomes infected, the sutures can be removed.

Bandages (p. 416) should be placed on all distal limb lacerations following repair. Splint or cast application may be necessary if the wound is over a highly mobile joint (see Chapter 2). Topical treatment is not usually applied. Systemic antimicrobial drugs should be administered, particularly in cases with deep structure involvement. Antimicrobial drugs should be administered immediately prior to wound debridement and closure. The duration of antimicrobial drug treatment depends on the extent of injury and should be unnecessary during the postoperative period in the case of superficial wounds.

Upper limb and body
Key points
- Lacerations to the upper limb and body heal well (eventually).
- The horse should be assessed thoroughly for deep structure involvement and the wound evaluated for any remaining foreign material.

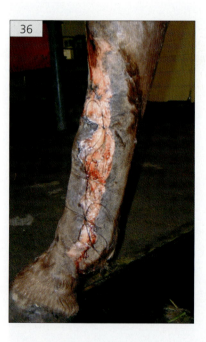

6.36 A distal limb laceration in which as much reapposition as possible was performed to protect the exposed bone and minimize the amount of area that needs to heal by second intention. (Courtesy Dr Ted Broome)

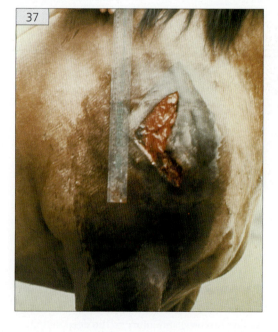

6.37 A full-thickness skin laceration to the upper limb that did not involve deep structures. This type of laceration will respond well to wound debridement, lavage, and primary closure. (Courtesy Dr Ted Stashak)

- Penetration of the thoracic or abdominal cavity is life-threatening and appropriate emergency treatment is critical.

Definition/overview

Lacerations to the upper limb (**6.37**) include those occurring above the carpus or tarsus and although these lacerations can on occasion be extensive and deep, they generally heal well. Proximal, cranial, antebracheal, lacerations and lacerations in the stifle region are among the most common upper limb lacerations. Puncture wounds can also occur to these regions and can affect underlying bone and joints (i.e. elbow, shoulder, stifle, and rarely hip joints). Similarly, lacerations to the body are often quite extensive (**6.37–6.42**) and are commonly in the axillary, pectoral, thoracic, and abdominal regions and in some cases can affect the underlying cavities (i.e. thoracic and abdominal) and organs (e.g. heart, lung, liver, spleen, diaphragm, and GI tract).[8,9]

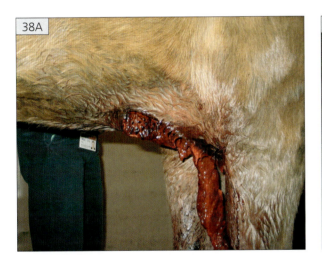

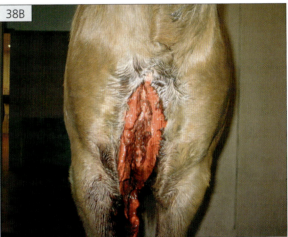

6.38A, B A laceration to the axilla and ventral thorax. The laceration extended approximately 60 cm in depth in a caudo-dorsal direction. The thoracic cavity was not penetrated. Lateral (cranial to right) (A) and cranial (B) views are shown.

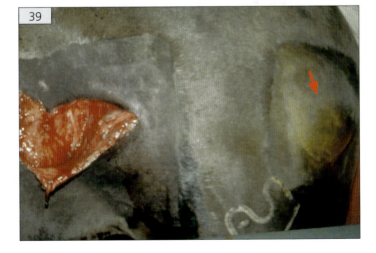

6.39 A deep puncture injury sustained when the horse impaled itself on a T-post. The head of the horse is to the left. The injury extended from the flank region (muscle flap) caudally (arrow).

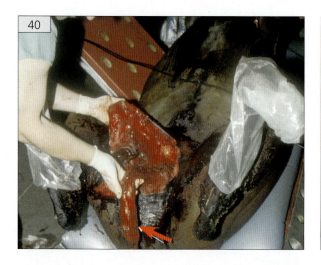

6.40 An injury to the inguinal region sustained by getting caught on a T-post. The penis (arrow) has been completely pulled out of its prepuce.

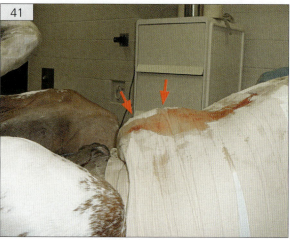

6.41 A laceration to the abdominal cavity with partial intestinal prolapse through the wound (arrows). A belly bandage was applied to protect the bowel from further injury. (Courtesy Dr David Freeman)

Etiology/pathogenesis

Lacerations to the upper limb and body occur commonly in horses. Most of these injuries happen when horses attempt to run through stationary objects (e.g. barbed wire or post and rail fence, stall door, or gate) or protruding sharp objects (e.g. gate hinge, bolt, or tree branch), are kicked by other horses, or misjudge the size of a jump. In addition, it is relatively common for horses to impale themselves on barn equipment such as handles from pitch forks, rakes, or brooms that are accidentally left in their stall.

Clinical features

The clinical features will vary depending on the location, depth, and severity of injury. Many horses will present with major tissue flaps that involve muscle, but do not extend deeper. Horses with injuries to these areas that do not involve deeper structures have minimal lameness; heart and respiratory rate, effort, and pattern are within normal limits; and oral mucous membranes are pink and moist and the CRT is <2 seconds.

The major considerations with injuries to the upper limb and body are: (1) hemorrhage (see Chapter 4 and Chapter 12); (2) mechanical lameness associated with extensive muscle injury (e.g. antebrachial injury with laceration of the extensor muscles of the carpus and distal limb); (3) penetration of or injury to deep limb structures (e.g. bone with fracture or septic osteitis/osteomyelitis or joints with septic arthritis); (4) subcutaneous emphysema, pneumomediastinum, and pneumothorax associated with axillary wounds; (5) thoracic cavity trauma or penetration with injury to the lung, heart, or great vessels, pneumothorax , hemothorax, and/or pleuritis/pleuropneumonia (see Chapter 3); and (6) abdominal cavity trauma or penetration with injury to the GI tract, diaphragm, liver, or spleen, hemoabdomen, and/or peritonitis (see Chapter 1).

Horses with puncture wounds to the axillary (pectoral) or inguinal regions may be difficult to identify. Many of these horses will present with emphysema of their entire body (**6.42**). This occurs because these wounds tend to act as a one-way valve in which air is sucked in as the limb is advanced, and then passes through the tissue planes. In addition, if the wound extends into the thorax, these horses may be dyspneic with a rapid and shallow respiratory pattern. Horses with injuries involving the heart will be tachycardiac and may have an arrhythmia or murmur and signs of heart failure (see Chapter 4).

Horses with deep penetrating wounds into the abdominal cavity may demonstrate signs of colic and/or endotoxic shock secondary to injury or puncture of the intestinal tract. In addition, some wounds will damage the abdominal wall causing evisceration (**6.41**).

Differential diagnosis

Lacerations to the upper limb and body are usually clinically apparent.

Diagnosis

A complete history and thorough physical examination should be performed. Information that should be obtained from the owner, trainer, or veterinarian includes:

- Type of structure on which the injury was sustained.
- Amount of blood loss (estimate).
- Removal of foreign objects including the direction and depth of penetration.
- Medication administered.

Horses with a completely normal physical and lameness examination are unlikely to have deeper structures injured. Horses with substantial blood loss or with hemorrhage into a body cavity will have signs of dull demeanor, tachycardia (>60 bpm), and pale, dry oral mucous membranes. Horses with a non-displaced fracture of the radius or tibia are usually lame at the walk and horses with lacerations or an avulsion injury to the antebracheal muscles will have difficulty extending their carpus and distal limb. Horses with joint involvement may not be lame initially. The wound should be explored thoroughly. Hematology (leukocyte count and differential and PCV) should be performed and TP, fibrinogen, and creatinine concentrations measured. Diagnostic tests specific for some common lacerations are outlined below.

Upper limb: The wound should be explored digitally or using a malleable probe and the depth and direction of the wound observed. If the wound extends toward the bone, palpation of bone defects or fragments should be noted. Radiographs should be taken in any case with an upper limb laceration or puncture wound because non-displaced fractures are not uncommon with kick injuries, and joint involvement can be determined based on the presence or absence of air within the joint. Radiographic contrast material or a malleable probe left in place can be used to assess communication of the wound with deeper structures. Sonographic examination can be used in some cases to assess injury to deep structures. Synoviocentesis should be performed in cases where joint involvement is suspected. The presence of foreign material can be difficult to identify in deep wounds; wound palpation, repeated lavage and debridement, as well as radiographic and sonographic examination, can be used to identify foreign material.

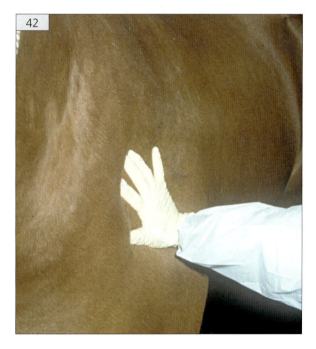

6.42 Subcutaneous emphysema of the entire body secondary to a deep axillary puncture wound. Cranial is to the left.

Axillary wounds: Axillary lacerations (**6.38A, B**) can usually be explored using a gloved hand. Care must be taken to explore the entire wound with particular attention to mediastinal and thoracic cavity involvement. Radiographic and sonographic examination may be necessary to explore the wound in addition to being particularly useful for assessing involvement of the thoracic cavity and associated organs.

Thoracic cavity: The respiratory rate, depth, and pattern should be observed closely in horses with penetrating wounds to the thoracic cavity. Respiration rate may be rapid and shallow, with signs of splinting. Rib fracture results in paradoxical movement of the thoracic cavity or flail chest (>3 ribs fractured in at least two locations). Rib fractures, as well as the initial trauma, can cause substantial damage to the underlying lung and heart and subsequent hemorrhage can be life-threatening.

Radiographic examination can be used to diagnose pneumothorax, rib fractures, and fluid accumulation within the thoracic cavity. Sonographic examination can be used to determine the depth of injury, assess damage to the lungs and heart, and diagnose pneumothorax or hemothorax. Rib fractures can also be diagnosed sonographically. It is important to determine whether any foreign body still remains in the horse (**6.43A, B**) and this can be accomplished with a combination of palpation and sonographic and radiographic examination.

Arterial blood gas analysis should be performed to assess oxygenation and ventilation and pulse oximetry can be used to monitor oxygenation in real time.

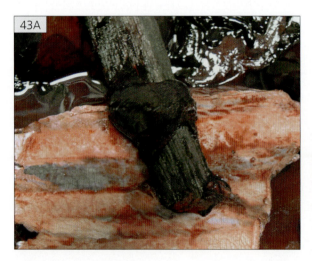

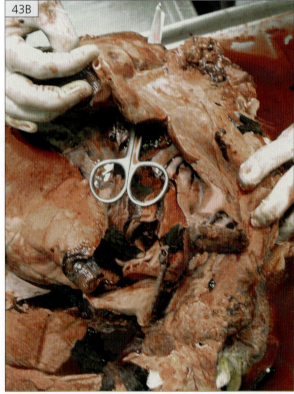

6.43A, B A piece of wood that penetrated the thoracic cavity (A) and became lodged within the heart (B). The wood was removed from the horse's chest; however, a large portion remained within the horse's thoracic cavity and had penetrated the heart. The scissors demonstrate the site of myocardial penetration.

Abdominal cavity: Abdominal palpation per rectum can be used to evaluate the caudal abdomen for viscus distension as well as caudal abdominal wall defects and herniation of abdominal contents through defects. Pneumoperitoneum can be appreciated with collapse of the rectal wall around the palpater's arm and a floating sensation because of loss of negative abdominal pressure.

Ultrasonographic examination can be used to assess the body wall defect, peritoneal fluid echogenicity that may be consistent with hemoabdomen, peritonitis, or contamination with ingesta, as well as diagnose pneumoperitoneum. Ultrasonographic examination can also be used to identify injured abdominal organs. Abdominal radiographs are unlikely to be useful in an adult horse.

Abdominocentesis can be used to diagnose hemoabdomen, peritonitis, and ingesta contamination of the peritoneal cavity.

Management/treatment

Most lacerations to the upper limb or body heal very well due to the relative lack of movement and good blood supply. However, many horses will sustain lacerations or major puncture wounds in these regions. Treatment depends mostly on the location and systemic status of the horse.

Some of these horses require immediate stabilization via invasive procedures such as a thoracocentesis to relieve pneumothorax or an exploratory celiotomy to diagnose and treat injury caused to the intestinal tract prior to addressing the laceration or puncture. Fluid therapy (see Chapter 12) (enteral or IV) is beneficial in many cases with extensive lacerations. Blood transfusion may be necessary in some cases (see Chapter 12). It is imperative to make sure that no foreign material remains in the wound. Some upper limb and body wounds can be closed primarily (completely or partially, **6.11**) or allowed to heal by second intention (**6.44**). Ventral drainage should be established (see Drains, **6.11**).

Antimicrobial drugs (e.g. trimethoprim sulfadiazine, ceftiofur, penicillin, and/or gentamicin) and NSAIDs are necessary in cases with extensive lacerations or deep puncture wounds. Antimicrobial drugs are not necessary in cases with small lacerations involving the skin and subcutaneous tissue only and their use should never replace meticulous debridement and lavage. The horse should be confined to a stall during the period of wound healing.

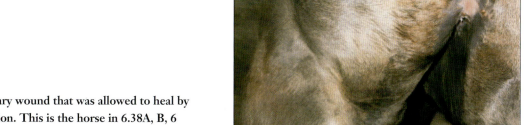

6.44 An axillary wound that was allowed to heal by second intention. This is the horse in 6.38A, B, 6 months later.

Upper limb: Upper limb lacerations should be debrided and lavaged (see Wound preparation). Muscle lacerations or avulsions where entire muscle bellies are transected can be repaired using large synthetic absorbable suture material in a vertical or horizontal mattress or near-far–far-near suture pattern. If blunt trauma was associated with the injury (e.g. hit by car), the muscle may slough and debridement may be necessary several days post injury. Synovial cavity lavage and local and systemic antimicrobial drug therapy is necessary in cases with joint involvement (see Chapter 2 and Chapter 16). All upper limb wounds should be closed as well as possible, but owners should be forewarned that dehiscence may occur due to the amount of motion present. These wounds can usually be closed at least partially using primary closure (see Suture techniques). Second intention healing, repeated debridement, and daily lavage may be necessary in some cases. Wounds that are healing by second intention become quite exudative. The skin below the draining wound must be protected from serum scald by frequent cleaning and application of petroleum jelly (Vaselin®) to the area. These wounds can be difficult to bandage. Small wounds can be covered with a stent bandage (see Bandaging). If bandaging is not possible, the wound can be left open and cleaned several times a day.

Wounds to the upper limb heal well with considerably less scarring compared with distal limb wounds. Occasionally, extensive muscle damage may result in an altered gait. A chronic draining tract may occur in some cases and is most often associated with foreign material, bone sequestration, or osteomyelitis.

Axillary wounds: Penetrating wounds to the axillary region that are not associated with substantial blood loss and do not penetrate the thoracic cavity can be managed in several ways. Gentle lavage is recommended to avoid pushing foreign material deeper into the wound. Stall confinement is important to minimize sucking and trapping of air into the wound, resulting in extensive subcutaneous emphysema and, in some cases, pneumo-mediastinum and pneumothorax. These wounds can be packed with gauze (e.g. 15-cm [6-in] rolled brown gauze), soaked in dilute povidone–iodine and knotted securely together, to eliminate dead space, prevent the entry of air into the thorax and/or subcutaneous tissues,

and provide a means for deep debridement of the tissue. It is absolutely critical to record the number of gauzes used to ensure that they are all removed. Stent bandages or adhesive drapes can also be used in an attempt to cover the wound. Extensive wounds, however, can be difficult to cover and packing often falls out. In these cases, the wound can be managed with daily or twice daily cleaning and lavage, strict stall confinement, cross-tying in some cases, and systemic antimicrobial drugs. Tap water through a hose can be used for daily cleaning of extensive wounds. Axillary wounds usually heal well (**6.44, 6.45**); however, they may take up to 6–8 months. A chronic draining tract may be associated with foreign material or a persistent deep infection.

Thoracic cavity: The site of a thoracic cavity penetration should be occluded ('plugged') immediately. This can be accomplished using packing and/or plastic adhesive drape or plastic wrap. In most cases of pneumothorax secondary to an injury that is managed with prompt wound packing, the pneumothorax resolves spontaneously with air resorption. Placement of a dorsal chest tube to remove the air may be necessary; however, in some cases patient stabilization involves intranasal oxygen (see Chapter 3) until patient oxygenation can be assessed, IV fluid therapy, and blood transfusion if necessary (see Chapter 12). Ventilation is not practical

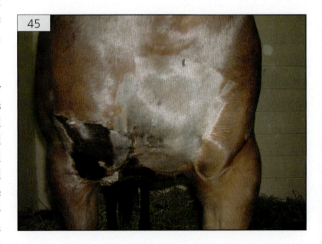

6.45 Healed axillary wound. This is a common location for deep punctures into the thoracic cavity.

except under general anesthesia in adult horses. Wound management can be performed following patient stabilization. These wounds are complicated by remaining foreign material, lung and heart injury, and pleuritis/pleuropneumonia (see Chapter 3). The prognosis is good if complications do not occur. Surgical removal of foreign material may be necessary following patient stabilization and initial wound healing. Horses with heart injury have a poor prognosis and euthanasia is indicated in most cases.

Abdominal cavity: Evisceration can be managed by sedating the horse following cardiovascular assessment. The omentum and small intestine are the most likely abdominal contents to herniate through a body wall defect. If omentum is occluding a body wall defect, it should be left in place until body wall repair is undertaken. Eviscerated intestine should be cleaned using sterile saline and returned to the abdomen and the abdominal wall bandaged. The defect can be temporarily closed using #2 or #3 suture material and/or be packed. Any packing should be secured to the skin to prevent it becoming free within the peritoneal cavity.

Antimicrobial drugs are indicated in any case where the peritoneal cavity is perforated. NSAIDs should be used conservatively because their use may delay early detection of fever or signs of abdominal pain. Fluid therapy, plasma, and/or blood transfusion may be indicated in cases of shock associated with endotoxemia or excessive blood loss.

Wound repair can be performed routinely on any wound that does not perforate the peritoneal cavity. In cases where the peritoneal cavity is perforated, wound closure can be performed with the horse either standing or under general anesthesia. The decision can be made based on wound location, risk of evisceration, availability of general anesthesia, and economic considerations. While general anesthesia will allow for better wound assessment, cleaning and debridement, and repair, there is a risk that the horse may tear the repaired tissue during recovery; therefore, meticulous surgical technique and bandaging is important. Based on the results of the diagnostic tests, abdominal exploration may be indicated and this is usually performed through a ventral midline celiotomy.

Head and neck
Key points
- It is important to thoroughly assess and determine all vital structures that are involved in head and neck wounds.
- After these structures have been addressed, the wound should be debrided and apposed.

Definition/overview
Lacerations and puncture wounds sustained to any location on the head or neck.[6,10,11]

Etiology/pathogenesis
Lacerations and puncture wounds to the head or neck can be life-threatening in a horse because they are often associated with severe trauma, such as running into a fixed inanimate object (**6.46**), flipping over, or car/truck

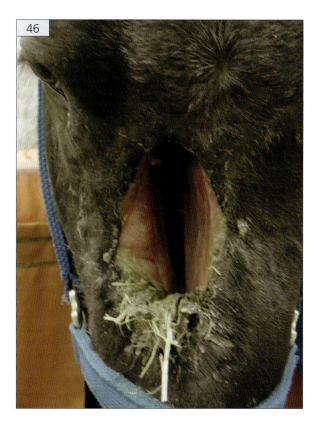

6.46 A horse that sustained a deep penetrating trauma to its skull by running into a stationary object. (Courtesy Dr Matthew Lane)

accidents (**6.47**). Many small head lacerations will be caused when horses that are in their stalls or tied to a trailer are startled and they react quickly by jerking their head. Often, they will lacerate themselves on the feeder, open windows, or other objects (**6.48**). Horses can also injure their head on a low ceiling if they rear upwards. Neck lacerations will often occur in horses housed on pasture with barbed wire fencing. Frequently, a horse will be found in the field with a head or neck laceration or puncture wound and the cause will be unknown.

Clinical features

The clinical features will vary depending on the location, depth, and severity of injury. Horses that have superficial lacerations of the skin and subcutaneous tissue will often have minimal hemorrhage or swelling. If the laceration is deeper, especially in the neck, there may be considerable hemorrhage. Neurologic deficits (especially CNs) present with both head and neck lacerations. Horses with lacerations of the head and neck may demonstrate secondary problems depending on the particular location and degree of further injury. Examples of this may be difficulty eating secondary to laceration of the tongue or esophagus, or fracture of the jaw.

Differential diagnosis

Lacerations and puncture to the head and neck are usually clinically apparent.

Diagnosis

A complete history and physical examination should be performed (see previous sections). It is imperative to determine the wound depth and extent of the vital structures that may be involved in the laceration. Structures that are commonly affected in cases with head lacerations or puncture wounds include: mandible or maxilla, which may be fractured or associated with incisor avulsion; sinuses (**6.46**), lips; tongue; nostrils; ear (**6.49A, B**); cornea and eyelids (**6.50A, B,** see Chapter 8)

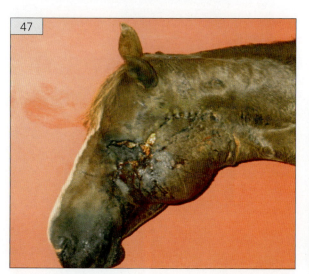

6.47 A horse that sustained severe head trauma and laceration after being hit by a truck.

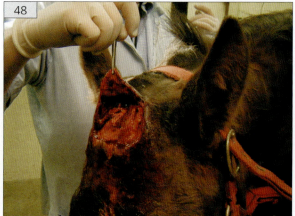

6.48 A horse that obtained a 'scalping' laceration from injury in the trailer. (Courtesy Dr Matthew Lane)

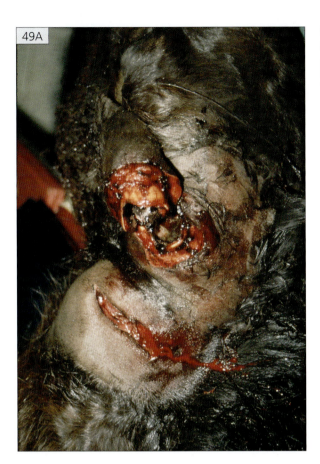
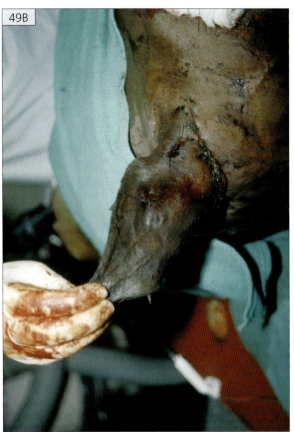

6.49A, B (A) Hemicircumferential laceration around the base of the ear involving approximately two-thirds of the circumference. The ear is bent in a rostral direction towards the top of the image. (B) The wound was debrided and the laceration repaired.

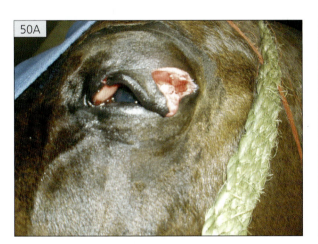
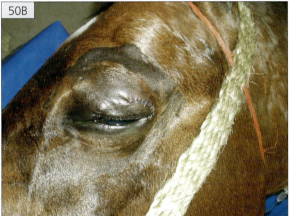

6.50A, B Eyelid laceration (A) and repair (B).

Neck lacerations most often involve the skin and muscle only; however, structures that could potentially be injured with neck lacerations or puncture wounds include: trachea, esophagus, jugular vein, carotid artery, vagus nerve, sympathetic trunk, vertebrae, and structures within the mediastinum and thoracic cavity.

Further diagnostics may be required including specialized examination of the eye and eyelid, sonographic and radiographic examination of the head and neck region, and endoscopic examination of the upper airway, guttural pouches, trachea, and/or esophagus.

Management/treatment

Treatment of the laceration depends mostly on the location and involvement of deeper structures. If the horse has suffered a severe injury to the head or neck, the horse should first be stabilized. Any deeper tissue trauma, such as fractures should be managed appropriately (see Chapter 2). In general, lacerations to the head heal very well due to good blood supply and inherent stability in most locations. Most lacerations can be apposed with one layer (i.e. skin) and often staples can be used instead of suture material. However, lacerations in locations with complex movements, such as the tongue, lips, nostrils, and eyelids, require closure in 2–3 layers.[11] Tongue lacerations can be particularly challenging to repair and require large full-thickness mattress sutures with stents to hold the tissue edges together, which can be combined with interrupted sutures apposing the mucosal edges. Large lacerations to the base of the neck can be difficult to close due to tension and many will partially dehisce because of the degree of motion. A martingale may be needed to limit motion. Deep puncture wounds should be debrided and lavaged, and ventral drainage established (**6.51**).

Antimicrobials and NSAIDs are necessary in cases of lacerations that involve deep structures and puncture wounds.

6.51 Puncture wound (arrow) associated with a piece of wood. The piece of wood was removed; however, the horse developed a severe anaerobic infection and was euthanized for economic reasons. It was difficult to establish ventral drainage in the wound at this location.

Cellulitis
Key points
- Severe limb cellulitis is a life-threatening condition requiring emergency care.
- Initial treatment involves broad-spectrum systemic and local antimicrobial drugs, anti-inflammatory and analgesic drugs, physical therapy, and laminitis prevention.
- The most serious complications are support limb laminitis and tissue necrosis.

Definition/overview

Cellulitis refers to a diffuse infection and inflammation in the subcutaneous tissue.[12] Cellulitis can occur at any location in the body and is often associated with an infected wound. Primary limb cellulitis can occur without an apparent wound and can be a severe and life-threatening problem.

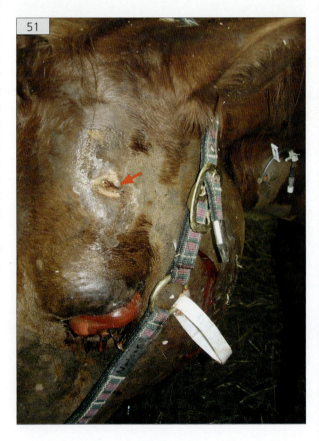

51

Etiology/pathogenesis

Cellulitis commonly occurs in association with an infected wound. Limb cellulitis can be primary or secondary. Primary limb cellulitis occurs without a history of skin penetration; these horses may have had a recent history of blunt trauma or dermatitis, but in many instances there is no known cause. Secondary limb cellulitis can occur following a wound, surgical procedure, or intra-articular injection.[13]

The most common organisms for primary limb cellulitis are coagulase-positive *Staphylococcus* spp. followed by β-hemolytic *Streptococcus* spp., *Escherichia coli*, coagulase-negative *Staphylococcus* spp., and *Enterobacter* spp.[13] Secondary limb cellulitis is most often associated with β-hemolytic *Streptococcus* spp., coagulase-positive *Staphylococcus* spp., and *Pseudomonas* spp.[13]

Infecting bacteria produce toxins that incite the inflammatory response through massive release of cytokines and cause tissue and vascular destruction. *Staphylococcus aureus*, for example, is one of the more common organisms involved and produces exotoxins including leukocidin (inducing leukocyte degranulation, cytokine release, and endothelial cell damage), toxic shock syndrome toxin-1, exfoliative toxins, and hemolysins ($\alpha, \beta, \delta, \gamma$), causing damage to erythrocytes, epidermal cells, and neurons, activating the arachidonic acid cascade, and increasing cell permeability.[12] The bacterial toxins and the patient's response to these toxins cause the clinical features observed with this disease.

Clinical features

Cellulitis is associated with swelling and edema, pain on palpation, heat, and redness. Severe limb cellulitis results in the limb becoming up to three times the normal size ('stove pipe'). A single limb is almost always affected and hindlimbs are affected most commonly.[13] Horses are markedly lame and the limb is hot and painful to the touch. Horses are often febrile and have a high fibrinogen concentration and normal or high leukocyte count.

Differential diagnosis

Septic synovial structure; osteomyelitis; lymphangitis.

Diagnosis

Radiographic examination of the affected area is recommended to identify any bone involvement. Ultrasonography is useful for differentiating primary cellulitis from a septic synovial structure and can also be used to evaluate the bone surface. Pockets of fluid accumulation can also be identified ultrasonographically and a sample of fluid collected for bacterial culture and sensitivity testing. Blood flow can be evaluated using Doppler imaging or flow-phase scintigraphy and may need to be repeated depending on the horse's initial response to therapy.[12]

Management/treatment

Aggressive therapy is required for severe cellulitis. Broad-spectrum systemic antimicrobial drugs are indicated (e.g. potassium penicillin and gentamicin) until results of bacterial culture and sensitivity testing become available. IV antimicrobial drugs are often necessary for at least 5–10 days and may be replaced with oral antimicrobials for up to several weeks' duration. Analgesia should be provided to encourage early weight bearing. Anti-inflammatory analgesic drugs (e.g. phenylbutazone or flunixin meglumine) are recommended. Other analgesic drugs include IV lidocaine, butorphanol, and epidural analgesia (e.g. morphine). Topical anti-inflammatory drugs (e.g. dimethylsulfoxide or diclofenac), hydrotherapy, and bandaging should also be used.

The skin can become devitalized and suppurate or slough. Laminitis, septic tendinitis or desmitis, thrombosis, bacteremia, and osteomyelitis are complications.[12]

The prognosis is fair to good for primary limb cellulitis and good to excellent for secondary limb cellulitis. Recurrence can be a problem. Horses can return to their intended use; however, the limb may not return to its normal contour.[13]

Thermal and chemical injuries
Burns
Key points
- Cool the burn site with running water.
- Protect the burn site(s).
- Administer fluid therapy.
- Analgesia is critical.
- Antimicrobial drug therapy is important for preventing infection.
- Owners need to be aware that the convalescent time may be long, the cost will be high, and the horse will be painful throughout the treatment process.

Definition/overview
Burns are defined, based on the cause, as thermal, chemical, or freeze. Burns are classified according to the depth of injury (grade 1 to 4) as well as the percentage of skin surface area affected.[14–16]

Etiology/pathogenesis
Burns are relatively uncommon in horses. Most burns requiring emergency care are sustained from barn or grass fires. Burns can be sustained to the skin from fire, heated objects or solutions, friction (e.g. rope), lightning strike or electricity, or sun exposure.[15] Chemical burns can be caused by overstrength topical medication, acids, alkalis, or other inappropriate chemicals (e.g. engine oil). Freeze burns are uncommon in horses and most often occur with freeze branding. The location of the wound can often be used to determine the etiology (e.g. grass fires often cause extensive limb burn injuries).

The extent of injury sustained from burns is related to the temperature and duration of exposure, and the regional blood supply. The injury location is also important (e.g. a mild corneal burn may result in loss of the affected eye or a distal limb burn may lead to loss of limb function depending on the deep structures affected). The initial skin injury will develop into three basic zones:
- Central zone of coagulation closest to the heat source.
- Intermediate zone of vascular stasis surrounding the central zone of coagulation.
- Outer zone of hyperemia.

Local tissue damage results from massive protein coagulation and cell death. Tissue ischemia can continue for 24–48 hours after the initial injury and the extent of the injury may not be apparent until later. Extensive full-thickness skin damage results in exudation with fluid and protein loss. Tissue necrosis results in delayed wound healing with a predisposition to infection.

In addition to the skin damage, most thermal injury patients have some degree of burn-related shock and smoke inhalation injury (see Chapter 3). Thermal injury-related shock resembles hypovolemic shock with a dramatic local and systemic increase in permeability of the capillaries resulting in fluid loss to the extracellular space and a decrease in cardiac output due to circulating myocardial depressant factors. This decrease in blood volume and cardiac output leads to increases in peripheral and pulmonary vascular resistance, resulting in decreased tissue perfusion and ultimately organ system failure. Smoke inhalation injury develops due to direct thermal injury of the airway resulting in edema and upper airway obstruction, combined with carbon monoxide poisoning and chemical insult. The carbon monoxide will interfere with oxygen delivery to the tissues. Chemical insult is related to the materials that are burned. Injury to the lower airway will occur due to chemical-covered carbon particles attaching to airway mucosa leading to peribronchial edema, mucosal sloughing, and bronchoconstriction. Neutrophil function of burned horses is compromised, making the horse predisposed to infection of the burn wound as well as the lower airway.

Clinical features

Clinical features vary based on the injury location, the surface area affected, and the depth of injury. The amount of injury is based on an estimate on the percentage of surface area of the skin that is affected (*Table 6.1*) combined with the depth (or degree) of injury (*Table 6.2*; **6.52–6.55**). Wound depth often varies across the affected skin.

Most horses sustain burn injuries on their back and face (**6.52–6.55**). Horses are usually lethargic, relatively reluctant to move, and febrile. Coughing secondary to smoke inhalation injury may be apparent (see Chapter 3). Blepharospasm, epiphora, or both may be present if ocular injury has occurred. The wounds may be extremely pruritic, causing the horse to demonstrate self-mutilation behavior.

Table 6.1 Classification of burn injuries based on the percentage of skin surface affected ('Rule of Nine')[17]

SITE	% SKIN SURFACE AREA
Forelimb	
Left	9
Right	9
Hindlimb	
Left	18
Right	18
Head	9
Neck	9
Thorax	9
Abdomen	9

Table 6.2 Classification of burn injuries based on depth of skin injury[14-16,18,19]

DEGREE	SKIN LAYERS	CLINICAL FEATURES	OUTCOME
First	Superficial epidermis (not germinal layer)	Painful; erythema, edema, desquamation of superficial skin layers	Heal without complication; no exudation; no scarring; good prognosis
Second	Superficial epidermis (stratum corneum, stratum granulosum, superficial basal layer)	Painful; erythema, edema, epidermal necrosis and sloughing	Heal rapidly within 2 weeks with minimal scarring
	Deep epidermis (all epidermal layers including basal layer)	Minimal pain; erythema and edema, epidermal necrosis, accumulation of leukocytes at basal layer of burn, eschar (slough from thermal injury) formation	Exposure of the dermis results in slow healing and scarring. May heal spontaneously within 3–4 weeks if care is taken to prevent further damage. Grafting may be necessary
Third	Dermal and epidermal layers plus adnexa (i.e. blood vessels and hair follicles)	No pain (loss of cutaneous sensation); white to black color; marked cellular response; eschar formation; substantial fluid and protein loss; shock; bacteremia and septicemia	Heal by contraction and epithelialization. Grafting may be necessary. Heal with scarring. Complicated by infection
Fourth	All skin, underlying muscle, bone, ligaments, fat, fascia	See third-degree burns	See third-degree burns. If on distal limb, euthanasia recommended because of loss of limb function

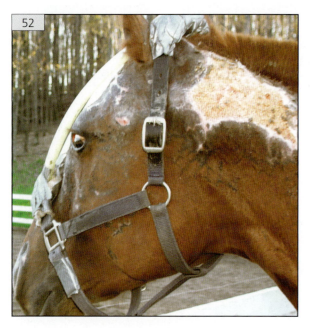

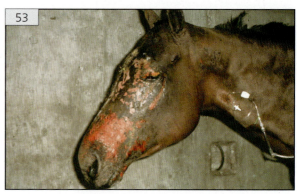

6.52 A horse that sustained first- and second-degree burns to its face and neck. Note the cicatricial ectropion of the right eye. (Courtesy Dr Dennis Brooks)

6.53 A horse that sustained a second-degree burn injury to its face. (Courtesy Dr Alioso Bueno)

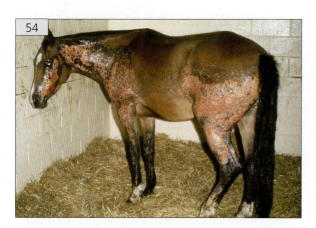

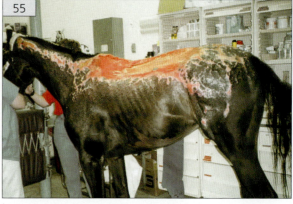

6.54 A horse that sustained second-degree burns to its face, neck, and limbs.

6.55 A horse that sustained a third-degree burn injury to its back. (Courtesy Dr Alioso Bueno)

Differential diagnosis
Thermal burn; chemical burn.

Diagnosis
A complete physical examination, with special focus on the cardiovascular and pulmonary status of the horse, should be performed prior to evaluating the burn.

It is usually difficult to assess accurately the amount of tissue damage because further damage will occur. The burn should be evaluated for the presence or absence of erythema, edema, and pain, which usually indicate viable tissue. In addition, the amount of blistering, eschar formation, and presence of infection should be assessed.

Hematology and serum or plasma biochemistry should be evaluated. Burn patients are often hypoproteinemic because of exudation from the burn wounds as well as loss of albumin from the intravascular space. Fibrinogen or serum amyloid A concentration should be measured initially to obtain a baseline value that can be used to monitor infection and also as an early indication of coagulopathy (hypofibrinogenemia). Similarly, leukocyte count and differential should be monitored. Electrolyte status should be checked regularly. Hyperkalemia is common as a consequence of massive cellular necrosis. Anemia occurs as a consequence of intravascular haemolysis and bone marrow suppression.[15] Thrombocytopenia is also common in patients with extensive burn injury. Blood lactate and serum or plasma creatinine concentrations can be used to assess tissue perfusion (see Chapter 11). Hemoglobinuria and renal failure can also occur; therefore, plasma or serum creatinine and BUN concentrations should be measured and monitored and urinalysis performed.

Thoracic radiographs and arterial blood gas analysis may be indicated as well as a complete ophthalmic examination.

Management/treatment

Burns should be treated immediately with cold running water for at least 15 minutes to prevent ongoing thermal injury and tissue necrosis because the skin is slow to dissipate heat. Once the skin is cooled, the burn wound can be lavaged with 0.05% sterile chlorhexidine solution. Water-based antimicrobial ointments (e.g. silver sulfadiazine) should be used to prevent loss of moisture and heat, as well as prevent against bacterial invasion. Full-thickness burns should be covered immediately with a fluid-proof dressing and a hydrogel applied to the wound.[15]

Initial assessment and management of burn patients should be directed at the cardiovascular and pulmonary status of the horse (see Chapter 3). An IV catheter should be placed and large volumes of balanced electrolyte solution (approximately 3–4 ml/kg for each percent surface area burned)[15] administered as soon as possible to prevent multiple organ system failure and bacterial translocation and sepsis from the intestinal tract. Airway patency needs to be identified and oxygen provided (see Chapter 3). The cardiovascular and pulmonary status needs to be monitored continuously and reassessed to determine the necessary changes. Plasma or a synthetic colloid is often necessary to maintain colloid oncotic pressure (COP) and may also have other benefits (see Chapter 12).

Analgesia is critical (see Chapter 14). NSAIDs can be used (e.g. phenylbutazone 2–4 mg/kg q12–24h, or flunixin meglumine 1.1 mg/kg q12h). Narcotics may also be used including butorphanol CRI and fentanyl patches. Other analgesics can also be used such as lidocaine and ketamine (see Chapter 14).

Assessment of the wound should involve clipping the surrounding hair and debriding devitalized skin; this is often performed after 24–36 hours. Necrosis can continue for several days to weeks and the extent of injury to deep structures (e.g. tendons and bone) may not be apparent for some time. Further treatment of the skin injury depends on the depth of injury. First-degree burns require only topical therapy and cold water baths as well as pain management. These wounds will heal without complication. Second-degree wounds can have blisters partially excised after the first 36–48 hours and topical dressing applied; however, the benefit of draining blisters is controversial.[15] Most second-degree burns will heal with minimal scarring in 14–17 days. Third-degree wounds can be treated in multiple different ways including use of occlusive dressings, wet dressings, open air exposure, or excision combined with skin grafting. One or all of these techniques may be utilized on each individual at some stage of the treatment. A non-adherent and absorbent dressing is necessary because burn wounds are usually exudative; a hydrogel dressing is recommended by some clinicians.[15] Bandages should be firm to provide support and avoid slippage; however, they should not cause further vascular compromise.[15] An eschar should be left *in situ* and natural sloughing allowed to occur.[15] Pruritus is most intense in the first few weeks, so horses need to be cross-tied or sedated to prevent self-mutilation. Skin grafting is often necessary.[20] The horse should be monitored closely for signs of laminitis (see Chapter 2). Burns to the eyelids and cornea (see Chapter 8) and respiratory tract (see Chapter 3) should also be addressed.

Systemic antimicrobial drugs are rarely of benefit for preventing wound infection in burn cases because of local vasculature compromise. However, systemic antimicrobial drugs may be beneficial to prevent complications such as sepsis and pneumonia from smoke inhalation. Topical antimicrobials, particularly silver sulfadiazine, are recommended. Oil- or fat-based ointments should be avoided.

Burn patients are often in a negative energy balance and nutritional support with the addition of corn oil to a good quality diet and/or parenteral nutrition may be beneficial (see Chapter 15).

Before initiating therapy it is important to note that the depth of the injury is associated with morbidity and the percentage total body surface area involved correlates with the mortality. Horses with partial or full-thickness burns to more than 10–15% of the body have a poor prognosis[15] and euthanasia should be considered for those horses with deep to full-thickness involvement of >30% of the total body surface area. The overall health of the horse, initial care and treatment, structures involved (e.g. tendon and bone), and complications (e.g. shock, renal failure, pneumonia, impaction colic, and laminitis) all affect the prognosis.

Frostbite

Key points

- Sick and debilitated animals and neonates are at risk of developing frostbite.
- Severe frostbite requires rapid thawing in warm water followed by application of antibiotic ointment and corticosteroids.
- Surgical debridement should not be performed until a clear line of demarcation is observed.

Definition/overview

Frostbite describes the metabolic, cellular, and vascular changes and subsequent tissue injury that occurs when extremities are exposed to extreme cold.

Etiology/pathogenesis

Frostbite occurs when a distal extremity is exposed to extreme cold.[21] Cold temperatures inhibit cell metabolism and cause tissue dehydration, cell disruption by ice crystals, ischemia, and vascular damage.[21]

Clinical features

The glans penis, ear tips, coronary bands, and heels are most commonly affected. Sick and debilitated animals and neonates have the highest risk of frostbite. Pale skin is initially observed followed by erythema, scaling, and hair and pigment loss. Severely affected animals have necrosis and dry gangrene.

Differential diagnosis

Traumatic injury; thermal or chemical burns.

Management/treatment

Mild cases do not require treatment.[21] Severely affected areas require rapid thawing in warm water (41–44°C [105.8–111.2°F]). Antibiotic ointment and corticosteroids should be applied to the area following rewarming. Necrotic areas should be managed with topical wet soaks and systemic and local antimicrobial drugs to prevent sepsis. Surgical debridement should be reserved until there is an obvious line of demarcation between viable and non-viable tissue.[21]

Other skin diseases
Pruritus
Key points

- Pruritic diseases are rarely a cause for emergency attention.
- A complete physical examination should be performed to ensure that there are no other apparent underlying problems requiring emergency management.
- If the horse appears to be stable, most diagnostic tests can wait to be performed on an elective basis.

Definition/overview

Pruritus is the sensation to rub, lick, scratch, or chew.[21]

Etiology/pathogenesis

Causes of pruritus include parasites, allergic reactions, and bacterial and fungal infections.

Clinical features

Horses typically rub the skin or hair coat when pruritic. Broken hairs, excoriations, hemorrhagic crusts, and alopecia can be seen with acute pruritus and lichenification (skin thickening) and hyperpigmentation are observed with chronic inflammation and pruritus.[21] Severe pruritus can cause ulceration and oozing crusts. Urticaria (hives) may be observed.

Differential diagnosis[21]

- Parasites: lice; mites; ticks; *Onchocerca* spp.; *Habronema* spp.; pinworms.
- Allergic reaction: insect hypersensitivity; food allergy; contact allergy; atopy.
- Bacterial or fungal infection: dermatophytosis; dermatophilosis; bacterial folliculitis.

Diagnosis

Obtaining a thorough history, particularly with regard to other horses (and people) on the premises with clinical signs, and management history of the individual patient can help eliminate some causes of pruritus. Careful examination of the skin and hair with a good light source, use of a fine tooth comb to look for lice, skin scrapings, cytology, and evaluation of skin biopsy are used to differentiate the various causes of pruritus.

Parasites: Biting lice (*Damalinia equi*) feed on epidermal debris along the dorsolateral trunk, whereas sucking lice (*Haematopinus asini*) feed on blood and lymph and predominantly infest the mane and tail and hair behind the pastern/fetlock region. Lice infestation is more commonly observed during the winter months. Diagnosis of biting lice infestation is made by observing adult lice or eggs, or both, on the hairs. Combing the hair with a fine tooth comb may be required to identify the lice or eggs.[21]

Mite infestations (mange) usually cause intense pruritus and are often associated with specific lesions on typical areas of the body. They can often be diagnosed based on the location and type of the lesion as well as with microscopic examination of skin scrapings. Mite infestations are often highly contagious to other horses and some species can be transmitted to humans. *Sarcoptes scabiei* (scabies, head mange) infestation primarily affects the skin around the ears, but can spread over the entire body. It is a reportable disease and has zoonotic potential. Scabies mites are difficult to identify on skin scrapings. Treatment is recommended if scabies is suspected. *Chorioptes equi* infest the distal limbs and perineum. Infestation during the winter months and in Draft breeds is more common. *Psoroptes equi* infestation is also a reportable disease but the mites do not infect humans. Infestations begin on the forelock, mane, and tail and spread to the trunk. *P. equi* can infest the ear canal causing otitis externa with associated signs of head shaking and rubbing. Trombiculidiasis (chiggers, red bugs, harvest mites) is larval infestation of free-living adult mites from the genus *Eutrombicula* or *Neotrombicula*, which live in grasses, forests, or swamps in late summer and fall. The natural hosts are rodents. Papular lesions or wheals with a small orange or red dot (larvae) are pathognomonic and infestations typically occur on the face, muzzle, distal limbs, ventral thorax, and abdomen. Infestation with *Pyemotes tritici* (straw itch mite) occurs from contaminated hay fed in overhead racks (*P. tritici* parasitizes larvae of grain insects) and causes maculopapular crusted eruption on the head, neck, and trunk that are not necessarily pruritic. Diagnosis is based on history and appearance of the lesion. *Dermanysus gallinae* (poultry mite) nymphs and adults can infest horses, causing pruritic papules and crusts on the head and limbs. Skin scrapings and tape preparations should be performed at night because the mite feeds at night. Demodicosis is rare in horses and usually associated with an underlying disease (chronic glucocorticoid use or equine Cushing's disease). *Demodex equi* infests the body and *Demodex caballi* the eyelids and muzzle and are easily identified on skin scrapings.[21]

Tick infestations (*Dermacentor*, *Ixodes*, and *Amblyomma* spp.) are most common in spring and summer and occur typically on the ears, face, neck, groin, distal limbs, and tail. Definitive diagnosis is by observing the ticks on the skin or in the ear canal.[21]

Onchocerciasis (*Onchocerca cervicalis*) causes lesions on the face, neck, and ventral midline (especially the umbilical area). Onchocerciasis is non-seasonal, but may be more severe in spring and summer. Definitive diagnosis is by identification of microfilaria on a skin biopsy with mince preparation or histological evaluation.[21]

Cutaneous habronemiasis (*Habronema muscae*, *H. majus*, and *Draschia megastoma*) causes ulcerative nodules on the limbs, urethral process of the penis, prepuce, medial canthus of the eye, or any area of trauma in the spring and summer. Lesions partially or completely regress in the winter. Lesions may appear similar to exuberant granulation tissue. Cytologic identification of larvae and histologic evaluation of biopsy tissue (granulomatous dermatitis with large numbers of mast cells and eosinophils and foci of coagulation necrosis) is diagnostic.[21]

Pinworms (*Oxyuris equi*) cause perianal puritis. Identification on pinworm eggs on a cellophane tape preparation is diagnostic.

Allergic reactions: Horses can have allergic reactions to insects (common) as well as feed and contact allergies (i.e. plants, bedding material, insect repellents, topical medications, tack) (rare). Diagnosis is made based on history and physical examination findings, skin biopsy, and intradermal skin testing. Methodical elimination of various potential allergens from the horse's environment (with or without repeating the skin biopsy) and then brief reintroduction or exposure can also be effective in determining the source of allergic reaction.[21] Atopy, a rare inherited dermatologic or respiratory condition causing seasonal or non-seasonal pruritus, is diagnosed by eliminating other causes of pruritus and observing a positive response to corticosteroids, and confirmed with skin testing and serum allergy testing.[21]

Bacterial or fungal infection: Bacterial or fungal infections are typically classified as crusting and exfoliative dermatoses. Dermatophilosis (rain scald) is caused by *Dermatophilus congolensis* (gram-positive, facultative anaerobic actinomycete).[21] Lesions can develop within 24 hours and have a follicular orientation appearing as crusted, moist mats of hair (small paintbrush appearance) often occurring along the back, gluteal area, face, neck, and distal extremities. Dermatophilosis is diagnosed by identification of the organism based on cytologic examination of the crust or skin biopsy.

Dermatophytosis (ringworm) is caused by the dermatophytes *Trichophyton* spp. and *Microsporum* spp. The lesions have a follicular distribution and begin as papular eruptions with erect hairs and rapidly progress to crusted papules that spread circumferentially (classical circular patch of alopecia with stubbly hairs on the margin and scaling).[21] The most reliable tests for confirming the diagnosis are fungal culture and skin biopsy.

Bacterial folliculitis caused by *Staphylococcus* spp. and *Streptococcus* spp. can be clinically indistinguishable from dermatophytosis, but are more likely to be painful. Diagnosis is based on cytology, bacterial culture, and skin biopsy.

Management/treatment

Parasites: Sucking lice can be treated with ivermectin (200 µg/kg PO every 2 weeks for 3 treatments). Biting lice do not respond to ivermectin treatment. Sucking and biting lice can be treated topically with lime sulfur or pyrethrins (recommended because of fewer adverse reactions); also methoxychlor, malathion, coumaphos, crotoxyphos, pyrethroids, lindane, permethrin, selenium sulfide, imidacloprid, phoxim, and fipronil can be used according to the manufacturer's instructions.[21] Topical treatments do not eliminate eggs and should be repeated every 2 weeks for 2–3 treatments. All horses on the farm should be treated to eliminate lice infestations. Cleaning and disinfecting tack, grooming supplies, equipment, and stabling areas using a commercial spray used to kill fleas is recommended.[21]

Sarcoptes scabiei, Chorioptes equi, Psoroptes equi, and *Dermanysus gallinae* are treated with ivermectin (200 µg/kg PO every 2 weeks of 2–3 treatments). Topical treatments, including lime sulfur, lindane, coumaphos, diazinon, malathion, and toxaphene, can be used every 7–10 days for 3–6 treatments. All horses in contact with the infected horse should be treated and equipment and the environment decontaminated. Trombiculidiasis and *Pyemotes tritici* infestation are self-limiting; however, topical treatments are recommended in horses with severe pruritus (lime sulfur dips or permethrin, pyrethrin, cypermethrin, or phoxim sprays). Hay contaminated with *Pyemotes tritici* should be removed. The horse's contact with poultry should be eliminated in instances of *Dermanysus gallinae* infestation. Management of demodicosis involves treating the underlying disease and topical treatment with 2% trichlorfon every other day. Amitraz is contraindicated in horses because it can cause colic. Ivermectin or doramectin have been used.[21]

Tick infestation is managed by applying pyrethrin or pyrethroid sponge-on dips to the body (usually one treatment only is necessary). Knowledge of local resistance patterns to insecticides is important.[18] Otic infestations can be treated by removing the ticks with one part rotenone and three parts mineral oil twice weekly, or with a pyrethrin otic prepation for small animals.[21]

Onchoceriasis is treated with ivermectin (200 μg/kg PO) usually once, but some horses require 2–3 monthly treatments. Clinical signs should resolve within 2–3 weeks of treatment. Prednisolone (0.5 mg/kg PO) may be necessary for the first week after treatment in some horses.[21] Because ivermectin does not kill adults in the ligamentum nuchae, signs may recur necessitating repeated treatment.

Cutaneous habronemiasis can be treated with ivermectin (200 μg/kg orally) or moxidectin (400 μg/kg orally) in combination with topical treatment. Topical treatment includes various combinations of dexamethasone or triamcinolone, 90% DMSO, nitrofurazone, and trichlorfon.[21] Hypersensitivity reactions can be treated with prednisolone (1 mg/kg PO q24h for 10–14 days).[21]

Pinworms can be treated with ivermectin, fenbendazole, or pyrantel pamoate.

Allergic reaction: Once the source of the allergic reaction is identified, the antigen should be removed from the horse's environment. Insect hypersensitivity should be managed with insect control.[21] Hydroxyzine hydrochloride (antihistamine) (200–500 mg/horse PO q8–12h) can be given. Side-effects include sedation or hyperactivity. If hydroxyzine hydrochloride is ineffective, prednisolone (1 mg/kg PO q24h) can be given until the pruritus resolves (usually 1–2 weeks) then taper the dose to the lowest effective every-other-day dose.[21]

Feed-related hypersensitivity is uncommon in horses. Once the feed source causing the reaction is identified it should be eliminated. Oats and grass hay tend to be less allergenic compared with other types of hay. Similarly, contact hypersensitivities are rare and managed by identification and avoidance of the offending material or substance. Atopy is extremely rare and treatment involves corticosteroids, fatty acid supplements, topical treatments, and hyposensitization.[21]

Bacterial and fungal infection: Dermatophilosis is treated topically by gently removing the crusts and using mild antibacterial shampoo (chlorhexidine or benzoyl peroxide), antibacterial sponge-on dips (chlorhexidine 1:32 dilution of 2% chlorhexidine stock solution or 1:32 dilution of lime sulfur stock solution), or chlorhexidine 2% lotion. Severely affected horses may require antimicrobial drugs (e.g. procaine penicillin [22,000 U/kg IM q12h for 5–7 days], trimethoprim sulfa [10–30 mg/kg PO q12h for 5–days], or doxycycline [10 mg/kg PO q12h for 5–7 days]).[21]

Dermatophytosis is a self-limiting disease. Treatment with antifungal shampoos and sponge-on dips is recommended to prevent spread:[21] (1) 2% miconazole shampoo followed by lime sulfur dip or (2) lime sulfur dip applied weekly for 4 weeks. Miconazole and chlorhexidine shampoo followed by rinsing is also effective. Systemic antifungal drugs (griseofulvin or itraconazole) are effective but expensive. IV injection of 20% sodium iodine can be used, but not in pregnant mares.[21]

Mild bacterial folliculitis may be self-limiting. Severely affected horses should be treated topically with antibacterial shampoos and antimicrobial drugs based on the results of culture and sensitivity testing.

Photosensitization
Key points

- Photosensitization can occur as a primary disease or secondary to liver impairment (hepatogenous photosensitization).
- The distribution of lesions is generally restricted to non-pigmented skin and the eyes.
- The prognosis is variable, especially in cases occurring secondary to liver damage.

Definition/overview

Photosensitization is a severe dermatitis resulting from a complex reaction induced by plant pigments exposed to ultraviolet wavelength sunlight.[22] The reaction is most severe in non-pigmented skin due to greater ultraviolet light penetration. The cornea, conjunctiva, and exposed mucosa are also affected.[23] Photosensitization is distinct from sunburn.

Etiology/pathogenesis

Ingestion of numerous plants has been associated with the occurrence of photosensitization.[23] Ingestion of moldy feedstuffs has also caused photosensitization. The occurrence of photosensitization is often sporadic and, in many cases, the underlying cause is not apparent.

Two types of photosensitization occur. Primary photosensitization occurs following ingestion of a photodynamic compound or its precursor originating outside the body. The compound or a metabolite reaches the skin as a result of normal physiologic processes, either directly by absorption through the epidermis following topical exposure or via systemic circulation following oral or parenteral exposure.[23] Relatively few plants or known compounds produce primary photosensitization. *Hypericum perforatum* (St. John's wort (**6.56**)) and *Fagopyrum esculentum* (buckwheat) produce the primary phototoxic compounds hypericin and fagopyrin, respectively.[22,23] Consumption of moldy-appearing dead leaves of *Cooperia pedunculata* (giant rain lily) has produced primary photosensitization in cattle and deer in Southeastern Texas.[23] Other plants causing primary photosensitization include *Ammi majus* (bishop's weed), *Cymopterus watsonii* (spring parsley), *Heracleum mentagazzianum*

(giant hog weed), and *Thamnosma texana* (Dutchman's breeches).[22,24] Phenothiazine, sulfonamide, and tetracycline use has also been associated with the occurrence of photosensitization.

Secondary or hepatogenous photosensitization occurs as a result of underlying liver or biliary dysfunction. The phototoxic compound is phylloerythrin, a metabolite of dietary chlorophyll, which is produced by microbial action in the GI tract.[23] Impaired biliary excretion of phylloerythrin results in increased circulating concentrations of phylloerythrin. Hepatogenous photosensitization is the most common form of photosensitization and ingestion of many hepatotoxic plants or other compounds can be associated with the disease. Examples of hepatotoxic plants that can cause photosensitization include those containing pyrrolizidine alkaloids (*Senecio* spp., *Crotalaria* spp., *Cynoglossum* spp., *Amsinckia* spp.), *Lantana camara* (lantana), *Agave lecheguilla* (lechuguilla), *Trifolium hydridum* (red clover), and *Tribulus terrestris* (puncture vine) (see Chapter 10).[22] A paper has been written that gives an extensive list of plants associated with the occurrence of photosensitization.[23]

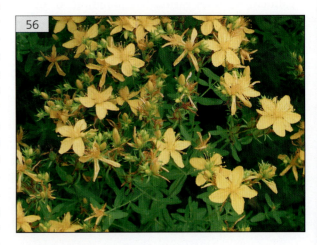

6.56 *Hypericum perforatum* (common St. John's wort) flowers. *H. peforatum* can cause primary photosensitization.

Clinical features

In horses, lesions are generally confined to white or light areas on the face, around the mouth, legs and coronary band, neck, underside of the abdomen, and on the udder (**6.57**).[23] Erythema, swelling, pruritus, exudation of serum, matting of hair, skin exfoliation, lacrimation, conjunctivitis, photophobia, keratitis, and partial blindness can occur. Vesicles and bullae can develop.[25] Skin lesions are generally more severe with photosensitization than with sunburn, but this is not always the case. Keratitis is also generally not associated with sunburn. This may be the only manifestation of photosensitization in animals with all-black coats.[23] Other signs referable to an underlying liver dysfunction, such as hepatic encephalopathy, can occur.

Differential diagnosis

Dermatitis: sunburn; irritant contact dermatitis. Liver disease: pyrrolizidine alkaloid intoxication; aflatoxicosis. Cholelithiasis: hepatic amyloidosis; chronic hepatic hypoxemia; chronic active hepatitis.

Diagnosis

Diagnosis is based on evidence of consumption of a primary photodynamic agent or detection of underlying liver disease along with characteristic clinical signs.

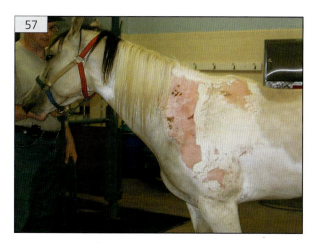

6.57 A horse with skin damage associated with photosensitization.

Management/treatment

Recommended treatment of photosensitization includes: (1) cessation of exposure to the source of the hepato- or phototoxic compound, (2) protection from direct exposure to sunlight, (3) treatment or prevention of secondary bacterial infection or fly strike, and (4) general supportive care including provision of good-quality feed.[23] Appropriate treatment of underlying liver disease also needs to be instituted. Topical or systemic glucocorticosteroids can be useful for controlling pruritus early in the course of the disease. The use of antimicrobial drugs can also be useful for preventing secondary bacterial infections. Gentle daily cleaning of affected skin with a mild antiseptic solution assists healing. Animals with primary photosensitization generally recover relatively quickly once the phototoxic compound is removed. However, recovery may be more prolonged in animals with an underlying liver disease.

Pemphigus foliaceus

Key point

- Pemphigus foliaceus is an uncommon reason for emergency care in horses.

Definition/overview

Pemphigus foliaceus is a rare autoimmune skin disease.[21]

Etiology/pathogenesis

An autoantibody against the glycocalyx of keratinocytes causes release and activation of keratinocyte proteolytic enzymes into the intercellular space. Hydrolysis of the glycocalyx causes loss of intercellular adhesion and acantholysis.[21] Insect hypersensitivity and drug reaction to trimethoprim sulfa have been suggested as possibly playing a role in the pathogenesis.[21]

Clinical features

The disease is characterized by severe crusting and matting of the hair coat with lesions typically beginning on the face and limbs and progressing over weeks or months to become generalized.[21] The disease may affect only the coronary band. Horses may have a dull demeanor with indications of systemic disease. Distal extremity and ventral edema and pain, lameness, and pruritus are also clinical features.

Diagnosis

Diagnosis is made based on routine histological evaluation of a skin biopsy.[21] **Note:** it is important to include intact crusts attached to the underlying skin or hair in the biopsy. Histologically, the disease is characterized by intragranular to subcorneal acantholysis.[21]

Management/treatment

The disease in horses <1 year old is self-limiting.[21] In adult horses, the disease is treated with prednisolone (1 mg/kg PO q12h) until no new lesions develop (usually 7–10 days), then 1 mg/kg PO q48h. Dexamethasone can also be used initially at immunosuppressive doses (0.05–0.1 mg/kg or 20–40 mg/horse). Chrysotherapy (gold salts) and azathioprine have also been used.[21] The prognosis is guarded.

Toxic epidermal necrolysis

Key point
- TEN is rare in horses.

Definition/overview

TEN ('Lyell's syndrome') is a rare, life-threatening dermatologic condition that is usually induced by a reaction to medications. It is characterized by the detachment of the epidermis from the dermis all over the body (>30%) including mucous membranes.[26] TEN is considered a more severe form of Stevens–Johnson syndrome (<30% of body surface area affected).[27]

Etiology/pathogenesis

TEN is a rare and usually severe adverse reaction to certain drugs. The drugs most often implicated in human patients are antimicrobial drugs (e.g. sulfonamides), NSAIDs, corticosteroids, anticonvulsants (e.g. phenobarbital, phenytoin), and allopurinol.[28] The disease is associated with necrosis of keratinocytes throughout the epidermis, including the mucosal surfaces.

Clinical features

Prodromal signs include macular exanthema, fever, mucositis, and pain on palpation of skin and mucocutaneous junctions.[29] These signs progress to denudation, bullae formation, and purpura. A positive Nikolsky's sign (slight rubbing of the skin resulting in epidermal exfoliation) is observed in most human patients.[29] The disease progresses to separation of the epidermis from most of the body surface area, including the mucous membranes. Clinical features that have been used to define the disease in human patients are epidermal detachment of >30% of the total body surface area and involvement of one or more mucosal surfaces (i.e. oral, genital, or ocular).[29]

Differential diagnosis

Burn injury; infection.

Diagnosis

Diagnosis is made based on the clinical features and histologic evaluation of biopsy tissue with full-thickness epidermal necrosis and dermoepidermal separation.[29]

Management/treatment

Management involves discontinuing treatment with any drugs that may be associated with the condition. Treatment is generally similar to that for burns (see Burns). Supportive care is important and should include analgesic drugs (see Chapter 14), intravenous fluids (see Chapter 12), and nutritional support (see Chapter 15) when necessary. Barrier nursing is recommended. Systemic antimicrobial drugs are only used to treat suspected active infection. IV immunoglobulin has been used in human patients.[29]

The mortality rate for TEN is high because of infection (local and systemic) associated with skin loss, with sepsis being the leading cause of death in human patients. Death can also be caused by respiratory distress, which is due either to pneumonia or to damage to the respiratory mucosa. Other complications include anemia, hypoproteinemia, hyponatremia, renal failure, ileus, and pulmonary embolism.[29]

CHAPTER 7

NEUROLOGY

Pamela A. Wilkins

GENERAL APPROACH TO THE HORSE WITH NEUROLOGIC PROBLEMS

- Differential diagnosis of neurologic disease in horses presenting on an emergency basis is simplified by specific knowledge of recent history, season, signalment, vaccination history, and geographic distribution of infectious diseases.
- Acutely neurologic patients should initially be examined with concerns for biosecurity and examiner safety, as some diseases are potentially zoonotic and horses with severe neurologic signs can be a danger to themselves and others. The examiner should wear gloves when performing the initial examination until rabies is effectively ruled in or ruled out, particularly in countries where rabies is an endemic disease.
- This chapter should not be considered exhaustive, but merely highlights several of the more common emergency presentations of neurologic disease in horses.

- Horses can present on an emergency basis with central nervous system (CNS) signs related to the spinal cord or within the cranial vault, or with both sites affected. Care should be taken to differentiate between the two anatomic regions of disease because emergency treatment may be different.
- The common presenting signs for horses with nervous system emergencies are listed in *Box 7.1*.
- The primary differential diagnoses for nervous system emergencies are presented in *Box 7.2*.

Box 7.2 Primary differential diagnoses for neurologic emergencies

Cerebral signs:
- Depression
- Seizure
- Coma
- Blindness
- Cranial nerve abnormalities
- Ataxia
- Weakness
- Recumbency
- Behavioral change

Cerebellar signs:
- Ataxia
- Intention tremor

Spinal cord and peripheral nerve/neuromuscular signs:
- Ataxia: symmetrical or non-symmetrical
- Weakness/extensor rigidity
- Muscle atrophy
- Loss of sensation
- Recumbency

Box 7.1 Common presenting signs of horses with neurologic emergencies

- Acute onset ataxia
- Seizures
- Depression
- Headpressing
- Coma
- Cranial nerve abnormalities such as facial paresis/paralysis, nystagmus, dysphagia
- Weakness
- Recumbency
- Behavioral change

- The most useful diagnostic tests for horses with nervous system emergencies are presented in *Box 7.3*.
- Control of seizure and preventing injury to the patient or to handlers are the key features of emergency treatment of horses with nervous system disease. The approach to immediate seizure control is presented in *Box 7.4*.

- Common diagnostic procedures are described on pages 455 to 460.
- Management of the recumbent horse is discussed in Chapter 21.
- Indications for immediate referral of horses with neurologic or neuromuscular emergencies are presented in *Box 7.5*.

Box 7.3 Useful diagnostic tests for horses presenting with neurologic emergencies

- Rabies is a serious potential zoonotic disease! Wear gloves during all initial examinations of horses showing neurologic signs until this disease can be ruled out
- Thorough history, meticulous physical examination, and a complete neurologic examination should result in an accurate localization of the lesion causing the clinical signs
- Knowledge of vaccination history should allow differentiation of viral encephalitis, tetanus, and botulism from other causes of clinical signs
- Cerebropinal fluid (CSF) sampling may be indicated
- Serology
- Imaging, including advanced modalities such as MRI and CT

Box 7.4 Immediate seizure control

- Any horse with uncontrolled seizures should be treated as quickly as possible to prevent new injury to itself, prevent injury to handlers, and minimize additional brain injury.
- Diazepam is commonly used for this purpose (0.01–0.4 mg/kg slow IV [approximately 5–10 mg to a 50 kg foal; start with 50 mg for an adult 450–500 kg horse]). Midazolam can be used (3–5 mg IV in neonates [~50 kg] and can be given IM). Phenobarbital (3–5 mg/kg slow IV over 20 minutes; repeat as necessary, effect seen in 30–40 minutes) or pentobarbital (2–10 mg/kg IV q8–12h) may be needed if the benzodiazipine drugs (diazepam, midazolam) fail to fully control seizure activity.
- Benzodiazipene drugs may cause respiratory arrest if given rapidly IV. It is important to be prepared to intubate and manually ventilate cases when these drugs are used. Other untoward side-effects include incoordination and hypotension.

Box 7.5 Indications for immediate referral of horses with neurologic emergencies

- Any horse with uncontrolled seizures, obvious head trauma, or that is recumbent should be considered a candidate for referral.
- In some cases, referral may not be immediately advisable and emergency stabilization and seizure control may be indicated prior to completing a physical examination and diagnostic tests.

COMMON PROCEDURES PERFORMED ON HORSES WITH NEUROLOGIC PROBLEMS

Neurologic examination
History and physical examination

The neurologic examination begins with a complete history and general physical examination.[1-8] The examiner should bear in mind that many suspected acute neurologic problems may, in fact, be of neuromuscular, musculoskeletal, metabolic, or other origin and these should always be considered initially. The purpose of the examination is to develop both a differential diagnosis list and to determine the neuroanatomic localization of any suspected abnormalities. The horse's signalment and management, the geographic location, and the season all play a role in considering the possible differential diagnoses for a presumptive neurologic condition. General physical examination may reveal areas of asymmetry, muscle mass loss, or evidence of unexplained trauma. Abnormal wear of the hooves or shoes may indicate abnormal gait, either due to neurologic abnormality or musculoskeletal disease.

Hematology and clinical chemistry testing

Hematology and clinical chemistry testing is generally performed to evaluate for the presence of possible inflammatory (increased fibrinogen concentration, increased total WBC count) or metabolic (e.g. hyponatremia, hypernatremia, hypokalemia, hypocalcemia, hypomagnesemia, altered liver enzymes, or liver function tests) conditions resulting in the observed clinical signs. Depending on the specific findings of the neurologic examination, additional blood testing may be performed later (e.g. virus isolation [EHV-1], serology [equine protozoal myeloencephalitis, EHV-1], bile acid concentration [liver disease], botulinum toxin in the feces or GI contents, PCR [EHV-1]).

Examination of the head

The head is generally examined first. In addition to assessing symmetry, the head is evaluated for specific nerve function. This examination includes an ophthalmologic examination to evaluate the retina and the optic nerve. Briefly, the tests described below examine the CNs:

Menace reflex: The examiner abruptly moves a hand toward the horse's eye without touching the eyelashes or creating air movement sensed on the cornea. An absence of the reflex indicates defective vision, paralysis of the eyelids, or serious depression of consciousness. The appropriate response is to blink the eye and, perhaps, move the head away. This reflex will not develop until approximately 2 weeks of age in the neonate and examines vision (afferent CN II) and CN VII, the facial nerve.

Palpebral reflex, corneal reflex: The examiner lightly touches the eyelid and the horse should close its eye, testing the ophthalmic branch of CN V and the auriculopalpebral branch of CN VII. Touching the cornea with a moistened cotton swab or ball should result in the same response plus, potentially, retraction of the globe. Sensation for the palpebrae and cornea is provided by a branch of CN V; globe retraction and eyelid closure require the abducent nerve (CN VI) and the auriculopalpebral branch of CN VII.

Pupillary light reflex: The examiner brings the horse into dim lighting and shines a bright light (point source) first into one eye, then the other, while observing both eyes for evidence of pupillary constriction. Pupillary constriction should occur directly and indirectly. This test examines CN II (the parasympathetic nucleus and fibers of CN II) and the visual pathways. Eye position is also evaluated; normal eye position requires intact CNs III, IV and VI.

Facial muscle symmetry: CN VII controls the muscles of expression. Problems with this nerve can result in apparent paresis or paralysis of facial muscles and/or loss of muscle mass. CN VII is also sensory to the ear.

Balance and hearing: Both require an intact CN VIII.

Gag reflex: This test examines CNs IX and X.

Tongue tone: This test examines CN XII (hypoglossal).

Prebension, chewing and swallowing: This test examines CNs IX, X and XII.

Examination of the neck

The neck is examined with particular attention paid to symmetry, abnormal sweating patterns, presence or absence of masses or deviations from normal anatomy, presence or absence of pain on manipulation, and flexibility. Loss of trapezius muscle mass may indicate a problem with CN XI. Abnormalities of the neck generally suggest a lesion within the bony cervical spinal column or calvarium.

Examination of the body

The body is examined next. Again, symmetry, strength, and presence or absence of muscle mass changes are important to evaluate. The panniculus reflex, performed by running a firm, relatively sharp object like a pen, down the length of the horse, bilaterally, from the neck to the tail just off the midline, will indicate if skin sensation and control of muscles underlying the skin is intact. Tail strength and appropriate perineal responses, including anal tone, are also tested.

Gait analysis

Gait analysis involves a standardized series of maneuvers including: backing the horse; circling the horse in large and small (tight) circles; walking the horse in a series of serpentines; walking the horse up and down an incline; walking with the head sharply elevated; and a tail pull, where the horse is walked forward while the examiner pulls the tail, which the horse should resist, as a test of strength. In cases where clinical signs and history suggest a vestibular problem, the horse may also be blindfolded and asked to walk forward. The examiner observes the horse for evidence of hypo- or hypermetria, circumduction, inappropriate limb placement (proprioceptive deficit), weakness, and also lameness. The symmetry and limbs involved provide clues for neuroanatomic localization; forelimb and hindlimb involvement suggests a cervical spinal cord problem, while hindlimb only involvement suggests a more caudal lesion or lesions, and asymmetry suggests a lateralizing lesion.

Genitourinary testing

In the more general neurologic examination, specific testing for genital, rectal, and bladder function is not necessary as during the course of evaluation many horses will both urinate and defecate voluntarily. However, evidence of urinary scalding, persistent penile prolapse, history of stranguria or dysuria, or history of poor reproductive performance (stallions particularly) may warrant further evaluation.

Ancillary tests

Ancillary testing includes imaging studies, CSF analysis (see below), specific blood and CSF serology, PCR for specific infectious agents on blood and CSF, nuclear scintigraphy, electromyelography (rarely), electroencephalography (rarely), and nerve conduction studies (rarely).

Skull and cervical plain/digital radiography are the most commonly performed imaging studies and are available at most large equine practices and referral centers, as is myelography. MRI and CT are less readily available, but can be found at many tertiary referral hospitals. These studies generally require general anesthesia, as does myelography. Endoscopy of the upper airway and guttural pouches is useful in cases of head trauma and suspected temporohyoid osteoarthropathy.

Cerebrospinal fluid collection and analysis

CSF is an ultrafiltrate of plasma that contains fewer cells, less protein, potassium, calcium, and glucose, and more sodium, chloride, and magnesium than plasma. Sixty to 70% of the total CSF is produced by the choroid plexus in the ventricles; the remainder arises from the brain parenchyma. Because CSF is in intimate contact with the CNS, neurologic disease may alter the composition of CSF. However, these changes rarely suggest a specific diagnosis, but rather allow diseases to be grouped into categories.

Cerebrospinal fluid collection

CSF can be collected from two sites: the lumbosacral (LS) space (**7.1**) and the atlanto-occipital (AO) space (**7.2**). In general, horses that present standing and remain standing are sampled via the LS space, although obtaining fluid from this site is more challenging.

If the horse presents recumbent and short-term general anesthesia is needed to safely remove the horse from the transport vehicle and/or obtain imaging studies (radiographs, MRI, CT), a CSF sample can be obtained from the AO space while the horse is anesthetized. AO sampling is not practical in the awake horse as the risk of iatrogenic injury to the CNS is too great. There may be qualitative differences between samples obtained at the two locations depending on the suspected underlying etiology, which may ultimately dictate the sample site.[9,10]

The risks of trauma and contamination of CSF with tissue or blood (potentially altering specific testing results) increase with multiple attempts to obtain CSF from the LS space, an anatomic challenge due to its depth and heavy musculature and/or fat in some cases (**7.3**).[11,12] Anatomic and position-dependent changes

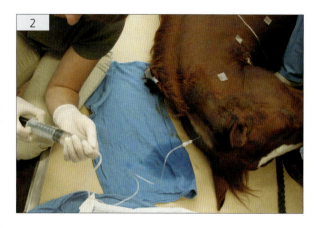

7.2 Collection of cerebrospinal fluid from the atlanto-occipital space. In this image the horse is under anesthesia and being prepared for a myleogram. CSF is collected prior to infusion of the radiodense marker for the myelogram. (Courtesy Dr Monica Aleman)

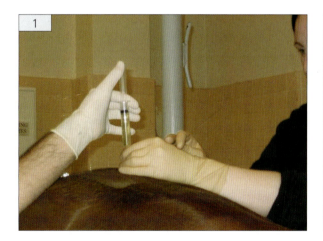

7.1 Collection of cerebrospinal fluid from the lumbosacral space in a standing horse. The collection site is generally on the midline approximately 0.5 cm cranial to the most superficial (dorsal) component of the tuber sacrale. The fluid being collected is xanthochromic. (Measurement from Aleman M, Borchers A, Kass PH *et al.* (2007) Ultrasound-assisted collection of cerebrospinal fluid from the lumbosacral space in equids. *J Am Vet Med Assoc* 230:378–84.) (Courtesy Dr Amy Johnson)

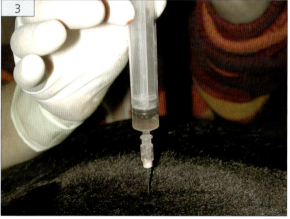

7.3 Blood contamination of a CSF tap performed at the lumbosacral space in a standing sedated horse. (Courtesy Dr Corinne Sweeney)

affect the alignment of the vertebral column and pelvis in recumbent horses and severely ataxic horses that cannot stand 'squarely', and further complicate the procedure. An ultrasound-guided technique for LS space CSF collection has been described (**7.4A, B**).[13]

Ultrasound-guided puncture of the AO area allows reduction of potential complications associated with blind percutaneous puncture, although AO punctures are generally 'cleaner' (**7.4A, B**).[14,15]

Performing standing LS space puncture in the adult horse can be a precarious undertaking and several individuals should be available to provide assistance and restraint. The horse will generally need to be sedated; choice of sedation may depend on the suspected underlying condition, but xylazine or detomidine are generally effective, perhaps combined with butorphanol. The horse should be sedated enough to stand quietly but not so sedated that it cannot stand as well as possible, given its underlying problem.

The adult horse has approximately 200 ml of CSF and approximately 20 ml can be safely removed at one time with minimal risk of herniation of the brain through the base of the skull, even in trauma cases where brain swelling, and increased intracranial pressure (ICP), is suspected.

CSF should be collected in several different tubes: EDTA tube for cytology; plain tubes with no coagulant for TP and serology and perhaps PCR testing; blood culture tubes for bacterial culture (1–2) if an infectious cause is suspected.

The procedure, whether LS or AO puncture, should be performed under sterile conditions, therefore the proposed puncture site must be surgically clipped (approximately 15 × 15 cm^2 area) and prepped in a routine manner using conventional pre-surgical cleaning and disinfecting fluids. The clinician performing the puncture should wear sterile surgical gloves and remain sterile throughout the procedure.

Atlanto-occipital tap

An AO tap is performed with the horse in lateral recumbency. The landmark is the dorsal midline where it intersects with a line imagined connecting the cranial borders of the wings of the atlas. Some clinicians use a 'guide hole' made through the skin with a 14-gauge needle, while others prefer either no hole or a small stab incision made with a #15 scalpel blade.

The horse's head is flexed to create a 90 degrees angle between the head and cervical vertebrae, and the nose is slightly elevated until the long axis of the head is parallel to the ground. A 3.5-inch, 19- or 20-gauge spinal needle is placed in the guide hole and directed towards the commissures of the lip with the bevel facing rostral. The needle is advanced slowly through the soft tissues. Entrance into the subarachnoid space will be accompanied by a 'popping' sensation. Once the 'pop' is felt, the stilette is removed and the needle hub observed for spontaneous flow of CSF. If no flow is observed, the stilette should be replaced and the needle advanced further. Each popping sensation should be checked for entrance into the subarachnoid space. If the needle hits bone, it should be withdrawn to the level of the skin, the landmarks re-evaluated, and the needle redirected appropriately.

When collecting CSF using this method, the fluid should be allowed to flow by gravity into the collection tubes.

Lumbosacral puncture

LS puncture is the most commonly performed method of CSF collection. Generally, this is performed in the standing but sedated horse. LS puncture is performed on the dorsal midline (determined from caudal vertebral structure, rather than skin, if possible) between and slightly cranial (generally 0.5 cm) to the cranial aspect of the tuber sacralis and intersecting with a line imagined connecting the caudal-most palpable edge of both tuber coxae. The dorsal spinous processes of the L6 and S2 vertebrae can generally be palpated.

The proposed puncture site is surgically prepped and scrubbed and infiltrated with local anesthetic. As with AO puncture, a guide hole or stab incision is generally made in the skin. Care should be taken to keep the needle perpendicular to the skin in the craniocaudal as well as the lateral plane. The needle is advanced slowly until a distinct 'pop' is felt when the interarcuate ligament is pierced. The horse may react somewhat violently to the puncture and handlers should be cautioned of this. Once the 'pop' is felt, the stilette should be removed and a sterile 10 ml syringe attached to the needle and gently aspirated to check for CSF. If the needle hits bone, it should be withdrawn, the landmarks re-evaluated, positioning checked, and the needle redirected appropriately. If no flow is observed, the stilette should be replaced and the needle advanced further. In some difficult cases, CSF flow/collection can be assisted by bilateral occlusion of the jugular veins and elevation of the horse's head. Repeated attempts at puncture increase the likelihood of blood contamination.

If gross blood contamination is observed during collection, the CSF should be aspirated in several sequential small (~2 ml) aliquots until it is grossly clear (**7.3**). Blood contamination is commonly occult, and several samples (approximately three sequential) should be removed before obtaining a 'clean' CSF sample for analysis.

Performing an LS puncture on an awake but recumbent horse carries its own set of problems beyond awkward positioning and loss of reliability of the usual landmarks. Sedation may still be required to limit what

movement the horse is capable of in order to ensure the safety of those around.

To facilitate the procedure, elevation of the upper hindlimb may improve alignment of the space with the palpable landmarks, and ultrasound can be used to more accurately identify the puncture site (**7.5**).

Cerebrospinal fluid analysis

Routine CSF evaluation usually includes determination of TP concentration, nucleated cell count, and RBC count. Iatrogenic contamination of CSF with blood is a common problem during collection of samples and causes high RBC counts that are not indicative of CNS disease. It may also cause increases in nucleated cell count and TP concentration, which may confound interpretation of results.[16,17] Blood contamination of

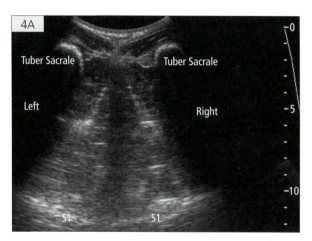

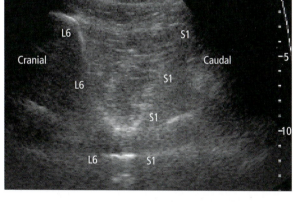

7.4A, B Transverse (A) and longitudinal (B) ultrasonographic images of the LS area (puncture site) approximately 0.5 cm (0.2 inches) cranial to the reference point. (Courtesy Dr Monica Aleman)

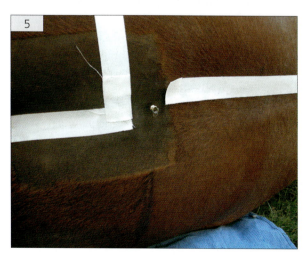

7.5 Cerebrospinal fluid tap performed in a recumbent horse with tape used to emphasize appropriate alignment of the landmarks. The needle hub can be seen over the lumbosacral puncture site. (Courtesy Dr Monica Aleman)

CSF has an effect on western blot analysis for detection of antibodies against *Sarcocystis neurona* and on albumin quotient and IgG index in horses.[12,18]

The most current recommendation is to collect 3–4 sequential 2–5 ml aliquots of CSF, changing the syringe between samples, with the first sample discarded even in apparently 'clean' punctures because of the high probability of iatrogenic blood contamination. The final sample should be submitted for both cytologic evaluation and specific antibody testing as it is less likely to have blood contamination. Cytologic evaluation should be performed within 1 hour of collection because the cellular component deteriorates rapidly in the low protein CSF milieu.

Many infectious diseases of the CNS are commonly associated with mononuclear pleocytosis, high protein concentration, or both. Acute Eastern equine encephalomyelitis (EEE) and Venezuelan equine encephalomyelitis (VEE) and equine herpesvirus myeloencephalopathy (EHM) are unique in that EEE and VEE are generally associated with neutrophilic pleocytosis and EHM is typically associated with marked xanthochromia (**7.1**) and increased protein concentration. Horses with acute onset of neurologic signs attributable to West Nile virus (WNV) encephalomyelitis commonly have mononuclear pleocytosis with lymphocytic predominance, with results of analysis of CSF collected from the LS tap more commonly abnormal than AO samples.[17]

In some cases, glucose, specific enzymes (LDH, AST, and creatine phosphokinase) and specific antibodies to EEE, WEE, EHV-1, and *S. neurona* are also evaluated. PCR testing for infectious agents is also performed by some examiners. Measurement of albumin in both CSF and serum or plasma can be performed in order to determine the albumin quotient (AQ), the ratio of CSF to blood albumin used by some to evaluate blood–brain or blood–CSF barrier dysfunction. Similarly, the IgG index can be determined as the (CSF IgG/serum of plasma IgG)/AQ. The antibody index (AI) is similar to the IgG index, but uses antigen specific antibody titers instead of total IgG.

DISEASE OF THE NERVOUS SYSTEM

Diseases producing cortical signs
Equine herpesvirus type 1 myeloencephalopathy
Key points

- EHM has a worldwide distribution and is a highly infectious disease of horses that can result in significant morbidity and mortality.
- EHM is a type of 'spinal stroke' and can have very acute onset.
- Fever may be the only prodromal sign.
- There currently are no vaccines labeled as protective for this form of EHV-1 infection and there is no widely accepted specific treatment.

Definition/overview
EHM has recently regained worldwide attention due to a perceived (or real) increase in both number and severity of outbreaks since 2000.[19,20]

Etiology/pathogenesis
There is a great deal of ongoing research into the underlying pathophysiology and epidemiology, with particular attention being paid to the identification of a specific single point mutation variant (the open reading frame 30 variant, or ORF30, at position 752) that displays what has been termed 'aggressive replicativity' and has been shown to be more commonly associated with neurologic form outbreaks of EHV-1 infection that have other variants.[20,21]

The neurologic manifestation of EHM is associated with CNS vascular endothelial infection and subsequent thrombosis of those vessels, making the condition a type of 'spinal stroke', which then leads to the acute onset of neurologic signs (**7.6, 7.7**)

Clinical features
Horses with EHM classically present as acute onset patients with symmetrical to slightly asymmetric spinal cords signs, generally worse in the hindlimbs than in the forelimbs.[19,22] Ataxia and weakness predominate and up to 50% of affected horses may have bladder dysfunction. Although rare, CN signs may be present. Frequently, horses are reported to have been normal

for up to a few hours before the onset of signs, although the horse may have had a mild to moderate fever several days beforehand.[19,22] There may have been a history of other horses with fever, respiratory signs and/or abortion at the patient's location. Alternatively, the patient may recently have experienced some type of stress, such as long distance transport or other illness, which subsequently has allowed recrudescence of latent infection.

Differential diagnosis

There are few differential diagnoses, primarily the other viral encephalitis diseases (EEE, WEE, VEE) and WNV. The rapid onset distinguishes EHM from equine protozoal myeloencephalitis (EPM).

Diagnosis

Diagnosis can be made in several ways:[19–21]

- Clinical signs and presentation: acute onset, symmetric spinal cord signs worse in the hindlimbs; history of, or current, fever; history of similarly affected horses on premises or horses affected by fever, respiratory disease or abortion.

- Virus isolation, PCR, paired serology: virus isolation and PCR are performed on nasopharyngeal swabs and whole blood, paired serology on serum collected 10–14 days apart; consult local laboratory.
- Necropsy: gross and histopathologic lesions are generally diagnostic (**7.7**); immunohistochemistry (IHC) is confirmatory (**7.6**).

Management/treatment

Horses suspected of having EHM should be considered infectious and potential sources of infection for other horses. Biosecurity protocols should be instituted. EHM is a reportable disease in many areas.[20]

Treatment is primarily supportive:[19]

- IV fluid support if needed.
- Systemic anti-inflammatory therapy: flunixin meglumine.
- Bladder catheterization if needed several times daily.
- If recumbent, manage as described in Chapter 21.

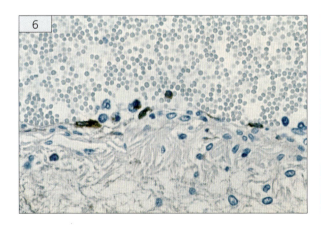

7.6 Immunohistochemistry labeling of equine herpesvirus type 1 in endothelial cells of a venule in the chorid plexus. Dark stained (golden brown) cells are endothelial cells, red blood cells are contained within the venule at the top of the image. (Courtesy Dr Fabio Del Piero)

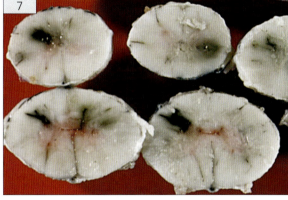

7.7 Cross-sections of the spinal cord of a horse severely clinically affected by the neurologic form of EHV-1. Darkened approximately triangular areas, with their points originating toward the central canal of the spinal cord, are areas of spinal cord infarction secondary to vascular occlusion resulting from thrombosis of vessels to the area caused by endothelial damage from EHV-1. (Courtesy Dr Fabio Del Piero and Dr Alexander de Lahunta)

- Antiviral treatment can be administered to affected horses and febrile 'in-contact' or 'at risk' horses if desired (e.g. acyclovir: 20–30 mg/kg PO q8–12h or 10 mg/kg in 1 liter crystalloid fluid over 1 hour IV q12h; or valacyclovir: 30 mg/kg PO q8–12h). The goal of this treatment is to decrease viremia and shedding of virus in the affected horse.[23,24]

Vaccination has not been demonstrated to be protective against EHM at this time, although efforts are underway to develop effective vaccination protocols.[19,20]

Most horses that do not become recumbent survive and fully recover, although residual neurologic deficits in gait and bladder function may remain in the rare individual. Recumbent adult horses have a guarded prognosis for survival.

The neurologic form of EHV-1 infection in horses has become a reportable disease in many states in the USA and Australia. Identification of EHM may lead to quarantine of the facility where it is currently located and the farm where the horse originated, if it has been evaluated at a referral hospital. Because the disease has been shown to be both infectious and contagious, isolation of affected animals is recommended, as is disinfection of any equipment used on the horse or in transport of the horse.

West Nile virus encephalomyelitis
Key points
- WNV is an arthropod (mosquito)-borne CNS viral disease that affects many species including the horse. It is NOT transmissible between affected animals.
- The disease is seasonal, but may occur year long in warm temperate climates that support mosquito populations.

Definition/overview
WNV has caused epidemic and endemic disease in humans and animals in Europe, Africa, Asia, and the Middle East for decades. WNV first appeared in the USA in 1999, causing illness and death in birds, horses, and humans.[22,25–27] While the initial outbreak of this sometimes deadly viral disease was limited to the northeastern USA, the virus had an inexorable migration across continental USA, causing huge losses among the affected species.

Etiology/pathogenesis
This disease is primarily limited to geographic regions and seasons with mosquito activity, as it is a mosquito-borne disease. The horse is essentially a dead-end host and poses no zoonotic or infectious risk.

Clinical features[25–28]
Fever may precede the onset of CNS signs or may be the only evidence of infection. Most infections remain asymptomatic or subclinical. Behavioral abnormalities were consistently present in cases described in Pennsylvania, USA.[25] Variable spinal cord involvement occurs, with signs ranging from ataxia and monoparesis to tetraparesis. Affected horses can be sensitive to stimulation, exhibiting extreme reactions to touch and sound. Sedation can be quite difficult, with larger than normal doses and very frequent administration of the chosen sedative and tranquilizer required to control them. Almost invariably, affected horses have muscular twitching of their head and neck, apparent at rest. Several cases exhibit a variety of abnormal postures, and may fall forward on their forelimbs while in the stall. CN signs are not unusual and facial paresis/paralysis and dysphagia may be commonly observed. In a report describing 48 horses with WNV presenting to a referral facility in Florida, blindness and paresis of the tongue were present in several cases.[29]

Differential diagnosis
Primary differential diagnoses include EEE, rabies, bacterial meningitis, EHM, and EPM.[22,28]

Diagnosis
Diagnosis of WNV has become relatively straightforward in areas where the disease is common in horses, although the diagnosis may be elusive in the occasional patient.

CSF findings are likely to be abnormal, exhibiting mononuclear pleocytosis.[22,28] Antemortem laboratory confirmation of a clinical diagnosis of WNV is primarily based on serology, although other tests, including monoclonal antibody capture ELISA, reverse transcriptase (RT)-PCR, and TaqMan tests, are also used.[26,28,30] Procedures for submitting diagnostic samples and reporting persons and animals with suspected WNV infection vary among states and jurisdictions.

The clinician should perform a thorough neurologic evaluation in order to provide the pathologist with a neuroanatomic diagnosis. Virus can be identified within the CNS using IHC (**7.8**).

Management/treatment

Treatment of horses with WNV infection is primarily supportive and symptomatic. The clinical course can be quite difficult to predict and reappearance of neurologic signs after apparent recovery has been anecdotally described and observed by the author.[22,25–28]

- IV crystalloid fluid support as needed.
- NSAIDs, such as flunixin meglumine and phenylbutazone, and IV administration of 10% solutions of DMSO.
- Corticosteroids, usually dexamethasone (10–20 mg/horse IV q24h), as an anti-inflammatory.

- Interferon (IFN) has been used in some cases (3 × 10^6 units SC q24h).
- Hyperimmune plasma and serum products are available and have been used.

Most horses that do not become recumbent survive and fully recover, although residual neurologic deficits in gait and behavior may remain in some individuals. Recumbent adult horses have a guarded prognosis for survival.[22,25,26,28]

Vaccination appears to be protective in the majority of cases, although older horses may mount less of a protective antibody (humoral) response with vaccination and thus remain more at risk. Debate exists regarding the frequency of revaccination, although vaccination at 6-month intervals in endemic regions appears reasonable once the initial vaccination series is complete.[27,29]

Alphaviruses

Key points

- Vaccination is protective against several equine encephalitis viruses, most notably EEE, WEE, and VEE.
- The horse is a dead-end host in these diseases and does not serve as a source of infection for other animals or people.

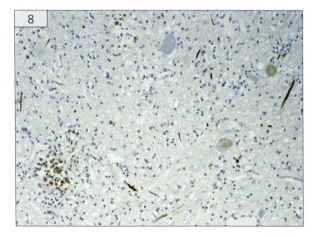

7.8 Immunohistochemistry labeling of neuron fibers in a glial nodule of a horse infected with West Nile virus. Dark stained (golden brown) areas are West Nile virus contained within the neurons. (Courtesy Dr Fabio Del Piero)

Definition/overview

The most common equine encephalitis viruses include EEE (**7.9A, B**), WEE, and VEE viruses. Other groups that may infect the horse, but prefer other hosts (such as humans), include the St. Louis and Japanese B encephalitis viruses.

Etiology/pathogenesis

Like WNV, these viruses threaten horses and humans. They are mosquito-borne viruses, displaying geographic specificity and seasonality. All of the encephalitides are reportable diseases in the USA and are notifiable diseases in the European Union. The horse is a dead-end host and poses no zoonotic or infectious threat.[22,28]

Clinical features

Non-specific fever, anorexia, and stiffness usually within 5 days of the initial infection. Hypersensitization of the skin (hyperesthesia), aggression, and excitability with continuous chewing movements. Propulsive walking, depression, sleepiness and loss of orientation. Head pressing, circling with a head tilt, and blindness.

Horses with VEE may develop diarrhea, become moribund, and die before they develop neurologic signs. Oral ulceration, nose bleed, and abortion may also be observed.

Differential diagnosis

Early in the course of disease EHM or EPM may be considered differential diagnoses.

Diagnosis

Diagnosis is based on clinical presentation, history of no recent vaccination, serologic testing, virus isolation, and necropsy findings.

Management/treatment

No known treatment exists for EEE, WEE, and VEE. Supportive treatment as described for EHM and WNV and support of the recumbent horse (see Chapter 21) should be provided.

Non-survivors are generally recumbent within 3–5 days. Survivors gradually improve over weeks to months and residual neurologic deficits are common. Mortality rates for EEE range from 75–90%, WEE from 19–50%, and VEE from 40–80%.

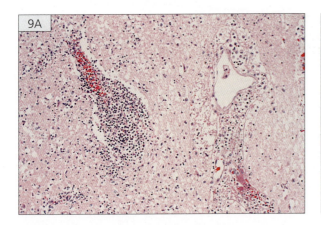
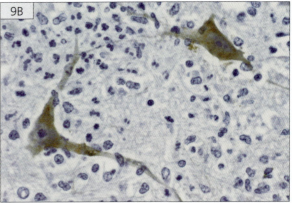

7.9A, B Eastern equine encephalitis. (A) Equine brainstem hematoxylin and eosin stain demonstrating the inflammatory encephalitis associated with Eastern equine encephalitis. (B) Immunohistochemistry demonstrating Eastern equine encephalitis virus (golden brown stained cells) within neurons of the brain and the associated inflammatory response. (Courtesy Dr Fabio Del Piero)

Prevention is based on control of intermediate host (generally bird) and insect vector (mosquito) populations and appropriate vaccination. Most currently marketed vaccination products against EEE, WEE, and VEE are considered effective and should be boosted yearly once the initial series is completed.

Bacterial meningitis/encephalitis and brain abscess

Key points

- Bacterial infections of the brain and spinal cord are not commonly encountered and may be associated with trauma or immunodeficiency.
- Meningitis is most commonly associated with sepsis in the neonatal foal.

Definition/overview

Infectious meningitis is considered to be a rare occurrence in adult horses.[22,31] Meningitis may arise from a disseminated bacterial infection of the meninges and subarachnoid space, or it may reflect inflammation secondary to a primary infection localized within the nervous tissue (e.g. brain abscess) (**7.10**).

Etiology/pathogenesis[22,31]

Reported routes of CNS infection of adult horses include hematogenous dissemination, direct contamination secondary to skull fractures, or extension from an adjacent site of infection (e.g. paranasal sinuses, periorbital tissues, retropharyngeal lymph nodes, guttural pouch). Meningitis secondary to brain abscess has been reported. Pituitary abscesses are common.

The cause of meningitis remains unknown in many cases. Pathogens isolated from septic foals include gram-negative enteric bacteria, *Streptococcus* spp., and *Staphylococcus aureus*. Pathogens isolated from adult horses with meningitis include *Cryptococcus neoformans*, *Streptococcus equi* subsp. *equi*, *Streptococcus equi* subsp. *zooepidemicus*, *Streptococcus suis*, *Actinomyces* spp., *Klebsiella pneumoniae*, *Escherichia coli*, *Actinobacillus equuli*, and *Pasteurella caballi*.

Clinical features

Systemic clinical signs are common and consist of lethargy, fever, anorexia, and generalized weakness. A wide range of neurologic signs, including CN abnormalities, have been described. Affected horses generally display ataxia that ranges in severity. Other abnormalities on physical examination include weight loss, cervical pain or stiffness and reluctance to flex the neck, an erratic breathing pattern, epistaxis, exophthalmos, enophthalmos and third eyelid protrusion, nasal discharge, and muscle fasciculations.

Differential diagnosis

Common variable immunodeficiency should be considered in adult horses with meningitis with no other obvious cause such as trauma or other head site infection. In the neonatal foal, generalized sepsis should be considered.

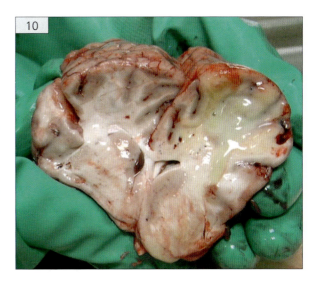

7.10 Bacterial meningitis/brain abscess in an adult horse.

Diagnosis

Diagnosis is based on history, clinical signs, and results of specific laboratory testing.[22,31] Mature neutrophilia and hyperfibrinogenemia are the most common abnormalities present on hematology. Blood culture is most rewarding in septic foals. The most common abnormalities identified on CSF analysis are neutrophilic pleocytosis and increased protein concentration. CSF should also be cultured.

Management/treatment[22,31,32]

Antimicrobial agents with good CNS penetration include fluoroquinolones, some third-generation cephalosporins, potentiated sulfonamides, doxycycline, chloramphenicol, rifampin, metronidazole, macrolides, tetracycline, and potentiated sulfonamides. Antimicrobial treatment should be based on the sensitivity of the isolate, with CNS penetration considered. Anti-inflammatory agents (flunixin meglume, phenylbutazone) may be administered to decrease CNS inflammatory responses and as pain management.

Use of dexamethasone as an anti-inflammatory agent has gained popularity for treatment of gram-positive meningitis in people, but no studies have been performed to date to support its routine use in horses with meningitis or brain abscesses. There are reports of surgical debridement and drainage of brain abscesses in horses, with variable result.

Outcome is dependent on effective early treatment and other associated diseases.[22,31]

Rabies
Key points
- Rabies is considered a reportable or notifiable disease worldwide.
- Vaccination is protective and should be performed in all geographic regions where rabies virus infection remains a possibility.
- Personal protective precautions should be taken against infection when working with rabies-suspect horses.

Definition/overview

Rabies virus (RABV) is an enveloped RNA rhabdovirus that induces lethal polioencephalomyelitis and ganglionitis in infected animals. The disease occurs in mammals and other warm-blooded vertebrates in many countries throughout the world.

Etiology/pathogenesis

RABV is transmitted to horses and other warm-blooded animals by bites from infected vectors such as foxes, raccoons, skunks, bats, and vampire bats.

Clinical features

Clinical signs may include spinal cord, cerebral and CN signs, apparent lameness, GI signs, genitourinary signs, and any combination of the above. Clinical signs become progressively more prominent. Death usually occurs by day 10 after the onset of clinical signs, with the average survival being around 5 days.

Differential diagnosis

Initial differential diagnoses are quite variable depending on clinical signs. Any horse presenting with acute neurologic signs should be treated as a rabies suspect until proven otherwise in countries where rabies is a possibility.

Diagnosis

There is no definitive antemortem test for rabies in horses. A minimum protocol for postmortem diagnosis of rabies can be found at the Center for Disease Control website.

Definitive diagnosis is made by specific testing of brain tissue. Handling and submission of materials for diagnosis should be performed following consultation with local and state public health officials, as regulations may vary.[33]

Management/treatment

There is no known effective therapy with clinical usefulness in unvaccinated or vaccinated horses with clinical rabies. Horses presenting with clinical signs of rabies should be isolated to prevent possible human exposure. Exposed vaccinated animals may be observed in isolation for a period of time; euthanasia is recommended for exposed unvaccinated horses.[33]

The mainstays of prevention are vaccination and exposure avoidance. Parenteral animal rabies vaccines should be administered only by or under the direct supervision of a veterinarian. This practice ensures that a qualified and responsible person can be held accountable to ensure that the animal has been properly vaccinated.

There is a zoonotic potential with rabies. The possibility of disease transmission is real and all equine rabies suspects must be handled as if a significant threat to human health exists.

Equine protozoal myeloencephalitis
Key points

- Horses throughout the Western hemisphere are affected by EPM, with cases identified in Canada, Panama, Brazil, and Mexico.
- Several cases of EPM have been identified in Britain and France in horses imported from the American continents.
- EPM is not a contagious disease, as the horse is a dead-end host.

Definition/overview

EPM is a neurologic disease, described in the latter half of the last century, affecting horses on the North and South American continents, although the occasional rare report appears from elsewhere in the world. The disease has many different neurologic manifestations, can present similarly to many other neurologic diseases of the horse, and can appear in any season, earning it the nickname 'the great imitator'.[22,34,35]

Etiology/pathogenesis

The parasite most commonly associated with EPM is *Sarcocystis neurona*, although *Neospora hughsei* has also been reported. The horse is a dead-end host of the parasite, with the opossum being the definitive host and other species, including the skunk, raccoon, and nine-banded armadillo, suggested as intermediate hosts in its two-host lifecycle.

The definitive host (opossum) sheds infective sporocysts in its feces which, when consumed by the horse, end up in its CNS and cause the resulting lesions in the brain and spinal cord (**7.11A, B**).

All breeds and ages can be affected, although most cases present under the age of 5 years. Stress, such as long distance transport, can be associated with development of clinical signs.[36] The distribution of the disease is associated with the range of the opossum, and many horses show evidence of silent infection, based on serologic surveys.[34,35]

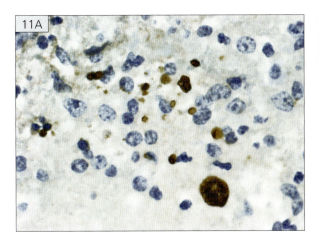
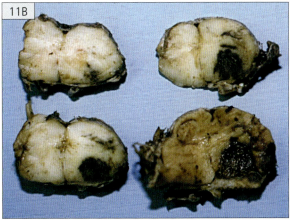

7.11A, B Equine protozoal myeloencephalitis. **(A)** Immunohistochemistry of equine brain from a horse with equine protozoal myeloencephalitis demonstrating zoites (gold brown stain) and cyst gliosis. **(B)** Brainstem from a horse with equine protozoal myeloencephalitis. Note the extensive areas of necrosis. Interestingly, this horse presented for necropsy in England, but had recently been imported from the USA. (Courtesy Dr Fabio Del Piero)

Clinical features[34,35]

EPM can mimic any other neurologic disease of the horse, but most usually the signs include ataxia, asymmetria, and muscle mass loss. Less commonly, dysphagia or head tilt are noted, while seizures and blindness are rare. The onset is generally insidious, but depending on owner acuity, EPM may present as an acute problem, making it an important rule-out for other neurologic disease.

Differential diagnosis

Includes EHM, WNV, trauma, and most other CNS diseases, as EPM can present with quite variable clinical signs.

Diagnosis

Diagnosis is based on the clinical presentation, effectively ruling out other causes of the clinical signs, and serologic testing of CSF (Western blot analysis, SAG-1, indirect immunofluorescent antibody test [IFAT]).[11,12,34,37] Diagnosis can sometimes be confirmed at necropsy by demonstration of classic gross and histologic lesions (**7.11A, B**).

Management/treatment[35]

Effective treatment is based on eradication of the organism from the CNS with the use of antimicrobial therapy. Recumbent horses should be treated and supported, as described elsewhere (see Chapter 21), with attention paid to hydration, nutrition, and excellent nursing care.

Initially, treatment is undertaken using sulfadiazine plus pyrimethamine. One antimicrobial treatment developed and marketed for treatment of EPM is ponazuril. Supportive treatment includes anti-inflammatory drugs and vitamin E.

Early treatment improves the possibility of good outcome.[22,34,35] Approximately 70% of horses will improve with treatment, with approximately 33% of those cases returning to normal neurologic status. Mild cases have the best chance of full recovery.

There is currently no proven effective vaccine against EPM, although a vaccine is currently available with its efficacy being studied. Prevention at this time is be based on decreasing exposure of horses to opossum feces, a daunting task in some geographic regions.

Head trauma
Key points
- Cases of head trauma are generally easily identified due to external evidence of trauma (e.g. wounds, epistaxis). Rarely, the traumatic incident will not have been observed and more careful evaluation is required.
- The traumatic events are frequently observed and result from halter-breaking or other training techniques.
- Trauma may be the result of another underlying CNS disease and other diseases should be ruled out as appropriate.

Definition/overview

Traumatic brain injury typically results from impact to the head, although acceleration–deceleration forces accompanying vigorous 'whiplash' head movements also have the potential to damage the brain.

Etiology/pathogenesis

The blow to the head causes transient bony deformation, which result in linear, stellate, compound, comminuted, and/or depressed fractures of the bones of the calvarium. The damaging effects of head trauma are usually focused on the portions of the brain adjacent to (coup) and opposite (contrecoup) the site of impact. Brain damage that occurs during the primary traumatic event is irreversible; however, there is a window of minutes to days in which equally important secondary injuries can theoretically be prevented or treated.[38,39]

There are three predominant types of injury to the head of horses that result in CNS signs:
- When a horse flips over backwards and strikes its poll (**7.12A–C**).
- When the frontal/parietal area of the head is impacted such as with a kick or by running into a fixed object.

- Petrous temporal bone fracture, associated with temporohyoid osteoarthropathy (THO), following movement of the hyoid apparatus (p. 472).

Clinical features[38]

Non-neurologic: Epistaxis (**7.12C**), respiratory distress (neurogenic pulmonary edema), systemic hypertension.

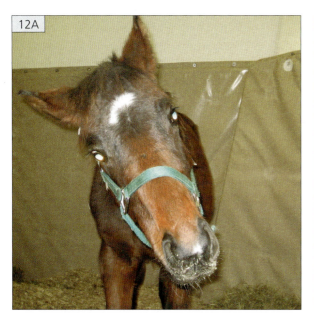

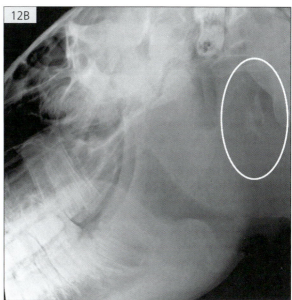

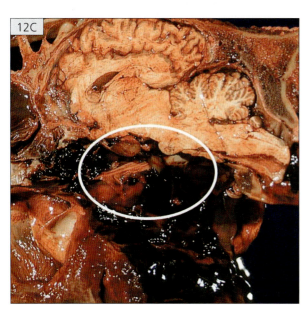

7.12A–C Head trauma. (A) Weanling foal with acute head trauma suffered while falling backward during halter training. Note the significant head tilt and bilaterally dilated pupils. The foal had ataxia, depression, vision loss, medial strabismus, and bilateral nystagmus that lasted for approximately 72 hours. Bilateral epistaxis was present 12 hours following presentation. This foal survived with treatment and the clinical signs resolved. (B) Lateral skull radiograph of the foal in 7.12A. Note the avulsion fracture from the basisphenoid region (outlined by the white oval). Also note the fluid line present in the guttural pouch, likely blood secondary to avulsion of the rectus capitis muscle from its insertion within the basisphenoid region. (C) Postmortem mid-saggital section of the skull of a foal with a basisphenoid fracture. Note the avulsion fracture present within the white oval and severe hemorrhage in the area of the fracture and the guttural pouches. (7.12A, B courtesy Dr Mike Karlin; 7.12C courtesy Dr Fabio Del Piero)

Neurologic

- **Forebrain syndrome**. Apparent concussion may occur immediately after the injury and last minutes to hours. Severely affected animals may lose all reflexes and initially appear dead. Altered behavior such as loss of suck in a foal. Impaired menace and vision with intact pupillary light reflex in the eye *contralateral* to injury. Generalized seizures. Coma.

- **Optic nerve syndrome**. Vision and pupillary light responses are impaired or absent and pupils are dilated immediately after the injury; visual function may progressively deteriorate during at least the first 24 hours post trauma (**7.12A**).

- **Midbrain syndrome**. This occurs immediately after the injury or can be secondary to subtentorial herniation of forebrain components, rostral herniation of the cerebellum, or intraparenchymal bleeding. Depression, coma. Ataxia and weakness of limbs bilaterally or contralateral to an asymmetric midbrain lesion. Neck, back, and limbs may be rigidly extended in a decorticate posture. Strabismus and a dilated unresponsive pupil.

- **Vestibular syndrome**. Is seen commonly in horses after poll trauma or THO. Clinical signs may arise because of injury centrally or, more commonly, because of involvement of the vestibular apparatus or nerve (CN VIII). Head tilt, neck turn, body lean, and staggering in tight circles, all toward the side of the lesion (**7.12A**). Signs can be revealed or exacerbated by blindfolding. With acute severe vestibular dysfunction secondary to THO, there may be sudden recumbency with flailing and thrashing movements that can be misinterpreted as seizures. Ipsilateral facial paralysis may be present. Central lesions can result in a paradoxical vestibular syndrome when the lesion is located on the side opposite to that which is expected from the clinical signs. Other signs of CN dysfunction (e.g. facial paralysis) on the side opposite to the direction of circling will be found if this is the case. Central vestibular disease signs are similar to those of peripheral injury but with additional signs of brainstem damage such as spontaneous vertical nystagmus, other CN dysfunction, mental depression, limb ataxia, and weakness (**7.12A**).

- **Hindbrain syndrome**. Is characterized by dysfunction of multiple CNs, mental depression, and limb ataxia/weakness. The gait may appear hypometric (spastic), similar to that seen in horses with compression of the cervical spinal cord. Signs of cerebellar injury occur rarely and are usually a result of poll trauma. Coarse head tremors are the most consistent sign.

- **Multifocal syndrome**. Is seen when multiple areas of brain injury become evident and may even incorporate spinal cord or cauda equina injury.

Differential diagnosis

Injury is usually obvious making other differential diagnoses unlikely. However, underlying CNS disease as a contributor to trauma should be investigated.

Diagnosis

Diagnosis is based on history, physical examination, neurologic examination, imaging studies (radiographs, CT, endoscopy, MRI) and CSF analysis.[38–40]

Management/treatment

Relevant treatments for brain injury can be classified into two levels according to evidence-based support for their use. All applicable level 1 treatments should be used in every case of clinically apparent brain injury, whereas level 2 treatments are less clearly indicated and can be considered optional.[38–40]

Level 1: These treatments should be practicable in a well-equipped equine referral hospital:

- **Treat other injuries or diseases**.
- **Treat hyperthermia**. High brain temperature accelerates all of the destructive forces unleashed during the secondary phase of brain injury so must be detected and treated vigorously. Rectal temperature should be checked frequently and efforts at cooling should begin when the

temperature exceeds 38.3°C (101°F). Antipyretic medication (e.g. flunixin meglumine, 1.1 mg/kg IV) is particularly useful when the horse has a fever, but should be tried in all cases of hyperthermia. NSAIDs have the additional advantages of analgesic and anti-inflammatory action.

- **Prevent or treat hypotension**. Blood pressure should be monitored frequently and heart base-adjusted systolic blood pressure maintained above 110 mmHg in adult horses. Blood volume should be maintained or expanded by IV infusion of isotonic (Normosol-R, Plasmalyte-A, lactated Ringer's solution) or hypertonic (Hypersaline) crystalloid or colloid (plasma, hetastarch) solutions. In the case of significant blood loss, cross-matched whole blood is the fluid of choice. If volume resuscitation alone is inadequate to restore normal pressure, pressor/inotropic drugs may be used (e.g. dopamine, dobutamine, norepinephrine). Remember that the effects of these drugs on cerebral vascular tone are difficult to predict.

- **Optimize oxygen content of blood**. Hypoxemia (PaO_2 <90 mmHg in this setting) should be treated by establishing airway patency, treating underlying pulmonary disease (e.g. head trauma-associated non-cardiogenic pulmonary edema), and beginning nasal or tracheal insufflation with oxygen. Hemoglobin concentration must be kept above 110 g/l (11 g/dl) (PCV of 0.33 l/l [33%]). Severe anemia can be treated with whole blood (preferable in the case of blood loss anemia), packed RBCs, or hemoglobin solutions.

- **Ensure adequate pulmonary ventilation**. High pCO_2 has the potential to exacerbate CNS acidosis and cerebral edema. In all horses with head trauma, pulmonary ventilation must be optimized by ensuring a patent airway and treating lung disease.

- **Control pain**. Alleviating pain in brain-injured horses is not only humane but also may reduce ICP. An NSAID can be used. Useful analgesic effects have also been seen with transdermal fentanyl patches or CRI of butorphanol or lidocaine.

- **Regulate blood glucose and maintain nutrition**. Blood glucose concentration should be kept >4.44 mmol/l (80 mg/dl) in order to provide adequate substrate for brain cells and <8.33 mmol/l (150 mg/dl) in order to prevent hyperglycemia-induced exacerbation of CNS acidosis and apoptosis of brain cells.

- **Prevent or treat brain swelling**. If possible, the neck should be free of constrictive wraps and only one jugular vein should be punctured or catheterized. Any recumbent horse should have its head elevated at least 10 degrees in order to facilitate blood flow. If the horse is significantly depressed or has signs of worsening brain function, a hyperosmolar infusion should be given to try to reduce the extravascular volume of the brain. Hypertonic saline (1,232 mmol Na/l) may be given as a continuous IV infusion of 1 ml (1.2 mmol)/kg/h for 6 hours and then 0.2 ml/kg for another 12 hours. Alternatively, boluses of 2 ml/kg can be given q4h for five infusions. Further treatment with hypertonic saline should be based on reassessment of clinical signs and plasma Na concentration (keep <150 mmol/l). Mannitol (20% solution) can also be used for this purpose as a series of bolus infusions of 0.25–1.0 g/kg q4–6h.

- **Treat seizures**. Seizures should be treated vigorously when they occur. They may be treated with diazepam (0.01–0.4 mg/kg slow IV) (or midazolam [3–4 mg slow IV] in neonates), phenobarbital (3–5 mg/kg slow IV over 20 minutes, repeat as necessary), or pentobarbital (2–10 mg/kg IV q8–12h). Once a horse has a seizure, anti-seizure medication (phenobarbital, 1–4 mg/kg PO divided q12h) should be continued for at least 7 days.

- **Decompress the skull**. After initial stabilization of the patient, depressed fractures of the frontal/parietal area that impinge on the cerebral cortex may be carefully elevated and reduced under general anesthesia. It is the author's opinion that horses with neurologic signs referable to THO should undergo some form of stylohyoid release surgery (removal of a portion of the hyoid apparatus on the affected side) in order to prevent or help stabilize skull fractures.

Level 2: These treatments are technically possible in horses and their use is supported either by strong anecdotal data from equine practice or by convincing experimental data in other species. These treatments either are impractical in an equine hospital or do not meet the standard of evidence-based medicine:

- **Treat with antioxidants**:
  - High-dose methylprednisolone sodium succinate (initial bolus dose of 30 mg/kg, followed by CRI of 5.4 mg/kg/hour for 24–48 hours) is effective treatment for spinal cord trauma in humans if given within the first 8 hours. High-dose steroids have not proven effective in humans with brain trauma.
  - DMSO (0.1–1.0 g/kg IV as a 10% solution) is very widely used by equine practitioners for treatment of CNS trauma. Potential advantages include antioxidant and diuretic actions, but there is virtually no evidence for effectiveness in the setting of brain injury.
  - Vitamin E (α tocopherol; 50 IU/kg PO q24h), vitamin C (ascorbic acid, 20 mg/kg PO q24h), mannitol (see above), and allopurinol (5 mg/kg PO q12h), are all antioxidant therapies that can be used in the horse and can be rationalized as part of the overall approach to brain trauma.
- **Give conventional doses of corticosteroids**. Traditional anti-inflammatory doses of dexamethasone (0.05–0.1 mg/kg IV or 0.1–0.2 mg/kg PO q12–24 h) or prednisolone (1–4 mg/kg PO q12h) likely inhibit the production and action of injurious mediators in the brain and may be of some value.
- **Place an intraventricular drainage catheter**. Core protocols for human head trauma all mandate transcalvarial insertion of a valved indwelling catheter into a lateral ventricle. The indwelling catheter is used both for monitoring of ICP and drainage of CSF in order to keep pressure <20–25 mm Hg. CSF drainage is technically possible in horses, but the clean conditions and prolonged head immobilization required likely make this procedure impractical in all but valuable neonates.

- **Give magnesium sulfate**. Magnesium sulfate ($MgSO_4$) has the potential to inhibit several aspects of the secondary injury cascade including glutamate release, activity of the N-methyl-D-asparate and calcium channels, and lipid peroxidation. Studies have shown that 250 μmole/kg improves neurologic outcome when given 30 minutes after brain impact injury. In light of these findings and its demonstrated safety in horses, it seems reasonable to give a single IV infusion of $MgSO_4$ at 50 mg/kg (approximately 250 μmole/kg). This dose (25 g in a 500-kg horse) can conveniently be administered with the first 5–10 liters of IV fluids.

In the past the prognosis for horses with severe head injury was thought to be guarded. Recent data suggest that with treatment, many horses with severe initial signs may survive and return to useful function. Even in horses initially recumbent and minimally responsive, a period of treatment, perhaps up to several weeks to months, is warranted, given evidence of continued improvement.[38,40]

Temporohyoid osteoarthropathy
Key points
- The most common emergency-related presenting complaints for THO relate to the eye and include corneal ulceration and excessive lacrimation due to exposure keratitis.

Definition/overview
THO is an inflammatory/infectious condition of the joint formed by the stylohyoid bone and the petrous temporal bone (**7.13**).

Etiology/pathogenesis
The pathogenesis remains speculative. A low-grade bacterial infection that affects the mucosal lining of the tympanic bulla may extend to involve adjacent structures (i.e. the stylohyoid and petrous temporal bones).[41] *Actinobacillus equuli* has been isolated from affected horses. The source of an infection may be hematogenous spread of bacteria, ascending respiratory tract infection, or extension from otitis externa or a guttural pouch infection.[42]

Clinical signs may be minimal to absent during this stage of disease. Bony proliferation and degenerative joint disease lead to ankylosis of the temporohyoid joint and clinical signs, if present, may temporarily improve at this time. However, with tongue movement and transfer of forces along the hyoid apparatus, acute fracture across the petrous temporal bone and/or stylohyoid bone may result. Fractures between the petrous temporal bone and the tympanic bulla may extend into the internal acoustic meatus. Infection can extend through the internal acoustic meatus, causing meningitis or encephalitis. The close association of CNs VII, VIII, IX, and X with the bony structures involved results in the clinical signs. Primary degenerative disease of the temporohyoid joint may occur without pre-existing infection.[42]

Clinical features

Early clinical signs may include head tossing/shaking, ear rubbing, resentment of the bit or bridle, pain over the base of the ear, and quidding. Head tilt, nystagmus, weak extensor tone, and facial nerve paralysis signs (ear droop, inability to close eyelids, collection of food in the buccal cavity [all ipsilaterally] and muzzle deviation to the unaffected side) are seen with progression of the disease (**7.14**).[41–44]

Following fracture an acute deterioration in clinical signs can be seen, with seizures, ataxia, and recumbency. Dramatic clinical signs may develop when the horse is being examined or treated for another problem and this is presumed to be secondary to fracture occurrence at that time.[42] Examples include post-dentistry and post-oropharyngeal intubation for general anesthesia.

Keratoconjunctivitis sicca and miosis may be noted because the parasympathetic efferent innervation of the eye that supplies the lacrimal gland courses with the facial nerve. Other conditions observed include laryngeal hemiparesis and megaesophagus. Purulent discharge from an infected ear may be present at the external ear canal.

Clinical signs are mostly unilateral but bilateral disease can be present, even with unilateral signs.[42]

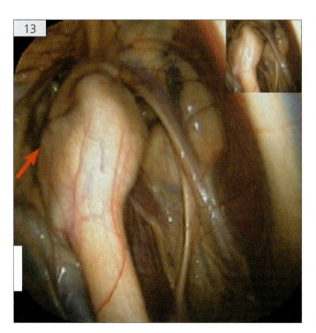

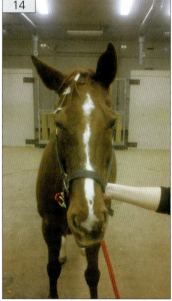

7.13 Enlarged right temporostylohoid articulation in the right guttural pouch of a horse with temporohyoid osteoarthropathy. (Courtesy Dr Jen Gold)

7.14 Right-sided ear droop and facial paralysis in a horse with temporohyoid osteoarthropathy of the right guttural pouch. This horse also has a subpalpebral catheter in place and has received a temporary tarsorrhaphy for treatment of exposure keratitis, the initial presenting complaint.

Differential diagnosis

Skull fracture/head trauma; otitis media/externa; guttural pouch mycosis; encephalitis; EPM; neoplasia.

Diagnosis

Physical, neurologic, radiographic, and endoscopic examinations are critical for accurate diagnosis.

Endoscopic examination of the guttural pouch is the most specific diagnostic method.[42] The stylohyoid bone appears enlarged at its junction with the petrous temporal bone (**7.13**). Radiographs can reveal abnormal appearing stylohyoid and petrous temporal bones (**7.15**) and tympanic bulla. A fracture may be seen in the shaft of the stylohyoid bone. CT and MRI provide a definitive method of diagnosing a fracture and assessing the temporohyoid joint, but the risks of general anesthesia must be considered.

Tympanocentesis to retrieve fluid for culture of bacterial pathogens in the middle ear is considered technically difficult, usually requires general anesthesia, and is not performed routinely.[43,44]

Management/treatment

Medical management with or without surgery is indicated. Horses with acute onset neurologic signs will require emergency care to prevent further injury and possibly seizure control (diazepam or midazolam *Box 7.4*).

Long-term systemic antimicrobial drugs are recommended to treat any possible infectious component of the condition and NSAIDs should be administered.

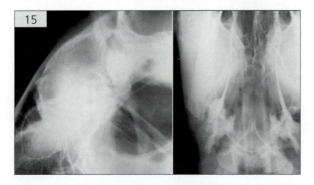

7.15 Lateral and DV radiographs of a horse with enlargement of the stylohyoid and temporostylohyoid articulation. (Courtesy Dr Tom Divers)

Immediate treatment of corneal ulceration (temporary tarsorrhaphy is useful) is mandatory.

Stylohyoid or ceratohyoid ostectomy performed under general anesthesia can prevent transfer of forces along the stylohoid that may result in a fracture at the petrous temporal bone/tympanic bulla level.[44,45]

Prognosis is guarded and based on the severity of clinical signs. In one study, however, 63% of horses were athletically usable following treatment.[42] Often neurologic deficits persist and managing recurrent eye problems is difficult.

Hepatic encephalopathy
Key points

- It is important that an attempt is made to distinguish between hepatoencephalopathy and intestinal hyperammonemia if at all possible, as the prognosis for intestinal hyperammonemia is better.
- It is important that precautions are taken to avoid/limit the potential for injury to both the patient and attending personel.
- Anti-seizure medication such as diazepam and midazolam should be avoided in these cases as they may exacerbate any underlying increased GABA activity.

Definition/overview

Hepatic encephalopathy (HE) is a frequently observed clinical syndrome in animals with liver dysfunction. HE is characterized by inappropriate behavior, impaired motor function, and alterations in mental status occurring secondary to hepatic insufficiency (or portosystemic shunting).[46,47]

Etiology/pathogenesis

The underlying pathophysiology of HE has not been fully elucidated, but is likely multifactorial.

The most widely accepted theory involves ammonia, produced by bacteria in the GI tract and transported to the liver for conversion to urea and glutamine. Failure of conversion allows ammonia accumulation in the systemic circulation. The brain has a limited capacity to remove ammonia, and ammonia acts as a neurotoxin, interfering with neurotransmission.

A second theory involves alteration in the branched chain amino acids (BCAAs) to aromatic amino acids (AAAs) ratio. BCAAs are metabolized by muscle and adipose tissue; AAA metabolism by the liver is decreased and results in a relative increase in AAAs and decrease in BCAAs. AAAs are preferentially transported into the brain where they act as precursors for serotonin, an inhibitory neurotransmitter, resulting in a net decrease in neuronal excitation (increase in neural inhibition).

A final theory suggests activation of the GABA/benzodiazepine/chloride ionophore complex on inhibitory postsynaptic neurons by endogenous benzodiazepine-like receptor ligands, whose source has yet to be identified. Activation of inhibitory neurons, as above, results in cerebral dysfunction.

Clinical features

Typical clinical signs include depression, head pressing (**7.16**), circling, aimless wandering, and persistent yawning, followed by recumbency and coma. Aggressive behavior and seizures may be observed, but are not typical. Fifty percent of horses with confirmed hepatic disease had clinical evidence of HE in one report.[48]

Differential diagnosis

The primary differential diagnosis is intestinal hyperammonemia.

Diagnosis

Diagnosis of HE is dependent on recognition of characteristic clinical signs, clinical or laboratory evidence of hepatic dysfunction, and elimination of other causes of cerebral dysfunction.[46–48] Increased blood ammonia concentration is supportive of a diagnosis of HE.

A primary rule-out is 'idiopathic (intestinal) hyperammonemia'. In these cases liver enzymes and function tests will be either within normal limits or close to normal limits, but ammonia concentration will be increased. This syndrome may carry an improved prognosis over HE.[49]

Management/treatment

Treatment is aimed at supporting the patient until liver function returns and involves general supportive measures such as correction of dehydration and acid–base abnormalities, as well as more specific therapies including reducing ammonia production:

- Intravenous fluids. Supplemented with potassium, as hypokalemia can exacerbate the condition by increasing formation of ammonia by the kidneys.
- Glucose supplementation in IV fluids. Unless the horse is hyperglycemic.
- Sedation. Low doses of the alpha-2 agonists xylazine or detomidine. Diazepam and other benzodiazepines should be avoided as they may enhance the effect of GABA on inhibitory neurons.
- Mineral oil and lactulose via nasogastric tube. Decreases GI transit time and limits absorption of ammonia.
- Oral administration of antimicrobials, such as neomycin or metronidazole, to reduce numbers ammonia-producing bacteria. Oral neomycin significantly alters the colonic bacterial population, and diarrhea commonly occurs. Metronidazole can result in neurologic disturbances, potentially exacerbating signs of HE.

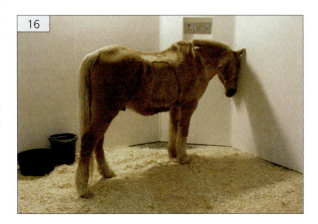

7.16 A horse with hepatoencephalopathy demonstrating head pressing behavior. (Courtesy Dr Brett Tennent-Brown)

Although HE is a potentially reversible syndrome, the prognosis remains guarded, as HE generally accompanies end-stage chronic liver disease (**7.17**).

Diseases producing cerebellar signs
Parasitic encephalitis
Key points
- *Halicephalobus* spp. infection can be seen more commonly in certain geographic regions.

Definition/overview
The genus *Halicephalobus* (previously known as *Micronema*) includes free-living nematodes of soil, manure, and decaying humus. *Halicephalobus gingivalis* (*deletrix*) invades and reproduces in tissues of horses and humans, with fatal outcomes. The most commonly involved organs in the horse include the brain, kidneys, oral and nasal cavities, mandible, lymph nodes, spinal cord, and mammary and adrenal glands.

Etiology/pathogenesis
The epidemiology of the disease is not understood because of the cryptic lifecycle of the organism and its rarity of presentation. Foals have been reportedly infected by exposure to their infected dams, perhaps through ingestion of milk from parasitized mammary gland.[50]

Clinical features
Clinical signs vary, as can the reported time of onset, but are frequently seen as referable to the cerebellum and/or the optic tract. Horses may be ataxic, with a base-wide stance, or present recumbent. Intention tremor may be present. Visual deficits, either apparent or suggested by loss of menace and pupillary light reflexes, are common. There may be concurrent lesions in the bones of the skull (mandible) and renal involvement is common.

Differential diagnosis
Includes all diseases that can result in acute onset ataxia and recumbency.

Diagnosis
Diagnosis is achieved by biopsy of a suspected non-CNS lesion and observation of the organism either as an adult female or larval form. CSF analysis may be abnormal with eosinophilia and increased protein concentration. Rarely, with renal involvement, the organism may be found in the urine.[50]

Management/treatment
There have been no reported cases of successful treatment, although various anthelmentic regimens have been attempted.

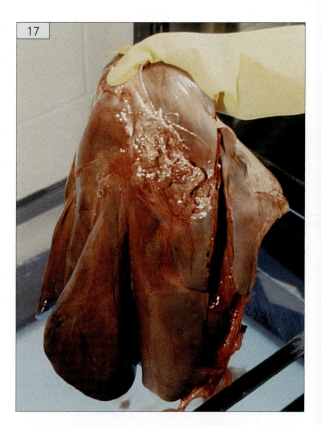

7.17 Classic 'dishrag liver' seen with Theiler's disease, a disease commonly associated with hepatoencephalopathy. (Courtesy Dr Fabio Del Piero)

Diseases producing spinal cord or peripheral nerve signs
Equine protozoal myeloencephalitis
See pp. 467–468.

Vertebral trauma
Key points
- A history of a traumatic incident may be present. Alternatively, the horse may be found suddenly recumbent.
- Unless trauma to the head has also occurred, affected horses frequently have normal CN signs and normal alert demeanor.

Etiology/pathogenesis
The pathophysiology of spinal cord injury comprises primary and secondary insults. The primary injury results from initial mechanical injury to the cord and consists of severed axons, physical damage to neurons and glial cells, and disturbed microvasculature (**7.18A, B**). Secondary injury, as with traumatic head injury, refers to the events that follow the primary insult including microvascular ischemia, oxidative stress, inflammation, excitotoxicity, ion dysregulation, and delayed demyelination.

Clinical features
To facilitate neuroanatomic localization, the spinal cord has been divided into five regions: (1) high cervical (C1 to C5), (2) cervicothoracic (C6 to T2), (3) thoracolumbar (T3 to L2), (4) lumbosacral (L3 to S2), and (5) sacrococcygeal (S3 to Cd5).

Clinical signs depend on the location of the lesion and the relative amount of damage to gray (cell bodies) and white (myelinated spinal cord tracts) matter. The white matter is usually more susceptible to compression than the gray matter. Animals with spinal cord disease and no central involvement usually have an intact sensorium and retain their appetite.

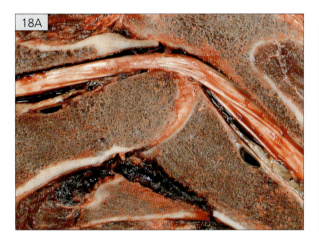
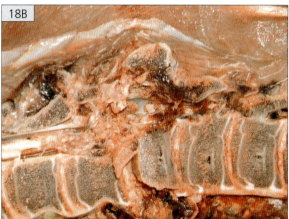

7.18A, B Spinal cord trauma. (A) Mid-saggital cross-section of a vertebral body fracture. Note the fracture of the cranial ventral body of the cudal vertebra, with compression of the spinal cord secondary to the dorsal luxation of the joint. There is severe local hemorrhage and hemorrhage within the spinal canal. (Courtesy Dr Fabio Del Piero) (B) Mid-saggital cross-section of a vertebral body compression fracture that has displaced dorsally and compressed the spinal cord. This foal was acutely affected following running into a tree.

Differential diagnosis

Includes all causes of acute recumbency unless trauma was observed.

Diagnosis

Diagnosis is based on history, clinical signs, thorough physical and neurologic examinations, and advanced imaging, where available. A thorough neurologic examination is required in an attempt to localize the lesion, which will direct additional diagnostics and enable formulation of a treatment plan.

The majority of the cervical spine is easily radiographed in the standing animal. In the anesthetized horse, additional radiographic views of the neck are possible and include lateral-flexed, lateral-extended, and ventrodorsal (C1 to C5 or C6) views. Detection of subtle lesions and fractures may be difficult unless there is significant displacement, particularly in large individuals. Minimal fracture displacement is common because of the extensive soft tissues supporting the spinal column. Significant injury to the spinal cord may occur without radiographic evidence of osseous damage. If history and clinical signs suggest a spinal fracture in a location that could be difficult to confirm with radiographs, or if radiography fails to reveal a definitive diagnosis, additional diagnostic modalities should be considered.

Myelography is a relatively safe, although not completely benign, procedure and may allow more accurate identification of lesions compressing the spinal cord. Although largely restricted to assessment of the cervical spine, myelography has been used to assess the integrity of more caudal structures.

The major limitation of CT and MRI is availability and requirement for a general anesthetic. Currently, there are physical limitations on what can be imaged. In most cases, CT imaging of the head and neck of adults is possible, MRI of adult equine heads has been described, and imaging of at least a portion of the neck is theoretically possible. In foals, CT of the entire spinal column may be possible. Broadly speaking, CT is preferred for imaging osseous structures and MRI for soft tissue assessment.

Sedation or short-term anesthesia will often be required in the initial management of trauma patients or to perform diagnostic procedures. Acepromazine and ketamine should be avoided in animals suspected of having head trauma or at risk for seizures. In healthy, conscious horses, the commonly used α_2-adrenergic agonists decrease CSF pressure. Xylazine (0.2–1.1 mg/kg IV) or detomidine (0.005–0.02 mg/kg IV) either alone or in combination with the opioid agionist-antagonist butorphanol (0.044–0.066 mg/kg IV) provides excellent sedation. The direct effects of opioids on cerebral blood flow and ICP are minimal, although they may indirectly increase CSF pressure as a result of respiratory depression and CO_2 retention.

Management/treatment

Treatment of spinal cord injuries in horses is generally not rewarding, but if undertaken, the therapies outlined for head injury (p. 468) may be appropriate. There is currently no evidence that high-dose corticosteroid therapy is of any benefit in horses, although its efficacy has been demonstrated in humans with spinal cord injury.[39,51]

Botulism

Key points

- Botulism is a flaccid paralysis of horses that may or may not progress to recumbency.
- Dysphagia is a common presenting complaint.
- Vaccination is protective and should be undertaken in endemic geographic regions.
- Death occurs due to respiratory failure.

Definition/overview

Botulism is a disease caused by the obligate anaerobe, gram-positive, spore-forming, toxin-producing organism *Clostridium botulinum*, although a few strains of *C. baratii* and *C. butyricum* may also cause disease. Reports describing botulism in horses can be found from the early 1950s. It occurs in adult horses and in foals, where it has been termed 'shaker foal syndrome'.[52–56]

Etiology/pathogenesis

Botulism is a flaccid paralytic syndrome caused by the neurotoxins produced by *Clostridium botulinum*. Botulinum toxin is referred to as the most potent toxin known to man. The organism produces eight distinct neurotoxins, depending on the isolate: A, B, Ca, Cb, D, E, F, and G. The toxin causes paresis and paralysis by interfering with acetylcholine release at the neuromuscular junction.[57] Death is usually attributed to respiratory failure. Botulism can result from the ingestion of preformed toxin or the growth of *C. botulinum* in anaerobic tissues. All types of botulinum toxin produce the same disease; however, the toxin type is important if antitoxin is used for treatment.[52]

Botulism has a world-wide distribution and the distribution of spore type is related to soil pH and temperature.[52,56] For example, there is a geographic distribution to the disease with a concentration of reported cases in Kentucky and the Mid-Atlantic region of the Eastern USA. Toxin types B and C most commonly affect horses and horses are extremely susceptible to minute amounts of toxin. In North America, type B is most commonly found in the Mid-Atlantic States and Kentucky. Type A is prevalent west of the Rocky Mountains and type C arises mainly in Florida.

Botulism intoxication occurs thorough a multistep process involving each of the toxin's functional domains and can be summarized as the outcome of three distinct stages:[57]
- Binding to the target cell and internalization.
- Translocation.
- Inhibition of neurotransmitter release.

Clinical features

Clinical findings are primarily those related to neuromuscular junction inhibition: dysphagia, flaccid paralysis, diminished pupillary reactivity, decreased eyelid (**7.19**), tongue and tail tone, and progressive flaccid tetraparesis/plegia.[52–56,58] The disease is characterized as affecting primarily the lower motor neurons of the general somatic efferent system, although some autonomic abnormalities may also occur.

Dyspnea and cyanosis may be present initially or terminally. Death is generally attributed to respiratory failure secondary to respiratory muscle paralysis. Horses that walk may have a stilted, short-strided gait without ataxia. Muscle trembling and/or weakness may be apparent, particularly in foals. There is normal sensation with depressed reflexes. Pharyngeal paralysis is frequently seen in adults. Abnormal prehension and pupillary dilatation are commonly seen. Adults and foals may rapidly progress to recumbency. Tachycardia is not uncommon, particularly in foals. Foals may appear or become constipated and dysuric.

Differential diagnosis

Differential diagnoses include, but are not limited to, severe electrolyte imbalance (hyponatremia), tick paralysis, and postanesthetic myasthenic syndrome.

Diagnosis

Diagnosis of botulism is first and foremost a clinical diagnosis after exclusion of other disease. Detection of circulating toxin by mouse innoculation is possible, but often too little toxin is circulating for detection in this manner. Isolation of *C. botulinum*, or toxin, from feedstuffs or GI contents (feces, or GI contents in the case of peracute death) or from lesions or wounds in the patient is strong circumstantial evidence of infection.[52]

Management/treatment

The efficacy of early administration of antitoxin in improving survival and decreasing hospitalization duration has been clearly demonstrated for humans and horses and is the mainstay of therapy.[52–56,58]

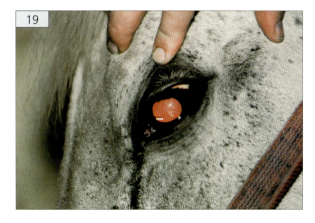

7.19 Botulism. Adult horse with botulism demonstrating decreased eyelid tone. Note the dilated pupil. (Courtesy Dr Robert Whitlock)

Adults and foals with mild respiratory failure and with normal pH in the face of mild to moderately increased $PaCO_2$ can frequently be treated with intranasal oxygen insufflation, positioning in sternal recumbency, and repeated arterial blood gas monitoring to detect worsening respiratory failure. Foals with botulism and respiratory failure can be successfully mechanically ventilated.[58]

Nutritional management must be considered in horses with botulism and can generally be achieved in foals by feeding milk or milk replacer via indwelling nasogastric or nasoesophogeal tubes, and, in adult horses, periodic nasogastic intubation of slurry meals can be provided. Parenteral nutrition is generally not necessary. IV fluid support may be required until patients are able to drink water safely. Recumbent patients should be managed as outlined (see Chapter 21).

Botulinum neurointoxication is a survivable disease for appropriately treated foals <6 months of age with survival rates of >90%.[55,56,58] Adult horses that remain standing carry a good prognosis for recovery, which may require several weeks to months before they return to work. Horses that become recumbent carry a poorer prognosis, even with antitoxin administration and excellent nursing care.[52–54,56]

Appropriate vaccination is protective for adults; vaccination of the pregnant dam will protect a foal as long as there is no failure of passive transfer and the foal receives its own vaccination at the appropriate age.[52–56,58]

Tetanus

Key points
- Tetanus is fully preventable by vaccination.

Definition/overview
Tetanus is a disease caused by *Clostridium tetani* infection.

Etiology/pathogenesis
The spores of *C. tetani* are found in the environment (soil) worldwide. When spores become inoculated into a wound, they germinate and the bacterium proliferates, eluting the tetanus toxin. Tetanus toxin is absorbed and travels to the CNS, via peripheral nerves, where it exerts an inhibitory effect on inhibitory internuncial neurons, resulting in an extensor spastic paresis.[57,59]

Clinical features
Skin wounds may be evident, but frequently the site of inoculation is a small puncture wound that is not definitively identified.

Spasm of voluntary muscles may appear anytime between 7 and 14 days post innoculation. The first signs are associated with chewing/swallowing difficulty and muscle spasm is progressive over the head/neck, trunk, and limbs; erect ears and flared nostrils are followed by limb rigidity and a sawhorse stance. Prolapse of the nictitans is an early prominent clinical sign. Muscle spasm increases until finally the respiratory muscles are paralyzed and death occurs.

Differential diagnosis
Hypocalcemia, hyponatremia.

Diagnosis
Diagnosis is based on the classic presentation of clinical signs. History of a recent wound (puncture in particular) is helpful.[59]

Management/treatment[59]
Administration of tetanus antitoxin (1,000–5,000 IU/500 kg body weight IV; 50 ml of 1,000 IU/ml antitoxin intracisternally after slow removal of 30 ml CSF has been anecdotally reported as useful), although this may be of little benefit as toxin is already bound.

If a wound can be found, it should be cleaned, debrided and lavaged. Antibiotic treatment (penicillin) is indicated. Supportive care such as IV fluids and nutritional support in addition to wound care. Provide a quiet, non-stimulating environment. Remove objects that could result in injury. Sedation if necessary. Acepromazine at 0.05–0.1 mg/kg IV q4–6h has been reported to be useful. Diazepam (0.01–0.4 mg/kg IV q2–8h has been used to quieten muscle spasticity by GABA enhancement.

Survival is possible if the condition is recognized early in the clinical course. As with most neurologic diseases of adult horses, recumbency decreases the prognosis.

Vaccination is protective.[59] Foals born to unvaccinated mares, or with failure of passive transfer of immunity, and unvaccinated horses with wounds or undergoing surgery, should be treated prophylactically with tetanus antitoxin.

Spinal cord abscess/vertebral osteomyelitis
Key points
- Bacterial infection of the spinal cord or vertebra with abscess formation is most commonly encountered in foals as a consequence of generalized sepsis that may have been previously unrecognized.
- Adult horses affected by the syndrome should be evaluated for underlying immune dysfunction.

Definition/overview
Osteomyelitis of a vertebral body is a rare condition in horses and has a grave prognosis, likely the result of the advanced stage of disease that is present when clinical signs and radiographic changes are identified.[60–62]

Etiology/pathogenesis
In foals, hematogenous spread of bacteria through slow-flowing vertebral capillaries is considered the most likely mechanism of infection. The most commonly reported isolated organism in foals is *Rhodococcus equi*.

Clinical features
Clinical signs most frequently observed in horses with vertebral body osteomyelitis are referable to pain and neurologic signs caused by extradural compression of the spinal cord. Fever and hyperfibrinogenemia may be present, as may other sites of infection, particularly in foals with *R.equi* infection.

Differential diagnosis
Meningitis.

Diagnosis
Diagnosis is made by identification of abscesses/osteomyelitis using imaging techniques, including plain radiography, myelography, CT, and MRI, of the affected area. CSF analysis may demonstrate inflammation or be within normal limits.

Management/treatment
Treatment, if undertaken, includes long-term administration of antimicrobials based preferably on the sensitivity pattern of isolated organisms and their ability to penetrate bone. Surgical debridement may be considered in cases where the infected vertebral body has reasonable surgical access, although this approach remains clinically untested.

Neoplastic disease producing cerebral, cerebellar, spinal cord, or peripheral nerve signs
Key points
- Neoplasia of the CNS is rare and always carries a guarded prognosis.

Definition/overview
Neoplasia affecting the spinal cord is a rare occurrence in the horse and clinical signs are generally referable to extradural compression of the spinal cord. The clinical course is generally insidious, although cases may rarely present as emergency admissions. Reported tumors involving the spinal cord of the horse have most commonly been metastases of non-neural origin with other

primary foci in the body. Reported neoplasms include melanoma, SCC, hemangiosarcoma, intestinal adenocarcinoma, plasma cell myeloma, fibrosarcoma, pheochromocytoma, lymphoma, and poorly differentiated sarcoma.[63]

Etiology/pathogenesis

Neoplasia of the brain can be divided into two main categories: non-pituitary CNS neoplasia and pituitary adenomas (**7.20A, B**). Non-pituitary tumors are generally compressive in nature, although some are also invasive. The majority of reported CNS tumors are secondary with only a few originating from nervous tissue. Pituitary adenomas predominantly occur in the pars intermedia of the older horse and will not be discussed further in this chapter beyond noting that if large, they may result in compressive lesions, primarily affecting the optic chiasm and hypothalamus.

Clinical features

The clinical signs exhibited are generally referable to single or multifocal asymmetric intracranial masses and can include seizure, ataxia, CN deficits, loss of vision, and depression among others. Behavioral changes (subtle and dramatic) are important indicators of potential intracranial disease.

Differential diagnosis

Any other CNS diseases resulting in similar clinical signs.

Diagnosis

Diagnosis is suggested by ruling out infectious or other causes of the clinical signs and is based on clinical signs and imaging studies, including plain radiography, myelography and MRI or CT where available.[63,64]

Management/treatment

Treatment is generally ineffective and unrewarding, although reports exist of surgical excision of solitary masses. Prognosis is uniformly grave.[63]

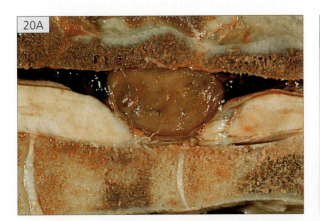
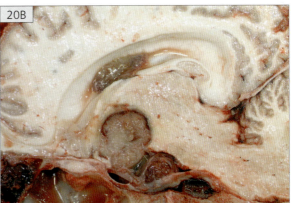

7.20A, B Neoplasia. (A) Mid-saggital section of spinal column showing spinal cord compressions secondary to an extradural schwannoma. (B) Mid-saggital cross-section of skull showing a pituitary primary lymphoma and adenoma compressing the midbrain region.

CHAPTER 8

EYE AND ASSOCIATED STRUCTURES

Elizabeth J. Davidson
and Mary Lassaline-Utter

GENERAL APPROACH TO THE HORSE WITH AN INJURY INVOLVING THE EYE OR ASSOCIATED STRUCTURES

- The most common ophthalmic emergencies in horses are related to injury to the eye and surrounding structures. The horse eye is prominently located along the lateral aspect of the head and is particularly susceptible to traumatic injury. Objects within stalls and fencing are frequently the source of blunt force trauma to the eye. Fortunately, eye injuries are often impressive in appearance and prompt immediate attention by the owner.
- Ophthalmic injuries are often painful. The patient can briefly be examined by observing the structures involved. Sedation as well as ophthalmic nerve blocks and topical local anesthesia is recommended prior to physically examining the eye.
- Initial examination involves determining the structures involved (i.e. eyelid, orbit, cornea, or intraocular structures) and the extent and type of injury to these structures.
- Specific treatments vary based on the structures involved and the type of injury; however, prompt emergency treatment is critical for a favorable outcome.

DEFINITIONS

- Blepharospasm: squinting
- Iridocyclitis: inflammation of the iris and ciliary body, also called anterior uveitis.
- Keratomalacia: 'melting' or collagenolysis of the cornea.
- Photophobia: greater than normal sensitivity to light.
- Epiphora: excessive lacrimation or tearing.
- Endophthalmitis: inflammation of the internal structures within the globe, often caused by infection; can be a complication of intraocular surgery.
- Hyphema: RBCs within the anterior chamber.
- Hypopyon: WBCs within the anterior chamber.
- Iridocyclitis: inflammation of the iris and the ciliary body.
- Synechia: adhesion between the cornea and iris (anterior) or the iris and lens (posterior).
- Seidel test: application of concentrated fluorescein, which appears orange, to the corneal surface to detect a perforation. A perforation, or leak, appears as dilute fluorescein (fluorescent green with a cobalt blue light) at the site of the leak, surrounded by the concentrated fluorescein.
- Uveitis: inflammation of the uvea, which is the middle layer of the eye between the sclera and retina including the iris, the choroid of the eye, and the ciliary body.

COMMON PROCEDURES PERFORMED ON HORSES WITH OPHTHALMIC EMERGENCIES

Ophthalmic nerve blocks
Indications
Auriculopalpebral nerve block: The auriculopalpebral nerve block provides akinesia of the orbicularis oculi muscle and can be used to prevent eyelid closure. Eyelid sensation persists. The auriculopalpebral nerve block can facilitate examination of a painful or fragile eye and is useful for diagnostic procedures including corneal culture and cytology. It can also be used for placement of subpalpebral lavage systems, as well as any other procedure in which a firmly closed lid would be prohibitive.

Supraorbital (frontal) nerve block: The frontal nerve, which innervates the medial and central upper lid, can be blocked at the supraorbital foramen, a depression medial to the narrowest aspect of the supraorbital process of the frontal bone. This block is performed prior to placement of an upper lid subpalpebral lavage.

Technique
Auriculopalpebral nerve block
- The palpebral branch can be palpated in two places, just lateral to the dorsal most border of the zygomatic arch and on the zygomatic arch caudal to the bony process of the frontal bone (**8.1**).
- Injection of lidocaine or mepivicaine at either of these sites, or at a third site just anterior to the base of the ear (where the nerve cannot be palpated), should paralyze the upper lid within several minutes and for several hours.
- Corneal dessication typically does not result from this temporary inability to blink.

Supraorbital (frontal) nerve block
- A 25-gauge needle is inserted into or just over the supraorbital foramen (**8.2**) and lidocaine or mepivicaine injected.
- It is not necessary for the needle to enter the foramen to achieve a good block.

Other nerve blocks
- The lateral upper lid is innervated by the lacrimal nerve, which can be blocked along the lateral aspect of the orbital rim.
- The infratrochlear nerve innervates the medial aspect of the lower lid as well as the medial canthus, and it can be blocked at the palpable trochlear notch, on the medial aspect of the orbital rim.
- The lateral lower lid is innervated by the zygomatic nerve, which can be blocked along the ventrolateral orbital rim.
- Anesthesia of the cornea and conjunctiva (including palpebral and bulbar conjunctiva, as well as that overlying the nictitans) can be achieved by topical application of tetracaine or proparacaine.

Complications
Complications are rare with these nerve blocks, with the most common being failure of the block to take effect.

Subpalpebral lavage catheter placement
Indications
A subpalpebral lavage catheter facilitates administration of topical ophthalmic medications. The catheter foot plate may be positioned through the upper or lower eyelid.[1]

Technique
- Catheters are typically placed in standing sedated horses.
- The horse is sedated and auriculopalpebral and frontal nerve blocks are performed (see Ophthalmic nerve blocks).
- The hair from the upper eyelid at the orbital rim is shaved (optional).
- The upper or lower eyelid is aseptically prepared.
- Local anesthetic is injected subcutaneously where the catheter will exit through the eyelid.
- Topical anesthetic (0.5% proparacaine) is placed in the eye.
- Using aseptic technique, a 10- to 14-gauge trochar is placed under the eyelid, then through the palpebral conjunctiva and eyelid skin at a point near the orbital rim and about midway along the length of the eyelid (**8.3**).

- With the trochar in place, the lavage tubing is inserted through the trochar going from the inner (conjunctival) to the outer (skin) side.
- The needle (trochar) and tubing are pulled through the skin.
- The tubing system is fed through braids in the mane and an injection port is attached at the distal end. The tube and port are taped to a tongue depressor to make the unit rigid (**8.4**).

- The lavage system should be pulled firmly into the fornix so the foot plate does not irritate the cornea.
- The tubing system is then anchored to the head by use of suture and tape (**8.4**).

Complications

Improper placement of a subpalpebral lavage catheter can result in corneal trauma with ulceration (p. 495). Therefore, care should be taken to ensure it is placed in the fornix near the orbital rim and secured in place.

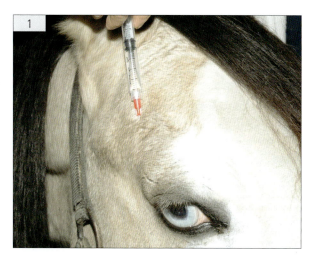

8.1 Auriculopalpebral nerve block. (Courtesy Dr Ralph Hamor)

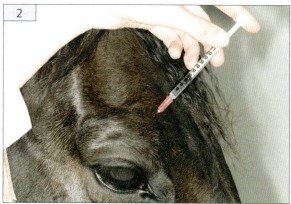

8.2 Frontal nerve block. A 25-gauge, 5/8 inch needle is inserted into the supraorbital foramen. (Courtesy Dr Ralph Hamor)

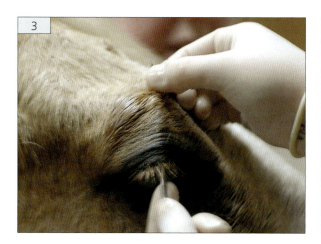

8.3 Trochar placement through the upper eyelid.

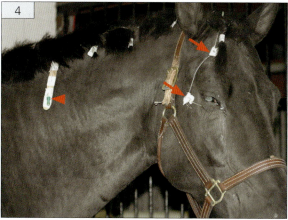

8.4 Subpalpebral lavage system. The injection port (arrowhead) is stabilized on a tongue depressor and the tubing is secured to the lower eyelid (arrows).

Conjunctival graft
Indications
Conjunctival grafts are used for deep corneal ulcers and other corneal wounds when the lesion extends to or close to Descemet's membrane. Grafts provide blood supply, fibroblasts, anticollagenases, and support for weakened corneal stroma. There are many types of conjunctival grafts; however, pedicle conjunctival grafts are the most frequently used and best suited technique.[2]

Technique
- The horse is anesthetized and the affected eye prepared using an aseptic technique.
- Necrotic, infected, or diseased cornea is removed. Keratectomy is best performed with a 6400 Beaver blade (**8.5**).
- Excised tissue samples are submitted for cytologic evaluation as well as bacterial and fungal culture and sensitivity testing.
- The conjunctiva is incised approximately 1 mm behind the limbus and extended parallel to the limbus (**8.6**). The incision is extended radially at 90 degrees to the limbus for a distance equal to the width of the ulcer (**8.7**).
- The conjunctival flap is completed by continuing the incision parallel to the initial incision to create a pedicle of conjunctiva with a wide base.
- A good, well dissected flap should be semitransparent.
- The flap is then rotated and placed over the ulcer (**8.8**).
- The flap is secured to the cornea with 6-0 to 8-0 absorbable suture material in a simple interrupted pattern (**8.9, 8.10**). The needle should penetrate one-half to two-thirds of the corneal depth.

Complications
Complications associated with a conjunctival graft include dehiscence and infection. If the conjunctiva used for the graft is too thick, extensive scarring can cause loss of vision.

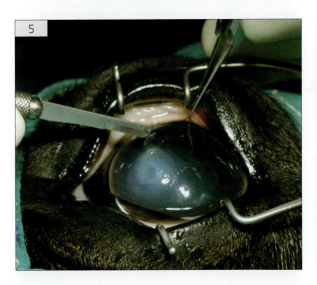

8.5 Intraoperative debridement of a melting corneal ulcer. A Beaver blade and handle are ideal instruments for debridement.

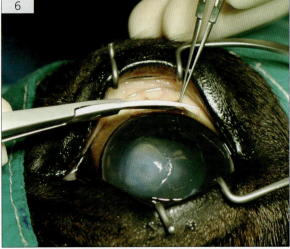

8.6 Initial incision in the dorsal bulbar conjunctiva.

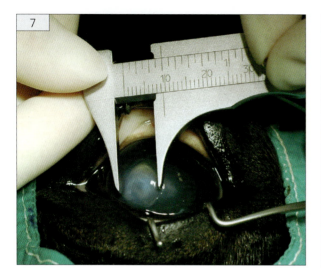

8.7 Intraoperative measurement of corneal ulcer diameter. The width of the conjunctival pedicle flap should be 2–3 mm wider than the ulcer.

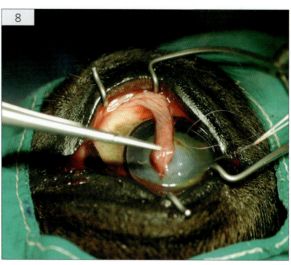

8.8 The distal part of the conjunctival flap is rotated medially.

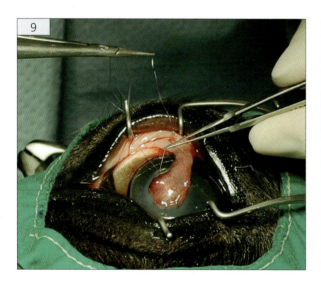

8.9 The conjunctival pedicle graft is secured to the cornea using 7-0 suture in a simple interrupted pattern.

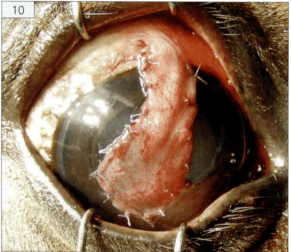

8.10 Conjunctival pedicle graft. Intraoperative placement of a conjunctival pedicle graft placed in the right eye of a horse with a deep corneal ulcer.

Tarsorrhaphy
Indications
A tarsorrhaphy, or surgical closure of the eyelid, can be partial or complete and temporary or permanent.[3] A temporary tarsorrhaphy is most commonly performed to facilitate corneal wound healing, to protect the cornea during recovery from anesthesia following corneal surgery, and to support the surgical site during healing following corneal surgery. A partial temporary tarsorrhaphy may also be performed to prevent corneal dessication in cases of facial nerve paralysis. Permanent tarsorrhaphies are rarely performed in horses.

Technique
- A temporary tarsorrhaphy is performed using 4-0 to 5-0 non-absorbable suture material in an interrupted horizontal mattress pattern, with the knot tied on a single lid, not crossing the lid margin (**8.11A**).
- Stents using split intravenous tubing or segments of rubber bands may be used to reduce tension on the eyelids and prevent the sutures from lacerating the lid margin. Rubber band stents are less likely to cause pressure necrosis than intravenous tubing because of their flat contour, which more closely approximates the lid contour (**8.11B**).

Complications
An improperly placed tarsorrhaphy can cause corneal injury with ulceration as a consequence of the suture material rubbing against the cornea.

Enucleation
Indications
Severe ocular trauma, infection, and endophthalmitis may necessitate removal of the eye. Surgical approaches include transpalpebral, which is indicated for infectious or neoplastic disease, and transconjunctival, which may be preferred for glaucomatous or uveitic globes. With both approaches, the conjunctiva, globe, and nictitating membrane are completely removed. Enucleation may be performed under general anesthesia or, for horses that are good candidates for standing orbital surgery, under standing sedation.[4,5] Horses can maintain a good quality of life following enucleation.[6]

Technique
Transpalpebral
- The horse is appropriately sedated or anesthetized and the affected eye prepared for removal using aseptic technique.
- The eyelids are sutured together.

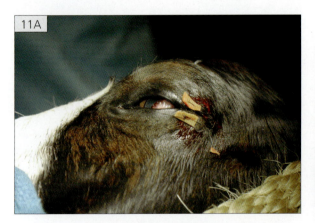
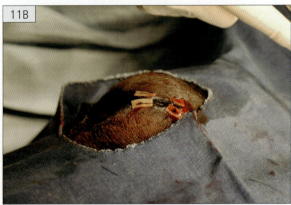

8.11A, B **(A)** A temporary tarsorrhaphy with the knot tied on a single lid, not crossing the lid margin. **(B)** A rubber band is used as a stent.

- A skin incision is made 5 mm from the eyelid margins (**8.12**).
- Blunt dissection with scissors is performed, taking care to avoid entering the conjunctival sac (**8.13**).
- The medial and lateral canthal ligaments are transected.
- The optic nerve and associated blood vessels are isolated, clamped, ligated, and transected.
- The globe and adnexa are removed and, when appropriate, submitted for histologic evaluation.

- To prevent a postoperative sunken eye socket (**8.14**), a silicone prosthesis can be inserted prior to closure.
- Subcutaneous tissues are closed using 3-0 absorbable suture material in a simple continuous pattern.
- The skin is apposed routinely with 3-0 nylon in a simple interrupted or cruciate pattern.

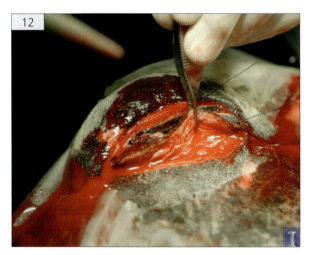

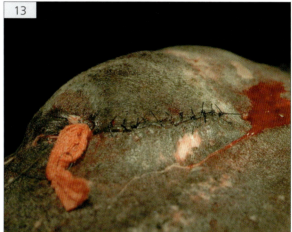

8.12 Transpalpebral approach for enucleation. The skin incision is 5 mm distal to the eyelid margin, which has been sutured closed. (Courtesy Dr Ralph Hamor)

8.13 Transpalpebral approach for enucleation. The globe was extracted from the socket by grasping the sutured eyelid margins with Allis tissue forceps and extending the dissection. The new eyelid edges have been sutured together and there is gauze packing evident at the medial margin of the incision. (Courtesy Dr Ralph Hamor)

8.14 This horse underwent enucleation 1 year previously. Note the sunken-in appearance of the left orbital area. An ocular prosthesis was not placed after enucleation.

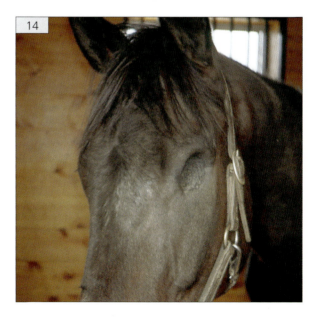

Transconjunctival

- As with the transpalpebral approach, the horse is appropriately sedated or anesthetized and the affected eye prepared for removal using aseptic technique.
- A lateral canthotomy is made to extend the palpebral fissure.
- A periotomy is performed with Stevens or Westcott tenotomy scissors by incising the bulbar conjunctiva circumferentially approximately 5 mm from the limbus.
- Blunt dissection with tenotomy scissors is performed to separate the bulbar conjunctiva from the globe and expose the tendinous insertions of the extraocular muscles, which are then transected.
- The optic nerve and associated blood vessels are isolated, clamped or ligated, and transected.
- The globe is removed and, when appropriate, submitted for histologic evaluation.
- The palpebral conjunctiva is excised using tenotomy scissors.
- The superior and inferior lid margins are excised.
- To prevent a postoperative sunken eye socket (**8.14**), a silicone prosthesis can be inserted prior to closure.
- Subcutaneous tissues are closed using 3-0 absorbable suture material in a simple continuous pattern.
- The skin is apposed routinely with 3-0 nylon in a simple interrupted or cruciate pattern.

Complications

The most common complication following enucleation is swelling, which may be associated with hemorrhage. Infection can occur and is managed with drainage. Complications associated with prosthesis placement include prosthesis shifting, surgical wound dehiscence, and prosthesis extrusion.[7,8]

LESIONS AND DISEASES AFFECTING THE EYE AND ASSOCIATED STRUCTURES

Eyelid
Eyelid laceration
Key points
- Diagnosis is obvious based on physical examination.
- Immediate surgical repair is indicated.
- Accurate surgical repair is imperative to restore normal eyelid function and prevent globe loss.

Definition/overview
An eyelid laceration is a traumatically induced wound involving the eyelid, most commonly extending to and disrupting the lid margin, resulting in a pedicle of lid tissue that must be replaced to preserve lid function.

Etiology/pathogenesis
Traumatic injuries to the eyelids are very common because of the prominent lateral location of the eyes and the horse's environment and temperament. Door latches, bucket handles, nails, or other pointed objects are often incriminated, although the actual event is frequently not witnessed. Upper eyelid damage is more important because the upper eyelid moves over more of the cornea than the lower lid. Immediate repair is recommended for restoration of eyelid function and cosmetics. The eyelids are well vascularized and heal well even in the face of infection, but improper eyelid laceration repair can be associated with loss of the eye, so attention to basic repair and healing principles is critical.

Clinical features
Loss of normal eyelid contour and, frequently, a hanging flap of skin will be seen (**8.15**). Lacerations often start at the medial canthus and extend laterally parallel to the lid margin. Blepherospasm, epiphora, hemorrhage, and ocular discharge are commonly present. Clinical signs will be more severe if corneal damage is also present.

Differential diagnosis[3]
Neoplasia; ulcerative eyelid blepharitis.

Diagnosis
Diagnosis is obvious based on physical examination. Ocular examination is recommended for identification of possible globe or orbit injury and additional evaluation using radiography (**8.16**), CT, or sonography may be necessary in some cases. If the laceration extends to the medial canthus, the nasolacrimal duct should be evaluated for patency.

Management/treatment
Eyelid lacerations should be repaired surgically as soon as possible. The wound should be minimally debrided without excising tissue. If the eyelid margin and palpebral fissure cannot be restored with available tissue, blepharoplastic procedures such as sliding skin grafts are warranted (**8.17**). Wounds should be closed in two layers to prevent dehiscence of the deep conjunctival layer and subsequent corneal ulceration from mechanical trauma. The deep conjunctival layer is closed using 5-0 or 6-0 absorbable suture material in a simple

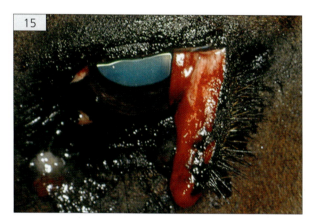

8.15 Upper eyelid laceration.

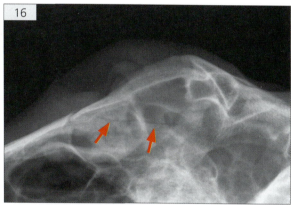

8.16 An oblique radiographic image of the orbit in a horse with an eyelid laceration. A non-displaced frontal bone fracture (arrows) extends rostrally to the lacrimal bone.

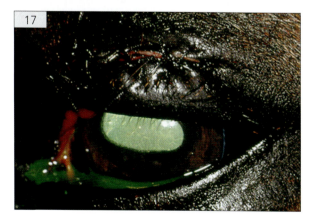

8.17 The upper eyelid laceration in 8.15 after surgical repair.

continuous pattern. The cornea should not be exposed to suture material, particularly knots. Routine skin closure using 4-0 or 5-0 non-absorbable suture material in a simple interrupted pattern is indicated. A figure-of-eight suture pattern at the eyelid margin is critical to achieve perfect apposition and prevent cicatricial entropion, secondary corneal damage, and potential globe loss (**8.18**). Suture placement should begin at the eyelid margin, or base of the wound, and work toward the apex of the laceration, to ensure perfect eyelid apposition.[3]

Postoperative care typically includes systemic antimicrobial therapy to prevent infection and should continue until sutures are removed. The use of topical antimicrobials can be associated with excessive granulation tissue and wound dehiscence if the upper eyelid is manipulated and, in particular, forced open when medication is applied; therefore, the use of topical antimicrobials is discouraged.

The prognosis for retention of lid function is typically good, but lid margin irregularities and mechanical or exposure keratitis may result, and if these are significant, globe loss is possible.

Entropion

Key points

- Entropion in horses is most common in recumbent, systemically ill foals and tends to resolve with systemic disease. Supportive care for associated corneal ulceration and temporary correction of entropion are both warranted in these cases.
- Entropion may occur as a primary anatomic disease, but this is rare in horses.
- Cicatricial entropion associated with lid laceration or lid mass excision warrants correction with a blepharoplastic procedure to restore normal lid margin and to avoid loss of the eye.

Definition/overview

Entropion (**8.19**) is a condition in which the eyelid margin turns in. It is of clinical concern when the eyelid margin contacts the cornea.

Etiology/pathogenesis

Entropion in horses is most common in the lower lid in recumbent neonatal foals with systemic disease that typically have impaired corneal sensitivity and enophthalmos secondary to dehydration, insufficient body fat, or abnormal globe position.[9] It can also occur as a primary anatomic disease, but this is extremely uncommon relative to the occurrence of primary anatomic entropion in dogs. Spastic entropion is also possible secondary to enophthalmos associated with corneal pain, as with corneal ulcers, but as with primary anatomic entropion, this is much less common in horses than in dogs. Cicatricial entropion can develop following alteration to the lid that results in an irregular lid margin, as with a lid laceration that is not adequately repaired or a lid tumor that is improperly excised.

Clinical features

Entropion can be diagnosed on visual inspection of the lid, although care must be taken to differentiate primary, or anatomic, entropion from secondary or spastic entropion. Instillation of a topical anesthetic can partially, although not completely, eliminate the spastic component.[10] Entropion is typically accompanied by signs of ocular pain, including epiphora and blepharospasm, as well as corneal ulceration secondary to lid contact with the cornea.

Differential diagnosis

Keratitis due to another eyelid anomaly (distichiasis[11], ectopic cilia[12]); enophthalamos (corneal pain, systemic disease, orbital fracture); eyelid neoplasia[3]; eyelid laceration.

Diagnosis

Corneal anesthesia is used to reduce the spastic component and more accurately assess the degree of anatomic entropion.

Management/treatment

Temporary surgical imbrication of the lower lid in foals with entropion secondary to systemic disease is typically all that is warranted. Supportive care to prevent infection and maintain corneal lubrication should be provided for any associated corneal ulceration. Entropion in these foals is generally self-correcting with the resolution of systemic disease. Imbrication is best performed using interrupted sutures in a vertical mattress pattern entirely on the lower lid (i.e. not crossing the lid margin from lower to upper lid). The risk of corneal or globe trauma with skin staples makes their use ill-advised. Subcutaneous injection of an inflammatory agent has been described, but is not recommended as lid position is difficult to precisely control with this technique.

To perform surgical imbrication in a recumbent foal, adequate and appropriate sedation and restraint must be based on systemic health, but local anesthesia is warranted even in obtunded patients, as their lack of response to stimulation does not necessarily imply lack of sensation.

Cicatricial entropion should be corrected with blepharoplastic procedures as dictated by the lid conformation, as with any other lid margin anomaly. These procedures are typically quite involved, as surgical correction must be precise and surgical wound healing is often unpredictable due to the presence of scar tissue from the underlying disease. General anesthesia is typically warranted for blepharoplastic procedures required to correct cicatricial entropion. Improper repair can be associated with impaired lid function, persistent corneal ulceration, and loss of the globe.

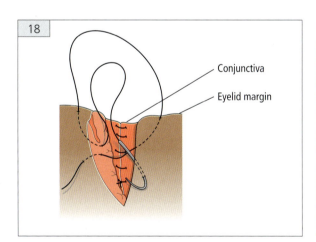

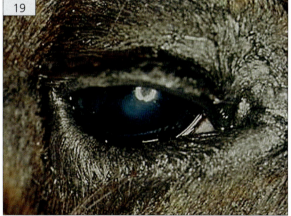

8.18 Schematic illustration of a figure-of-eight suture pattern used at the eyelid margin.

8.19 Entropion of the lower eyelid causing corneal ulceration

Orbital fracture
Key points
- Orbital rim fractures rarely require surgical treatment.
- Large fractures causing extensive facial deformity and/or impinging or entrapping the globe should be surgically repaired.

Definition/overview
Fracture of the orbital rim, zygomatic arch, or supraorbital process (**8.20**).[13]

Etiology/pathogenesis
Orbital and periorbital fractures generally occur as a result of blunt force trauma with the horse colliding with a solid object or receiving a kick from another horse.

Clinical features
Asymmetry of the globe or face is typically observed along with a depression or concavity of the periorbital region (**8.20**). Eyelid and/or conjunctival swelling is common. Crepitus and pain on palpation is found during examination. Horses with orbital fractures may also have epistaxis, exophthalmos, or proptosis. In any horse with an orbital fracture, damage to the intraosseous nasolacrimal duct, globe, optic nerve, or paranasal sinuses should be considered during the examination.[13] Examination of the fracture site should include palpation at the conjunctival fornix.

Differential diagnosis
Neoplasia; foreign body.

Diagnosis
Radiographic and ultrasonographic examination is recommended to confirm the diagnosis and determine the fracture configuration. Ultrasonography can also be useful for further assessing surrounding soft tissue structures.

Management/treatment
Minor orbital rim fractures rarely require surgical treatment. Open fractures should be debrided and lavaged. Small bone fragments should be removed to avoid sequestrum formation.

Large fractures causing extensive facial deformity and/or impinging or entrapping the globe should be surgically repaired. Surgical repair should be performed within days of injury because fibrous union occurs within 1 week, which can make fracture reduction difficult. Surgical repair involves elevating the fragments into the normal position and stabilizing the fracture with monofilament stainless steel (20- to 22-gauge), cerclage wire, small pins, or orthopedic bone plates.[13] Perioperative antimicrobials and NSAIDs are indicated. Concurrent corneal ulcers, uveitis (p. 504), and lid lacerations (p. 490) should be treated.

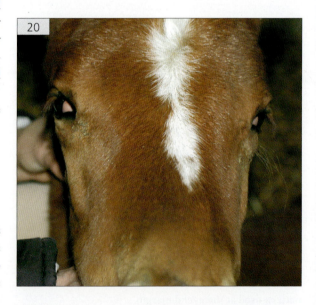

8.20 Fracture of the left orbit in a young horse. Note the asymmetry between the left and right orbit.

Ophthalmic complications associated with orbital fractures include corneal ulcers, iridocyclitis, entrapment of the globe by bone fragments, and blindness (p. 510).[13]

Cornea
Corneal ulceration
Key points
- Corneal ulceration is a frequently encountered injury.
- Most ulcers are uncomplicated and heal quickly.
- Aggressive medical therapy is recommended for any type of corneal ulceration.
- In severe, deep, or poorly responding ulcers, surgical treatment should be considered.

Definition/overview
Corneal ulceration is any loss of corneal epithelium resulting in exposed corneal stroma.

Etiology/pathogenesis
Corneal ulcers are common and result from traumatic injuries. Most ulcers are superficial and heal quickly without complication. However, the conjunctiva and cornea of the equine eye are constantly bathed in bacteria and fungus, which quickly adhere to exposed stroma. Secondary infections are common and should always be considered, especially in ulcers that do not improve or worsen within a few days.[14] Microbial and ubiquitous tear film proteinases may contribute to the progression of the corneal injury, resulting in keratomalacia characterized by a 'melting' cornea.[15]

Clinical features
Clinical features are diverse and depend on the duration and severity of the disease. Non-specific signs include epiphora, ocular discharge, conjunctival hyperemia, blepharospasm, photophobia, and corneal edema. Ulcer depth can range from superficial abrasions (**8.21**) to extremely deep erosions (**8.22**). A descemetocele

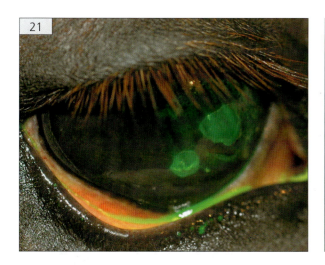

8.21 Superficial corneal ulcer. Positive fluorescein stain uptake in the exposed corneal stroma.

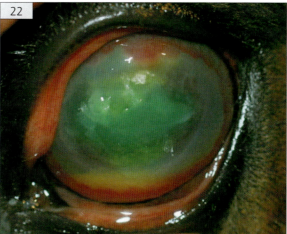

8.22 Deep corneal ulcer. The presence of a crater in the ventral cornea indicates the presence of a stromal corneal ulcer.

(**8.23, 8.24**) is the result of complete stroma loss and exposure of the thin Descemet's membrane. Keratomalacia (**8.25**) and corneal neovascularization (**8.26**) may also be apparent.

Differential diagnosis

Corneal laceration; iris prolapse; corneal stromal abscess; corneal foreign body, non-ulcerative keratouveitis[2]; esoinophilic keratoconjunctivitis[2]; equine herpesvirus[2]; corneal degeneration.[2]

Diagnosis

Positive uptake of fluorescein stain is diagnostic for a corneal ulcer and will appear green in the exposed stroma with a cobalt blue light. Rose Bengal dye positively stains degenerate or dead epithelial cells and can be used to identify early disease. Descemet's membrane does not stain with fluorescein, so a descemetocele will have a fluorescein-stained outer ring of exposed stroma with a non-staining center. A corneal scraping should be obtained with a cotton swab or the blunt end of a scalpel blade and submitted for (1) bacterial culture and sensitivity testing, (2) fungal culture and sensitivity testing, and (3) cytology.

Management/treatment

Healing of uncomplicated superficial ulcers occurs by migration and mitosis of epithelial cells and is completed in 5–7 days.[14] Complicated ulcers may deteriorate quickly despite treatment; therefore, any corneal ulcer should be treated aggressively.

Medical therapy: Medical therapy should be broad until targeted toward specific etiologic agents based on cytology and culture results. The frequency of each topical medication is determined by clinical signs. Broad-spectrum antimicrobial drugs such as triple antibiotic (bacitracin–neomycin–polymyxin B) can be used prophylactically for simple ulcers or in initial treatment.[2] Natamycin is commercially available, but other antifungal medications, including miconazole, itraconazole, and voriconazole, can be compounded for ophthalmic use and may be indicated in addition to, or instead of, natamycin, based on geographic trends in fungal culture and sensitivity.[16–18]

Atropine ophthalmic solution is used to treat uveitis by reducing ciliary spasm and preventing iris to lens adhesions, which can occur with prolonged miosis.

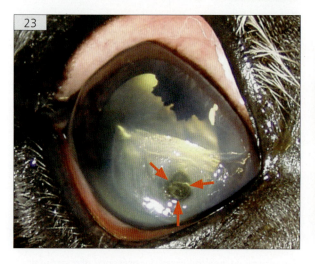

8.23 Deep corneal ulcer with a transparent descemetocele (arrows).

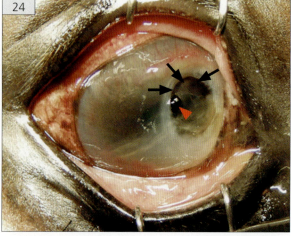

8.24 Descemetocele (black arrows) with iris prolapse (arrowhead). The prolapsed iris was resected, the integrity of the anterior chamber re-established, and a pedicle conjunctival flap applied. The horse retained its eye and had limited vision.

Autologous serum is a broad-spectrum anticollagenase that should be used to inhibit proteinases released by infectious organisms and WBCs, and in the tear film. Systemic NSAIDs should be administered as needed to control pain and inflammation. More specific therapies are based on cytology, as well as the results of culture and sensitivity tests.

A subpalpebral lavage system (p. 484) is recommended for the horse that is difficult to treat, particularly when multiple medications are administered frequently, or to treat an eye that is at risk for rupture with lid manipulation.

Duration of therapy is dictated by clinical signs but in general, topical antimicrobials should be continued until the cornea has completely epithelialized.

Surgical therapy: Corneal grafts are indicated in cases of severe and deep ulcers and those not responding to medical therapy.[2] Various biomaterials are available to use in corneal grafting, including conjunctiva, cornea, amnion, and commercially available materials such as porcine submucosa (BioSIS®) and extracellular matrix derived from porcine bladder (Acell®). The biomaterial best indicated in each case is determined by the reason for the graft: optical, to restore or improve vision; therapeutic, to control medically refractory corneal disease; tectonic, to preserve or restore the structural integrity of the globe when tissue is missing; and cosmetic, to improve the appearance of the globe without necessarily improving vision. Conjunctival grafts are indicated to bring a blood supply to the ulcerated cornea both for therapeutic and tectonic reasons, but can be associated with significant scarring.

Pedicle conjunctival grafts are the most commonly used type of conjunctival graft. Briefly, the diseased cornea is debrided and the graft is rotated over the defect and secured to the cornea using absorbable 7-0 to 8-0 suture material in a simple interrupted pattern. Hood or bipedicle (bridge) conjunctival grafts may be used to bring a blood supply to larger ulcers. When the stromal defect is deep, or an iris prolapse has developed, a corneal graft (fresh or frozen) may be used underneath the conjunctival graft to replace missing tissue. In cases of extreme keratomalacia or for ulcers with a large surface area, an amniotic membrane transplant may be warranted.[19,20] Amnionic membrane can provide significant structural support, as this tissue is very strong. In addition, amnion has antiangiogenic, anti-inflammatory, and antimicrobial properties that contribute to healing. Amnion typically sloughs off as the underlying cornea heals.

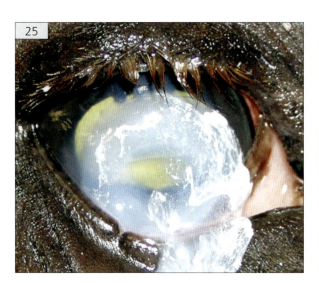

8.25 Melting corneal ulcer (keratomalacia). Necrotic stroma streaming ventrally. The dilation of the pupil is a result of previous atropine treatment and the white substance is topical natamycin.

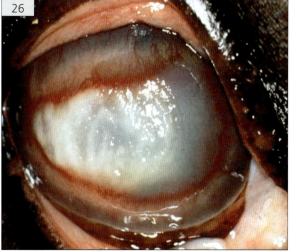

8.26 Fungal keratitis. Cake-like fungal plaque located centrally and neovascularization.

Postoperative care is as for medical therapy of corneal ulcers, typically including topical antimicrobial drugs, antifungals, anticollagenases, atropine, and systemic NSAIDs. Treatment should be continued until the cornea is completely epithelialized and the graft material (conjunctiva, cornea, or amnion) has become incorporated into or sloughed from the recipient cornea. This is typically at least 2 weeks postoperatively. Anti-inflammatory therapy is sometimes required longer term (weeks to months) to control keratitis and uveitis associated with grafting procedures.

Prognosis for retention of vision depends on the resulting corneal scar as well as the presence of a pupillary opening. The prognosis for retention of the globe depends on maintenance of structural integrity of the globe.

Corneal burns

Key points
- Alkali burns are worse than acid burns because of their rapid progression.
- Immediate copious lavage with saline, or tap water if no saline is available, is critical to stop corneal damage.

Definition/overview
A corneal burn occurs with corneal exposure to a chemical or naturally occurring substance, including ultraviolet light, which causes a corneal ulcer (**8.27**).

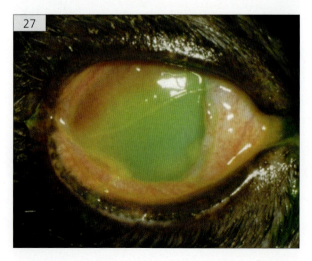

27

8.27 Corneal burn.

Etiology/pathogenesis
Corneal burns can occur following corneal exposure to any substance that is irritating, an acid or base (chemical burn), or to ultraviolet light (i.e. flash burn). The severity of a corneal burn depends on the cause, duration of contact between the causative agent and the cornea, and the initial treatment. Alkali burns caused by a substance with a pH >7 are the most dangerous because these substances react with fat in the cornea to form soap and so the damage can rapidly progress to Descemet's membrane and result in perforation. Acids, in contrast, which have a pH <7, precipitate with stromal proteins so these burns are typically self-limiting.[2] Irritants with a neutral pH tend to cause more discomfort to the eye than actual damage. Household detergents and pepper spray are examples of irritants that can cause significant ocular pain but typically do not affect vision or damage the eye. Corneal burns can also occur as a result of thermal injury (e.g. barn fires).

Clinical features
Damage resulting from a corneal burn is typically limited to the cornea and conjunctiva, but in severe cases the globe may rupture. Signs of a corneal burn include blepharospasm, blepharitis, conjunctival hyperemia and chemosis, and epiphora.

Differential diagnosis
Corneal ulcer not caused by a burn.

Diagnosis
Fluorescein stain should be applied to determine whether an ulcer is indeed present and, if so, evaluate the depth of the ulcer.

Management/treatment
Immediate copious lavage with sterile saline, or clean water if saline is not available, is critical to stop chemical degradation of the cornea. The longer a chemical is in contact with the ocular surface, the more damage may occur. Medical treatment should include a topical broad-spectrum antimicrobial, a mydriatic, and anticollagenase therapy. Systemic NSAIDs should be used at the minimum amount and frequency necessary to control ocular pain to avoid interfering with prostaglandin-mediated corneal vascularization and subsequent healing.

Corneal laceration
Key points

- Corneal lacerations are easily diagnosed on clinical examination.
- Aggressive medical management is necessary for superficial lacerations.
- Immediate surgical repair is important for deep or full-thickness (iris prolapse) lacerations.
- Enucleation is recommended for a large laceration and a severely traumatized eye.

Definition/overview

A corneal laceration is a tear or rent in the cornea or sclera.

Etiology/pathogenesis

The etiology of a corneal laceration is blunt or sharp force trauma. It is a common injury because of the environment of the horse and the prominent position of the eye. Penetrating foreign bodies, such as wood, glass, metal, and plant material, can be found embedded in the cornea or in the anterior chamber when the laceration occurs. Blunt trauma from whips, buckets, tree branches, and fences can also result in a corneal laceration. Sharp force corneal injuries have a better prognosis than blunt force injuries and injuries involving the sclera.[21,22]

Clinical features

Loss of corneal surface contour is apparent and often the wound edges will be irregular (8.28). The affected eye is frequently cloudy, red, and painful. Blepharospasm, lacrimation, and corneal edema at the wound margins are common. In an eye with a full-thickness laceration or corneal perforation, iris prolapse, anterior chamber collapse, and severe iridocyclitis (i.e. anterior uveitis) will be present (8.29, 8.30).

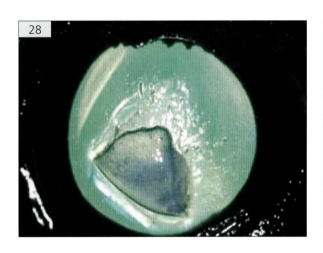

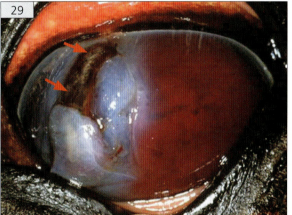

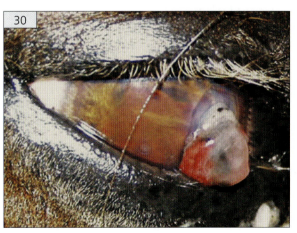

8.28 Superficial corneal laceration. A triangular tear in the corneal stoma is plainly visible.

8.29 Full-thickness corneal laceration. Iris prolapse (arrows) and hyphema.

8.30 Full-thickness corneal laceration. Protrusion of the iris and fibrin and mild hyphema are apparent. The prolapsed iris was resected, the corneal defect repaired, and a pedicle conjunctival flap applied. The horse retained the globe and regained vision.

Differential diagnosis

Corneal ulceration; corneal foreign body; anterior synechia; corneal neoplasia.[2]

Diagnosis

Diagnosis is usually obvious. Sedation and nerve blocks to immobilize the eyelids and desensitize the cornea are necessary for further evaluation in the standing awake horse (see Ophthalmic nerve blocks). For identification of the depth and extent of the laceration, topical fluorescein stain is applied to the corneal wound margins. A Seidel test is used to test the integrity of the cornea. In this test, after application of a topical anesthetic, the fluorescein strip is applied directly to the cornea to deliver concentrated fluorescein, which appears orange. With full-thickness laceration, leakage of aqueous humor causes the concentrated fluorescein to become dilute and turn from orange to fluorescein green under the cobalt blue filter. If additional damage to the orbit is suspected, ultrasonographic evaluation of the eye through a transpalpebral approach can be performed for assessment of the lens, retina, vitreal contents (hemorrhage, foreign debris), and corneal margin. Radiography and CT are useful for identifying the presence of metallic debris or bony orbital fractures.[23]

Management/treatment

Superficial corneal lacerations can be managed with medical treatment (see Corneal ulceration). Surgical repair is indicated for deep lacerations or corneal perforation and should be performed as soon as possible. Primary closure of the cornea is recommended and covering the laceration with a conjunctival graft may be warranted. If the iris is prolapsed, the necrotic tissue should be sharply removed and the remaining iris pushed back into the eye. Wound closure can be accomplished with 7-0 to 9-0 absorbable suture material in a simple interrupted pattern. Sutures should be placed 1–2 mm apart and should not incorporate the inner endothelial corneal surface. The anterior chamber may be re-established with sodium hyluronate, irrigation solution, or an air bubble. In severely infected or severely traumatized eyes, enucleation should be considered.

Postoperative care is as for a corneal ulcer (p. 495), with antimicrobial, antifungal, anticollagenase, and anti-inflammatory therapy as dictated by clinical signs, cytology, and culture results.

Prognosis depends on the chronicity, size, and location of the laceration. Full-thickness wounds >15 mm, corneal ulcers older than 2 weeks, and lacerations that extend along or past the limbus carry a poorer prognosis.[21]

Corneal stromal abscess

Key points

- A corneal stromal abscess is a focal abscess in the stroma covered by epithelium.
- Aggressive medical and surgical treatment is indicated.

Definition/overview

A corneal stromal abscess is a cellular infiltrate within the stromal layer covered by epithelial cells.

Etiology/pathogenesis

A corneal stromal abscess is formed by the migration of epithelial cells over a corneal injury, which seals infected material in the corneal stroma.[2,24,25] The lack of blood vessels and lymphatics within the cornea slows the recognition and removal of foreign material by the immune system.[26] The abscess may be bacterial, fungal, or sterile; however, epithelial cells are more likely to cover fungal hyphae and 56% of stromal abscesses are fungal in origin.[27] Treatment of an epithelialized ulcer with topical corticosteroids to reduce the resultant scar is a risk factor for development of a stromal abscess because even though the epithelium may have completely migrated over an ulcer, infectious organisms may still be present within the stroma and infection can be exacerbated by corticosteroid treatment.

Clinical features

A focal white or yellow opacity within the corneal stroma is highly suggestive of stroma abscessation.[2] Stromal abscesses are typically disproportionately painful relative to the apparent severity of the lesion (i.e. an abscess may not look bad, but may be very painful).

The abscess is commonly singular and centrally or paracentrally located, although multiple and peripheral lesions (**8.31**) have also be noted. Clinical signs include corneal edema, blepherospasm, epiphora, photophobia, aqueous flair, and anterior uveitis. Variable corneal vascularization is noted in chronic lesions (**8.32**).

Differential diagnosis

Corneal foreign body; corneal neoplasia[2]; calcific band keratopathy[2]; parasitic infiltrate.[2]

Diagnosis

Diagnosis is based on clinical signs. Fluorescein dye retention will be typically negative. Sampling of a deep abscess tissue is only achieved with surgery. Tissue samples should be submitted for cytology, culture, and sensitivity testing.

Management/treatment

Medical therapy: Topical medications are similar to those used for corneal ulceration (p. 495) and include broad-spectrum antimicrobial drugs, antifungal drugs, and 1% atropine. Although concern has been expressed regarding the ability of topical antimicrobial drugs to penetrate the corneal epithelium, the inflamed cornea may allow adequate penetration even through an intact epithelium; therefore, debridement of the corneal surface may not be necessary and indeed may create an open wound and a potential site of secondary infection. Since most abscesses are centrally located and healing is not complete until vascularization, the duration of treatment can be long (weeks to months). Placement of a subpalpebral catheter is recommended (p. 484). Systemic antimicrobial or antifungal drugs may be useful if there is a good corneal blood supply. Systemic NSAIDs (e.g. flunixin meglumine) are typically warranted.

Surgical therapy: When medical therapy is inadequate, surgical intervention is indicated. Corneal debridement with or without a conjunctival graft can be successful in cases of superficial lesions; however, most stromal abscesses are deep. With deep lesions, abscess removal and replacement with donor cornea using a penetrating keratoplasty, posterior lamellar keratoplasty, or deep endothelial lamellar keratoplasty is recommended

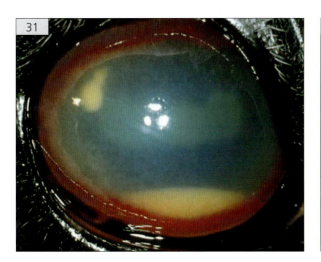

8.31 Multiple paracentrally located stromal abscesses. The associated anterior uveitis is recognized by the corneal edema, the hypopyon, and the miotic pupil.

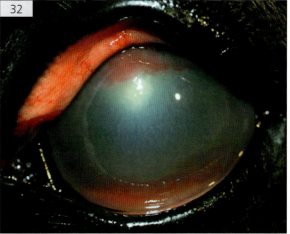

8.32 Corneal stromal abscess. Neovascularization along the dorsal aspect of the abscess is noted in this chronic lesion.

(**8.33A–C**).[28–30] Postoperative care, duration of treatment, and prognosis for retention of vision and of the globe is similar to that for corneal ulcers requiring grafting.

Immune-mediated keratitis
Key points
- Immune-mediated keratitis (IMK) is a clinical diagnosis based on history, appearance, and response to immunosuppressive therapy.
- Differentials include stromal abscess, which is often infectious and typically associated with severe pain, and non-ulcerative keratouveitis,

which while non-infectious is also typically painful and accompanied by uveitis.
- Therapy with immunosuppressive medication may control the condition, but surgical keratectomy to remove corneal antigens may be curative.

Definition/overview IMK is a clinical condition defined by a corneal opacity (**8.34**) or infiltrate that is typically non-infectious, not associated with severe pain or uveitis, and responds to varying degrees, based on the depth of the infiltrate, to anti-inflammatory therapy.[31,32]

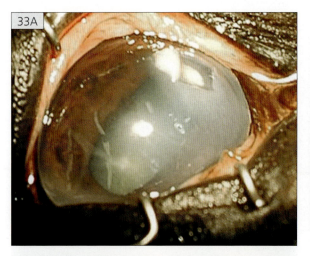

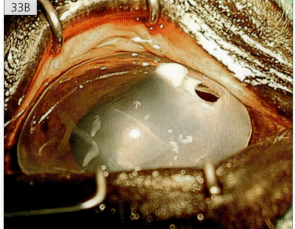

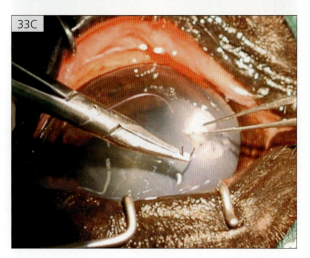

8.33A–C (A) Penetrating lamellar keratoplasty for a corneal stromal abscess. A three-sided rectangular incision is made in the cornea adjacent to the abscess. The corneal flap has been reflected to the left. (B) The corneal stromal abscess has been removed. (C) Donor cornea has been placed in the corneal defect and the rectangular flap sutured back into place.

Etiology/pathogenesis

The inciting cause of IMK is not known, but may be a self-antigen or a foreign protein that stimulates an immune response. Histology of keratectomy specimens from horses diagnosed with IMK reveals lymphoplasmacytic inflammation, stromal fibrosis, and vascularization, with neutrophils also evident in more acute (i.e. <12 months) cases and mineralization identified in more chronic (i.e. >24 months) cases.[31]

Clinical features

IMK typically manifests as a white or yellowish-white corneal opacity at varying depths in the stroma (**8.34**), which may or may not be accompanied by corneal edema and vascularization (**8.35**). Features of uveitis, such as blepharospasm, epiphora, aqueous flare, and miosis, are typically not seen.

Differential diagnosis

Corneal stromal abscess, band keratopathy[2]; corneal dystropohy[2]; corneal degeneration[2]; eosinophilic keratitis[2]; bullous keratopathy[2]; non-ulcerative keratitis.[2]

Diagnosis

IMK is diagnosed based on clinical signs seen on complete ophthalmic examination, including measurement of intraocular pressure (IOP), as well as by response to anti-inflammatory therapy. By definition, bacterial and fungal culture, cytology, and histology from excised keratectomy specimens do not reveal the presence of microorganisms. Serology for *Leptospira* serovars is typically negative.

Management/treatment

Medical management consists of topical anti-inflammatories, including corticosteroids and immunosuppressive drugs such as cyclosporine. Extreme caution must be used to differentiate IMK from potentially infectious keratidites, such as stromal abscess, because of the risk of exacerbation of infectious disease with immunosuppressive therapy. Superficial and mid-stromal lesions are more likely to respond to topical therapy than deep endothelial lesions. Surgical intervention via keratectomy to remove the infiltrate may be curative.[2,31]

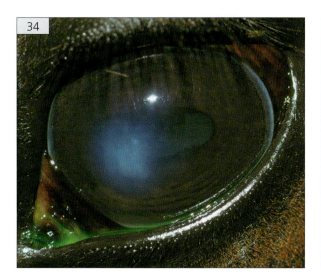

8.34 Immune-mediated keratitis with a white or yellowish-white corneal opacity.

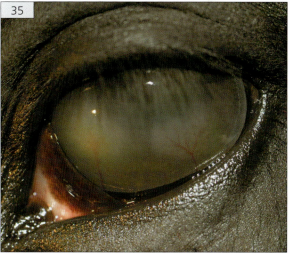

8.35 Immune-mediated keratitis with corneal edema and vascularization.

Intraocular
Equine recurrent uveitis
Key points
- Blepharospasm, epiphora, conjunctival hyperemia, and miosis are common sign of uveitis.
- Topical steroids and systemic NSAIDs are the mainstay treatments.
- Cyclosporine implants can help reduce the frequency and severity of uveitis flare-ups and thereby help maintain vision in affected eyes.

Definition/overview
Equine recurrent uveitis (ERU) is characterized by multiple episodes of intraocular inflammation. It is also known as 'moon blindness' or 'periodic ophthalmia'.

Etiology/pathogenesis
The specific inciting causes of ERU are often unknown. The preponderance of T lymphocytes suggests that ERU is an immune-mediated, delayed-type hypersensitivity reaction.[33] *Leptospira* spp. are commonly incriminated[34,35], although other bacteria and EHV have been implicated as possible causes.[36] Appaloosas are 8.3 times more likely than other breeds to develop ERU.[34]

Clinical features
Clinical signs of ERU can be acute or chronic and depend on the location (anterior or posterior globe) of the inflammation.[36] Blepharospasm, miosis, and excessive lacrimation are common. In acute episodes, corneal edema, conjunctival hyperemia, and ciliary injection may be noted (**8.36**). Aqueous flare (cloudy anterior chamber) and hypopyon or hypema may also be present. In chronic cases, corneal scarring, copra nigra atrophy, posterior synechia (iris to lens adhesion), and cataract formation can be noted (**8.37**).

Differential diagnosis
Uveitis due to another etiology (trauma; infectious disease; endotoxemia; septicemia; neoplasia; cataract [lens induced]); corneal ulcer; corneal stromal abscess; IMK; glaucoma; herpesvirus[23]; intraocular neoplasia.[23]

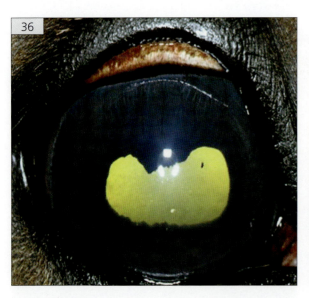

8.36 Equine recurrent uveitis. Corneal edema and miosis.

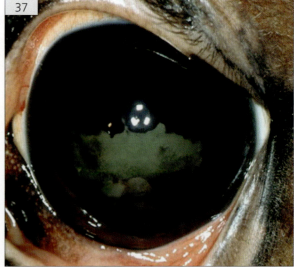

8.37 Chronic equine recurrent uveitis. Mild corneal edema, posterior synechia, iris hyperpigmentation, and dense cataract are visible.

Diagnosis

Diagnosis is based on clinical signs and recurrence of uveitis. Careful ocular examination should be performed to rule out corneal disease. Fluorescein dye retention is typically negative, although secondary corneal disease, such as calcific band keratopathy, can complicate ERU[2] and IOP is typically low, although secondary glaucoma can develop if cells and protein accumulate in the iridocorneal angle.[37] Leptospiral serology is useful for assessment of previous exposure to this risk factor.[38–40]

Management/treatment

The goals of therapy are to reduce pain, preserve vision, and minimize recurrence. Specific prevention is difficult since the underlying inciting factor cannot be identified in many cases. Topical atropine and corticosteroids (prednisolone acetate 1% and dexamethasone hydrochloride 0.1%) and systemic NSAIDs (e.g. flunixin meglumine) are typically indicated. Cyclosporine implants have been developed to decrease the frequency and severity of uveitis flare-ups. These implants tend to have the best results when placed in a quiet eye in which uveitis is controlled at the time of surgery. Surgical placement of cyclosporine implants in horses with ERU was associated with retention of vision long term, although repeat implants may be warranted after depletion of drug from the implant, at about 4 years.[41]

Hyphema

Key points

- Hyphema has many underlying causes, although trauma and uveitis are the most common in horses.
- IOP should be monitored in horses with hyphema because secondary glaucoma can develop as RBCs settle in and occlude the iridocorneal angle.
- Atropine use should be cautious and accompanied by IOP measurement.
- Long-term sequelae of hyphema, including synechia formation and cataract development, can lead to eventual blindness even following resolution of hyphema.

Definition/overview

Hyphema is the presence of RBCs in the anterior chamber (**8.38**). It may be partial or complete.

Etiology/pathogenesis

Causes of hyphema include causes of third compartment bleeds elsewhere in the body, most notably trauma, inflammation, coagulopathy, and neoplasia. Traumatic hyphema and hyphema secondary to severe uveitis are most common in the horse. Traumatic hyphema may result from direct trauma to vascular structures, as in the case of a scleral rupture, or be an indirect result of trauma, as with a corneal perforation associated with ocular hypotony and bleeding from the drainage angle, or blunt trauma resulting in retinal detachment and leakage of blood into the anterior chamber. Hyphema secondary to uveitis develops when uveal vessels leak cells into the anterior chamber.

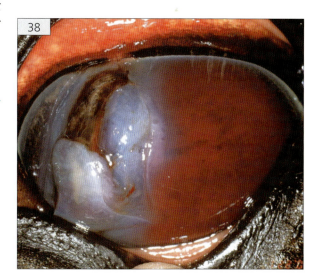

8.38 Hyphema associated with corneal trauma.

Clinical features

Hyphema is characterized by a red appearance behind the cornea, which may be partial or complete. Hyphema is often accompanied by corneal edema associated with inflammation of and damage to the corneal endothelium. Active bleeding is associated with a dynamic appearance, such that the amount of blood may increase and the anterior chamber appears red. Once bleeding has stopped, red cells will typically settle in the ventral anterior chamber with the result that a gravity line develops and the color will often become darker. Secondary glaucoma is a concern as red cells can occlude the iridocorneal angle; therefore, measurement of IOP is critical to direct medical therapy.

Differential diagnosis

Uveal neoplasia; foreign body.

Diagnosis

A complete ophthalmic examination including assessment of indirect pupillary light reflex from the affected to the non-affected eye should be performed. Evaluation of the indirect pupillary light reflex can help establish the potential for return of vision once the hyphema resolves, although absence of an indirect pupillary light reflex can be the result of failure of light to reach the retina due to obstruction by dense anterior chamber blood, rather than truly reflecting absence of retinal function in the affected eye.

IOP should be measured, as secondary glaucoma can develop when blood coagulates in the iridocorneal angle. If corneal edema or hyphema precludes evaluation of structures posterior to the cornea, ocular ultrasound should be performed. Retinal detachment, lens luxation, or intraocular neoplasia may be underlying etiologies for hyphema and can potentially be identified ultrasonographically.

Management/treatment

Therapy should be directed at stopping the bleeding, for sources that are amenable to therapy (e.g. foreign body, corneal or globe rupture), reducing inflammation associated with frank blood in the anterior chamber, and facilitating resorption of blood. Topical and systemic anti-inflammatory drugs are the primary medical therapies. Caution in the use of topical corticosteroids is warranted, as corneal ulceration is potentially associated with hyphema either directly as a result of trauma or indirectly as a result of endothelial damage by RBCs in the anterior chamber. In some cases the cornea may appear fluorescein negative on initial examination but become fluorescein positive within 1–2 days of the development of hyphema as endothelial function becomes impaired.

Caution is also advised with the use of mydriatics, such as atropine, when hyphema is present, because IOP can increase rapidly as RBCs occlude the iridocorneal drainage angle. IOP may change dynamically as the amount of hyphema and the size of the pupil changes over time. Atropine should only be used if IOP can be monitored throughout therapy.

Anti-inflammatory and mydriatic therapy may need to be continued long term, even after hyphema has apparently resolved, to reduce synechia formation and decrease the likelihood of cataract formation, both of which are long-term complications of hyphema that can be associated with eventual blindness.

Retinal detachment
Key point
- Retinal detachment is an uncommon complication of intraocular inflammation.

Definition/overview

Retinal detachment is separation of the neurosensory retina from the retinal pigmented epithelium.

Etiology/pathogenesis

Retinal detachment occurs when the interface between the retinal pigmented epithelium and the neurosensory retina is disrupted. This may be accomplished by fluid accumulation, hemorrhage, or during blunt force trauma. Retinal detachment may also be a complication of ERU.[36]

Clinical features

Evaluation of the fundus will reveal an elevated hazy area in the retina in partial tears or a gray, floating veil of tissue extending into the vitreous in complete tears. Acute blindness or slowly progressing loss of vision may be appreciated. In many cases of concurrent uveitis and retinal detachment, miosis will preclude fundic examination.[42]

Differential diagnosis

Fibrin strands within the vitreous; vitreal degeneration; neoplasia.

Diagnosis

Induced mydriasis using 1% atropine is helpful to fully evaluate the fundus (**8.39**). If the cornea is opaque, the vitreous is cloudy or bloody, or a cataract is present, ultrasonographic examination may be necessary to obtain a diagnosis (**8.40**). The classic 'seagull sign' may be noted on ultrasonographic examination in a complete detachment.[43]

Management/treatment

Treatment of the underlying source of inflammation is indicated. Prognosis for retinal reattachment and return of vision in the detached area is poor.[43]

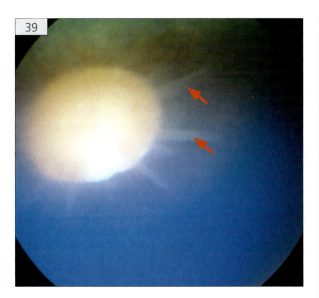

8.39 Partial retinal detachment. Hazy, gray veil of tissue (arrows) around the optic nerve.

8.40 Ultrasonographic image of retinal detachment. The detached retina (arrows) is identified as hyperechoic lines within the vitreous. This horse also has a cataract.

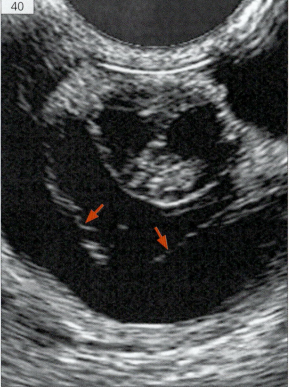

Glaucoma

Key points

- Equine glaucoma may be primary, which is not clearly defined, or secondary, potentially associated with uveitis, lens luxation, intraocular neoplasia, or intraocular infection.
- Glaucoma is a painful, potentially blinding disease.
- Glaucomatous globes can be intractably painful, warranting enucleation.
- Options for medical therapy in the horse are limited.
- Medical therapy targets reduction of aqueous production via topical beta blockers such as timolol and carbonic anhydrase inhibitors such as dorzolamide.
- Medical therapy (e.g. prostaglandin analogs such as latanoprost) that is effective in other species (e.g. dogs and humans) is not effective in horses. More research is warranted in this area.
- Options for surgical therapy are also limited and include two general categories of therapy: reduction of aqueous production by destruction of the ciliary body (e.g. transcleral cyclophotocoagulation) and increase in aqueous outflow (e.g. anterior chamber shunt).
- Removal of the globe is, unfortunately, all too often the end stage of glaucoma in the horse.

Definition/overview

Glaucoma is an optic neuropathy associated with abnormal aqueous outflow resulting in elevated IOP.[37]

Etiology/pathogenesis

Glaucoma results when outflow of aqueous humor is impaired. This can occur as primary disease associated with abnormal conformation of the iridocorneal angle, or as secondary disease. Primary disease as it occurs in dogs and humans, which is generally bilateral but asymmetric in onset and typically results in permanent blindness, is not well described in the horse. Secondary glaucoma has numerous mechanisms, including contraction of preiridal fibrovascular membranes (which form as a result of uveitis), occlusion of the iridocorneal angle by cellular debris or protein (as with uveitis or hyphema), posterior synechia (adhesion of the iris to the cornea) causing pupillary block, or mechanical obstruction as with lens luxation, intraocular tumor (e.g. melanoma), or infectious endophthalmitis.

Clinical features

Glaucoma is associated with increased IOP, although pressure in a uveitic eye with secondary glaucoma may be normal. The normal range of IOP in horses is generally given as 18–28 mmHg.[44–47] Glaucoma typically manifests clinically as corneal edema with a dilated pupil, but may also be accompanied by signs of uveitis such as corneal vascularization, aqueous flare, and miosis. Haab's striae are breaks in Descemet's membrane that can be seen histologically but appear clinically as curvilinear endothelial opacities, most often occurring roughly horizontally in the cornea.

Increased IOP may be accompanied by buphthalmos (an increase in the size of the globe), but this does not develop in horses until IOP is extremely high. Once bupthalmos develops, it typically does not resolve, even when IOP decreases, because of poor scleral elasticity.

The iridocorneal angle, visible using slit lamp biomicroscopy and appearing without magnification as a gray stripe between the iris and limbus (junction of cornea and sclera), may be abnormal in glaucomatous eyes as well as those predisposed to glaucoma. In the normal iridocorneal angle, the pectinate ligament appears as a gray moth-eaten band where the iris meets the cornea. Aqueous humor flows through holes in the ligament and eventually into the bloodstream. In glaucomatous globes, the pectinate ligament may appear thin with few holes or even as a solid band without holes. Sometimes, pigment migrates over the iridocorneal angle, making it difficult to see.

Horses appear to tolerate increases in IOP even up into the 50s and 60s mmHg without the degree of corneal edema seen in dogs and without the apparent discomfort. However, the improvement in attitude that often follows enucleation of a glaucomatous globe believed to be non-painful suggests that glaucoma pain may manifest in more subtle ways in horses than the tearing, squinting, or obvious behavioral changes such as vocalizing seen in dogs. In addition, horses do not seem to develop corneal edema at the IOPs associated with corneal edema in dogs, and do not appear to lose functional vision at IOPs associated with vision loss in dogs. Nonetheless, equine glaucoma is still considered a painful, vision-threatening disease.

Differential diagnosis

Exophthalmos, as seen with retrobulbar tumor, abscess, or cellulitis; uveitis; anterior lens luxation, which may give the appearance of mydriasis and be associated with artifactually increased IOP when tonometry is performed directly over the luxated lens; artifactually increased IOP not associated with true disease, as when profound blepharospasm affects measurement.

Diagnosis

Measurement of IOP is necessary but not sufficient to diagnose glaucoma. IOP measurements must be interpreted in the context of the remainder of the ocular examination, including globe size, globe position, and pupil size. The iridocorneal angle should be examined using slit lamp biomicroscopy. Additional diagnostics that may provide more information about visual prognosis include ocular ultrasound, which is useful for detecting intraocular masses that may affect IOP measurement, and electroretinography, which is used to evaluate retinal function.

Several types of tonometers are available, including applanation and rebound, both of which are easily used in the horse.

Management/treatment

As in other species, management of glaucoma is directed at decreasing IOP and controlling any associated primary disease process that underlies secondary glaucoma. Medical therapy for IOP control is generally directed at one of two mechanisms: decrease in the rate of aqueous production or increase in the rate of aqueous outflow. Drugs that decrease aqueous production and are effective in horses include beta-blockers such as timolol and carbonic anhydrase inhibitors such as dorzolamide.[48–50] Prostaglandin analogs such as latanoprost, which increase aqueous outflow and thereby profoundly reduce IOP in other species (e.g. dogs, humans), unfortunately are not shown to be effective at lowering IOP in horses.[51,52] Use of atropine in horses with glaucoma is controversial. It does not appear to decrease IOP, but may decrease uveitis by stabilizing the intraocular vasculature in glaucoma secondary to uveitis; therefore, it should be used only when IOP is carefully monitored.[37,53,54]

Surgical therapy for equine glaucoma includes procedures targeted towards decreasing aqueous production and those intended to increase aqueous outflow. Aqueous production can be decreased by damaging the ciliary body, either with cryotherapy or laser therapy. Cryotherapy is associated with severe postoperative inflammation and is best reserved for use in permanently blind eyes.[37] Transcleral cyclophotocoagulation with a diode laser is used commonly in clinical ophthalmology and can be associated with reduction in IOP, although even following laser ciliary body ablation, topical medical therapy must often be continued to maintain IOP in a comfortable range.[55] Transcleral cyclophotocoagulation works by applying a diode laser, which is preferentially absorbed by pigmented tissue and thus passes through the conjunctival and sclera with minimal damage, to the ciliary body epithelium and stroma of the pars plicata. Sites for transcleral laser ciliary body ablation have been well defined.[56,57] Endolaser cyclophotocoagulation has been used in canine and human ophthalmology, but is still in the developmental stages in equine ophthalmology.

Increased aqueous drainage from the eye can be accomplished via a gonioimplant, which bypasses the obstructed iridocorneal angle and directs aqueous humor to the subconjunctival space, from where it is absorbed into the bloodstream. These implants are experimental in the horse.[37]

Acute blindness

Key points

- Acute blindness can have many potential underlying causes.
- Retinal blindness can be identified using electroretinography.
- The best prognosis for return of vision with acute blindness is for optic neuritis, which responds to corticosteroid therapy.

Definition/overview

Acute blindness, or loss of vision, may be unilateral or bilateral, partial or complete, and temporary or permanent.

Etiology/pathogenesis

Acute blindness is often traumatic, but can result from many causes including: (1) an obstruction in the normally clear ocular media (e.g. complete and severe corneal edema, hyphema, profound miosis, cataract, or vitreal hemorrhage); (2) bullous separation of, or a tear in, the neurosensory retina from the outer retinal pigmented epithelium (i.e. retinal detachment); (3) acute glaucoma; (4) optic nerve ischemia related to acute blood loss; or (5) optic neuritis.

Blunt trauma to the head can result in compression of or hemorrhage around the optic nerve or neuropraxia of retinal ganglion cell axons resulting from pull of the brain away from the optic nerve.

Surgical ligation of the internal or external carotid artery, used as a treatment for guttural pouch mycosis and associated epistaxis, can cause ischemic optic neuropathy and acute, permanent blindness. Optic neuritis can be caused by parasites, recurrent uveitis, encephalomyelitis, and neoplasia.[58]

Clinical features

The clinical appearance of acute blindness depends on the underlying etiology, but in cases where blindness is retinal in origin, or involves structures involved in the pupillary light reflex including the optic nerve, mydriasis is the hallmark. Horses with central or cortical blindness but normal retinas and optic nerves will typically have intact pupillary light reflexes, but still be blind.

Differential diagnosis

Non-ocular neurologic disease (i.e. that may not affect vision but may affect behavior); lameness; behavioral problems.

Diagnosis

Electroretinography can be used to evaluate retinal function and differentiate between retinal and non-retinal (i.e. optic nerve or cortical) blindness.[59] Electroretinography can be performed in the standing horse.[60,61] Ocular ultrasound examination can be used to identify retinal detachment.[62]

Management/treatment

Treatment of acute blindness is directed at the underlying disease process. If optic neuritis is diagnosed or suspected, treatment with systemic corticosteroids may help control inflammation and result in a return of vision.[58] Prognosis for return of vision depends on the nature of the underlying disease and the response to treatment. Safe adaptation to blindness can be facilitated by owners and other handlers by providing a safe environment and training the blind horse to use nonvisual cues like voices, smell, and touch.[63]

CHAPTER 9

NEONATOLOGY

Jane E. Axon, Catherine M. Russell, and Pamela A. Wilkins

GENERAL APPROACH TO THE CRITICALLY ILL EQUINE NEONATE

- The equine neonate is highly vulnerable to the systemic manifestations of disease. Frequently, *in-utero* challenges result in the delivery of a systemically ill foal with a significantly compromised ability to make the transition from fetus to neonate. Rapid deterioration and death will occur if early recognition and emergency treatment of the sick neonate does not occur.
- Effective treatment and management of the critically ill equine neonate is often time-consuming and expensive. Many therapies can be successfully completed on the farm with experienced and dedicated personnel; however, the specialized expertise, equipment, and personnel available only at an equine intensive care unit (ICU) are frequently required to achieve a desirable outcome.

COMMON PROCEDURES PERFORMED ON HORSES WITH NEONATAL EMERGENCIES

Stabilization of the neonate is aimed at supporting the cardiovascular and respiratory system to ensure good tissue perfusion and oxygenation, with subsequent treatment of the primary problem. Many critically ill neonates require stabilization prior to a physical examination being performed. Recumbent foals are immediately placed on intranasal oxygen (INO$_2$) (see Chapter 3) insufflation and an IV catheter is placed. During this time, a minimum data base of heart and respiratory rate,

peripheral pulse strength, body and distal extremity temperature, blood pressure, arterial blood gas analysis, and glucose and lactate concentrations is obtained. If required, fluid resuscitation is started and if there is no response, inopressor therapy is initiated. Further therapies are then implemented as a result of the physical examination.

Respiratory support

The majority of critically ill neonates need some form of respiratory support. An arterial blood gas (ABG) sample (see Chapter 3) obtained from the dorsal metatarsal or decubital artery will help assess the respiratory function and metabolic status of the foal (**9.1**).

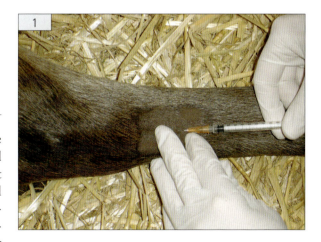

9.1 Collection of an arterial blood gas sample from the dorsal metatarsal artery with a heparinized syringe.

Intranasal oxygen insufflation

(See also Chapter 3)

INO_2 is administered to any recumbent foal or foal <24 hours of age while other procedures are performed, as the stress of manipulating an already compromised neonate can be fatal.[1] Foals that have an elevated respiratory rate, cyanotic mucous membranes, increased respiratory effort, PaO_2 of <60 mmHg or SaO_2 <90% should also be started on INO_2. Therapy is aimed at maintaining the PaO_2 between 80 and 110 mmHg, SaO_2 >92%, decreasing respiratory effort and rate, and improving the mucous membrane color and demeanor of the foal.[2]

INO_2 is initiated at 5 liters/minute and adjusted according to physical examination and laboratory findings (**9.2**). The usual flow rates required to maintain an adequate PaO_2 are 2–15 liters/minute, although higher flow rates may be required in severely affected foals.[3]

Respiratory stimulants

Respiratory stimulants are useful in foals with a blunted central CO_2 receptor sensitivity, which seems to most commonly occur with hypoxic ischemic encephalopathy (HIE) as part of the manifestation of neonatal encephalopathy (NE).[2] Caffeine is a commonly used stimulant, although recent work suggests it is of no additional benefit over constant rate infusion (CRI) of doxapram.[4,5] Recent experimental data in anesthetized normal foals suggest that continuous IV infusion of doxapram may also be useful (*Table 9.1*).[4,5] If ventilation does not improve and results in significant acidemia, mechanical or assisted ventilation may be required.

Mechanical ventilation

Mechanical or assisted ventilation is usually indicated when $PaCO_2$ is >70 mmHg, acidemia is present, INO_2 fails to correct hypoxemia, or where there is respiratory muscle fatigue.[2] A $PaCO_2$ of 60–65 mmHg may be appropriate if respiratory acidosis is compensating for metabolic alkalosis and pH is maintained within an appropriate range (>7.35). Increased $PaCO_2$ may also be tolerated if the foal has significant lung pathology and where mechanical ventilation may worsen lung injury. Manual ventilation (following nasotracheal intubation) using a self-inflating resuscitation bag with an attached source of humidified oxygen can be used in temporary short-term situations. Sustained ventilation is achieved with mechanical ventilation (*Table 9.1*). The aim is to keep the PaO_2 between 80 and 120 mmHg with SaO_2 >92% and pH between 7.34 and 7.42.[2]

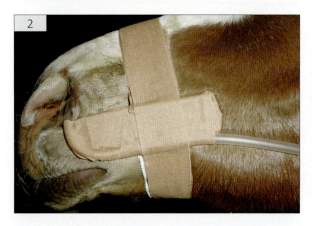

9.2 Intranasal oxygen tube placement. Flexible tubing with a fenestrated tip is placed up the ventral meatus to the level of the medial canthus of the eye. The tubing is wrapped around the curved end of a tongue depressor, run along the side of the face, and held in place with tape. Oxygen is run through a sterile water (not saline)-filled humidifier.

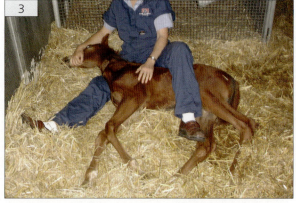

9.3 Positioning a foal for catheter placement. This holding position is also used for other procedures.

The details of prolonged mechanical ventilation beyond emergency manual ventilation are beyond the scope of this emergency based text.

Other therapies

Foals with upper airway obstruction from pharyngeal collapse may require temporary nasotracheal tube placement; however, intubation may increase opportunistic lung infection. Suctioning of airways to remove meconium or copious secretions is not generally recommended.[6]

Cardiovascular support

Fluid loading, inotrope, and vasopressor therapy are utilized to improve tissue perfusion.

Fluid therapy

Catheters are placed aseptically in the jugular or cephalic vein with the foal in lateral recumbency (**9.3**). Over-the-wire polyurethane catheters are used as they are flexible, less thrombogenic, and easier to place in hypovolemic foals. A blood culture and blood for laboratory samples are collected aseptically after placement.

Table 9.1 **Drugs used for stabilization of foals**

THERAPY	DOSE	COMMENTS
Intranasal oxygen	5–10 liters/minute	
Balanced electrolyte solution (warm)	20 ml/kg over 20 minutes	50 kg foal: 1 liter fluid bolus. Maximum of 4 liters
10% dextrose	4 mg/kg/minute (8 mg/kg/hour)	50 kg foal: 120–180 ml/hour. 10% dextrose = 100 ml 50% dextrose in 1 liter of 5% dextrose
Insulin	0.00125–0.2 IU/kg/hour (usually start at 0.05 IU/kg/hour)	Use glass bottle. Prime lines for 20 minutes. Do not increase by >0.05 IU/kg/hour. Attach to glucose/parenteral nutrition line
Dobutamine	2–15 µg/kg/minute. (Normally start at 2 µg/kg/minute and increase to 5 µg/kg/minute. If no improvement seen, other vasopressors are used)	Lower doses: inotrope through β_1 effects. Used on patients with adequate tissue perfusion. Discontinue if tachycardia develops
Norepinephrine	0.1–0.3 µg/kg/minute	β_1 and α_1 activity. Main effect vasoconstriction through α_1 effects
Dopamine	2–10 µg/kg/minute	Low doses: may improved renal blood flow. Medium doses: support cardiac function. High doses: increase BP but reduce renal and splanchnic blood flow
Vasopressin	2–10 µg/kg/minute	If no response to adrenergic pressor
Ventilator: initial settings	Tidal volume: 5–10 ml/kg FIO_2: 0.5 (0.3–1.0) PEEP: 4–5 cm H_2O Breath rate: 20–30 breaths/minute Pressure support: 8–12 cm H_2O	Settings adjusted as per discussion by Palmer 2005[2]
Caffeine	Loading dose: 10 mg/kg PO/PR Maintenance: 2.5 mg/kg PO/PR q12–24h	Side-effects: tachycardia, general stimulation. Therapeutic levels: 5–25 µg/ml. Effects seen in 2 hours
Doxapram infusion	400 mg total dose infused at 0.05 mg/kg/minute	Irregular/apneic foals

PR, per rectum.

Fluid therapy for perfusion deficit due to hypovolemia:
Fluid boluses of warmed isotonic balanced electrolyte solutions are given under pressure at 20 ml/kg over 20–30 minutes ('shock' fluid bolus therapy) with clinical re-evaluation between each bolus. Improved perfusion is recognized clinically as improved pulse quality, increased temperature of distal extremities, improved arterial and central venous blood pressure, return of borborygmi, urine production, and improved demeanor.[7,8] An appropriate fluid resuscitation 'target' (e.g. urine production, increased CVP to a pre-specified target) should be chosen above which additional boluses are not administered and inopressor therapy considered instead. This will avoid potential fluid overload in cases where septic shock exists and further fluid administration will not be beneficial.[8]

Colloid therapy (hetastarch, 5–10 ml/kg/day) should be considered as part of the volume resuscitation especially if there is concurrent hypoproteinemia. There is debate as to whether synthetic colloids are beneficial in volume resuscitation in the neonate due to increased movement of colloid molecules through damaged endothelium into the interstitium, which promotes edema formation.[9] Plasma is the ideal colloid as it provides immunoglobulins, coagulation factors, and other proteins in addition to albumin and is cost-effective in foals. Recent data suggest that plasma administered at admission in compromised foals will not greatly increase albumin levels, but even small increases in oncotic pressure may be beneficial.[10]

Fluid therapy for dehydration: After hypovolemia has been treated, dehydration should be evaluated. An estimation of fluid replacement for dehydration should be obtained. Estimating dehydration in neonates is different from adults as neonates have a larger interstitial volume.

Mild dehydration is equivalent to 5% dehydration (a deficit of 50 ml/kg body weight) and may only be recognized by slightly decreased urine production; moderate dehydration is equivalent to 10% dehydration (a deficit of 100 ml/kg body weight) and is characterized by dry buccal mucous membranes, tachycardia, little or no urine output, lethargy, sunken eyes, and loss of skin turgor; severe dehydration is equivalent to 15% dehydration (a deficit of 150 ml/kg body weight) and is characterized by dry buccal mucous membranes,

tachycardia, little or no urine output, lethargy, sunken eyes, and loss of skin turgor plus a thready pulse, cyanosis (secondary to poor cardiac output), rapid breathing, delayed capillary refill, hypotension, mottled mucous membranes/skin, and possibly coma. In these cases laboratory abnormalities would include polycythemia, azotemia and, possibly, increased urine SG. Electrolyte abnormalities commonly accompany severe dehydration.

Treatment is best approached by considering the fluid resuscitation requirements, current deficit, ongoing losses, and maintenance requirements separately. The volume (e.g. amount of fluid), composition, and rate of replacement differ for each. Formulas and estimates used to determine treatment parameters provide a starting place, but treatment requires ongoing monitoring of vital signs, clinical appearance, urine output and SG, weight, and, sometimes, serum electrolyte levels. Ideally, deficits should be made up within the first 12 hours of treatment.

As an example a moderately dehydrated 50 kg foal would need 5 liters of IV crystalloid fluids. The fluid deficit (~5 liters over 12 hours or ~417 ml/hour) plus 'dry' maintenance requirements (~104 ml/hour) would result in a fluid rate of about 520 ml/hour following resuscitation, assuming no large ongoing losses. This would be in addition to fluids used for resuscitation. For ease of treatment, fluid therapy is sometimes administered as a further fluid bolus administration; in this case a 1 liter bolus every 2 hours would accomplish the task.

Inopressor therapy

If no improvement is seen after the fluid boluses, inotrope and vasopressor therapy needs to be considered. The aim of therapy is to achieve tissue perfusion, not to obtain a specific blood pressure value.

As a guide, the MAP should be >60 mmHg; however, adequate tissue perfusion can occur at lower values (more common in premature foals), therefore other factors such as L-lactate concentration[11–13] and examination findings discussed above should also be evaluated.[14,15]

Direct and indirectly measured blood pressures may not be in agreement depending on the technique(s) used. It is important to understand the frailties of any equipment used for measuring blood pressure.[16]

Dobutamine (3–10 µg/kg/minute) and norepinephrine (0.3–1.0 µg/kg/minute) are commonly used (*Table 9.1*). Recently, vasopressin (0.25–1.0 mU/kg/minute) has been used to provide support for adrenergic pressors, especially in septic patients, although support for this approach in human medicine remains controversial with the Vasopressin and Septic Shock Trial failing to demonstrate a clear advantage for vasopressin use.[14,17] The goals of treatment are improved demeanor, improved perfusion, improved pulse pressure, improved ABG parameters, and improved urine production.

Glucose support

All critically ill neonates benefit from exogenous IV glucose support.[7] The initial rate of supplementation using 5% dextrose in water begins at 4 mg/kg/minute (2.2 mmol/kg/minute) and increases to 8 mg/kg/minute (4.4 mmol/kg/minute) depending on response as monitored by serial blood glucose determinations and clinical condition. Supplementation begins at 6 mg/kg/minute with severe hypoglycemia (<2.8 mmol/l [50 mg/dl]). As the volume of fluid required for glucose supplementation often exceeds fluid requirements, up to 10% dextrose can be used (*Table 9.1*).

To determine the fluid rate required to administer 4 mg/kg/minute to a 50 kg foal :

$$[(4 \text{ mg/kg/minute}) \times (50 \text{ kg})] \times 60 = 12{,}000 \text{ mg/hour}$$
$$(12 \text{ g/hour}) = 240 \text{ ml/hour of 5\% dextrose}$$

(Note: There are 50 g dextrose/liter in 5% dextrose.)

The rate can also be estimated rapidly using the following formula:

$$(\text{Body weight in pounds} \times 2) + [0.1 \times (\text{body weight in pounds})] = \text{ml/hour 5\% dextrose}$$
$$(110 \times 2) + 0.1 \times (110 \times 2) = 220 + 22 = 242 \text{ ml/hour of 5\% dextrose}$$

The response to glucose supplementation varies with each individual's physiological condition. Compromised neonates that become hyperglycemic may benefit from insulin therapy (0.00125–0.2 U/kg/hour; begin at the lower dose and increase slowly by doubling q4–6h until glucose control is achieved) and thiamine supplementation (5–20 mg/kg added to IV fluids/day); those remaining hypoglycemic secondary to SIRS or sepsis may need rates as high as 20 mg/kg/minute.

Monitoring blood glucose using handheld glucometers requires knowledge of the accuracy of those monitors. Their accuracy and reliability is quite variable and each hospital should know the performance limitations of any monitor they use.[18,19]

Glucose solutions should **not** be given as a bolus. The resultant hyperglycemia may result in loss of infused electrolytes, fluids, glucose in the urine (osmotic diuresis), and rebound hypoglycemia. Hyperglycemia of any duration may have deleterious effects on the CNS of neonates with HIE.[20] Initial hypoglycemia can be treated by adding 1% glucose (2 ml 50% dextrose/liter) to fluid resuscitation bolus(es), which essentially results in a CRI of approximately 4–8 mg/kg/minute to a 50 kg foal, assuming two boluses and reassessment take 1 hour to complete. CRI of 5% glucose at a rate of 4 mg/kg/minute should be instituted as soon as possible. Infusion of 10% dextrose solution over several minutes at a dose of 10 ml/kg has also been used, but carries greater risk of inadvertent hyperglycemia.[21]

Electrolyte therapy

Electrolyte replacement or restriction should be considered if life-threatening abnormalities are present; however, many abnormalities will correct after fluid therapy and improved tissue perfusion. The newborn neonate's electrolytes are a reflection of the *in-utero* environment and, with normal renal function, should correct over the following 24 hours.

Potassium

Hyperkalemia usually only occurs with uroperitoneum in neonates, although it can be recognized with severe muscular injury (gastrocnemius tendon rupture, nutritional myodegeneration) and 'sick cell syndrome' where cellular injury results in leakage of potassium extracellularly.

Drainage of urine from the abdomen is the definitive treatment for hyperkalemia associated with uroperitoneum (see Urinary tract disruption). If uroperitoneum is suspected on admission, non-potassium fluids such as 0.9% NaCl and 5% dextrose should be used. Although rare under modern management conditions, if severe or symptomatic hyperkalemia is present (>6.2–7.0 mmol/l), abdominal drainage is highly recommended. If no further improvement in potassium concentration is noted, then 1 ml/kg IV slowly of 10% calcium gluconate, 1–2 mEq/kg IV of $NaHCO_3$ and/or 1 g/kg IV glucose has been recommended.[22] Potassium-binding resins can be administered intrarectally or intragastrically to manage hyperkalemia (20–60 g/day to a 50 kg [110 lb] foal). Calcium polystyrene sulfonate (e.g. Sorbisterit®, Ca-Resonium®), sodium polystyrene sulfonate (e.g. Kayexelate®, Anti-Kalium-NA®), and administration of β-agonist medications such as terbutaline can treat life-threatening hyperkalemia temporarily because of their action on the sodium-potassium ATPase pumps.[23]

Hypokalemia is common. If potassium is <2.5 mEq/l, IV supplementation should be given. Potassium supplementation can be estimated using the following formula:

$$potassium\ replacement\ (mEq) = 0.4 \times body\ weight\ (kg) \times potassium\ deficit\ in\ mEq$$

The potassium can be added to the glucose as long as the rate of administration is not >0.5 mEq/kg/hour. Moderate to severe hypokalemia that is unresponsive to potassium supplementation may require magnesium supplementation to resolve.

Sodium

Foals can present with hypo- and hypernatremia. Both can have fatal neurologic consequences if not corrected properly. Sodium concentrations in neonates with neurologic deficits and moderate to severe hyponatremia can be corrected fairly rapidly up to 115–120 mEq/l and then corrected more slowly at approximately 0.5 mEq/hour.[24] In foals with hypernatremia, sodium concentration should also be decreased slowly (not faster than >0.5 mEq/hour).

Severe (<120 mEq/l) hyponatremia is generally seen with advanced uroperitoneum, diarrhea, and inap-propriate antidiuretic hormone (ADH) secretion. Mild to moderate hyponatremia may be seen with any of the above and also with sick cell syndrome where hyponatremia is due to redistribution.

Hypernatremia is seen with dehydration (free water loss) or with mixing errors when milk replacers are fed. Rarely, hypernatremia is seen when saline instead of water is used for humidification of intranasally administered oxygen or in mechanical ventilator circuits.

Acid–base disturbances

It is difficult to predict the source of disturbance without an ABG analysis. Bicarbonate or TCO_2 measurements are influenced by strong ions and may compensate for respiratory abnormalities. Therefore, correction of the acid–base disturbance is aimed at correcting the primary disturbance. In cases of compensatory metabolic alkalosis, improving ventilation will help reduce respiratory acidosis. In cases of diarrhea, correction of electrolyte abnormalities and improving tissue perfusion will help resolve metabolic and lactic acidosis.

If possible, all foals should have an ABG obtained at the time of admission in order to assess respiratory function and acid–base status. Portable blood gas monitors that may be useful for the equine neonate are commercially available.

Immune therapy

IV plasma is often given as part of fluid stabilization of the foal and supplementation should be considered in any critically ill neonate (see Chapter 12).

Antimicrobial therapy

Critically ill neonates require antimicrobial therapy (see Chapter 16). In human medicine it has been demonstrated that early administration of appropriate antimicrobial therapy improves survival. Antimicrobials such as ceftiofur sodium (5–10 mg/kg IV q6–12h), which are broad spectrum with few toxic adverse effects, may be administered at the time of admission after blood culture samples have been obtained. Ceftiofur sodium may be added to the first liter of resuscitation fluids with minimal concern for adverse effect. This will provide initial antimicrobial coverage until an antimicrobial plan can be clearly determined.

Nutritional support

All recumbent foals and those showing signs of colic should be checked for nasogastric reflux, as debilitated and compromised foals often show no signs of colic, perhaps due to cerebral dysfunction (**9.4**). The nasogastric tube is left in place to check for reflux or to assist with feeding foals with no suckle reflex and a functional GI tract (**9.5**).

Feeding is withheld until the foal's temperature is >37.5°C (99.5°F), borborygmi are present, meconium is passed, and tissue perfusion has improved. IV glucose (p. 515) is used for short-term energy supplementation during stabilization until a complete nutritional plan can be instituted.

Temperature

The foal should be warmed gradually. Rapid warming should be avoided until fluid resuscitation is performed in order to prevent peripheral vasodilation and cardiovascular collapse prior to the foal being euvolemic. Warming is facilitated by the use of specialized blankets that surround the foal with warmed air. The foal should be placed on a mat and not on the ground in order to prevent additional heat loss.

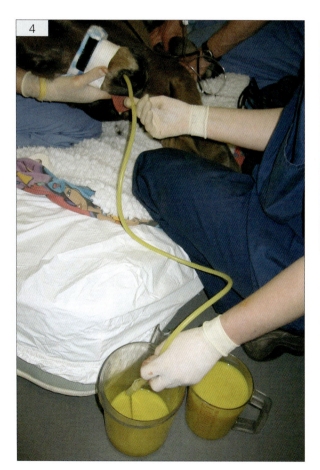

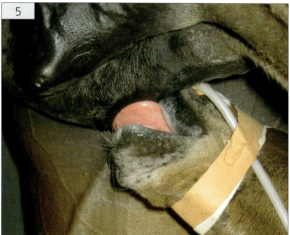

9.5 Nasogastric tubes are attached to the non-cartilaginous nares with suture material and held in place around the muzzle with tape. Foals are able to learn to nurse with the nasogastric tube in place. This foal also shows an excellent tongue seal.

9.4 Nasogastric reflux from a newborn foal with hypoxic ischemic syndrome that had been fed 1 liter of fluids via a stomach tube just after birth. Only gentle negative pressure should be applied to the end of the tube to avoid damaging mucosa of stomach.

Eyes

Corneal and eyelid trauma are common in recumbent neonates. Both eyes should be examined at admission and at least daily during treatment. Superficial corneal ulceration should be treated initially with topical antimicrobial ointment every 4–6 hours. If no response is seen, the eye is deteriorating, or a deep ulcer is present, corneal cytology and culture should be considered.

Lower lid entropion is common in critically ill neonates. If still present after rehydration, vertical mattress sutures are placed along the entire lower lid with 4/0 polyglactin 910 mattress sutures extending from the medial to the lateral canthus.

Umbilicus

The umbilicus is examined for the presence of excessive bleeding, trauma, or herniation. It is ligated if bleeding and 2.5% povidone–iodine or dilute chlorhexidine solution applied topically to the external umbilical remnant only. Exuberant treatment of the external umbilical remnant can lead to significant scalding of the surrounding skin and promote development of patent urachus.

DISEASES OF THE EQUINE NEONATE

Failure of passive transfer

Key points

- Failure of passive transfer (FPT) of immunity is common in sick foals.
- Early treatment of FPT is considered optimal as foals with FPT are prone to infection and other neonatal diseases.

Definition/overview

FPT occurs when there is insufficient absorption of immunoglobulins from colostrum resulting in serum IgG concentrations <4 g/l (400 mg/dl) after 24 hours of age.[25,26] Foals with adequate immunoglobulin transfer have an IgG concentration >8 g/l (800 mg/dl). Foals with FPT are at greater risk of sepsis.

Etiology/pathogenesis

FPT can be due to ingestion of poor quality colostrum, loss of colostrum by premature lactation, failure to ingest or absorb colostrum, or increased immunoglobulin consumption (*Table 9.2*).

The diffuse epitheliochorial nature of the equine placenta does not permit *in-utero* transfer of immunoglobulins to the fetus, therefore foals are essentially agammaglobulinemic at birth. Although foals are immunocompetent at birth, they rely on immunoglobulins and immune factors provided by colostrum for protection in the first 4–8 weeks of life. Colostrum is usually produced in the last 2–3 weeks of pregnancy. It contains primarily IgG, although other factors and immunoglobulins are present, which are also important in the foal's immune protection. Immunoglobulins are absorbed via pinocytosis by specialized enterocytes. Maximal absorption occurs within 8 hours of birth and there is minimal absorption after 24 hours.

The minimum amount of IgG necessary to provide adequate immunity is generally recognized to be >8 g/l (800 mg/dl).[27] However foals with IgG concentrations <8 g/l (800 mg/dl) can remain healthy, therefore other factors, such as exposure to and virulence of environmental pathogens, management factors, and colostral antibody titers to specific pathogens, all play a role in the susceptibility of the foal to infection.[26]

Table 9.2 **Causes of failure of passive transfer**	
Premature lactation	Placentitis
	Twins
	Premature placental separation
Failure of lactation	Fescue toxicosis
	Maternal systemic illness
Poor quality colostrum	Age of mare (>15 years old)
	Individual or breed variation
	Seasonal weather and climate change
Failure to nurse	Neonatal weakness
	Musculoskeletal abnormalities
	Rejection by dam
	Colic
	Hepatic encephalopathy
Failure to absorb	Enteritis
	Hypoxic damage of specialized enterocytes
Increased consumption	Sepsis

Clinical features

FPT does not directly cause any clinical signs of disease.

Differential diagnosis

Sepsis can cause an increase consumption of immunoglobulins. Malnutrition can result in protein catabolism and subsequent FPT.

Diagnosis

There are several tests available for measuring IgG concentration, which is usually measured at 18–24 hours when maternal serum immunoglobulins have reached their peak. The single radial immunodiffusion test is the most quantitatively accurate test; however, results are not available for 18–24 hours. Glutaraldehyde coagulation and the zinc turbidity test are quick, inexpensive tests. They are best used as screening tests to detect the foal that is likely to have FPT; these tests have low specificity, therefore a positive test may not indicate FPT.[28] Immunoassays are convenient and easier to use. Both currently available assays have similar sensitivity but higher, though not ideal, specificity.

Management/treatment

Treatment depends on the systemic condition of the foal and the environmental conditions. Healthy foals with an IgG concentration between 400 and 800 mg/dl on well managed farms with low disease prevalence may not require treatment. However, foals with an IgG concentration <8 g/l (800 mg/dl) that are systemically ill or in poor environmental conditions should have immunoglobulin supplementation.

Foals with an IgG concentration <4 g/l (400 mg/dl) should have immunoglobulin supplementation, regardless. Immunoglobulin supplementation is by oral or IV administration depending on GI function and the age of the foal. Foals 12–24 hours of age with a functional GI tract can be given oral immunoglobulin supplementation. Efficacy of absorption is decreased after 12 hours of age. Foals >18 hours of age or with GI dysfunction require IV supplementation. Immunoglobulin levels should be re-evaluated after any supplementation to ensure concentrations are >8 g/l (800 mg/dl).

Oral immunoglobulin supplementation: Equine colostrum is the ideal supplement. Oral or nasogastric administration of 1–2 liters of good quality colostrum divided into 200–400 ml increments is recommended if complete FPT is suspected. Breeders should store frozen good quality colostrum. After the newborn foal has nursed from one side, 200–250 ml of colostrum can be milked from the other side and stored.

Bovine colostrum can be used but is not ideal as bovine immunoglobulins have a short half-life in foals and are not directed against equine pathogens.[29] Concentrated equine serum and lyophilized immunoglobulin result in detectable IgG levels; however, levels are <8 g/l (800 mg/dl) with recommended doses.[30]

Intravenous immunoglobulin supplementation: Many commercially available licensed plasma products are available that have a guaranteed IgG concentration and are free of anti-equine antibody. Generally, 1 liter of normal equine plasma containing 12 g/l (1,200 mg/dl) will increase a 45 kg foal's IgG by about 2 g/l (200 mg/dl).[27,31] Some commercial products have an IgG concentration >25 g/l (2,500 mg/dl) and are sold as hyperimmune products. Septic foals may need larger amounts due to continued utilization of immunoglobulins and/or protein catabolism and should be retested every few days while under treatment. Plasma can also be harvested from a local donor who is negative for alloantibodies, infectious diseases and, ideally, Aa and Qa alloantigens, but carries an increased risk of exposure to non-cell red cell antigens.

Fresh frozen plasma should be thawed slowly in warm water to prevent denaturing proteins. Plasma should always be administered using a blood administration set with an in-line filter. Plasma transfusions should be monitored closely for any sign of transfusion reaction, characterized by piloerection, fever, tachycardia, and/or tachpnea. It is important that plasma is administered very slowly for the first 10–15 minutes in order to monitor for plasma reactions. Vital signs should be obtained at 5-minute intervals throughout the initial transfusion. Should a plasma transfusion reaction occur, **stop the transfusion immediately**. If signs continue or the foal exhibits respiratory distress, administer IV epinephrine (0.3–0.7 ml 1:1,000 dilute with sterile saline to 3–7 ml at 1:10,000).

Prevention

The IgG concentration of foals should be measured at 12 hours of age and, if needed, oral supplementation given. The quality of the colostrum can be assessed and the foal supplemented at birth if required.

Good quality colostrum should have an IgG concentration of >30 g/l (3,000 mg/dl). Colostral immunoglobulin levels can be measured using a Colostrometer or BRIX 0-50% sugar refractometer; the latter is easier and more reliable to use (**9.6, 9.7**).[32] A SG >1.060 corresponds to an IgG concentration >30 g/l (3,000 mg/dl) and a reading of >23% on the sugar scale corresponds to an IgG concentration of >60 g/l (6,000 mg/dl).

Neonatal isoerythrolysis
Key points

- Foals with neonatal isoerytholysis (NI) will not also have FPT.
- The owner should be made aware that the dam is at risk for producing foals with NI in the future.
- Large volume and repeated transfusion may result in kernicterus and/or liver injury in severe cases of NI and the foal should be closely monitored for these complications.

Definition/overview

NI is an alloimmune hemolytic anemia of newborn foals caused by antibodies against the foal's erythrocytes in the mare's colostrum. NI usually occurs in foals from multiparous mares and involves Aa and Qa factors.

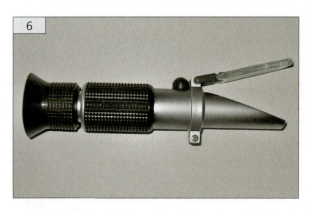

9.6 BRIX 0-50% sugar refractometer. A drop of milk is placed on the platform and a reading taken from the Brix scale in the eyepiece.

9.7 Colostrometer. A milk sample is suspended in distilled water and specific gravity measured from increments on a suspended rod.

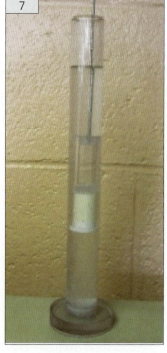

Etiology/pathogenesis

Aa and Qa factors (surface antigens) are the most immunogenic factors and account for approximately 90% of NI cases.[33,34] The Ca blood group appears to influence the incidence of NI as Aa-negative mares with anti-Ca antibodies do not produce antibodies against Aa factors. In mule foals a specific donkey factor has been identified. The prevalence of NI in Thoroughbred and Standardbred populations is low.[33] All mares bred to donkeys are at risk of producing foals that develop NI; however, only about 10% of mule foals develop NI.[35]

There are prerequisites for the development of NI (*Table 9.3*). The absorbed alloantibodies bind to the foal's RBC surface antigen, resulting in hemolysis.[25,34] If hemolysis is severe, decreased tissue oxygenation and cardiovascular collapse can occur, resulting in seizures and multiorgan failure. Toxic hepatopathy from severe hemolysis or hepatic necrosis from hypoxia can occur.[36] Severe hyperbilirubinemia can result in deposition of unconjugated bilirubin in the CNS, resulting in kernicterus.[36]

Clinical features

Typically, foals are clinically normal at birth and develop signs after ingestion of colostrum. Clinical signs vary depending on the rate and severity of hemolysis and resulting anemia and can occur from 5 hours to 7 days after birth. Peracute cases occur at a younger age.

Clinical signs in mild, slow-onset NI include lethargy, tachypnea, tachycardia, and pale icteric mucous membranes (**9.8**). In more severe acute-onset cases the foals may be febrile, stop nursing, and develop pigmenturia. Peracute cases may be found dead or present with signs of multiorgan failure and seizures and may not have developed icterus. Depression and neurological signs associated with kernicterus may be present.

Differential diagnosis

Sepsis; meconium impaction; liver disease; hypoxic ischemic syndrome (HIS); EHV-1; internal or external hemorrhage.

Table 9.3 Prerequisites for the development of neonatal isoerythrolysis

- The mare must be negative for the offending RBC antigen
- The mare is exposed to and produces antibodies against RBC antigens. This occurs in:
  - Multiparous mares with exposure to fetal RBCs during previous pregnancies
  - Primiparous mares that have had a blood transfusion or developed placental abnormalities that allow exposure to fetal RBCs
- The foal from the current pregnancy must inherit the specific RBC antigen from the stallion
- The foal ingests and absorbs alloantibodies from the colostrum

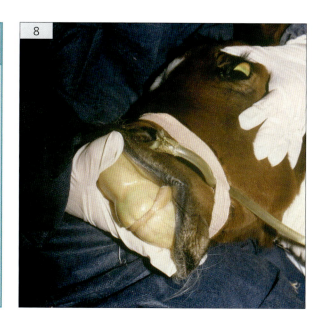

9.8 Typical pale jaundiced mucous membranes and sclera in a horse with neonatal isoerthyrolysis.

Diagnosis

Diagnosis is based on clinical signs and demonstration of maternal alloantibodies on the foal's RBCs (*Table 9.4*). Typically, the foal has anemia and hyperbilirubinemia. Severely affected foals may also have increased L-lactate concentrations, metabolic acidosis, pigmenturia, and elevated liver enzyme activites. Alloantibody thrombocytopenia and neutropenia may be present.

Hemolytic cross-match is the most reliable test. A positive test for NI is recognized by a strong hemolytic reaction in the minor cross-match – mare serum against foal erythrocytes. The alloantibodies responsible for NI are stronger hemolysins than agglutinins, therefore tests for agglutination are not as reliable.

The jaundiced foal agglutination (JFA) assay can be performed in the field and in experienced hands correlates well with the hemolytic test.[37] In this test, the foal's RBCs are mixed with the mare's blood and evidence of agglutinating (or clumping) confirms anti-RBC antibody is present.

Management/treatment

Treatment of NI depends on the severity of clinical signs. If clinical signs are present before 24 hours of age, the mare's colostrum should be withheld. If only mild hemolysis occurs, specific treatment may not be necessary. In more severe cases, a blood transfusion and supportive therapy may be necessary.

If the foal has not been nursing and is hypovolemic, fluid therapy is instituted to improve tissue perfusion and oxygenation. INO_2 insufflation can be carried out to improve oxygen saturation.

The decision for a blood transfusion depends on the clinical signs (weakness, tachypnea, and tachycardia) and laboratory findings.[36,38] Indicators of impaired tissue perfusion are used as PCV is unreliable. A combination of indicators of impaired tissue perfusion, PCV <0.12 l/l (12%) and hemoglobin <50 g/l (5 g/dl) are used by the authors (*Table 9.5*). Washed dam's RBCs are the ideal choice for transfusion. A Qa/Aa-negative blood donor or Standardbred, Morgan, or Quarter horse gelding with no prior history of blood transfusion is also suitable. The optimal volume required can be calculated, or 2–3 liters can be given empirically (*Table 9.6*).[33] Deferoxamine mesylate may prove helpful for iron elimination in these cases.[39]

Table 9.4 Laboratory tests available for diagnosis of neonatal isoerythrolysis

Hemolytic cross-match test	Exogenous complement, foal RBCs, mare serum*	Hemolysis
Minor cross-match	Mare serum, foal RBCs	Agglutination
Coombs test	Foal RBCs, mare serum* Coombs reagent	Agglutination

* Needed for the presuckle test.

Table 9.5 Laboratory values used in assessing tissue oxygenation

Lactate concentration	>4 mmol/l
PvO_2	<30 mmHg
SvO_2	<50%
Oxygen exchange ratio ($[SaO_2-SvO_2/SaO_2] \times 100$)	>50%

Table 9.6 Volume of blood required

$$\frac{(PCV\ desired - PCV\ observed) \times body\ weight\ (kg) \times blood\ volume\ (liters/kg)*}{PCV\ of\ donor}$$

(*150 ml/kg is blood volume of 2-day-old foal)

The prognosis is favorable for uncomplicated cases.[36] Foals have a poorer prognosis if there is continued hemolysis after blood transfusions and are at risk of developing kernicterus and severe degenerative hepatopathy, both which carry a grave prognosis.[36]

Prevention

NI is a preventable disease. At-risk brood mares, Aa- and Qa-negative mares, and mares that have produced NI foals can be identified. These mares can be bred to Aa/Qa-negative stallions; however, due to the high prevalence of these antigens in the population, this is impractical. Thus the 'at-risk mare' should be screened for anti-RBC antibodies, which are produced in the last month of pregnancy. If anti-RBC antibodies are present, a hemolytic or JFA test should be done on the foal prior to nursing. If positive, foals should be supplemented with colostrum from another source and should not nurse from the mare for 48 hours, or as determined by the JFA test. The mare should be milked frequently and milk/colostrum discarded.

Sepsis

Key points

- Foals with sepsis that progresses 25 to septic shock have a significantly increased risk of non-survival.
- Sepsis remains the leading cause of death in sick neonatal foals.
- Sepsis in foals can be occult and present as acute collapse.

Definition/overview

Sepsis is the systemic inflammatory response to infection and is a leading cause of morbidity and mortality in the equine neonate.[40]

Etiology/pathogenesis

Foals can acquire an infection *in utero* or during or after delivery. Predisposing factors include maternal illness, placentitis, abnormal gestational length, FPT, and poor environmental conditions.[41] *In-utero* infection is usually associated with a bacterial placentitis. Post-natal infection occurs through the GI or respiratory tract or umbilicus. Currently, translocation of bacteria across the GI tract, not the umbilicus, is believed to be the most important route of entry.[41,42]

The predominant bacteria involved in neonatal sepsis vary with different studies and geographic locations. The majority of infections are due to gram-negative bacteria, in particular *Escherichia coli*; however, an increasing number of gram-positive bacteria are being isolated.[17,41–45] *Candida albicans* is isolated more commonly from immunocompromised foals with prolonged hospitalization. EHV-1 and equine arteritis virus can also cause sepsis.

Invasion of the body by an infectious organism normally results in a local inflammatory response at the site of insult. This response is a combination of pro-inflammatory responses that are 'balanced' by anti-inflammatory responses. Both have the aim of containing the infectious agent, destroying and repairing damaged tissue.[46] If the initial insult is overwhelming or the reaction spills over into the systemic circulation, there is activation of multiple systemic pro-inflammatory (SIRS) and anti-inflammatory (compensatory anti-inflammatory response syndrome [CARS]) pathways and pathologic changes remote from the original insult occur. The disease syndrome and clinical signs resulting from the cascade of systemic mediators depends on the balance between SIRS and CARS. Multiple organ dysfunction syndrome results when there is evidence of organ dysfunction. Severe sepsis results when there is organ dysfunction, hypoperfusion, or hypotension. The foal develops septic shock if the sepsis-induced hypotension is not responsive to fluid therapy and is accompanied by organ dysfunction. Manifestations of organ dysfunction in the foal can include coagulopathies, cardiovascular, pulmonary, renal, GI, or hepatic dysfunction.[46] Neonates can also develop acute lung injury or ARDS as part of the systemic response to sepsis.[47,48] Microorganisms can also be disseminated throughout the body and localize in different body systems, resulting in clinical diseases such as pneumonia, enteritis, meningitis, or infectious orthopedic disease.

Clinical features

Clinical signs depend on the duration and severity of illness and the competency of the foal's immune system. Initial clinical signs can be subtle and non-specific; however, if left untreated, clinical signs of septic shock can rapidly develop.

Initial signs include decreased nursing, depression and increased recumbency. The foal often has a milk-stained face as a result of standing under the mare and not nursing (**9.9**). The rectal temperature is variable; a normal temperature does not preclude the foal from having sepsis. Heart rate and respiratory rates can initially be normal, but can become elevated or slower as the disease progresses. Hyperemic and injected mucous membranes with a rapid CRT accompanied by scleral injection and hyperemic coronary bands are classic findings in early sepsis (**9.10A–C**).[1] Jaundice is often seen and is distinguished from jaundice associated

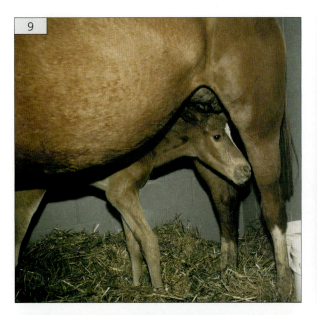

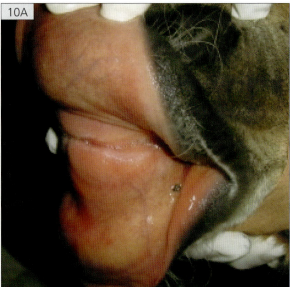

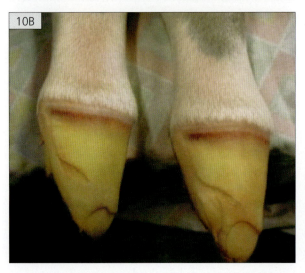

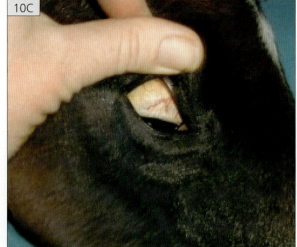

9.9 This foal standing under the mare is not nursing and has a milk-stained face and sunken eyes.

9.10A–C (A) Injected mucous membranes with a hint of jaundice. (B) Coronitis. This can also be seen in pigmented coronary bands. (C) Injected sclera with a hint of jaundice.

with NI by the presence of injected mucous membranes. Petechiae can be seen on mucous membranes and within the pinnae. Uveitis is often present in foals that have become septic *in utero* (**9.11**).[49]

Dehydration and hypoglycemia will develop if the foal is not nursing. The foal will develop tacky mucous membranes and sunken eyes with possible lower lid entropion. If the disease progresses, recumbency, muddy mucous membranes with a slow CRT, poor to no palpable peripheral pulses, cold extremities, and organ dysfunction may be seen as the foal develops septic shock.

Clinical signs associated with localization of infection may also be present; those associated with enteritis and pneumonia are the most common. Clinical signs of enteritis include diarrhea, colic, ileus, and/or abdominal distension. Early clinical signs of pneumonia include an increased respiratory rate and effort; however, pneumonia may be present with no signs of respiratory disease. Other clinical signs of localizing infection are joint effusion with or without lameness, lameness with or without edema and pain over a physis, cellulitis, subcutaneous abscess, and altered demeanor including seizures and omphalitis.[40]

Differential diagnosis
HIS; NI; prematurity/dysmaturity; Tyzzer's disease.

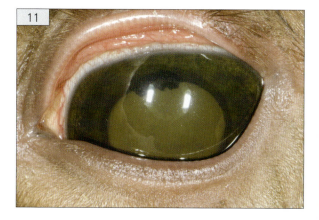

9.11 Uveitis in a newborn foal with characteristic green discoloration of the iris.

Diagnosis
Diagnosis of sepsis relies on perinatal history, clinical examination findings, laboratory data, and cultures of samples from blood or sites of localized infection (joint, CSF, abscess, umbilicus, peritoneum). Clinical signs, historical information, and laboratory data are initially used in the diagnosis of sepsis as culture results are typically not available for at least 48 hours.

Leukopenia characterized by a neutropenia with toxic changes and a degenerative left shift is the most common hematologic finding in acute sepsis.[41] Later in the disease process, leukocytosis with neutrophilia occurs. Fibrinogen concentration is normal in the acute stages and increased in advanced cases. If increased at birth, *in-utero* infection should be suspected. Hypogammaglobulinemia is a common finding due to FPT and increased consumption of immunoglobulins with sepsis. Abnormal blood glucose concentrations are common. Other biochemical abnormalities that may be present are azotemia, hyperbilirubinemia, lipemia, increased lactate concentration, and altered coagulation times.[41]

Respiratory function is best evaluated through ABG analysis and thoracic radiographs, as auscultation of the foal's thorax is not reliable in detecting the presence of disease and cyanotic mucous membranes do not occur until significant hypoxemia is present (PaO_2 <40 mmHg). Transtracheal aspiration may be too stressful to perform on the septic neonate unless the clinican is very experienced and the procedure is performed rapidly.

Ultrasonographic examination assists with the diagnosis of internal umbilical remnant infections, osteomyelitis, subcutaneous abscesses, and cellulitis. Radiographs and joint fluid analysis should be performed if infectious orthopedic disease is suspected.

The sepsis score was developed in the 1980s to help clinicians identify a septic foal.[50] Later studies from other institutions, however, have found it not to be accurate in predicting sepsis and results may be very institution/hospital specific.[41,51]

Management/treatment
Therapy is aimed at stabilizing the foal, eliminating the infection, and treating the localized manifestations.

Eliminating the infection

Antimicrobial therapy: Broad-spectrum IV bactericidal therapy should be instigated immediately in any foal with suspected sepsis. The choice is generally dictated by antimicrobial sensitivity patterns of local common isolates and the clinician's experience. Therapy can then be altered according to culture and sensitivity results. A minimum of 10–14 days is recommended for blood culture-positive foals without localizing signs.

If localizing signs are present, antimicrobials may be necessary for a prolonged period of time. A combination of penicillin and an aminoglycoside is the most commonly recommended regimen in neonates with normal renal function. In cases where renal function is not normal or unknown, high-dose ceftiofur sodium, trimethoprim-sulfonamides, ticarcillin/clavulanic acid, or a third-generation cephalosporin can be used (see Chapter 16). Fluconazole (8 mg/kg PO loading dose followed by 4 mg/kg PO q24h) can be used for fungal infections. Acyclovir (16–30 mg/kg PO q6–8h; 10 mg/kg diluted in 1 liter isotonic crystalloid over 1 hour q12h) has been used in foals with EHV-1 sepsis.

Immune system support: This can be given by colostrum or plasma. Colostrum is ideal if the neonate has a functional GI tract and is <12 hours old. Plasma is administered to foals with a normal or low IgG concentration to provide immunoglobulins and other immunoprotective substances. More than normal amounts of plasma may be required in septic foals because of the sepsis-induced catabolism of immunoglobulins.

Anti-endotoxin therapy: Flunixin meglumine, polymyxin B, and pentoxifylline have been used in adult horses but have not been evaluated in treatment of endotoxemia in foals. Flunixin meglumine is ulcerogenic and polymyxin B sucralfate and NSAIDs are potentially nephrotoxic and should be used with caution. However, the anti-endotoxin dose of polymyxin B is one-tenth the nephrotoxic antimicrobial dose and nephrotoxicity occurs with accummulation,

suggesting that one or two doses should not be harmful and may be beneficial in foals with suspected endotoxin exposure.

E. coli J5 or *Salmonella typhimurium* hyperimmune plasma or serum are safer options for anti-endotoxin therapy as well as having benefits for colloid therapy and providing other immune factors.[40] Most commercially available hyperimmune equine plasma products intended for the treatment of FPT in foals also have high anti-endotoxin titers.

Localized infection

Respiratory: Foals with bacterial pneumonia may develop respiratory failure unless intensive therapies are instituted (see Chapter 3). Recumbent foals have a poorer prognosis, although once the foal begins to stand the prognosis improves. Adjunctive therapies, such as frequent standing and coupage (every 1–2 hours) and nebulization with saline and antimicrobials (ceftiofur sodium and gentamicin), can be utilized. Foals with EHV-1 pneumonia have an extremely poor prognosis.

Gastrointestinal: The treatment of enteritis is symptomatic (see Chapter 1) and usually resolves with systemic improvement of the foal. Septic foals without enteritis can also show signs of ileus and colic. Approximately 50% of all foals with enteritis will also be bacteremic.[42]

Umbilical: An ultrasonographic examination of the internal umbilical remnants should be performed as infection is often present without external signs (**9.12, 9.13**). Long-term antimicrobial therapy results in resolution of the majority of cases. Occasionally, surgical resection is necessary if there is a large discrete abscess or when seeding of infection from the remnant is suspected.

Septic arthritis/osteomyelitis: Infectious orthopedic disease is a frustrating complication of neonatal sepsis as it often occurs after 7–10 days of expensive treatment. Early aggressive treatment is critical for a successful outcome. There are a variety of therapies including joint lavage, arthroscopy, and IV and IO perfusion (**9.14**).[52] Joint lavage assists with removing damaging inflammatory products and regional limb perfusion increases local concentration of antimicrobials (see Chapter 16).

Meningitis: Meningitis is rare in septic foals. Third-generation cephalosporins (e.g. cefotaxime), which pass the blood–brain barrier into the CSF, are recommended. The prognosis for recovery is poor.

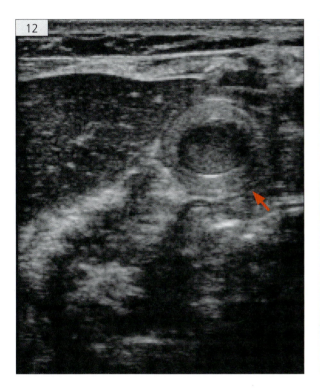

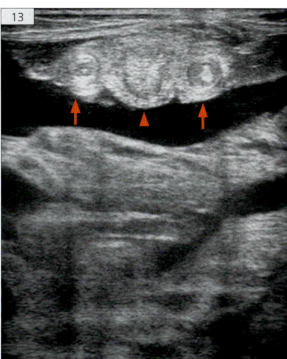

9.12 Sonogram of an infected enlarged umbilical vein (arrow) near the liver. The diameter of the umbilical vein should be <1 cm.

9.13 Sonogram of the internal umbilical arteries (arrows) and urachus (arrowhead) highlighted by an increase in anechoic peritoneal fluid. This view is commonly known as 'ET'. The diameter of 'ET' (from the extremities of the umbilical arteries) should be <2.5 cm.

9.14 Intraosseous bone perfusion using minimum volume tubing with a male luer end inserted into a 4 mm unicortical bone portal.

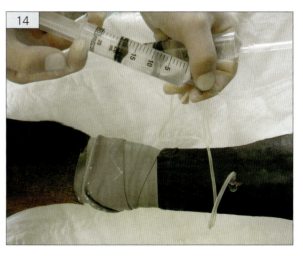

Prematurity

Key points

- Prematurity does not have a specific gestation length as a cut-off; rather the diagnosis is based on physical characteristics and duration of gestation in relation to previous gestations by the dam.
- Foals born prematurely because of interventions such as elective cesarian section or induction of parturition may not have gone through the final steps of readiness for birth and are less likely to survive.
- Foals born prematurely following successful treatment of placentitis may have improved survival.
- Musculoskeletal abnormalities are common and, in particular, cuboidal bone immaturity may be athletically limiting if not recognized early.

Definition/overview

A premature foal has a gestational length that is less than the normal gestation length for the dam and displays physical characteristics of prematurity. These foals have a classic clinical appearance of small size, domed head, floppy ears, soft silky coat, and increased joint and tendon laxity. Dysmaturity is used to describe a foal that has experienced some form of intrauterine growth retardation. These foals have a normal or prolonged gestational age, but have signs such as poor muscle mass in relation to skeletal mass and immaturity of body systems.

Management of premature foals is often complicated and involves multiple organ systems. Premature foals exposed to intrauterine stresses such as placentitis appear to have a better chance of survival.[53]

Etiology/pathogenesis

Fetoplacental causes of prematurity include placental insufficiency (twins, premature placental separation), placentitis, or fetal malformations. Severe maternal illness or medical/surgical conditions requiring premature removal of the foal and mistimed induction of parturition are also causes.[53] Fetal unpreparedness for extrauterine life should be a major consideration

in any decision involving removal of the fetus from the uterus due to convenience or significant medical problems of the dam as these particular foals have a poor chance for survival even with intensive care.

Maturation of the hypothalamus–pituitary–adrenal (HPA) axis plays a vital role in ensuring fetal viability by controlling the final maturation of various organ systems. During most of gestation there are various mechanisms in place to restrict fetal exposure to cortisol.[53] The trigger that results in an increase in fetal cortisol so final maturation can occur is not known. However, in the last 3–5 days of gestation the adrenal glands are more sensitive to adrenocorticotropic hormone and there is an increase in production of cortisol and prostaglandins from the placenta. These changes result in increased fetal cortisol levels 48–72 hours before parturition. The surge of cortisol coincides with maturation of the hemopoetic system with changes in the red and white blood cell parameters and an increase in the neutrophil to lymphocyte ratio to more than 2:1.[54] Tri-iodothyronine (T_3) also increases in late gestation. Thyroid hormones regulate thermogenesis, skeletal developments and, with glucocorticoids, assist with lung maturation.[53]

There are several factors that can induce premature maturation of the fetal HPA axis:

- Exogenous corticosteroids used in humans to hasten maturation of the fetal HPA axis do not appear to be effective in the mare at doses that are safe to administer.[55,56]
- Placental or fetal infection through stimulation of prostaglandins stimulates maturation of the fetal HPA axis. This is commonly seen in foals that are born before term from mares with placentitis. However, maternal problems in late gestation do not appear to have a significant effect on maturity and foals are born with an immature HPA axis.[53]

Lack of maturity of organs and subsequent multiorgan failure is common in foals with an immature HPA axis. Respiratory failure develops due to poor lung compliance, weak respiratory muscles, and a soft thoracic cage; however, it is rarely due to surfactant deficiency and hyaline membrane disease unless foals are <300 days of gestation. Pulmonary hypertension often results in reversion to fetal circulation. Immature hormonal responses and enzyme activity result in inconsistent responses to normal vasoactive therapy and glucose supplementation. Hypoglycemia is common due to inadequate glycogen stores and poor gluconeogenic enzyme activity.[53]

Clinical features

Characteristically, premature foals are small in body size and weight with varying degrees of tendon and periarticular laxity, incomplete ossification of cuboidal bones, domed head, floppy ears, and a soft silky coat (**9.15**). Foals may have generalized weakness and be unable to stand, poor thermoregulatory control, and intolerance to enteral feeding. Respiratory distress, paradoxical respiration, and subsequent respiratory fatigue and failure can occur (**9.16**).

Foals removed from the *in-utero* environment before final maturation of the organ systems has occurred often show clinical progress for up to 12–18 hours – giving the naive attending veterinarian and owner false hope – and then develop a range of progressive abnormalities including respiratory failure, glucose intolerance, feeding intolerance, cardiovascular collapse, and renal failure. These foals have low blood cortisol levels, no response to exogenous ACTH administration (0.125 mg IM) and no increase in WBC count after 2 days.[53] However, foals that have maturation hastened with intrauterine stress are frequently born with mature cardiopulmonary and hemopoietic systems. These foals may not have a suckle reflex, may be weak, need assistance to stand, and have poor glucose and temperature regulation; however, with appropriate supportive care these foals may show clinical improvement in a 24-hour period and have an improved chance of survival despite physical immaturity.[57] A primary limiting aspect in these cases is cuboidal bone immaturity and residual musculoskeletal abnormalities. Foals may have concurrent signs of HIS and sepsis.

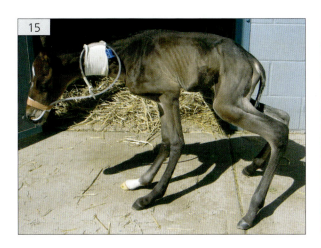

9.15 Classic appearance of a premature foal.

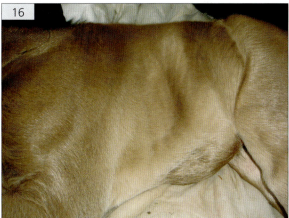

9.16 Paradoxical respiration with collapse of the thorax during inspiration.

Differential diagnosis

Sepsis; neonatal EHV-1.

Diagnosis

Clinical signs are usually diagnostic. Thoracic radiographs and ABG analysis will assist in evaluating the function and maturity of the pulmonary system. Neonatal equine respiratory distress syndrome is a primary surfactant deficiency different from the equine neonatal acute lung injury/respiratory distress syndrome and has a classic diffuse alveolar pattern with air bronchograms. Premature foals with dependent lung atelectasis have an interstitial pattern without air bronchograms, which is difficult to distinguish from inflammatory lung disease.[48,53] Radiographs of the carpi and hocks will assess the degree of ossification of cuboidal bones and skeletal maturity (**9.17A–C**).

Premature foals have a leukopenia with a neutropenia and neutrophil to lymphocyte ratio <2:1. There is no evidence of a degenerative shift or neutrophil toxicity as seen with sepsis; however, these abnormalities may be present if the foal has concurrent sepsis.

Fibrinogen concentration may be increased if the foal has *in-utero* sepsis and is considered a good prognostic indicator.[53] Creatinine concentration may be increased associated with renal failure or placental insufficiency, termed 'spurious hypercreatininemia'.[58] Hypoglycemia is common.

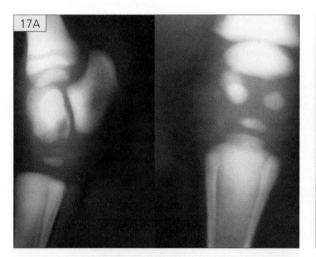

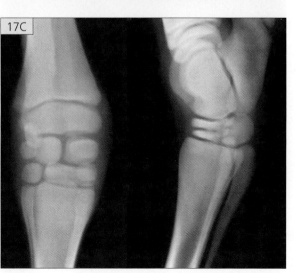

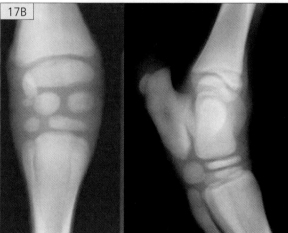

9.17A–C Dorsopalmar radiographs of the carpus and lateromedial radiographs of the tarsus highlighting changes used in the skeletal ossification index. (A) Grade 1: some cuboidal bones have no radiographic evidence of ossification. (B) Grade 2: all the cuboidal bones show some radiographic evidence of ossification. (C) Grade 3: the cuboidal bones are small with rounded edges. The tarsal bones have a wedge shape. Joint spaces are wide.

Management/treatment

The cause of the premature delivery should be established, as this not only affects the treatment and management of the foal, but helps with prognosis. Many premature foals with hastened *in-utero* maturation require minimal treatment apart from nasogastric tube feeding and management of orthopedic problems. Foals with incomplete maturation of the HPA axis require intensive management and often die. IV broad-spectrum bactericidal antimicrobial therapy should be started if there was evidence of placentitis and if the foal is septic or compromised. If there is FPT or evidence of sepsis, IV plasma should be given.

Respiratory support: The degree of ventilatory support is dependent on the severity of respiratory dysfunction. Most premature foals have some degree of respiratory insufficiency.

INO$_2$ insufflation (see Chapter 3) (5–10 liters/minute) is the most commonly administered form of therapy to improve hypoxemia (PaO$_2$ <60 mmHg; SaO$_2$ <90%). The PaO$_2$ should be maintained between 80 and 110 mmHg and SaO$_2$ >92%.[2] The foal's PCV should also be monitored and if it is <0.24 l/l (24%), a blood transfusion may be considered to improve loading of oxygen from the lungs.[2]

Mechanical positive pressure ventilation (PPV) is the ideal treatment for hypoventilation. PPV should be considered in foals with severe hypercapnia (PaCO$_2$ >65 mmHg) and acidemia or where INO$_2$ insufflation fails to correct the hypoxemia or to decrease the work of breathing.[2] PPV and nitric oxide (NO) (added to ventilator gas at 5–40 ppm) has been used in the treatment of persistent pulmonary hypertension.[59] Recently, sildenafil has been used to maintain pulmonary vessel dilation, which decreases the amount of NO required and reduces potential side-effects.[53]

Intratracheal instillation of bovine or synthetic surfactant has been used in newborn foals <300 days of age with severe respiratory distress associated with hyaline membrane disease. This therapy, however, is extremely expensive and of questionable benefit. Nursing care involves maintaining sternal recumbency, which may improve PaO$_2$ by up to 30 mmHg, and alternating sides of recumbency to minimize atelectasis.[60]

Cardiovascular support: Failure of the cardiovascular system is common and is difficult to manage due to inconsistent responses to the vasoactive agents in premature foals. Successful treatment depends on early detection of falling systemic pressures. Falling mean arterial blood pressure and urine output, reduction in intensity of peripheral pulses, and edema formation are indicative of falling systemic blood pressure. If not aggressively treated or if treatment is unsuccessful, secondary renal and GI failure usually follows. Initial therapies include ionotrope and vasopressor therapy (see Chapter 13) and avoiding over administration of sodium containing fluids (see Chapter 12).

Glucose support: Monitoring blood glucose concentrations is important as glucose regulation may be poor and insulin therapy may be required. (See p. 515 for details of glucose administration to foals.)

Gastrointestinal support: The GI tract is usually not mature and most foals have some form of dysmotility and are at risk of developing necrotizing enterocolitis.[53] Feeding is withheld until the foal's temperature is >37.5°C (99.5°F), borborygmi are present, meconium is passed, and tissue perfusion has improved. IV glucose is used for short-term energy supplementation while the foal is stabilized and then parenteral nutrition provided to meet energy requirements (see Chapter 15).

Thermoregulatory support: Premature foals are susceptible to hypothermia and will require closer attention to environmental temperature and body temperature control than other ill foals. (See also Chapter 20.)

Musculoskeletal support: Skeletal maturity is assessed by radiographic examination of the ossification of the hocks and carpi.[61] Management of foals with incomplete ossification is controversial.[53] Exercise restriction is recommended; however, enforced recumbency can predispose or exacerbate pneumonia and limit weight bearing, which encourages ossification.

The foal's weight needs to be closely monitored to ensure there is not excessive weight gain. Increased periarticular and joint laxity are common (**9.18**). Stall rest and time improves the majority of laxity problems (**9.19A, B**). The limbs should not be supported in bandages or casts as this exacerbates the laxity. Braces and splints have been used to maintain even loading on the joints in foals with increased periarticular laxity.[62] Foot trimming and corrective shoeing to maintain a proper weight-bearing axis are also important.

Urinary tract disruption
Key points
- The actual emergency associated with uroabdomen is correction of hypokalemia, which is life-threatening. Anesthesia and definitive surgical correction should be delayed until potassium concentration is 5.0 mmol/l (5 mEq/l) or less.
- Correction of hyperkalemia requires removal of urine from the abdomen.

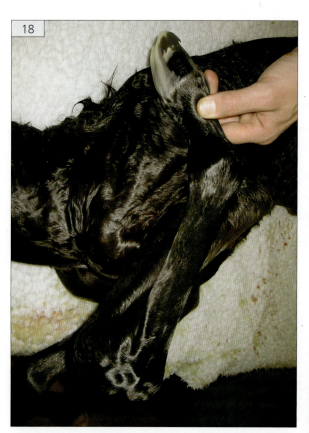

9.18 Increased tendon and periarticular joint laxity.

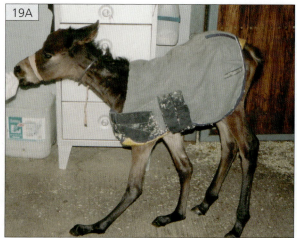

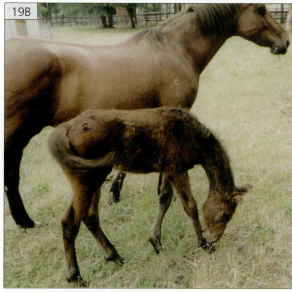

9.19A, B (A) Premature foal with hyperextension. (B) The same foal as in 9.19A at 3 months of age after stall rest until complete ossification of the cuboidal bones had occurred.

- Many foals with uroperitoneum are hypoxemic and will remain so for a day or two following definitive correction. Oxygen supplementation as INO_2 insufflation should be provided routinely to foals with uroperitoneum until their oxygenation status can be confirmed as within normal limits without supplementation.

Definition/overview

Disruption of the urinary tract can occur at any site. The most common sites are the bladder and urachus, which result in uroperitoneum. Ruptures can occur less commonly in the extra-abdominal urachus, retroperitoneal ureter, and urethra.[63] Affected foals are usually <7 days old, although older foals can be affected.[63] Recent reports have shown no sex predilection.[64,65]

Etiology/pathogenesis

Proposed causes of urinary tract disruption include increased pressures exerted on the bladder during parturition, external trauma, congenital defects, and urachal infection. Recent reports have highlighted localized ischemia, sepsis, and necrosis as significant factors.[64]

The pathophysiology is not fully understood, although disruption from infection, sepsis, and local malperfusion – perhaps secondary to 'stretch' applied to the umbilical cord during parturition – with resulting necrosis is becoming a more favored mechanism.[64] Uroperitoneum develops when urine accumulates in the abdominal cavity following disruption of the urinary tract.

If urinary tract disruption is in the retroperitoneal space, fluid drainage into the abdomen may occur or, if retained in the space, perineal edema or perivaginal swelling may occur. As the urine accumulates in the peritoneal cavity, there is equilibration of urine electrolytes and water across the peritoneal membrane with the systemic circulation. This results in hyponatremia, hypochloremia, and hyperkalemia, reflecting the foal's diet of mare's milk, which is low in sodium and high in potassium. Systemic absorption of creatinine results in azotemia.

Foals can develop respiratory distress with compression of the thorax by abdominal distension (abdominal compartment syndrome), accumulation of pleural fluid, and lung atelectasis or ARDS.[48,66,67]

Clinical features

Clinical signs vary depending on the location and duration of disruption. These foals may also present with a primary complaint of suspected meconium impaction/retention (p. 545).

Initial signs include straining to urinate, dribbling urine, and stretching out frequently. Foals developing uroperitoneum in hospital may only show decreased urine production and increased abdominal volume and may not demonstrate the classic electrolyte disturbance apart from increasing creatinine and potassium concentrations.[64,65] Abdominal distension becomes evident as urine accumulates and ballottement may detect a fluid wave.

The foal becomes lethargic, depressed, and disinterested in nursing as the metabolic status deteriorates. Other clinical signs of systemic disease may be present. Affected foals may have clinical signs of respiratory distress due to pneumonia or effects of the uroperitoneum. Subcutaneous edema around the umbilicus, preputial edema, or perineal edema can be seen with ruptures in the extra-abdominal urachus, urethra, and ureter, respectively, and are not associated with altered metabolic status unless uroperitoneum develops (**9.20**).

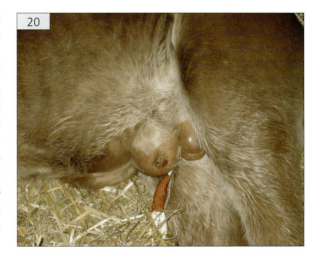

9.20 Swelling of the umbilicus and surrounding area due to urine leakage from an extra-abdominal tear of the urachus.

Differential diagnosis

Urachitis; meconium impaction; ileus; enteritis; renal disease.

Diagnosis

Diagnosis of uroperitoneum is relatively straightforward and should not be challenging.

Abdominal ultrasonography is the most useful diagnostic aid for uroperitoneum. Findings include an excessive amount of anechoic peritoneal fluid and visualization of the defect in the bladder wall or urachus (**9.21, 9.22**). Increased echogenicity of the fluid can be indicative of concurrent peritonitis. Excessive fluid accumulation around the kidney is seen secondary to ureteral tears.

Laboratory value abnormalities depend on the duration of uroperitoneum, diet of the foal, concurrent fluid administration, and other existing clinical problems. Classically, hyperkalemia, hyponatraemia, hypochloremia, and azotemia are seen; however, uroperitoneum should not be discounted if electrolyte values are normal.[64,65] Peritoneal fluid analysis should include cytologic analysis, culture, and creatinine concentration. A peritoneal to serum creatinine ratio greater or equal to 2:1 is diagnostic for uroperitoneum.[68] Ratios of subcutaneous urine to serum can also be used.[63]

Cytologic evaluation identifies peritonitis secondary to infected umbilical remnants or concurrent GI disease.

Injection of non-toxic dye through a urinary catheter can help identify a bladder or urachal defect. Contrast radiography can help identify lesions, in particular ureteral tears, although results are inconsistent.[63,68]

Management/treatment

Initial treatment is aimed at stabilizing the patient, correcting electrolyte and acid–base abnormalities, and providing fluid volume replacement. 0.9% or 0.45% NaCl and 5% dextrose should be used until laboratory results are available.

Some foals may have marked hyponatremia, which will need slow correction if the hyponatraemia has been of several days' duration. Potassium concentrations

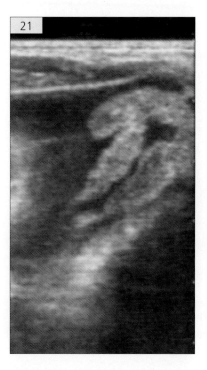

9.21 Sonogram of the ventral abdomen of a 3-day-old foal with uroperitoneum and a bladder defect highlighting the 'ghost' appearance of the bladder that can occur.

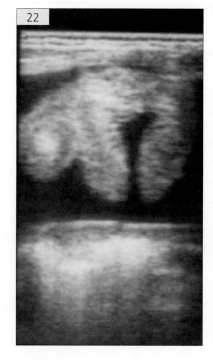

9.22 Sonogram of the ventral abdomen of a 4-day-old foal with uroperitoneum and a bladder defect.

>5.5 mmol/l can be life-threatening. Glucose, sodium bicarbonate, or insulin have been used to decrease serum potassium levels by moving potassium into the cells; however, this does not decrease total body potassium.[21] Hyperkalemia >5.5 mmol/l should be corrected prior to induction of anesthesia if surgical repair is undertaken. While anesthetic complications are less common with the advent of isoflurane inhalant anesthesia than reported with halothane, they may still occur and are generally identified as cardiac dysrhythmias associated with hyperkalemia.[64] Limiting milk intake will limit the intake of potassium. Abdominal drainage via teat cannula, Foley or mushroom catheter, and human peritoneal dialysis catheters has been described to assist in removing potassium from the body. An aseptically placed urinary catheter can be used to drain urine that accumulates in the bladder and assist with drainage of the peritoneal space.

Broad-spectrum antimicrobial treatment should be initiated immediately after blood and peritoneal fluid samples for culture have been obtained. INO_2 insufflation is administered to foals with compromised ventilation.

Once the foal has been stabilized surgical repair can be considered. Details of surgical repair are beyond the scope of this text.

The prognosis is closely related to the presence or absence of sepsis; foals with no clinical signs of sepsis have an excellent prognosis.[65]

Hypoxic ischemic syndrome
Key points
- HIS is a multisystemic disorder most generally characterized with CNS dysfunction but also with fairly predictable involvement of other body systems, particularly the GI and renal systems.
- Uncomplicated HIS carries a good prognosis both for life and athletic function.

Definition/overview
HIS is a multisystemic disorder that results from decreased oxygenation and tissue perfusion in the perinatal period. A variety of clinical signs are seen; the most commonly recognized are neurologic and behavioral abnormalities. These foals were referred to as 'barkers' or 'dummies', which resulted in the terminology 'neonatal maladjustment syndrome'. The new terminology of HIS or perinatal asphyxia syndrome reflects the multisystemic nature of the disease and suspected underlying etiology.[69,70]

Etiology/pathogenesis
HIS can result from any adverse periparturient event that results in decreased oxygen delivery to tissues or other fetal compromise (*Table 9.7*).[69,71] The potential role for inflammatory mediators – possibly associated with subclinical placentitis – is being explored in both veterinary and human medicine and is gaining credence.[72]

Table 9.7 Causes of hypoxia and ischemia in the fetus and neonate

Maternal causes	Reduced maternal oxygen delivery
	Anemia
	Pulmonary disease
	Cardiovascular disease
	Reduced uterine blood flow
	Hypotension (endotoxemia)
	Hypertension (painful conditions)
	Increased vascular resistance
Placental causes	Premature placental separation
	Placental insufficiency
	Placentitis
	Reduced umbilical blood flow
Intrapartum causes	Dystocia
	Premature placental separation
	Cesarean section
	Uterine inertia
	Oxytocin induction of labour
Neonatal causes	Prematurity
	Recumbency
	Pulmonary disease
	Irregular breathing patterns
	Septic shock
	Anemia
	Congenital cardiovascular disease

One proposed and commonly accepted pathophysiologic theory is based on similarities between the neurologic manifestations of HIS in the foal and those seen in other species.[69] A combination of hypoxemia and ischemia (asphyxia) is necessary for tissue damage to occur. A failure of compensatory mechanisms in the fetus or foal in maintaining adequate tissue perfusion is also necessary. The extent of tissue injury depends on the length and severity of the insult and fetal and foal maturity. The most commonly affected organ systems are the CNS, GI tract, and kidneys.

Central nervous system: HIE, also known as neonatal encephalopathy, is a result of acute and delayed neuronal cell death. Mild transient asphyxia usually results in reversible changes. More severe asphyxia can lead to disruption of tight junctions in the capillary endothelium with subsequent vasogenic edema. There is, however, debate over the role of extracellular edema in HIE.[20] Glutamate, an excitatory neurotransmitter, is an important mediator in CNS injury. Asphyxia results in increased synaptic concentrations of glutamate, which opens glutamate-regulated ion channels. This allows sodium and subsequently water into the cells, resulting in cellular edema and possible death. Glutamate is also involved in delayed cellular death through mediation in opening of calcium channels and stimulation of N-methyl-D-aspartate (NMDA) receptors, which open additional calcium channels. The high concentrations of intracellular calcium cause activation of calcium-dependent enzyme systems and subsequent cell death.

Gastrointestinal tract: Asphyxia results in reduced splanchnic and mesenteric blood flow, resulting in decreased production of the protective mucosal layer. This allows autodigestion of the mucosa by intraluminal proteolytic enzymes.[69] Bacteria within the lumen then invade the intestinal wall and are absorbed, resulting in severe sepsis. Gas production from bacterial colonization of the intestinal wall can result in pneumatosis intestinalis.

Ileus and maldigestion, manifested as intolerance to oral/enteral feeding, are characteristic of injury to the GI tract and can prolong hospitalization for days to weeks. GI abnormalities may not manifest for several days following the intitial insult and feeding should be approached cautiously in these patients.

Renal: Redistribution of blood flow away from the kidneys results in decreased perfusion and glomerular filtration and acute tubular necrosis.[69] Other syndromes, such as incomplete transition from fetal renal physiology, water/sodium retention, and mild tubular dysfunction, have been attributed to mild hypoxic ischemic damage.[72] Foals may have spurious hypercreatininemia associated with HIS and this should not be confused with renal failure.[58]

Clinical features

The clinical signs and organs affected depend on the length and severity of the insult and when it occurred in relation to either fetal or neonatal life. Clinical signs of SIRS can occur if there is severe hypoxic ischemic damage. Clinical signs of HIS are usually seen from 24–72 hours after birth, although signs may be present at birth. The foal can appear clinically normal prior to the onset of clinical signs.

Central nervous system: A large range of signs are associated with HIE from mild behavioral abnormalities to seizure-like activity. Behavioral abnormalities include loss of affinity for the mare and inability to find the udder. Neurologic abnormalities most commonly include loss of suckle reflex and uncoordinated swallowing resulting in dysphagia (**9.23**). Other signs include hyperresponsiveness, which may progress to intermittent opisthotonus, extensor rigidity, and grand mal seizures. After seizure activity there is a typical pattern of hypotonicity followed by a gradual return to normal function. The suckle reflex is the last function to return.

A variety of other neurologic abnormalities have been attributed to HIE. They include: focal seizure-like activity; lack of pharyngeal tone resulting in guttural pouch tympany, dysphagia, and respiratory stridor; head tilt; central blindness; and limb deficits (**9.24**).

Central respiratory system damage can result in irregular breathing patterns, tachypnea, and periods of apnea.

Kidneys: Clinical signs include decreased urine production, edema formation, isosthenuric urine, and decreased creatinine clearance (**9.25**). These signs are often subtle and transient; however, anuric renal failure can occur.[72]

Gastrointestinal tract: Clinical signs range from mild indigestion with gas distension and signs of colic to severe forms of the disease (necrotizing enterocolitis) with hemorrhagic diarrhea, sepsis, and possible intestinal rupture (**9.26**).[69,72]

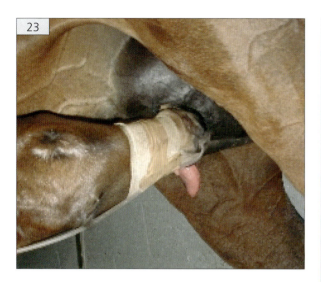

9.23 Foal with an uncoordinated suckle reflex. This photo highlights the importance of bending down and watching the foal nurse to ensure a good tongue seal is formed around the teat.

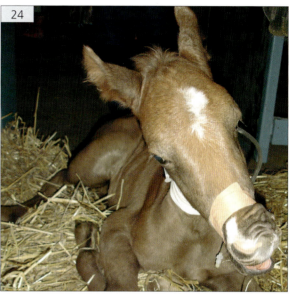

9.24 Foal with residual focal seizure activity and head tilt.

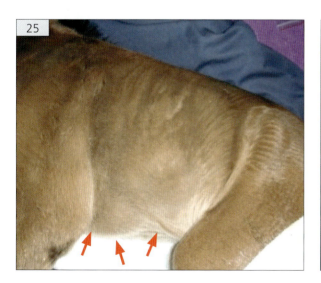

9.25 Edema (arrowed) developing in the ventral midline and axilla region because of renal dysfunction.

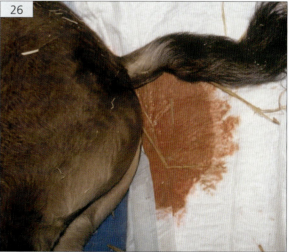

9.26 Hemorrhagic diarrhea seen with necrotizing enterocolitis, which needs to be differentiated from clostridiosis.

Other: The cardiovascular system, lungs, liver, and endocrine function can all be affected by hypoxic ischemic insults. Insults to the cardiovascular system can result in reduced myocardial function, arrhythmias secondary to focal cardiac lesions, and reduced responsiveness of blood vessels to endogenous and exogenous adrenergic agents.[69]

Hypoxia and acidemia increase pulmonary vascular resistance, which can result in conversion back to fetal circulation.[69,70]

Hypoxic ischemic liver damage results in a moderate elevation of liver enzymes and bilirubin concentrations. Endocrinopathies are poorly characterized and have been associated with hypocortisolemia, syndrome of inappropriate ADH secretion, and abnormal parathyroid hormone secretion.[69,70,72]

Differential diagnosis

- Central nervous system: metabolic disorders (hypo/hypernatremia, hypo/hyperglycemia, hypocalcemia); sepsis, meningitis; CNS malformations; trauma; other causes of dysphagia.
- Gastrointestinal: bacterial enteritis, especially clostridiosis; sepsis, SIRS; meconium impaction; surgical lesions.
- Renal: toxic nephropathy; congenital abnormalities; syndrome of inappropriate ADH secretion, spurious hypercreatininemia.

Diagnosis

Diagnosis is based on clinical signs and lack of evidence of other disease processes. It is important to remember that HIS often occurs concurrently with, and is complicated by, sepsis and prematurity. There are no laboratory findings pathognomonic for HIS and abnormalities reflect the organ system(s) involved.

HIE is supported with normal serum values, which eliminate metabolic disorders, and a normal CSF analysis, WBC count, and fibrinogen concentration, which eliminate sepsis and meningitis.

Radiography, CT, and MRI can be used to further evaluate the CNS if trauma or congenital anomalies are suspected. Abdominal ultrasonography assists with differentiation of HIS from other causes of colic and helps evaluate intestinal motility and kidney structure.

Table 9.8 Medications used for hypoxic ischemic encephalopathy or in foals with suspected birth asphyxia

DRUG	DOSE	ACTION
Allopurinol	40 mg/kg PO within 2–3 hours of birth	Xanthine oxidase inhibitor, prevention of free-radical formation
Ascorbic acid	100 mg/kg/day IV	NMDA-receptor blockade, antioxidant
Dimethyl sulfoxide	0.5–1.0 g/kg IV as 10% solution over 1 hour Can repeat every 12 hours	Free-radical scavenger and other anti-inflammatory effects
Magnesium sulfate	50 mg/kg/hour loading dose over 1 hour 25 mg/kg/hour maintenance	NMDA-receptor blockade
Mannitol	0.25–1.0 g as 20% solution q6–12h as IV bolus over 20 minutes	Osmotic agent for cerebral edema, antioxidant
Thiamine	10–20 mg/kg IV q12–24h	Supports cerebral energy metabolism
Vitamin E	500 IU PO q24h 68 IU/50 kg IV q24h	Antioxidant

Endoscopy will differentiate dysphagia from other causes. Thoracic radiographs should be taken if aspiration pneumonia is suspected.

Management/treatment

There is no specific treatment for HIS, therefore treatment is aimed at supporting the neonate while damaged tissues are repairing. General systemic support of the cardiovascular and respiratory system and provision of energy requirements is necessary (see Chapter 15). Prophylactic broad-spectrum antimicrobial therapy should be used in compromised foals (see Chapter 16). Immune support is given to foals with FPT or that have concurrent sepsis. Specific therapies for the different systems are outlined below.

Central nervous system: Maintaining cerebral perfusion with IV fluid therapy and maintaining adequate blood pressure is the most important therapy for CNS support. Blood transfusions may be required if the foal has mild anemia (<0.24l/l [24%]) to ensure optimal tissue oxygenation.[7] There are a variety of therapies

recommended for the prevention and treatment of HIE; however, the efficacy of any prophylactic treatment not been proven (*Table 9.8*).[73]

Seizures need to be controlled to prevent recurrence of CNS ischemia and to prevent self-trauma (*Table 9.9*). Diazepam (0.1–0.2 mg/kg; 5–10 mg for a 50 kg foal) and midazolam (3–5 mg for a 50 kg foal) are most useful for immediate seizure control; however, their effects are short lived (about 20 minutes) and repeated dosing can cause respiratory depression, as can rapid IV administration. Recently, midazolam has been used for longer-term seizure control as a CRI (1–5 mg/foal/hour).[74] The advantages of its short half-life and ability to reverse its actions with flumazenil (Romazecon®; 0.01 mg/kg IV over 15 seconds) allow for repeated evaluation of the foal's neurologic status. It is especially useful in hyperresponsive thrashing newborn foals where the side-effects and prolonged half-life of phenobarbital are of concern. There are, however, concerns of potential altered cerebral perfusion in patients with severe head trauma.[75] If seizure activity continues, phenobarbital or midazolam CRI may be used. The half-life of phenobarbital is about 100 hours and it can cause marked respiratory depression, hypothermia, and exacerbation of hypoperfusion.

Nursing care is important to minimize self-trauma. Restraining the foal on a mattress with foam wall supports, leg wraps, and foam helmets are all beneficial. Ocular lubricants reduce the risk of corneal ulceration.

Foals without a coordinated suckle and swallow reflex are fed via a nasogastric tube if the GI tract is functional. Occasionally, a foal will take over a month for a coordinated suckle to develop; however, these foals can usually be taught to drink from a bucket.

Gastrointestinal: All foals with suspected GI tract hypoxic ischemic damage should be fed very cautiously or started on parenteral nutrition due to the high risk of developing necrotizing enterocolitis. Foals with mild intestinal dysmotility may respond to limited access to the mare. Foals with ileus and gaseous distension should have oral feeding withheld and parenteral nutrition provided.

Table 9.9 **Drugs used to control seizures in hypoxic ischemic encephalopathy**	
DRUG	**DOSE**
Diazepam	0.11–0.44 mg/kg IV (5–10 mg bolus for 50 kg foal)
Midazolam	Loading dose: 0.1 mg/kg IV (5 mg/50 kg) Maintenance: 0.02–0.1 mg/kg/hour (usually see effect with 0.03–0.06 mg/kg/hour)
Phenobarbital	2–10 mg/kg IV q12–24h (usually 4–8 mg/kg) Given slowly over 20 minutes to effect
Phenytoin	5–10 mg/kg loading dose; 1–5 mg/kg q4h for first 24 hours

Motility stimulants are not routinely recommended as they have been associated with intussusceptions and intestinal motility usually returns once the intestinal tract has healed. Enema administration may stimulate distal colonic function. Oral administration of sucralfate (10–20 mg/kg PO q6h) may provide some GI protection and has been shown to decrease bacterial translocation in some animal experimental models.[76,77]

Renal: Urine volume and SG should be closely monitored to assess renal function and avoid overhydration. Particular attention should be paid to fluid therapy and sodium balance. If renal dysfunction is suspected, bladder catheterization is recommended for accurate assessment of urine production (**9.27**).

Dopamine and furosemide have been used to manage fluid volume overload.[20] Dopamine (2–5 µg/kg/minute) enhances urine production through natriuresis. Furosemide can be used as a bolus (0.25–1.0 mg/kg) or CRI (0.25–2 mg/kg/hour). Once diuresis begins, electrolytes need to be monitored carefully.

Prognosis: The prognosis for complete recovery is 70–80%. A poorer prognosis is given to foals with concurrent sepsis, prematurity, prolonged neurologic abnormalities, necrotizing enterocolitis, or anuric renal failure.

Pneumonia
Key points
- Pneumonia is a common problem in sick neonates and also a common complication of other neonatal diseases.
- Aspiration pneumonia should be a concern in all sick foals, particularly if they are weak, depressed, or recumbent.

Definition/overview
Pneumonia is a leading cause of mortality and morbidity in foals and is most commonly seen in neonates and 1–6-month-old foals. Pneumonia is most commonly caused by bacterial infection; however, predisposing factors and other infectious agents (viral and fungal) may play a role in the development of disease. A single individual can be affected or outbreaks can occur.

Etiology/pathogenesis
In neonates, pneumonia is caused by the same bacteria and viruses as those causing neonatal sepsis. In older foals, pneumonia is commonly caused by opportunistic bacteria, with *Rhodococcus equi* and *Streptococcus zooepidemicus* reported most frequently. Anaerobic bacteria are not commonly involved. Influenza, EHV-1, EHV-2, EHV-4, adenovirus, and rhinovirus commonly cause respiratory tract disease, but are rarely reported as the primary cause of pneumonia.[78] Predisposing factors include environmental and management factors and parasite and viral infections.

In neonates, pneumonia is usually associated with sepsis, aspiration during nursing, and prolonged recumbency. In 1–6-month-old foals, infection is most likely by inhalation of aerosolized or dust-borne organisms.[78] Colonization occurs when pulmonary defense mechanisms are overwhelmed by organisms or compromised by predisposing factors. The pathogenesis of *R. equi* relies on the organisms' ability to replicate within alveolar macrophages.[79] Virulence is associated with expression of plasmid coded virulence-associated protein (Vap) antigens. Viral infections damage respiratory tract epithelium and reduce mucociliary clearance and alveolar macrophage function, thus compromising pulmonary defense mechanisms. The development of pleuropneumonia in foals is uncommon.

The cause of ARDS in older foals is not fully understood, but has been associated with *R. equi*, *Pneumocystis carinii*, or viral infection and possible immune dysfunction.[78]

Clinical features
Clinical signs vary depending on the etiology, severity, and chronicity of disease. Signs range from tachypnea (>40 breaths/minute) and altered breathing pattern to nostril flaring with increased abdominal lift to respiratory distress with cyanosis and reluctance

to move (**9.28**). Foals are often febrile and may have a nasal discharge or cough. Auscultation findings vary from increased audibility and harshness of inspiratory and expiratory breaths sounds to a plethora of abnormal sounds, which are highlighted in foals with severe *R. equi* pneumonia.

R. equi pneumonia usually has an insidious onset and severe lung changes are often present when the foals show clinical signs of disease. Foals with *R. equi* pneumonia usually do not have a nasal discharge or pleural effusion, but may cough. Clinical signs associated with extrapulmonary lesions may also be present.

Differential diagnosis

Rib fracture; diaphragmatic hernia; pneumothorax; hemothorax; hyperthermia/tachypnea seen with HIE and draft breeds.

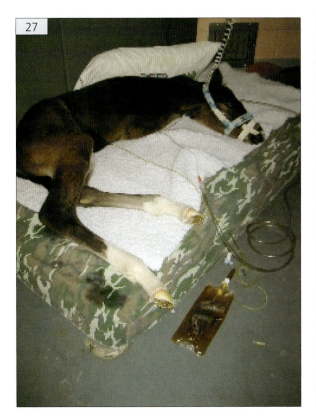

9.27 Urine collection system used to monitor urine production.

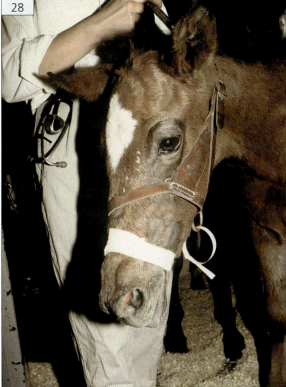

9.28 Foal with acute respiratory distress syndrome showing flared nostrils and depression.

Diagnosis

Diagnosis is based on physical examination, laboratory findings, and ancillary diagnostic procedures. WBC count and fibrinogen concentration are typically elevated, fibrinogen concentration being a more reliable indicator. Ultrasonography and radiography are both used in evaluating foals with pneumonia (**9.29, 9.30**). Ultrasonography is used in combination with WBC count and fibrinogen concentrations in screening foals on farms with endemic *R. equi*.[80] ABG analysis is useful in assessing ventilation and response to treatment.

Blood cultures from neonates are recommended. A transtracheal aspirate is recommended in older foals that do not have respiratory distress. While not feasible to perform on every foal from a farm with an endemic problem, it can be used to assist with initial diagnosis and management of individuals failing to respond to therapy.[78] Virus isolation and paired serology can be performed for suspected viral etiologies. Serology can be performed for *R. equi*; however, a positive result may not be indicative of infection.

Management/treatment

Treatment is aimed at eliminating infection, providing respiratory and systemic support, reducing the influence of predisposing factors, and preventing spread to other foals or horses.

Antimicrobial therapy is based on culture and sensitivity results, but has to be initiated prior to results being available. Broad-spectrum IV bactericidal therapy should be used in neonates (see Chapter 20). In older foals, penicillin G is the first line choice as β-hemolytic *Streptococcus* spp. are the most common isolate. *R. equi* pneumonia is treated with a combination of a macrolide and rifampin (see Chapter 16).

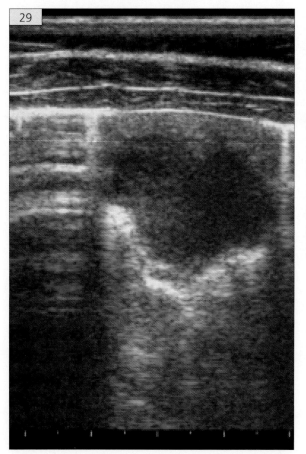

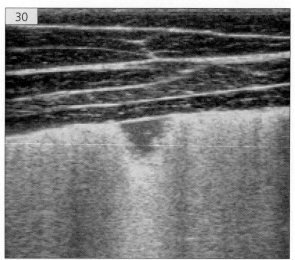

9.30 Sonogram of the thorax of a foal with *R. equi* acute respiratory distress syndrome showing a small area of consolidation and complete loss of normal air echo in surrounding tissue giving the appearance of 'sheets of rain'. This sonographic finding is common in foals with acute respiratory distress syndrome.

9.29 Sonogram of the thorax of a foal with *R. equi* pneumonia showing a discrete area of superficial consolidation surrounded by normal air echo of lung.

INO_2 insufflation is indicated in foals with severe respiratory distress and hypoxemia. When tolerated, nebulization can be used to assist with moistening secretions, bronchodilation, and administration of antimicrobials.[78,81] Mucolytics have been used in cases with mucopurulent material in airways. NSAIDs are commonly used to assist with controlling fevers; however, care needs to be taken to avoid toxicity.

Steroidal anti-inflammatory therapy is used in foals with ARDS (dexamethasone, 0.2mg/kg IV q12h for 3 days then tapered dose; methylprednisolone, 2 mg/kg IV q12h for 3 days then tapering over 3 days). Antimicrobial therapy is aimed against *P. carinii* and *R. equi*. The foal's environment should also be kept cool and well ventilated.

Rib fractures
Key points
- Thoracic trauma is common in neonatal foals and is more usually associated with maiden mares and dystocia, although it can be present in foals without that history.
- Displaced rib fractures are potentially life-threatening and have been reported as a common contributor to mortality in sick neonatal foals.

Definition/overview
Rib fractures in newborn foals are most commonly associated with trauma during parturition. Rib fractures in older foals are usually due to external trauma such as a kick or paddock accident. The resulting costochondral dislocation or rib fracture can be subclinical or cause a variety of clinical signs including sudden death.

Etiology/pathogenesis
Rib fractures are more common in foals from primiparous mares and dystocias.[82] Contributing factors have included shape of the thoracic cage, retention of an elbow during parturition, manipulation during delivery, and an abnormally narrow pelvic canal.[82] The foal's weight or thoracic circumference are not believed to be a factor and there does not appear to be a sex predilection.[83,84]

The fracture or osteochondral dislocation appears to be caused by pressure on the thorax during passage through the pelvic canal. The most common site of injury is the cranioventral half of the thorax at the costochondral junction or adjacent proximal area.[82,85] The majority of fractures are subclinical; however, the periosteal damage and surrounding muscle damage and blood vessel disruption can result in hematomas and pain. If the fracture extremities displace axially, parietal pleura can be perforated and underlying structures damaged, resulting in bruising or laceration of the heart, lung, diaphragm, and major vessels (**9.31**). Fatal myocardial lacerations can occur with fractures on either the right or left side and there is a higher risk of death with a higher number of fractured ribs.[84]

Clinical features
Clinical signs are variable and depend on the number and location of ribs affected and severity of the damage to the adjacent structures. Less severe clinical signs include crepitation on rib palpation, a 'clicking' sound on auscultation, and edema localized over or ventral to the fractured ribs. Signs of pain include increased heart and respiratory rates and grunting or groaning when manipulated or lying on the affected side. Auscultation of the thorax may reveal ventral dullness and lack of breath sounds if a hemothorax is present or lack of breath sounds dorsally if a pneumothorax is present. Respiratory distress can be seen in foals with multiple rib fractures and a flail chest, pneumothorax,

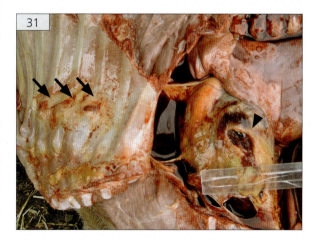

9.31 Fractured ribs (arrows) with fatal laceration in the myocardium (arrowhead).

hemothorax, or diaphragmatic hernia. Subcutaneous emphysema over the sides of thorax or axilla region may be present. Pale mucous membranes can be indicative of internal hemorrhage into the pleural or abdominal cavities. Tachycardia may reflect primary cardiac disease such as myocardial bruising, laceration, or hemopericardium. Sudden death is not uncommon and occurs when a major vessel, a coronary vessel, or the myocardium is lacerated.

Differential diagnosis

Diaphragmatic hernia; pneumonia; NI; umbilical remnant hemorrhage.

Diagnosis

Palpation of crepitus over the fracture site is not a consistent finding and rib fractures are often not detected on physical examination. The ribs should be palpated by sliding the hand up cranially under the elbow and using gentle pressure with flat fingers. Radiographs are not reliable for detection of fractured ribs in neonates.[84,85] Ultrasonographic examination is more reliable and allows visualization of the fracture site and displaced extremities, and evaluation of the adjacent structures (**9.32, 9.33**).[84,85] Analysis of pleural fluid should be performed if a concurrent infectious component is suspected.

Management/treatment

Conservative treatment with box rest for 3–4 weeks is successful in the majority of uncomplicated rib fractures. Analgesics may be used judiciously; however, providing pain relief may increase the foal's level of activity and chance of a fatal movement of a fractured end. Sedation may be needed to encourage decreased activity. Although different positioning is recommended for improved ventilation, foals are more settled if allowed to find their own side of comfort. Prophylactic broad-spectrum antimicrobial coverage is recommended if the foal is compromised or a hemothorax

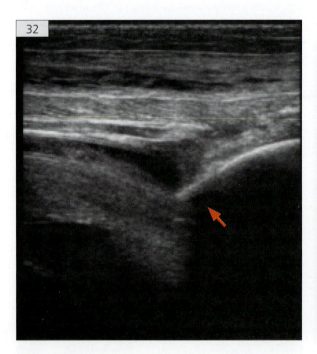

9.32 Sonogram of the thorax of a 2-day-old foal showing the displaced end of a fractured rib and the underlying heart (arrowed). Note the edema and disruption in surrounding tissues. Sagittal view, left is dorsal.

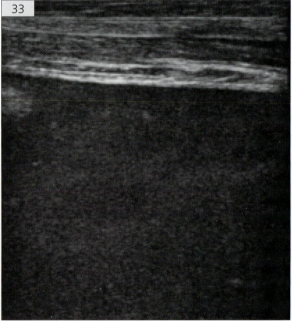

9.33 Sonogram of a foal with hemothorax secondary to displaced rib fracture. Sagittal view, left is dorsal.

is present. Surgical repair has been advocated in cases with multiple rib fractures or those with potential for severe internal injury.[83,86]

Initial treatment of complicated fractures with damage to underlying structures is aimed at stabilization of the foal by ensuring adequate ventilation and treatment of hypovolemic shock. INO_2 insufflation should be administered if hypoxemia is present and specific treatment of the pneumothorax and hemothorax should be instigated if the foal exhibits respiratory distress.

Meconium impaction/retention

Key points

- Meconium impaction is a common cause of neonatal colic and can generally be resolved medically.
- Uroperitoneum has been reported in association with meconium impaction/retention.
- Foals with HIS may be more prone to meconium impaction/retention due to GI dysfunction.

Definition/overview

Meconium impaction/retention is one of the most common causes of colic in the neonatal foal. The foal normally begins passing meconium within the first few hours after birth and it is usually passed within 48 hours. If retained, the impaction and subsequent gas accumulation can cause tenesmus and mild to severe signs of abdominal pain.

Etiology/pathogenesis

Meconium is formed throughout fetal development and is a mixture of swallowed amniotic fluid and intestinal secretions including bile. Meconium has a characteristic olive brown color and can be thick and tarry or in pellets (**9.34**).

Meconium impaction can result from impaired GI motility, failure to ingest colostrum, dehydration, and prolonged recumbency. There is an increased incidence of meconium impaction in colts.[87] The impaction can lead to complete intestinal obstruction and gaseous abdominal distension.

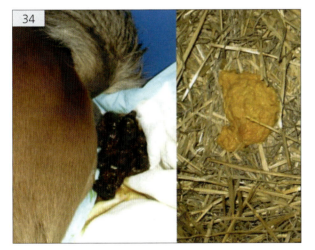

34

9.34 Dark pellets of meconium (left). Note the normal softer, yellow to orange milk feces that follows meconium (right).

Clinical features

Signs of colic can begin within a few hours to 36 hours after birth, although they most commonly occur 12–24 hours after birth. Early signs are restlessness, standing under the mare not nursing, aimless wandering, tail swishing, and posturing to defecate (**9.35**). The signs of discomfort are often after nursing and the foal is usually bright in between colic episodes. More advanced cases have gaseous abdominal distension and more severe clinical signs of colic.

Differential diagnosis

Intestinal atresia or agangliosis (lethal white syndrome); ileus (sepsis, HIS, prematurity); enterocolitis; rectal irritation from enemas; strangulating intestinal lesions; uroperitoneum; intussusception.

Diagnosis

History, clinical signs, and age will assist with diagnosis. Digital examination of the rectum with a well-lubricated finger may, but not always, detect meconium. Meconium can be palpated through the abdominal wall in relaxed recumbent foals. Abdominal ultrasonography is used to identify meconium and help rule out other causes of colic (**9.36**). Meconium is visualized as intraluminal masses. Fluid distension of proximal segments and an increase in anechoic peritoneal fluid may be present. Contrast radiography can be used to help identify the impaction.[88]

Management/treatment

Treatment is aimed at resolving the impaction, providing pain relief, and systemic support. The majority of meconium impactions/retentions respond to medical treatment.[87] In extreme cases surgical removal may be required; however, this carries a poor prognosis.

Gentle digital manipulation may be able to remove retained meconium; however, usually an enema is required. Initially, either a warm soapy water enema or a commercial phosphate-based enema (e.g. Fleet®) can be used. The foal needs to be adequately restrained and the tubes well lubricated to avoid rectal damage. Fleet® enemas are convenient and work well. Warm soapy water gravity enemas (300–500 ml/50 kg foal) can be used with a non-irritant soap such as Ivory®. Repeated enema administration can cause rectal irritation, edema, and tenesmus. If initial enemas are not successful, an acetylcysteine retention enema should be given. It is important to have the foal relaxed and sedated so

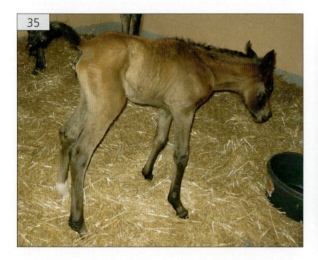

9.35 Foal straining to defecate. Note the elevated tail position and arched back.

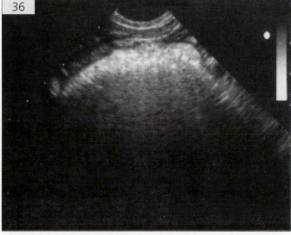

9.36 Ultrasonographic image of meconium highlighting the hyperechoic particles.

the enema fluid is not pushed out prematurely. The foal is placed in lateral recumbency with its hindquarters moderately elevated and a 30 Fr Foley catheter with a 30 ml balloon is inserted 5–10 cm into the rectum and slowly inflated to avoid straining. The acetylcysteine solution is administered slowly and left in place for 30–45 minutes (*Table 9.10*).[87,89] The enema can be repeated after 12–24 hours. INO$_2$ insufflation (5 liters/minute) is provided to foals with abdominal distension or systemic compromise while the enema is being given. Oral laxative therapy (120–160 ml mineral oil) is used in proximal impactions if no reflux is present. The use of dioctyl sodium sulfosuccinate, glycerin, and castor oil is not recommended. The use of metal instruments and repeated digital manipulation should be avoided. Percutaneous bowel trocharization should only be considered in extreme circumstances.

Butorphanol (0.01–0.04 mg/kg IM or IV; 2–4 mg/50 kg foal) is the preferred analgesic as it also provides sedation, which assists with enema administration. Flunixin meglumine (1.1 mg/kg) can be given; however, repetitive doses should be avoided because of the potential for toxicity. Xylazine needs to be used cautiously as it can cause respiratory depression and ileus in compromised foals.

Table 9.10 Two formulations for 4% acetylcysteine solution

Option 1:

8 g N-acetyl-l-cysteine powder

20 g sodium bicarbonate*

200 ml water

Option 2:

40 ml of 20% solution of Mucomyst® 10ml vials

160 ml water

20 g sodium bicarbonate*

* The mucolytic effect of acetylcysteine improves with increasing pH, so the addition of sodium bicarbonate is recommended. However, it is often not added as it provides a large amount of sodium which may be systemically absorbed.

IV fluid therapy is given if needed to restore circulating volume. If the foal does not respond to the initial enema, restriction of milk intake may be required until the impaction resolves. During this time energy and maintenance fluid requirements are met with IV fluids with glucose or parenteral nutrition. It may be necessary to provide INO$_2$ insufflation to foals with severe abdominal distension.

Antimicrobial therapy may be necessary as disruption of the mucosal barrier can predispose to increased bacterial translocation and foals may have ingested insufficient quantities of colostrum while painful. Patent urachus, bleeding umbilical remnant, bladder rupture, and scrotal hernia are secondary complications that may occur from straining.[90]

Diarrhea/enterocolitis
Key points
- There are many causes of diarrhea in neonatal foals.
- Foals with diarrhea may be severely dehydrated with significant electrolyte abnormalities.
- Half of all foals with diarrhea will be blood-culture positive for bacteria and all young foals with diarrhea should receive broad-spectrum antimicrobial treatment.

Definition/overview
Diarrhea is one of the most common medical conditions in foals. There are a variety of infectious and non-infectious causes; however, identifying the exact cause can be difficult as many potential enteric pathogens are isolated from normal foals. The episode of diarrhea can be mild and self-limiting or life-threatening with severe dehydration and marked electrolytes abnormalities.

Etiology/pathogenesis
Infectious organisms invade different areas of the intestinal tract and their effects depend on where the organism invades (crypt/villous), depth of invasion (mucosa/submucosa), and subsequent inflammatory reaction. The diarrhea results from a combination of malabsorption and increased secretion. The infectious organism can also produce endo- and exotoxins, which cause altered electrolyte and fluid movement

across the mucosa. Establishment of normal GI flora is the proposed cause of foal heat diarrhea. (See also *Table 9.11* [24,91–93].)

Clinical features
Clinical signs can range from mild, self-limiting diarrhea, as seen with foal heat and mild rotaviral infection, to hemorrhagic diarrhea with severe sepsis as seen with clostridial infections. Common signs include fever, depression, dehydration, and not nursing. Often, signs of colic are present even before the foal develops diarrhea.

Differential diagnosis
Strangulating obstruction; ascarid or foreign body impaction; intussusception.

Table 9.11 **Causes of diarrhea in the foal**

CAUSE	COMMENT	AGE
Sepsis	GI tract is common site for localizing infection	<4 days
Hypoxic ischemic syndrome	Asphyxial injuries can result in necrotizing enterocolitis	<4 days
Foal heat	Coincides with the mare's foal heat cycle. Due to development changes in the GI tract.	6–12 days
Nutritional		
Orphan foal	Milk formulas and overfeeding	Any age
Lactose intolerance:		Any age
Primary	Rare	
Secondary	Common with small intestinal infections	
Foreign material	Sand, dirt	Older foals
Parasites		
Helminths	Uncommon, *Strongyloides westerii*, cyathostomiasis	1 week to 6 months
Cryptosporidia	Severe life-threatening in immunocompromised foals	<4 days
	Protracted diarrhea	2–3 weeks
	Self-limiting/chronic intermittent diarrhea	Older foals
Bacteria		
Clostridium perfringens biotype C	Hemorrhagic diarrhea, abdominal distension, shock, and death	<4 days
C. perfringens biotype A	Transient hemorrhagic diarrhea	<4 days
C. difficile	Severe watery to hemorrhagic diarrhea	<4 days
Salmonella spp.	Neonatal septicemia	<4 days
	Enterocolitis	All ages
Rhodococcus equi	Intestinal form	Older foals
Escherichia coli	Common cause of sepsis	<1 month
	Rarely associated with primary diarrhea	
Virus		
Group A rotavirus	Most common cause of infectious diarrhea	1–6 months
Other		
Gastroduodenal ulcer syndrome	Rare primary cause, often present in foals with diarrhea	Older foals

Diagnosis

Diagnostic tests for infectious agents are outlined in *Table 9.12*.[93] The significance of organisms isolated from feces should be based on clinical signs and farm history. Lactose tolerance testing, withholding milk, and evaluating feces/rectum for foreign material can be undertaken if nutritional causes are suspected. Ultrasonographic examination of the abdomen helps distinguish enteritis from other causes of colic (**9.37, 9.38**). Clinicopathologic data can be useful in the diagnosis

Table 9.12 **Tests available for diagnosis of enteric pathogens**		
PATHOGEN	**PROCEDURE**	**COMMENTS**
Cryptosporidium	Acid-fast staining Flow cytometry IFA	Experience beneficial in identifying stained oocysts
Clostridium perfringens	Culture ELISA enterotoxin Multiplex PCR	Toxin should also be identified
Clostridium difficile	Culture ELISA toxin A or B Gram stain of fecal smear PCR for toxigenic genes	Toxin should also be identified
Cyathostomiasis	Fecal egg and larval count Rectal biopsy	
Salmonella spp.	Fecal culture and PCR	Repeat cultures are necessary
Rotavirus	Fecal ELISA[a] Fecal LA[b] Electron microscopy	
Lawsonia intracellularis	PCR and IPX on feces Intestinal biopsy	

PCR, polymerase chain reaction; IFA, immunofluorescent antibody assay; ELISA, enzyme-linked immunosorbent assay; IPX, immunoperoxidase stain; LA, latex agglutination; [a] Rotazyme®; [b] Virogen Rotatest®

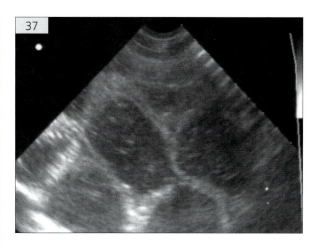

9.37 Sonogram highlighting the moderately distended loops of small and large intestine with particulate contents commonly seen in enteritis.

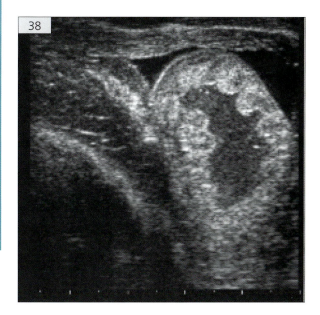

9.38 Sonogram highlighting the thickened small intestinal wall and small increase in anechoic peritoneal fluid seen with enteritis.

and is necessary in the management of the foal. Leukopenia, left shift, and toxic neutrophils are seen in septic neonates or with primary bacterial or viral infections. Hypoproteinemia, electrolyte abnormalities, and metabolic acidosis are often present.

Management/treatment

Many therapies used in the treatment are similar regardless of the etiology. The foal may need stabilization prior to determining the cause of the diarrhea. Strict hygiene and isolation protocols should be adhered to when treating foals with infectious diarrhea. Often diarrhea is part of a farm problem therefore, where possible, control and preventive measures on the farm should be instigated.

Fluid and electrolyte therapy: Restoring circulatory volume and correcting dehydration, electrolyte, and metabolic abnormalities are essential. Initially, hypovolemia and dehydration should be treated then fluid therapy can be tailored as laboratory information becomes available (see Chapter 12). Plasma is the best colloid to use if hypoproteinemia is present, as it also provides immune factors. Synthetic colloids should be used with caution in septic neonates. Once hypovolemia and dehydration are corrected, therapy is aimed at providing maintenance and ongoing loss requirements. Improvement of tissue perfusion will improve metabolic acidosis in many foals. Further therapy with IV and/or oral sodium bicarbonate may be necessary.[24] Electrolyte replacement therapy is based on severity of electrolyte deficits and ongoing losses. As individual responses to electrolyte supplementation are varied, half the estimated deficit is replaced and then supplementation is re-evaluated. IV supplementation is used if the GI tract is not functional or there are marked abnormalities (K^+ <2.5 mmol/l, Na^+ <120 mmol/l, HCO_3 <15 mmol/l).

Oral fluid and electrolyte supplementation can be used in mild to moderate dehydration where there is a functional GI tract.

Antimicrobial therapy: Broad-spectrum antimicrobial therapy should be used in foals <7days old because of the high risk of translocation of bacteria and an infectious etiology. Its use in older foals is determined by the suspected etiologic agent. If clostridial enteritis is suspected, penicillin and metronidazole are recommended.

Gastrointestinal rest and nutrition: Nutritional support is an important part of management of the foal with diarrhea as many foals respond to milk restriction. Foals with ileus, abdominal distension, and colic should be withheld from feeding until these signs resolve. Many foals benefit from GI rest with a brief period of 6 (3-day-old foal) to 12 (older foal) hours' rest followed by slow reintroduction back onto the mare over 12 hours. During this time the foal should be given IV fluid and glucose supplementation (4–8 mg/kg/hour). If the diarrhea or colic recurs after this period, or the foal is debilitated, parenteral nutrition is recommended.

Other therapies: Protectants such as kaolin/pectin, bismuth subsalicylate, and sucralfate can be used (*Table 9.13*). Other therapies such as di-tri-octahedral smectite, loperamide, and yogurt have been described. The benefits of probiotics are questionable.[24]

The use of antiulcer medications is controversial; however, their use is recommended by some in older (>7 day old) foals. Use of H_2 receptor antagonists (ranitindine, cimetidine) and proton pump inhibitors (omeprazole) appear to be associated with diarrhea in neonatal foals.[94] Supportive therapies, such as regular cleaning and application of protective cream and fly repellants over the rump and vulva, are important.

Table 9.13 Supportive therapies for foals with enteritis

DRUG	DOSE	COMMENT
Loperamide	0.1–0.5 mg/kg PO q6h 4–6 mg to 12–14 mg q6h not to exceed 20 mg/ day	Watch for gas retention, constipation
Di-tri-octahedral smectite	30 g with 30 ml of water q6–12h	Toxin absorption
Bismuth subsalicylate	0.5–2.0 ml/kg PO q4–6h	Causes dark feces
Omeprazole	Treatment: 4 mg/kg PO q24h Prevention: 2 mg/kg PO q24h	Proton pump inhibitor
Ranitidine	2 mg/kg IV q6h 6.6 mg/kg PO q8h	H_2 receptor antagonist
Sucralfate	10–20 mg/kg PO q6–8h	Useful in foals <7 days of age
Isotonic bicarbonate (1.3%)	12.5 g in 1 liter of sterile water	Administer slowly

Limb deformities

Key points

- Unless severe, most cases of flexural limb deformity and angular limb deformity (ALD) in the equine neonate will resolve with time, physical therapy, or medical management.
- All premature and dysmature foals should be evaluated for cuboidal bone immaturity.
- Nursing care is intensive and important in foals with limb deformities that limit their ability to stand.
- Many foals with severe flexural deformities are born following a dystocia. Their clinical course may be complicated by HIS.

Definition/overview

Foals can present with a variety of flexural limb deformities and ALDs. These are congenital or acquired after birth. Severe limb deformities and those incorrectly managed can result in euthanasia.

Etiology/pathogenesis

Flexural deformities include hyperextension and contractural deformities.[95] Hyperextension is common in premature/dysmature foals that have generalized poor muscle tone and increased tendon and periarticular laxity. Term foals can be born with flexor tendon laxity, the cause of which has not been identified.[52] Foals with long-standing systemic illness develop generalized muscle and tendon weakness and hyperextension. Laxity can develop from increased loading in the supporting limb in a lame foal.

Congenital contractural deformities are a major cause of dystocia. The suspected causes include movement restriction *in utero*, exposure to influenza, and ingestion of plant toxins.[96] Acquired contracture can be related to rapid growth or a mild lameness resulting in less weight bearing on the contracted limb. Rupture of the common digital extensor tendon is a common complication through knuckling forward onto the fetlock.

ALD can also be congenital or acquired. Congenital causes include movement restriction *in utero* and toxin, hormonal, or nutritional insults.[52] Acquired ALD can be associated with excessive loading of the limb due to contralateral limb lameness, damage to the physis with infection, inflammation, or trauma. Premature/dysmature foals with incomplete ossification and excessive periarticular laxity are born with or develop ALD.

Clinical features

Hyperextension in premature foals can involve multiple joints (**9.39**). The laxity may be so severe that the foal is unable to stand. Tendon laxity in term foals usually involves the fetlock joint in the forelimbs and/or the hindlimbs.

Contracture can be unilateral or bilateral and most commonly involves the carpus and fetlock in the forelimb and hindlimb fetlocks. Presentation can vary from mild and able to stand to recumbent where the leg can be straightened with manipulation to severe contracture that does not respond to manipulation

(**9.40**). A soft fluid swelling over the dorsolateral carpus may be present associated with rupture of the common digital extensor tendon (**9.41**). Foals that develop a unilateral contracture should be evaluated for an underlying lameness.

Visual inspection of the foal from front and behind and while walking will assist in identifying ALDs.[97] A mild to moderate degree of carpal valgus is present in most newborn foals. The hoof should be evaluated for evenness of wear. ALDs in premature foals are usually associated with periarticular laxity, which can be confirmed with manipulation of the joint.

Differential diagnosis

Traumatic musculoskeletal injuries; infectious orthopedic disease.

Diagnosis

Physical examination and manipulation of the legs will help identify the deformity. Lameness work-up should be performed on foals that develop a unilateral

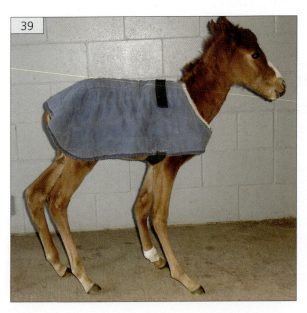

9.39 Premature foal highlighting laxity in the carpi, fetlocks, and coffin joints.

9.40 Contracted frontlimbs extended after manipulation.

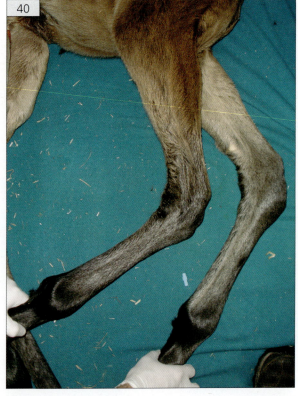

contracture after birth. Radiographs will help identify incomplete ossification, the site of the ALD, and abnormalities in the physis and are recommended for joints involved in severe contractural deformities.

Management/treatment

Hyperextension: The use of bandaging and splinting should be avoided as it results in increased laxity. Stall confinement and time will improve the majority of foals. A small protective wrap may be necessary over the heel bulb region. Foals with continued distal limb hyperextension benefit from hoof trimming and heel extension (**9.42A, B**).

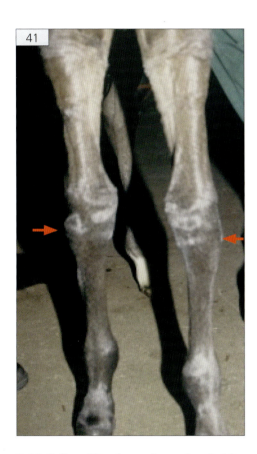

9.41 Soft swelling (arrows) associated with rupture of the common digital extensor tendon.

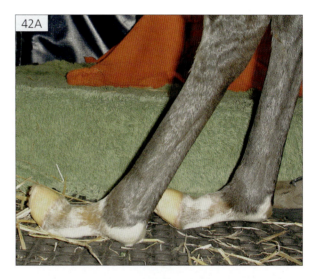

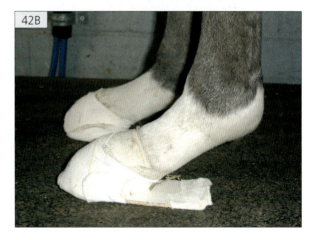

9.42A, B Limb hyperextension. (A) Hyperextension of the fetlock and coffin joint. (B) Shoe with heel extensions to assist with weight bearing on the hoof. Ply wood cut to shape can also be used temporarily. Bandages around the distal pastern and coronary band need to be closely monitored and changed frequently.

Contraction: Foals with mild to moderate contracture may initially require physiotherapy, bandaging, and possibly splinting (**9.43**). PVC piping or fiberglass cast material is used to create a splint. Oxytetracycline therapy (44 mg/kg IV q24h for 1–3 days; diluted and given slowly) can be used in foals with normal renal function and those without laxity in other joints. If there is no response in 3 days, casting may be considered. Because of the continual growth of foals, these should be left on for a maximum of 3–5 days. In severe cases or where casting fails, surgery can be considered; however, the chances of producing an athletic individual are reduced.[52] Contracture in rapidly growing foals is managed by diet restriction or early weaning. Lameness evaluation should be performed on older foals with acquired unilateral contracture.

Angular limb deformity: Time, stall confinement, and proper foot care are successful in many foals. Shoes with extensions or acrylic hoof extensions can be used and are often used in combination with periosteal elevation and transection.[95] Transphyseal bridging is used in severe deformities in older foals.

Nursing care: Increased periods of recumbency predispose foals to the development of decubital ulcers. Pressure sores associated with improper bandaging, splinting, and casts can also occur. It is important to ensure that underlying soft tissues are well padded. Splints and bandages should be replaced every day and if applied tightly, should be left on only for short periods (4–6 hours) of time.

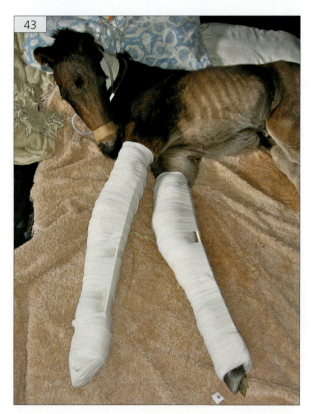

9.43 The foal in 9.40 after 2 days of splinting, bandaging, and oxytetracycline. Initially, molded fiber glass splints were used down the front of the leg.

TOXICOLOGY

Robert H.Poppenga

GENERAL CONSIDERATIONS FOR HORSES WITH INTOXICATION

- Horses are less commonly intoxicated than other species such as dogs and cattle. A lower incidence of intoxication may be due to several factors such as:
  - More observant and conscientious owners.
  - Confinement in a more controlled environment.
  - More selective dietary habits.
  - Continuous feeding habits and the relatively small stomach size of horses, which would result in ingestion of a smaller dose of a potential toxicant per unit of body weight.

- There are many toxicants that cause serious intoxication of horses. Horses are more sensitive than other species to many toxicants (e.g. ionophores [p. 603]) and are uniquely affected by several (e.g. fumonisin mycotoxins [p. 585] and *Centaurea* spp. [p. 579]).
- Horses with intoxication can present with a variety of clinical signs. The clinical signs associated with some of the more common intoxications are listed in *Tables 10.1–10.4*. The most common or important causes of intoxication in the horse are presented in this chapter, with additional causes of intoxication listed in *Table 10.7* [p. 607] and *Table 10.8* [p. 610].

Table 10.1 **Gastrointestinal signs associated with common causes of intoxication in horses**

CLINICAL SIGNS	TOXICANT
Abdominal pain	Maples, oleander, aflatoxins, slaframine, cantharidin, snake venom, botulinum toxin, iron, mercury, selenium, NSAID, ionophore
Excessive salivation	Oleander, slaframine, algal toxins, cantharidin, snake venom, botulinum toxin, cholinesterase-inhibiting pesticides
Oral erosions	Cantharidin
Dysphagia	Locoweeds, yellow-star thistle and Russian knapweed[1], snake venom, botulinum toxin, lead
Choke	White snakeroot
Constipation	Pyrrolizidine alkaloids, botulinum toxin
Diarrhea	Pyrrolizidine alkaloids, slaframine, algal toxins, cantharidin, snake venom, botulinum toxin, mercury, selenium, NSAID, ionophore, cholinesterase-inhibiting pesticides
Hematochezia	Aflatoxins, cantharidin
Melena	Iron, NSAID
Involuntary defecation	Cyanogenic glycoside-containing plants, snake venom

[1] Equine nigropallidal encephalomalcia (chewing disease)

Table 10.2 **Nervous system signs associated with common causes of intoxication in horses**

CLINICAL SIGNS	TOXICANT
Disorientation[1]	Pyrrolizidine alkaloids, fumonisin mycotoxins[3], iron
Belligerence/circling[1]	Pyrrolizidine alkaloids, mycotoxins
Head pressing[1]	Pyrrolizidine alkaloids, aflatoxins
Dull demeanor	Locoweeds, pyrrolizidine alkaloids, white snakeroot, yellow-star thistle and Russian knapweed[2], mycotoxins, fumonisin mycotoxins[3], cantharidin, iron, lead, mercury, selenium
Weakness	Algal toxins, botulinum toxin[4], mercury, selenium, cholinesterase-inhibiting pesticides
Muscle fasciculations/tremors	Cyanogenic glycoside-containing plants, locoweeds, tremorogenic mycotoxins, algal toxins, cantharidin, snake venom, botulinum toxin, lead, cholinesterase-inhibiting pesticides
Ataxia	Cyanogenic glycoside-containing plants, locoweeds, white snake root, mycotoxins, fumonisin mycotoxins[3], tremorogenic mycotoxins, lead, ionophore
Hypermetria	Tremorogenic mycotoxins
Stiff gait	White snakeroot, yellow-star thistle and russian knapweed, ionophore
Excitement	Locoweeds, oleander, fumonisin mycotoxins[3]
Rigid paralysis	Algal toxins
Flaccid paralysis	Snake venom, botulinum toxin
Seizures	Cyanogenic glycoside-containing plants, oleander, aflatoxins, tremorogenic mycotoxins, cholinesterase-inhibiting pesticides
Blindness	Locoweeds, pyrrolizidine alkaloids, aflatoxins, fumonisin mycotoxins[3]
Synchronous diaphragmatic flutter	Cantharidin

[1] Consistent with hepatic encephalopathy

[2] Equine nigropallidal encephalomalcia (chewing disease)

[3] Leukoencephalomalacia (moldy corn disease)

[4] Decreased tongue and tail tone are 'classic' signs of botulinum toxin

Table 10.3 **Clinical signs associated with common causes of intoxication in horses**

BODY SYSTEM	CLINICAL SIGNS	TOXICANT
Musculoskeletal	Laminitis	Black walnut, snake venom, mercury, selenium
	Fetal limb malformation, muscle fasciculations (see *Table 10.2*)	Locoweeds
Respiratory	Dyspnea	Cyanogenic glycoside-containing plants, maples, oleander, white snakeroot, snake venom, lead, selenium, ionophore, cholinesterase-inhibiting pesticides
	Laryngeal hemiplegia/stridor	Lead
	Aspiration pneumonia	Yellow-star thistle and russian knapweed, botulinum toxin, lead
Cardiovascular	Bradycardia	Oleander, slaframine, cholinesterase-inhibiting pesticides
	Cardiac arrhythmias	Oleander, white snakeroot, snake venom, ionophore
Blood	Cherry red blood	Cyanogenic glycoside-containing plants
	Brown discolored blood	Maples
	Hemolytic anemia	Maples, snake venom, iron, selenium
	Anemia	Maples, snake venom, lead, selenium
	Icterus	Alsike clover, maples, pyrrolizidine alkaloids, aflatoxins, fumonisin mycotoxins, iron
Urogenital	Involuntary urination	Cyanogenic glycoside-containing plants, snake venom
	Polyuria	Slaframine, algal toxins, selenium, NSAID, ionophore, cholinesterase-inhibiting pesticides
	Pollakiuria	Cantharidin
	Oliguria	Maples, mercury, ionophore
	Hematuria	Cantharidin, white snakeroot
	Red-brown urine	Maples
	Abortion	Locoweeds, maples, ergot alkaloids
	Agalactia, prolonged gestation, dystocia, placental abnormalities, poor neonate viability, subfertility	Ergot alkaloids
Skin	Photosensitization	Secondary (most common): pyrrolizidine alkaloids, alsike clover, algal toxins
	Local swelling, hemorrhage, ecchymoses/petechiation	Snake venom
	Dermal erosion, ulceration, crusting	Mercury (topical)
	Alopecia, dystrophic hoof growth	Snake venom
Ophthalmology	Excessive lacrimation	Slaframine, algal toxins, cholinesterase-inhibiting pesticides
	Paralysis of third eyelid	Botulinum toxin
	Miosis	Cholinesterase-inhibiting pesticides

Table 10.4 General signs associated with common causes of intoxication in horses

CLINICAL SIGNS	TOXICANT
Severe sweating	White snakeroot, cantharidin, ionophore
Fever	Maples, aflatoxins
Peripheral edema	NSAID
Anorexia	Maples, aflatoxins
Weight loss and anorexia	Alsike clover, locoweeds, pyrrolizidine alkaloids, yellow-star thistle and Russian knapweed[1], fumonisin mycotoxins, lead, selenium, ionophore
Shock	Maples, oleander, algal toxins, cantharidin, snake venom, iron
Sudden death	Cyanogenic glycoside-containing plants, oleander, white snakeroot, fumonisin mycotoxins, algal toxins, cantharidin, snake venom, botulinum toxin, ionophore

[1] Equine nigropallidal encephalomalcia (chewing disease)

GENERAL APPROACH TO TREATING HORSES WITH INTOXICATION

The recognition of a possible intoxication and the identification of specific toxicants can be challenging, especially in the absence of historical clues to specific toxicant exposure. Obtaining a comprehensive history that includes possible toxicants in a horse's environment is critical. The mere presence of a toxicant, however, does not mean that there has been exposure to the compound. Evidence of exposure, occurrence of compatible clinical signs, and possible laboratory testing are necessary components to a toxicologic diagnosis.

A thorough and detailed examination of the horse's environment is critical. Walking pastures, examining grain and hay, assessing housing and feed storage facilities, and identifying products used on a premise can provide important clues (e.g. detection of insects in alfalfa hay should make one think of possible exposure to blister beetles [p. 591]). It is important for equine clinicians to be aware of local factors that can contribute to an increased risk of intoxication (e.g. occurrence of toxic plants, common local or regional use of specific pesticides).

Although there are specific and sensitive tests available to detect a wide variety of toxicants in environmental, feed, and biological samples, test results may not be available for several days after sample submission. Therefore, with a few exceptions, treatment of a suspected intoxication needs to be undertaken in the absence of a firm diagnosis. Since antidotes are either unavailable or not readily obtainable for the majority of toxicants, successful case outcome depends on appropriate decontamination procedures and good symptomatic, supportive, and nursing care. A general approach to treating the intoxicated or suspected intoxicated patient should adhere to the principles shown in **10.1**.[1–3]

Stabilize vital signs

Stabilization generally focuses on maintaining respiratory, cardiovascular and neurologic function. It is important to keep in mind that many toxicants affect more than one critical organ system:

- Airway patency and normal ventilation can be impaired by a number of toxicants (e.g. localized swelling and edema secondary to snake bites [p. 592], increased bronchial secretions secondary to cholinesterase enzyme inhibitors [organophosphorus (OP) or carbamate insecticides, p. 605], or respiratory muscle failure due to neuromuscular blockade secondary to nicotine exposure [p. 615]).

- Several toxicants impair heart function (e.g. taxine, cardiac glycosides and ionophores) or cause circulatory shock (e.g. cantharidin).
- Toxicants can cause significant CNS stimulation or depression. In particular, CNS stimulation often requires therapeutic intervention.

Obtain a history and clinically evaluate the patient

Whenever possible, an exposure assessment should be performed. Necessary information includes:
- The toxicant to which the animal may have been exposed.
- The amount of exposure (known or estimated toxicant dose).
- A measure of the toxicity of the toxicant (e.g. minimum lethal dose or the lethal dose that would result in death of 50% of exposed animals [LD_{50}]).
- The body weight of the animal.

A proper exposure assessment, especially in an asymptomatic animal, can help a clinician decide whether observation of the patient is indicated (exposure to a non-toxic amount of a toxicant) or whether GI tract decontamination should be instituted (exposure to a potentially toxic amount of a toxicant). An exposure assessment can also be useful in a symptomatic animal from the standpoint that exposure to a non-toxic amount of a chemical might rule out intoxication in situations where both toxic and non-toxic differentials are being considered. In many cases an exposure assessment cannot be done because adequate information is not available.

Prevent continued systemic absorption of the toxicant

Preventing continued absorption of a toxicant following oral exposure is discussed under Gastrointestinal tract decontamination (p. 562).

While less frequent than oral exposure, dermal, inhalational, or ocular exposure to toxicants can also occur. Bathing an animal with soap and water, flushing eyes with copious amounts of saline or tap water, and provision of fresh air minimize continued systemic absorption via these routes.

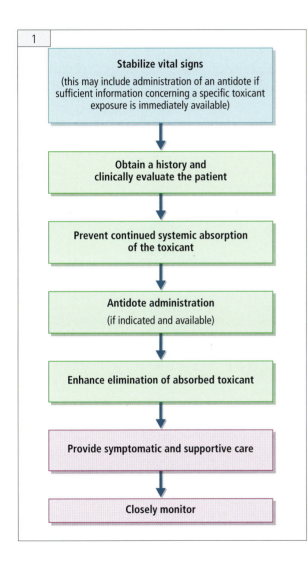

10.1 A general approach to treating the intoxicated or suspected intoxicated patient. Obviously, each situation is unique and one or more of the steps may be eliminated or their priority changed depending on the circumstances of the case.

Antidote administration

The timely administration of an antidote can be life-saving (e.g. the initial administration of atropine in horses intoxicated by OP or carbamate insecticides [p. 605] can buy precious time to then allow appropriate GI tract or dermal decontamination procedures to be undertaken). Unfortunately, there are relatively few antidotes for toxicants and their availability and expense may preclude their use in horses. *Table 10.5* lists several antidotes for use in horses.

Enhance elimination of absorbed toxicant

There are a variety of techniques available to enhance the clearance of already absorbed toxicants. These include:

- Increasing renal clearance by fluid +/– diuretic administration or ion-trapping.
- Multiple doses of activated charcoal to interrupt enterohepatic circulation or to enhance movement of a toxicant from the blood into the GI tract (gut 'dialysis') (p. 563).
- Employing techniques such as hemoperfusion, peritoneal dialysis or hemodialysis, or plasma and blood exchanges.[2,4,5]

Table 10.5 **Decontamination and common antidotal agents**

DECONTAMINATION AGENT OR ANTIDOTE	INDICATION	DOSAGE	COMMENTS
Activated charcoal	Gastrointestinal decontamination	Single dose: 1–4 g/kg PO as aqueous slurry (~ 1 g per 5 ml). Multiple doses: 1–4 g/kg PO as aqueous slurry q4–6h	Other adsorbents are available, but binding efficacy is generally less than AC; few side-effects reported following use
Atropine sulfate	OP/carbamate insecticides	0.1–0.5 mg/kg (given until muscarinic signs controlled), ¼ initial dose given IV with the remainder given IM or SQ. Administered as needed	Low-dose trial to assess response may be warranted since high doses are generally required for OP/carbamate intoxication. Narrow therapeutic index and short duration of action. Glyopyrrolate can be used in lieu of atropine. Onset of action is slower than that of atropine, but the duration of action is longer. Drug of choice for use in horses
CaNa$_2$EDTA	Lead, zinc	25 mg/kg SC q6h as a 1% solution (in 5% dextrose/water) for 5 days. Provide 5–7 day rest period between courses of treatment to minimize potential for nephrotoxicity	No veterinary formulation; use in large animals requires compounding
Calcitonin	Cholecalciferol	Not determined for horses	Used for treating hypercalcemia. Biphosphonates such as pamidronate may be more efficacious, convenient and associated with fewer side-effects

Table 10.5 *(continued)*

DECONTAMINATION AGENT OR ANTIDOTE	INDICATION	DOSAGE	COMMENTS
Crotalid antivenom (polyvalent equine-derived, serum globulin-based antivenin)	Crotalid snake envenomation	Not determined for horses; empirically, 10–50 ml (1 to 5 vials)	Antivenin doses vary in people and depend on several factors including severity of symptoms, size of snake and, therefore, venom dose, size of animal, and time after bite
Deferoxamine mesylate	Iron	Not determined; for humans a suggested dose is 5 g of a 5% solution given PO, then 20 mg/kg IM q4–6h. If shock is present, dose is 40 mg/kg by IV drip over 4 hours, which is repeated 6 hours later and then 15 mg/kg by IV drip q8h	Little clinical benefit if treatment is begun >12 hours after iron ingestion. Recommended that chelation therapy continue until serum iron concentration is <53.7 µmmol/l (300 µg/dl) or serum iron binding capacity. Urine will turn reddish-brown
Digoxin Fab fragments	Cardiac glycosides (i.e. digoxin, plants such as *Digitalis* and *Nerium* spp., *Bufo* spp.)	Dosing in animals is empiric. In humans it is suggested that 1.7 ml (of Digibind®) is administered IV per mg of digoxin ingested. If unknown dose ingested, then 400 mg Digibind is given IV	Administered over 30 minutes unless cardiac arrest is imminent, in which case a bolus is given. Monitor for anaphylaxis and hypokalemia. Based on human use, patient should improve quickly
D-penicillamine	Copper, lead	Copper: 10–15 mg/kg/day PO (for treatment of chronic copper storage disease in dogs). Lead: 110 mg/kg/day PO for 1–2 weeks, re-evaluate animal 1 week after initial course, additional treatment may be necessary	Not approved for use in food animals
Pralidoxime chloride (2-PAM)	OP Insecticides	20 mg/kg IM, SC or slow IV q12h	Not necessary in carbamate intoxications. If in doubt as to whether exposure to OP or carbamate, administer 2-PAM (except carbaryl). Probably not cost-effective for use in livestock
Sodium nitrite	Cyanide	16 mg/kg of a 1% solution IV, given once only	No withdrawal time in food animals
Sodium or magnesium sulfate (Glauber's or Epsom salt, respectively)	Cathartics	1 g/kg dissolved in 4 liters of warm water PO	Only one dose of a cathartic should be administered; more effective at inducing catharsis than mineral oil
Sodium thiosulfate	Arsenic, cyanide	30–40 mg/kg of a 20% solution IV, may be repeated	No withdrawal time in food animals
Succimer	Lead, arsenic	10 mg/kg PO q8h for 5 days followed by 10 mg/kg PO q12h for 2 weeks	Orally effective chelator, which makes its use on an out-patient basis possible
Vitamin K_1	Anticoagulant rodenticides	1st generation anticoagulants: 1 mg/kg PO for 4–6 days. For 2nd generation anticoagulants: 2.5–5.0 mg/kg PO for 2–4 weeks	Close monitoring for recurrence of coagulopathy is critical following cessation of vitamin K_1. Vitamin K_3 is not effective and is potentially toxic

OP = organophosphorus

From a practical standpoint, diuresis, urinary ion-trapping, and multiple doses of activated charcoal are likely to be the only techniques used in horses. Diuresis and urinary ion-trapping are only useful for toxicants that are primarily eliminated via the kidneys. Urinary alkalinization is only useful for a few weak acids (salicylates) and urinary acidification to trap weak bases is never indicated.[4–6] The use of diuresis can be associated with hyponatremia, fluid overload, pulmonary edema, cerebral edema, hypokalemia, and either alkalemia or acidemia, depending on the agent used.[5] The ability to alkalinize urine sufficiently to affect clearance of weak acids can be difficult with an underlying acidemia. Severe alkalemia can cause dysrhythmias. As an aside, urinary alkalinization may potentially minimize renal damage in intoxicated animals with rhabdomyolysis.[7] The goal of any of these techniques is to substantially increase toxicant clearance; modest increases in clearance are unlikely to alter case outcome. Evidence that any of these approaches alter case outcome in the intoxicated horse is lacking.

Provide symptomatic and supportive care and closely monitor

Good symptomatic and supportive care will likely have a greater influence on case outcome than any other factor:

- Effective correction of fluid, acid–base, and electrolyte abnormalities.
- Controlling seizures and muscle tremors (see Chapter 7).
- Treating cardiac arrhythmias (see Chapter 4).
- Maintaining pulmonary function (see Chapter 3).
- Protecting animals from self-induced trauma.
- Providing adequate nutritional support (see Chapter 15).

Close monitoring of either asymptomatic or symptomatic animals is needed to identify correctable problems as early as possible.

COMMON PROCEDURES PERFORMED IN HORSES WITH INTOXICATION

Gastrointestinal tract decontamination
Indications

GI tract decontamination is a critical component of case management. Appropriate and timely decontamination may prevent the onset of clinical signs or lessen the severity or shorten the course of intoxication. GI tract decontamination consists of three components: (1) gastric evacuation, (2) administration of an adsorbent, and (3) catharsis.[3]

Technique
Gastric evacuation

- Approaches to gastric evacuation include induction of emesis with emetics and gastric lavage. Since horses do not vomit, induction of emesis is not a viable option in this species. Gastric lavage may be used as an alternative depending on the condition and temperament of the horse.
- Gastric lavage requires the placement of a nasogastric tube and the repeated instillation of water or normal saline to remove stomach contents.[2] Airway protection is essential whenever gastric lavage is performed. As large a nasogastric tube as possible with terminal fenestrations is introduced into the stomach. Tube placement is confirmed by aspiration of gastric contents or air insufflation with a stethoscope placed over the stomach. Tepid tap water or normal saline (5–10 ml/kg) is introduced into the stomach with minimal pressure application and is withdrawn by aspiration or allowed to return via gravity flow. The procedure is repeated until the last several washings are clear. Numerous cycles may be required. Activated charcoal +/– a cathartic can be administered via the tube just before its removal. The initial lavage sample should be retained for possible toxicologic analysis.

Administration of an adsorbent

- Realistically, the only adsorbent routinely used in veterinary medicine is activated charcoal. Activated charcoal is produced in a two-step process. The first step involves the pyrolysis of carbonaceous materials, such as wood, coconut, or peat, followed by high temperature treatment with activating agents such as steam or carbon dioxide.[8] The activating step increases the adsorptive capacity of the material by increasing its total surface area as a result of the formation of a maze of internal pores. The rate of toxicant adsorption is dependent on the external surface area, while the adsorptive capacity is dependent on the internal surface area. Adsorption is believed to be due to hydrogen bonding, ion–ion, dipole, and van der Waal's forces and is, therefore, reversible.[8]

- Activated charcoal is likely to be an effective adsorbent for most organic toxicants, although the adsorptive capacity of activated charcoal for most has not been determined. Non-polar, poorly water soluble organic substances are more likely to be adsorbed and adsorption is enhanced as the molecular size of the toxicant increases.[8] Small, polar, water-soluble organics are less well adsorbed. In-vitro studies have demonstrated that adsorption begins almost immediately after instillation of activated charcoal, but may not reach equilibrium for 10–25 minutes. Activated charcoal has been shown to decrease the systemic absorption of a number of drugs including aspirin, acetaminophen, barbiturates, glutethimide, phenytoin, theophylline, cyclic antidepressants, and most inorganic and organic chemicals.[8] However, activated charcoal does not adsorb alcohols, strong acids and alkalies, iron, and lithium.

- Activated charcoal is available as a powder, as an aqueous slurry, or combined with cathartics such as sorbitol. If using a powder, 1–4 grams of activated charcoal should be mixed with tepid tap water (approximately 1 gram of activated charcoal to 5 ml of water) to form a slurry.[4] Administration via nasogastric tube is recommended for horses.

- Multiple dose activated charcoal is effective in interrupting enterohepatic recycling of a number of toxicants and the continued presence of activated charcoal in the GI tract may allow the tract to serve as a sink for trapping toxicant passing from the circulation into the intestines.[9] There is little hazard to repeated administration of activated charcoal, although cathartics should be given only once.

- Other possible adsorbents include bentonite clay and aluminum silicates such as kaolin. A commercial clay product (BioSponge®) marketed to support healthy intestinal function has been suggested as a good adsorbent for various toxicants and has been used by clinicians to treat *Nerium oleander*-intoxicated horses. Although the product reportedly adsorbs *Clostridium difficile* and *Clostridium perfringens* toxins, its efficacy for other toxicants is likely to be considerably less than that of activated charcoal. However, if activated charcoal is not available, other adsorbents may be better than no adsorbent.

- Although commonly recommended and administered, mineral oil has not been shown to be efficacious for decreasing the systemic absorption of toxicants in horses and, therefore, cannot be recommended for routine GI tract decontamination. If mineral oil is administered with activated charcoal, theoretically the oil may decrease the adsorptive ability of the activated charcoal. Therefore, the combination is not recommended. In addition, if catharsis is desired, saline or saccharide cathartics will be more effective than mineral oil.

- Activated charcoal is relatively safe. In humans, emesis with resultant aspiration pneumonia secondary to activated charcoal administration has been the most serious complication.[8,10] Intestinal obstruction has been reported following repeated administration of activated charcoal in the presence of dehydration and prior bowel adhesions.[8]

Catharsis: Both saline (sodium sulfate [Glauber's salt] or magnesium sulfate [Epsom's salt] or citrate) and saccharide (sorbitol) cathartics are available for GI tract decontamination. The mechanism of cathartic action is not entirely known. Traditionally, the cathartic effect of sodium and magnesium sulfate was attributed to the creation of an osmotic gradient within the lumen of the GI tract, thus increasing water retention and intestinal pressure and resulting in an increase in intestinal motility. However, other mechanisms may contribute to catharsis. Magnesium releases cholecystokinin from the duodenal mucosa, which stimulates intestinal motor activity and alters fluid movement.[11] Presumably, sorbitol, found naturally in many ripe fruits and synthesized industrially from glucose, works by osmotic action, but the mechanisms causing its cathartic action have not been thoroughly investigated.

In general, cathartics are safe, particularly if used only once.[4,10] However, repeated administration of magnesium-containing cathartics can lead to hypermagnesemia manifested as hypotonia, altered mental status, and respiratory failure. Also, repeated administration of sorbitol can cause fluid pooling in the GI tract, excessive fluid losses via the stool, and severe dehydration. Mineral oil has a laxative, not cathartic, effect and can be used when saline or saccharide cathartics are unavailable. However, mineral oil is not as effective in inducing bowel evacuation and, as mentioned, it has the potential to interfere with the adsorptive capacity of activated charcoal if given concurrently. Contraindications to the use of cathartics include adynamic ileus, pre-existing or anticipated diarrhea, abdominal trauma, and intestinal obstruction.[10]

The recommended dosage of sodium or magnesium sulfate is 1 g/kg body weight dissolved in 4 liters of warm water and given orally.[2] A recommended dose of sorbitol (70%) is 3 ml/kg.[4] Formulations of activated charcoal with a cathartic should be administered only once and if multiple doses of activated charcoal are given, those subsequent to the first should not include a cathartic. Make sure that the horse is adequately hydrated following cathartic administration. Under no circumstances should a cathartic be given alone to achieve GI tract decontamination.[10]

In recent years, a critical reappraisal of GI tract decontamination approaches in human intoxications has occurred that is relevant for the management of intoxicated animals.[12,13] In human patients, there has been movement away from gastric evacuation (induction of emesis or gastric lavage) followed by the administration of an adsorbent toward administration of only the adsorbent, especially in mild to moderate intoxications. Early administration of activated charcoal alone has been shown to be as efficacious as the combination of gastric evacuation followed by activated charcoal. Therefore, from a practical, logistical, and economic standpoint, initial use of activated charcoal in lieu of gastric evacuation is recommended for most cases of intoxication involving horses.

The case for or against the inclusion of a cathartic with activated charcoal is less clear-cut, but the administration of a single dose of a cathartic along with the initial dose of activated charcoal is currently recommended. Again, those activated charcoal formulations that include a cathartic such as sorbitol should be administered only once, followed by activated charcoal alone if repeated doses are indicated.

Complications
See above.

TOXICITIES

Naturally occurring toxins
Plants

The more selective eating behavior of horses compared with other livestock and the relative unpalatability of many toxic plants make the incidence of plant intoxication relatively infrequent.[14] However, there are situations that can predispose horses to toxic plant ingestion:

- Horses introduced into new areas are more likely to ingest injurious plants compared with animals habituated to their environment.
- The confinement of horses to small areas combined with inattention can lead to sampling any available greenery.
- The palatability of plants and, in some cases, their toxicity can increase if treated with herbicides.[14] Therefore, herbicide treated areas should not be grazed until potentially toxic plants are completely dead.
- Incorporation of toxic plants into hay can expose horses as a result of loss of the ability to be selective. In addition, many toxic plants retain their toxicity when dry.
- The unavailability of alternative forage in arid areas or during periods of drought can force animals to consume toxic plants that otherwise would not be consumed.[15]

Most plant poisonings have no specific treatments and favorable outcomes rely on good nursing and supportive and symptomatic care. Unfortunately, with few exceptions, toxic plant ingestions are most often recognized long after exposure, which lessens the efficacy of decontamination procedures such as administration of activated charcoal. The best prevention for toxic plant problems is for owners to know what potentially toxic plants are in their animal's environment and to examine feed sources, especially hay, for contamination.

Alsike clover
Key points

- Alsike clover (*Trifolium hybridum*) ingestion should be considered in any cases presenting with signs of anorexia and weight loss, hepatic encephalopathy (HE), or photosensitization.
- Diagnosis relies on elimination of other causes of chronic liver or CNS disease and a history of ingestion of implicated plants.
- Treatment is mostly supportive.
- The prognosis is poor.

Definition/overview

Alsike clover (**10.2**) is a bovine forage crop that grows in a wide range of soils in northern latitudes and at high elevations.

Etiology/pathogenesis

Two disease syndromes have been associated with grazing alsike clover: (1) an irreversible liver disease that may be accompanied by neurologic abnormalities due to HE and (2) hepatogenous photosensitization.[16] Generally, horses have to graze the plant for extended periods of time for adverse effects to occur. Alsike clover is reportedly not particularly palatable to horses.[14]

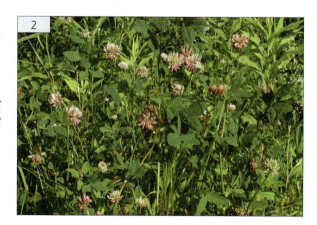

10.2 *Trifolium hybridum* (alsike clover).

The toxin in the plant has not been identified, although toxicity has been hypothesized to be due to a bacterial endophyte. Occurrence of disease is more common in years with high rainfall and humidity.[17] Other forages, such as red clover (*Trifolium pratense*) and alfalfa (*Medicago sativa*), have been associated with hepatogenous photosensitization.[18]

Clinical features
Clinical signs associated with alsike clover intoxication are due to liver damage and include anorexia, loss of condition, icterus, HE, and death. Photosensitization (**10.3**) occurs secondary to the inability of the liver to eliminate phylloerythrin, the principal breakdown product of chlorophyll.

Differential diagnosis
Central nervous system signs: pyrrolizidine alkaloid exposure; locoism; fumonisin mycotoxicosis; rabies; EPM; viral encephalitides; brain abscesses or meningitis. Chronic active hepatitis: cholelithiasis; hepatic amyloidosis; chronic hepatic hypoxemia; narcoplepsy; neoplasia. Photosensitization: Common St. Johnswort exposure; Buckwheat exposure; Spring parsley exposure. Chronic liver disease.

Diagnosis
Diagnosis is primarily based on ruling out other causes for the clinical signs based on routine diagnostic tests such as clinical pathology, serology, CSF evaluation, ultrasonographic examination of the liver and liver biopsy, along with known exposure to implicated plants.

Management/treatment
The reported irreversibility of liver damage makes long-term management of affected animals challenging. Access to the offending plant should be stopped and, if photosensitization is present, exposure to sunlight should be minimized. Topical and systemic glucocorticoids may alleviate inflammation and pruritis associated with photosensitization. Antimicrobial drugs can be given if skin infections are present. Provision of dry hay is recommended to decrease chlorophyll intake.[14]

Supportive treatment needs to be provided until the liver regenerates sufficiently to provide adequate function. Agitated, restless, and uncontrollable horses with HE will require sedation. Drugs need to be selected judiciously since their metabolism can be impaired and neurologic signs exacerbated. Xylazine or detomidine in small doses are recommended.[19] Diazepam is contraindicated because of possible exacerbation of CNS signs as a result of its GABAergic effect. Fluid and electrolyte abnormalities need to be corrected. Anorexia can cause hypoglycemia, therefore initial administration of 5% dextrose IV can be beneficial.

Lowering production and absorption of toxic protein metabolites by enteric bacteria should be attempted. Treatment approaches have included administration of mineral oil or magnesium sulfate, antimicrobial drugs (e.g. neomycin), lactulose, and probiotics such as *Lactobacillus acidophilus* or *Enterococcus faecium*.[19] Provision of low-protein diets is also recommended.

A number of drugs have been evaluated in human patients with hepatic insufficiency to stimulate hepatic regeneration, reduce hepatic fibrosis, or ameliorate clinical signs. These drugs include flumazenil, bromocriptine, pentoxyfylline (8–16 mg/kg q8–12h), cholchicine, and cyclosporine.[19] Unfortunately, most have not been shown to alter case outcome in human patients or have not been critically evaluated in horses.

Cyanogenic glycoside-containing plants
Key points
- Cyanogenic plants are common and are the most likely source for cyanide intoxication in horses.
- Cyanide intoxication is an acute disease that is most likely to be associated with sudden death.

- Effective antidotes are available, but the rapidity of onset of signs and death or the relatively rapid recovery following exposure most often precludes their use.

Definition/overview

A variety of plants contain cyanogenic glycosides (*Table 10.6*).[16] The most common cyanogenic plants belong to the *Prunus* genus and include chokecherries

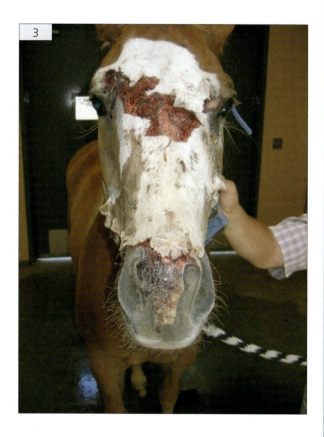

10.3 Photosensitization of the non-pigmented facial skin. Note the sloughing of affected skin.

Table 10.6 **Cyanogenic plants**

COMMON NAME	SCIENTIFIC NAME
Catclaw, acacia	*Acacia* spp.
Service, june or Saskatoon berry	*Amelanchier alnifolia*
Bahia	*Bahia oppositifolia*
Cassava, manihot, tapioca	*Mannihot esculentum*
Mountain mahogany	*Cercocarpus montanum*
Flowering quince	*Chaenomales* spp.
Star grass	*Cynodon* spp.
Eucalyptus, gum tree	*Eucalyptus* spp.
Tall manna grass	*Glyceria grandis*
Toyon, tollon, Christmas berry, Christmas holly	*Heteromeles arbutifolia*
Hydrangea	*Hydrangea* spp.
Flax	*Linum* spp.
Bird's foot trefoil	*Lotus* spp.
Crab apple, apple	*Malus* spp.
Heavenly or sacred bamboo	*Nandina domestica*
Lima bean	*Phaseolus lunatus*
Christmas berry	*Photinia* spp.
Chokecherry, wild black cherry, pin cherry, apricot, peach, cherry laurel, almond	*Prunus* spp.
Bracken fern	*Pteridium aquilinum*
Crabapple, pear	*Pyrus* spp.
Elderberry	*Sambuccus* spp.
Johnson grass, Sudan grass	*Sorghum* spp.
Indian grass	*Sorghastrum nutans*
Texas Queen's delight	*Stillingia texana*
Poison suckleya	*Suckleya suckleyana*
White clover	*Trifolium repens*
Arrow grass	*Triglochin maritima*
Common vetch	*Vicia sativa*
Corn, maize	*Zea mays*

(**10.4, 10.5**), wild black cherries (**10.6**), cultivated cherries, almonds, peaches and apricots.[14,20] In addition, grasses such as Johnson grass (**10.7**), sorghum, and Sudan grass (**10.8**) are also cyanogenic.

Etiology/pathogenesis

When plants are stressed by drought, frost, stunted growth, or wilting, or when plants are masticated and ingested by an animal, cyanogenic glycosides are hydrolyzed to release free cyanide. Forage cyanide concentrations of 200 parts per million or greater are considered to be potentially toxic.[20]

Cyanide is rapidly absorbed from the GI tract. The major route of cyanide detoxification is via the addition of a sulfur atom from a sulfur donor by rhodanese, an enzyme that is widely distributed in the body.[21] The resulting thiocyanate is eliminated via the kidneys. The rate-limiting step in cyanide detoxification is the availability of adequate quantities of sulfur donors.

Cyanide is an inhibitor of multiple enzymes including succinic acid dehydrogenase, superoxide dismutase, carbonic anhydrase, and cytochrome c oxidase.[21] Cytochrome c oxidase is an iron-containing metalloenzyme found within mitochondria and required for oxidative phosphorylation. Cyanide combines with iron in cytochrome c oxidase to prevent terminal electron transfer resulting in inhibition of cellular respiration. Oxygen cannot be utilized by the cell and adenosine triphosphate is not formed. Hydrogen ions that are normally combined with oxygen are not utilized and contribute

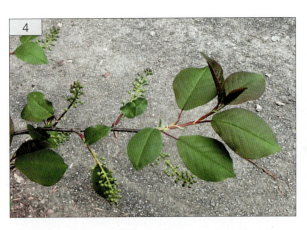

10.4 *Prunus virginiana* (chokecherry) leaves.

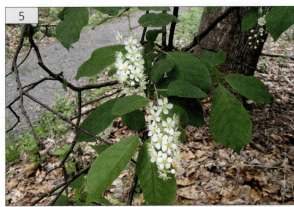

10.5 *Prunus virginiana* (chokecherry) flowers and leaves.

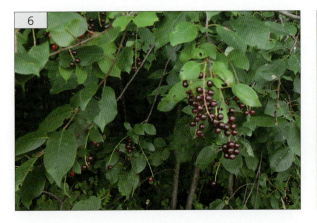

10.6 *Prunus serotina* (wild black cherry) fruit and leaves.

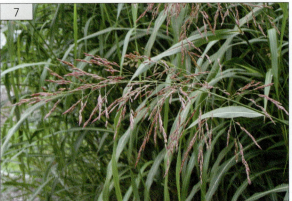

10.7 *Sorghum halepense* (Johnsongrass).

to acidemia.[21] Cyanide is also a potent neurotoxin. It has an affinity for areas of the brain with high metabolic activity. CNS injury occurs via impaired oxygen utilization, oxidant stress, and enhanced excitatory neurotransmitter release.[21]

Clinical features
Onset of clinical signs is often within minutes. Signs are related to dysfunction of oxygen-sensitive organs, especially the central nervous and cardiovascular systems. Because oxygen is not released from oxyhemoglobin, hemoglobin in RBCs becomes saturated, leading to a bright cherry red appearance to the blood (**10.9**) and mucous membranes.[20] Animals become dyspneic with flaring nostrils and exhibit involuntary urination and defecation, hypotension, trembling, ataxia, seizure, prostration, struggling, and death.[14,20]

Differential diagnosis
Sudden death: ionophore intoxication; insecticide intoxication; *Taxus* spp. intoxication; *Conium maculatum* (poison hemlock) intoxication; *Nerium oleander* (oleander) intoxication; cardiac electrical conductance disturbances; cardiac tamponade; acute hemorrhage; embolic events; malicious intoxication; electrocution.

Diagnosis
Diagnosis of cyanide intoxication relies on a history of exposure to and consumption of a cyanogenic plant and measurement of cyanide in GI tract contents or blood samples. Since free cyanide is volatile, it is important that samples for analysis are frozen quickly and remain frozen prior to analysis.

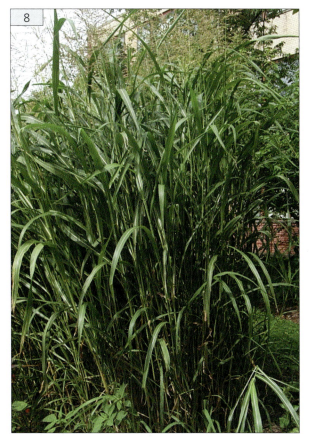

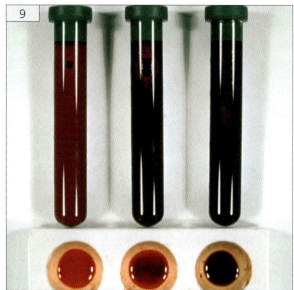

10.9 Bright red blood (left) as a result of cyanide intoxication. The blood sample in the middle is from a control animal and the blood sample on the right is from an animal with methemoglobinemia.

10.8 *Sorghum sudanense* (Sudan grass).

Management/treatment

The rapidity of onset of clinical signs and death often precludes effective treatment. However, when treatment is possible, sodium nitrite (20%) should be administered rapidly IV at 10–20 mg/kg.[20] The nitrite forms methemoglobin, which has a greater affinity for cyanide than does cytochrome c; this results in the formation of cyanmethemoglobin. Care needs to be taken to avoid excessive formation of methemoglobin, hypotension, and tachycardia. The administration of sodium thiosulfate (20%) IV at <600 mg/kg provides a source of sulfur that enhances the formation of thiocyanate.

Hydroxycobalamin, a vitamin B_{12} precursor, has been used effectively in human and experimental animal intoxications.[8,22] It is a metalloprotein that complexes with cyanide to form cyanocobalamin, which is eliminated via the kidneys. The standard dose for an adult human is 4 g.[21]

More general treatment involves ventilatory support or oxygen administration, provision of crystalloid fluids and vasopressors for hypotension, and administration of sodium bicarbonate based on ABG and bicarbonate monitoring.[21]

Black walnut
Key points

- Black walnut (*Juglans nigra*)-associated laminitis is caused by exposure to fresh walnut shavings, most often when incorporated into bedding.
- The toxin in black walnut has not been identified.
- Outbreaks often involve multiple horses and occur within 12–24 hours following use of new bedding.
- Confirmation of exposure relies on microscopic identification of black walnut in suspect bedding.

Definition/overview

Black walnut (**10.10**) is a hardwood tree that is native to the eastern and central USA and has been introduced into Europe.[23]

Etiology/pathogenesis

Exposure to black walnut heartwood (the older, non-living central wood of a tree or woody plant that is usually darker and harder than the younger sapwood, **10.11**) can cause severe laminitis in equids within 10–12 hours.[24] The most common exposure occurs when black walnut shavings are inadvertently included in horse bedding. The responsible toxin has not been identified, although it is present in aqueous extracts of the heartwood.[25] It is not clear whether exposure occurs via ingestion, skin contact, or inhalation. Horses do not have to eat the shavings to develop laminitis.[16]

The underlying pathogenesis of the laminitis is not entirely clear. *In-vitro*, crude aqueous extracts of the heartwood enhance the ability of epinephrine to cause contraction of digital arteries and veins.[26] The response of laminar veins was significantly reduced in response to phenylephrine and 5-hydroxytryptamine in horses given

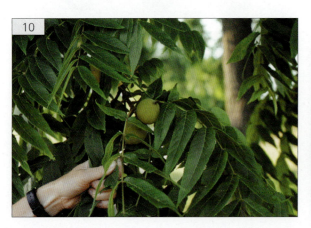

10.10 *Juglans nigra* (black walnut) fruit and leaves.

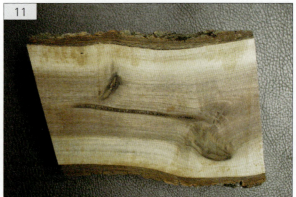

10.11 Sagittal section through the wood of *Juglans nigra* (black walnut) showing the darker heartwood.

an aqueous extract of black walnut.[27] The later study suggested a selective dysfunction of laminar veins. Laminar microvascular blood flow has been shown to decrease significantly by 1 hour after administration of an aqueous extract, but rebound by 3 hours post dosing.[28] A significant decrease in microvascular blood flow reoccurred by 8 hours post dosing. Clinical signs of laminitis were noted 8–12 hours after dosing. Thus, low-flow ischemia followed by reperfusion injury could play an important role in black walnut-induced laminitis.[28] The condition is also associated with an upregulation of cyclooxygenase-2 mRNA, molecule possessing ankyrin-repeats induced by lipopolysaccharide mRNA, interleukin-6 mRNA, and interleukin-1 beta mRNA during the prodromal stage of the intoxication.[29–31] These findings are consistent with the hypothesis that local digital proinflammatory cytokine expression may be an initiating factor in black walnut-associated laminitis. The systemic activation of leukocytes and induction of inflammation may also play a role in disease pathogenesis.[32]

Clinical features

Experimentally, horses given crude aqueous extracts orally develop a transient leukopenia and pyrexia 4–8 hours after administration.[26] This is followed by a pounding digital pulse, dependent edema of the forelimbs, and mild lethargy within 12 hours of administration. Clinical signs in spontaneous cases include hyperthermia, tachycardia, tachypnea, lower limb edema, palpable increases in coronary band and hoof temperatures, and bounding digital pulses.[33,34] The incidence and severity of clinical signs vary within a group of horses.[35]

Differential diagnosis

Laminitis: salmonellosis; Potomac horse fever; acute metritis; acute septic peritonitis; acute pleuropneumonia; ingestion of hoary alyssum (*Beteroa incana*); ingestion of lush pasture; grain overload; concussion to the foot; Cushing's syndrome.

Diagnosis

Confirmation of black walnut-associated laminitis requires documentation of exposure to wood shavings from the tree. This generally entails microscopic examination of implicated bedding and identification of the wood.

Management/treatment

Exposed horses should be removed from the suspected bedding immediately. If exposure is recognized before the onset of clinical signs, administration of activated charcoal is warranted. Although the route of toxin exposure has not been identified, washing of the lower legs should be considered. Once clinical signs are evident, standard treatment protocols for laminitis should be instituted (see Chapter 2).

The mainstays of treatment include: (1) ensuring sufficient plasma oncotic pressure via administration of colloidal solutions such as hydroxyethyl starch or plasma (see Chapter 12); (2) improvement of digital blood flow via administration of drugs such as acepromazine, isoxsuprine hydrochloride, or glyceryl trinitrate; (3) administration of anti-inflammatory drugs such as phenylbutazone, flunixin meglumine, or ketoprofen; and (4) reduction of mechanical forces and stabilization of the distal phalanx.[36]

In an experimental model of black walnut-induced laminitis, topical application of 15 mg of glyceryl trinitrate to digital arteries in the pastern region of all four limbs in combination with 4 mg/kg phenylbutazone IV after the onset of laminitis did not improve blood flow.[28] There was no advantage to giving the combination of glyceryl trinitrate plus phenylbutazone over the use of phenylbutazone alone. More controversial interventions include soaking affected feet in crushed ice or cold water and administration of DMSO. Severe sequelae such as rotation or prolapse of the third phalanx are associated with a poor prognosis.

Locoweeds
Key points

- Locoism results following the chronic ingestion of swainsonine-containing plants (*Astragalus* spp., *Oxytropis* spp., and *Swainsona* spp.).
- Ingestion of locoweeds can be addictive.
- Disease is due to accumulation of incompletely metabolized oligosaccharides in a variety of cells.
- Clinical signs are reversible if exposure is stopped early after the onset of signs, although affected horses are generally considered to be unsound.

Definition/overview

Numerous species of locoweeds grow in western North America and Australia (**10.12**, **10.13**) and their ingestion is associated with several disease syndromes in livestock including locoism, 'cracker heals', and selenosis.[16,23,37] However, some locoweeds are considered to be non-toxic.

Etiology/pathogenesis

Locoism is caused by an indolizidine alkaloid called swainsonine.[14] Swainsonine inhibits α-mannosidase, a lysosomal enzyme necessary for cellular processing of oligosaccharides. Incompletely metabolized oligosaccharides accumulate in lysosomes, eventually disrupting normal cell function. Onset of clinical signs varies from as short as 2 weeks to up to 2 months after consumption begins. The toxin is transferred through the milk. Animals that begin eating locoweeds often become 'addicted' or 'habituated' to the plant and will eat the relatively unpalatable plant in preference to other forage.

Clinical features

Clinical signs are generally neurologic in nature and include CNS depression, excitement when disturbed, trembling, ataxia, slow staggering gait, behavioral changes, and visual impairment.[14,24] Other signs include unthrifty appearance, weight loss, difficulty eating and drinking, poor libido, immunocompromise, and abortion. Foals born to pregnant mares can have limb malformations.

Differential diagnosis

Toxicants causing CNS stimulation: tremorgenic mycotoxins (lolitrems and paspalitrems); cholinesterase-inhibiting insecticides (OP and carbamate insecticides); strychnine; metaldehyde; fumonisin mycotoxins; 4-aminopyridine; lead; plants such as poison hemlock (*Conium maculatum*) and water hemlock (*Cicuta maculata*). CNS diseases: rabies; EPM; viral encephalitides; brain abscesses; meningitis; chronic liver diseases associated with hepatic encephalopathy.

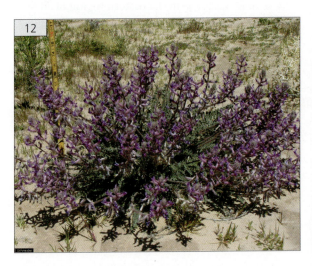

10.12 *Astragalus molissimus*. **(Courtesy Dr Asheesh Tiwary)**

10.13 *Astragalus* spp. **(Courtesy Dr Asheesh Tiwary)**

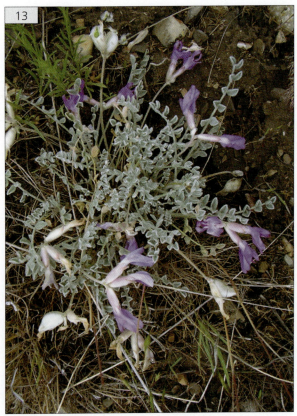

Diagnosis

Diagnosis is primarily based on ruling out other causes for the clinical signs based on routine diagnostic tests such as clinical pathology, serology, CSF evaluation, liver ultrasonographic examination, and liver biopsy along with known exposure to locoweeds.

Management/treatment

If exposure to the plant is stopped sufficiently early (approximately 30 days or less), cell damage is reversible and affected horses can make an uneventful recovery within several weeks. However, if neurologic signs are present, full recovery is unlikely due to altered synaptic formation in nervous tissue.[15] Because of the irreversibility of neurologic lesions, horses are believed to be unpredictable and, therefore, unsafe for riding. Animals that have aborted should be able to be successfully rebred.[16]

Maples
Key points

- Ingestion of wilted leaves from red maples (*Acer rubrum*) is associated with an acute hemolytic anemia due to an unidentified toxin.
- Diagnosis relies on the occurrence of a hemolytic anemia and evidence of leaf consumption.
- Treatment is symptomatic and supportive; renal function should be monitored closely.

Definition/overview

Acer spp. (particularly *Acer rubrum*) intoxication results from the ingestion of wilted or dried leaves of the tree (**10.14**). Red maples are especially common in Eastern North America.[23]

Etiology/pathogenesis

Although there is limited information that *Acer* spp. other than *Acer rubrum* are associated with intoxication, there is some *in-vitro* evidence that leaf extracts from *Acer saccharum* (sugar maple) and *A. saccharinum* (silver maple) contain components that cause damage to RBCs and hemoglobin similar to that caused by *Acer rubrum* extracts.[38] Therefore, all trees in the *Acer* genus, including hybrids, should be considered potentially toxic.

The toxicity of red maple leaves is not well established. Ponies given dried red maple leaves orally at 1.5 g/kg became ill.[39,40] The toxicity of red maple bark has also not been established. Although the toxicant or toxicants responsible for clinical signs have not been positively identified, oxidant damage to RBC membranes and hemoglobin occurs. Experimental work *in vitro* has identified several potential oxidants including gallic acid and 2, 3-dihydro-3,5-dihydroxy-6-methoxy-4H-pyran-4-one.

Clinical features

Initial clinical signs result from hemolysis, methemoglobin formation, and tissue hypoxia and generally occur within 48 hours of exposure.[39–42] Signs include icterus, tachypnea, dyspnea, tachycardia, fever, weakness, lethargy, depression, anorexia, scleral petechiation, dehydration, cyanosis, colic, reddish-brown urine, and brown discoloration of the blood. Pregnant mares can abort.[43] Secondary renal damage can result in oliguria and anuria.

Hematologic changes associated with red maple intoxication include methemoglobinemia, Heinz body anemia, decreased PCV, increased mean corpuscular hemoglobin concentration, free plasma hemoglobin, anisocytosis, poikilocytosis, eccentrocytes, ghost RBCs, agglutination, increased RBC fragility, and neutrophilia. Clinical pathologic changes can include

10.14 *Acer rubrum* **leaves (left is the underside of the leaf and right is the top of the leaf).**

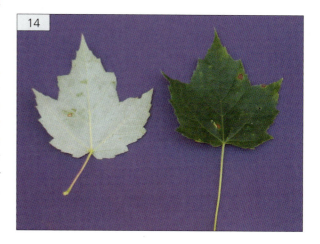

increases in total, conjugated and unconjugated bilirubin, creatinine, blood urea nitrogen, aspartate aminotransferase, sorbitol dehydrogenase, creatine phosphokinase, gamma glutamyl transferase, calcium, and glucose. A mild metabolic acidosis can occur. Hemoglobinuria, methemoglobinuria, proteinuria, bilirubinuria, and urobilinogenuria may be noted on urinalysis. Clinical presentation can be variable. For example, Heinz bodies are not always noted in intoxicated animals.[44]

Differential diagnosis

Immune-mediated hemolytic anemia; equine infectious anemia; equine granulocytic ehrlichiosis; piroplasmosis; familial methemoglobinemia; equine glucose-6-phosphate dehydrogenase deficiency; phenothiazine poisoning; wild onion poisoning; hepatic failure; microangiopathic hemolysis; iatrogenic hemolysis due to hypertonic or hypotonic fluid; hemolysis secondary to some bacterial toxins or crotalid snake venom.

Diagnosis

Diagnosis relies on a history of exposure to red maple, identification of red maple leaves in stomach contents, and ruling out other causes of acute hemolytic anemia based on historical clues and diagnostic testing.

Management/treatment

The efficacy of activated charcoal to prevent onset of clinical signs in asymptomatic animals or shorten the course of intoxication in symptomatic animals has not been evaluated, but its administration should be considered within a reasonable time of exposure.

Treatment of affected animals is symptomatic and supportive. Dexamethasone may be useful for RBC membrane stabilization and decreasing phagocytosis of damaged RBCs. Ascorbic acid has been given to reduce oxidant damage to RBCs, but its efficacy has not been determined.[45] While methylene blue effectively reverses methemoglobin in many species, it is not efficacious in horses.[46] Severely anemic horses (PCV, 0.01–0.12 l/l [10–12%] or less) should be given blood transfusions and supplemental oxygen should be administered to horses that are hypoxic.

It is important to maintain renal perfusion in affected animals because of the potential for renal damage secondary to hemoglobinuria. However, care should be taken when administering IV fluids due to the presence of anemia. In cases of renal failure, administration of furosemide, dopamine, or mannitol should be considered. Administration of potentially nephrotoxic drugs such as NSAIDs should be avoided.

Unfortunately, the mortality rate in symptomatic animals is high (up to 60–65%).[40,41] Other than a return of mucous membrane and urine color to normal, no clinical variable has been identified as a useful prognostic indicator.[42]

Oleander

Key points

- Oleander (*Nerium oleander*) contains cardiotoxic components and is highly toxic to horses; it is one of the most common plant intoxications in areas in which it is found.
- Intoxication is often associated with sudden death due to myocardial damage and cardiac arrhythmias.
- Diagnosis can be facilitated by detecting the toxin (oleandrin) in serum or GI tract contents.
- Mortality is high, but intoxicated horses can be treated effectively if the intoxication is recognized early.

Definition/overview

Oleander (**10.15, 10.16**) is an introduced ornamental evergreen shrub that is commonly found in the southern USA, throughout California, and in other Mediterranean climates.[47]

Etiology/pathogenesis

All parts of the plant are toxic. Fresh oleander is not palatable, although clippings or dried leaves appear to be much more palatable.[14] Ingestion of clippings from the plant or inadvertent incorporation of leaves into hay are two common exposure scenarios. Toxicity is retained in dried plant tissues.[16]

The toxicity of oleander results from the presence of several cardiac glycosides in the plant, the most important of which is oleandrin. Cardiac glycosides such as oleandrin cause intoxication as a result of inhibition of Na$^+$-K$^+$ ATPase.[48] Oleander is among the more toxic plants; ingesting as little as 0.005% body weight (equivalent to 10–20 leaves for an adult horse) can be lethal.[47] Horses given 40 mg/kg body weight of green oleander leaves consistently develop clinical signs.[49]

Cardiac glycosides are found in a variety of other unrelated plants including foxglove (*Digitalis purpurea*), summer pheasant's eye (*Adonis aestivalis*), lily-of-the-valley (*Convallaria majalis*), dogbane (*Apocyanum* spp.), and some species of milkweed (*Asclepias* spp.).[23]

Clinical features

Clinical signs of intoxication generally develop within 2 hours and include abdominal pain, weakness, and excessive salivation. Cardiac signs include bradycardia or tachycardia, weak and irregular pulse, heart block, and ventricular arrhythmias. Excitement, periodic seizures, dyspnea, and coma precede death. Myocardial damage (**10.17**) results in high serum creatinine kinase activity.[50] Animals ingesting oleander are often found dead without premonitory signs.

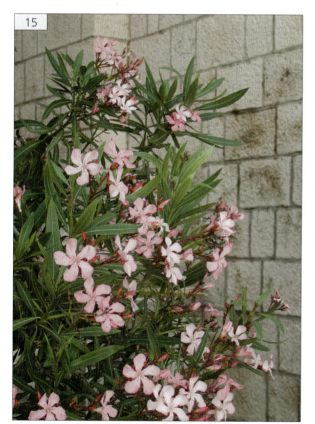

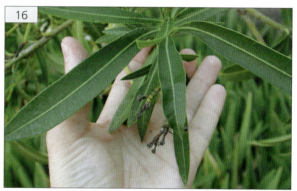

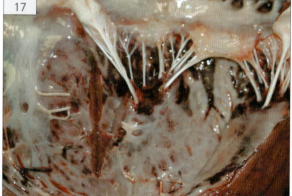

10.15 *Nerium oleander* (oleander) flowers and leaves.

10.16 *Nerium oleander* (oleander) leaves.

10.17 Heart from an oleander intoxicated horse showing significant endocardial hemorrhage, especially associated with the papillary muscle. (Courtesy Dr Francisco Uzal)

Differential diagnosis

Ionophore intoxication; cyanide intoxication; OP or carbamate insecticide intoxication; exposure to neurotoxic plants such as poison hemlock (*Conium maculatum*), water hemlock (*Cicuta maculate*), tree tobacco (*Nicotiana glauca*), lupine (*Lupinus* spp.); *Taxus* spp. intoxication; Star-of-Bethlehem (*Ornithogalum* spp.) intoxication; myocarditis; endocarditis; intestinal compromise (e.g. volvulus, intussusception).

Diagnosis

Diagnosis of oleander intoxication relies on evidence of exposure to the plant, consistent clinical signs, evidence of myocardial damage (ECG or cardiac-specific clinical pathologic changes), and detection of oleandrin in serum or GI tract contents.

Management/treatment

Early recognition of exposure is critical to case outcome. Administration of repeated doses of an adsorbent such as activated charcoal is recommended. Although activated charcoal is preferred over other adsorbents, such as bentonite, they should be given if activated charcoal is not available.

If possible, continuous monitoring of heart rate and rhythm is recommended. Cardiac arrhythmias are treated according to their nature (see Chapter 4).

Antidigoxin fragment antigen binding (Fab) fragments have been shown to cross-react with oleandrin and are a safe and effective treatment for cardiac arrhythmias[51,52]; however, the expense may be prohibitive.

Pyrrolizidine alkaloids
Key points

- A number of plants contain pyrrolizidine alkaloids. Disease is most often associated with chronic ingestion of pyrrolizidine alkaloid-containing plants.
- There are a large number of pyrrolizidine alkaloids, which vary in their toxicity.
- The target organ is the liver. Often, by the time that liver damage is noted, it is extensive and the prognosis is poor.
- The antemortem diagnosis of pyrrolizidine alkaloid intoxication is difficult since exposure to pyrrolizidine alkaloid-containing plants may have been many weeks prior to the onset of clinical signs.

Definition/overview

Over 350 pyrrolizidine alkaloids have been identified in a wide variety of plant species; approximately half of the pyrrolizidine alkaloids are considered to be toxic. Important pyrrolizidine alkaloid-containing genera include *Senecio* spp. (**10.18**), *Amsinckia intermedia* (**10.19**), *Cynoglossum officinale* (**10.20**), and *Crotalaria* spp. (**10.21**).[53]

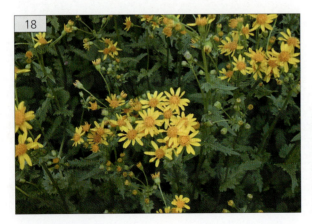

10.18 *Senecio* spp. (ragwort).

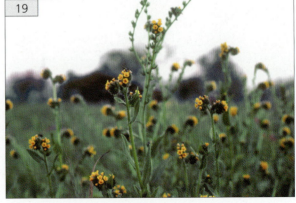

10.19 *Amsinckia* spp. (fiddleneck).

Etiology/pathogenesis

The palatability of many pyrrolizidine alkaloid-containing plants is variable along with the concentration of pyrrolizidine alkaloids. While animals are often exposed to pyrrolizidine alkaloid-containing plants in pastures, contaminated hay or grains contaminated with pyrrolizidine alkaloid-containing seeds are other exposure scenarios.[14]

Pyrrolizidine alkaloids require bioactivation for toxicity.[14] Bioactivation occurs in the liver and results in the formation of reactive electrophilic pyrroles, which cross-link with DNA, proteins, amino acids, and glutathione, forming pyrrolizidine alkaloid adducts. Depending on the extent, importance, and location of the reaction with cellular components, adduct formation causes the cytotoxic and antimitotic effects of pyrrolizidine alkaloids. With more chronic exposure, affected hepatocytes grow without dividing, resulting in megalocytes. As hepatocytes die they are replaced by fibrosis, which is irreversible.[14] More acute exposure results in hemorrhage and hepatocyte necrosis.

The toxicity of pyrrolizidine alkaloids is species specific; goats and sheep are relatively resistant, while pigs are very susceptible. Cattle and horses are intermediate in sensitivity.[53] Pyrrolizidine alkaloid toxicity is also dependent on age, sex, and nutritional status of an animal.

Clinical features

Acute and chronic intoxications occur, although chronic intoxications are more common. In most species, the liver is the target organ and clinical signs

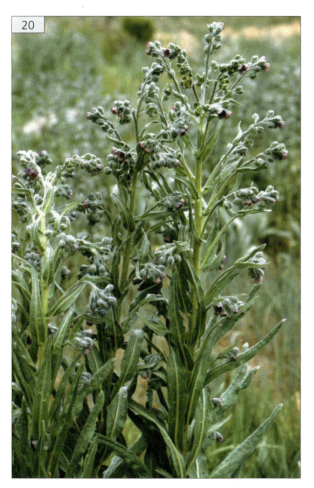

10.20 *Cynoglossum officinale* (hound's tongue).

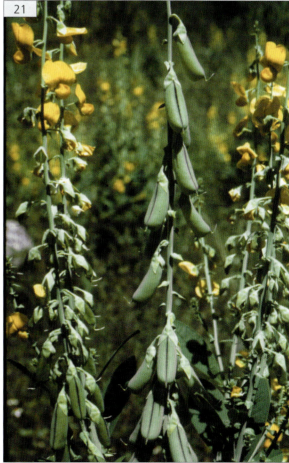

10.21 *Crotalaria spectabilis* (rattlebox).

include photosensitivity, icterus, unthrifty appearance with poor hair coat, diarrhea or constipation, weight loss and HE, disorientation, unawareness of surroundings and external stimuli, head pressing, blindness, and aggression.[54–56] Clinical signs often do not become apparent until many months after exposure has ceased. Animals with chronic disease develop transient increases in concentration of aspartate aminotransferase, sorbitol dehydrogenase, alkaline phosphatase, and gamma glutamyl transferase, along with mild increases in the concentration of serum bilirubin and bile acids.

Acutely affected animals show signs consistent with acute liver failure including anorexia, dullness, icterus, visceral edema, and ascites. Liver-specific clinical chemistry changes are much more dramatic than in the chronically affected animal.

Differential diagnosis

Alsike (*Trifolium hybridum*) or red (*Trifolium pretense*) clover intoxication; fumonisin intoxication (equine leukoencephalomalacia); aflatoxicosis; nigropallidal encephalomalacia (*Centaurea* spp. intoxication); viral encephalitides; EPM; numerous hepatotoxic chemicals; acute hepatitis (Theiler's disease); liver abscess; cholilithiasis.

Diagnosis

An antemortem diagnosis of pyrrolizidine alkaloid intoxication can be difficult if exposure occurred well before the onset of clinical signs. Examination of pastures and hay for the presence of pyrrolizidine alkaloid-containing plants should be performed. Gamma glutamyl transferase is the earliest and most consistent enzyme to increase following toxic exposures.[57,58] However, the best diagnostic aid is a liver biopsy, since pathologic liver lesions (megalocytosis, centrilobular and periportal fibrosis, and biliary hyperplasia) are highly suggestive of intoxication.[57]

Management/treatment

The progressive nature of chronic pyrrolizidine alkaloid intoxication often makes treatment unrewarding. Feeding a good-quality, low-protein diet is recommended. Administering branched chain amino acids to patients with HE may help alleviate signs, at least temporarily.[56]

White snakeroot (*Eupatorium rugosum*)
Key points

- White snakeroot (*Eupatorium rugosum*) is a common plant species that is adaptive to different growing conditions and can be found in open shady areas with open bare ground.
- Intoxication requires large ingestions over days to weeks.
- The toxin is passed in milk and can intoxicate nursing foals.
- Treatment is symptomatic and supportive; the prognosis is poor.

Definition/overview

White snakeroot (**10.22, 10.23**) is found in open shady areas with open bare ground in well-drained, rich soils of wooded areas (e.g. the eastern USA).[23]

Etiology/pathogenesis

The toxin in white snakeroot, called tremetol, is a high molecular weight, fat-soluble alcohol. Tremetol is cardiotoxic, although its mechanism of toxic action is not known. Necrosis of the myocardial and skeletal muscle cells occurs. The lipophilic nature of the toxin leads to a relatively long half-life, accumulation of the toxin in the body with continued intake, and its excretion into milk. The plant retains its toxicity when dry.[59] Consumption of the dried plant equivalent to 0.5–2.0% body weight on a dry matter basis or 1–10% on a wet matter basis is lethal.[14]

Clinical features

Clinical signs can occur within several days to several weeks of consumption. Stress appears to precipitate clinical signs. Clinical signs include dullness, sluggishness, stiff gait, ataxia, crossing of the hindlimbs, wide stance, partial throat paralysis and choke, severe sweating, dyspnea, possible hypothermia, cardiac arrhythmias, and death[14,59–61] Atrioventricular block, ventricular premature beats, and marked ST segment depression have been noted clinically.[59] Clinical pathologic findings can include hematuria, hemoglobinuria, proteinuria, mildly high serum alkaline phosphatase concentration, high aspartate aminotransferase concentration, and markedly high creatinine kinase activity.[24]

In horses, myocardial damage is generally more severe than skeletal muscle damage. In addition to myocardial necrosis, moderate to severe hepatic centrilobular vacuolation and myoglobinuric nephrosis have been noted.[14]

Death generally occurs within 1–2 days of the onset of clinical signs.[23] Marked myocardial fibrosis can be a long-term sequela in horses that survive.[61]

Differential diagnosis

Ionophore intoxication; gossypol intoxication; blister beetle intoxication; botulism; cholinesterase-inhibitor (OP/carbamate insecticide) intoxication; selenium or vitamin E deficiency.

Diagnosis

Diagnosis relies on evidence of consumption of the plant and consistent clinical findings. Although the toxin has been identified, tests for its detection are not routinely available.

Management/treatment

Treatment is symptomatic and supportive. The prognosis is poor.[24] Horses should be immediately removed from access to the plant. The cumulative nature of the toxin generally precludes effective GI tract decontamination, although a dose of activated charcoal is probably indicated. Since tremetol is excreted in milk and nursing animals are at risk for intoxication, nursing foals can be affected even though the dam is asymptomatic.[23]

Yellow-star thistle and Russian knapweed
Key points

- Horses need to ingest a fairly large amount of yellow-star thistle and Russian knapweed (*Centaurea* spp.) for clinical signs to occur.
- The plant toxin has not been conclusively identified.
- Signs are associated with a sudden lack of coordination of the facial and oral muscles.
- Death is due to dehydration, starvation, or aspiration pneumonia.
- There is no effective treatment.

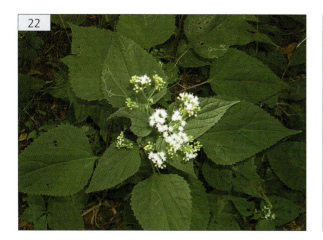

10.22 *Eupatorium rugosum* (white snakeroot) leaves and flowers.

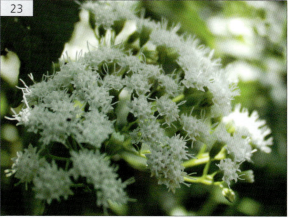

10.23 *Eupatorium rugosum* (white snakeroot) flowers.

Definition/overview

Species of *Centaurea* (*C. solstitialis* [yellow-star thistle, **10.24, 10.25**]; *C. repens* [Russian knapweed]; *C. melitensis* [Malta-star thistle]) cause equine nigropallidal encephalomalcia (chewing disease).[14] *Centaurea* spp. exhibit the greatest diversity in the Mediterranean region, although a few species are native to the Americas and Australia.[23]

Etiology/pathogenesis

Intoxication requires continuous ingestion of large quantities of the plant for several weeks. Only horses are affected and younger horses seem more susceptible than older animals. Experimentally, horses eating at least 60% up to 200% of their body weight of *Centaurea* spp. over 3–11 weeks exhibit clinical signs.[62] The responsible plant constituent has not been identified, although the sequiterpene lactone, repin, has been implicated.[63] Plants retain their toxicity in hay.

Clinical features

Signs of intoxication include a sudden lack of coordination of the facial and oral muscles necessary for effective eating and drinking.[14,23] Swallowing can still occur and animals are often noted to put their muzzle deeply into water troughs or buckets. Facial muscles become hypertonic and a characteristic fixed facial expression is noted. There may be constant but ineffective chewing movements. Weight loss and dullness are seen. The gait is initially normal, although there can be aimless walking and circling, intermittent stiffness, slowness, ataxia, and proprioceptive deficits. Animals eventually die from dehydration, starvation, or aspiration pneumonia.

Differential diagnosis

EPM; guttural pouch mycosis; dental or oral disease.

Diagnosis

An antemortem diagnosis of equine nigropallidal encephalomalcia is dependent on a history of exposure to *Centaurea* spp. and the characteristic clinical signs. MRI to identify the brain lesion (**10.26, 10.27**) has been used successfully.[64] Diagnosis is confirmed at necropsy, with characteristic malacic lesions in the substantia nigra and globus pallidus of the brain.

Management/treatment

Once clinical signs occur, animals do not recover. Euthanasia of affected horses is recommended.

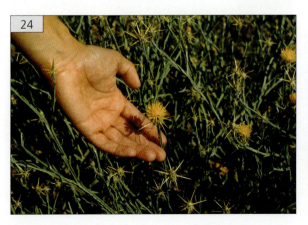

10.24 *Centaurea solstitialis* (yellow star thistle).

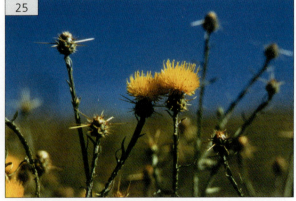

10.25 *Centaurea solstitialis* (yellow star thistle) flower.

Mycotoxins

Aflatoxins

Key points

- Aflatoxins are sporadically found in grains; however, aflatoxicosis is a relatively rare intoxication of horses.
- Chronic intoxication is more likely than acute intoxication.
- The liver is the primary target organ.
- Diagnosis is generally confirmed by analysis of feed, although obtaining a representative feed sample is critical.
- Treatment is symptomatic and supportive; the prognosis is generally poor.

Definition/overview

Aflatoxins (B_1, B_2, G_1, and G_2) occur in grains such as corn, milo cottonseed, and peanuts.[65] They are produced by *Aspergillus flavus* and *Aspergillus parasiticus*, which are most commonly found in warm, humid regions.

Etiology/pathogenesis

Aflatoxin B_1 is of most toxicologic concern. It is metabolized in the liver to a reactive epoxide that binds covalently to nucleic acids and proteins in the liver, producing the characteristic liver lesions of fatty change and necrosis. Although natural cases of aflatoxicosis in horses are infrequently reported, certainly the risk for exposure is present.[66–68] Acute or chronic intoxication can occur depending on the degree and length of exposure. Dietary concentrations of total aflatoxins of 0.5–1.0 parts per million can cause weight loss and liver damage.[69] Single, oral doses of aflatoxin B_1 as low as 2 mg/kg can be lethal.[70] Experimentally, dietary concentrations of approximately 3.8 parts per million caused death in ponies dosed for 37–39 days.[71] Chronic exposure to dietary concentrations of total aflatoxins >200 parts per billion is likely to be associated with adverse effects.[65]

Clinical features

Clinical signs of aflatoxicosis are dependent on whether acute or chronic liver disease is present. Acutely, signs can include fever, anorexia, ataxia, colic, tachycardia, seizures, icterus, hematochezia, and tenesmus.[65,72] HE, manifested as belligerence, somnolence or dullness, circling, blindness, and head pressing is more likely to be associated with chronic aflatoxicosis.

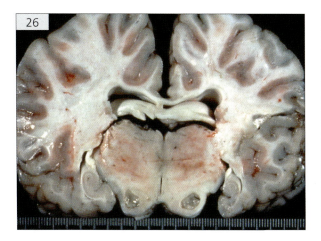

10.26 Cross-section through the brain of a horse with nigropallidal encephalomalacia showing bilaterally symmetric foci of malacia in the substantial nigra.

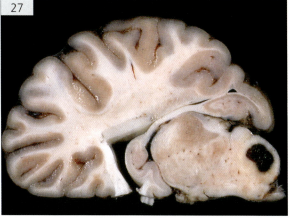

10.27 Sagittal section through the brain of a horse with nigropallidal encephalomalacia showing bilaterally symmetric foci of malacia in the substantial nigra.

Differential diagnosis

Acute: iron and fumonisin mycotoxin intoxications; drug-induced hepatopathy; Theiler's disease; Tyzzer's disease; hyperlipemia; infectious necrotic hepatitis; cholangiohepatitis; acute biliary obstruction; parasite-induced hepatitis; virus-induced hepatitis. Chronic: pyrrolizidine alkaloid intoxication; pasture-associated hepatopathy (alsike clover or Klein grass); chronic active hepatitis; cholelithiasis; neoplasia; amyloidosis; chronic hypoxia.

Diagnosis

Diagnosis of aflatoxicosis depends on the presence of hepatic disease and detection of potentially toxic concentrations of aflatoxins in representative feed samples. Unfortunately, as with other mycotoxins, failure to detect aflatoxins in a feed sample does not rule out animal exposure, since the offending feed may have already been consumed or non-representative samples may have been collected for analysis. A liver biopsy may be highly suggestive of aflatoxin exposure.

Management/treatment

There is no antidote for aflatoxicosis. Often, by the time aflatoxicosis is suspected, liver damage is severe. Affected feed should be removed immediately. Supportive treatment for either acute or chronic liver failure should be instituted. IV fluids (acetated Ringers solution with 20–40 mEq/l KCl) and dextrose (50 g/l) should be given continuously.[73] Correction of fluid and acid–base deficits may be necessary. Animals that are anorectic and/or hypoglycemic should receive 5% dextrose (2 ml/kg/hour) initially followed by 2.5–5.0% in 0.45% saline.

Horses with HE may need sedation if dysphoric or demented (xylazine, 0.2–0.4 mg/kg IV).[74] Neomycin (10 g/500 kg) should be given orally mixed in molasses via a syringe q8h for 2 days.[73] High-carbohydrate, low-protein diets should be offered frequently in small amounts. Coagulopathy should be treated with vitamin K_1 at 0.5–1.0 mg/kg.[65] Horses with moderate to severe hepatic fibrosis have a guarded to poor prognosis for surviving more than 2 years.[73]

Ergot alkaloids
Key points

- Ergot alkaloids are associated with classical ergotism following ingestion of ergotized grains or reproductive problems due to grazing endophyte infected tall fescue.
- Classical ergotism in horses is rare.
- Tall fescue intoxication is a problem associated with mares grazing the grass during late pregnancy.
- The most serious consequences of pregnant mares grazing tall fescue is the occurrence of dystocia and/or birth of dysmature and non-viable foals.
- Prevention of intoxication relies on removal of the mare from tall fescue pastures late in gestation. Pharmacologic intervention using dopamine antagonists is also possible to prevent the occurrence of clinical signs

Definition/overview

A number of ergot alkaloids have been identified. They are produced by *Claviceps purpurea*, which infests cereal grains such as rye, triticale, wheat, barley, and oats, and *Neotyphodium coenophialum*, an endophytic fungus of tall fescue. Ergot alkaloids can be divided into two categories: (1) the ergopeptine alkaloids including ergotamine, ergocristine, ergosine, ergocryptine, ergocornine, and ergovaline and (2) the ergoline alkaloids including lysergic acid, lysergol, lysergic acid amide, and ergonovine.[75]

Etiology/pathogenesis

Claviceps purpurea has a fairly complex life-cycle. It produces visible dark brown, purple or black sclerotia or 'ergot' bodies that replace the ovarian tissue of infected cereal grains.[76] In addition to affected grains, a number of grasses are infested by *Claviceps purpurea* and can be associated with ergot alkaloid intoxication. Ergot alkaloids are also produced in tall fescue grass (*Festuca arundinacea*, **10.28**) by a fungal endophyte called *Neotyphodium coenophialum* (**10.29**).[77] Thus, classic 'ergotism' following ingestion of ergot-contaminated grains and tall fescue toxicosis associated with ingestion of endophyte-infested tall fescue pasture or hay should perhaps be more appropriately termed ergot alkaloid intoxication. It appears that the ergopeptine alkaloids are primarily responsible for the clinical signs associated with ergotism and play a major role in the pathogenesis of intoxication from tall fescue, although other compounds may contribute to the latter syndrome.[77]

Ergopeptine alkaloids cause vasoconstriction secondary to D_1-dopaminergic receptor inhibition and partial agonism of α_1-adrenergic and serotonin receptors.[75] Additionally, stimulation of D_2-dopamine receptors decreases prolactin secretion by lactotropes in the anterior pituitary.[78] A number of ergot alkaloids have also been shown *in vitro* to stimulate the release of dopamine in the brain.[79] Vasoconstriction and hypoprolactinemia are directly or indirectly associated with the pathogenesis of ergot alkaloid intoxication syndromes.[75] Progesterone concentrations are also lowered in mares grazing tall fescue; this likely exacerbates the effects of hypoprolactinemia.[80] Ergot alkaloids also compromise fetal production of corticotropin-releasing hormone, adrenocorticotropic hormone, and cortisol.[80,81] These alterations may be responsible for the prolonged gestation noted in mares.

Tall fescue toxicosis is by far the most common syndrome produced by ergot alkaloids in horses. A number of ergot alkaloids have been isolated from endophyte-infested tall fescue, but ergovaline accounts for over 80% of the total ergot alkaloid content of tall fescue.[82] Ergovaline concentrations >200 parts per billion are likely to be associated with adverse effects in mares.[80] The most critical time for exposure to endophyte-infested tall fescue is during the last 30 days of pregnancy.[83] Mares removed from the pasture before gestation day 300 foal normally.

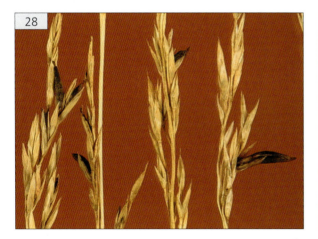

10.28 Ergot bodies replacing the seed heads in rye grass.

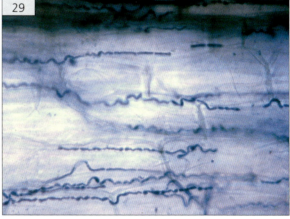

10.29 Photomicrograph of *Neotyphodium coenophialum*, the endopyte of *Festuca arundinacea* Shreb. (tall fescue grass).

Clinical features

Tall fescue toxicosis of horses is most commonly manifested as a disease syndrome of mares during late gestation and the early postpartum period. The clinical signs of intoxication are almost exclusively limited to impairment of reproductive function and poor fetal and neonatal viability.[77,84] Agalactia, prolonged gestation, dystocia, abortion, placental abnormalities (premature placental separation, thickening and edema of fetal membranes, and retained placenta) and subfertility are associated with ergot alkaloid intoxication in pregnant mares. Signs of impending parturition such as rapid increase in udder development and waxing are often minimal. Prolonged gestation results in large fetal sizes, which, in turn, contributes to a high incidence of dystocia (**10.30**). Potentially life-threatening maternal tissue trauma, metritis, septicemia, endotoxemia, and laminitis are also common sequelae.[85,86]

Fetal asphyxia can occur. This may be secondary to edema, fibrosis, and mucoid degeneration of placental arteries in affected mares.[87] Stillbirths are common and stillbirths in experimental studies have ranged from 50 to 86%.[80] FPT, neonatal septicemia, and decreased viability commonly occur in foals born alive. Affected foals are also dysmature, which is characterized by long and lanky bodies with a prominent skeleton and poor musculature, long fine hair coats, overgrown hooves, and non-erupted or irregular incisor teeth (**10.31**).[80] Foals may be hypothyroid at birth, which may contribute to poor suckling, hypothermia, incoordination, and poor righting reflexes.[80]

Differential diagnosis

Classical ergotism: frostbite. Tall fescue intoxication: dystocia (fetal malpositions or deformities [e.g. ankylosis or hydrocephalus]; small pelvic opening; uterine inertia; incomplete cervical dilation; trauma; uterine torsion. Placentitis: bacterial infection; viral infection; fungal pathogens. Foal dysmaturity: severe maternal illness; placental insufficiency; congential hypothyroidism.

Diagnosis

Diagnosis of classical ergotism is based on classical signs of extremity gangrene, visual detection of ergot bodies in infected grains, and measurement of ergot alkaloids. Tall fescue-associated reproductive problems are associated with pasture ergovaline concentrations of 200 parts per billion or greater. The presence of *Neotyphodium coenophialum* can be determined in tall fescue microscopically. The combination of clinical signs in mares and foals is relatively unique. Pathologic examination of foals that die and their placentas may be useful to rule out infectious etiologies.

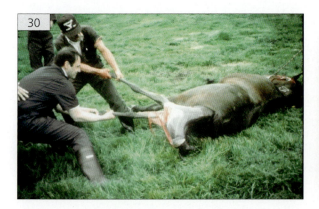

10.30 Dystocia in a mare that had grazed endophyte-infected tall fescue prior to parturition. (Courtesy John Dascanio)

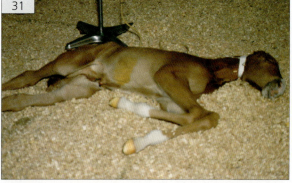

10.31 Foal born to a mare that had grazed endophyte-infected tall fescue prior to parturition. The foal is long and lanky and was born weak.

Management/treatment

Gravid mares past their foaling date should be removed from fescue pasture or hay as soon as possible. Udder development and relaxation of the tail-head and vulva can be expected within 48 hours. Dopamine D_2-receptor antagonists such as domperidone (1.1 mg/kg PO q24h) can be given to mares past their foaling date to stimulate milk production.[80] If only a few doses of domperidone are given pre-partum, it can be continued post-partum (1.1 mg/kg PO q12h) to ensure maximum milk production. Agalactic mares that have already foaled can be given domperidone (1.1 mg/kg PO q12h) for several days to try to stimulate milk production. A variety of other dopamine D_2-receptor antagonists, such as perphenazine, sulpiride, and acepromazine, have also been used successfully.[88,89] Reserpine, which decreases brain concentrations of dopamine, serotonin, and norepinephrine, can be effective. The advantage of domperidone is that CNS function is not altered in the mare since it does not cross the blood–brain barrier.[80,88] Mares with dystocia (see Chapter 5) and affected neonates (see Chapter 9) generally require intensive therapy. Affected foals should be closely monitored. Colostrum or plasma should be given to provide needed immunoglobulins. If colostrum is used, serum IgG should be monitored to ensure adequate absorption.[90] Administration of fluids and antimicrobial drugs are generally necessary.[77,86]

Exposure to higher concentrations of ergot alkaloids in *Claviceps pupurea*-infested grains, as compared with concentrations typically found in *Neotyphodium coenophialum*-infested tall fescue, can cause gangrenous ergotism and death of horses.[75] Fortunately, the occurrence of gangrenous ergotism is rare.

Fumonisin mycotoxins

Key points

- Fumonisins are a group of mycotoxins, produced by the fungus *Fusarium verticillioides* (formerly *Fusarium moniliforme*), which are responsible for the sporadically-occurring disease equine leukoencephalomalacia, also referred to as moldy corn disease.

- The most toxic fumonisin is fumonisin B_1.
- Equine leukoencephalomalacia is a fatal disease characterized by rapidly progressing neurologic impairment in horses and other equids. Other target organs include the liver and, possibly, the heart.
- Distinctive lesions include softening and necrosis of cerebral white matter, as well as swollen and discolored livers.
- Once clinical signs are apparent, the prognosis is poor.
- There is no specific treatment for affected horses.

Definition/overview

Fumonisin mycotoxins cause equine leukoencephalomalacia (also called moldy corn disease), a rapidly progressing and generally fatal neurologic disease of horses.[91,92]

Etiology/pathogenesis

The mycotoxins are produced on corn that has been infected by *Fusarium verticilliodes* (formerly *Fusarium moniliforme*) and *Fusarium proliferatum*, which are ubiquitous throughout the world.[65,93] Several fumonisins have been identified (B_1, B_2, and B_3); fumonisins B_1 and B_2 are the most toxic. Equine leukoencephalomalacia is a sporadically occurring disease most commonly noted in temperate, humid climates after a dry summer and wet harvest season. Horses are the most sensitive species. Development of disease depends on the concentration of fumonisin in the feed and the length of exposure. Concentrations in feed of 10 parts per million fed for 30 days can be lethal.[94,95]

Fumonisins interfere with sphingolipid metabolism, which results in vascular endothelial damage in the brain and hepatotoxicity.[96] Cardiovascular dysfunction may also play a role in the pathogenesis of equine leukoencephalomalacia.[97] Neurotoxicity is more common than hepatotoxicity, but both can occur simultaneously.[98] Hepatotoxicity is more likely to be associated with short-term, high-level exposures, while neurotoxicity is more likely with long-term, low-level exposures.[98]

Clinical features

Neurologic signs include anorexia, depression with lack of response to stimuli or, alternatively, hyperexcitability, progressive ataxia with proprioceptive deficits, delirium, blindness, aimless wandering, recumbency, coma, and death from as little as 12 hours to as much as 1 week after the onset of clinical signs.[65] Signs associated with hepatotoxicity include icterus, mucous membrane petechiae, and swelling of the lips and muzzle.[99]

Differential diagnosis

Locoism; tremorgenic mycotoxins; cholinesterase-inhibitor (OP or carbamate insecticide) intoxication; strychnine intoxication; metaldehyde intoxication; 4-aminopyridine intoxication; levamisole intoxication; rabies; equine encephalomyelitis; equine herpesvirus myeloencephalopathy; hepatoencephalopathy; head trauma; bacterial meningioencephalitis.

Diagnosis

Antemortem diagnosis of equine leukoencephalomalacia relies on detection of potentially toxic concentrations of fumonisins in representative feed samples (more than 5 parts per million in the grain ration or more than 1 part per million in the total ration) and the presence of acute neurologic disease. Increases in serum sphinganine:sphingosine ratios are perhaps the earliest manifestation of intoxication, but few laboratories offer the analysis.[100]

Management/treatment

Severe and irreversible cerebral necrosis (**10.32**) is generally present in animals with neurologic signs. The prognosis is poor and euthanasia should be considered.[101] Although less common, horses with only hepatic affects have a more favorable outcome. Contaminated feed should be removed immediately. There is no antidote for equine leukoencephalomalacia, therefore treatment is exclusively supportive. Hyperexcitable horses should be sedated. Feed and water can be given via a nasogastric tube if horses are not able to eat or drink on their own. Mannitol or DMSO may help alleviate cerebral edema. GI tract decontamination is generally not useful because by the time of onset of clinical signs, exposure has been over days to weeks.

Slaframine

Key points

- Slaframine, produced by *Rhizoctonia leguminicola* in several clovers, causes a hypersalivation syndrome in horses.
- The disease occurs sporadically and is generally self-limiting once animals are removed from affected pastures or hay.
- Treatment is often not necessary.

Definition/overview

Rhizoctonia leguminicola is a ubiquitous soil fungus that parasitizes red clover (*Trifolium pratense*, **10.33**) and, less frequently, other legume forages.[65,102]

Etiology/pathogenesis

Fungal infection occurs in cool, high-moisture conditions, resulting in the plant disease 'black-patch' (**10.34**). The fungus elaborates a toxin called slaframine, which is responsible for the disease called 'slobbers' in horses. The occurrence of slaframine is most often associated with second cutting red clover hay.[65] The toxin slowly degrades in hay over a several month period.[103]

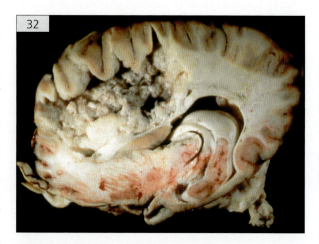

10.32 Brain from a horse that died from equine leukoencephalomalacia showing extensive white matter liquefactive necrosis.

Clinical features

Slaframine is bioactivated by the liver to a metabolite with acetylcholine-like activity. Clinical signs are due to muscarinic receptor stimulation and include excessive salivation, lacrimation, polyuria, and diarrhea.[65] Bradycardia and bradypnea also occur. Affected animals are often anorectic and can experience mild colic. Signs can begin within several minutes of ingesting infected red clover and last for several days following cessation of exposure. While the clinical signs are dramatic, mortality is rare and most animals recover uneventfully once removed from infected pastures or hay. Interestingly, once signs occur, atropine (and presumably other antimuscarinic drugs) is not effective.[65]

Differential diagnosis

Cholinesterase-inhibiting insecticides (OP and carbamate insecticides); foreign objects, such as awns, in the oropharyngeal region; choke; dental disease; stomatitis.

Diagnosis

The fungus can be identified on infected clovers. However, diagnosis generally relies on a history of exposure to susceptible clovers, the occurrence of typical clinical signs, and the relatively rapid cessation of signs once removed from suspect pastures or hay. Detection of slaframine is possible, but few laboratories offer such testing.

Management/treatment

Affected horses are generally successfully managed by removing them from infected pastures. Response to atropine is often poor and is generally not indicated or advisable.

Tremorgenic mycotoxins
Key points

- Several families of tremogenic mycotoxins have been characterized including the lolitrems and paspalitrems.
- Mycotoxin occurrence is due to the presence of invasive fungi in susceptible plant species.
- As the name implies, tremogenic mycotoxins cause nervous system stimulation, especially when animals are excited or stressed. Signs resolve once animals calm down.
- Mortality is low and is generally associated with trauma during a tremorgenic episode.
- Animals generally recover following cessation of exposure to infected plants.

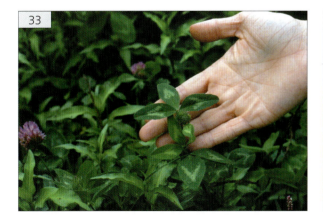

10.33 *Trifolium pretense* (red clover), a common host for the fungus *Rhizoctonia leguminicola*, which produces slaframine.

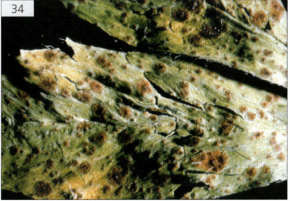

10.34 Black-patch disease of *Trifolium pretense* (red clover). Note the dark patches of fungal infection on the leaves.

Definition/overview

There are two families of tremorgenic mycotoxins, called paspalitrems and lolitrems.[65] Paspalitrems (paspalinine, paspalitrems A and B) are produced by *Claviceps paspali*, which invades seed heads of dallis grass (*Paspalum dilatatum*) and bahia grass (*Bahia oppositifolia*). Lolitrems (lolitrems A, B, C, and D) are produced by a fungal endophyte of perennial ryegrass (*Lolium perenne*) called *Neotyphodium lolii*. Intoxication occurs most commonly in animals at pasture, although a complete pelleted ration containing perennial ryegrass straw caused tremorgenic disease in ponies.[104] Feeding perennial ryegrass seed screenings has also caused intoxication in horses.[105]

Etiology/pathogenesis

Tremorgenic mycotoxins cause CNS stimulation, possibly as a result of reduction in inhibitory neurotransmitter concentrations (GABA, glycine) in the brain or increases in excitatory amino acids.[65,106] *In vitro*, lolitrem B is a potent inhibitor of large conductance, calcium-activated potassium channels, which may mediate some of the signs associated with perennial ryegrass staggers.[107] The toxicity of the compounds is not well defined, but plant concentrations of lolitrem B exceeding 2 parts per million (dry weight) are associated with the occurrence of clinical signs.

Clinical features

Clinical signs are generally mild when animals are at rest, but when stimulated or forced to move, signs initially include fine muscle tremors around the head and neck, stiffness, ataxia, and hypermetria. More severe tremors, seizures, and opisthotonus follow the initial clinical signs.[65] During tremorgenic episodes, animals can become belligerent and dangerous. If left undisturbed, signs subside quickly. Signs caused by paspalitrems are considered to be less severe than those caused by lolitrems. Morbidity is high with low mortality. Death is most likely to occur due to self-induced injury.

Differential diagnosis

Locoism (*Astragalus* spp. or *Oxytropis* spp.) intoxication; white snakeroot (*Eupatorium rugosum*) intoxication.

Diagnosis

Diagnosis of disease due to tremogenic mycotoxins generally relies on the occurrence of typical clinical signs associated with the consumption of infected grasses. The endophytic fungi associated with mycotoxin production can be identified. Testing forage for lolitrems is possible, but such testing is not widely available. A mouse bioassay for lolitrems has been used for diagnostic purposes.

Management/treatment

Treatment of affected animals primarily consists in ceasing exposure to toxic pasture or hay. Keeping the animal quiet is important to reduce tremorgenic episodes. Although the lolitrems have a long duration of action and produce tremors that last for many hours, their neurotoxic effects are completely reversible in mice.[108]

Algal toxins
Key points

- Toxigenic blue-green algae produce several potent toxins that affect either the liver (microcystin) or the nervous system (anatoxin-a and anatoxin-a$_s$).
- Toxin production is associated with certain environmental conditions that result in the rapid proliferation of algae in bodies of water.
- The toxicity of the toxins and the peracute nature of intoxications often precludes effective treatment.
- Initial treatment for microcystin-associated liver damage should focus on treating hypovolemic shock, whereas controlling muscle tremors or providing ventilatory support and controlling cholinergic signs should be the initial concern following exposure to anatoxin-a and anatoxin-a$_s$, respectively.

Definition/overview

Although there are no literature reports of intoxication of horses as a result of blue-green algal (**10.35**) toxin ingestion, the occurrence of toxin-producing algae in fresh surface waters is common.

Etiology/pathogenesis

There are a variety of blue-green algae that are toxigenic. The three toxins of most concern are the hepatotoxic microcystins (many individual microcystins have been identified, but microcystin LR is the most prominent) and the neurotoxic anatoxin-a and anatoxin-a$_s$.[24,109,110] Microcystins are produced by *Microcystis* spp. (**10.36**), *Anabaena* spp. (**10.37**), and *Planktothrix* spp. among others. Anatoxin-a and anatoxin-a$_s$ are produced by *Anabaena* spp., *Plankothrix* spp., *Oscillatoria* spp., *Microcystis* spp., *Aphanizomenon* spp., *Cylindrospermum* spp., and *Phormidium* spp.[110] Anatoxin-a and anatoxin-a$_s$ are toxins produced primarily by cyanobacteria in the *Anabaena* genus. Toxins are elaborated following rapid growth of the algae (algal blooms), which occurs under appropriate environmental conditions. Warm weather and slow moving or stagnant, nutrient-rich waters are especially prone to bloom development.[111] Toxic blooms are most likely to occur from late spring to early fall.

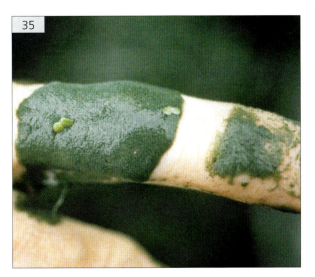

10.35 *Microcystis aeruginosa* bloom material.

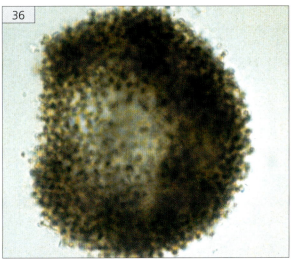

10.36 *Microcystis aeruginosa* colony identified from an intoxicated animal's stomach contents.

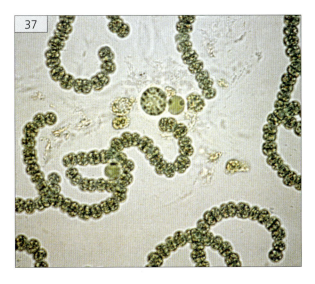

10.37 *Anabaena flos-aquae* colony identified from water containing an algal bloom.

Clinical features

Microcystins: Acute hepatotoxicosis results following exposure to microcystins. Onset of clinical signs can be rapid with death occurring within several hours of exposure. Initial signs include diarrhea, weakness, and pale mucous membranes. There is massive hemorrhage into the liver, which leads to circulatory shock.[110,111] Coagulopathies are possible. Animals that survive can develop hepatogenous photosensitization.

Anatoxin-a: Anatoxin-a is a potent cholinergic agonist at nicotinic acetylcholine receptors in neurons and at neuromuscular junctions.[110] Anatoxin-a ingestion causes rigidity, muscle tremors, cyanosis, and paralysis as a result of nicotinic receptor stimulation.[110] A depolarizing blockade at neuromuscular junctions results in muscle paralysis and death due to respiratory failure. As with microcystins, the onset of clinical signs is rapid.

Anatoxin-a$_s$: Anatoxin-a$_s$ irreversibly inhibits cholinesterase activity and causes a clinical syndrome similar to that caused by OP and carbamate insecticides.[110] However, anatoxin-a$_s$ does not penetrate the blood–brain barrier so signs are due to peripheral muscarinic and nicotinic receptor stimulation. Muscarinic signs include hypersalivation, lacrimation, urination, and defecation. Nicotinic receptor stimulation at neuromuscular junctions causes muscle tremors initially followed by a depolarizing blockade. Death is due to paralysis of respiratory muscles.

Differential diagnosis

Microcystins: Theiler's disease; Tyzzer's disease; hyperlipemia; infectious necrotic hepatitis; cholangiohepatitis; acute biliary obstruction; viral hepatitis; toxic hepatopathy (plants, aflatoxins, iron); parasitic hepatitis.

Anatoxin-a: Nicotine intoxication (most often following exposure to *Nicotiana* spp.); cholinesterase-inhibiting insecticides (OP and carbamate insecticides); tremorgenic mycotoxin intoxication; tetanus; hypocalcemic tetany.

Anatoxin-a$_s$: Cholinesterase-inhibiting insecticides (OP and carbamate insecticides); bacterial or viral gastroenteritis; slaframine intoxication; arsenic intoxication.

Diagnosis

Microcystins: The diagnosis of microcystin intoxication relies on a history of exposure to water sources in which algal blooms have occurred, detection of microcystins in water or samples of GI tract contents, and evidence of a peracute or acute liver disease. Characteristic algal colonies can be identified in water samples or stomach contents. Alternatively, a mouse bioassay can be used to assess the toxicity of bloom material.[111]

Anatoxin-a: As is the case with the microcystins, detection of anatoxin-a in water or samples of GI tract contents will help confirm intoxication. Characteristic algal colonies can be identified in water samples or stomach contents. Alternatively, a mouse bioassay can be used to assess the toxicity of bloom material.[111]

Anatoxin-a$_s$: Diagnosis of anatoxin-a$_s$ intoxication is dependent on identification of toxigenic algae in bloom material or in samples of GI tract contents and detection of anatoxin-a$_s$ in the same samples.[110] Alternatively, a mouse bioassay can be used to assess the toxicity of bloom material.[111]

Management/treatment

Microcystins: The peracute nature of microcystin intoxication often precludes effective treatment. Activated charcoal can be administered to prevent continued absorption of the toxins. Hypovolemic shock should be treated with normal saline with or without dextrose. Vasopressors such as dopamine or dobutamine (see Chapter 13) may be needed. Other therapy is symptomatic and supportive.

Anatoxin-a: Peracute death often precludes effective treatment. There is no effective antidote for anatoxin-a. Administration of activated charcoal to prevent further absorption of the toxin is warranted. Specific measures to control muscle tremors include administration of a benzodiazepine or methocarbamol. Monitoring body temperature and correction of hyperthermia are important if severe muscle tremors are present. Ventilatory support may be needed in cases with respiratory muscle paralysis.

Anatoxin-a$_s$: The rapidity of onset of clinical signs and sudden death often precludes effective treatment. If given early, activated charcoal should be administered. Atropine should be tried in anatoxin-a$_s$-intoxicated animals. However, close monitoring of anticholinergic effects is necessary and the lowest possible dose to control muscarinic signs should be used.

Zootoxins
Cantharidin
Key points

- Cantharidin is a vesicant toxin that is found in the hemolymph of blister beetles (*Epicauta* spp. and *Pyrota* spp.).
- Blister beetles are almost exclusively found in baled alfalfa hay.
- Horses poisoned by cantharidin display clinical signs of severe colic and damage to the GI tract (also the urinary bladder and heart).
- Intoxication can result in hypocalcemia, hypomagnesemia, renal failure, and cardiac abnormalities.
- Intoxicated horses should be treated aggressively; in the absence of intense treatment mortality is high.

Definition/overview

Cantharidiasis or blister beetle poisoning is a common equine intoxication.[112–115] Blister beetles (**10.38**) are most commonly found in alfalfa fields. The majority of blister beetles are found at the periphery of hay fields. Intoxication of horses most often occurs following the ingestion of alfalfa hay or alfalfa products containing blister beetles.[116] Blister beetles are trapped in alfalfa hay in large numbers when the hay is crimped and baled. Cantharidin retains its toxicity in hay.

Etiology/pathogenesis

Cantharidin is a vesicant found in the hemolymph of blister beetles (*Epicauta* spp. and *Pyrota* spp.). It is reportedly lethal to horses at dosages of 1 mg/kg body weight or less. The cantharidin content of beetles varies from 1–5% dry weight. A 500 kg horse would need to consume from 100–500 beetles to reach a lethal dose.[116]

Cantharidin is rapidly absorbed from the GI tract following blister beetle ingestion, with rapid excretion via the kidneys. Cantharidin inhibits phospholipase-2A, which controls cell proliferation, modulates phosphatases and protein kinases, and plays a role in the activity of cellular membrane channels and receptors.[117] Cantharidin is also a vesicant, causing cell damage on contact.

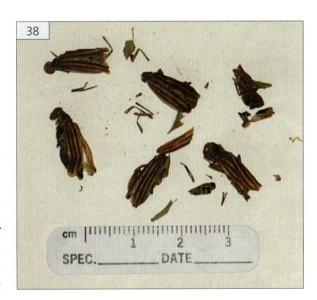

10.38 *Epicauta spp.* (blister beetles) collected from a sample of hay associated with intoxication.

Clinical features

Onset of signs is generally rapid. The most commonly reported signs exhibited by intoxicated horses include abdominal pain, CNS depression, pollakiuria, mucous membrane congestion, anorexia, sweating, fever, tachycardia, tachypnea, delayed CRT, submerging muzzle in water, and diarrhea with or without blood.[114,115] Less frequently reported signs include hematuria, hemoglobinuria, oral erosions, salivation, stiff gait, synchronous diaphragmatic flutter, muscle fasciculations, and sudden death.[114]

Differential diagnosis

Multiple causes of colic; ionophore intoxication; endotoxic shock. Neurologic signs: rabies; viral or bacterial encephalitides; HE; equine leukoencephalomalacia; thiamine deficiency; OP insecticide intoxication; organochlorine intoxication; trauma.

Diagnosis

While clinical pathologic findings are variable, hypocalcemia and hypomagnesemia are frequently reported. Total serum calcium can be as low as 1.12 mmol/l (4.5 mg/dl) and serum magnesium is usually <0.6 mmol/l (1.5 mg/dl).[114] Serum ionized calcium is often normal to slightly decreased. Azotemia is also common.[115] Many affected horses develop hypovolemic shock.

A diagnosis of blister beetle intoxication should be considered in any horse with a sudden onset of abdominal pain or dullness that has been given alfalfa hay or alfalfa products. It is important to examine representative hay samples for the presence of blister beetles, keeping in mind that contamination can affect only a limited portion of hay. Stomach contents and urine can be tested for the presence of cantharidin.[113]

Management/treatment

All symptomatic horses require close monitoring and intensive treatment. The focus of treatment includes: (1) enhancing fecal and urinary elimination of cantharidin; (2) correcting hypotension and dehydration; (3) correcting electrolyte abnormalities (especially calcium and magnesium); and (4) controlling pain. If exposure is recognized early, activated charcoal should be administered. Although administration of mineral oil has been suggested, the reasoning for its use over activated charcoal is dubious.[114] Balanced polyionic fluids should be given for dehydration and hypovolemia. Fluid diuresis may enhance urinary clearance of cantharidin, although its effect on case outcome has not been determined.

Serum calcium concentrations should be monitored frequently. If hypocalcemic, adult horses can be given 500 ml of a commercial calcium-containing fluid (not exceeding 23 g of calcium compound per 100 ml) slowly IV.[117] The calcium solution should be diluted in isotonic fluids to decrease the chance of an adverse cardiac effect. Dilute calcium 1:4 with saline or dextrose if there is a need to administer calcium frequently to control synchronous diaphragmatic flutter or muscle fasciculations. Supplemental magnesium may be needed to correct hypomagnesemia.

Glucocorticosteroids should be administered for shock (prednisolone sodium succinate, 50–100 mg IV). If typical analgesics are inadequate to control pain, detomidine (20–40 µg/kg IV), xylazine (1.1 mg/kg IV), or butorphanol tartrate (0.02–0.1 mg/kg IV q3–4h not to exceed 48 hours) can be used. Broad-spectrum antimicrobial drugs can be given if there is a concern about sepsis as a result of GI tract ulcerations or erosions.

Although the prognosis is guarded for symptomatic animals, relatively good survival rates can be achieved with aggressive supportive care. In one case series, 36 of 70 equids diagnosed with blister beetle intoxication survived.[115] Three to 10 days of treatment were required. Early recognition of intoxication is critical for a successful case outcome.

Snake venoms
Key points

- Most clinically important snake bites in horses are due to snakes in the *Crotalidae* spp. or pit viper family.
- Most snake bites occur from April to October (northern hemisphere) and result from accidental encounters. It is estimated that several hundred horses per year are bitten by pit vipers.
- Most horses are bitten on or near the muzzle, which results in a severe local reaction and commonly airway obstruction. (See also Chapter 3.)

- Snake venoms are complex mixtures of chemicals that can cause a number of systemic pathophysiologic effects.
- Immediate attention is warranted and bitten animals should be taken to a veterinary facility for appropriate monitoring and treatment.
- Attention should be paid to maintaining the airway and cardiovascular function in addition to local wound management.

Definition/overview

Most clinically important snake bites in horses are due to snakes in the *Crotalidae* spp. or pit viper family. Due to the shyness and nocturnal nature of coral snakes, along with their relatively small mouth and fixed fangs, bites to livestock are rare. It has been estimated that 99% of all snake bites to animals are due to pit viper bites.[118] Most snake bites occur from April to October (northern hemisphere) and result from accidental encounters. Horses in the western USA are most likely to be bitten by rattlesnakes.

Etiology/pathogenesis

As with most venoms, pit viper venom is a complex mixture of enzymes and non-enzymatic polypeptides.[119] Proteins include myotoxins, proteases, hyaluronidase, bradykinin-releasing enzyme, and phospholipase A_2. These proteins cause marked local tissue destruction and act systemically to increase capillary permeability. Loss of plasma volume, peripheral pooling of blood, decreased cardiac output, hypoproteinemia, hypotension, and a metabolic acidosis result.[119] Ultimately, acute deaths are due to respiratory and circulatory collapse. In horses, death following snake bites is often attributed to more chronic problems such as heart disease, laminitis, myopathy, and hepatopathy.[120]

Clinical features

Most horses are bitten on or around the muzzle, leading to local tissue damage, edema, and possible airway obstruction (**10.39**).[119] Horses are also bitten on the legs. Trunk bites are uncommon. Due to the size of horses, many animals are not severely affected except for local tissue destruction at the bite site. In addition, snakes that bite defensively inject less venom than offensive or agonal bites; this is more likely to be the case when snakes encounter horses than with more aggressive species such as dogs.

Local reactions are rapid; however, systemic signs can be delayed for several hours. Locally, there is painful swelling, hemorrhage, ecchymoses, and petechiation. Bites around the muzzle can lead to dyspnea. Tachypnea and dyspnea can occur from the systemic effects of the venom as well. There can be tachycardia, dysrhythmias, fever, pyrexia, lethargy, diarrhea, salivation caused by dysphagia, flaccid paralysis, incontinence, tremors, coagulopathy, laminitis, colic, circulatory shock, and coma.[118–120] Clinical pathologic changes include high creatinine kinase, aspartate aminotransferase, and sorbitol dehydrogenase activity, leukocytosis, hyper- or hypofibrinogenemia, hypoproteinemia, thrombocytopenia, hyperglobulinemia, and azotemia. An initial hemoconcentration is followed by a hemolytic or coagulopathy-induced anemia. A metabolic acidosis can be present.

Differential diagnosis

Angioedema secondary to insect stings or bites; trauma; foreign bodies or abscesses; botulism; *Centaurea* spp. intoxication; purpura hemorrhagica.

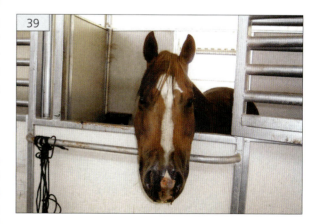

10.39 Facial swelling following rattlesnake envenomation.

Diagnosis

In some cases, the snake bite may be witnessed. In cases where a bite has not been witnessed, close inspection of areas of soft tissue swelling can be used to identify bite wounds. Although there are a number of clinical pathologic changes associated with clinically important snake bites, they are often not specific for snake envenomation. The presence of an initial hemoconcentration followed by a hemolytic or coagulopathy-induced anemia is suggestive of snake envenomation. There are no routinely available tests for snake venoms.

Management/treatment

Horses bitten by snakes should be taken to a veterinary facility as soon as possible after the bite. Immediate goals of treatment involve: (1) stabilizing the patient; (2) neutralizing the venom; (3) minimizing local tissue reaction; and (4) preventing secondary bacterial infections. Stabilization includes correcting hypotension and treating circulatory shock, providing an open airway, and correcting electrolyte and acid–base abnormalities. Since most snake bites occur around the muzzle, assuring a patent airway is a top priority. If there is marked swelling, a rigid tube can be inserted in the nostril to prevent complete occlusion.[2] An emergency tracheostomy may be required.

The administration of crystalloid fluids to treat shock and hypotension and to increase tissue perfusion is warranted.[2,119] This may be followed by whole blood or blood products to correct anemia, thrombocytopenia, and coagulopathies. Local wounds are treated with regular cleaning, hydrotherapy, and debridement. NSAIDs can be given to help control pain and swelling. Corticosteroids should not be used since a high mortality has been associated with their administration.[118] A broad-spectrum antimicrobial drug such as a cephalosporin should be given for up to 7–10 days.

Two antivenins are available (in the USA) for crotalid venom: an equine-derived serum globulin-based polyvalent antivenom (Antivenin®) and an ovine-derived Fab polyvalent antivenom (CroFab®). The equine-derived antivenin is approved for use in horses and is considerably cheaper than the ovine-derived product. However, adverse reactions are less likely with the ovine-derived product.[2,118] Antivenom is most effective if given soon after envenomation.

Antivenom administration can be especially important in small and/or young horses and ponies. An initial dose of antivenin should be 5 vials given IV.[119] Administration can be facilitated by mixing each vial with approximately 200 ml of crystalloid fluid. This allows for more controlled infusion and the infusion can be stopped if an allergic reaction is noted.[118] Administration of subsequent doses should be based on the nature and progression of clinical signs, the degree of hypotension, and the bite site. Antivenin should not be given IM or into the bite.[119] Although adverse effects following antivenom administration are infrequent, they can occur.[118]

Recovery may take several weeks. In one retrospective study of 27 horses bitten by rattlesnakes, the mean duration of hospitalization was 6.2 days.[120] The 27 horses were approximately equally divided among those with rather mild clinical signs and uncomplicated recoveries ($n = 9$), those with moderate-to-severe local reactions with multiple physical and laboratory abnormalities ($n = 8$) and those with moderate-to-severe local reactions with multiple, severe systemic signs of intoxication ($n = 10$). The overall mortality rate was 25%.

Botulism
Key points

- Botulism is a gradually progressive, symmetric muscular weakness in horses characterized initially by dysphagia and progressing to recumbency.
- Botulism in horses is most often due to toxin types A, B, and C, with type B responsible for the large majority of cases.
- Exposure to botulinum toxin is most often due to ingestion of preformed toxin, but toxin production can occur within the GI tract (toxicoinfectious botulism of foals) or in wounds.
- Ingestion of preformed toxin can occur following contamination of feed with animal carcasses or following its formation in poorly ensiled, small grain haylage or hay.
- Diagnosis of botulism in horses is most often based on the occurrence of typical clinical signs, but detection of the toxin in source material should be attempted.
- The prognosis in symptomatic horses is guarded unless specific antitoxin is administered.

Definition/overview

Botulism is a disease characterized by a progressive flaccid paralysis and is caused by exotoxins from *Clostridium botulinum*.[121] *C. botulinum* is an obligate anaerobe that is gram positive and forms spores. It produces eight different botulinum toxins designated A, B, C_1, C_2, D, E, F, and G. Botulinum toxin is one of the most toxic compounds known, with a mouse median lethal dose of 0.005 µg/kg body weight.[122] Toxin types A, B, and C are most commonly associated with equine botulism, with type B responsible for >85% of the cases.[123] Types A and B are associated with forage, while type C is found associated with carrion.

Etiology/pathogenesis

Horses are affected by botulinum toxin as a result of ingesting pre-formed toxin, most often as a result of contamination of feed, or as a result of enteric or wound infection with *C. botulinum* with resultant toxin formation.[121] Ingestion of pre-formed toxin can occur following contamination of feed with animal carcasses or following its formation in poorly ensiled, small grain haylage, or hay. Hay stored in plastic bags or in large round bales is a common factor in many outbreaks of botulism in the USA and UK.[123] Ingestion of processed alfalfa hay cubes has also caused botulism in horses.[124]

Toxicoinfectious botulism (also called shaker foal syndrome) results from production of toxin within the GI tract and occurs in foals. Toxicoinfectious botulism only occurs in neonates because the intestinal microflora of adults prevents the intraintestinal growth of *C. botulinum* spores.[123] Equine grass sickness, a form of dysautonomia in horses, has been hypothesized to be due to toxicoinfection.[125]

Wound botulism results following infection of a wound in which an anaerobic environment is present. It has been reported in association with castration sites, umbilical hernia repairs, or deep puncture wounds.[126,127]

Botulinum toxins, with the exception of type C_2 toxin, prevent the release of acetylcholine from presynaptic terminals of cholinergic neurons. C_2 toxin alters membrane permeability.[121] Toxin that reaches the systemic circulation binds to the surface of targeted neurons and penetrates the plasma membrane by receptor-mediated endocytosis and endosome membranes by pH-induced translocation.[122] The toxin acts as a metalloendoprotease to cleave polypeptides that are critical for the release of acetylcholine.

Clinical features

Depending on the dose of botulinum ingested, paralysis and death can occur as quickly as 24 hours following exposure or develop and progress over a period of at least 2–3 weeks.[121,123] Initial clinical signs in adult horses include exercise intolerance, weakness and paralysis of the third eyelid, and muscle tremors. Horses can have a noticeable twitch in the triceps region of the forelimbs and carpal buckling. Additional signs include mydriasis, ataxia, muscle weakness, paralysis (most often progressing from the hindlimbs forward), labored breathing, anorexia, hypersalivation, hypomotile intestinal borborygmi, constipation, and dysphagia. Decreased tongue tone (**10.40**) and strength and decreased tail tone are

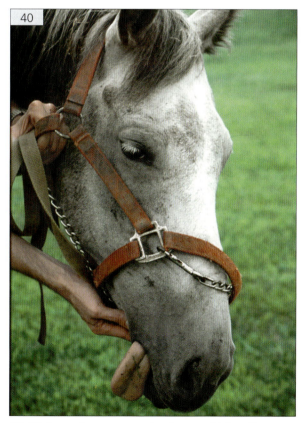

10.40 Loss of tongue tone in a horse with botulism. (Courtesy Dr Robert Whitlock)

'classic' signs of botulism.[123] Diarrhea can develop following exposure to type C_2. The cause of death is usually from respiratory paralysis and heart failure.[128]

Signs in foals with toxicoinfectious botulism can initially be vague, with the chief complaint being that the foal is lying down more than usual.[123] When forced to stand, affected foals develop muscle tremors and drop to the ground in lateral recumbency. They may drool milk when suckling. Otherwise, foals are bright and alert with no other abnormalities noted.

Differential diagnosis
Equine herpesvirus myeloencephalopathy; ionophore intoxication (especially salinomycin); EPM.

Diagnosis
Diagnosis is based on consistent clinical signs and detection of botulinum toxin in source material. Assessing tongue tone and strength is one of the most sensitive and early tests that can be performed.[123] Another clinical test that can be used consists of offering 226 grams (8 ounces) of sweet feed in a large flat feeding tub on the floor and determining the time required to consume the feed (normal time should be <2 minutes).[123] The extreme sensitivity of horses to the toxins (speculated to be anywhere from 1 to 10,000 time(s) more sensitive than mice) generally precludes toxin identification in biological specimens using the mouse bioassay.[121,124] Identification of *C. botulinum* in intestinal contents is also possible, but the organism is commonly found in the environment and as part of the GI tract flora from many animals.[121]

Management/treatment
The prognosis for symptomatic horses is guarded unless specific antitoxin is administered.[123] In one study, only 2 of 91 affected foals survived without antitoxin.[129] In contrast, over 90% of foals given antitoxin and good nursing care survived.[130] Possible sources of contaminated feed should be identified and removed. Specific or multivalent antitoxin should be given to foals and adults at 200 ml (30,000 IU) and 500 ml (70,000 IU), respectively.[123] A single administration is sufficient.

It is important to minimize physical activity, since stores of acetylcholine are further depleted and signs exacerbated with activity. Animals that struggle can be sedated with xylazine or diazepam.[121,131]

Antimicrobial drugs effective against gram-positive bacilli should be given if wound botulism is suspected or to treat possible complications such as aspiration pneumonia. Aminoglycosides and metronidazole are contraindicated.[123] Foals should be given H_2 receptor blockers and sucralfate to help prevent gastric ulcers.

Mineral oil should be administered to facilitate passage of feces and avoid impaction colic. Foals may accumulate fluids in their stomachs, which should be relieved by nasogastric intubation. Affected males cannot urinate and require regular bladder catheterization.[121,123] Muzzling animals to prevent aspiration of bedding in recumbent patients who attempt to eat is advised. Eye ointments can be useful to help protect the corneas. Foals require frequent turning to prevent decubital ulcers from occurring.

Supplemental alimentation is generally required. Alfalfa meal gruel with adequate water can maintain an adult animal for 2 weeks or more.[123] Affected foals require intragastric feeding with mare's milk, goat's milk, or a commercial milk replacer.

Severely affected animals with respiratory paralysis require assisted ventilation.[121,130] Recovery can occur in mildly affected horses, although muscle wasting, if present, can take months to resolve. Adult horses that are recumbent for more than 24 hours have a poor prognosis.[123]

Metals
Iron
Key points
- There are a large number of forms of iron designed for parenteral or oral use and their toxicity is variable.
- Two syndromes are associated with iron intoxication in horses: (1) acute intoxication resulting in acute liver damage and (2) chronic intoxication resulting in hepatic hemochromatosis and fibrosis.

- Measurement of free serum iron (iron in excess of iron binding capacity) can help confirm intoxication.
- Treatment is primarily symptomatic and supportive; however, the iron chelator, deferoxamine mesylate, effectively binds iron.

Definition/overview

Iron is available for oral administration in various salt forms that vary in their iron content.[132] Injectable iron (iron dextran, iron dextrin, iron polysaccharide, iron sorbitol, and ferric ammonium citrate) and iron salts (large number including ferrous sulfate, ferrous chloride, ferris fumarate, and chelated forms [e.g. iron combined with amino acids]) for oral administration are also available.[24] Iron intoxication of horses is less common since the removal in the 1980s of products containing ferrous fumarate (33% iron by weight) intended for administration to neonates.[133,134] The dietary iron requirement of horses has not been established, but is estimated to be approximately 40 mg/kg (expressed on a dry matter basis).[135]

Etiology/pathogenesis

Two syndromes associated with excessive exposure to iron are possible: (1) acute to subacute iron intoxication in which large doses of iron are given and acute liver damage results and (2) exposure to lower doses of iron can result in chronic liver damage characterized by hemochromatosis and hepatic fibrosis.[136,137] However, high liver concentrations of iron and resulting hemochromatosis occur secondary to other liver diseases.

The toxicity of iron is variable. Chelated forms of iron are less toxic than other forms of iron. There is no mechanism for the excretion of iron and susceptibility to intoxication is dependent on the amount of iron already present in the body.[132] Ferrous fumarate administered over 5 days orally to a 400 kg gelding (total dose of approximately 390 mg/kg body weight of iron) was lethal.[138] A Thoroughbred gelding given a vitamin/mineral supplement containing ferrous sulfate (0.6 mg/kg body weight of iron per day) for 6 weeks developed a hepatopathy.[139] In contrast, ponies given ferrous sulfate daily per os (50 mg/kg of iron) for 8 weeks did not develop toxicosis.[140]

Iron is very reactive with tissues and causes oxidative damage to cells. Oral exposure to sufficient iron causes a corrosive-like effect in the GI tract. Systemically absorbed iron in excess of the ability of the body to bind it to proteins allows reactive iron to damage membranes of cellular organelles. The liver, brain, and heart are particularly susceptible to damage.[132] Multiple organ failure can occur, although mortality is primarily a result of acute, fulminant hepatic failure.

Hepatic failure is one of the more common complications in foals requiring blood transfusion to treat NI (see Chapter 9). Iron intoxication is likely the cause of hepatic injury.[141]

Clinical features

Clinical signs following acute oral exposure are initially associated with GI tract damage including abdominal pain and melena.[142] Classically, clinical improvement can be noted before the onset of signs related to liver and cardiovascular damage. Hypotension and hypovolemia result from cardiovascular damage. Hyperglycemia, hyperammonemia, icterus, coagulation defects, and HE can occur as a result of hepatic damage. High activities of serum liver enzymes, bilirubin, and bile acids are seen.

Differential diagnosis

Numerous other acute hepatotoxicants such as microcystins, aflatoxins, and pyrrolizidine alkaloids; Theiler's disease; Tyzzer's disease; cholangiohepatitis; causes of hemolytic anemia such as red maple (*Acer rubrum*) intoxication and equine hemolytic anemia; immune-mediated thrombocytopenia; NI or septicemia in foals; equine herpesvirus myeloencephalopathy.

Diagnosis

A recent history of administration of iron along with the onset of acute liver disease, gastrointestinal tract signs, and hemolysis is consistent with iron intoxication. Routine clinical pathologic changes are not specific for iron. It is important to try to demonstrate serum iron concentrations in excess of total serum iron-binding capacity. Liver biopsies for histopathologic evaluation and determination of iron concentration can be useful.

Management/treatment

Gastrointestinal tract decontamination (p. 562) is questionable since activated charcoal does not bind iron.[8] Oral sodium bicarbonate (25%) given as a gastric lavage has been suggested as a way to decrease iron absorption.[132] Hypovolemic patients require fluid therapy. Electrolyte and acid–base status needs to be assessed and corrected appropriately.

The metal chelator, deferoxamine mesylate, has the highest affinity for iron, but is only available in a formulation for human patients.[143] The recommended dosage for human patients is 15 mg/kg/hour by CRI. GI tract protectants such as sucralfate, cimetidine, or misoprostol may be useful. General approaches to treat acute or chronic liver disease are required. Continuous IV fluids such as acetated Ringer's solution (20–40 mEq KCl/l) and dextrose (50 g/l) should be given.[73] A high-carbohydrate, low-protein diet with branched chain amino acids and neomycin (10 g/500 kg) PO mixed in a molasses q8h for 2 days is indicated if signs of HE are present.[73,74]

Prevention of hepatic damage with iron intoxication in foals receiving blood transfusion may be achieved with deferoxamine.[141] Deferoxamine (1 g q12h for 14 days) enhances urinary iron elimination and decreases hepatic iron accumulation after blood transfusion in foals.

Lead
Key points
- Lead is a widely distributed environmental contaminant, especially in urban environments and associated with industrial operations such as mining and smelting.
- The occurrence of lead intoxication in horses is much less than for dogs and cattle, with most reports associated with chronic ingestion.

- The toxicity of lead is quite variable and is dependent on a number of factors.
- Lead intoxication in horses is manifested as central and peripheral neurologic dysfunction, GI tract disturbance, and impairment of erythropoeisis.
- Successful treatment relies on the chelation of tissue lead with subsequent renal elimination of the lead–chelate complex.
- The source for lead exposure should be identified and further access prevented.

Definition/overview

Lead is a widely distributed environmental contaminant, especially in urban environments, and is associated with industrial operations such as mining and smelting.[142] In horses, lead exposure is more likely to occur from environmental contamination of habitat associated with mining and smelting activities (**10.41**), discarded lead-acid batteries, and old lead-based paints. The occurrence of lead intoxication in horses is much less than for dogs and cattle with most reports associated with chronic ingestion.[144–149]

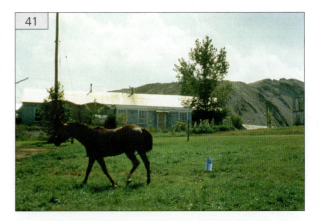

10.41 Lead mine tailings adjacent to a horse pasture contaminated with lead.

Etiology/pathogenesis

The toxicity of lead is quite variable and depends on the form of lead as well as the diet and age of the horse. A minimum toxic dose of lead in horses is reported to be 15.3 mg/kg following chronic oral administration.[150]

Most cellular damage due to lead is caused by the ability of lead to substitute for a variety of polyvalent cations, especially calcium and zinc, in their binding sites.[151] The roles that metal ions play in biological systems are numerous and diverse. They serve as charge carriers, intermediates in catalyzed reactions, and as structural elements in the maintenance of protein conformation. Metal transport, energy metabolism, apoptosis, ionic conduction, cell adhesion, inter- and intracellular signaling, diverse enzymatic processes, protein maturation, and genetic regulation can all be affected.[151] Lead produces oxidative damage to lipids and proteins as a result of release of iron, disruption of antioxidant mechanisms, and direct oxidative damage.[151-153]

The neurotoxicity of lead is most likely due to such diverse mechanisms as lipid peroxidation; excitotoxicity (i.e. cell damage secondary to receptor overstimulation due to excitatory neurotransmitters such as glutamate); alterations in neurotransmitter synthesis, storage, and release; alterations in expression and functioning of receptors; interference with mitochondrial metabolism; interference with second messenger systems; and damage to astroglia and oligodendroglia.[151]

Clinical features

Lead intoxication in horses is manifested as both central and peripheral neurologic dysfunction, GI tract disturbance, and impairment of erythropoeisis.[142] Common clinical signs include laryngeal hemiplegia, stridor, dysphagia, secondary aspiration pneumonia, ataxia, muscle fasciculations, hyperesthesia, dullness, and weight loss. Laryngeal dysfunction can result in inspiratory dyspnea, exercise-induced pulmonary hemorrhage, and nasal discharge.[142] Mild to moderate anemia can be present and a high number of nucleated red blood cells in proportion to the anemia is consistent with lead intoxication.

Differential diagnosis

Laryngeal hemiplegia or paralysis ('roaring'); esophageal obstruction ('choke'); exercise-induced pulmonary hemorrhage not associated with lead; rabies; equine leukoencephalomalacia; viral encephalitides; botulism; intoxications by *Centaurea* spp.; arsenic toxicosis; equine motor neuron disease and equine degenerative myeloencephalopathy.

Diagnosis

Diagnosis of lead intoxication can be made by analysis of whole blood. Whole blood lead concentrations >0.35 parts per million, along with compatible clinical signs, are sufficient to make a diagnosis. Blood lead concentrations do not correlate well with the severity of clinical signs.[148]

Management/treatment

Successful treatment relies on the chelation of tissue lead with subsequent renal elimination of the lead-chelate complex. Calcium disodium edetate ($CaNa_2$EDTA) and succimer are effective lead chelators. For horses, $CaNa_2$EDTA is given at 75 mg/kg/day by slow IV infusion divided into 2 daily doses.[154] A 6.6% solution is prepared in normal saline or 5% dextrose. Chelation is continued for 3–5 days followed by a 2–3 day rest period.[155] Additional courses of chelation therapy may be needed, but this should be guided by blood lead determinations just before starting another course. Alternatively, succimer is an orally effective chelator that has a good margin of safety. Doses for horses are empiric, but 10 mg/kg PO q8h for 10 days is recommended for other mammals. Again, the continuation of chelation therapy should be guided by whole blood lead determinations.

General supportive care includes maintaining adequate hydration and urination, providing a good quality diet, controlling CNS excitation, and monitoring for aspiration pneumonia. Thiamine (250–1,000 mg q12h for 5 days) has been reported to be useful in lead-intoxicated cattle.[155] The source for lead exposure should be identified and further access prevented.

Mercury

Key points

- Mercury intoxication is uncommon in horses. Intoxication has been associated with the use of mercury salts as blistering agents.
- Inorganic forms of mercury damage the GI tract and are nephrotoxic.
- Chelators are available to bind to mercury and facilitate its excretion. Other treatment is symptomatic and supportive.

Definition/overview

Mercury intoxication has been reported in horses associated with the use of inorganic mercury salts, such as mercuric iodide and mercuric chloride, as blistering agents.[156,157] Other inorganic and organic forms of mercury have historically been used for a variety of purposes, but exposure of horses is unlikely.

Etiology/pathogenesis

The pathophysiologic effects of mercury are due to its covalent binding to sulfhydryl groups of different cellular enzymes, which cause disruption of cell metabolism and function.[158] Inorganic forms of mercury damage the GI tract and are nephrotoxic.

Clinical features

Clinical signs of intoxication include CNS depression, colic, diarrhea, weakness, dehydration, and oliguria. Dermal application of mercury salts causes skin erosions, ulcerations, and crusting. Laminitis has also been reported.

Differential diagnosis

Lead intoxication; arsenic intoxication; NSAID intoxication; cantharidin (blister beetle) intoxication; oak intoxication; colitis (salmonellosis, ehrlichial colitis, clostridial colitis, acute cyathastomiasis, antimicrobial-associated colitis).

Diagnosis

Diagnosis of intoxication relies on measurement of mercury in urine or blood samples.

Management/treatment

Dermally exposed skin should be washed with mild soap and water. Specific treatment involves administration of the chelator dimercaprol. A loading dose of 4–5 mg/kg is given by deep IM injection followed by 2–3 mg/kg q4h for 24 hours then 1 mg/kg q4h for 2 days.[159] Alternatively, N-acetyl-DL-penicillamine has been used to treat a mare with mercury intoxication at 3 mg/kg PO q6h.[157] Other therapeutic interventions are supportive and symptomatic. Abdominal pain should be ameliorated, but NSAIDs should be avoided because of the potential for exacerbating renal damage. Butorphanol tartrate (0.1 mg/kg IV q3–4h for up to 48 hours) can be given. IV fluids are recommended to treat dehydration and maintain urine output. GI tract demulcents can be used and a bland diet containing reduced amounts of high-quality protein is recommended.

Selenium

Key points

- Acute and chronic forms of selenium intoxication occur in horses.
- Signs of acute intoxication include dullness, muscular weakness, anorexia, and a progressively worsening dyspnea.
- Chronic intoxication is a slowly progressing, debilitating disease characterized by bilaterally symmetric alopecia and dystrophic hoof growth.
- There are no proven therapies for acute selenium intoxication.

Definition/overview

Selenium salts (e.g. sodium selenite) are administered to animals to supplement selenium-deficient diets. Selenium intoxication in horses can be manifested either by an acute intoxication that affects primarily the cardiorespiratory systems or a chronic intoxication affecting skin, hooves, and hair.

Etiology/pathogenesis

Excessive administration of selenium salts via feed or injection can cause acute selenium intoxication. An acutely toxic oral dose of sodium selenite for horses is between 3.3 and 6 mg/kg.[24] Vitamin E- and selenium-deficient animals are more susceptible to acute selenium intoxication.[160] In addition, some plants (e.g. *Xylorrhiza* spp. [woody astor], *Oonopsis* spp. [golden-weed], *Stanleya* spp. [princess plume], and *Astragalus* spp. [locoweeds]) can accumulate high concentrations of selenium in organic forms that, when ingested over a protracted period of time (30–90 days), cause chronic selenium intoxication or 'alkali disease'.[24,160] Horses are more sensitive to chronic selenium intoxication than ruminants.

Clinical features

Signs of acute intoxication include dullness, muscular weakness, anorexia, and a progressively worsening dyspnea.[160] Signs can begin from 1 to 24 hours after exposure. Colic, diarrhea, tachycardia, tachypnea, cyanotic mucous membranes, weak pulse, fever, polyuria, and hemolytic anemia are also reported. Symptomatic animals become comatose and die within 12–48 hours. Death is generally attributed to myocardial damage that results in CHF and pulmonary congestion and edema.

Chronic intoxication is a slowly progressing, debilitating disease that is characterized by bilaterally symmetric alopecia and dystrophic hoof growth (**10.42**).[160] Alopecia typically involves the mane and tail. Hoof involvement begins as lameness, erythema, and swelling of the coronary bands. This is followed by circumferential cracking just distal to the coronary band. Hoof separation and lameness increase until the damaged hoof is displaced by new, underlying growth. The damaged hoof can be shed or remain attached, resulting in an upwardly curled toe that results in abnormal stresses on the appendicular skeleton. Affected animals can become so lame that they cannot eat or drink and eventually die from dehydration and/or starvation.

Differential diagnosis

Acute: arsenic intoxication; endotoxemia; cantharidin (blister beetle) intoxication. Chronic: *Leucaena leucocephala* intoxication; ergotism; laminitis due to a variety of causes; thallium intoxication.

Diagnosis

An antemortem diagnosis of acute or chronic selenium intoxication is based on characteristic clinical signs and possibly measuring selenium concentrations in whole blood samples. Blood values >1 part per million are high. However, blood selenium concentrations are variable and should not be relied on for confirming intoxication.[160]

Management/treatment

There are no proven therapies for acute selenium intoxication. Uncomplicated chronic selenosis can be treated with palliative measures including appropriate shoeing and hoof trimming and good nursing care. Analgesics and NSAIDs are usually required to keep a chronically affected horse moving and eating.

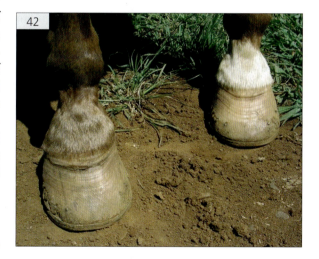

10.42 Circular cracks in the hooves of a horse with chronic selenosis. (Courtesy Dr Asheesh Tiwary)

Non-steroidal anti-inflammatory drugs
Key points
- The GI tract and renal toxicity of NSAIDs is well recognized.
- Toxicity generally depends on both the dose and duration of exposure.
- Diagnosis relies on a history of administration and the occurrence of signs consistent with intoxication.
- Treatment involves discontinuing NSAID administration, maintenance of urine flow, and other symptomatic and supportive care.

Definition/overview
NSAIDs are among the most commonly prescribed agents for use in horses.[161] Phenylbutazone and flunixin meglumine are the most commonly used, although others have also been used.

Etiology/pathogenesis
The GI and renal toxicity of NSAIDs is well recognized. Toxicity generally depends on both the dose and duration of exposure.[161] Damage to GI mucosa is primarily a result of inhibition of protective prostaglandin production, but direct irritation may play a role. The glandular portion of the stomach is particularly sensitive to damage. Horses given flunixin (1.1 mg/kg), ketoprofen (2.2 mg/kg), and phenylbutazone (4.4 mg/kg) q8h for 12 days developed significant GI tract ulceration.[162]

Nephrotoxicity also relates to inhibition of prostaglandin synthesis and resultant alterations of renal blood flow.[163] Nephrotoxicity is associated with the administration of high NSAID doses or administration of therapeutic doses to horses that are volume depleted, hypotensive, or have underlying renal or hepatic disease.[161,164] Renal papillary necrosis is more common when NSAIDs are administered to animals with decreased renal perfusion or dehydration.[161] There is a high risk of nephrotoxicity with the concurrent administration of other highly protein-bound drugs. Young and old animals are also at a high risk.[163] The administration of two or more NSAIDs concurrently, even at reduced dosages, increases the risk of NSAID intoxication.[164] All NSAIDs have the potential to induce hepatotoxicity, although this has not been documented in horses.[161] A protein-losing enteropathy had been noted in ponies and horses given phenylbutazone at 8–12 mg/kg over 8–10 days.[165]

Clinical features
Clinical signs are referable to adverse effects on the GI tract or kidneys. GI tract signs include anorexia, dullness, abdominal discomfort, diarrhea, and melena.[24] Colonic involvement can be manifested by weight loss and peripheral edema secondary to hypoproteinemia.[24,164] Signs associated with renal damage include oral ulcerations, proteinuria, hyposthenuria, and polyuria.[164] (See also Chapter 1.)

Differential diagnosis
Colic due to a variety of other causes; diarrhea due to a variety of other causes (e.g. salmonellosis or Potomac horse fever); peripheral edema due to a variety of other causes (e.g. CHF or protein-losing enteropathies); polyuria due to a variety of other causes (e.g. renal disease, hyperadrenocorticism, or diabetes insipidus).

Diagnosis
Diagnosis relies on a history of administration of NSAIDs and the occurrence of signs consistent with intoxication (**10.43, 10.44**). In the absence of a history of administration, it is possible to detect commonly used NSAIDs in appropriate samples such as serum/plasma or urine.

Management/treatment
Treatment involves discontinuing NSAID administration, maintenance of urine flow, and other symptomatic and supportive care. GI tract effects can be treated with H_2-receptor antagonists such as ranitidine (7 mg/kg PO q8h) or omeprazole (4 mg/kg PO q24h) along with sucralfate (10–20 mg/kg PO q8h).[164] IV fluid diuresis is recommended if renal damage is present. Hypoproteinemia can be treated with plasma or a synthetic colloid (see Chapter 12). Potential complications from NSAID intoxication include chronic recurrent colic, chronic diarrhea, chronic poor body condition, and chronic polyuria and polydipsia.

Feed additives (ionophores)
Key points
- Several ionophore compounds are routinely used in animal agriculture. Horses are particularly sensitive to the toxic effects of these compounds.
- Ionophore intoxication results in physiochemical or pathologic disruption of skeletal and cardiac muscle cells and nerve cells.
- The onset of clinical signs is most often peracute or acute, but delayed onset of clinical signs is possible.
- Antemortem diagnosis of ionophore intoxication relies on detection of an ionophore in the feed or stomach contents and compatible clinical signs.
- Treatment is primarily symptomatic and supportive.
- Animals that survive intoxication often have permanent damage to the heart, nerves, or muscles.

Definition/overview
Ionophores are commonly used feed additives and include monensin, lasalocid, salinomycin, narasin, maduramicin, and laidlomycin. Ionophores are biologically active compounds produced by *Streptomyces cinnamonensis*. They are classified as polyethers. Initially, ionophores were developed as poultry coccidiostats. In ruminants, ionophores enhance propionic acid production by altering rumen microflora and subsequent rumen fermentation.[166]

Etiology/pathogenesis
These compounds were given the name ionophore because of their ability to bind and transport cations down concentration gradients through biologic membranes.[166] Monovalent ionophores such as monensin transport Na^+ and K^+, while divalent ionophores such as lasalocid can also transport Ca^{++}. Ion movement into mammalian cells sets up a cascade of events that

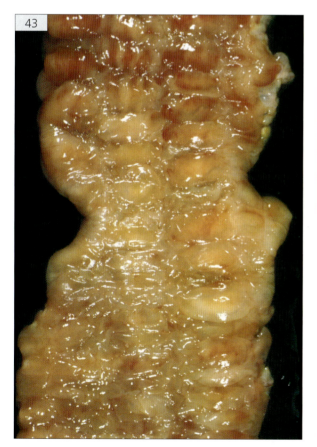

10.43 Submucosal edema and hemorrhage in a foal with phenylbutazone intoxication.

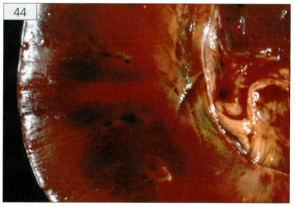

10.44 Renal papillary necrosis in a horse with phenylbutazone intoxication.

attempt to re-equilibrate the ion gradients. In cases of ionophore intoxication, transmembrane ion gradients and electrical potentials required for normal cell function are disrupted.[167] Excitable cells of the myocardium, skeletal muscles, and nervous tissue are particularly vulnerable. Lipid peroxidation may also play a role in the pathogenesis of cell damage.[168]

Horses are the most susceptible species for ionophore intoxication. The reported lethal dose that would kill 50% of exposed animals (LD_{50}) for monensin, lasalocid, and salinomyin (2–3 mg/kg, 15–21.5 mg/kg, and 0.6 mg/kg, respectively) are much lower than those for other livestock species.[167] Horses can be poisoned by feed containing 100 parts per million of monensin (i.e. the poultry feeding level) and have been killed by eating feed containing 300 parts per million (i.e. the premix level). Salinomycin concentrations of 130 parts per million in a commercial feed concentrate and 230 parts per million in commercially prepared horse and pony 'nuts' have been associated with intoxication.[167,169] The reason for the sensitivity of horses is not known. The most common scenario of intoxication for horses is the inadvertent inclusion of an ionophore into the diet (e.g. feeding a treated ration intended for use in ruminants or poultry).

Clinical features

The clinical course associated with ionophore intoxication can be peracute, acute, or chronic.[167,170,171] High-dose exposures can result in death within minutes of ingestion. More typically, clinical signs occur within several hours to days following exposure. Acute clinical signs in horses include partial to complete anorexia (feed refusal is often the earliest observed sign), uneasiness, and profuse, intermittent sweating.[166] Fever is variable. Polyuria occurs early, followed by a terminal oliguria. Intermediate signs include progressive ataxia (12–36 hours post exposure) followed by colic and stiffness ('tying up'). Posterior paresis and intermittent recumbency and standing occur as signs of progress. Advanced signs include tachycardia, hypotension, hyperventilation, and dyspnea. Chronically affected horses exhibit weight loss, lethargy, poor performance, cardiac arrhythmias, edema, diarrhea, and polyuria.[167] Chronic signs are due to chronic heart failure.

Delayed onset of clinical signs has been reported.[170] Interestingly, although cardiac and skeletal muscles are considered to be the tissues most commonly affected by ionophores, lesions restricted to the nervous system have been reported in salinomycin-intoxicated horses.[167]

Clinical pathologic changes are primarily related to cardiac and skeletal muscle damage.[166,167] High serum activities of creatine kinase, alkaline phosphatase, aspartate aminotransferase, alanine transaminase, and lactate dehydrogenase occur within 24 hours of exposure. Increases in indirect bilirubin, blood urea nitrogen, glucose, PCV, serum osmolality, and phosphorus have been noted.[166] Myoglobinuria may occur. Electrolyte abnormalities (low serum Ca^{++} and K^+ concentrations) can occur. However, a lack of these changes does not rule out exposure in an individual horse due to the variable nature of their occurrence.[167] Measurement of plasma or serum troponin I concentrations holds promise for better quantifying cardiac muscle damage.[172] Echocardiographic examination may also be useful.

Differential diagnosis

White snakeroot (*Eupatorium rugosum*) intoxication; oleander (*Nerium oleander*) intoxication; vitamin E deficiency; selenium deficiency.

Diagnosis

Diagnosis of intoxication relies on documenting the presence of an ionophore in representative feed samples or stomach contents along with the occurrence of compatible clinical signs. Obtaining representative samples of feed can be challenging, especially if the onset of signs is delayed or the ionophore was not evenly distributed in a batch of feed.

Management/treatment

There is no specific treatment for ionophore intoxication. Prompt GI tract decontamination should be performed using activated charcoal and a saline cathartic. Feed should be removed to prevent further exposure. Fluids and electrolytes should be administered to correct changes in the PCV, serum potassium, and serum calcium. Early administration of selenium and vitamin E may lessen the severity of muscle damage, although these antioxidants have demonstrated efficacy only if administered prior to ionophore exposure.[168] Extended stall rest is recommended in horses that survive acute intoxication. However, residual heart damage makes the horse susceptible to long-term performance problems, heart failure, and sudden death.[166] The short- and long-term prognosis for affected horses is guarded. However, some horses exposed to sublethal doses may not develop permanent myocardial disease and a return to athletic/reproductive use is possible.[173] Exercise stress testing, echocardiography, and electrocardiography can be used to assess cardiac function and the possibility of return to athletic function.[173]

Cholinesterase-inhibiting insecticides

Key points
- There are many cholinesterase-inhibiting insecticides belonging to the OP or carbamate families that are used in the environment of horses, although the number of products for use on horses has declined.
- The toxicity of the various insecticides is variable.
- The OP and carbamate insecticides bind to and inhibit cholinesterase enzymes, the most clinically important of which is acetylcholinesterase.
- Clinical signs result from overstimulation of muscarinic, nicotinic, and CNS acetylcholine receptors.
- Diagnosis of intoxication can be difficult, but the presence of a parasympathetic toxidrome along with demonstration of low whole blood cholinesterase activity (generally >50% inhibition of normal activity) is sufficient for a tentative diagnosis.
- Treatment begins by stabilizing animals exhibiting seizures or respiratory distress.
- Atropine and pralidoxime hydrochloride are antidotal.

Definition/overview
OP and carbamate insecticides are found in a variety of products for use on or around horses including oral anthelmintics, fly baits, dips, dusts, sprays, and pour-ons.[174] OP and carbamate products for use on animals or in their environment have decreased in number over the years and have been replaced by other generally less toxic pesticides. Therefore, intoxication is less likely today than in the past. However, potent OP and carbamate insecticides are still commonly used in agriculture and, therefore, are potentially found in the vicinity of horses. Accidental grain or forage contamination with agriculturally used OP and carbamate insecticides can occur as well as overdosing with oral parasiticidal products or malicious poisoning.[175]

Etiology/pathogenesis
The OP and carbamate insecticides bind to and inhibit cholinesterase enzymes, the most clinically important of which is acetylcholinesterase.[174,176] Inhibition of acetylcholinesterase results in the accumulation of acetylcholine at postsynaptic receptors in the parasympathetic and sympathetic nervous systems and at neuromuscular junctions. OPs are considered to be irreversible inhibitors of acetylcholinesterase, while carbamates are reversible inhibitors, which allows for spontaneous regeneration of enzyme activity. Once an OP irreversibly binds acetylcholinesterase, in a process called 'aging', spontaneous enzyme regeneration cannot occur.

Clinical features
Clinical signs result from overstimulation of muscarinic, nicotinic, and CNS acetylcholine receptors.[174,176] The most commonly observed clinical signs are due to muscarinic cholinergic receptor stimulation and can be remembered by the mnemonic SLUD (increased salivation, lacrimation, urination, and defecation). Other muscarinic signs include miosis and bronchospasm. Bradycardia, excessive bronchial secretions, and dyspnea can occur. While signs caused by parasympathetic stimulation generally predominate, signs associated with sympathetic stimulation can occur and be opposite to those expected (e.g. tachycardia or mydriasis).[174] Nicotinic cholinergic receptor stimulation can cause muscle tremors and fasciculations, weakness, and paresis leading to paralysis as a result of a depolarizing blockade. CNS signs such as seizure and hyperactivity can also occur and are more commonly associated with ingestion of high doses or from ingestion of extremely

toxic compounds. Bilateral laryngeal paralysis has occurred in foals after dosing with an OP anthelmintic.[175]

Differential diagnosis

Bacterial or viral enteritis; intestinal compromise (e.g. volvulus or intussusception); peritonitis; arsenic intoxication; mercury intoxication; slaframine intoxication (slobbers).

Diagnosis

Diagnosis of intoxication can be difficult, but the presence of a parasympathetic toxidrome along with demonstration of low whole blood cholinesterase activity (generally >50% inhibition of normal activity) is sufficient for a tentative diagnosis. Detection of a specific OP or carbamate in feed or GI tract contents is also useful, but results of such testing are rarely available to aid in initial case management. Another useful clue is the clinical response to a pre-anesthetic dose of atropine (0.02 mg/kg IV). If such a dose elicits a heart rate increase and mydriasis, then exposure to an OP or carbamate can be ruled out (i.e. it takes a much higher dose of atropine to control muscarinic signs in an intoxicated animal).[177]

Management/treatment

Treatment begins by stabilizing animals with seizure activity or respiratory distress. Bronchoconstriction and pulmonary edema may respond to bronchodilator (aminophylline, 4–7 mg/kg PO q8h) and diuretic (furosemide, 0.25–1.0 mg/kg IV) therapy, respectively. Early after exposure, GI tract decontamination should be performed with activated charcoal +/– a cathartic. Atropine competitively blocks muscarinic receptor stimulation. Atropine sulfate (0.1–0.2 mg/kg, one quarter of the dose given IV and the remainder given IM) can control muscarinic signs (although the dose of atropine should be tailored to the individual and should only be given to effect).[174] Nicotinic signs are not reversed by atropine. Because of the low margin of safety of atropine in horses, it should be used judiciously and primarily to reverse bradycardia and bronchial and pulmonary secretions. GI tract motility should be monitored closely. Diazepam (25–50 mg IV in adults and 0.05–0.4 mg/kg IV in foals) can help alleviate anxiousness and help control muscle tremors or seizures.

Pralidoxime hydrochloride is considered to be antidotal for OP intoxication because it regenerates acetylcholinesterase by promoting its release from the OP.[177] Pralidoxime hydrochloride is considered to be more effective when combined with atropine. A recommended dose is 20 mg/kg IV q4–6h. Discontinue pralidoxime hydrochloride if there is no improvement within 48 hours. Pralidoxime hydrochloride is effective prior to acetylcholinesterase aging, therefore it is best administered as soon after onset of clinical signs as possible. However, pralidoxime hydrochloride administration several days following exposure is recommended to see if a clinical improvement occurs. Pralidoxime hydrochloride is not considered to be useful following intoxication with carbamates because of the rapid and spontaneous regeneration of acetylcholinesterase.

Recovery from carbamate intoxication is relatively rapid. However, recovery following OP exposure may be prolonged, especially if enzyme aging has occurred.

Other toxic plants potentially affecting horses

See *Table 10.7*.

Other potential causes of intoxication in horses

See *Table 10.8*.

Table 10.7 Additional toxic plants potentially affecting horses

PLANT	TOXIN	PATHOPHYSIOLOGIC MECHANISM	CLINICAL SIGNS	TREATMENT	COMMENT
Black locust (*Robinia pseudoacacia*)[16,23]	Not entirely clear; robin and possibly other biologically active constituents	Robin inhibits protein synthesis	Anorexia, diarrhea, colic, depression, weakness, irregular pulse	Early decontamination with activated charcoal (1–2 g/kg PO); fluid and nutritional support	Honey locusts in the genus *Gleditsia* are not toxic
Castor bean (*Ricinus communis*)[23]	Ricin, ricinine	Ricinine is a GABA receptor antagonist; ricin inhibits protein synthesis	Colic, profuse and watery diarrhea, fever, incoordination, depression, sweating, terminal convulsions	Early decontamination with activated charcoal (1–2 g/kg PO); flunixin meglumine (1.1 mg/kg IV); xylazine for sedation (0.4 mg/kg); fluids (hypertonic saline solution initially followed by polyionic isotonic solution)	Seeds and foliage are poisonous; seeds need to be macerated to be toxic; horses reportedly one of the most sensitive species
Bracken fern (*Pteridium aquilinum*)[23]	Thiaminase (type 1): forms an inactive analog of thiamine that competitively inhibits thiamine cofactor activity	Disruption of cell energy production and metabolic processes (especially pyruvate metabolism)	Weight loss soon after beginning consumption, progressive ataxia, forelimbs occasionally cross, wide-based stance, arched back, muscle fasciculations, tremors, clonic spasms, opisthotonus, death	Thiamine (0.25–0.5 mg/kg IV, SC, or IM q24h); initial dose of 5–10 mg/kg can be given IV, but dilute dose in fluids and give slowly; keep animal quiet	Chronic ingestion of relatively large amounts of the plant is necessary; plant retains toxicity after drying; prognosis good if animal not recumbent
Hoary alyssum (*Berteroa incana*)[178]	Unknown	Unknown	Pyrexia, distal limb edema and laminitis	Lactated Ringer's solution; NSAIDs (phenylbutazone or flunixin meglumine); cool water hydrotherapy and/or icing of the feet	Not all horses ingesting plant are affected; recovery within 2–4 days of treatment; pasture or hay exposure
Jimsonweed, thornapple (*Datura stramonium*)[23]	Tropane alkaloids: atropine and scoplamine	Muscarinic receptor antagonism; anticholinergic effect	Tachycardia, tachypnea, mydriasis, excessive thirst, sweating, increased urination, GI atony, abdominal pain	GI tract decontamination with activated charcoal +/− cathartic; prevent further ingestion of the plant; recovery gradual when no further ingestion of the plant	Intoxications from ingestion of contaminated hay and ingestion of grain contaminated with seeds; fresh plant considered unpalatable
Oaks (*Quercus* spp.)[179]	Tannins and/or tannin metabolites (especially pyrogallol)	GI tract and kidneys are primary target organs	Colic, tachycardia, hyperpnea, abdominal borborygmus, tenesmus, hemorrhagic diarrhea	GI tract decontamination with activated charcoal +/− cathartic; lactated Ringer's solution; pain relief	Young leaves and green acorns most toxic part of tree; a long-term sequela is chronic renal failure

(continued overleaf)

Table 10.7 *(continued)*

PLANT	TOXIN	PATHOPHYSIOLOGIC MECHANISM	CLINICAL SIGNS	TREATMENT	COMMENT
Onions (*Allium* spp.)[14]	N-propyl disulfide or related compound	Not clear; oxidant damage to red blood cells resulting in a hemolytic anemia	Hemolytic anemia, icterus, hemoglobinuric nephrosis	Whole blood or packed cell transfusions as needed; fluid diuresis to prevent or treat renal impairment; avoid drugs that are potentially nephrotoxic	Can occur when horses ingest large amounts of culled farm-raised onions or wild onions
Poison hemlock (*Conium maculatum*)[14,180]	Piperidine alkaloids (conine, N-methyl conine, and γ-coniceine among others)	Akaloids have a nicotine-like effect. Initially stimulate neuromuscular activity followed by neuromuscular blockade	Rapid onset of signs (30 minutes to 2 hours): apprehensive, ataxic, weakness, recumbency, coma, respiratory failure	Rapidity of onset of clinical signs often precludes effective decontamination	Widely distributed plant found in a variety of habitats; 4 to 5 leaves sufficient to kill a horse; teratogenic following sublethal ingestion by pregnant animals
Japanese or English yews (*Taxus* spp.)[23]	Taxine alkaloids (taxine B especially toxic)	Death due to peracute cardiac failure; cause decreased cardiac contractility, maximal rate of depolarization and coronary blood flow	Horses typically collapse and die in a matter of minutes; signs prior to death may be only muscle tremors and fasciculations	Very early decontamination with activated charcoal +/− cathartic; continuous cardiac monitoring and treatment of dysrhythmias (atropine, lidocaine), external cardiac pacing	Dried or stored leaves retain toxicity for several months
Pokeweed (*Phytolacca americana*)[23]	Plant contains saponins and oxalates	Irritant action	Sometimes the only sign is diarrhea that occurs several hours after ingestion	Decontamination with activated charcoal (cathartics not needed due to spontaneous diarrhea); GI demulcents; fluid therapy	Limited toxicity reported in animals
Nightshades (*Solanum* spp.)[23]	Alkaloids, steroidal glycoalkaloids, cholinesterase-inhibitor	Primary glycoalkaloid (solanine) is an irritant	Anorexia, salivation, abdominal pain, diarrhea. Also, mydriasis, depression, weakness, progressive paralysis, prostration	Early decontamination with activated charcoal (1–2 g/kg PO); fluid and nutritional support	Sprouted potatoes reportedly toxic; true toxicity of *Solanum* spp. to horses is not well defined

Table 10.7 *(continued)*

PLANT	TOXIN	PATHOPHYSIOLOGIC MECHANISM	CLINICAL SIGNS	TREATMENT	COMMENT
Oxalate-containing plants: *Rumex* spp. (beets and dock), *Halogeton glomerulatus* (halogeton), *Sarcobatus* spp. (greasewood), *Rheum* spp. (rhubarb), *Chenopodium* spp. (lambsquarters)[14,24]	Soluble oxalates: sodium and potassium oxalate	Complex with calcium to form calcium oxalate; hypocalcemia and calcium oxalate crystal deposition in kidneys	Hypocalcemia, ileus, synchronous diaphragmatic flutter, depression, twitching, ataxia, incoordination, seizures	Dicalcium phosphate:sodium chloride ratio of 1:3 can bind soluble oxalates in the GI tract; correct hypocalcemia with calcium gluconate; closely monitor serum calcium concentrations; balanced electrolyte solutions and possibly furosemide to aid diuresis	Rare intoxication; plants are unpalatable
Sorghum spp. (Sudan grass, Johnson grass, sorghum)[14,24]	Not known. Hypothesized to be due to low level exposure to hydrocyanic acid or lathyrogenic nitriles	Not known. Axonal degeneration and demyelination of nerve fibers in the lumbar and sacral spinal cord	Posterior ataxia and urinary incontinence. Progression from urine dribbling and scalding of dependent skin to complete rear paresis. Distended and atonic urinary bladder, moderate to severe cystitis, and ascending pyelonephritis. Mares can abort and foals can be born with arthrogryposis	Remove from plant; gradual improvement can occur within weeks to months of supportive care; antibiotics for urinary infections; topical treatment for urine scalding of skin; catheterization with frequent urine aspiration or manual decompression of urinary bladder	
Wild or day-blooming jasmine (*Cestrum diurnum*)[181]	1,25-dihydroxy-cholecalciferol	Hypercalcemia with metastatic tissue calcification	Progressive loss of condition and weight over weeks to months with normal appetite, lameness, hunched appearance, choppy gait, lie down frequently, tender tendons and suspensory ligaments; infrequently renal failure	Prevent plant consumption; symptomatic and supportive; hypercalcemia may respond to saline diuresis, furosemide, and prednisone administration. Biphosphonates (e.g. pamidronate) have been effective in lowering high serum calcium concentrations in dogs	Signs associated with prolonged plant ingestion; signs can resolve over time after plant consumption ceases

Table 10.8 **Additional toxicants of concern for horses**

TOXICANT	USES/SOURCES	MOST LIKELY EXPOSURE	PATHOPHYSIO-LOGIC EFFECT	CLINICAL SIGNS	TREATMENT
Ammonia[182]	Decomposition of excrement in confined areas; disinfectant; fertilizer (anhydrous ammonia)	Ocular or inhalational exposure	Direct irritant action on mucosa of eyes and respiratory tract; tracheitis and pulmonary edema	Excessive tearing, shallow breathing, clear or purulent nasal discharge. Anhydrous ammonia: signs are more severe and can include acute death due to apnea, laryngospasm, and fluid in lungs; surviving animals can have permanent corneal and pulmonary damage	Ocular and dermal decontamination. Obtain admission blood gas and co-oximetry data. Provide supplemental oxygen. Consider intubation if difficulty breathing. Observe animal for at least 24 hours for onset of pulmonary edema
Aminoglycoside antibiotics: neomycin, gentamicin, kanamycin, amikacin, streptomycin[183]	Used to treat gram-negative bacterial infections	Therapeutic use	Reabsorption by pinocytosis along microconvoluted and straight portions of renal proximal tubules; intracellular accumulation of drug with damage to lysosomes, apical plasma membrane, and mitochondria	Signs consistent with acute kidney injury: depression, anorexia, polyuria, or oliguria	Stop further use of drug; polyionic alkalinizing fluids to induce volume diuresis
4-aminopyridine[184]	Avicide®; bait is often a treated grain	Oral exposure; feed contamination	Enhances acetylcholine release from motor nerve terminals, prolongs action potential by preventing K+ conductance during depolarization, directly or indirectly increases Ca++ influx	Apprehension, backing movements, sweating, rapid third eyelid fluttering, severe muscle tremors, exaggerated response to external stimuli, sensory discomfort manifested as wiggling or curling of lips and tongue, arching or stretching of the neck, snorting, squealing, coughing, seizures	GI decontamination, activated charcoal, xylazine reportedly has variable efficacy

Table 10.8 *(continued)*

TOXICANT	USES/SOURCES	MOST LIKELY EXPOSURE	PATHOPHYSIO-LOGIC EFFECT	CLINICAL SIGNS	TREATMENT
Amphotericin B[185]	Antifungal: effective for *Candida* and *Cryptococcocus* spp.	Therapeutic use	Nephrotoxic: renal vasoconstriction with subsequent glomerular filtration rate decrease; also possible direct damage to renal epithelial cells. Lipid-based amphotericin B less nephrotoxic	Signs consistent with acute kidney injury: depression, anorexia, polyuria, oliguria; also, tachycardia, tachypnea, fever, restlessness, anemia, phlebitis, collapse	Polyionic fluid diuresis, furosemide, mannitol
Anticoagulant rodenticides: first generation (warfarin, diphacinone, chlorophacinone) and second generation (brodifacoum, bromodiolone, difethialone)[186]	Rodent control	Accidental access to large amounts of product, contamination of food, malicious poisoning; warfarin has been used for navicular disease, laminitis, venous arteritis, disseminated intravascular coagulopathy, and thrombophlebitis	Causes coagulopathy as a result of inhibition of vitamin K_1 epoxide reductase with a subsequent inability to activate clotting factors II, VII, IX, and X	Bleeding diathesis: mild to severe. Signs generally 3–5 days post exposure	Early decontamination with activated charcoal and cathartic. Fresh frozen plasma to replace clotting factors. Whole blood to provide clotting factors and red blood cells. Vitamin K_1 at 2.5 mg/kg SC q12h for first 3 days then PO for 3–5 weeks (with long-acting second generation anticoagulants)
Arsenic[187]	Herbicide, insecticide, wood preservative, feed additive	Arsenic-containing pesticides, arsenic-contaminated soils and burn piles; contaminated feed and water	Pathophysiology is form dependent; acute intoxication with arsenic salts inhibits cellular respiration and damage capillaries	Sudden death. Intense abdominal pain, hypersalivation, severe, watery/bloody diarrhea, decreased abdominal sounds, muscle tremors, circulatory shock, ataxia, depression, recumbency. Renal failure if animal survives for several days	Remove animal from known source. Fluids and corticosteroids for circulatory shock. Control abdominal pain (flunixin meglumine at 1.1 mg/kg IV q12–24h or butrophanol tartrate at 0.1 mg/kg IV q3–4h up to 48 hours. Demulcents. Dimercaprol: 4–5 mg/kg by deep IM injection, followed by 2–3 mg/kg q4h for 24 hours, followed by 1 mg/kg q4h for 2 days or succimer at 10 mg/kg PO q8h *(continued overleaf)*

Table 10.8 (continued)

TOXICANT	USES/SOURCES	MOST LIKELY EXPOSURE	PATHOPHYSIO-LOGIC EFFECT	CLINICAL SIGNS	TREATMENT
Atropine (tropane alkaloids: scopolamine, hyoscyamine)[188]	Anticholinergic drug; tropane alkaloid-containing plants: *Datura stramonium* (Jimsonweed); *Atropa belladonna* (belladonna); *Convolvulus* spp. (bindweed)	Therapeutic use; ingestion of alkaloid-containing plants in pasture or hay	Competitive antagonists of acetylcholine at muscarinic receptors	Increased thirst, skin flushing, dry mucous membranes, ileus, mydriasis, visual disturbances, restlessness, tachycardia, muscular twitching, incoordination, paralysis, delirium, convulsions	Remove from source. GI tract decontamination (activated charcoal may be useful even if delayed administration due to decreased gastric emptying). Fluid and nutritional support. Control neurologic signs with diazepam (0.01–0.04 mg/kg IV), xylazine (4–20 µg/kg IV), or detomidine (5 µg/kg IV loading dose followed by 3.5 µg/kg/hour CRI)
Carbon disulfide[189]	Manufacture of rayon, cellophane, semiconductors; fumigant of boxcars of grain	Most likely exposure following use as fumigant (in combination with carbon tetrachloride)	Irritating to mucous membranes and respiratory tract; corrosive effect on skin	Signs referable to respiratory and mucous membrane irritation; corrosive burns with erythema and blistering; CNS signs include agitation, delirium, lethargy, blurred vision, hallucinations, seizures; hypotension, muscle spasms, coma	Decontamination of skin and mucous membranes. Symptomatic and supportive care. Monitor heart
Carbon tetrachloride[190]	Fumigant in combination with carbon disulfide or ethylene dichloride	Careless disposal; contamination of drinking water; inhalational exposure	Classic hepatotoxicant; nephrotoxicant; toxicity due to metabolism to phosgene	Signs associated with fulminant hepatic failure; inhalational exposure can result in depression and ataxia	Provide fresh air if inhalational exposure; symptomatic and supportive care appropriate for liver failure
Chlorates[191]	Chlorate salts (sodium or potassium) used as herbicide and defoliant	Careless disposal or chlorate salt mistaken for sodium chloride	Strong oxidant chemical; causes oxidation of hemoglobin to methemoglobin; Heinz body formation	Incoordination, abdominal pain, dyspnea, cyanosis and/or brownish discoloration to blood and mucous membranes	Gastric lavage with 1% sodium thiosulfate; demulcents; methylene blue considered ineffective in horses

Table 10.8 *(continued)*

TOXICANT	USES/SOURCES	MOST LIKELY EXPOSURE	PATHOPHYSIO-LOGIC EFFECT	CLINICAL SIGNS	TREATMENT
Chlorinated hydrocarbon insecticides (DDT, methoxychlor, dicofol, cylcodienes (aldrin, dieldrin, endrin, chlordane, hepatachlor), toxaphene, lindane)[192]	Most no longer used (limited use of lindane and methoxychlor)	Access to or spillage from old containers; accidental food contamination	DDT affects peripheral nerves and brain by slowing Na+ influx and K+ efflux; cyclodienes competitively inhibit GABA receptors	Neurologic signs: agitation, apprehension, hyperexcitability, incoordination, tremors, clonic–tonic seizures, hyperthermia	Decontamination of GI tract or skin; control seizures with diazepam or barbiturate; long half-life of the insecticides can delay recovery
Cyanide[193]	Cyanide salts (e.g. potassium cyanide); cyanogenic glycosides in plants; hydrogen cyanide gas; cyanide gas-containing smoke (from burning of nitrogen containing polymers: vinyl, polyurethane, silk)	The most common source for exposure would be ingestion of plant material containing cyanogenic glycosides; smoke inhalation	Binds to ferric iron of mitochondrial cytochrome oxidase resulting in inability of cells to utilize oxygen. This results in tissue anoxia, anaerobic metabolism, and lactic acidosis	Onset of clinical signs is rapid: tachypnea, dyspnea, weakness, tachycardia, bright red mucous membranes, recumbency; terminal seizures	Rapidity of onset of intoxication often precludes treatment. Decontamination with activated charcoal. Sodium nitrite causes methemoglobin, which binds cyanide; sodium thiosulfate helps convert cyanide to thiocyanate, which is rapidly excreted. Sodium nitrite and sodium thiosulfate can be given as a mixture of 1 ml and 3 ml of 20% solutions, respectively, and administered IV at 4 ml/45 kg body weight; supplemental oxygen may be useful after antidote administration
Dimethyl sulfoxide	Only approved use as a topical application to reduce acute swelling due to trauma; treatment of transient ischemia, nervous system trauma, skin ulcers, wounds or burns,	Therapeutic use		Generally considered to be safe. Can cause hemolysis and hemoglobinuria in horses following IV administration; diarrhea, muscle tremors and colic; possible hepato- and nephrotoxicity rarely	

(continued overleaf)

Table 10.8 *(continued)*

TOXICANT	USES/SOURCES	MOST LIKELY EXPOSURE	PATHOPHYSIO-LOGIC EFFECT	CLINICAL SIGNS	TREATMENT
	enhancement of drug penetration of skin			reported; overdosage can cause CNS and pulmonary effects following high IV doses	
Dioctyl sodium succinate (DSS or docusate sodium, calcium or potassium)[194]	Surfactant stool softener	Therapeutic use	Reduce surface tension and allow water and fat to penetrate ingesta and stool; increase cAMP concentrations in colonic mucosal cells with resultant increase in ion secretion and cell permeability	Colic, diarrhea, dehydration, electrolyte disturbances; intestinal mucosal damage	Monitor hydration and electrolyte status and treat appropriately
Fluoride[195]	Acute and chronic fluoride intoxication possible, but chronic much more likely; generally an environmental contaminant resulting from industrial activities	Contamination of forages from airborne or soil contamination; drinking water with high concentrations; feed supplements and mineral mixtures with high fluoride content	Fluoride accumulates in calcified tissues; inadequate matrix and defective mineralization or altered matrix crystallization	Chronic fluorosis is a progressive, debilitating disease involving bones and teeth. Signs include lameness, difficult mastication, weight loss, dry and rough haircoat	Identify and remove from source of exposure; good quality diet; possibly anti-inflammatory drugs for pain relief; slow recovery expected
Heparin[196,197]	Used to promote re-epithelialization in chronic refractory ocular ulceration in the horse; adjunctive treatment of DIC, circulatory shock, and laminitis	Therapeutic use	Acts on coagulation factors in both the intrinsic and extrinsic coagulation pathways; overdose is associated with bleeding	Hematuria, tarry stools, petechiae, bruising, thrombocytopenia; high IV doses in horses cause RBC agglutination and decreased PCV	Protamine sulfate complexes with heparin to form stable salt (administered at 1 mg protamine/100 units heparin to be inactivated by slow IV injection followed by ½ the previous dose every 30 minutes that has lapsed since heparin administration)
Imidocarb dipropinate[198]	Antiprotozoal useful against *Babesia* and related parasites	Therapeutic use		Horses given high therapeutic doses (4 mg/kg) develop lacrimation, sweating and serous nasal discharge ~30 minutes following treatment; cholinergic signs	Symptomatic and supportive care. Anticholinergic (atropine) if severe cholinergic signs

Table 10.8 (continued)

TOXICANT	USES/SOURCES	MOST LIKELY EXPOSURE	PATHOPHYSIO-LOGIC EFFECT	CLINICAL SIGNS	TREATMENT
Iodine[199]	Essential element; germicides (teat dips, dairy sanitizer, general antiseptics for dermal and mucosal infections); seaweed	Overzealous use of germicide; dietary exposure	Altered thyroid function; stimulates vagus nerves causing expectorant action	Lacrimation, salivation, increased respiratory secretions, non-productive cough, dry, scaly skin, anorexia, tachycardia, abortion, infertility, goiter, decreased cell and humoral-mediated immunity	Remove from source of exposure; relatively short half-life; generally recover unless complicating factors such as pneumonia
Lincomycin, clindamycin[24]	Broad-spectrum antibiotics; contraindicated in horses	Accidental administration	Toxic action not precisely known: (1) possible bacterial overgrowth of pathogens such as *Salmonella*, *Clostridium perfringens* and *C. difficile*; (2) direct damage to GI tract mucosa; (3) hypersensitivity	Signs begin 2–4 days following exposure and include abdominal pain, tachycardia, mucous membrane congestion, loose to watery feces +/– blood, fever, dehydration, circulatory shock, laminitis	Laxatives and GI tract protectants may decrease colonization and invasion by pathogenic bacteria; maintain hydration and electrolyte balance; treat laminitis
Metaldehyde[175, 200,201]	Molluscicide: slugs or snails	Accidental feed contamination; mistaking bait for feed; malicious posioning	Decreased GABA brain concentrations; altered brain neurotransmitter concentrations	Salivation ataxia, tremors, dyspnea, hyperpnea, colic, nystagnmus, seizures	Decontamination if early after exposure. Control CNS excitation: diazepam (0.05–0.44 mg/kg IV), methocarbamol (4.4–22 mg/kg IV to effect for moderate conditions up to 22–55 mg/kg IV for severe conditions)
Nicotine[24]	Alkaloid derived from *Nicotiana* spp.; nicotine sulfate used in older insecticide formulations	Direct ingestion of plant or contamination of forage with plant material	Stimulates sympathetic and parasympathetic nicotinic receptors; depolarizing blockade at neuromuscular junctions	Rapid onset of hyperactivity, salivation, tremors, dyspnea, tachycardia, weakness, and paralysis	Decontamination if early after ingestion; assisted ventilation if respiratory distress

(continued overleaf)

Table 10.8 *(continued)*

TOXICANT	USES/SOURCES	MOST LIKELY EXPOSURE	PATHOPHYSIO-LOGIC EFFECT	CLINICAL SIGNS	TREATMENT
Nitrate/nitrite[202]	No documented cases in horses; ruminants reduce nitrate in plants or fertilizers to toxic nitrite	Exposure to concentrated nitrate sources such as fertilizers	Nitrite oxidizes hemoglobin to methemoglobin	Polypnea, dyspnea, cyanotic or brownish mucous membranes, weakness, muscle tremors, reluctance to move, terminal seizures	Methylene blue is the treatment of choice in ruminants, but is not effective in horses; antioxidants such as vitamin C theoretically useful, but efficacy not shown
Petroleum distillates[24]	Crude oil and refined products; often used as carriers for other chemicals, especially insecticides	Environmental contamination; excessive application or misapplication of products with subsequent systemic absorption from skin	Petroleum products are complex mixtures of aliphatic and aromatic hydrocarbons; highly volatile, low viscosity petroleum products such as petroleum distillates, gasoline, and kerosene are easily aspirated; many are irritating to mucous membranes; some have anesthetic-like actions	Signs generally involve GI tract upset and colic, respiratory signs if aspirated including tachypnea, dyspnea, fever, and CNS signs including depression	Decontamination: washing of skin with mild soap and water; administration of activated charcoal +/– cathartic if oral exposure; GI tract protectants; antibiotics if pulmonary aspiration
Pentachlorophenol (PCP) and other chlorophenols[203]	Restrictions on use of PCP make exposure unlikely; wood preservative, acute and chronic intoxications reported but chronic intoxication may be due to PCP contaminants	Possible exposure to old products or treated fences or feedbunks; volatility of PCP can result in inhalational exposure	Uncouples oxidative phosphorylation; directly irritating to skin and respiratory tract	Acute signs: hyperthermia, restlessness, tachypnea, increased GI tract motility, weakness, seizures, collapse. Chronic signs: anorexia, weight loss, alopecia, skin cracks and fissures, dependent edema, joint and hoof problems, conjunctivitis, hematuria, immunocompromise, and increased suspceptibility to infections	Following acute exposures decontamination with activated charcoal +/– cathartic; symptomatic and supportive care

Table 10.8 *(continued)*

TOXICANT	USES/SOURCES	MOST LIKELY EXPOSURE	PATHOPHYSIO-LOGIC EFFECT	CLINICAL SIGNS	TREATMENT
Phenothiazine[24,204]	Anthelmintic	Therapeutic use has resulted in acute and unpredictable adverse effects in horses; rarely used	Oxidant; the metabolite phenothiazine sulfoxide is a photodynamic agent	Hemolytic anemia, hemoglobinuria, icterus, anorexia, weakness, CNS disturbances, and photosensitization	Whole blood transfusions if anemia is severe; antioxidants such as ascorbic acid, monitor renal function; treat photosensitization
Phosphine[205]	Gas produced following fumigation of feed with aluminium phosphide for insect and rodent control or ingestion of zinc phosphide used as a rodenticide	Absorbed across respiratory epithelium and mucous membranes	Not fully understood. Gas inhibits cytochrome C oxidase, leading to disruption of mitochondrial oxidative phosphorylation, which leads to rapid cell death and multiorgan failure	Profuse sweating, tachycardia, tachypnea, pyrexia, ataxia, seizures, and widespread muscle tremors. High mortality	Gastric lavage, DTO-smectite, atropine, IV fluids, sedatives, flunixin meglumine
Phosphorus[24,206]	Elemental phosphorus (red and white forms); red form used in fertilizers and matches; white form use as a rodenticide	Direct exposure or accidental feed contamination	Toxic mechanism of action not clear; yellow phosphorus is corrosive and has a direct effect on myocardium, kidney, and peripheral vessels	GI signs due to corrosive effect: oral burns, colic, diarrhea +/− blood; CNS signs can include restlessness, irritability, depression, stupor, coma; hypotension, circulatory shock; liver and renal impairment; hypoglycemia	Decontamination with activated charcoal; gastric irrigation with 1:5,000 potassium permanganate has been suggested to form non-toxic phosphorus oxides (efficacy not proven); supportive care
Piperazine salts (adipate, citrate, monohydrochlo-ride)[24,207]	Anthelmintic; wide margin of safety, but some variation reported for the different salts (adipate perhaps less toxic than other salt forms)	Accidental overdose	Not certain; anthelmintic efficacy due to neuromuscular blockade ('curare-like' effect)	Depression, incoordination, hyperesthesia, mydriasis, muscle tremors, constipation, anorexia	Decontamination if early after exposure (activated charcoal +/− cathartic); symptomatic and supportive care

(continued overleaf)

Table 10.8 *(continued)*

TOXICANT	USES/SOURCES	MOST LIKELY EXPOSURE	PATHOPHYSIO-LOGIC EFFECT	CLINICAL SIGNS	TREATMENT
Propylene glycol[24,208]	Drug diluent and glucose precursor for treating hypoglycemia in ruminants	Accidental administration of product intended for ruminant use	Lactic acidosis as a result of metabolism to acetate, lactate, and pyruvate	Salivation, profuse sweating, ataxia, depression, tachypnea, cyanosis, seizures, diarrhea	Early decontamination with activated charcoal +/– cathartic; treat severe acidemia and hypovolemia: IV fluids with added sodium bicarbonate; frequent monitoring of acid–base status
Reserpine[24,209]	Alkaloid from *Rauwolfia serpentina* and other *Rauwolfia* spp.; has been used in horses for prolonged tranquilization	Low therapeutic index	Sympatholytic agent that acts at presynaptic nerve terminals of postganglionic adrenergic nerves to deplete norepinephrine, dopamine, and serotonin in the brain	Marked depression, generalized profuse sweating, flatulence, sporadic episodes of violent, colic-like behavior followed by abrupt onset of somnolence and recumbency; other signs include increased borborygmi, diarrhea, muscle tremors, sinus bradycardia, 2nd degree AV block, miosis, and ptosis	Symptomatic and supportive, long-half life so signs can persist for 2–3 days
Sodium fluoroacetate (compound 1080)[210]	Rodent and predator control	Strict limits on availability and use; unlikely exposure of horses unless maliciously used	Forms fluorocitrate, which inhibits aconitase in the tricarboxylic acid cycle. This results in energy depletion, citrate and lactate accumulation, and metabolic acidosis	Rapid onset of clinical signs related to CNS, GI tract, and cardiovascular system: excitation, anxiety, hypesthesia, increased salivation and urination, diarrhea, cardiac arrhythmias, terminal convulsions	Rapid onset of clinical signs and death often precludes treatment; early decontamination with activated charcoal +/– cathartic; IV fluids with added sodium bicarbonate; monitor calcium and potassium concentrations

Table 10.8 *(continued)*

TOXICANT	USES/SOURCES	MOST LIKELY EXPOSURE	PATHOPHYSIO-LOGIC EFFECT	CLINICAL SIGNS	TREATMENT
Strychnine[24,211]	Rodenticide; generally grain-based baits	Accidental feed contamination; ingestion of baits; malicious poisoning	Competitively inhibits glycine binding to receptors in the CNS; glycine is an inhibitory neurotransmitter	Rapid onset of signs including apprehension, nervousness, muscle stiffness, tetanic seizures often induced by external stimuli, apnea, anoxia	Rapid onset of signs and death often precludes effective therapy; early decontamination with activated charcoal +/- cathartic; barbiturates or chloral hydrate to control seizures; methocarbamol (150 mg/kg IV) or quaifenesin (100 mg/kg IV) repeated as needed to control muscle tremors; assisted ventilation and/or oxygen administration
Sulfonamides: variety[212]	Used to treat bacterial and coccidial infections	Therapeutic use, overdose	Physiochemical properties allow precipitation within renal tubules; alteration of normal GI tract microflora (decrease folate production, which can lead to reversible aplastic anemia); hypersensitivity reaction; inhibition of vitamin K epoxide reductase, which can lead to coagulopathy	Dehydrated animals more likely to have renal tubular crystal formation; signs associated with acute kidney injury including oliguria or anuria, crystalluria, hematuria, anorexia, depression; signs related to coagulopathy; aplastic anemia (reversible)	Discontinue medication; fluid therapy to maintain hydration and to promote urine production; alkalinization of the urine by administering sodium bicarbonate may increase drug elimination
Tetrachloro-dibenzodioxin (TCDD)[190]	Industrial chemical by-product that is environmentally and metabolically stable	Exposure to contaminated products: waste oil; possible oral, inhalational, or dermal exposure	Metabolic enzyme induction	Vague clinical signs including conjunctivitis, skin ulceration, anorexia, weight loss, laminitis, colic, polydipsia, oral mucous membrane hyperemia, stiffness, ataxia, and alopecia	Identify source of exposure and remove; symptomatic and supportive care

(continued overleaf)

Table 10.8 *(continued)*

TOXICANT	USES/SOURCES	MOST LIKELY EXPOSURE	PATHOPHYSIO-LOGIC EFFECT	CLINICAL SIGNS	TREATMENT
Zinc salts[24,213,214]	Variety of salts such as zinc acetate, zinc sulfate, zinc oxide	Chronic syndrome in young horses has been reported secondary to environmental zinc contamination of pastures/feed	Manifestations of chronic zinc exposure may in part be due to copper deficiency; copper is an essential co-factor for lysyl oxidase, which is important for collagen formation	Swelling at physeal region of long bones, lameness and stiffness, swollen joints with synovial effusions, weight loss, unthrifty appearance, anemia	Identify source of exposure and remove; supplementary copper (dietary concentration of 250 parts per million on a dry weight basis)

CHAPTER **11**   Monitoring

CHAPTER **12**   Fluid therapy

CHAPTER **13**   Inotrope and vasopressor therapy

CHAPTER **14**   Sedation and analgesia

CHAPTER **15**   Nutritional support

CHAPTER **16**   Antimicrobial drugs

CHAPTER **17**   The systemic inflammatory response

CHAPTER **18**   Postoperative colic patient

CHAPTER **19**   The pregnant mare

CHAPTER **20**   The neonate

CHAPTER **21**   The recumbent horse

CHAPTER 11

MONITORING

*K. Gary Magdesian and
Louise L. Southwood*

GENERAL APPROACH TO MONITORING

- The goal of managing critically ill patients is to provide the necessary support of cellular and organ function to enable healing from the primary disease. Cardiovascular, respiratory, and metabolic support may be necessary.
- Monitoring of critically ill patients should be performed every 1–6 hours depending on the severity of illness and specific type of monitoring used.
- Decisions about treatment should not be made based on an individual measurement at one point in time, but based on observed trends over time and using various monitoring methods.
- Goal-directed therapy involves close patient monitoring, with adjustment of therapy to maintain tissue perfusion and organ function. Clinicians should aspire to using a goal-directed approach when managing critically ill patients.
- Some of the main types of monitoring for equine critically ill patients are:
  - Patient examination.
  - Hematology.
  - Plasma protein concentration.
  - Urine output and urinalysis.
  - Serum and plasma biochemistry.
  - Blood gas analysis.
  - Arterial blood pressure.
  - Central venous pressure.
  - Coagulation profile.
  - Cardiac output.
- Monitoring levels can be established for the hospital with the daily hospitalization charges to the client being adjusted depending on the level of care. For example:
  - Level I: physical examination, PCV, TPP.
  - Level II: physical examination, PCV, TPP, indirect arterial blood pressure, urinalysis, quantification of nasogastric reflux and/or diarrhea.
  - Level III: physical examination, PCV, TPP, indirect arterial blood pressure, urinalysis, quantification of nasogastric reflux and/or diarrhea, direct arterial blood pressure, CVP, lactate, and COP.
- It is important for the clinician to be fiscally responsible during the care of a critically ill equine patient by optimizing care without unnecessary monitoring and treatment, because this can add considerable expense to case management and lead to patient euthanasia for 'economic reasons'.
- This section will focus on general principles and monitoring of the critically ill adult horse. Monitoring of neonatal foals is discussed further in Chapter 20.

MONITORING

Patient examination
Key points

- Maintenance of meticulous medical records is important for monitoring critically ill patients.
- Monitoring trends over time using various physical and laboratory measurements is more useful for patient assessment than using a single value at one time point.
- Critically ill patients should be examined every 1–6 hours depending on the severity of illness. The examination may vary from walking by the stall to look for signs of colic to measurement of vital signs and specific body system examination. The findings on examination should be recorded in the medical record in a way that trends can be observed (**11.1**). The patient's body weight should be measured daily for neonates and every few days where possible for adult horses.

General appearance

The general appearance of the horse is a critical part of patient assessment. Critically ill patients should be observed at least every hour. Any abnormalities should be identified and the cause determined. Some of the key points to observe are:

- Is the patient bright or quiet, alert, and responsive or dull?
- Is the patient standing or recumbent?
- Is the patient's appetite good? Has the patient been drinking?
- Is there a normal amount of feces and urine in the stall?
- Does the patient come to the front of the stall when approached?
- Is the patient sweating?
- Is the patient showing signs of colic?
- Does the patient have abdominal distension?
- Is the patient standing and walking normally?
- Does the patient have an exaggerated respiratory effort or nostril flaring (**11.2**)

Vital signs

The rectal temperature, pulse rate and quality, respiratory rate, oral mucous membrane color and moistness, and CRT can provide considerable information about patient status.

Rectal temperature

Fever can be an early indication of an infection and rectal temperature should be monitored closely in any hospitalized horse. Common sites of infection include IV catheter site, URT and LRT, deep or superficial surgical site infection, and enterocolitis. Some surgical patients may have a mild fever in the early postoperative period (within 48 hours) and this may be from inflammation associated with the surgical procedure. If a horse develops a fever, all possible sites of infection should be examined and the infection site localized. Hematology and fibrinogen or serum amyloid A concentration should be measured. The IV catheter site should be examined and the catheter removed if any abnormalities are noted. A rebreathing examination should be performed. Surgical site infections can be investigated using radiographic or ultrasonographic examination, endoscopy, and/or cytology depending on the site. Culture and sensitivity testing is recommended.

Heart rate, pulse rate, and pulse quality

Heart rate, pulse rate, and pulse quality can be used to assess the cardiovascular system. Tachycardia can be attributed to pain, cardiovascular compromise (shock), and occasionally an arrhythmia. Analgesia should be provided (see Chapter 14). An ECG should be performed on any horse with persistent tachycardia with no apparent reason. Additional monitoring using PCV, lactate, creatinine, urinalysis, CVP, and blood pressure in a horse that is persistently and severely tachycardic and has poor pulse quality can be used to assess fluid requirements and in some cases the need for additional support using inotropes and vasopressors (see Chapter 13).

Respiratory rate

Respiratory rate and effort are often variable, but a high respiratory rate and an exaggerated effort can be an indication of pain (e.g. colic, laminitis), fever, or respiratory tract or thoracic disease and warrant further diagnostic tests. Horses in pain will often have tachypnea with nostril flare (11.2). During periods of high ambient temperatures horses can have tachypnea (50–60 breaths/minute) with no underlying problems. A rebreathing examination should be performed on any horse with a high respiratory rate. The character of respiration should also be observed (i.e. rapid shallow breathing versus an exaggerated expiratory effort).

Oral mucous membranes

Oral mucous membranes should normally be pink and moist with a CRT <2 seconds. Endotoxemic horses will initially have bright pink or injected oral mucous membranes (hyperdynamic phase of shock), which will progress to dark purple (hypodynamic phase of shock). (See also Chapter 17.) Tacky or dry oral mucous membranes are a sign of dehydration (total body water loss) and a prolonged CRT is a sign of hypovolemia, and both indicate the need for fluid therapy. The cardiovascular system and hydration status should also be assessed using jugular refill and extremity temperature. Skin tent may also be used to assess hydration; however, this is not always reliable in the horse.

Gastrointestinal system

Borborygmi should be monitored in all abdominal quadrants and recorded. A horse from which feed is withheld and inappetent horses will usually have borborygmi that are decreased compared with normal. Once feed is reintroduced or the appetite returns, borborygmi should return to normal. Absent borborygmi generally reflect serious underlying GI tract disease and will often be associated with signs of colic and lack of defecation. Horses showing these signs should also be monitored for signs of colic and abdominal distension, and checked for gastric accumulation of fluid by passing a nasogastric tube.

Musculoskeletal system

Any critically ill horse should be monitored closely for signs of laminitis, which include an increase in digital pulses, warm hooves, and lameness when walked around the stall. Foals should be monitored for lameness, periarticular edema, and joint effusion associated with septic physitis and arthritis. (See Chapter 2, Chapter 9, and Chapter 20.)

Hematology

Key points

- Leukopenia is always associated with pathology and severe leukopenia (<2,000 cells/µl) is usually associated with serious diseases.
- PCV should be monitored frequently in critically ill patients as a crude assessment of intravascular volume and the need for more or less IV fluids and to allow for early identification of anemia.

Definition/overview

Hematology is the assessment of the leukogram and RBC indices. The leukogram refers to the total leukocyte (WBC) count, differential analysis, and WBC morphology. Mature WBCs are categorized as granulocytes, which are produced in the bone marrow (neutrophils, eosinophils, and basophils) and mononuclear leucocytes, which are produced in the bone marrow (monocytes) or bone marrow and lymphoid tissue (lymphocytes). Immature WBCs that may be in the peripheral circulation in response to severe infection and overwhelming inflammation are band or non-segmented neutrophils, metamyelocytes, myelocytes, and progranulocytes.[1]

RBC indices include the PCV, RBC count, hemoglobin (Hb) concentration, mean corpuscular volume (MCV), mean corpuscular hemoglobin (MCH), and mean corpuscular hemoglobin concentration (MCHC).[2]

A platelet count is also performed with hematology and will be discussed under Coagulation profile (p. 638).

Indications

Hematology should be performed on any emergency admission as part of the standard of care to identify any underlying disease and obtain baseline values. Any abnormalities detected at admission should be reassessed until the values return to within normal limits for the laboratory. Hematology should also be performed preoperatively on horses undergoing general anesthesia to detect early underlying disease such as pneumonia.

EQUINE INPATIENT TREATMENT RECORD – LEVEL I

FRONT PAGE

Example Template Only

Parameters to contact clinician:

1. If painful, acute diarrhea, dyspnea, or laminitis
2. If temperature ≥ _____
3. If pulse ≥ _____
4. If PCV > _____
5. If catheter or NG tube problems _____
6. Other: _____

DATE: _____ PAGE: _____

BODY WEIGHT: _____

CLINICIAN SIGNATURE: _____

	TIME	12 pm	1 pm	2 pm	3 pm	4 pm	5 pm	6 pm	7 pm	8 pm	9 pm	10 pm	11 pm
Monitoring	*Initials (student/nurse)*												
	Walk By ~q 1 hr												
	ATTITUDE/PAIN												
	FECES (character/volume)												
	VITAL SIGNS q ___ hr												
	TEMPERATURE												
	PULSE (rate/strength)												
	RESPIRATION												
	MUCOUS												
	MEMBRANES (CRT/color)												
	ABDOMINAL q ___ hr AUSCULT -upper -lower	L R	L R	L R	L R	L R	L R	L R	L R	L R	L R	L R	L R
	DIGITAL q ___ hr PULSES -fore -hind	L R	L R	L R	L R	L R	L R	L R	L R	L R	L R	L R	L R
	PCV/TP q ___ hr												
	GASTRIC REFLUX q ___ hr												
Treatment	q ___ hr												
	q ___ hr												
	q ___ hr												
	q ___ hr												
	q ___ hr												
	q ___ hr												
	q ___ hr												
	q ___ hr												
	CATHETER q ___ hr √ vein & flush												
	FEEDING q ___ hr Type/amt:												
Fluids	q ___ hr												
	q ___ hr												
	q ___ hr												
	q ___ hr												
	q ___ hr												
	q ___ hr												
	q ___ hr												

EQUINE INPATIENT TREATMENT RECORD – LEVEL I

Example Template Only

PAGE: _____

	TIME	12 am	1 am	2 am	3 am	4 am	5 am	6 am	7 am	8 am	9 am	10 am	11 am
Monitoring	*Initials (student/tech)*												
	Walk By ~q 1 hr												
	ATTITUDE/PAIN												
	FECES (character/volume)												
	VITAL SIGNS q ____ hr												
	TEMPERATURE												
	PULSE (rate/strength)												
	RESPIRATION												
	MUCOUS												
	MEMBRANES (CRT/color)												
	ABDOMINAL q ____ hr AUSCULTATION -upper -lower	L R	L R	L R	L R	L R	L R	L R	L R	L R	L R	L R	L R
	DIGITAL q ____ hr PULSES -fore -hind	L R	L R	L R	L R	L R	L R	L R	L R	L R	L R	L R	L R
	PCV/TP q ____ hr												
	GASTRIC REFLUX q ____ hr												
Treatment	q ____ hr												
	q ____ hr												
	q ____ hr												
	q ____ hr												
	q ____ hr												
	q ____ hr												
	q ____ hr												
	q ____ hr												
	CATHETER q ____ hr √ vein & flush												
	FEEDING q ____ hr Type/amt:												
Fluids	q ____ hr												
	q ____ hr												
	q ____ hr												
	q ____ hr												
	q ____ hr												
	q ____ hr												
	q ____ hr												

11.1 An example of a monitoring and treatment sheet.

WBC count and differential should be performed on any horse with a fever of unknown origin or a known infection site. WBC count and differential can be monitored every few days in patients with abnormal values.

PCV should be monitored in critically ill horses every 6–12 hours because trends can be used as an indication of intravascular volume changes and to guide fluid therapy (i.e. an increase in PCV [hemoconcentration] can indicate hypovolemia and the need to increase fluid administration). PCV should also be monitored routinely in these patients for early detection of acute anaemia (e.g. a postoperative colic patient that has intra-abdominal hemorrhage or a critically ill patient with hemolytic anemia). PCV, Hb, and RBC count should be monitored every 1–2 days or more often in any case with historical hemorrhagic or hemolytic anemia.

Technique

- A blood sample is collected from the jugular or other peripheral vein (lateral thoracic, cephalic, or saphenous vein) using an 18- to 20-gauge 1½ – 2 inch needle.
- The blood is placed immediately into an evacuated EDTA tube (Vacutainer®). The tube should be filled to capacity to ensure an appropriate amount of anticoagulant and the tube inverted several times to ensure proper mixing of blood and EDTA. Alternatively, blood can be collected directly into the evacuated EDTA tube using a Vacutainer® needle (**11.3**).

- Samples should be processed immediately or refrigerated at 4°C (39.2°F)for up to 24 hours. An air-dried blood smear should be prepared immediately to preserve cell morphology if processing is to be delayed by more than 2 hours, after which it can be held for several days. Hematology samples should be shipped on ice in an insulated container.
- WBC count and RBC indices can be measured manually using a hemocytometer or an automated cell counter.
- The differential WBC count can be performed by making a blood smear and staining with Wright's or a modified Romanovsky's stain. Generally, 100–200 cells are counted and categorized and the percentages of the different WBCs calculated.
- Blood for measurement of PCV can be collected from the jugular or other peripheral vein or the facial venous sinus either into an EDTA tube or directly into a heparinized microhematocrit tube (**11.4**). The microhematocrit tube is centrifuged and the PCV measured from the reference card (**11.5**).

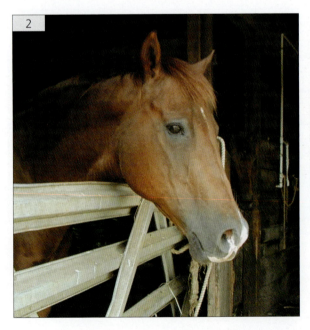

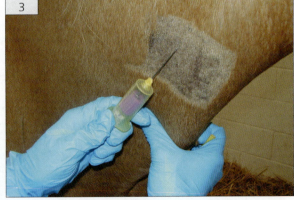

11.3 Collection of blood directly into a Vacutainer® tube. Note: The Vacutainer tabe should not be punctured until the needle is in the vein.

11.2 A horse showing exaggerated respiratory effort with nostril flaring.

- MCV, MCH, and MCHC can be calculated from the PCV, Hb, and RBC count:

SI units

$$MCV \text{ (fl/cell)} = \frac{PCV \text{ (1/1)} \times 10^3}{RBC \text{ count } (10^{12} \text{ cells/l})}$$

$$MCH \text{ (pg/cell)} = \frac{Hb \text{ (g/l)}}{RBC \text{ count } (10^{12} \text{ cells/l})}$$

$$MCHC \text{ (g/l)} = \frac{Hb \text{ (g/l)}}{PCV \text{ (1/1)}}$$

Conventional units

$$MCV \text{ (fl/cell)} = \frac{PCV \text{ (\%)} \times 10}{RBC \text{ count } (10^6/\mu l)}$$

$$MCH \text{ (pg/cell)} = \frac{Hb \text{ (g/dl)} \times 10}{RBC \text{ count } (10^6/\mu l)}$$

$$MCHC \text{ (g/dl)} = \frac{Hb \text{ (g/dl)} \times 100}{PCV \text{ (\%)}}$$

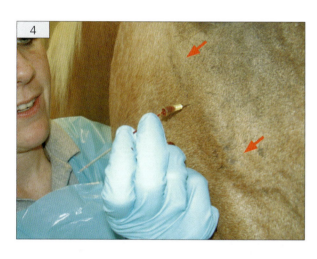

11.4 Collection of blood from a facial venous sinus directly into a hematocrit tube. Arrows, facial crest.

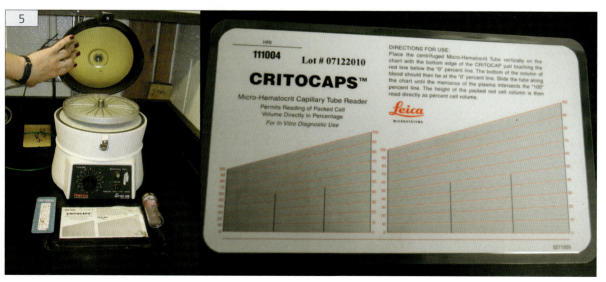

11.5 Hematocrit tube, centrifuge, and reference card for measuring packed cell volume. (Courtesy Wendy Hitchens)

Interpretation

Normal values for the leukogram and RBC indices are shown in *Table 11.1*.[3] Each laboratory, however, should establish normal values. A leukocytosis in horses can be physiological (stress, excitation, anxiety, exercise) or pathophysiological and a leukopenia is always pathophysiological. Common causes of a neutrophilia are: excitement, stress, or exercise; exogenous corticosteroid administration; chronic pneumonia or pleuropneumonia; *Streptococcus equi* infection; chronic peritonitis; internal abscess; chronic salmonellosis or colitis; thrombophlebitis; or vasculitis (purpura hemorrhagica). Common causes of neutropenia are: acute colitis (e.g. salmonellosis, ehrlichial colitis [Potomac horse fever]); necrotic intestine; GI tract perforation and acute severe peritonitis; endotoxemia; septicemia; acute severe pleuropneumonia; acute metritis; duodenitis-proximal jejunitis; or viral diseases. A lymphocytosis is most often caused by excitement or exercise and a lymphopenia by stress, exogenous corticosteroid administration, endotoxemia, septicemia, GI tract perforation, or some viruses.[1] Monocytosis and eosinophilia are uncommon in emergency and critical care cases.[2]

A left shift (increase in non-segmented [band] neutrophils is always abnormal and typically indicative of an infection). A degenerative left shift is uncommon in adult horses.

PCV, RBC count, and Hb are the most commonly measured RBC indices. While PCV is not the 'gold standard' for monitoring hydration or intravascular volume because it can be influenced by confounding problems such as blood loss, changes in PCV can be used to guide fluid therapy (e.g. an increase in PCV in a postoperative colic patient that is refluxing or has diarrhea should prompt an increase in intravascular fluid administration and close monitoring with necessary fluid therapy adjustments). An acute decrease in PCV compared with previous values, particularly in combination with a decrease in Hb and RBC count, should prompt a thorough examination for evidence of hemorrhage or hemolysis.

Table 11.1 Normal hematology values in adult horses

LEUKOGRAM AND ERYTHRON INDICES	VALUES
WBCs ($\times 10^9$/l) [/µl]	5.4–14.3 [5,400–14,300]
Segmented neutrophils ($\times 10^9$/l) [/µl]	2.3–8.6 [2,300–8,600]
Non-segmented neutrophils (bands) ($\times 10^9$/l) [/µl]	0–0.1 [0–100]
Lymphocytes ($\times 10^9$/l) [/µl]	1.5–7.7 [1,500–7,700]
Monocytes ($\times 10^9$/l) [/µl]	0–1 [0–1,000]
Eosinophils ($\times 10^9$/l) [/µl]	0–1 [0–1,000]
Basophils ($\times 10^9$/l) [/µl]	0–0.29 [0–290]
Neutrophil:Lymphocyte ratio	0.8–2.8
PCV (l/l) [%]	0.32–0.53 [32–53]
Hemoglobin (g/l) [g/dl]	110–190 [11–19]
RBCs ($\times 10^{12}$/l) [10^6/µL]	6.7–12.9 [6.7–12.9]
MCV (fl)	37–58.5
MCH (pg)	12.3–19.7
MCHC (g/l) [g/dl]	310–386 [31–38.6]

Other RBC indices are not routinely monitored in horses and cannot be used alone to interpret changes in the erythron because erythrocytes are retained in the bone marrow until hemoglobin synthesis is complete. MCV can be increased (macrocytosis) in some horses with regenerative anemia and in older horses and decreased (microcytosis) with iron-deficiency anemia. MCH can increase with reticulocytes (immature erythrocytes) in the peripheral blood or intravascular hemolysis and decrease with iron-deficiency anemia. MCHC will be increased with hemolysis and decreased with reticulocytosis or iron deficiency. Other changes in the erythron can be observed using cytology and are uncommon.[2]

Plasma proteins
Key points
- Critically ill patients are often hypoproteinemic/hypoalbuminemic.
- Hypoalbuminemia can lead to hypovolemia and tissue edema formation.
- Monitoring COP directly may be indicated in critically ill patients and patients treated with synthetic colloids.

Definition/overview
The major plasma proteins are albumin, fibrinogen, and the globulins. TPP refers to the combined quantity of the plasma proteins. The plasma proteins, in particular albumin, are responsible for maintaining COP, which is the force that maintains the intravascular volume.

Indications
TPP should be monitored regularly (i.e. every 6–12 hours) with PCV in critically ill patients because hypoproteinemia (hypoalbuminemia) is common, can have detrimental effects on the COP, and can also indicate other underlying disease.

Technique
- A blood sample can be collected from any vessel using a needle and syringe or evacuated tube containing heparin or EDTA. Excessive EDTA can falsely increase the TPP concentration.

A blood sample for measurement of fibrinogen using the nephelometry method (see below) should be collected into sodium citrate.
- TPP is measured on the plasma following centrifugation of blood in a microhematocrit tube using a refractometer. Mild hemolysis or icterus does not interfere with the accuracy of TPP concentration when a refractometer is used. Turbidity and lipemia may alter light transmission, leading to inaccurate measurements of TPP.
- TPP can also be measured using the colorimetric Biuret technique used in automated chemical analyzers.[3]
- Fibrinogen can be measured using the Schalm technique, which involves subtracting the protein concentration in plasma following fibrinogen precipitation from that prior to fibrinogen precipitation. This can be performed by collecting EDTA blood in two microhematocrit tubes, centrifuging both samples for 3 minutes, measuring the TP following centrifugation in one sample (albumin, globulins, fibrinogen), heating the second sample (56°C [132.8°F] for 3 minutes) to precipitate the fibrinogen, repeating the centrifugation, and then measuring the TP (albumin and globulins).
- The Miller technique for measurement of fibrinogen concentration requires a specially equipped microscope.
- Fibrinogen can also be measured using the nephelometry method, which is a light scatter technique used in clinical laboratories and provides more accurate measurements of fibrinogen concentration.
- Albumin and globulins (alpha, beta, gamma) are measured using serum protein electrophoresis.[3]
- COP can be measured indirectly using equations.[4] For example, the Landis–Pappenheimer equation, which provides a reasonable estimate in healthy foals:

$$COP = 2.1TP + 0.16TP^2 + 0.009TP^3$$
(TP = total plasma protein; COP = colloid osmotic pressure)

- Other equations that correlate with direct COP measurement in healthy adult horses are listed below:

$$COP = 0.986 + 2.029A + 0.175A^2$$
$$COP = -0.059 + 0.618G + 0.028\,G^2$$
$$COP = 0.028 + 1.542P + 0.219P^2$$
$$COP = -1.989 + 1.068Pr + 0.176Pr^2$$
$$COP = -4.384 + 5.501A + 2.475G$$

(A = albumin; G = globulin; P = protein; Pr = protein measured using refractometry)

- COP can be measured directly using a colloid osmometer. Use of this technique should be considered in critically ill patients, because equations are not as accurate, and in patients administered synthetic colloids. However, TPP can provide an estimate of COP.

Interpretation

Normal values for plasma proteins are shown in *Table 11.2*.[3]; however, reference values for each laboratory should be used. Normal COP values in adult horses range from 15 to 22 mmHg and in neonates from 19 to 30 mmHg.[4]

Hypoproteinemia is a common concern in critically ill equine patients, with hypoalbuminemia being the most common cause for hypoproteinaemia. Albumin accounts for 75% of the plasma COP and binds to and transports plasma components that do not have a specific transport protein.[3] Adequate COP is necessary to maintain intravascular volume and edema formation occurs with albumin concentrations <15 g/l (1.5 g/dl). It is critical to provide appropriate rates of IV fluids to avoid overhydration in hypoproteinemic/hypoalbuminemic patients (see Central venous pressure and Arterial blood pressure); however, fluid administration should not be restricted to maintain plasma protein >40 g/l (4 mg/dl) or albumin >15 g/l (1.5 g/dl). In cases where the required IV fluid rate causes hypoproteinemia/hypoalbuminemia, either synthetic (e.g. hetastarch) or natural (e.g. plasma) colloids should be administered (see Chapter 12) to maintain COP.

Common causes of hypoalbuminemia in critically ill patients are loss through the vascular wall because of endothelial changes. This can occur in response to the systemic inflammatory response or actual vascular injury. Loss into the intestinal lumen or wall because of mucosal damage and inflammation can also occur. Inadequate protein intake and increased metabolic demands associated with fever, trauma, and surgery should also be considered as causes of hypoalbuminemia in critically ill patients. Hypoalbuminemia is common in patients with enterocolitis, right dorsal colitis, strangulating intestinal lesions, extensive burns, and acute hemorrhage following fluid resuscitation. Other less common causes of hypoalbuminemia in horses are protein losing nephropathy, chronic hepatic fibrosis, infiltrative bowel diseases, and parasitism.

Acute hyperproteinemia is most often associated with hypovolemia (loss of water from the intravascular space) and dehydration (loss of total body water). Common causes in critically ill equine patients include GI disease (e.g. enterocolitis, strangulating intestinal obstruction) with loss of fluid into the intestinal lumen or wall and inadequate intake because of illness or dysphagia (e.g. botulism, esophageal obstruction, guttural pouch mycosis). Dehydration and hypovolemia can be assessed clinically (see Patient examination). Hyperglobulinemia can also cause hyperproteinemia and is associated with chronic infections (e.g. abdominal or pulmonary abscessation, pleuropneumonia), immune-mediated disease, or neoplasia.

Table 11.2 **Normal plasma protein concentrations in adult horses**	
PLASMA PROTEIN	**VALUES**
Total protein (g/l) [g/dl]	62–79 [6.2–7.9]
Albumin (g/l) [g/dl]	26–37 [2.6–3.7]
Globulin (g/l) [g/dl]	26–40 [2.6–4.0]
Albumin:Globulin ratio	0.6–1.5
Fibrinogen (g/l) [mg/dl]	2–4 [0.2–0.4]

Hyperfibrinogenemia occurs in patients with generalized or localized inflammation, including any type of infection (e.g. abscess, enterocolitis, peritonitis, pleuropneumonia, septic arthritis/osteomyelitis, and cellulitis), and following accidental or surgical trauma. Fibrinogen concentration in a patient with an untreated internal abscess will often be >10 g/l (1,000 mg/dl) and in a postoperative colic patient 5–7 g/l (500–700 mg/dl). SAA is an adjunct to the use of fibrinogen for identification of infection. It is a more sensitive marker, but its increase is short lived.

Hypofibrinogenemia can result from severe, diffuse liver failure and an absolute or relative hypofibrinogenemia from DIC. In the latter case, the fibrinogen concentration may be within normal limits because of the combination of increased fibrinogen production from inflammation and increased consumption from DIC (see Coagulation profile).

Serum and plasma biochemistry

Key points

- Serum biochemistry profiles can be broken down into the following segments for analyses: (1) acid–base and electrolytes; (2) creatinine and BUN; (3) liver enzymes and bilirubin; (4) muscle enzymes; (5) serum proteins; and (6) glucose.
- Serial monitoring of creatinine is important to prevent and treat renal failure.
- Close monitoring of blood glucose concentrations may aid in improved regulation of normoglycemia, a finding that has resulted in improved survival in critically ill human patients.
- Blood lactate concentrations are a rapid and practical means of monitoring perfusion and tissue metabolic status. Serial monitoring of lactate can aid fluid and inotrope/vasopressor therapy.

Definition/overview

Serum chemistries and electrolytes are important monitoring tools for critically ill patients in evaluating for development of organ dysfunction syndromes including renal disease, hepatic dysfunction, and GI disorders. Additional chemistries that are useful in the ICU include plasma magnesium (total and ionized), ionized calcium, blood glucose, and serum triglyceride concentrations. The basic chemistry profile can be broken down into the following categories: (1) acid–base and electrolytes; (2) creatinine and BUN; (3) liver enzymes and bilirubin; (4) muscle enzymes; (5) serum proteins; (6) glucose. Normal values are shown in *Table 11.3*.

Table 11.3 Normal serum and plasma biochemistry values for adult horses

BIOCHEMISTRY MEASUREMENT	VALUE*
Sodium	130–140 mmol/l (mEq/l)
Potassium	3.0–5.6 mmol/l (mEq/l)
Chloride	91–104 mmol/l (mEq/l)
Lactate	<2.0 mmol/l
Calcium (total)	2.9–3.5 mmol/l (11.4–14.1 mg/dl)
Phosphorus	0.6–1.5 mmol/l (2.1–4.7 mg/dl)
Magnesium (total)	0.78–1.23 mmol/l (1.9–3.0 mg/dl)
Total carbon dioxide	23–32 mmol/l
Creatinine	80–177 µmol/l (0.9–2.0 mg/dl)
Blood urea nitrogen	4.28–9.64 mmol/l (12–27 mg/dl)
Sorbitol dehydrogenase	0–8 U/l
Aspartate aminotransferase	168–494 U/L
Gamma glutamyltransferase	8–22 U/l
Alkaline phosphatase	86–285 U/l
Blood ammonia	3.65–43.07 µmol/l (5–59 µg/dl)
Bile acids	0–20 µmol/l (0–7.8 µg/ml)
Creatine kinase	119–287 U/l
Glucose	4.44–5.94 mmol/l (80–107 mg/dl)

*These values will vary with the laboratory technique used. Refer to your specific laboratory references.

Indication

Serum or plasma biochemistry should be performed based on the expected underlying disease. A chemistry profile can be used in emergency and critically ill cases as a screening test to detect underlying disease (e.g. renal disease).

Technique

- Venous blood can be collected from the jugular or other peripheral vein into a plain evacuated tube or syringe (serum) or into a heparinized evacuated tube (plasma).
- Most serum or plasma biochemistries are measured using automated chemical analyzers.

Interpretation

Acid–base and electrolytes: Electrolytes and total CO_2 provide important information for evaluating acid–base balance, particularly as they pertain to strong ion difference. The clinically relevant strong ion difference formula is: $(Na + K) - (Cl + lactate)$, with a high value (>40) being consistent with a strong ion metabolic alkalosis and a low value (<40) with a strong ion acidosis. Knowledge of electrolytes is useful for guiding supplementation of fluids with electrolytes. Total CO_2 can be used to estimate base deficit. Because the major contributor to total CO_2 is bicarbonate ion, bicarbonate concentration can be calculated as $0.9 (TCO_2)$.

Calcium and phosphorus are often decreased in anorexic and hypoalbuminemic animals. Magnesium is speculated to be associated with ileus in horses. In neonates with peripartum asphyxia, magnesium supplementation, as an NMDA receptor antagonist, has been suggested by some, although this is somewhat controversial. Monitoring of ionized magnesium concentrations is important to avoid overdose in these foals.

Creatinine and blood urea nitrogen: Renal failure is a common complication in critically ill horses and serial monitoring of serum creatinine is very important. An incremental increase in serum creatinine with time, even if still in the normal range, reflects a trend toward decreasing GFR and is an earlier marker of renal dysfunction than waiting for azotemia to develop.

Liver enzymes and bilirubin: Liver enzymes can be used to evaluate hepatic and biliary health. SDH and AST are hepatocellular, whereas GGT and ALP are biliary in origin. Of these, SDH is liver-specific and GGT is nearly biliary-specific, although pancreatitis can cause increases as well. SDH has a short half-life (2–3 hours) and reflects active disease; at the opposite end of the spectrum is GGT, with a very long half-life (~3 days) allowing it to stay increased for prolonged periods. Liver function can be monitored through blood ammonia and serum bile acid concentrations. Hyperammonemia is associated with hepatic and GI-associated encephalopathies. Bile acids increase with liver dysfunction, biliary stasis, and secondary to GI disorders such as colitis.

Muscle enzymes: Muscle enzymes (CK and AST) may increase with tissue hypoperfusion, as occurs with septic shock and peripartum asphyxia in foals. Genetic myopathies may become clinically apparent in horses with other primary disorders, including polysaccharide storage myopathy, and recurrent exertional rhabdomyolysis. Neonates with markedly increased muscle enzymes compared with normal should be evaluated for selenium deficiency.

Serum proteins: Serum proteins are listed on biochemistry profiles as albumin and globulin concentrations. Albumin is a negative acute phase protein and is often low in critically ill horses. Also, losses occur through the gut and kidneys with protein losing enteropathies such as colitis and glomerular diseases, respectively. Albumin concentrations can trigger the need for plasma transfusions or administration of colloids, especially when albumin concentrations are <15 g/l (1.5 g/dl).

Glucose: Serum or whole blood glucose concentrations should be monitored frequently in ICU patients. This is particularly important in neonates and horses at risk for lipid derangements including ponies, donkeys, miniature horses, horses with Cushing's disease or metabolic syndrome, and pregnant mares. Both hypo- and hyperglycemia are detrimental to critically ill patients. Moderate regulation of blood glucose concentrations has shown promise in improving outcome in human critical care patients.[5] Guidelines for maintenance of glucose concentrations are not available for horses. The author targets 4.44–8.32 mmol/l (80–150 mg/dl) for adults and 4.44–9.99 mmol/l (80–180 mg/dl) for foals.

Lactate: Blood lactate concentration is a very informative and rapid monitoring tool. It is one of the most useful tools introduced to clinical equine practice in recent years. Lactate is produced from anaerobic metabolism when the oxygen demands of tissues are greater than the supply. Examples of states of increased lactate production include exercise, seizure activity, and hypoperfusion. Blood or plasma lactate concentration reflects a balance between production and clearance. The primary organ of clearance is the liver, with the kidneys playing a secondary role. Type A lactic acidosis occurs in association with evidence of poor tissue perfusion or oxygenation, as with hypotension or hypovolemia. Type B lactic acidosis is when no evidence of poor tissue perfusion or oxygenation exists. Other causes of increased lactate, other than reduced oxygen delivery, include sepsis (through inhibition of pyruvate dehydrogenase by activation of pyruvate dehydrogenase kinase), catecholamine surges, thiamine deficiency, cyanide toxicity, alkalosis, seizures and exercise, hyperglycemia, liver failure, kidney failure, lymphosarcoma, cytopathic hypoxia, and administration of drugs such as salicylates, acetaminophen, ethanol, isoniazid, ethylene glycol, sorbitol, nitroprusside, lactulose, niacin, and theophylline. Cytopathic hypoxia refers to a state of cellular and mitochondrial dysfunction where oxygen cannot be utilized even if present.

Serial blood lactate concentrations are helpful in monitoring response to fluid and vasopressor therapy. Normalization of lactate serves as an end point to these therapies. Lactate response to therapy also has prognostic abilities. Using blood lactate concentration to determine the prognosis for survival is controversial; however, it may be useful for horses with specific causes of colic (e.g. large colon volvulus or colitis). It should be kept in mind that persistent increases in lactate do not necessarily equate to hypoperfusion. Sepsis and SIRS states, as well as other causes listed above, may be responsible for hyperlactatemia. This is particularly true in neonatal foals, which often have persistent hyperlactatemia, despite resolution of hypovolemia, due to sepsis and SIRS. Normal lactate values for adult horses are <2 mmol/l, although most are <1 mmol/l.[6,7] Hospitalized horses on IV fluids should have a lactate concentration of <1 mmol/l. Neonatal foals have decremental values after birth, with concentrations of 4.9 ± 1.02, 2.25 ± 0.6, and 0.89 mmol/l at birth, 12 hours, and 24 hours of age, respectively. In a study performed by one of the the authors (KGM), foals had values of 2.3 ± 0.9, 1.2 ± 0.3, and 1.1 ± 0.3 at 0 to 2 hours, 24 hours, and 48 hours of age, respectively, compared with 0.6 ± 0.2 mmol/l in adult horses.[8]

Blood gas analysis

Key points

- ABG analysis provides monitoring of pulmonary oxygenation efficiency and ventilatory status.
- Venous and central venous blood gas analyses provide information about metabolic status (oxygen extraction efficiency).
- Both arterial and venous blood gas analyses can be used to estimate acid–base status.
- Expected compensation of primary metabolic or respiratory acid–base disorders can be calculated. Comparison of expected to actual values can determine whether responses are compensatory or primary.

Definition/overview

Blood gas analysis refers to measurement of arterial, venous, or central venous pH, oxygen tension (PaO_2, PvO_2, and $PcvO_2$ respectively), carbon dioxide tension ($PaCO_2$, $PvCO_2$, and $PcvO_2$ respectively), and oxygen saturation (SaO_2, SvO_2, and $ScvO_2$). Venous samples are taken from the jugular, cephalic, or saphenous vein and central venous samples from the cranial vena cava (see Central venous pressure). Mixed venous samples are taken from the pulmonary artery using a pulmonary artery catheter and are rarely used in equine patients.

Indications

ABGs are usually analyzed in patients with pulmonary, thoracic, or respiratory disease, patients under general anesthesia, and in critically ill neonates. Venous blood gases can be analyzed in any critically ill patient to assess and monitor metabolic status.

Technique

- In horses, arterial samples can be obtained from the transverse facial (standing), dorsal metatarsal, facial, or carotid arteries. Other arteries that can be sampled in neonatal foals include the brachial, median, decubital, and femoral arteries. A venous blood sample can be routinely taken from the jugular or any other peripheral vein. If a CVP catheter is placed in the cranial vena cava, a CVP sample can be collected.
- The selected site should be cleaned and prepared; a lidocaine bleb can reduce movement during the arterial stick.
- The blood sample should be collected anaerobically into a heparin-coated syringe and kept on ice until analysis.
- After elimination of air bubbles, the syringe should be sealed with a rubber stopper or cap.
- The sealed blood sample may be stored on ice for up to 2–3 hours without significant alterations.
- Analysis should occur within 10 minutes of collection if maintained at room temperature.
- Temperature correction of blood gas results, for individual patient body temperatures, is controversial. The complex effects of changes in body temperature on cardiovascular function and respiration are unknown. Both corrected and uncorrected blood gas values may, therefore, have uncertainties in interpretation for febrile or hypothermic patients. Interpretation of corrected values demands deviation from familiar and better understood guidelines for interpreting uncorrected values. In most cases, corrected and uncorrected values are similar and all samples should be treated the same (either corrected or not corrected) for comparison purposes and for the sake of consistency.
- Accidental introduction of room air into the sample will artificially increase the PaO_2, decrease the $PaCO_2$, and raise the pH slightly.
- Blood gas analysis can be performed using automated blood gas analyzers such as the ABL 700 Series Analyzers.
- A number of portable stallside analyzers have also been evaluated for horses and include the i-STAT, the StatPal II, and the IRMA.[9,10]

Interpretation

Blood gas analysis requires different interpretation for venous and arterial samples. Blood gas tensions in arterial samples reflect pulmonary function, whereas in venous samples they are more representative of tissue metabolism. Normal values are shown in *Table 11.4*.

Table 11. 4 **Normal blood gas values in adult horses and foals >24 hours old and standing**

BLOOD GAS INDICES	ADULT HORSES	FOALS
PaO_2 (mmHg)	$90.2 \pm 2.2 - 101.7 \pm 1.6$	$81 \pm 6.0 - 84.6 \pm 6.9$ For foals >12 hours old
$PaCO_2$ (mmHg)	$41.5 \pm 1.0 - 43.0 \pm 0.7$	45.2 ± 2.5
SaO_2 (%)	≥95	≥95
PvO_2 (mmHg)	45.6 ± 4.7 (jugular)	
$PvCO_2$ (mmHg)	3–6 mmHg higher than $PaCO_2$	52.9 ± 4.0
SvO_2 (%)	65–75 (jugular)	
$PmvO_2$ (mmHg) (mixed venous)	37–38	37.1 ± 0.5
$PmvCO_2$ (mmHg)	47–48	51.9 ± 0.9

PaO_2 reflects pulmonary oxygenating function and is independent of Hb concentration. Values <80 mmHg indicate hypoxemia and correlate with an SaO_2 <95%. Values <60 mmHg (SaO_2 approximately 90%) indicate severe hypoxemia (**11.6**). Clinically healthy neonatal foals in lateral recumbency may have PaO_2 values <80 mmHg during the first 12–24 hours of life.[11] Reported values for PaO_2 in immediately postpartum, recumbent foals are 40–50 and 39.7 ± 2.1 mmHg.[11,12] By 24 hours of age, PaO_2 is reported to be 81 ± 6 and 83.2 ± 3.1 mmHg.[11,13] Positioning alters blood gas interpretation as PaO_2 increases from 72.7 ± 14.2 to 84.6 ± 6.9 mmHg in the same foal when changed from lateral recumbency to a standing position.[11] Reported values for PaO_2 in adults horses include 96.0 ± 8.0 and 90.2 ± 2.2 to 101.7 ± 1.6 mmHg.[14,15]

The $PaCO_2$ reflects ventilatory status. Hypoventilation (a $PaCO_2$ value >60–65 mmHg) may warrant intervention in the form of positive pressure ventilation or chemical stimulation with caffeine or doxapram. Treatment of hypoventilation is indicated if blood pH is affected by respiratory acidosis (pH <7.25) or if signs of intracranial hypertension develop or worsen. Severe hyperventilation ($PaCO_2$ <30 mmHg), on the other hand, may cause respiratory alkalosis and a reduction in cerebral blood flow and should also be avoided. Arterial CO_2 tension in normal adult horses is 41.5 ± 1.0 – 43.0

± 0.7 mmHg.[14] In 24-hour-old foals, $PaCO_2$ is 45.2 ± 2.5 (standing) and 48.1 ± 3.82 (recumbent) mmHg. Other reported values include similar numbers, including 42.2 ± 1.8, 44.5 ± 1.2, and 42.4 ± 1.0 mmHg for 1–12-hour, 12–48-hour, and 48–168-hour-old laterally recumbent foals, respectively.[11,13]

Venous blood gas analysis provides an evaluation of metabolic status. $PvCO_2$ is usually 3–6 mmHg higher than $PaCO_2$ and reflects tissue metabolism in addition to ventilatory status. In 1-day-old foals, $PvCO_2$ was reported to be 52.9 ± 3.97 (standing) and 54.0 ± 2.6 mmHg (lateral).[11] PvO_2 primarily reflects tissue PO_2 rather than pulmonary function. When systemic oxygen demands exceed supply, as with low peripheral oxygen delivery, oxygen extraction efficiency increases; this causes a reduction in PvO_2. A sustained and marked increase in central SvO_2 (>80%) in a patient breathing room air may be associated with impaired systemic oxygen extraction or utilization, as occurs with cytopathic hypoxia, and is an ominous sign. Mixed venous (right atrial or pulmonary arterial) samples are ideal for evaluation of PvO_2, because jugular samples may not be representative of global oxygen extraction. However, mixed venous samples require a pulmonary artery catheter. Cranial vena cava (central) samples can be used to estimate mixed venous PvO_2 and only require central lines rather than pulmonary arterial catheters. Central venous blood samples usually have higher PvO_2 or SvO_2 than mixed venous samples during shock states, but are reasonable estimates. Normal jugular PvO_2 is reported to be 45.6 ± 4.7 mmHg and SvO_2 is 65 to 75% in adult horses.[14] Mixed venous oxygen tension in neonatal foals is 40.5 ± 0.4 and 35.9 ± 0.4 mmHg in recumbent and upright foals, respectively.[16]

In addition to oxygen and carbon dioxide tensions, blood gas analysis also provides pH, bicarbonate concentrations, and base deficit, other markers of tissue oxygenation, and acid–base status. Whereas the $PaCO_2$ defines the respiratory component of acid–base balance, base deficit (BD) or base excess (BE) defines the metabolic component of acid base balance. BD is the difference between patient bicarbonate concentration and the median normal value of 24 mmol/l. A negative value represents a metabolic acidemia, and a positive value is alkalemia. Normal BD is –1 to +6. Neonatal foals tend to have positive BD (i.e. base excess).

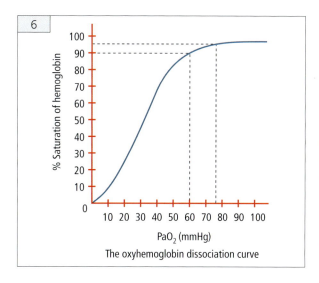

The oxyhemoglobin dissociation curve

11.6 Oxygen–hemoglobin dissociation curve.

In evaluating acid–base status, expected metabolic and respiratory compensations can be estimated as shown in *Table 11.5*. If compensation is disproportionate to these expected calculated values, a mixed acid–base disorder or two primary disorders should be suspected. For example, if the actual $PaCO_2$ on the blood gas result is lower than the calculated value from the formula for a given metabolic acidosis, then a primary respiratory alkalosis should be suspected in addition to the primary metabolic acidosis. In other words, the respiratory alkalosis is above and beyond that expected for a simple compensatory response.

Coagulation profile

Key points

- Coagulopathy is common in critically ill equine patients.
- A coagulation profile should be performed on any patient with clinical signs of a coagulopathy, relative hypofibrinogenemia, or thrombocytopenia.

Definition/overview

A coagulation profile includes platelet count, plasma fibrinogen, prothrombin time (PT), activated partial thromboplastin time (APTT), and serum fibrin/fibrinogen degradation products (FDPs). Plasma fibrinogen concentration is discussed under Plasma proteins (p. 631).

Indications

Plasma fibrinogen and platelet count should be measured as part of the admission minimal data base in critically ill patients, particularly patients that may undergo general anesthesia and surgery. A coagulation profile should be performed on any patient with hypofibrinogenemia or thrombocytopenia.

Coagulopathy is common in critically ill equine patients (e.g. horses with enterocolitis, large colon volvulus, liver disease, or clostridial infection and horses that have had substantial blood loss). In most cases, the coagulopathy is subclinical. Clinical signs of a coagulopathy that should prompt performing a coagulation profile include: petechial hemorrhages on the mucous membranes, nictitans, sclerae, or pinnae; hemorrhage or hematoma formation at a venipuncture or catheter site; prolonged hemorrhage from the nose following passage of a nasogastric tube; as well as hemarthrosis, scleral hemorrhage, spontaneous epistaxis, melena, hyphema, or hematuria. Venous thrombosis (e.g. jugular, intestinal) can also be a sign of a hypercoagulable state and warrants further investigation into the patient's coagulation status.

Table 11. 5 Calculations the expected metabolic and respiratory compensation in equine patients with acid–base abnormalities

ACID–BASE ABNORMALITY	EXPECTED COMPENSATION
Acute respiratory acidosis	HCO_3^- increases by 1 mEq/l for every 10 mm Hg increase in $PaCO_2$
Chronic respiratory acidosis	HCO_3^- increases by 3–4 mEq/l for every 10 mm Hg increase in $PaCO_2$
Acute respiratory alkalosis	HCO_3^- decreases by 1–3 mEq/l for every 10 mm Hg decrease in $PaCO_2$
Chronic respiratory alkalosis	HCO_3^- decreases by 5 mEq/l for every 10 mm Hg decrease in $PaCO_2$
Metabolic acidosis	$PaCO_2$ decreases by 1.2 mm Hg for every 1 mEq/l decrease in HCO_3^-
Metabolic alkalosis	$PaCO_2$ increases by 0.6–1 mm Hg for every 1 mEq/l increase in HCO_3^-

Technique

- Blood samples used for a coagulation profile should be collected via clean venipuncture because even a small amount of tissue thromboplastin can activate clotting factors and invalidate the coagulation profile.
- Blood should be collected into sodium citrate (3.8% aqueous solution).
- When using a Vacutainer® tube, the first sample may be discarded to ensure that there are no tissue fluids containing tissue thromboplastin.[17]
- Samples should be kept on ice and analyzed within 1 hour of collection. Platelet counts should be performed immediately. The platelet count can be estimated by comparing platelet to WBC or RBC numbers per high power field on a smear.[17]
- If immediate analysis is not possible, plasma should be collected immediately by centrifugation (800–1000 g for 15 minutes), harvested with a plastic pipette, and frozen at –70°C. The coagulation profile should be performed within a few days. Defrosted plasma should be tested immediately.[17]
- Two or more normal controls should be used for comparison or normal values for the laboratory used.

Interpretation

The most common cause of alterations in the coagulation profile in horses is DIC, which can occur as a result of a severe inflammatory response in cases of trauma, anaphylaxis, sepsis, endotoxemia, neoplasia, acute haemorrhage, and neonatal hypoxemia-ischemic syndrome.[18] Examples of cases in which DIC is commonly a complication are colitis, large colon volvulus, and clostridial infection. DIC is defined by abnormalities in multiple coagulation tests and can be clinical or subclinical.

Thrombocytopenia: Thrombocytopenia (platelet count <100,000/µl) is caused by inadequate production (e.g. bone marrow disease and immune-mediated destruction of megakaryocytes), platelet sequestration (e.g. splenomegaly in acute and chronic infections; inflammation and splenic congestion associated with intestinal displacements and CHF), and excessive platelet consumption (e.g. DIC, overwhelming endotoxemia or septicemia, vasculitis, and some viral diseases) or destruction (e.g. immune-mediated thrombocytopenia). Prolonged bleeding following minor trauma and hematoma formation at venipuncture sites occurs with platelet counts <40,000/µl and spontaneous hemorrhage can occur when the platelet count is <10,000/µl.

Prothrombin time: PT measures the extrinsic and common coagulation pathways (**11.7**). Causes of prolonged PT include hypofibrinogemia (<1 g/l [100 mg/dl]) or <50% of the normal concentration of prothrombin and/or clotting factors V, VII, and X. Clotting factor functional abnormalities or inhibitors can also cause a prolonged PT. Increased clotting factor consumption (e.g. DIC) and insufficient hepatic production (e.g. liver disease, vitamin K deficiency) are the most common reasons. Thrombocytopenia and prolonged APTT also occur with DIC.

Activated partial thromboplastin time: APTT measures the intrinsic coagulation pathway (**11.7**). Causes of prolonged APTT include deficiency or abnormal activity of clotting factors VIII, IX, XI, XII (+/– prekallikrein and high-molecular weight kininogen[17]). The activated clotting time (ACT) can be used as a simplified APTT. DIC and hepatic insufficiency are the most common reasons for prolonged APTT in horses.

Fibrin/fibrinogen degradation products: FDPs indicate increased fibrinolysis compared with normal in response to hypercoagulation (e.g. DIC). Causes of an increase in FDPs include DIC, thrombophlebitis, postoperative states, severe inflammation, immune-mediated thrombocytopenia, and massive internal hemorrhage.[17] High FDPs can cause hypocoagulation by interfering with thrombin activity and fibrin monomer polymerization and causing platelet dysfunction.

Antithrombin III: ATIII is the most important inhibitor of coagulation and acts by neutralizing thrombin-activated factors IX, X, XI, and XII (**11.7**). Heparin is a necessary cofactor for ATIII. Causes of reduced ATIII include DIC (e.g. endotoxemia, trauma), protein-losing enteropathy (e.g. intestinal lymphosarcoma, right dorsal colitis) or nephropathy (e.g. glomerulonephritis), acute hepatic necrosis, and starvation or sepsis resulting in protein catabolism.

Hypofibrinogenemia: Hypofibrinogenemia can result from increased consumption during DIC, acute hepatic necrosis or severe fibrosis, or massive hemorrhage. Fibrinogen is produced exclusively in the liver and is rapidly released in response to inflammation and procoagulant stimuli. Hypofibrinogenemia is uncommon, most likely because the liver is capable of producing vast quantities and has a large reserve and hyperfibrinogenemia, which occurs during inflammation, may overshadow a relative hypofibrinogenemia in cases of DIC (i.e. a postoperative large colon volvulus patient may have a fibrinogen concentration of 3.5 g/l [350 mg/dl], which may indicate a relative hypofibrinogenaemia because the fibrinogen concentration should be 5–7 g/l [500–700 mg/dl]).

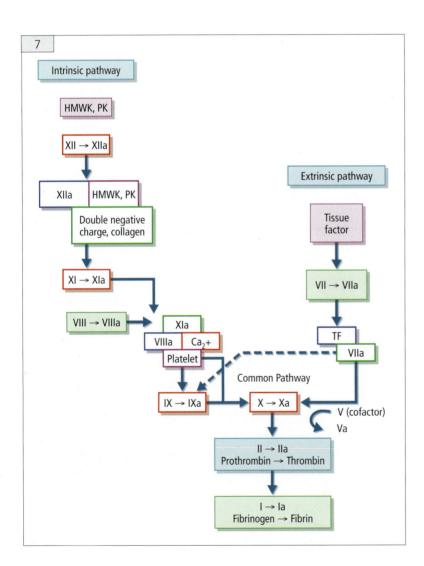

11.7 Coagulation cascade.

Thromboelastography: Thromboelastography (TEG) provides data about the entire coagulation system from initiation of coagulation through clot formation and finally fibrinolysis. TEG provides information on both the quality of the clot as well as the dynamics of its formation.[19] The apparatus consists of a plastic cup and a pin that is suspended by torsion wire; blood is placed into the cup, the wire lowered into the cup, and the cup oscillated. The pin begins to oscillate with the cup when the clot begins to form and generates torque. The torque is transmitted to the TEG tracing on a computer terminal through a mechanical-electrical transducer.[19] Four standard measurements are made from the TEG tracing (**11.8A, B**):

- The reaction time (R) or precoagulation time evaluates the intrinsic pathway (factors VIII, IX, XI, and XII).[19]
- The clot formation time (K) is an arbitrary point corresponding to the maximal divergence obtained in normal platelet-poor plasma and measures the rapidity of clot formation from the beginning of the visible phase of coagulation to a defined clot strength. K assesses factors II, VIII, platelet count and function, thrombin formation, fibrin precipitation, fibrinogen concentration, and PCV.

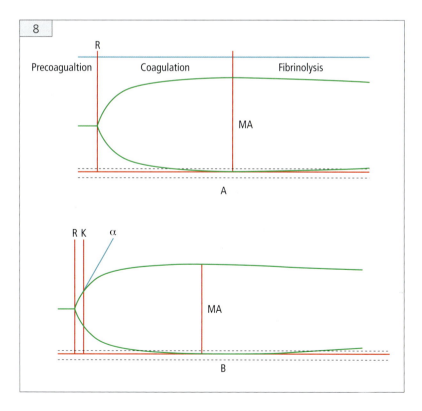

11.8A, B Thromboelastography. (A) Thromboelastograph tracing showing precoagulation, coagulation, and fibrinolysis. (B) Measurements that can be taken from the thromboelastograph. R (reaction time), the distance (mm) from the start of the tracing to the point where the lines have diverged 1 mm. K (clot formation time), the distance (mm, with a tracing speed of 2 mm/minute) between the end of R and the point at which the distance between the two branches reaches 20 mm. MA (maximal amplitude), maximal distance (mm) between the two diverging branches. α (angle), the angle between the midline and the tangent to the curve drawn from the 1 mm wide point.[19]

- Maximal amplitude (MA) reflects clot strength and assesses fibrin and fibrinogen concentration, platelet count and function, thrombin concentration, factor XIII, and PCV.[19]
- The angle (α) is an indication of the rate of clot formation and provides similar information to K.[19]

The coagulation index (CI) can be calculated as follows:

$$CI = 0.1227(R) + 0.0092(K) + 0.165(MA) - 0.0241(\alpha) - 5.002$$

Normal CI in humans is +3.0 to −3.0; values >+3.0 are consistent with hypercoagulability and <−3.0 with hypocoagulability.[19]

Urine output and urinalysis
Key points
- Urine output should be monitored at least subjectively in any critically ill patient.
- Urinalysis should be performed on any patient with signs of renal disease (persistent azotemia or very high serum or plasma creatinine, inappropriate urine production).
- Persistent azotemia, urine casts, and a high fractional excretion of sodium are indications of primary renal disease.

Definition/overview
Urine output is the amount of urine voided per day or per hour. Urinalysis involves measurement of urine SG, pH, protein, glucose, occult blood, myoglobin, cells, casts, crystals, bacteria, and urine creatinine clearance ratios.

Indications
Urine output should be monitored quantitatively or qualitatively in any critically ill patient because it is an indicator of renal blood flow and can be used to indirectly assess end-organ perfusion and the adequacy of fluid therapy. Urinalysis should also be performed on any critically ill patient to monitor:
- Urine SG to determine the appropriateness of fluid therapy.
- Urine glucose concentration, particularly in patients on glucose-containing fluids (i.e. dextrose or parenteral nutrition).

- Urine SG, casts, cells, and creatinine clearance, as well as occult blood and bacteria, to diagnose renal damage or urinary tract infection in any patient that is persistently azotemic (high creatinine or BUN; see Serum and plasma biochemistry).
- Myoglobin in any patient with muscle damage.

Technique
- Urine output can be monitored subjectively by observing the frequency and amount of voided urine and assessing the amount of urine in the stall (**11.9**). Subjective assessment is usually used in adult horses.
- Urine output in neonates can also be performed by observation. It can be estimated by placing an absorbent pad under the foal and weighing the pad following urination, or by measuring water 'ins and outs' in a patient with a bladder catheter.[4] Bladder catheterization in neonatal foals can be performed using an 8–10 French human infant feeding tube or a 12 French Foley catheter (fillies 33 cm, colts 64 cm).[4] Bladder catheterization with measurement of 'ins and outs' is rarely performed in adult horses because of the difficulty with catheter maintenance and the risk of ascending infection.
- Urinalysis can be performed on a voided urine sample collected into a small clean cup. A urine catcher can be placed on male and castrated male horses to facilitate sample collection (**11.10**).
- Bladder catheterization can be performed in male and castrated male horses using a 'stallion catheter' or in female horses using a 26–30 French Foley catheter if a sterile urine sample is necessary or collection of a voided sample is unsuccessful. Routine aseptic preparation of the glans penis or vulva should be performed prior to catheterization and sterile gloves should be worn. The catheter should be adequately lubricated and passed gently until urine is obtained.
- Urinalysis should be performed immediately following urine collection or at least within 30 minutes.
- Urine SG is measured using a refractometer and a urine dipstick can be used to measure pH, protein, glucose, bilirubin, occult blood, and myoglobin.

- Urine should be analyzed in a laboratory in any horse suspected of having renal disease (azotemia, inappropriate isosthenuria, consistent abnormal findings on the urine dipstick).
- Fractional excretion (FE) of sodium can be calculated as follows:

$$FE = \frac{Urine\ [sodium]}{Serum\ [sodium]} \times \frac{Serum\ [creatinine]}{Urine\ [creatinine]} \times 100$$

Interpretation

Urine output is a measurement of renal blood flow and an indirect indicator of tissue perfusion and can be used to adjust fluid therapy. Horses on IV fluids should have several moderately sized wet areas throughout the stall; a soaking wet stall or a dry stall that has not recently been cleaned is an indication of over- and underhydration, respectively, and should prompt adjustment in fluid therapy and measurement of serum or plasma creatinine. It is important to be sure that the wet areas are not from other sources (e.g. water from a water bucket or hose, reflux, leakage from IV fluids). Adult horses generally produce urine at a 0.6–1.25 ml/kg/hour (i.e. 300–625 ml/hour or 7.2–15 liters/day for a 500 kg horse).[20] Normal neonatal foals should produce urine at 4–8 ml/kg/hour (i.e. 200–400 ml/hour or 4.8–9.6 liters/day for a 50 kg foal). Urine production in critically ill neonates is different to that in normal neonates and should reflect fluid balance (i.e. 'ins and outs'; enteral and parenteral fluid input and insensible and sensible [urine] losses). Urine production ('outs') should be >50% of 'ins'.[4] Prerenal, renal, and postrenal renal disease can be reasons for disparity between fluid 'ins and outs'. (See also Chapter 20.)

Urine SG is the weight of urine relative to the weight of distilled water (i.e. an estimation of the number of particles dissolved in the urine) and reflects the changes in the glomerular filtrate made by the renal tubules and collecting ducts. Serum and the glomerular filtrate have a SG of 1.010 and normal urine SG is 1.020–1.050 (adult horse) and <1.010 (neonate). Isosthenuria (urine SG 1.008–1.012) or dilute urine in a dehydrated animal reflects primary renal disease or, less commonly, glucosuria, medullary washout, or nephrogenic diabetes insipidus.[21]

Urine SG can be used to monitor fluid therapy in adult horses. Normal horses on maintenance IV fluids usually have a urine SG of 1.010–1.020. Except for horses with renal failure, which are isosthenuric, adult horses with a urine SG <1.008 may be overhydrated and diluting their urine and the IV fluid rate should

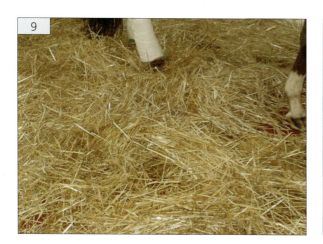

11.9 Urine output is usually measured subjectively in adult horses by assessing the amount of urine in the stall.

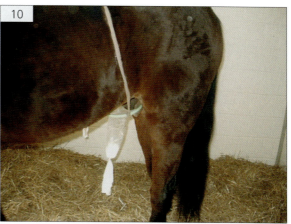

11.10 Urine catcher used on male and castrated male horses.

be slowed. Adult horses with a urine SG >1.030 are concentrating their urine and may benefit from a higher rate of IV fluid administration if there are also other indications.

The normal pH of equine urine is 7–9 and is <7 in neonatal foals and in some cases of metabolic acidosis.

Proteinuria is abnormal; however, false-positive results on a urine dipstick can be obtained with strongly alkaline or concentrated urine. Reasons for proteinuria include glomerular protein loss (glomerulonephritis or amyloidosis), urinary tract sepsis, or urogential tract hemorrhage or inflammation.[21]

Glucosuria is abnormal except when blood glucose exceeds the renal threshold of 8.9–10.0 mmol/l (160–180 mg/dl). Reasons for glucosuria include Cushing's syndrome, stress, catecholamine or glucocorticoid hormone release, and iatrogenic with administration of glucose-containing fluids.[21] Glucosuria in patients receiving glucose-containing fluids warrants re-evaluation of the glucose administration rate and, if appropriate, insulin administration (see Chapter 15).

Positive occult blood on a dipstick can be caused by myoglobin or hemoglobin. Myoglobinuria should be associated with evidence of muscle injury. Hemoglobinuria is usually associated with intravascular hemolysis. An increase in the number of erythrocytes in the urine (hematuria) is associated with neoplasia, trauma, inflammation, or coagulopathy, and an increase in leukocytes (pyuria) with inflammation and sepsis.

Casts are formed by accumulations of protein and cellular material in the renal tubules and indicate renal damage or tubular disease (**11.11A, B**).[21] Crystalluria (calcium carbonate crystals) is normal in the horse. Small numbers of bacteria can be surface contaminants; however, bacuria in combination with pyuria warrants collection of a urine sample for culture and sensitivity testing.

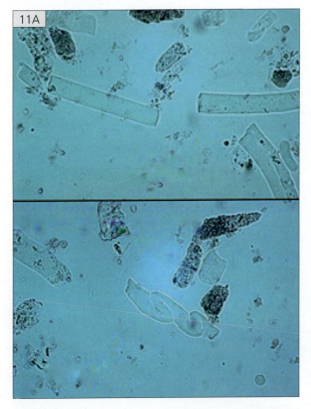
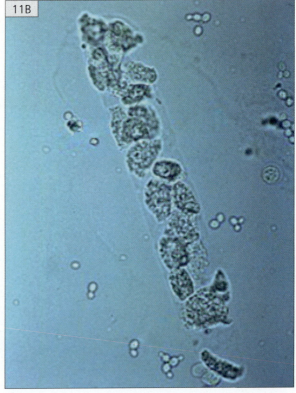

11.11A, B Urinary casts showing waxy and granular casts (A). Granular casts at higher magnification (B). (Courtesy Dr Raquel Walton)

Fractional excretion of sodium should be <1% in normal horses that are not receiving IV fluid therapy. A high FE of sodium indicates renal tubular damage and impaired sodium resorption. Horses that may be azotemic because of dehydration have a low sodium FE.[21]

Arterial blood pressure

Key points

- MAP can be used as an estimate of organ and tissue perfusion and is most commonly measured using an oscillometric (indirect) technique.
- Use of an appropriate sized cuff, correct patient positioning, creation of a quiet environment, checking that the reported heart rate is the same as the actual patient heart rate, and checking consistency by performing consecutive measurements should be used to ensure accurate MAP measurement using the oscillometric technique.
- A MAP <65 mmHg in combination with other indications of poor perfusion warrants re-evaluation of fluid therapy and possible use of inotropes and vasopressors.

Definition/overview

Arterial blood pressure is the product of cardiac output and systemic vascular resistance (SVR). Cardiac output is the product of heart rate and stroke volume (SV). SVR reflects vascular capacity (vasomotor tone). Mean (MAP), systolic (SAP), and diastolic (DAP) arterial pressures are measured. MAP is more important than SAP or DAP for organ and tissue perfusion. Arterial blood pressure is used as an estimate of blood flow.

Indications

Arterial blood pressure is a marker of circulatory status and should be measured in any critically ill patient. Hypotension in horses may result from hypovolemia, hemorrhagic shock, SIRS, cardiac failure, anaphylaxis, and acute trauma.[22] Hypertension is less common, but may occur from increased sympathetic responses (stress, pain, pheochromocytoma), thermal injury, and some forms of head trauma.

Technique

Direct measurement

- Direct monitoring provides for a continuous display of pressure waveforms using intra-arterial catheters, a pressure transducer, and a recorder.
- Catheterization of the transverse facial artery with a 20-gauge catheter is feasible in the standing adult horse (**11.12**).
- Neonatal foals can be instrumented with a 20-gauge catheter in the great metatarsal artery, especially if recumbent.
- Other sites of catheterization in foals include the radial and caudal auricular arteries.
- The transducer should be maintained at the sternal level.

Indirect measurement

- Advantages of indirect measurements include ease and non-invasiveness, although they are less accurate.
- Indirect methods include sphygmomanometry, Doppler, and oscillometric methods.

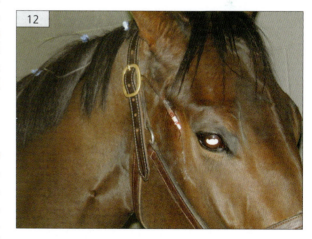

11.12 Direct arterial blood pressure measurement using the transverse facial artery.

- Occlusion cuffs are placed over an artery such as the coccygeal (**11.13**). Other sites include the dorsal metatarsal, median, or palmar digital arteries.
- Oscillometric techniques (e.g. Dinamap® Veterinary Blood Bressure Monitor) are most commonly used in the equine ICU. Whereas other techniques only provide systolic pressure, oscillometric monitors determine systolic, mean, and diastolic pressures and provide pulse rate. The displayed pulse can be used to evaluate the accuracy of the monitor by comparing it with the actual pulse rate.
- Another means of confirming indirect blood pressure measurements is to repeat them serially (e.g. three times).
- Falsely low indirect readings occur when cuffs are too tight and internal bladders are too wide. Loose cuffs and narrow bladders result in falsely high readings. The width of the bladder should be 25–34% and 40–50% of the tail and limb, respectively, in adult horses.

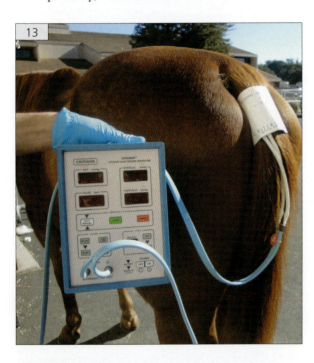

11.13 Indirect arterial blood pressure measurement using the coccygeal artery in an adult horse.

- The head should be in a resting position when performing indirect coccygeal blood pressure measurements. Lowering the head decreases and raising the head increases the measured blood pressure. The horse should be kept quiet with minimal restraint.
- Blood pressure values may be corrected to heart level or stated as unaltered for coccygeal values. Because the tail base is higher than the level of the heart, recorded pressures will be 15–20 mmHg lower than actual pressures.
- Whether correcting for position or not, consistency of methodology should be maintained between readings.

Interpretation

MAP is more important than SAP or DAP for organ perfusion and a minimum of 65 mmHg is required for cerebral, pulmonary, and coronary blood flow. Normal blood pressure values for neonatal foals vary with gestational age, size, and breed of foal. Normal values for direct and indirect arterial blood pressure for foals and adult horses are shown in *Table 11.6*.

The exact blood pressure at which intervention for hypotension should occur in horses is unknown. Isolated blood pressure readings should not be the sole criteria. Rather, trends in blood pressure, used in conjunction with clinical perfusion parameters, urine output, blood lactate concentration, and central venous oxygen saturation, should determine the need for treatment. Foals and adult horses with a MAP <60–69 mmHg in combination with low urine output, hyperlactatemia, and low central venous oxygen saturation should be supported with IV fluids and inotrope and/or vasopressor therapy.

Central venous pressure
Key points
- CVP can be used to guide fluid therapy in critically ill adult and neonatal patients.
- Patients in which CVP monitoring may be particularly beneficial include hypotensive and hypoproteinemic patients and patients with renal or heart failure.

Definition/overview

CVP is the intraluminal blood pressure within the thoracic vena cava. The CVP is an estimate of preload and right ventricular filling pressure (right atrial pressure), and is an approximation of the ratio of blood volume to blood volume capacity (vessel capacity). CVP is determined by central venous blood volume, venous tone, and cardiac function. Values for CVP increase with fluid overload and right-sided heart failure and decrease with hypovolemia.

Indications

CVP should be measured in any case where providing appropriate fluid therapy is critical. Examples of such cases include patients with oliguric or anuric renal failure, cardiac failure and severe hypoalbuminemia where excessive administration of IV fluids is detrimental. CVP can also be measured in critically ill patients with diseases where it is difficult to predict the fluid requirements (e.g. severe colitis, postoperative large colon volvulus, postoperative ileus). In horses with the latter diseases, excessive fluid administration may exacerbate intestinal edema, but the intestine will be poorly perfused with inadequate IV fluids; therefore, providing the optimum amount of IV fluids is vital.

Technique

- CVP is measured through catheters that terminate in the intrathoracic vena cava.
- These pressures are transferred from the vena cava, through the jugular, catheter and extension tubing to a column of water (plastic manometer for intermittent measurement) or pressure transducer (for continuous monitoring).
- Central catheters can easily be placed in neonatal foals through the use of 20–30 cm central catheters. Catheter placement can be confirmed in foals through thoracic radiography.
- Either commercial CVP catheters or polytetrafluorethylene/polyethylene tubing (30–55 cm length) passed through a 10-gauge jugular catheter can be used in adult horses. Confirmation of intrathoracic placement of adult central venous catheters is made through the finding of small oscillations in the fluid meniscus with breathing or from pressure magnitudes and waveforms. Large pressure fluctuations suggest intraventricular placement and the catheter should be backed out until the fluctuations disappear. During spontaneous respiration, CVP is maximal at expiration. With mechanical ventilation CVP increases with inspiration. In either case, CVP should be measured at end expiration.
- Use of multilumen catheters allow for concurrent administration of fluids and measurement of CVP.
- An important aspect in accurately measuring CVP is the establishment of a reference point. The point of the shoulder or the sternal manubrium can be utilized as the 'zero' or reference point.

Table 11. 6 **Indirect and direct arterial blood pressure measurements in foals and horses**

	MEAN ARTERIAL PRESSURE (MMHG)	SYSTOLIC ARTERIAL PRESSURE (MMHG)	DIASTOLIC ARTERIAL PRESSURE (MMHG)
Pony foals (indirect)[23]	85 ± 10	128 ± 17	64 ± 10
Thoroughbred foals (indirect)[23]	95 ± 13	144 ± 15	74 ± 9
Full-term foals (indirect)[24,25]	–	80–125	60–80
1-day-old foals (direct)[26]	84.4 ± 3.7	–	–
14-day-old foals (direct)[26]	101.3 ± 4.4	–	–
Adult horse (indirect)[27]	–	111.8 ± 13.3	67.7 ± 13.8
Adult horse (direct)[28–30]	110–133	126–168	85–116

- Patient positioning should be the same during each measurement. CVP can be measured in either laterally or sternally recumbent foals, while adult horses are usually standing (**11.14**). Positioning of horses under anesthesia has been shown to cause increases in CVP, especially during lateral recumbency.

Interpretation

Normal CVP values in neonatal foals are 2.1–8.9 mmHg (2.8–12 cmH$_2$O).[26] Adult values have been reported as 7.5 ± 0.9 cm H$_2$O and 5–15 cm H$_2$O.[7,31]

CVP recordings (**11.15**) demonstrate a, c, and v waves and x and y descents. The 'a' wave represents atrial contraction, the 'c' wave is caused by tricuspid valve closure and bulging of the valve back into the right atrium, and the 'v' wave is generated by filling of the atrium from venous return. The x descent occurs after the 'a' wave and represents the pressure drop associated with atrial relaxation. The 'c' wave occurs within the x descent. The y descent occurs after the 'v' wave, representing a decrease in CVP due to ventricular relaxation and opening of the A-V valves. Simultaneous recording of an ECG allows for accurate interpretation of the CVP pressure tracing. The 'a' wave starts during the P-R interval, corresponding to atrial contraction. The most precise CVP measurement is the mean of the 'a' wave at the end of expiration. The 'v' wave starts early in the T-P interval of the ECG strip. As with arterial blood pressure, CVP trends and changes over time are much more informative than single measurements. Serial or continuous monitoring is useful in evaluating the outcome of fluid volume administration and heart failure intervention.

In using CVP as an end point to volume loading, once maximum allowable CVP is reached (10–12 cm H$_2$O in neonates; 15 cm H$_2$O in adults), inotrope and/or vasopressor therapy is indicated as further administration of fluids will result in edema. A normal CVP (5–15 cm H$_2$O for adults; 2–12 cm H$_2$O for neonates) does not necessarily indicate euvolemia, as hypovolemic animals can have CVP values within the normal range. However, low to negative CVP values suggest either vasodilation or hypovolemia. Lack of an increase in CVP in response to fluid boluses is consistent with hypovolemia. In addition to right heart dysfunction

and volume overload, increases in CVP may be due to vasoconstriction, pericardial or pleural effusion, positive pressure ventilation, patient positioning, catheter occlusion, inadvertent ventricular catheterization, and air within the manometer or lines.

Cardiac output
Key points

- A number of techniques have been validated for measurement of cardiac output in horses.
- Lithium dilution and echocardiographic techniques are currently the most practical means of monitoring cardiac output in clinical horse and foal patients.
- Measurement of cardiac output is useful in optimizing the hemodynamic physiology of equine patients, particularly when vasopressors and inotropes are administered.

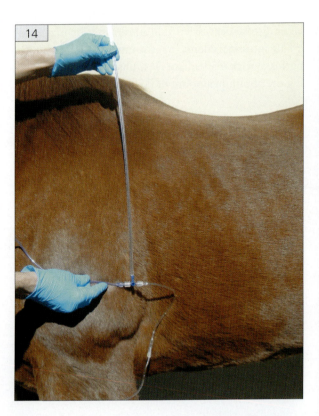

11.14 Measurement of central venous pressure in an adult horse.

Definition/overview
Cardiac output is the amount of blood in liters pumped through the heart in one minute (liters/minute) and is the product of heart rate (beats/minute) and stroke volume (liters/beat).

Indications
Measurement of cardiac output in clinical equine cases has been increasing in recent years with the development of more practical methods. Cardiac output measurements may be beneficial in critically ill neonates and adult horses, particularly hypotensive patients that do not respond to IV fluid boluses. Cardiac output can be used to determine whether hypotension is due to inadequate stroke volume or cardiac output (see Arterial blood pressure). Measurement of cardiac output in patients being treated with pressors can be used to ensure that cardiac output is not decreasing with an increase in SVR.

Technique
Indicator dilution methods
- Indicator dilution methods rely on injection of an indicator in a vein upstream of the heart, which is subsequently measured downstream in a pulmonary or peripheral artery.
- Cardiac output can be determined from knowledge of the volume and concentration of indicator added to the blood and the concentration of indicator once diluted by the blood.
- The area under the time–concentration curve of the diluted indicator is used to determine cardiac output; the greater the cardiac output, the smaller the area under the curve (**11.16**).

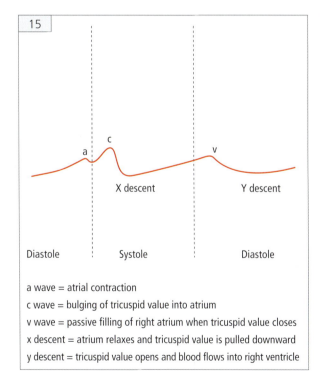

a wave = atrial contraction
c wave = bulging of tricuspid value into atrium
v wave = passive filling of right atrium when tricuspid value closes
x descent = atrium relaxes and tricuspid value is pulled downward
y descent = tricuspid value opens and blood flows into right ventricle

11.15 Central venous pressure wave forms.

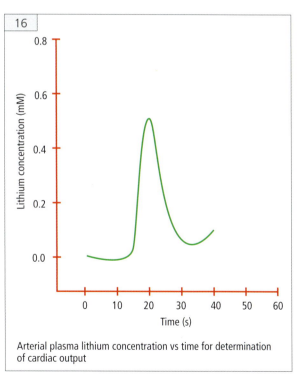

Arterial plasma lithium concentration vs time for determination of cardiac output

11.16 Time–concentration curve for measurement of cardiac output using the lithium dilution method.

- The indicator must be injected instantly as a rapid bolus in order to minimize errors in interpretation.
- Indicators studied in horses include indocyanine green, thermal, and lithium dilutions.
- The problem with indocyanine green is that of calibration: the densitometer requires calibration with each individual patient's blood.
- Thermodilution is the most common method of cardiac output monitoring in human critical care and has been used in equine research. This technique relies on a change in blood temperature detected by a thermistor in the pulmonary artery after bolus injection of saline or 5% dextrose at 4°C (or at room temperature for foals) into the right atrium or vena cava. Computer programs calculate cardiac output from the area under the curve of the temperature change. Advantages of thermal dilution include the ability to perform multiple measurements without accumulation of indicator. The disadvantages, however, include variable accuracy in horses due to difficulty in performing immediate bolus injections (due to volume), temperature alterations due to handling of the syringe, and the need for placement of a pulmonary arterial catheter. Complications of right heart catheters include cardiac and pulmonary endothelial fibrinous lesions and thrombi, as well as ventricular arrhythmias. These complications make the use of this technique in the clinical setting somewhat impractical.
- Lithium dilution precludes the need for right heart catheters. With this technique a small bolus of lithium chloride solution is injected into a peripheral vein or the vena cava. Next, arterial blood is sampled at a constant rate through a lithium electrode, which generates a lithium concentration–time curve. Cardiac output is calculated from the area under the curve for lithium. Advantages of lithium dilution include relative non-invasiveness, good accuracy in horses, and requirement for small volumes of injectate.[32] Disadvantages include the need for continuous arterial blood and lithium accumulation.

Volumetric echocardiography

- Volumetric echocardiography refers to non-invasive cardiac output measurements through a variety of methods including cubic, Teichholz, Bullet area-length, and single and biplane modified Simpson formulas.
- In comparing these measurements with lithium dilution in anesthetized foals, the Bullet method had the lowest relative bias and appears to provide an accurate estimate of cardiac output with no invasive procedures.[33]
- The Bullet method requires the following measurements:

$$SV = (5/6 \times LVAd \times LVLd) - (5/6 \times LVAs \times LVLs);$$

LVAd = left ventricular area in diastole (in short axis)
LVLd = left ventricular length in diastole (in long axis)
LVAs = left ventricular area in systole (in short axis)
LVLs = left ventricular length in systole (in long axis)

Doppler echocardiography

- Doppler echocardiography is another non-invasive means of determining cardiac output through determining velocity of blood flow.
- Velocity is calculated based on changes in frequency between emitted and reflected ultrasound waves after striking moving RBCs.

- The area under the velocity curve yields an estimate of SV, which determines cardiac output along with aortic cross-sectional area and heart rate.
- Doppler echocardiography can be performed transthoracically or transesophageally, with the latter providing better agreement with thermodilution techniques.

Partial carbon dioxide rebreathing

- Partial CO_2 rebreathing has been studied in anesthetized foals, but had a relatively high bias compared with lithium dilution and requires specialized equipment.[33]
- In addition, it would be difficult to perform under circumstances other than general anesthesia.

Pulse contour analysis

- Pulse contour analysis uses arterial pressure waveforms from peripheral arterial catheters to generate cardiac output from the area under the curve and the shape of the arterial pressure tracing.
- Advantages include relative non-invasiveness and beat-to-beat, continuous measurement of cardiac output.
- Disadvantages include the need for frequent and individualized calibration.
- Pulse contour analysis has been evaluated in anesthetized horses and found to be reliable.[32]

Bioimpedance

- Bioimpedance is a non-invasive technique where imperceptible electric currents are applied to the thorax, and electrodes detect tissue conductivity.

- The pulsatile flow of blood changes the thoracic impedance, and the magnitude of change corresponds to cardiac output.
- Disadvantages include the need for development of algorithms designed for horses of different sexes and ages. Accuracy and precision are variable when thoracic fluid compartments are altered, as with pulmonary edema or pleural effusion. Electrical impedance measured in a peripheral artery has been shown to be a reasonable means of estimating cardiac output in horses.
- The advantage of this technique is the lack of requirement for a pulmonary arterial catheter.

Interpretation

Cardiac output in healthy horses (400–500 kg) is 32–40 liters/minute. Cardiac index (cardiac output divided by body weight) is a means of comparing cardiac output between individuals. The normal cardiac index in adult horses is 72–88 ml/kg/minute. Cardiac output is reported to be 7.1 ± 0.4 liters/minute (cardiac index = 155.3 ± 8.1 ml/kg/minute) in 2-hour-old foals. At 24 hours of age cardiac output was determined to be 9.0 ± 0.5 liters/minute (cardiac index = 197.3 ± 12.0 ml/kg/minute) using cardiac catheters. This increased to 15.7 ± 1.5 liters/minute (cardiac index = 222.1 ± 21.6 ml/kg/minute) at 14 days of age.[26] A general guide for neonatal foals is a cardiac index of 100–300 ml/kg/minute.

Low cardiac output may be due to a decreased SV associated with low preload (hypovolemia) or cardiac contractility, or increased afterload. Concurrent monitoring of MAP allows calculation of peripheral vascular resistance (= MAP/CO).

CHAPTER 12

FLUID THERAPY

Vanessa L. Cook and
Louise L. Southwood

GENERAL APPROACH TO FLUID THERAPY

- Fluid therapy can be used to maintain water and electrolyte balance in critically ill patients as well as correct measured or estimated deficits.
- Deficits should be calculated based on the estimated percentage dehydration and replaced.
- Maintenance fluid rate for an adult horse is approximately 2 ml/kg/hour (i.e. 1 liter/hour for a 500 kg horse). Polyionic isotonic replacement crystalloid solutions (p. 658) are most often used.
- Ongoing losses (e.g. GI, such as diarrhea and gastric reflux) should be estimated and replaced in addition to the maintenance requirements. The patient's cardiovascular status should be monitored closely in cases with large-volume fluid losses and altered water distribution (e.g. colitis, postoperative large colon volvulus). (See also Chapter 11.)
- Electrolyte abnormalities should also be identified and corrected appropriately. Close monitoring of plasma electrolytes is important in critically ill patients.
- In patients with hypoproteinemia, specifically hypoalbuminemia, plasma (p. 669) or synthetic colloids (p. 666) may be necessary to maintain the COP.
- Whole blood transfusion (p. 671) is necessary in patients with anemia, particularly anemia associated with clinical signs.

COMMON PROCEDURES PERFORMED FOR FLUID THERAPY

Intravenous catheterization
Indications
Obtaining and maintaining vascular access is one of the most important aspects of emergency medicine and critical care. Vascular access is important for administration of fluids and medications, particularly if a horse is difficult to handle due to pain, shock, or neurologic signs.

Technique
Two important considerations when placing an IV catheter are (1) using an aseptic and atraumatic technique and (2) ensuring that the catheter is secured in place to avoid complications.

Intravenous catheterization sites
- The jugular vein is most commonly used and the easiest site for catheterization, but jugular vein catheters are often rubbed (and dislodged) by the horse and there can be problems with thrombophlebitis (see Chapter 4).
- It is important to place the jugular vein catheter in the upper third of the neck because the omohyoideus muscle lies between the jugular vein and the carotid artery at this site. Lower in the neck the carotid artery is immediately deep to the jugular vein.

- The cephalic and lateral thoracic veins are alternative sites. If the cephalic vein is to be used, a 16-gauge, 7.6-cm (3-in) catheter should be placed and the catheter secured and bandaged. The lateral thoracic vein is often difficult to identify and catheterization can be facilitated using ultrasonographic guidance to identify the vein. The lateral thoracic vein should be used if jugular vein thrombophlebitis develops.

Intravenous catheters

- Short-term, polytetrafluoroethylene (Teflon®) catheters are inexpensive and easy to place because they are relatively stiff. These catheters should not be left in longer than 72 hours. Teflon® catheters kink and they can break off at the hub and are more likely to cause thrombophlebitis/cellulitis.
- The use of silastic or polyurethane material for long-term (>72 hours) IV catheterization is recommended (e.g. Arrow®, Milacath®). Long-term catheters are not as stiff as Teflon® catheters and can be more difficult to place, particularly if rapid venous access is needed.
- Catheter sizes commonly used for jugular vein catheterization are 12.5-cm (5-in) long, 16-, 14-, 12-, or 10-gauge catheters. Large-bore catheters (14- to 10-gauge) are used if large volumes of fluids are needed for resuscitation of an adult horse, and are more likely to cause thrombophlebitis and/or cellulitis. Small-bore catheters (16-gauge) are used for foals and for administration of medication in adult horses. The most commonly used catheter size in an adult horse is a 14-gauge catheter.

Jugular vein catheterization – over-the-needle (stylet) technique:
An area (approximately 10 cm × 10 cm) in the cranial third of the jugular groove should be clipped and aseptically prepared (**12.1**). The catheter and extension set should be filled with sterile heparinized saline. Sterile gloves should be worn. The protective sleeve and cap on the stylet are removed and discarded. It is important to touch only the stylet and the hub of the catheter and avoid touching the

white catheter shaft that will be placed within the vein. Distend the jugular vein by placing fingers in the jugular groove distal to the site of catheter placement (**12.2**). Angle the catheter so that it is following the flow of blood in the vein. Insert the catheter through the skin at a 45-degree angle (**12.3**) and advance the catheter and stylet until blood appears at the hub (i.e. the catheter is in the vein, **12.4**). It is important to avoid removal of the stylet from the catheter at this point because it will result in damage to the catheter tip. Then angle the catheter parallel to the jugular groove and advance the catheter and stylet a few centimeters. Separate the catheter and stylet and slide the catheter over the stylet and

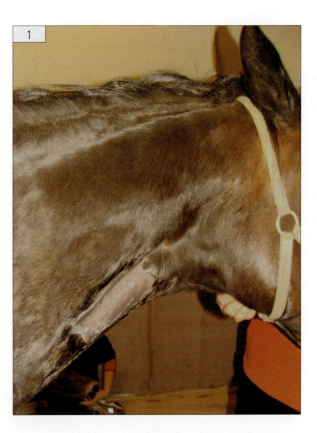

12.1 An area (approximately 10 cm × 10 cm) in the cranial third of the jugular groove is clipped and aseptically prepared.

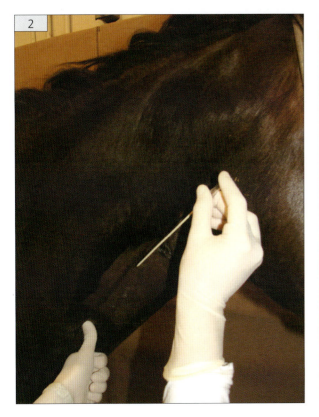

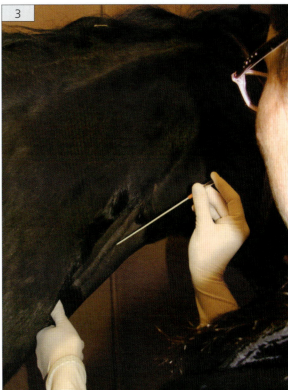

12.2 The jugular vein is distended by placing fingers in the jugular groove distal to the site of catheter placement. The catheter is angled so that it is following the flow of blood in the vein.

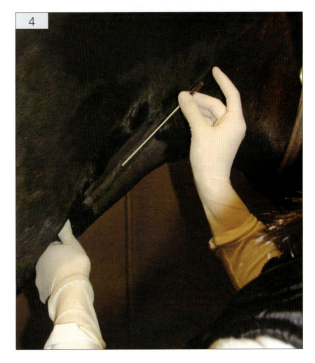

12.3 The catheter is inserted through the skin at a 45-degree angle.

12.4 The catheter and stylet are advanced until blood appears in the hub, indicating that the catheter is in the vein.

down the vein, holding the stylet in place (**12.5**). There should be no resistance. Remove the stylet. Attach the extension tubing or injection cap (**12.6**). The catheter and extension set can be secured to the skin in several places using suture (**12.7**). Cyanoacrylate adhesive can be used in addition to sutures.

It should be easy to flush sterile heparinized saline through the catheter and draw blood into a syringe from the catheter. Extension tubing is used to facilitate fluid and drug administration (e.g. extension set (7-inch or 30-inch) or large animal extension set (large-bore, 7-inch)). An injection cap is placed on the end of the extension tubing when it is not being used for fluid administration. Alternatively, an injection cap can be placed directly onto the end of the catheter.

Placement of long-term intravenous catheters: Long-term catheters can be placed routinely using a stylet or a guide wire (Seldinger technique; Guide wire catheters: (14- or 16-gauge, 8-inch). Placement of the softer polyurethane catheter over the stylet can be more difficult than a commonly used Teflon® catheter; however, creating a stab incision through the skin as well as inserting the catheter with the stylet in place further down the vein until about half of the catheter is in the vein, and then sliding the catheter over the stylet, facilitates this placement.

Placement of a catheter using a needle and guide wire (**12.8**) is performed by first inserting the needle into the vein to the hub. The guide wire is then fed through the needle into the vein. It is important not to let go of the wire at any time during catheter placement. The needle is removed from the vein with the wire left in place. The wire is removed, leaving the catheter in place. Both of these types of catheter have holes adjacent to the hub of the catheter where it can be sutured to the skin to secure it in place. There is also an indentation in the catheter that can be used to place a third suture to prevent the catheter slipping in and out of the vein.

Intravenous catheter maintenance and removal: The catheter should be checked and flushed regularly (every 6 hours) and not left in longer than necessary. Blood should not be left in the extension tubing or cap. The catheter site should be kept clean and free of blood.

Fluid lines and short-term catheters should be changed every 72 hours. The catheter and catheter site should be monitored closely for complications (see below).

IV catheters are removed by cutting the sutures securing the catheter in place with suture scissors, holding a sterile or clean gauze sponge over the catheter insertion site, and then sliding the catheter from the vein. Pressure should be applied to the vein and the horse's head kept upright for about 30–60 seconds. Catheter site monitoring should be continued for 24 hours following removal.

Complications

The main complication during jugular vein catheter placement is penetration of the carotid artery, which results in extensive hematoma formation. Pressure should be applied to the area and the hematoma usually resolves without complication. Occasionally, the carotid artery can be lacerated and result in fatal hemorrhage.

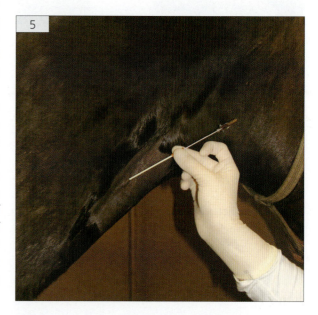

12.5 The catheter is separated from the stylet and the catheter is slid over the stylet and down the vein, holding the stylet in place. Note that the fingers are on the catheter hub. The stylet is not being held in place in this photograph in order to show the separation of the stylet and the catheter.

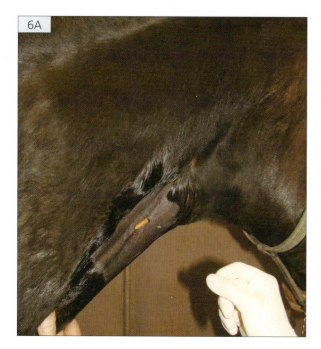

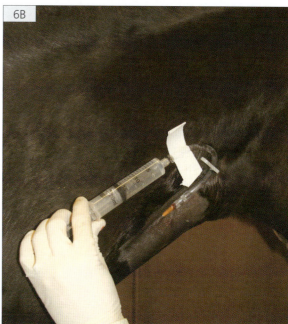

12.6A, B The stylet is removed (A) and the extension tubing or injection cap attached (B).

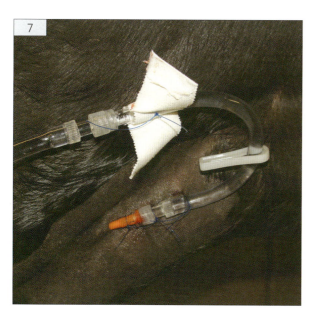

12.7 The catheter and extension tubing are secured to the skin in several places using sutures.

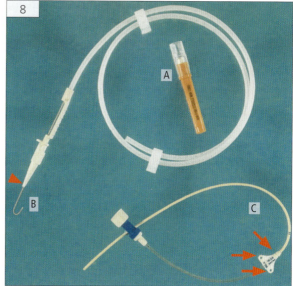

12.8 Placement of a catheter using a needle and guide wire is performed by first inserting the needle (A) into the vein to the hub and the guide wire (B) is then fed through the needle into the vein. The needle is removed from the vein with the wire left in place and the catheter (C) is fed over the wire. The wire is removed. The catheter is sutured in place using the holes and groove (arrows).

Difficulty with jugular vein catheter placement can result in the catheter being placed in subcutaneous tissue, which will cause fluids and drugs to be administered perivascularly. Perivascular administration of certain drugs is irritating to the tissues. Recommendations are to remove the incorrectly placed catheter, dilute the site of administration of the drug, and apply topical anti-inflammatory medication (e.g. DMSO or 1% doclofenac sodium).

Occasionally, an IV catheter will break off and the catheter will be lost into the jugular vein. This can occur (1) during catheter placement if the stylet inadvertently transects the catheter; (2) during removal if a scalpel blade is used to cut the suture securing the catheter in place and the catheter is inadvertently transected with the blade; or (3) during catheter maintenance with repeated kinking. In most instances the catheter becomes lodged in the lung without complication. Radiographic and sonographic evaluation should be performed to determine the location of the catheter and retrieval may be necessary.

Complications during catheter maintenance are common. The catheter should be monitored for kinking, local signs of thrombophlebitis/cellulitis, clotted blood, and loosening of the attachment between the catheter and extension tubing or injection cap. If the catheter is kinking, it should be replaced because this affects the fluid rate (i.e. the catheter is 'positional'), medication can leak around the catheter, and medication and fluid can go into the subcutaneous tissue. Catheters that are kinking are also predisposed to breaking. If there are signs of thrombophlebitis or cellulitis, the catheter should be removed or replaced. A different vein should be used if catheterization is still necessary. The affected area should be hot packed and culture and sensitivity performed on the part of the catheter that was in the vein. Loosening between the cap and an extension set can result in either bleeding or air aspiration. While air aspiration is uncommon, it can cause neurologic signs and ultimately be fatal, although this is uncommon.

FLUIDS

Crystalloids

- Fluids are classified as crystalloids based on their ability to cross the capillary membrane and move from the intravascular to the extravascular (interstitial) fluid compartment.
- Crystalloid fluids are composed primarily of water and electrolytes (mainly sodium chloride) and are classified as isotonic or hypertonic. (See also Chapter 15: 5% dextrose.)
- Crystalloids are the most commonly used IV fluids for resuscitation of equine patients because of their availability, low cost, and effectiveness in correcting dehydration. While there are several potential advantages with colloid solutions, controversy remains regarding the benefit of colloid over crystalloid solutions for resuscitation, with the clearest indication for use of colloids in equine patients being hypoalbuminemia.

Isotonic crystalloids
Key points
- Isotonic crystalloids are most beneficial for correcting whole body fluid deficits.
- A typical resuscitation regimen is to administer isotonic crystalloids in 20 ml/kg boluses (10 liters for a 500 kg horse or 1 liter for a 50 kg foal) and then reassess the patient. Boluses are continued until the patient is volume resuscitated. Total body deficit (liters) is determined by multiplying the estimated percentage dehydration by the body weight (kg).
- Maintenance fluid rates are typically 2 ml/kg/hour (1 liter/hour for a 500 kg horse). (See also Chapter 20.)
- TPP and plasma electrolyte concentrations should be monitored during administration of isotonic crystalloids.

Definition/overview

Isotonic crystalloids are fluids composed of water and electrolytes, principally sodium, with an osmolality similar to that of plasma (isotonic). Isotonic crystalloids are the principal IV fluid type used. The composition of the principal crystalloid fluids is listed in *Table 12.1*.

Indications

The goal of fluid therapy is to restore intravascular volume and improve cardiac output. Ultimately this increases tissue oxygenation and maintains aerobic metabolism. The principal electrolyte in crystalloid fluids is sodium at isotonic concentrations. This is also the principal electrolyte in extracellular fluid; therefore, crystalloids freely distribute across the entire intravascular and interstitial (extravascular) fluid space. The intravascular space comprises only about

Table 12.1 Electrolyte composition (mEq/l) of different crystalloid fluids

FLUID	Na^+	Cl^-	K^+	Ca^{2+}	Mg^{2+}	COMMENT
Normal equine clinical laboratory reference ranges	134–140	97–105	3.2–4.9	1.33–1.85	1.7–2.5	Reference range, North Carolina State University College of Veterinary Medicine, Clinical Pathology Laboratory
0.9% NaCl	154	154	0	0	0	Slightly hypertonic. Prolonged use may result in hyperchloremic metabolic acidosis
0.45% NaCl	77	77	0	0	0	Slightly hypotonic
7.2% NaCl	1232	1232	0	0	0	Very hypertonic. Follow with large volumes of isotonic crystalloids
Lactated Ringer's solution	130	109	4	3	0	Contains calcium, therefore cannot be given with citrated blood
Normosol R, Plasma-Lyte A	140	98	5	0	3	Additional K^+ supplementation required for long-term use
Normosol M and 5% Dextrose	40	40	13	0	3	Not available in 5-liter bags. Contains dextrose

one-quarter of the extracellular fluid space; therefore, crystalloids primarily expand the interstitial fluid space, with only 28% of their volume remaining in the vascular space 30 minutes after infusion (**12.9A, B**).[1] Therefore, they are most suitable for correcting whole body fluid deficits and maintaining hydration, but not for treatment of acute hypovolemia.

Clinical use

Three factors are considered when determining crystalloid administration rate:

- The existing volume deficit based on the estimated percentage of dehydration (*Table 12.2*). This should be replaced over the first few hours of administration.
- Maintenance requirements to allow for sensible (urine) and insensible (fecal and respiratory) water losses.
- Provision for ongoing losses. These are fluid requirements above those expected and include losses due to nasogastric reflux and diarrhea.

A sample calculation for formulation of a fluid therapy plan is shown in *Table 12.3*.

The balanced electrolyte solutions Plasma-Lyte A and Normosol R, and lactated Ringer's solution, have a similar osmolality to plasma and are considered isotonic. Plasma osmolality is 300 milliosmoles (mOsm)/kg and a fluid is described as hypertonic if its osmolality is higher than that of plasma and hypotonic if its osmolality is lower than that of plasma. The osmolality of crystalloid fluids can be estimated at twice the sodium concentration:

SI units:
plasma osmolality (mOsm/kg)
= 2 Na + Glucose + Urea (all in mmol/l)

Conventional units:
plasma osmolality (mOsm/kg)
= 2[Na] + [glucose]/18 + [BUN]/2.8

where, Na is sodium concentration in mmol/l (mEq/l); glucose is glucose concentration in mg/dl; and BUN is blood urea nitrogen concentration in mg/dl.

Table 12.2 Clinical signs in patients that can be used to estimate the percentage of dehydration

PERCENTAGE DEHYDRATION	HEART RATE (BEATS/MINUTE)	CRT (SECONDS)	PCV/TPP (%/g/dl)	Cr (µmol/l)[mg/dl]	ADDITIONAL CLINICAL SIGNS
<5%	30–40	<2	WNL	WNL	Not detectable
6	40–60	2	40/7	133–177 [1.5–2]	
8	61–80	3	45/7.5	177–265 [2–3]	Possible dry mucous membranes; eyes possibly sunken in orbits
10	81–100	4	50/8	265–354 [3–4]	Definite dry mucous membranes; eyes sunken in orbits; possibly signs of shock (cool extremities, rapid and weak pulse)
12	>100	>4	>50/>8	>354 [>4]	Definite signs of shock; imminent death

WNL, within normal limits for the laboratory; CRT, capillary refill time; PCV, packed cell volume; TPP, total plasma protein; Cr, serum or plasma creatinine concentration.
(Adapted from Hardy 2004[2] and DiBartola 2000[3])

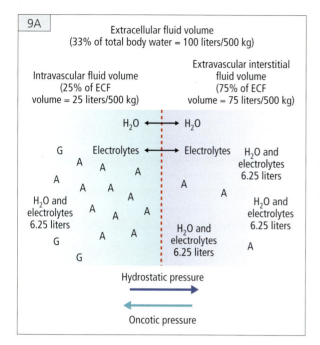

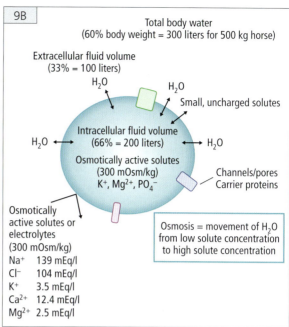

12.9A, B Schematic illustration of the distribution of isotonic crystalloids throughout the body. **(A)** Isotonic crystalloids (water [H_2O] and electrolytes) are distributed across the capillary wall (dotted red line) throughout the extracellular fluid space (intra- and extravascular spaces). **(B)** Water moves freely across the cell membrane between the intra- and extracellular fluid space by osmosis, based on the osmotic gradient. Electrolytes do not move freely across the cell membrane and the intra- and extracellular electrolyte concentrations are different; however, the osmolality in the intra- and extracellular fluid space is 300 mOsm/kg. A, albumin; G, globulin.

Table 12.3 A sample calculation for determining the rate of crystalloid administration: patient is a 400 kg pony with estimated 10% dehydration and 6 liters nasogastric reflux every 2 hours

REQUIREMENTS	FORMULA	CALCULATION	HOURLY RATE
Volume deficit (liters)	% dehydration x body weight (kg)	10% x 400 kg = 40 liters. Replace over next 4 hours	10 liters
Hourly maintenance requirements	2 ml/kg/hour	2 ml x 400 kg	1 liter (approximately)
Ongoing losses	Amount of loss (liters)/ time collected (hours)	6 liters/2 hours	3 liters
Total hourly rate for first 4 hours			14 liters
Total hourly rate after the first 4 hours, once fluid deficit is corrected	Maintenance rate + ongoing losses	1 liter + 3 liters	4 liters

The effective plasma osmolality is as above minus the BUN factor because it is freely diffusible across cell membranes. Thus normal saline (0.9% NaCl) is slightly hypertonic (154 mmol/l [mEq/l]) and half strength saline (0.45% NaCl) is hypotonic (77 mmol/l [mEq/l]).

The balanced electrolyte solutions also contain potassium and magnesium. The inclusion of magnesium may be beneficial as hypomagnesemia has been documented to occur in nearly half of hospitalized horses.[4] Magnesium sulfate can be used at 8–32 mg/kg over 12–24 hours administered in the IV fluid.[4a] The amount of potassium supplied by these fluids is too low to provide maintenance requirements in an inappetent horse. Therefore, during prolonged use, potassium should be supplemented by addition of 20 mEq KCl per liter of crystalloids. Commercially available maintenance fluids that contain a higher concentration of potassium and a lower concentration of sodium (e.g. Normosol M with 5% dextrose), are not available in 5-liter bags, which makes administration to adult horses difficult. Calcium can be added to the fluids in the form of calcium borogluconate 23% at 20 ml per liter of fluid.

Complications

There are minimal recognized complications associated with isotonic crystalloid administration. Patients that are predisposed to hypoproteinemia (e.g. horses with GI disease) should have their TTP monitored closely.

Electrolytes should also be monitored during fluid administration and corrected as necessary. In patients with chronic hyponatremia (>48 hours), increasing the plasma sodium concentration by <10–12 mEq/liter/day or <0.5 mEq/liter/hour using crystalloid solutions in a volume calculated to replace the patient's volume deficit is recommended to avoid osmotic demyelination syndrome.[5] The syndrome has been documented best in human and small animal patients. Osmotic demyelination occurs because during periods of hyponatremia (hypo-osmolality), potassium and organic osmolytes are lost from the cells in the brain in order to adapt to the low osmolality (<300 mOsm/kg); rapidly increasing the plasma osmolality following this adaptation results in brain dehydration and injury. Clinical signs develop 3–4 days after correction of hyponatremia and include

lethargy, weakness, and ataxia, which may progress to hypermetria and quadriparesis. Lesions have been reported in the thalamus and pontine region.[5] Similarly, in patients with hypernatremia, the brain adapts to hypertonicity by producing osmolytes or idiogenic osmoles that prevent cellular dehydration. Cerebral edema may occur if the plasma osmolality is rapidly decreased. Correction of the serum sodium concentration at a rate of <0.5 mEq/liter/hour minimizes the risk of neurologic signs associated with water intoxication in human patients.[6] The serum or plasma sodium concentration should be monitored closely during rehydration in patients with hypo- or hypernatremia. While resuscitation with fluids containing a high concentration of potassium is uncommon, the clinician should remember that potassium chloride should not be infused at rates >0.5 mEq/kg/hour to avoid cardiac side-effects.

Patients that are at risk for cerebral (e.g. head trauma) or pulmonary edema (e.g. CHF) and patients in renal failure should have fluid therapy monitored closely (see Chapter 11).

Hypertonic saline
Key points

- Hypertonic saline does not improve the overall hydration status of the patient and should be rapidly followed with large volumes of isotonic fluids.
- Recommended dose rates are 2–4 ml/kg.
- Hypertonic saline should not be administered in patients with uncontrolled hemorrhage and sodium concentrations should be taken into consideration and monitored.

Definition/overview

Technically, hypertonic saline is any saline solution with an osmolality greater than plasma. However, the usual strength that is used clinically is 7.2% NaCl (see *Table 12.1*).

Indications

The different effects of hypertonic saline are summarized in *Table 12.4*. Hypertonic saline is mostly indicated to rapidly expand the intravascular volume and improve cardiac output in an emergency situation. Hypertonic saline has the greatest intravascular volume expanding efficacy of any fluid, with administration resulting in an increase in blood volume of nearly three times the volume infused.[1] This occurs because of the osmotic shift of water from the intracellular space, which results in cellular dehydration (**12.10**). Therefore, hypertonic saline does not improve the overall hydration status of the horse and should be rapidly followed with large volumes of isotonic fluids. The intravascular volume expanding effects of hypertonic saline are short-lived because the sodium will rapidly distribute across the entire extracellular fluid space.

In addition to expanding the intravascular volume, hypertonic saline has other effects that are potentially beneficial in horses with shock or sepsis.[7] Hypertonic saline results in an increase in myocardial contractility, probably due to the direct effect of hyperosmolality on the myocardium. It also reduces edema in endothelial cells, which reduces resistance to flow and hence improves tissue perfusion. The increase in tonicity it produces may also suppress neutrophil activation and thus reduce tissue damage in inflammatory conditions. T cells are usually suppressed during trauma due to the effect of anti-inflammatory mediators such as interleukin (IL)-4 and IL-10. However, treatment with

Table 12.4 Mechanisms of action of hypertonic saline and its advantages and disadvantages in critical patients[1,7,8]

SITE OF ACTION	ADVANTAGES	DISADVANTAGES
Intravascular space	Rapid volume expansion. Small volume resuscitation. Reduced viscosity increases oxygen delivery	Causes cellular dehydration. Short-lived effect. Hypertension. Hypernatremia
Myocardium	Increases contractility	May increase myocardial oxygen consumption
Endothelium	Reduces edema. Increased capillary diameter	May reduce systemic vascular resistance
Neutrophils	Decreases migration into inflamed tissue. Reduces respiratory burst. Reduces cytokine release	May cause immunosupression in already compromised patients

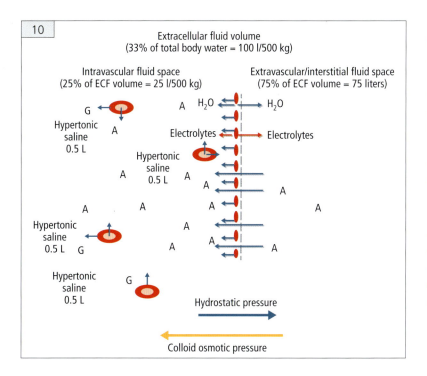

12.10 Schematic illustration of the intra- and extravascular fluid space illustrating the effects of hypertonic saline. Hypertonic saline increases the extracellular (intravascular) fluid tonicity and draws water via osmosis from the endothelium, erythrocytes, and the interstitial fluid into the intravascular space, which increases the intravascular volume. There is an increase in hydrostatic pressure and a relative decrease in colloid osmotic pressure that results in the redistribution of hypertonic saline throughout the extracellular (extravascular and intravascular) fluid space.

hypertonic saline can increase IL-2 production and restore the function of suppressed T cells, which could prevent sepsis.[8]

Hypertonic saline can lower ICP following head trauma with brain injury. Its action is likely achieved through the creation of an osmotic gradient. Therefore, the blood–brain barrier, which is relatively impermeable to sodium, must be intact. In contused areas of brain tissue, the blood–brain barrier is open and treatment with hypertonic saline actually increases the volume of contused tissue.[9] Thus its primary effect in reducing brain volume is in areas of uninjured brain tissue, resulting in an overall decrease in ICP.

Clinical use

The use of hypertonic saline in different clinical scenarios is summarized in *Table 12.5*. Hypertonic saline is usually given at a dose of up to 4 ml/kg and should be rapidly followed by 10 liters of isotonic fluids for each liter of hypertonic saline given. For preoperative resuscitation, synthetic colloids result in a more sustained increase in blood volume and improvement in cardiac index than hypertonic saline.[1,10] Hypertonic saline is also indicated in the treatment of acute head trauma. Administration of 1.5 ml/kg has been shown to reduce ICP in people with traumatic brain injury of <72 hours duration.[11]

Complications

Complications that can be associated with the use of hypertonic saline are shown in *Table 12.5*. Hypertonic saline is contraindicated in situations of uncontrolled hemorrhage. In such cases, a rapid increase in intravascular volume, and hence MAP, could exacerbate hemorrhage and dislodge clots that have already formed. Repeated doses of hypertonic saline can result in hypernatremia; therefore, serum electrolyte concentrations should be monitored. In traumatic brain injury, a rebound phenomenon can occur as serum sodium decreases, which can increase ICP again.

Colloids

- Colloid solutions contain particles that are too large to pass freely across the capillary endothelium into the interstitial space. Therefore, they exert a pressure in the intravascular space, the COP, which opposes the hydrostatic pressure forcing water out of the capillary (**12.11**).
- Several factors contribute to the overall capillary fluid balance and are combined in Starling's equation (*Table 12.6*, **12.11**). Alterations in all of these factors can occur in critically ill horses, but a decrease in plasma COP is most commonly observed. This results in a net increase in the filtration of fluid out of the capillary, which causes tissue edema.

Table 12.5 Examples of scenarios in which hypertonic saline may be used, its appropriate administration, and potential problems

SCENARIO	ADMINISTRATION	POTENTIAL PROBLEMS
Preoperative colic with severe hypovolemia	4 ml/kg immediately prior to induction of general anesthesia. Follow immediately with 10 liters of crystalloids for every liter administered	Short-lived effect. Hemodilution may result in hypokalemia
Acute traumatic brain injury	1.5 ml/kg. Administer crystalloids at maintenance rate to support cerebral perfusion	Influx of sodium if BBB is not intact. Increase in volume of contused areas. Increased ICP due to rebound phenomenon possible as serum sodium declines
Acute uncontrolled hemorrhage	Administration of half calculated dose while monitoring MAP. Aim for permissive hypotension (MAP 70–90 mmHg)	Rapid increase in MAP may dislodge clots and restart hemorrhage
Acute renal failure	4 ml/kg while monitoring urine output. Follow with 0.9% NaCl. Monitor electrolyte concentrations	If anuric, volume overload may result. Monitor MAP and CVP carefully

BBB, blood–brain barrier; ICP, intracranial pressure; MAP, mean arterial pressure; CVP, central venous pressure. (See also Chapter 11.)

11

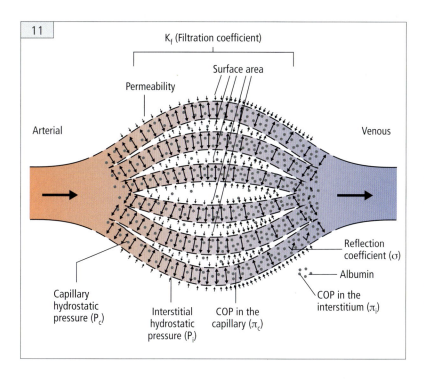

K_f (Filtration coefficient)

Surface area

Permeability

Arterial

Venous

Reflection coefficient (σ)

Albumin

COP in the interstitium (π_i)

Capillary hydrostatic pressure (P_c)

Interstitial hydrostatic pressure (P_i)

COP in the capillary (π_c)

12.11 Schematic illustration of Starling's equation. There is normally a net movement of fluid across the capillary membrane from the intravascular to the interstitial fluid space on the arterial side of the capillary bed because of the higher intravascular hydrostatic pressure compared with the interstitial hydrostatic pressure. On the venous side of the capillary bed, there is a net movement of fluid into the capillary because of the higher intravascular oncotic pressure compared to the interstitial oncotic pressure. Overall, there is a net movement of fluid from the intravascular to the interstitial fluid that is ultimately returned to the intravascular fluid space by the lymphatic system.

Table 12.6 **Starling's equation and alterations in each component that may occur in critically ill horses**

$$J_v = K_f [(P_c - P_i) - \sigma (\pi_c - \pi_i)]$$

FACTOR	DEFINITION	ALTERATIONS POSSIBLE
J_v	Net movement of fluid across the capillary membrane	If positive, fluid tends to leave the capillary. If negative, fluid tends to enter the capillary
K_f	Filtration coefficient. Determined by capillary surface area and permeability to water	Increased permeability to water occurs in inflammatory conditions
P_c	Capillary hydrostatic pressure	Decreased with hypovolemia. Increased if overly aggressive fluid therapy
P_i	Interstitial hydrostatic pressure	Increased due to tissue edema
σ	Reflection coefficient	Decreased towards 0 (less reflection of particles) due to endothelial damage
π_c	COP in the capillary	Decreased due to capillary leak, decreased production, increased losses
π_i	COP in the interstitium	Increased due to leakage of plasma proteins

COP, colloid osmotic pressure.

- Correction of COP to normal values can be achieved by administration of colloid fluids. The ultimate effect is to expand the plasma volume in an amount proportional to its COP.
- The ability of colloid molecules to hold water in the circulation is enhanced by their negative charge, which holds mobile positively charged ions around them. This is called the Gibbs–Donnan effect and results in the COP being about 50% greater than it would be from the proteins alone.
- When choosing a colloid solution, several factors should be considered:
  - Large colloid molecules stay in the vascular space longer, but due to their size, each liter of solution contains fewer colloid molecules and, therefore, has a lower COP.
  - Solutions with smaller colloid particles exert a greater oncotic effect, but that effect is shorter lasting.
  - Particle size is a particularly important consideration when there is damage to the capillary endothelium from inflammatory conditions such as endotoxemia.[12] The increased distance between capillary endothelial cells allows smaller colloid particles to leak out into the interstitium, increasing interstitial oncotic pressure and potentiating tissue edema formation.[13]
- Synthetic colloids include hydroxyethyl starch (hetastarch and pentastarch), dextrans, and gelatines and natural colloids include plasma, albumin, and blood.

Synthetic colloids
Hydroxyethyl starch
Key points
- Hydroxyethyl starch products are primarily administered to improve COP to help maintain water within the vascular space.
- Recommended dose rates are 10 ml/kg/day.
- Hydroxyethyl starch products have been associated with coagulopathy at high doses.
- Recently, in human critical care patients the use of synthetic colloids has been reported to be associated with an increase in acute kidney injury and the need for renal replacement therapy, as well

as hemorrhage and the need for blood products. There has been no clear survival benefit to their use in human patients.[13a-h] These and similar products are no longer available in Europe and carry a Black Box Warning Label in the United States following a ruling by the FDA. The clinical relevance of these findings to equine patients is not known.

Definition/overview
Hetastarch is a hydroxyethyl starch that is derived by introducing hydroxyethyl groups into the glucose units of amylopectin. The current formulations have a high degree of substitution at 0.75, which means that there are approximately 75 hydroxyethyl groups for every 100 glucose units. The higher the substitution with hydroxyethyl groups, the slower the rate of degradation and elimination.[14] Hetastarch is polydisperse, with a wide range of molecular sizes and a weight average molecular weight of 450 kDa. Thus, the standard hetastarch formulation can be written as 450/0.75 (average molecular weight/degree of substitution).[14a]

Pentastarch is also a hydroxyethyl starch, but with a slightly different formulation to hetastarch. It has a lower degree of substitution at 0.5, a lower molecular weight at 200 kDa, and a narrower range of particle sizes compared with hetastarch.

Indications
Hydroxyethyl starch products are primarily indicated to increase the COP and expand the intravascular fluid volume.

Clinical use
Hetastarch is available as a 6% solution in either 0.9% NaCl (HESpan®) or a lactated electrolyte solution containing potassium, magnesium, and calcium (Hextend®). A comparison of hetastarch, pentastarch, and dextrans is found in *Table 12.7*. A dose of 10 ml/kg has been shown to increase COP in normal ponies.[15] Thirty minutes after administration of hetastarch, there is expansion of the blood volume as the increase in COP causes a redistribution of fluid into the intravascular space.[1] The overall effect on plasma volume expansion lasts approximately 24 hours. Hetastarch has been shown to increase COP for approximately

12 hours in hypoalbuminemic dogs.[16] Therefore, it should be administered twice daily in order to maintain COP, although the total 24-hour dose should not exceed 20 mg/kg in order to avoid the side-effects on coagulation. After administration, hetastarch is eliminated in two phases. First, molecules smaller than the renal threshold are rapidly excreted in the urine. The remaining molecules are metabolized by α-amylase in the blood to smaller fragments, which are then renally excreted. Therefore, a rise in serum amylase level can be found after hetastarch administration, although serum lipase levels remain constant.

Pentastarch is available as a 6% or 10% solution (HAES-Steril [200/0.5] and Voluven [130/0.4]) and can be administered at a dose rate up to 15 ml/kg/day. Due to the smaller size molecules, pentastarch induces a higher COP than hetastarch, but its effects are shorter lasting. Another advantage of pentastarch is the presence of medium molecular weight molecules, which may seal leaky capillary endothelium and help maintain plasma volume in the presence of albumin leakage.[17,18] As with hetastarch, smaller molecules are rapidly eliminated by renal excretion. Approximately 70% of the total dose administered is eliminated within the first 24 hours. The effect on plasma volume expansion lasts for approximately 12 hours and dosing can, therefore, be repeated twice daily. Administration of pentastarch to preoperative colic patients at a dose of 4 ml/kg resulted in a significant improvement in cardiac index compared with the same dose of hypertonic saline.[10] This effect lasted at least 3 hours after administration, although obviously the cost differential may outweigh the benefits of it use. (**Note:** Pentastarch is not currently approved for use in the USA, but is routinely used in other countries.)

Recent investigations have examined the effect of a low molecular weight and substitution hydroxyethyl starch solution (130/0.42; Vetstarch™) in 0.9% sodium chloride. This solution was found to be even more effective at reducing capillary leakage of albumin than pentastarch in a porcine model of hemorrhagic shock.[19] Its use in horses has not been evaluated; however, it has been used clinically.

When using colloid solutions, knowledge of the horse's serum COP is helpful to guide administration, and may be more accurate than relying on TPP concentration. This is especially true when synthetic colloids are used because measurement of TPP on a refractometer underestimates the increase in COP from synthetic colloids.[20] COP can be estimated from the Landis–Pappenheimer equation using TPP

Table 12.7 **Comparison of the synthetic colloids hetastarch, pentastarch, and dextran**

COLLOID	MEAN MOLECULAR WEIGHT	DEGREE OF SUBSTITUTION	AMOUNT ELIMINATED IN 24 HOURS	EFFECT ON VOLUME EXPANSION	HEMOSTATIC ABNORMALITIES
Hetastarch	450 kDa	0.75	33%	Less expansion immediately, but more prolonged effect	Greater
	130 kDa	0.42		Should be greater volume expansion	Fewer
Pentastarch	200 kDa	0.5	70%	Greater immediate effect, but shorter lasting	Less
Dextran 40 and 70	40 kDa and 70 kDa	N/A	70%	Very high volume expansion immediately, but rapidly eliminated	Greatest effect: interferes with cross-matching and inhibits coagulation

(see Chapter 11), but this appears to be inaccurate in animal species.[21] Additionally, in critically ill foals, the correlation between the calculated and directly measured COP value is poor when lactate concentration is increased compared with normal.[22] Therefore, in critically ill horses, direct measurement of COP using a colloid osmometer is recommended. COP should be approximately 19 mmHg in foals and 21 mmHg in adult horses.[23]

Complications

The most widely recognized side-effect of hetastarch in horses is a trend towards an increase in bleeding time.[15] This occurred at a dose of 20 ml/kg and is likely due to a decrease in factor VIII and von Willibrand factor antigen activity. Hetastarch formulations with a lower degree of substitution have less of an effect on coagulation[24]; however, the mechanism behind the decrease in coagulation factors is not known. No adverse effects on coagulation have been documented in surgical equine patients administered hetastarch. However, it should be used with caution in horses with an abnormal coagulation profile and probably avoided in cases with uncontrolled hemorrhage.

Pentastarch had less effect on hemostasis than hetastarch at a dose of approximately 20 ml/kg in healthy human subjects.[25] This is likely due to the absence of highly substituted molecules that persist in the circulation and interfere with several clotting factors.[26] However, in horses with a surgical condition of the large colon, administration of pentastarch at 10 ml/kg did significantly increase APTT.[27] Further investigation is necessary to distinguish the effect of the drug from the underlying disease process.

Dextrans
Key points
- Due to their small particle size, dextrans have a high COP, but their effect is short lived.
- Dextrans are associated with more complications compared with hydroxyethyl starch products, which has limited their use in the horse.

Definition/overview
Dextrans are glucose polymers produced by the fermentation of sucrose by the bacterium *Leuconostoc mesenteroides*. Several formulations are available; the most commonly used include Dextran 40 and Dextran 70, where the number corresponds to the average molecular weight.

Indications
Dextrans can be administered to improve COP. Due to their small particle size, dextrans have a high COP, but their effect is short lived. They tend to be less expensive than hydroxyethyl starch solutions; however, they are associated with more complications, which has limited their use in the horse.

Clinical use
Dextran is available as a 6% solution in 0.9% saline (Gentran 40 and 70). Administration results in an increase in blood volume that is not significantly different to that seen with hetastarch administration.[1] Dextrans have also been used as carriers for other therapeutic agents, to extend the effect of that drug in the plasma and reduce its toxicity. This is achieved by conjugation of hydroxyl groups in the dextran molecule to the desired treatment.[28] In horses, dextran 70 conjugated to polymyxin B was effective in ameliorating the signs of endotoxemia, although mild adverse systemic effects of the infusion including transient sweating and elevation in heart rate, respiratory rate, blood pressure and temperature were seen.[29] Hypertonic saline dextran (HSD) (6% dextran 70, 7.5% NaCl) is available in Europe as a small volume resuscitation fluid to provide rapid plasma volume expansion (RescueFlow®).

Complications
Dextran 70 has been shown to significantly reduce the concentration of von Willebrand factor antigen and factor VIIIC in healthy dogs[30] and is considered to cause more disturbances in coagulation than hydroxyethyl starch. Additionally, the small particle size allows them to adhere to red cells, which interferes with cross-matching.

Low-molecular weight dextrans (i.e. dextran 40) have been reported to cause AKI. High concentration of the small dextran molecules is thought to cause obstruction of the renal tubules or osmotic nephrosis.[5]

In one study, hypertonic saline with dextran (25% NaCl with 24% dextran) caused hemolysis in horses due to the extremely high osmolality of the solution.[31] A less hypertonic saline with dextran solution has not been examined in horses.

Gelatins
Key point
- The main indication for use of gelatins is acute resuscitation of severely hypovolemic horses.

Definition/overview
Gelatins (proteins derived by chemical modification of bovine collagen) are low-weight, average molecular weight products (~30–35 kDa) available in some countries (e.g. Australia, New Zealand, Europe, and some Asian Countries, but not in the USA).

Indications
The main indication for use of gelatins is for acute resuscitation of severely hypovolemic horses.[32]

Clinical use
Gelatins available for use in horses include succinylated gelatin (Gelofusine®) and urea-linked gelatin (Haemacell®).[32] Gelatins have a high osmotic pressure (342 mmHg) and can therefore increase the intravascular volume by drawing fluid from the interstitial and intracellular fluid spaces (see Hypertonic saline). Gelatins are administered at a rate of 2–4 ml/kg and administration should be followed up with large volumes of isotonic crystalloid fluids (>10–20 ml/kg).[32] Because of their low molecular weight (<55 kDa), they are freely filtered by the renal glomerulus and rapidly eliminated.[32]

Complications
Because of their small molecular size compared with other colloids, gelatins are easily extravasated, which can predispose to edema formation. The high osmotic pressure can also lead to fluid overload and pulmonary edema. Allergic reactions have been reported in human patients but not in horses.[32]

Naturally occurring colloids
Plasma and albumin
Key points
- Hypoalbuminemia is the main indication for plasma use in horses.
- Because the principle colloid in plasma is albumin, it may be less effective than synthetic colloids in increasing the COP.
- Administration of plasma, however, provides advantages other than increased COP.
- Plasma is typically more expensive than synthetic colloids, requires thawing, and can be associated with transfusion reaction. Horses should, therefore, be monitored closely during administration.

Definition/overview
Plasma is a blood substitute prepared by removing the cells and corpuscles from donated sterile blood and freezing the resulting fluid until it is needed. The principal colloid in plasma is albumin, which provides approximately 75% of the normal COP. Plasma is most effective if it is separated and frozen within 6 hours of collection and used within 1 year. This is considered fresh frozen plasma and contains the labile coagulation factors V and VIII, which are degraded with longer storage. Plasma also contains globulins, fibronectin, antithrombin III, and the stable coagulation factors, making it useful for treatment of endotoxemia and clotting defects and not simply as a volume expander.

Indications
Hypoalbuminemia is the main indication for plasma use in horses. Hypoalbuminemia can occur through loss of albumin via the GI tract, decreased synthesis by the liver, or third spacing into the interstitium due to increased vascular permeability. When supplementing albumin, it is important to consider the underlying cause of the initial loss. Albumin has a molecular

weight of 69 kDa and is therefore a relatively small colloid molecule. The gaps between normal capillary endothelial cells are only slightly smaller than the albumin molecule. Therefore, if capillary permeability is increased, albumin can leak into the interstitium and cause the formation of edema. In such situations, it may be beneficial to initially administer a larger molecular weight colloid to maintain COP. However, if capillary permeability is not affected, supplementation of albumin itself may be justified. When plasma albumin is lost, it is initially replaced by a shift of albumin from the interstitial space, primarily the skin and skeletal muscle, into the circulation.[33] Thus, when exogenous albumin is supplemented, it is the interstitial stores that are first replenished and an increase in serum albumin concentration may not occur.

Administration of plasma provides advantages other than increased COP. Albumin itself not only maintains COP, but is important as a carrier molecule. It is involved in the transportation of bilirubin, drugs, fatty acids, and free radicals.[34] Therefore, it is important to maintain albumin concentration at or above 20 g/l (2 g/dl) for these functions to occur. Plasma contains immunoglobulins and is also given to neonatal foals with FPT of maternal immunoglobulins (see Chapter 9).

Clinical use

Plasma is the colloid solution that is most frequently administered to horses. It is used to provide colloid support, replenish albumin, and provide clotting factors. Because it is stored frozen, advanced planning for its use is necessary. Frozen plasma should only be defrosted in warm water and not in the microwave, as this will denature the proteins. There is no specific dose of plasma; several liters are usually given until the desired effect on TPP, COP, and albumin concentration are documented. Approximately 10 liters of plasma are required to increase the plasma albumin concentration by 5 g/l (0.5 g/dl) in a 450 kg horse. In reality, even more

may be required due to replenishment of the interstitial stores and continued losses. Plasma is not very effective at improving COP, as it has the same COP as normal blood. Additionally, in horses with increased capillary permeability, much of the albumin may extravasate into the interstitial space. Therefore, it is often combined clinically with a synthetic colloid (e.g. hetastarch) to improve COP.

Concentrated human albumin is available as a 5%, 20%, or 25% solution (Buminate®, Flexbumin®, Plasbumin®). In critically ill dogs and cats it has been used at an average dose of 2 ml/kg to increase COP or blood pressure after other colloid products were ineffective.[35] Administration significantly increased serum albumin concentration, total solids, and blood pressure in these cases.[35] When albumin is administered to critically ill human patients, an increased risk of death has been documented.[36,37] The most recent review found no benefit of albumin compared with cheaper alternatives such as saline, but acknowledges that it may be beneficial in a select population of critically ill patients.[37] Given the expense that would be associated with the use of concentrated albumin in horses, it is advisable to use synthetic colloids combined with plasma to maintain serum albumin concentration until there is documentation of its efficacy in horses.

Complications

The main complication with plasma administration is a transfusion reaction. Horses should be monitored during transfusion for signs of tachycardia, fever, and urticaria. If these signs are observed, the transfusion should be stopped. Short-acting corticosteroids (e.g. dexamethasone sodium phosphate or methylprednisolone succinate) and an antihistamine can be administered in cases with urticaria. Usually, transfusion reactions are mild compared with those that occur with whole blood transfusions (see Whole blood administration and also Chapter 4).

Blood and oxygen carrying solutions
Key points

- Whole blood is primarily administered to improve tissue oxygenation after red cells have been lost through hemorrhage or hemolysis.
- Horses should be monitored closely while receiving an allogenic whole blood transfusion for signs of a transfusion reaction.
- Alternatives to allogenic whole blood transfusion should be considered in patients undergoing surgical procedures during which excessive blood loss is anticipated.

Definition/overview

Whole blood is essentially a colloid, but the presence of RBCs allows it to carry oxygen. It is primarily administered to improve tissue oxygenation after red cells have been lost through hemorrhage or hemolysis. Due to the presence of red cells and plasma proteins it exerts an oncotic pressure and primarily remains in the intravascular space after administration resulting in expansion of the intravascular volume.

Oxygen carrying solutions also have the ability to carry oxygen through their binding to free hemoglobin in the solution and, therefore, improve tissue oxygenation. Much of their purported clinical effect may be due to their impressive oncotic properties. However, they cannot be thought of as blood substitutes, as they do not the contain the platelets, WBCs, and clotting factors that are present in whole blood. They do not require a cross-match to be performed prior to use and are instantly available off the shelf. Unfortunately, these products are relatively expensive to use as the sole replacement for lost red cells, especially when considering the volume that would be needed for treatment of an adult horse. Availability may also be extremely limited.

Indications

Whole blood transfusion: Allogeneic transfusion of whole blood is used to improve oxygen delivery to the tissues. Whole blood also exerts oncotic pressure and, therefore, will expand the intravascular volume. Signs of acute blood loss are usually seen when >15% of the blood volume (approximately 6 liters) has been lost. The initial response is tachycardia, followed by hypovolemic shock and circulatory collapse as the volume lost increases (*Table 12.8*). Following acute hemorrhage, it takes between 4 and 12 hours for fluid to redistribute from the interstitial space into the intravascular space and reduce the PCV. Therefore, PCV is not an accurate indicator of the severity of blood loss in acute hemorrhage. However, when red cell loss is more chronic, for example due to hemolysis, PCV and Hb concentration are useful indicators of the need for a transfusion. Other indicators that can be used to assess acute blood loss are tachycardia, hypotension, and signs of decreased tissue oxygenation, such as a high anion

Table 12.8 Relationship between the volume of blood loss, clinical effect, and transfusion requirements in a 450 kg horse

PERCENTAGE OF BLOOD VOLUME LOST	APPROXIMATE AMOUNT LOST (LITERS)	CLINICAL EFFECT	VOLUME OF BLOOD TO TRANSFUSE (LITERS)
15	6	Mild loss, little effect	Unnecessary
15–30	12	High heart rate	6
30–40	14	Hypovolemic shock	7
>40	16	Circulatory collapse	8

gap and hyperlactatemia (see Chapter 11). Preoperative blood collection, normovolemic hemodilution, and autotransfusion can be used as an alternative to allogenic blood transfusion in surgical cases where a large volume of blood loss is anticipated (*Table 12.9*).

Hemoglobin-based oxygen carrying solutions: An alternative to whole blood is the use of a hemoglobin-based oxygen carrying (HBOC) solution (e.g. Oxyglobin®). This is not a blood substitute because it does not contain the platelets, WBCs, and clotting factors that are present in whole blood, but it does increase oxygen carrying capacity by increasing the total Hb concentration.

Because of the cost of HBOC solutions, its use is only feasible in miniature horses and foals. It should be considered when a suitable donor cannot be found, as reported in a miniature horse with ovarian hemorrhage that had suffered two previous transfusion reactions.[38] It is also suitable for use when ongoing hemolysis is occurring, as reported in a miniature horse and a pony with red maple toxicosis[39], and in a foal with neonatal isoerythrolysis.[40] In a canine model of hemorrhagic shock, HBOC solutions were not as effective as whole blood in restoring oxygen delivery[41], but were shown to improve oxygen delivery and utilization parameters in a normovolemic anemia model in ponies.[42] Therefore, in situations of acute hemorrhage, whole blood transfusion should remain the treatment of choice.

Table 12.9 Options available for replacement of shed blood

METHOD	TECHNIQUE	ADVANTAGES	DISADVANTAGES
Allogeneic transfusion	Transfusion of blood collected from a different individual	Large volume of blood can be obtained	Risk of transfusion reaction. Short half-life of transfused red cells. Risk of disease transmission
Autotransfusion	Collection and reinfusion of the patients own shed blood	Less risk of transfusion reaction. Blood is immediately available and warm. Longer life span of transfused red cells	Blood must be shed into a body cavity, or collected intraoperatively. Risk of hemolysis and sepsis. Blood cannot be stored
Preoperative autologous deposit	Blood collected 7–10 days prior to surgery and stored until use	Erythropoiesis already stimulated. Less risk of transfusion reaction	Time and transportation costs of an additional hospital visit. Lower preoperative PCV. Lower 2,3-DPG concentration
Acute normovolemic hemodilution	Blood collected after induction of anesthesia, volume replaced with crystalloids, blood reinfused in surgery as needed	Fewer red cells lost in surgery. Fresh autologous blood available for transfusion. Improved tissue perfusion	Lower intraoperative PCV. Not feasible if there is pre-existing anemia. Excellent anesthetic monitoring essential
HBOC solution	Administered at rate of 10–15 ml/kg	Immediately available. Cross-matching unnecessary	No clotting factors or platelets. Expensive. Interferes with colorimetric chemistry assays

HBOC, hemoglobin-based oxygen carrying; PCV, packed cell volume; DPG, diphosphoglycerate.

Clinical use

Allogenic whole blood transfusion

Cross-match: Horses have over 30 serologically relevant RBC antigens resulting in over 400,000 blood types and, therefore, there is no universal donor or perfect cross-match. However, the most immunogenic antigens are Qa and Aa, so hospital-owned donors ideally lack these antigens and antibodies against them. Even with cross-matching, 80% of transfused red cells may be lost within days. This is in contrast to humans, where transfused cells have the same life span as autologous red cells. Thus, in horses, transfusion of whole blood provides support while erythropoiesis is stimulated.

If the situation allows, major (donor red cells and recipient serum) and minor (donor serum and recipient red cells) cross-matches for agglutination and lysis should be performed. If this is not available, the most suitable donor is a gelding and preferably a Standardbred or Quarter Horse, because they have a lower incidence of Aa and Qa antigens. A first transfusion usually does not incite a transfusion reaction; however, a cross-match is highly recommended prior to subsequent transfusions.

Blood collection: A donor can donate approximately 15% of its blood volume, averaging 6–8 liters, without adverse effects, although heart rate and respiratory rate should be monitored carefully. It is unnecessary to transfuse the entire volume lost, as movement of fluid from the interstitial space will expand the intravascular volume. Therefore, collection and transfusion of approximately half the shed blood is usually adequate. Blood should be collected using strict aseptic techniques into bags pre-filled with 100 ml of anticoagulant per liter of blood. Collection into glass bottles results in loss of the platelets, which rapidly adhere to the glass. Acid-citrate dextrose is an acceptable anticoagulant if the blood is to be used immediately. However, if longer term storage is anticipated, citrate-phosphate-dextrose with adenine (CPD-A) will preserve 2,3-diphosphoglycerate concentration and adenosine triphosphate levels, resulting in longer survival of red cells.[43]

Whole blood administration: Whole blood should be administered slowly for the first 30 minutes through a filter administration set while observing for hypersensitivity or anaphylaxis (see below). No calcium containing fluids, such as lactated Ringer's solution, should be administered concurrently.

Preoperative autologous deposit

Alternatives to allogeneic transfusion are possible, especially if blood loss is anticipated in advance, and are summarized in *Table 12.9*. For example, prior to elective sinus surgery, a preoperative deposit of blood can be made 7–10 days in advance and stored refrigerated with CPD-A as the anticoagulant. The stored blood is then administered as needed at surgery as an autologous transfusion. This reduces the risk of a transfusion reaction, but also lowers the PCV at the time of surgery and incurs the cost of an additional hospital visit for the horse prior to surgery for blood collection.

Acute normovolemic hemodilution

Another alternative is acute normovolemic hemodilution. With this technique in people, blood is collected from the patient after induction of anesthesia until the PCV is 0.28 l/l (28%). This blood is replaced with 1 liter of hetastarch and crystalloids at three times the collected volume. The harvested blood is then reinfused at surgery to maintain an acceptable PCV.[44] Blood lost in surgery thus contains fewer red cells per ml. The patient's residual blood is also less viscous due to dilution with crystalloids, which improves blood flow and tissue perfusion.[45]

Autotransfusion

The patient's own shed blood may also be collected and reinfused as an autotransfusion. The shed blood can be collected by suction as it is lost, for example during sinus surgery, or by simply draining it from the cavity in which it has collected, for example with hemothorax or hemoabdomen. Commercially available 1-liter collection systems are available for intraoperative or postoperative use (e.g. Autovac IO and Autovac TC) (**12.12A, B**), which are extremely convenient, although expensive. Alternatively, a cannula can be placed into the abdomen and the blood collected into a glass jar primed with anticoagulant. Shed blood is usually defibrinogenated by contact with body surfaces and, therefore, less anticoagulant is required than with routine blood collection, so an anticoagulant:blood ratio of 1:15 is usually used. Blood for autotransfusion is immediately available and warm. There is less risk of an immune reaction and the red cells have a longer life span than allogeneic red cells. Excessive suction pressure can result in hemolysis and there is a greater risk of sepsis, so the collected blood should be used within 4 hours.

Hemoglobin-based oxygen carrying solutions

Oxyglobin® contains 13 g/dl of polymerized bovine hemoglobin in modified lactated Ringer's solution. Polymerization of the hemoglobin molecule reduces the renal toxicity of free hemoglobin and also prolongs its effect. Due to the absence of antigenic red cell membranes, cross-matching is not necessary and immunogenic transfusion reactions should not occur.

Oxyglobin® is currently only licensed for the treatment of anemia in dogs, although its use has been investigated in horses. In six ponies with normovolemic anemia, 15 ml/kg significantly increased CVP, oxygen extraction, and SVR compared with treatment with hetastarch.[42] One pony did have an anaphylactic reaction, most likely to the hemoglobin in the solution. The observed increase in CVP in this study is due to the high COP (43 mmHg) of the solution. Volume overload is less of a problem in horses than in small animals; however, clinicians should be cognizant of this fact when administering this product to foals. The observed increase in SVR could occur by two different mechanisms: (1) direct scavenging of nitric oxide in the blood by HBOC solutions or (2) by free hemoglobin inhibiting the action of nitric oxide on guanylate cyclase, which in turn inhibits the intracellular increase in calcium that is required for smooth muscle contraction.[46]

Complications

Signs of a transfusion reaction with an allogenic whole blood transfusion include piloerection, restlessness, and fasciculations. There are two basic categories of transfusion reactions, immune and non-immune. An immune response can occur to any component of the transfused blood, the most common being acute hemolysis and anaphylaxis due to the presence of preformed antibodies against the transfused red cells. Non-immune reactions are due to improper collection or processing of the blood, and are preventable. They include hemolysis due to osmotic shear stress on the cells, bacterial contamination, and hypocalcemia.

If signs of a transfusion reaction are observed, administration of the blood should be stopped immediately. The remainder of the blood should be stored in case further analysis to determine the cause of the reaction is necessary. If an acute anaphylactic reaction is seen, epinephrine should be given IV at a dose of 0.01 ml/kg of 1:1,000 epinephrine (approximately 5 ml for an adult horse). If hypersensitivity is seen, an antihistamine should be given (e.g. diphenhydramine, 1 mg/kg PO). A sample of blood from the recipient should be centrifuged to detect intravascular hemolysis.

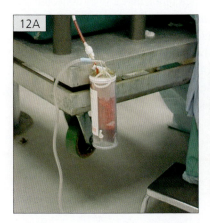
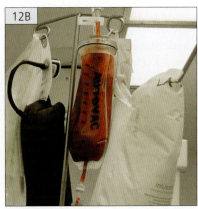

12.12A, B (A) A commercially available autotransfusion system in use during elective sinus surgery in a horse with an ethmoid hematoma. (B) The blood is collected into a bag primed with acid-citrate dextrose, which can be removed from the rigid outer container for immediate administration to the horse.

CHAPTER 13

INOTROPE AND VASOPRESSOR THERAPY

Brett S. Tennent-Brown
and Janyce Seahorn

GENERAL APPROACH TO USE OF INOTROPE AND VASOPRESSOR THERAPY

- The ultimate goal of fluid resuscitation and inotrope and vasopressor therapy is to restore perfusion and oxygen delivery to the tissues.[1]
- Although most emergency equine patients will respond to volume replacement alone, some cases, particularly foals, will require additional therapies to support cardiovascular function.
- The most common cause of cardiovascular disturbances in equine patients is severe sepsis usually as a consequence of gram-negative infection and endotoxemia. In treating these animals, it is critical to identify the underlying cause of sepsis or endotoxemia and institute appropriate therapy.
- It is crucial that affected animals are adequately volume resuscitated before initiating inotrope and vasopressor therapy, as many of the adverse effects of these drugs are exacerbated by hypovolemia.
- Indications for inotrope or vasopressor therapy include persistence of the following despite appropriate volume replacement:
  - Hypotension (MAP <65 mmHg).
  - Tachycardia.
  - Oliguria.
  - Hyperlactatemia.
- Additional clinical signs of inadequate tissue perfusion include:
  - Cold distal extremities and poor peripheral pulses.
  - Obtundation.
  - Decreased GI activity.
- Biochemical or blood-gas indicators of poor organ perfusion include:
  - Increases in serum creatinine concentration.
  - Increases in muscle and liver enzyme activities.
  - Decreases in central venous hemoglobin saturation or increases in oxygen extraction ratios.
- The drugs used to support cardiovascular function generally have a number of physiological effects depending on:
  - Patient species.
  - Disease condition and severity.
  - Receptor specificity and tissue distribution.
  - Drug administration rate.
- The minimum information necessary to select an appropriate inotrope or vasopressor includes heart rate and rhythm and an indirect measure of arterial blood pressure. Continual or repeated measurement of multiple cardiovascular parameters is essential to monitor and guide therapy. More accurate titration of these agents and enhanced safety can be achieved with measurement of:
  - Central venous pressure.
  - Direct arterial blood pressure.
  - Pulse oximetry.
  - Central venous or pulmonary artery hemoglobin-oxygen saturation.
  - Cardiac output.

- Therapeutic goals will vary based on the disease process, patient, clinical signs, and monitoring capabilities. However, a reasonable goal for inotrope and vasopressor therapy is:
  - An increase in MAP to 65–75 mmHg; sufficient to increase urine output without inducing tachycardia or arrhythmias. It is important to realize that improvements in blood pressure do not necessarily translate into improved tissue oxygen delivery.
  - There should also be an improvement in the clinical and biochemical indicators of inadequate tissue oxygen delivery (e.g. low pulse oximetry values [low hemoglobin saturation] and high serum creatinine and blood lactate concentrations).
  - When using vasodilators, the goal is to reduce MAP to <120 mmHg without inducing hypotension, tachycardia, or acidosis.
- A decision tree for treatment of hypotension and poor organ perfusion with suggested goals and indications for inotrope and vasopressor use is shown (**13.1**). *Table 13.1* shows the receptor affinities for the various catecholamine drugs.

PREPARATION AND ADMINISTRATION

- Inotropes and vasopressors have short half-lives and must be administered as a CRI for the treatment of hypotension or poor cardiac output.
- Electronic infusion pumps are recommended for accurate delivery of inotropic and vasopressor drugs.
- Many of these agents, particularly dopamine and norepinephrine, can cause severe tissue injury if extravasation should occur; each should be diluted for administration, which will also allow more accurate delivery.
- Most are compatible with commonly used fluid types (bicarbonate-containing or other strongly alkaline fluids are an exception); however, some of these agents are incompatible with other commonly used drugs. Possible incompatibilities should be checked before use and IV delivery sets carefully monitored.
- Although not applicable to most equine veterinary patients, one must avoid delivery of excessive fluid volumes to very small patients when vasopressor administration rates are increased.

Table 13.1 **Receptor affinity of various catecholamine drugs**

DRUG	ADRENERGIC				DOPAMINERGIC	
	α_1	α_2	β_1	β_2	1	2
Dobutamine	+	+	+ + +[1]	+ +	0	0
Norepinephrine	+ + +	+ + +	+ + +	0[2]	0	0
Dopamine[3]	+ +	(+)	+ +	+	+ + +	+ +
Phenylephrine	+ + +	+	(+)	0	0	0
Epinephrine	+ + +	+ + +	+ + +	+ + +	0	0

+ + + strong affinity, + + moderate affinity, + weak affinity, (+) possible affinity, 0 no affinity

[1] Inotropism greater than chronotropism

[2] β_2 effects are present but not seen clinically

[3] Effects are markedly dose dependent

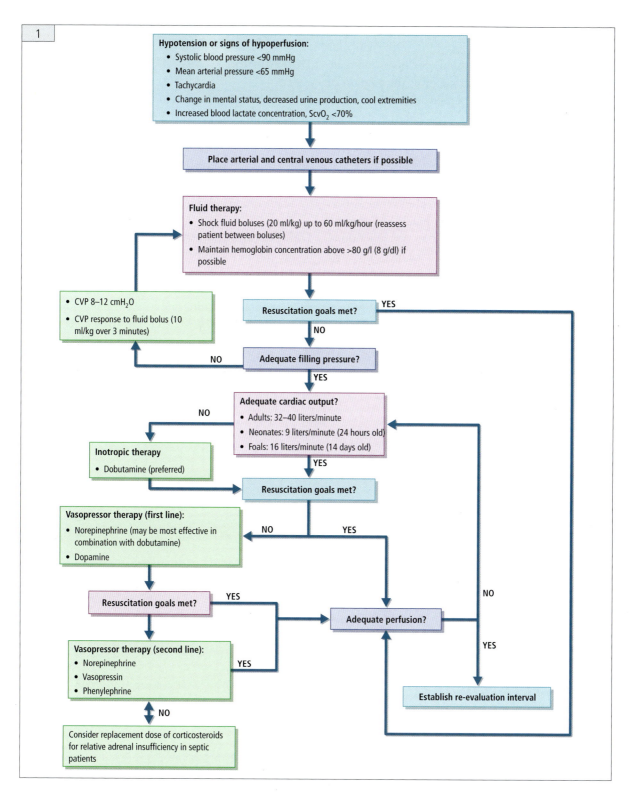

13.1 An algorithm for the treatment of hypotension and tissue hypoperfusion with suggested goals and indications for inotrope and vasopressor use.

The 'rule of 6' may be used to prepare solutions for CRI of drugs that are dosed in micrograms per kilogram per minute (µg/kg/min). Six times the body weight in kilograms (6 × bwt kg) gives the amount of drug in milligrams (mg) that should be added to 100 ml of carrier solution. **Note:** An equal volume of carrier solution should be removed prior to adding the drug. The infusion rate volume in ml/hour will then equal the µg/kg/min dose ordered.

Example. You wish to administer dobutamine at a rate of 3 µg/kg/min to a 55 kg foal in septic shock. The concentration of the dobutamine is 12.5 mg/ml, which is available as 250 mg in a 20 m vial. Therefore, 330 mg (6 × 55 kg) of dobutamine (26.4 ml of 12.5 mg/ml dobutamine) is added to 100 ml of isotonic sodium chloride (0.9% NaCl). **Note:** 26.4 ml of 0.9% NaCl should be removed prior to adding the drug. Infusion of this solution at 3 ml/hour will administer 3 µg/kg/min of dobutamine to the foal.

INOTROPES AND VASOPRESSORS

Dobutamine
Key points
- Dobutamine primarily increases cardiac output by increasing myocardial contractility.
- Dobutamine administration should be titrated to effect.
- 'Low-dose' dobutamine may preserve splanchnic perfusion when used with other vasopressors (e.g. norepinephrine).

Definition/mechanism of action
Dobutamine is considered a direct β_1-adrenergic agonist with mild β_2 and α_1 activity. The drug's primary effect is to increase cardiac output via an increase in myocardial contractility and stroke volume subsequent to β_1 stimulation (*Table 13.2*). The drug is also mildly chronotropic and can cause arrhythmias. The vasodilatory effects of β_2 stimulation generally offset α_1-mediated vasoconstriction and dobutamine may improve splanchnic circulation.

Table 13.2 **Summary of indications, mode of action, and suggested dose ranges for dobutamine**

INDICATIONS	ACTION[1]	SUGGESTED DOSES[2]	COMMENTS
Shock (septic, cardiogenic) not responsive to fluid resuscitation. Low cardiac output	β_1: inotropic (chronotropic) β_2: (mild) vasodilation α_1: (mild) vasoconstriction[3]	**Equine** 0.5–1.0 µg/kg/minute 1.0–3.0 µg/kg/minute 1.0–5.0 µg/kg/minute	Adult starting dose range Foal starting dose range 'Low dose' used with a vasopressor
		Human 0.5–1.0 µg/kg/minute 5–10 µg/kg/minute 2–20 µg/kg/minute	Adult human starting dose Pediatric starting dose Typical human dose range

[1] Ranked on subjective order of importance

[2] Suggested dose rates are for treatment of hypotension and/or poor cardiac output unless otherwise stated

[3] Off-set by β-effects

Indications

Dobutamine is usually the first drug used in hypotensive horses, particularly if cardiac output monitoring is not available. This is because without a measure of cardiac output, the clinician has no estimate of SVR and it is probably safer to increase cardiac output rather than vascular tone. Specific indications for the use of dobutamine include low cardiac output and decreased central venous oxygen saturation ($S_{cv}O_2$) (or increased oxygen extraction ratio [O_2ER]). A decreased $S_{cv}O_2$ (or increased O_2ER) indicates increased oxygen utilization by the tissues as a result of low cardiac output and sluggish tissue blood flow. In practice, indications for the use of dobutamine are often limited to low blood pressure values, low urine output, low pulse oximeter readings, and poor peripheral pulse quality.

Dobutamine may be particularly useful in preserving splanchnic circulation when using vasopressors to maintain blood pressure.[2]

Clinical use

Dobutamine is unavailable orally and is rapidly metabolized by the liver and other tissues following IV administration, therefore a CRI is required. Recommended administration rates are given in *Table 13.2*. Dobutamine is compatible with most fluid types but should not be administered in sodium bicarbonate solutions or other strongly alkaline fluids. Incompatibilities have been reported with commonly used drugs and infusion lines should be carefully checked for precipitates when dobutamine is administered. Dobutamine should only be used in patients who have been adequately volume repleted.

Complications

Cardiac arrhythmias are the most common complication when using dobutamine. Patients should be monitored for the presence of ectopic beats and increases in heart rate >10% of baseline should be avoided.

Norepinephrine

Key points

- Norepinephrine primarily increases SVR, with relatively mild effects on myocardial function.
- Advanced cardiac monitoring techniques (e.g. cardiac output) should be considered when using norepinephrine.

Definition/mechanism of action

Norepinephrine is a strong α-adrenergic agonist with moderate β_1-adrenergic activity and no demonstrable β_2 effects (*Table 13.3*). The drug is primarily a powerful

---

Table 13.3 **Summary of indications, mode of action, and suggested dose rates for norepinephrine**

INDICATIONS	ACTION[1]	SUGGESTED DOSES[2]	COMMENTS
Hypotension refractory to fluids and other agents	α: potent arterial and venous vasoconstriction	**Equine**	
		0.1 µg/kg/minute	Suggested starting dose
Low SVR (with normal or increased cardiac output)	β_1: (mild) inotropic		
		Human[3]	
		1–30 µg/minute	Typical human dose range (note units)

SVR, systemic vascular resistance.

[1] Ranked on subjective order of importance.

[2] Suggested dose rates are for treatment of hypotension and/or poor cardiac output unless otherwise stated.

[3] Note that careful attention should be paid to units used; the suggested human dose range is given per individual rather than per kg of body weight.

venous and arterial vasoconstrictor. By increasing afterload, norepinephrine has the potential to decrease cardiac output; however, this is generally offset by the β_1 effects. The β_1-adrenergic agonistic effects of norepinephrine are similar in potency to those of epinephrine and increase both myocardial contractility and stroke volume.

Indications

Norepinephrine should be considered in patients that have not responded to dobutamine or have a documented increase in cardiac output and yet remain hypotensive (*Table 13.3*). Norepinephrine is considered a more effective vasopressor than dopamine in human septic shock patients.[3] The drug is often used in combination with 'low-dose' dobutamine (<5 µg/kg/minute); the β_2 activity of dobutamine may preserve perfusion of splanchnic and other tissue beds.[3,4]

Clinical use

The use of norepinephrine requires careful monitoring. Inappropriate dosing may cause excessive vasoconstriction, reducing cardiac output and organ perfusion. In particular, norepinephrine will increase myocardial workload without a compensatory increase in coronary blood flow. Urine output should be monitored and more advanced cardiovascular monitoring techniques (e.g. cardiac output measurements) should be considered if available. Norepinephrine should be diluted in a 5% dextrose solution (protects against oxidation) for administration. Clinical effects may be seen in some patients at dose rates as low as 0.01 µg/kg/minute. Recommended administration rates are given in *Table 13.3*.

Complications

As with many of the catecholamines, norepinephrine has arrhythmogenic potential. Excessive vasoconstriction may occur with inappropriate doses of norepinephrine, which can reduce cardiac output and organ perfusion.

Dopamine
Key points
- Dopamine has inotropic, vasopressor, and vasodilatory properties.
- The effects of dopamine are dose dependent and there is considerable overlap; therefore, dopamine administration must be titrated to effect.

Definition/mechanism of action

Dopamine is an agonist for dopaminergic receptors and also acts at α-, β_1-, and β_2-adrenergic receptors (*Table 13.4*). Dopamine is a precursor to norepinephrine and stimulates the release of norepinephrine from nerve terminals, which contributes to the drug's effects. The activity at these various receptors is dose dependent, with different effects predominating at different doses.[3]

Indication

Dopamine has inotropic, vasopressor, and vasodilator properties depending on the dose (*Table 13.4*). In equine medicine, dopamine is most commonly employed to increase cardiac output and improve vascular tone. Dopamine may improve perfusion to some tissue beds (kidneys, GI tract, heart, and brain), although these effects can be difficult to predict.

Clinical use

Unfortunately, there is considerable overlap in the doses at which particular receptors are stimulated and it is difficult to accurately predict plasma concentrations of dopamine from a given infusion rate.[5] The drug's complex profile coupled with a number of potentially adverse effects may limit its usefulness and dopamine is now less commonly used by equine clinicians.[4]

At very low doses (0.5–2.0 µg/kg/minute), dopamine primarily acts at dopaminergic (DA-1) receptors, producing vasodilation particularly of the coronary, renal, cerebral, and splanchnic vasculature. At moderate doses (2–10 µg/kg/minute), β_1 stimulation occurs and dopamine displays inotropic activity. The extent of β_2 stimulation is debated, but appears to be limited if present at all. Dopaminergic-mediated vasodilation is overridden at higher doses (>10–12 µg/kg/minute) by α-adrenergic-mediated vasoconstriction, which increases SVR and may decrease tissue perfusion. Dopamine can be administered in most commonly used fluids, but is incompatible with sodium bicarbonate solutions or other strongly alkaline fluids. There are some incompatibilities reported with other drugs.

Complications

In septic human patients, dopamine may cause vasoconstriction of the colonic arteries (generally at higher doses) and reduce mucosal perfusion.[2,3] For this reason it has been suggested that dopamine should not be used in GI disease in horses.[4] Dopamine may also disrupt normal equine GI motility. At very high doses (>20 µg/kg/minute), intense vasoconstriction can compromise limb circulation. Dopamine may cause cardiac arrhythmias such as PVCs, supraventricular tachycardia, and ventricular tachycardia. The role of dopamine in the treatment of renal disease has also been questioned.[3]

Vasopressin

Key points

- Vasopressin acts at V1a receptors in the peripheral vasculature to cause vasoconstriction.
- Vasopressin may be particularly effective in the management of shock, especially shock that is refractory to treatment with conventional catecholamines.
- Clinically, vasopressin has been shown to reduce the requirements for other vasopressor agents.
- Controversy exists as to whether vasopressin can be used as the sole vasopressor.

Table 13.4 **Summary of indications, mode of action, and suggested dose ranges for dopamine**

INDICATIONS	ACTION[1]	SUGGESTED DOSES[2]	COMMENTS
Hypotension in absence of hypovolemia	DA: vasodilation (renal, mesenteric)	**Equine**	
		2–5 µg/kg/minute	Inotropic starting dose
	β: inotropic, chronotropic, NE release (indirect)	5–10 µg/kg/minute	Vasopressor starting dose
	α_1: vasoconstriction	**Human**	
		0.5–2.0 µg/kg/minute	Dopaminergic (low) dose – vasodilation
		2.0–10.0 µg/kg/minute	β_1-adrenergic – inotropic
		10–20 µg/kg/minute	α-adrenergic – vasopressor
		6–25 µg/kg/minute	Typical human dose range

DA, dopaminergic receptors; NE, norepinephrine.
[1] Effects of dopamine are listed in the order in which they occur with increasing dose.
[2] Suggested dose rates are for treatment of hypotension and/or poor cardiac output unless otherwise stated.

Definition/mechanism of action

Vasopressin (arginine vasopressin [AVP] or anti-diuretic hormone [ADH]) is a non-catecholamine vasopressor (*Table 13.5*). It acts on V1a receptors in the peripheral vasculature to cause vasoconstriction and at V2 receptors in the renal collecting tubules to promote water reabsorption.

Indications

In acute shock states, serum vasopressin concentrations increase rapidly but then decrease during prolonged illness. Endogenous vasopressin levels are significantly lower in adult humans with severe sepsis and this is thought to contribute to their hypotension. Additionally, loss of catecholamine vasopressor ability is well recognized in sepsis; vasopressin administration restores some of the vasoconstrictor effects of circulating catecholamines. Furthermore, the vasopressor effects of vasopressin appear to be enhanced during septic shock.[6]

Because vasopressin can cause smooth muscle contraction through non-catecholamine-mediated pathways, it represents an attractive adjunct to the management of septic shock, especially when conventional catecholamines have been ineffective.

Clinical use

In clinical trials with human patients, vasopressin has usually been used in combination with other inotropes and vasopressors and allows the dose of these agents to be reduced. Most evidence from human research does not support the use of vasopressin alone or as a replacement for more conventional catecholamines. There are currently no published reports of vasopressin use in equine patients, but anecdotal accounts suggest that low doses of vasopressin (0.25–0.5 mU/kg/minute) are effective in reducing the need for other inotropes and vasopressors in the hypotensive neonate.[4]

Current evidence suggests that vasopressin should be used in combination with a catecholamine (e.g. dobutamine); however, further studies are needed to establish the exact role of this agent in cardiovascular support.[8]

Complications

Potential side-effects of vasopressin range from ischemic skin lesions to possible intestinal ischemia. There is some concern that V1 agonists may decrease cardiac output and reduce hepatosplanchnic oxygen delivery.[2,7] These effects may be related to the volume status of the patient and, as with any inotrope or vasopressor therapy, it is critical to ensure adequate fluid resuscitation.

Table 13.5 Summary of indications, mode of action, and suggested dose ranges for vasopressin

INDICATIONS	ACTION	SUGGESTED DOSES[1]	COMMENTS
Hypotension, especially if non-responsive to catecholamines	V1a: vasoconstriction V2: water reabsorption in renal collecting tubules	**Equine** 0.25–0.5 mU/kg/minute	Suggested dose for foals (note units)[2]
		Human[3] 0.01–0.04 U/minute	Typical human dose range (note units)

[1] Suggested dose rates are for treatment of hypotension unless otherwise stated.

[2] Doses of 0.3 and 1.0 mU/kg/minute used in healthy, anesthetized, neonatal foals with induced hypotension.[7]

[3] Note that careful attention should be paid to units used; the suggested human dose range is given per individual rather than per kg of body weight.

Phenylephrine

Key points

- The primary effect of phenylephrine is to cause vasoconstriction and an increase in diastolic and systolic blood pressure.
- Phenylephrine is used clinically to increase SVR and MAP without altering cardiac output.
- A CRI is required to treat hypotension and the infusion rate is titrated to effect.

Definition/mechanism of action

Phenylephrine is a selective α_1-adrenergic agonist; there is negligible β-adrenergic activity at normal doses, although some β effects may occur at higher doses (*Table 13.6*). The primary effect is vasoconstriction with a resultant increase in diastolic and systolic blood pressure. There is usually a small decrease in cardiac output and a reflex bradycardia may occur. The bradycardia in conscious horses can be quite dramatic and may necessitate slowing or stopping the infusion. Most vascular beds are constricted (renal, splanchnic, pulmonary, and cutaneous), but coronary blood flow is increased.

Indications

Phenylephrine may be used in the treatment of hypotension and shock after adequate fluid replacement. It may be of particular benefit when cardiostimulation is undesirable.[3] Historically, phe-nylephrine has been recommended for the treatment of hypotension secondary to drug overdoses or idiosyncratic hypotensive reactions to drugs. In septic human patients, infusion of phenylephrine has been shown to cause an increase in SVR and MAP with no change in cardiac output. In normal adult horses and anesthetized neonatal foals, SVR and MAP were increased and cardiac output decreased (heart rate decreased but stroke volume was unchanged).[4] It has been suggested that if phenylephrine is to be used as a vasopressor, it should be combined with an agent with β-adrenergic activity (e.g. dobutamine).

Clinical use

Phenylephrine is metabolized within the GI tract following oral administration and a constant IV infusion is required for treatment of hypotension (*Table 13.6*). Infusion rate should be titrated to desired end-points. Effects begin almost immediately after IV administration and persist for 20–30 minutes after the infusion has been discontinued. The agent should be diluted in 0.9% NaCl or 5% dextrose solutions for administration. Recommended administration rates are given in *Table 13.6*.

Complications

Mild neurologic signs (restlessness, excitement) may be seen at usual doses in conscious patients. Phenylephrine rarely causes arrhythmias, although they may occur

---

Table 13.6 Summary of indications, mode of action, and suggested dose ranges for phenylephrine

INDICATIONS	ACTION	SUGGESTED DOSES[1]	COMMENTS
Hypotension – may be beneficial when cardiostimulation is undesirable	α: potent vasoconstriction	**Equine**	
		0.1–0.2 µg/kg/minute	Suggested initial pressor dose
		Human[3]	
		100–180 µg/minute	Typical human initial dose (note units)
		40–60 µg/minute	Typical maintenance rate (note units)
		0.4–9.1 µg/kg/minute	Dose range used in one human trial[2]

[1] Suggested dose rates are for the treatment of hypotension unless otherwise stated.

[2] Human clinical trials reviewed in Hollenberg *et al.*, 2004.[3]

[3] Note that careful attention should be paid to units used; the first two suggested human dose rates are given per individual rather than per kg of body weight.

more frequently in patients anesthetized with halothane or receiving digoxin. Administration may cause a pronounced bradycardia.

Epinephrine

Key points
- Epinephrine is most commonly administered as a bolus during resuscitation.
- Occasionally, epinephrine is used as a CRI for the treatment of refractory hypotension by increasing cardiac output.
- The dose of epinephrine must be very carefully titrated to effect.
- Epinephrine may have detrimental effects on splanchnic perfusion.

Definition/mechanism of action
Epinephrine is a potent α- and β-adrenergic agonist with no dopaminergic activity (*Table 13.7*).

Indications
In human and veterinary medicine, epinephrine is used most often in resuscitation or treatment of life-threatening allergic reactions. Infusions of epinephrine are occasionally used to improve tissue perfusion in patients that are refractory to fluid resuscitation and the more commonly used catecholamines. However, the rationale for this has been questioned because epinephrine acts at the same group of receptors as the other catecholamines.[4]

Clinical use
Rapid IV injection of epinephrine produces a sudden increase in blood pressure as a result of direct myocardial stimulation (increases both the rate and force of contraction) and vasoconstriction of a number of vascular beds. When given by slow IV injection, there is usually only a moderate increase in systolic pressure and a decrease in diastolic pressure. Cardiac output is increased, but MAP is usually only slightly increased as a result of compensatory reflexes. Total peripheral resistance is decreased secondary to of β_2-mediated vasodilation; however, although vasodilation occurs within some tissue beds (e.g. skeletal muscle), vasoconstriction occurs in others. CRIs of epinephrine to treat hypotension should only be used in patients with stable cardiac rhythms. Recommended administration rates are given in *Table 13.7*.

Complications
Cardiac arrhythmias, particularly supraventricular and ventricular tachycardia, may occur. Of particular concern is the vasoconstriction and decrease in splanchnic circulation observed in some sepsis models and septic human patients.[9] GI function should be monitored closely. Careful attention must be paid to the concentration of epinephrine used to formulate infusions. Care should be taken when combining epinephrine with other inotropes or vasopressors, as the effects can be unpredictable.

Table 13.7 Summary of indications, mode of action, and suggested dose rates for epinephrine

INDICATIONS	ACTION[1]	SUGGESTED DOSES[2]	COMMENTS
Resuscitation	α: vasodilation, vasoconstriction[3]	**Equine**	Suggested starting dose
Hypotension – in the face of volume repletion and stable cardiac rhythm	β: inotropic, chronotropic, bronchodilation	0.1 µg/kg/minute	
		Human[4]	Typical human dose range (note units)
		1–10 µg/minute	

[1] Ranked on subjective order of importance.

[2] Suggested dose rates are for the treatment of hypotension and/or poor cardiac output unless otherwise stated.

[3] Effect will depend on tissue bed examined.

[4] Note that careful attention should be paid to units used; the suggested human dose range is given per individual rather than per kg of body weight.

GENERAL APPROACH FOR USING SEDATION AND ANALGESIA

It has been suggested that pain assessment be added as the 'fourth vital sign' when evaluating equine patients.[1] Knowledge of pain mechanisms supports a pre-emptive, multimodal, and mechanism-based therapeutic approach.[2] Analgesic protocols should be tailored to the individual, response to treatment should be frequently assessed, and synergistic and adjunctive approaches utilized to maximize effectiveness.

A multimodal approach to alleviation of anxiety and pain in equine patients, including administration of sedative–analgesic combinations in subclinical dosages and incorporation of diverse delivery techniques, improves safety, versatility, and effectiveness of therapy.

Agents currently available for equine sedation and analgesia include: alpha-2 agonists, opioids, acepromazine, benzodiazepines, NSAIDS, lidocaine, ketamine, and gabapentin.

More novel delivery methods, including CRI, transdermal absorption, and regional administration, enhance the versatility and effectiveness of these agents compared with more traditional administration routes and interval protocols.

Equine mortality rates associated with general anesthesia increase 3–5-fold when systemically ill horses are included in the analyses.[3–7] While this suggests that critically ill horses are more susceptible to adverse effects associated with sedative/analgesic agent administration, sedation and analgesia are essential components of successful management of these patients.

COMMON PROCEDURES PERFORMED WHEN USING SEDATION AND ANALGESIA

Epidural catheterization

Epidural catheterization facilitates long-term analgesic therapy. Currently available epidural catheter kits (**14.1**) are convenient to use and relatively inexpensive. Minimal complications have been reported in horses with epidural catheters for up to 14 and 20 days, respectively.[8,9]

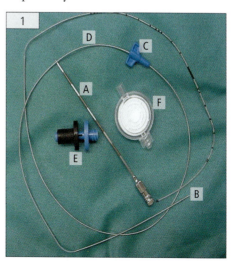

14.1 Epidural catheter kit. (Arrow International). The Tuohy spinal needle (A) is placed in the caudal epidural space and the epidural catheter is inserted through the needle to a predetermined length using the centimeter markings on the catheter. (B) Epidural catheter tip; FlexTip catheters are used most commonly. (C) Threading assist device (TAD) to facilitate catheter insertion through the needle without kinking the catheter. Once the catheter is positioned, the TAD is removed along with the needle. The catheter can be secured to the skin using a white tape butterfly at the entry site. The excess catheter is used as extension tubing (D) and is secured to the patient using an adhesive dressing. (E) SnapLock™ – catheter-syringe adapter. (F) Filter (0.2 micron flat).

The catheter is introduced through a spinal needle inserted into the first intercoccygeal space and advanced cranially 2–4 cm beyond the tip of the needle into the vertebral canal. The catheter is secured and a protective cover applied to minimize contamination (**14.2**).

Constant rate infusion

A syringe pump (**14.3**), which accommodates programming of a desired infusion rate and initial bolus dose (when needed), is the most convenient method for delivering a CRI. Other methods, including volumetric infusion pumps or direct delivery through an IV infusion line, require dilution of the infused agent in isotonic crystalloid fluid (usually saline) and calculation to determine the appropriate infusion rate.

The following protocol describes one method for calculation of the infusion drug volume to add to a specific quantity of IV fluids for administration of a desired CRI:

- Assign a fluid administration rate (ml/hour).
- Calculate how many minutes the IV fluids will last: fluid volume in bag ÷ administration rate (ml/hour) × 60 (minutes/hour).
- Calculate the total amount of drug that will be needed: milligrams of drug needed = drug infusion rate (µg/kg/minute) × body weight (kg) ÷ 1,000 (µg/mg).
- Calculate the volume of infusion drug to add to the fluid bag: milliliters of drug = mg needed ÷ drug concentration (mg/ml).

Example

- A 500 kg horse; lidocaine infusion rate = 50 µg/kg/minute; fluid volume = 1,000 ml; fluid administration rate = 500 ml/hour; lidocaine concentration = 20 mg/ml.
- Minutes fluid will last = 1,000 ml ÷ 500 ml/hour × 60 = 120 minutes.
- Total amount of lidocaine needed (mg) = 50 µg/kg/minute × 500 kg × 120 minutes = 3,000,000 µg ÷ 1,000 µg/mg = 3,000 mg.
- Lidocaine volume to add to fluids (ml) = 3000 mg ÷ 20 mg/ml = 150 ml.
- Remove 150 ml of fluid from bag and add the lidocaine.

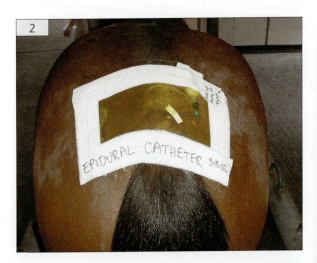

14.2 Epidural catheter in position.

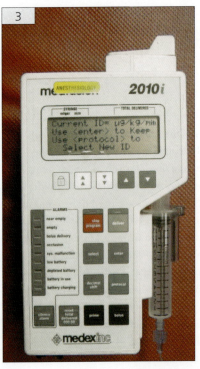

14.3 A syringe pump can be used to accommodate programing of a desired infusion rate and initial bolus dose (when needed) and is the most convenient method for delivering a constant rate infusion.

SEDATIVES AND ANALGESICS

Alpha-2 agonists

Key points

- Alpha-2 agonists, including xylazine, detomidine, and romifidine, are the most commonly used agents for equine chemical restraint, providing analgesia, sedation, and muscle relaxation.
- Many body systems, including cardiovascular, GI, and hormonal, are altered by alpha-2 agonists. Their use in critically ill patients, while necessary, should be accompanied by objective monitoring.
- Alternative administration techniques, including epidural administration and CRI, should be considered when using these agents in critically ill patients.

Definition/mechanism of action

These agents act on alpha adrenergic receptors in the CNS and peripheral tissues. The adrenergic nervous system is integral in modulating levels of consciousness and processing sensory stimuli. Alpha-2 adrenoceptor activation results in inhibition of neuromodulators including norepinephrine and dopamine. Sympathetic tone is decreased and vagal tone is increased. The result is sedation, analgesia, and muscle relaxation. Three agents are currently available (xylazine, detomidine, and romifidine) and have been extensively described in the literature.[10–18]

Indications

Alpha-2 agonists are the most commonly used agents for equine chemical restraint.[17] While these agents are most commonly used to provide sedation, the profound analgesic activity makes them effective for short-term control of visceral pain. These agents also provide excellent analgesia when administered epidurally. Sedative effects are not present with epidurally administered xylazine, but do occur with detomidine.

Clinical use

Dosages for alpha-2 agonists are listed in *Table 14.1*. Maximal effect following IV injection is 15 minutes, with xylazine possessing the shortest duration of effect.[17] Ataxia is a predictable and dose-dependent side-effect; however, quick and precise reaction to external stimuli (i.e. targeted kicking) may occur with all three agents.[18] One study reported the safe and effective use of detomidine CRI for standing procedures in horses.[19]

An advantage of the alpha-2 agents is reversibility with alpha-2 antagonists. Yohimbine, tolazoline, and atipamezole have been reported to reverse the effects of alpha-2 agonists in horses safely and effectively.[20–24] Dosages for alpha-2 antagonists are listed in *Table 14.1*.

Table 14.1 Dosages for alpha-2 agonists and antagonists in critically-ill equine patients

DRUG	DOSAGE
Alpha-2 agonists	
Xylazine	0.1–0.5 mg/kg IV
Detomidine	0.005–0.02 mg/kg IV
Detomidine (CRI)[19]	6-9 µg/kg (bolus)
	0.6 µg/kg/minute (CRI)
	↓ rate by 50% every 15 minutes
Romifidine	0.04–0.06 mg/kg IV
Antagonists	
Yohimbine	0.05 mg/kg IV
Tolazoline[24]	4 mg/kg IV
Atipamezole[24]	0.05–0.1 mg/kg IV

Dosages reflect recommendations of the author or specific references.

Alpha-2 agonists administered epidurally, alone or in combination with local anesthetic agents or opioids, provide excellent regional analgesia. Epidural dosages are listed in *Table 14.2*. One study demonstrated a synergistic effect when xylazine was used with lidocaine to provide perineal anesthesia and analgesia.[25] Epidurally administered detomidine produces sedation, ataxia, cardiopulmonary depression, and diuresis similar to systemic administration.[26] Ataxia and recumbency, requiring subsequent general anesthesia, have been reported in a horse administered epidural detomidine for elective surgery.[27] The systemic side-effects of epidurally administered detomidine are effectively reversed with atipamezole or yohimbine.[28,29]

Complications

Alpha-2 agonists have the potential to exacerbate cardiopulmonary instability. Low-end or subclinical dosing, when combined with supplemental techniques, can provide effective sedation for procedural intervention as well as long-term analgesic management.[30] Cardiopulmonary monitoring is important when these agents are administered.

Cardiopulmonary effects are dose dependent and include decreased respiratory rate and tidal volume, decreased arterial oxygen tension, cough reflex suppression, bradycardia, atrioventricular block, transient hypertension followed by hypotension, and decreased cardiac output.[14,31] Critically ill horses are more likely to develop arrhythmias, hypotension, and hypoxia following alpha-2 agent administration. A comparison of detomidine and romifidine as premedication to general anesthesia concluded that arterial blood pressure was better maintained in detomidine-premedicated horses during the anesthetic period.[32] One study concluded that romifidine should be used judiciously in horses with cardiovascular compromise.[33]

Alpha-2 agonists reduce propulsive motility in the jejunum, cecum, pelvic flexure, and right dorsal colon[34–36], inhibit gastric emptying in a dose-related manner[37], and alter myoelectrical activity of the proximal small intestine.[38]

Other side-effects that can impact the critically ill horse include hyperglycemia and decreased insulin secretion (adults only), increased urine output with or without glucosuria, transient anorexia, and altered thermoregulation (sweating, transient hyperthermia, hypothermia).[31] One study concluded that administration of xylazine or detomidine to water deprived horses may exacerbate dehydration.[39] Uterine tone increases following xylazine or detomidine administration; however, an increased incidence of abortion has not been demonstrated.[31,40]

Because of the profound impact on cardiac performance and the widespread effects on homeostasis, alpha-2 agonists should only be used intermittently, judiciously, and with close monitoring for short-term sedation and analgesia in compromised equine patients.

Table 14.2 **Epidural alpha-2 agonist dosages**	
DRUG	**DOSAGE**
Xylazine	0.17 mg/kg qs saline to 1 ml/50 kg
Detomidine	5–10 µg/kg qs saline to 1 ml/50 kg
Morphine/xylazine	Morphine (0.1 mg/kg)/xylazine (0.17 mg/kg) qs saline to 1 ml/50 kg
Morphine/detomidine	Morphine (0.1 mg/kg)/detomidine (5–10 µg/kg) qs saline to 1 ml/50 kg
Lidocaine/xylazine	Lidocaine (0.22 mg/kg)/xylazine (0.17 mg/kg)

qs, quantum satis (as much as is enough) (i.e. bringing up the volume to the final measurement [e.g. 1 ml/50 kg]).

Opioids

Key points

- Opioid agents provide several options for pain management in critically ill horses.
- Epidurally administered morphine, CRI of butorphanol, and transdermal fentanyl are options that minimize adverse side-effects.
- While not well-documented, intra-articular injection of morphine may represent an additional avenue for pain intervention in equine patients.

Definition/mechanism of action

Opioids are chemically related compounds, including naturally occurring, semisynthetic and synthetic, derived from opium. They act on membrane-bound receptors, including mu, delta, and kappa, located in the brain, spinal cord, and periphery.

Indications

Opioids are used in horses as an adjunct to general anesthesia, in combination with sedatives or tranquilizers to enhance analgesia and sedation for standing restraint, and for long-term pain management. Opioids provide a versatile option or adjunct for treating moderate to severe pain.

Clinical use

Dosages, including CRI, for opioids are listed in *Table 14.3*. The most relevant opioid agents for equine use include morphine, butorphanol, buprenorphine, and fentanyl. Effects vary between opioids because of differences in opioid receptor affinity and activity. Effects also vary between dosages of the same agent and between individuals. Opioid effects in horses include analgesia, sedation, excitement, dysphoria, increased locomotor activity, hyperresponsiveness to external stimuli, respiratory depression, tachypnea, and decreased GI propulsive motility.[31,41] Advantages of opioid agents include minimal effect on heart rate, cardiac output, and arterial blood pressure and reversibility with opioid antagonists.[31]

Opioids are effective when administered epidurally for analgesia without causing locomotor and behavioral effects associated with systemic administration. Epidural dosages for several opioids have been reported for horses[42–46]; however, morphine is the most commonly used and the most effective.

The finding of opioid receptors in equine synovial membranes[47] suggests that intra-articular morphine may also be an effective analgesic adjunct in the management of equine pain (*Table 14.3*). No detrimental effects were reported when morphine was injected into the tibiotarsal joint of ponies.[48]

Morphine: Morphine was one of the first opioids described for treatment of equine pain and it remains cost-effective for use in horses. The undesirable excitatory effects of morphine and the need for stringent record keeping have limited widespread clinical use. Recent studies have failed to demonstrate clearly a beneficial analgesic effect when morphine is used as an adjunct to inhalation anesthesia.[49–51]

Table 14.3 Dosages for opioids and the opioid antagonist

DRUG	DOSAGE	
Opioids		
Morphine	0.05–0.1 mg/kg IV	
Morphine (intra-articular)	50 mg total dose	
Butorphanol	0.01–0.02 mg/kg IV	
Butorphanol (CRI)	13 µg/kg/hr	
Buprenorphine	0.005 mg/kg IV	
Fentanyl (transdermal)	>115 kg:	2 × 10 mg patches
	50–115 kg:	1 × 10 mg patch
	< 50 kg:	1 × 5 mg patch
Antagonist		
Naloxone[31]	0.005–0.02 mg/kg IV	

Dosages reflect recommendations of the author or specific references.

While compelling evidence for the benefits of systemic morphine administration remains equivocal, use of epidural morphine in horses is clearly beneficial. Despite case reports of complications associated with epidural morphine[52,53], several studies have reported beneficial effects with minimal adverse side-effects.[8,54–57] Epidural dosages for morphine are listed in *Table 14.4*.

Butorphanol: Butorphanol, an agonist–antagonist opioid, is presently the most commonly used opioid in horses. Studies have reported beneficial analgesic effects of butorphanol when administered concurrently with an alpha-2 agonist.[58–60] There have been conflicting results regarding analgesic effects, with visceral analgesia more consistently demonstrated than somatic analgesia.[61–63] However, clinical studies strongly support the benefit of butorphanol as an analgesic agent, at least in postoperative colic cases.[64] Butorphanol is an effective agent for critically ill horses as both a short-term and longer-term analgesic adjunct.

Buprenorphine: Buprenorphine in combination with alpha-2 agonists has sedative and analgesic effects.[23,65] Buprenorphine is a partial opioid agonist and, like other opioids, can induce excitement when used alone in normal horses.[66–68] Hoof withdrawal reflex latency was increased by up to 11 hours following 10 µg/kg buprenorphine.[68]

Fentanyl: Fentanyl is an opioid agonist with a short duration of effect when administered systemically. Early studies on the effects of IV administered fentanyl in horses reported analgesia and locomotor and sympathetic stimulation typical of opioid agonists.[69] The pharmacokinetics of IV and transdermal fentanyl have been reported.[70–73] Despite reported variability in serum concentrations[71] and increased variability in serum fentanyl concentrations in sick horses compared with normal horses[72], transdermal fentanyl appears to be an effective analgesic adjunct for critically ill equine patients. Dosage and site of application vary; reported sites of application include lateral or medial antebrachium (**14.4**), lateral neck (**14.5**), and mid-dorsal thorax. Hair should be clipped prior to application. The most commonly used dosage is one or two 10-mg patches (Duragesic®, 100 µg/hour), depending on body weight (*Table 14.3*).

Complications

Morphine: The effect of morphine on equine cardiovascular and respiratory parameters is variable. Decreased alveolar ventilation was reported following morphine administration to isoflurane anesthetized horses, while respiratory values did not change significantly when morphine was administered with xylazine[50] or administered alone to halothane anesthetized horses.[51] Two clinical studies reported a significant decrease[74] and no significant change[51] in arterial

Table 14.4 **Epidural opioid dosages**	
DRUG	**DOSAGE**
Morphine	0.1 mg/kg qs saline to 1 ml/50 kg
Morphine/xylazine	Morphine (0.1 mg/kg)/xylazine (0.17 mg/kg) qs saline to 1 ml/50 kg
Morphine/detomidine	Morphine (0.1 mg/kg)/detomidine (5–10 µg/kg) qs saline to 1 ml/50 kg

qs, quantum satis (as much as is enough) (i.e. bringing up the volume to the final measurement [e.g. 1 ml/50 kg]).

oxygen tension following morphine administration to halothane anesthetized horses. Cardiovascular stimulatory effects were reported in awake ponies.[62] However, significant cardiovascular changes following morphine administration to anesthetized horses have not been reported.[49–51,74,75]

Concern over the excitatory effects of morphine and potential adverse effect on equine recovery quality may have historically limited the use of perioperative morphine.[74] Morphine administration was identified as a significant risk factor for development of colic in the postoperative period.[76] However, a subsequent study[77] did not identify morphine administration as a risk factor for colic following general anesthesia. In a retrospective study, morphine administration was not found to increase postoperative complications such as colic and 'box-walking'.[75] In fact, a significantly better quality of recovery with a similar or decreased recovery time was reported in horses receiving morphine at both 0.1 and 0.2 mg/kg.[74] Conversely, an 'undesirable and dangerous' recovery was reported in horses receiving morphine.[49] This disparity in results is most likely dose related.

Butorphanol: Butorphanol is less likely to produce undesirable excitement and locomotor activity compared with morphine. Initial studies utilized dosages of 0.1–0.4 mg/kg, which caused several adverse side-effects including moderate excitement with increased motor activity, shivering, ataxia, and restlessness.[30,61,78] Butorphanol has been reported to significantly, though transiently, affect GI motility.[30,36,79] However, administration of butorphanol by CRI effectively reduced adverse GI effects[30] and it was suggested in a subsequent study that these effects on intestinal motility were probably not clinically detrimental.[64]

Buprenorphine: Like butorphanol, systemic administration of buprenorphine is less likely to cause excitatory effects compared with morphine. However, hemodynamic stimulation for at least 2 hours and decreased abdominal auscultation scores for 4 hours after administration of 10 µg/kg of buprenorphine has been reported.[67] While a longer duration of analgesia may be desirable, the prolonged effect of buprenorphine on intestinal motility could be detrimental in some critically-ill horses.

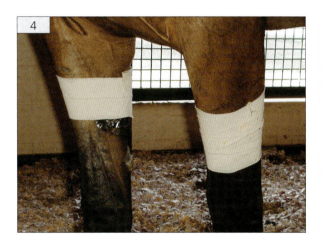

14.4 A fentanyl patch applied to the medial aspect of the antebrachium.

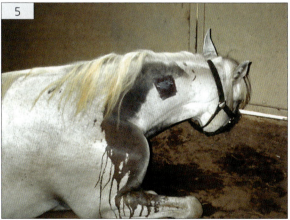

14.5 A fentanyl patch applied to the lateral aspect of the neck.

Fentanyl: IV administration of fentanyl produces adverse effects similar to morphine; side-effects and short duration of effect limits its usefulness as an injectable agent. Adverse effects associated with transdermal delivery have not been reported.[72]

Acepromazine
Key points
- Acepromazine has non-reversible, relatively long-lasting effects on the equine cardiovascular system, including hypotension and occasionally tachycardia.
- Acepromazine should be avoided in critically ill equine patients, especially if cardiovascular instability or hepatic dysfunction is present.
- Potential use of acepromazine in equine critical care includes horses with acute laminitis and mares with postpartum uterine hemorrhage.

Definition/mechanism of action
Acepromazine is classified as a phenothiazine sedative (or tranquilizer) producing sedation and some muscle relaxation at relatively low doses. Behavior and the autonomic nervous and endocrine systems are affected by this agent; these effects are mediated by blockade of dopaminergic, alpha-1 adrenergic, muscarinic, serotonin, and histamine receptors.[80]

Indications
Acepromazine has been used in horses for several decades to provide a calming effect; there is no analgesic activity. Because of the diverse receptor activity, acepromazine also produces antihistaminic, antiarrhythmic, and antipyretic effects. Acepromazine is best avoided in horses with cardiovascular instability, common in critically ill patients. The drug depends on hepatic metabolism for elimination and should be avoided in horses with clinical signs of hepatic dysfunction.

Clinical use
Clinical use of acepromazine is usually limited to healthy horses. Response to acepromazine administration is variable from no effect to profound sedation with ataxia. The dosage of acepromazine used by the author is 0.02 mg/kg SC or IM. Concurrent administration of an opioid or alpha-2 agonist provides a more predictable response.[31,65] Peak effect after IV administration is 30 minutes with sedation lasting 2–3 hours.

Two situations involving critically ill horses in which acepromazine may have application include acute laminitis (to encourage vasodilation and peripheral blood flow) and uterine hemorrhage (to promote quietude and to lower blood pressure to facilitate clot formation). In other situations, acepromazine should be reserved for use in horses that are hemodynamically stable.

Complications
The hypotensive effect of acepromazine is due to alpha-adrenergic blockade. Hypotension may be accompanied by tachycardia, which is more likely to occur in horses with high circulating catecholamines.[31] Critically ill patients are more likely to have high catecholamine levels associated with pain, stress, and anxiety.

The most relevant adverse effects limiting its use in critically ill horses, besides hypotension, include decreased PCV and TPP, decreased GI peristalsis and secretions, and augmentation of hypothermia.[31] Although uncommon, priapism can occur following acepromazine administration.

Interestingly, a study identifying risk factors for mortality associated with equine anesthesia found acepromazine premedication reduced risk of death.[81] One study reported improved hemodynamic variables and arterial oxygenation when acepromazine was added to a romifidine–butorphanol combination.[82] However, these findings involved healthy horses; horses with cardiopulmonary compromise may not respond in a similar manner.

Benzodiazepines
Key points
- Benzodiazepines provide muscle relaxation and short-term control of seizure activity. Analgesia is not an effect of the benzodiazepines and sedative effects are unpredictable, with paradoxic excitement a potential adverse effect.
- Other than the potential use as an appetite stimulant and as an anticonvulsant agent, benzodiazepines should be avoided in critically ill adult horses because of the profound effect on muscle strength.

Definition/mechanism of action

Diazepam and midazolam produce muscle relaxant, anticonvulsant, and sedative effects by depressing the brainstem reticular formation, blocking spinal polysynaptic reflexes, and potentiating the effect of GABA, the primary inhibitory neurotransmitter in the mammalian nervous system.[31,80]

Indications

Like acepromazine, the benzodiazepines have no analgesic effect but do cause profound muscle relaxation and CNS effects, which vary from minimal calming to paradoxic excitement when administered alone. Benzodiazepines are effective anticonvulsant agents. They do stimulate appetite in horses[83], which represents one potential indication for use in critically ill horses.

Clinical use

The dosages used for diazepam and midazolam are listed in *Table 14.5*. Benzodiazepines are not reliable sedatives, but provide profound relaxation. With the exception of seizure management, benzodiazepines should not be used alone and are best avoided in equine adults.

Flumazenil, a benzodiazepine antagonist, has been observed to reverse midazolam sedation effectively in foals without adverse side-effects. Studies in adult horses are lacking.

A midazolam CRI dosage has been reported (*Table 14.5*); however, in this study midazolam was administered concurrently with medetomidine and ketamine CRI to sevoflurane anesthetized horses.[84] The effect of midazolam CRI in awake horses has not been reported.

Complications

Cardiopulmonary effects of benzodiazepines are minimal.[85] Some horses become apprehensive or excited approximately 5–10 minutes following IV administration of diazepam.[31] Profound muscle weakness, ataxia, and recumbency has been reported with diazepam administration (the latter effect occurred at 0.4 mg/kg dosage).[85] One study compared three protocols for anesthetic induction and found that addition of midazolam to the induction protocol significantly increased ataxia during the recovery period.[86] The profound muscle weakness is less problematic in equine neonates.

Nystagmus is a side-effect of benzodiazepine administration. In horses with neurologic disease, benzodiazepines should be avoided due to the profound muscle relaxation that will exacerbate pre-existing ataxia and because the resulting nystagmus may complicate interpretation of clinical signs.

Ketamine
Key points

- Ketamine at subanesthetic dosage as a CRI provides a useful analgesic technique for horses that fail to respond to other therapeutic protocols.
- Epidural and perineural administration of ketamine has also been reported to provide analgesia.
- Horses receiving ketamine by CRI or by epidural administration should be closely monitored for excitatory effects.

Definition/mechanism of action

Ketamine is a dissociative anesthetic agent producing dose-related unconsciousness and analgesia. Antagonism of the NMDA receptor is the most likely mechanism for the anesthetic, analgesic, psychotomimetic, and neuroprotective effects of the drug.[87] The NMDA receptor plays a significant role

Table 14.5 **Dosages for benzodiazepines and the benzodiazepine antagonist**	
DRUG	**DOSAGE**
Benzodiazepines	
Diazepam	0.01–0.02 mg/kg IV
Midazolam	0.005–0.01 mg/kg IV
Midazolam[84]	0.02 mg/kg/hour CRI
Antagonist	
Flumazenil	0.005–0.01 mg/kg IV

Dosages reflect recommendations of the author or specific references.

in pain mechanisms including central sensitization ('wind-up').[2] Analgesia produced by ketamine occurs at subanesthetic dosages and appears to be more effective for somatic pain than for visceral pain.[88]

Indications

Ketamine has gained attention as an analgesic adjunct agent in addition to its established role as an equine induction agent. Ketamine CRI reduced the halothane minimum alveolar concentration requirement in horses in one study.[89] More recently, a study reported the use of ketamine CRI in awake horses with a variety of painful lesions including septic arthritis, osteomyelitis, and burns.[90] The clinical response between patients was variable, but attitude and appetite improved in the majority of patients.

Clinical use

The dosage for ketamine CRI is 0.4–0.8 mg/kg/hour.[90] Two recent studies reported the pharmacokinetics and clinical effects of ketamine CRI at multiple subclinical dosages[91,92]; side-effects were not observed. Ketamine CRI has been combined with a morphine (or butorphanol) and lidocaine CRI.

Epidural administration of ketamine in awake[93,94] and in halothane anesthetized[95] horses has been reported; adverse side-effects were not observed in either study. The dosage for epidural ketamine is 1 mg/kg qs with saline to 1 ml/50 kg. Ketamine administered epidurally and by CRI appears to be a beneficial analgesic adjunct in horses refractory to more traditional therapy.

A regional analgesic effect was reported when 5 ml of 2% or 3% ketamine was injected as an abaxial sesamoid block.[96] Duration of effect was 15 minutes, which makes this technique of limited practicality for long-term pain management.

Complications

Side-effects associated with IV administered ketamine bolus may include excitement, delirium, muscle fasciculations, and ataxia; these undesirable effects are more likely when sedation is inadequate. Horses receiving ketamine CRI should be closely monitored. An excitatory reaction should respond effectively to alpha-2 agonist administration.

Lidocaine
Key points
- Lidocaine CRI provides analgesic, anti-inflammatory, and prokinetic effects that may be beneficial for the critically ill horse.
- Side-effects are minimal but may include dullness, muscle fasciculations, and ataxia; these effects resolve with discontinuation of the infusion.

Definition/mechanism of action

Lidocaine is classified as a local anesthetic that reversibly binds sodium channels and blocks impulse conduction in nerve fibers. Interruption of sensory afferent nerve transmission effectively prevents nociceptive input. Analgesia of the desensitized area is complete when administered by local and regional techniques; central sensitization ('wind-up') to a painful stimulus is prevented.[97] The precise mechanism of action has not been elucidated, but theories include the surface-charge theory, the membrane-expansion theory, and the specific-receptor theory.[97] Lidocaine may also inhibit substance P binding and inhibit GABA uptake.

Indications

Lidocaine CRI has been reported to reduce halothane[98] and isoflurane[99] minimum alveolar concentration without adverse cardiopulmonary effects. In addition to analgesia, studies have reported an antimicrobial effect, a GI prokinetic effect, improved wound healing, and an anti-inflammatory effect.

Lidocaine has been used to treat postoperative ileus without adverse effects.[100] One report described the application of 5% lidocaine patches (Lidoderm®) for alleviation of lameness associated with the carpus, fetlock, or distal limb.[101]

Clinical use

Lidocaine CRI may be a beneficial analgesic adjunct in critically ill horses, especially those with GI disease. The dose rate for a lidocaine CRI is 1.3 mg/kg as a slow bolus followed by a CRI at 0.05 mg/kg/minute.[100] Lidocaine and other local anesthetic agents are often used epidurally and dosages are listed in *Table 14.6*.

Complications

The toxic effects of lidocaine are dose dependent and include agitation, convulsions, coma, respiratory arrest, and cardiovascular collapse.[97] Muscle fasciculation, dullness, and mild to severe ataxia have been reported in horses receiving lidocaine CRI.[102] Muscle fasciculations were reported in one of 28 horses receiving lidocaine CRI for postoperative ileus.[100] These signs resolved with cessation of lidocaine delivery.

Non-steroidal anti-inflammatory drugs

Key points

- NSAIDs play a significant role in the antipyretic, analgesic, and anti-inflammatory management of critically ill equine patients.
- NSAIDs possess significant potential for life-threatening side-effects (GI and renal), which are more likely to occur in critically ill equine patients.
- NSAID use in critically ill equine patients requires close monitoring, which should include serial assessment of fluid and electrolyte homeostasis, TPP concentration, and urinalysis.

Definition/mechanism of action

NSAIDs comprise a large group of agents with anti-inflammatory, analgesic, and antipyretic effects. These drugs act by inhibition of the COX isoenzymes 1 and 2 and 5-lipooxygenase, thus preventing prostaglandins and leukotriene production, respectively.

Prostaglandins act both to protect and to potentially injure the body. Historically, it has been accepted that COX-1 (constitutive) prostaglandins tend to promote homeostasis/protection while COX-2 (inducible) prostaglandins tend to promote inflammation and pain. However, with increased knowledge, selection of NSAIDs with selective COX-2 inhibition is no longer straightforward; prostaglandins produced by both isoenzymes appear to play a role in nociception.[103] Additionally, diversion of arachadonic acid to the 5-lipooxygenase pathway by COX inhibition, with subsequent leukotriene production, may also promote inflammation and has been incriminated in NSAID-induced ulcers.[104] However, it is also recognized that some leukotrienes possess anti-inflammatory activity. Therefore, the ideal NSAID for use in equine patients is not clearly elucidated.

Indications

Flunixin meglumine, phenylbutazone, and ketoprofen are commonly used in horses to treat fever and traumatic and post-surgical pain and inflammation. NSAIDS are effective in the treatment of mild to moderate acute and chronic pain. Severe pain is not adequately managed with NSAIDs alone.

Clinical use

Dosages for commonly used NSAIDs are listed in *Table 14.7*. Phenylbutazone is commonly used to treat both acute and chronic musculoskeletal pain. Flunixin

---

Table 14.6 Epidural local anesthetic dosages

DRUG	DOSAGE
Lidocaine	0.26–0.35 mg/kg
Mepivicaine	0.22 mg/kg
Bupivacaine	3 ml (0.5%)/450 kg
Ropivicaine	0.02 mg/kg (mid-sacrum)
Lidocaine/xylazine	Lidocaine (0.22 mg/kg)/xylazine (0.17 mg/kg)

Dosages reflect recommendations of the author or specific references.

Table 14.7 Non-steroidal anti-inflammatory drug dosages

DRUG	DOSAGE
Phenylbutazone	2.2 mg/kg IV or PO q12 or 24h
Flunixin meglumine	0.25–1.1 mg/kg IV q12 or 24h
Ketoprofen	2.2 mg/kg IV q12 or 24h
Carprofen[106,110]	0.7 mg/kg IV q24h
Meloxicam[108]	0.6 mg/kg IV q12 or 24h
Firocoxib	0.27 mg/kg initial loading dose; 0.09 mg/kg IV or PO q24h

Dosages reflect recommendations of the author or specific references.

meglumine has been used more often to treat acute visceral pain and fever. Ketoprofen is also effective in temperature management. Increased severity of GI lesions was reported when phenylbutazone and flunixin were administered concurrently.[105] The practice of combined therapy has been anecdotally reported to improve efficacy of treatment, but there is limited supportive evidence. Combined therapy should not be used in critically ill equine patients. NSAID use requires close monitoring to avoid the well-documented adverse side-effects.

The effective use of either flunixin meglumine or phenylbutazone in combination with transdermal fentanyl in horses with moderate to severe pain has been reported.[72]

Dosages for more selective COX-2 or COX-1-sparing inhibitors are shown in *Table 14.7*. Studies regarding safety and efficacy of these newer NSAIDs are limited at this time.[106–110] Superior efficacy and safety compared with the currently approved NSAIDs has not been definitively established.

Complications

NSAIDs exert toxic effects on the renal and GI systems. Toxicity in horses is dose dependent and is greatest in foals and hypovolemic patients and with extended use.[111] Critically ill horses certainly require the beneficial effects of anti-inflammatory agents; however, these patients are more susceptible to their adverse effects. There are no safe NSAIDs; only conscientious use in critically ill horses will minimize risk of complications. One study compared the three most commonly used agents, using greater than recommended dosages, and found the toxic potential was greatest for phenylbutazone and least for ketoprofen.[112] COX-1-sparing NSAIDs should be considered in patients with renal disease or GI ulceration.

Conservative dosing, appropriate renal (i.e. serum or plasma creatinine and urine creatinine:GGT ratio) and GI (i.e. TPP and albumin) monitoring, and prophylactic GI protectant therapy is essential when using NSAIDs in critically ill horses.

Gabapentin

Definition/mechanism of action

Gabapentin was originally approved as a human anticonvulsant agent and later identified as an analgesic agent in the control of neuropathic pain. The mechanism of its analgesic effect is unknown, but may involve inhibition of glutamate synthesis.[113]

Indications/clinical use/complications

Gabapentin may have application in the management of intractable pain associated with peripheral neuropathy in horses.[114] While published information for horses remains sparse, anecdotal communication supports the benefit of gabapentin use in horses for treatment of neuropathic pain. No adverse side-effects have been reported for gabapentin administration. Controlled studies are needed to confirm the benefit, to provide research-based dosage, and to assure lack of adverse effects. Currently, dosages used are 2.5 mg/kg PO q12h or q8h.[114]

CHAPTER 15

NUTRITIONAL SUPPORT

Brett S. Tennent-Brown

GENERAL APPROACH TO PROVIDING NUTRITIONAL SUPPORT

- Equine patients may have their feed intake reduced either as part of their treatment or as a consequence of their disease state.
- Malnutrition (defined as a diet that contains all the essential nutrients but in suboptimal quantities) has been shown to impair immune function and increases morbidity and mortality.[1]
- Non-pregnant and non-lactating adult horses in good body condition (neither underconditioned nor overconditioned) will comfortably tolerate at least 2–3 days of fasting.
- Foals, severely ill horses, and horses in poor body condition may be intolerant of even brief periods of malnutrition and some form of nutritional support should, therefore, be considered early in their therapeutic regimen.
- Any animal that fails to consume sufficient energy and protein for more than 48 hours is a candidate for nutritional intervention.

COMMON PROCEDURES PERFORMED FOR PROVIDING NUTRITIONAL SUPPORT

Body condition scoring

Indications

Body condition scores are a semi-quantitative method of evaluating body fat and, to a lesser extent, muscle mass. Although body condition scoring lacks the sensitivity required to monitor acute changes in weight, it provides an immediate assessment of long-term nutritional adequacy and current reserves. Furthermore, body condition scores are less affected by differences in body frame than weight tapes and can be useful when weight scales are not readily available.

Technique

- The technique of body condition scoring is described in *Tables 15.1* and *15.2* and illustrated in **15.1**.

Complications

None.

Table 15.1 **Body condition scoring for adult horses (15.1)**[2]

	SCORE	DESCRIPTION
1	Poor	Extremely emaciated; spinous processes, ribs, tail head, tuber coxae, and ischii prominent; bone structure of withers, shoulders, and neck easily noticeable; no fatty tissue can be felt
2	Very thin	Emaciated; slight fat covering over base of spinous processes; transverse processes of lumbar vertebrae feel rounded; spinous processes, ribs, tail head, tuber coxae, and ischii prominent; withers, shoulders, and neck structure faintly visible
3	Thin	Fat build-up halfway on spinous processes; transverse processes cannot be felt; slight fat cover over ribs; spinous processes and ribs easily discernible; tail head prominent but individual vertebrae cannot be identified visually; tuber coxae appears rounded but easily discernible; tuber ischii not distinguishable; withers, shoulders, and neck accentuated
4	Moderately thin (ideal)	Slight ridge along back; faint outline of ribs discernible; tail head prominence depends on conformation but fat can be felt around it; tuber coxae not discernible; withers, shoulders, and neck not obviously thin
5	Moderate	Back flat; no crease or ridge; ribs not visibly distinguishable but easily felt; fat around tail head beginning to feel spongy; withers appear rounded over spinous processes; shoulders and neck blend smoothly into body
6	Moderately fleshy	May have slight crease down back; fat over ribs spongy; fat around tail head soft; fat beginning to be deposited along the sides of the withers, behind shoulders, and along sides of neck
7	Fleshy	May have crease down back; individual ribs can be felt but noticeable filling between ribs with fat; fat around tail head soft; fat deposited along withers, behind shoulders, and along neck
8	Fat	Crease down back; difficult to feel ribs; fat around tail head very soft; area along withers filled with fat; area behind shoulders filled with fat; noticeable thickening of neck; fat deposited along inner thighs
9	Extremely fat	Obvious crease down back; patch fat appearing over ribs; bulging fat around tail head, along withers, behind shoulders, and along neck; fat along inner thighs might rub together; flank filled with fat

Table 15.2 **Modified Henneke body condition scoring for foals**[3]

	SCORE	DESCRIPTION
1	Extremely emaciated	Spinous processes, ribs, tuber coxae, tail head, and tuber ischii very prominent; shoulder and neck structures evident
2	Emaciated	Slight fat covering of base of the spinous processes; slightly rounded feel to transverse processes and ribs; shoulder and neck structures barely noticeable
3	Thin	Fat build-up mid-way down the spinous processes; slight fat cover over ribs; individual vertebrae not discernible
4	Moderately thin	Slight ridge along back; faint outline of ribs; fat can be felt over tail head and withers; shoulder and neck structures not thin
5	Moderate (normal)	Back flat, ribs not visible but easily palpable; fat around tail head spongy; withers rounded over spinous process; shoulder and neck structures blend well into body

Placement of an esophagostomy feeding tube

Indications

Animals that are unable or unwilling to voluntarily consume sufficient calories can often be fed via a nasogastric tube. In cases where nasogastric intubation is not possible, an esophagostomy may be performed and animals fed through an indwelling cervical esophagostomy tube (**15.2**).

Technique

- The procedure is performed in the standing horse under light sedation using local anesthesia.
- The surgical site is at the junction between the upper and middle thirds of the neck (**15.3**). A generous area is clipped and prepared aseptically.
- A nasogastric tube is passed (if possible) beyond the surgical site to facilitate identification of the esophagus.

- A ventrolateral approach is preferred for placement of a feeding tube because it allows the tube to lie comfortably on the patient's neck and permits better anchorage of the tube to the skin. This approach also provides better access to the middle and distal cervical esophagus.
- A 5–8 cm incision is made to the left of midline, just ventral to the jugular vein.
- The sternocephalicus and brachiocephalicus muscles are separated and retracted.
- The deep cervical fascia is dissected bluntly until the tube within the esophagus is palpated. The esophagus is then gently separated from the surrounding soft tissue.

- A 3-cm full-thickness incision is made into the esophagus.
- The nasogastric tube is removed and a second tube inserted through the esophagostomy. The tube may be secured with a finger trap and butterfly bandages of tape (**15.3**).

Postoperative care

- A mild cellulitis inevitably develops at the surgery site and broad-spectrum antimicrobial therapy should be considered.
- The tube should remain in place until a mature fistula has formed (10–14 days).
- The surgical site should be cleaned several times daily and petroleum jelly may be applied to protect the skin.

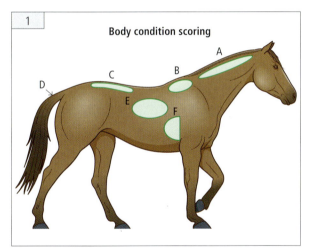

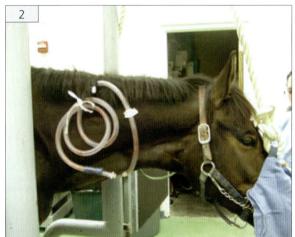

15.1 Sites used to assess the body condition score of adult horses. A, neck; B, withers; C, transverse processes of lumbar vertebrae; D, tail head; E, ribs; F, area behind shoulders.

15.2 A horse with dysphagia associated with guttural pouch mycosis that received enteral nutrition via a nasogastric tube placed through an esophagostomy.

15.3 An esophagostomy is performed at the junction of the upper and middle thirds of the neck using local anesthetic and with the horse standing and sedated.

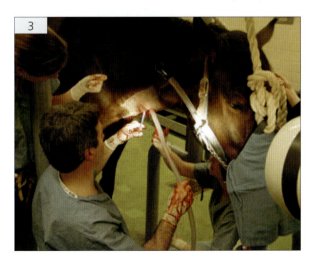

- The tube should be capped between feedings to prevent aerophagia.
- If a mature fistula has been allowed to form, this will heal spontaneously over 2–3 weeks once the tube has been permanently removed. If the tube is removed prior to formation of a mature fistula, healing of the incision can be prolonged.

Complications

A mild cellulitis generally develops at the surgical site; this may be more pronounced if the feeding tube is removed prematurely. Laryngeal hemiplegia is a common complication of esophageal surgery.

Calculation of parenteral nutrition formulation

Indications

Parenteral nutrition is often indicated to meet the needs of critically ill equine patients (see Parenteral nutrition).

Technique

An example of a form that can be used to prepare parenteral nutrition is shown (15.4):

- Determine the rate at which dextrose:amino acids:lipids are being provided in g/kg/day (15.4, A). Ratios of 10 g/kg/day of dextrose, 2 g/kg/day of amino acids, and 1 g/kg/day of lipids (i.e. 10:2:1) for neonatal foals and 2.8 g/kg/day of dextrose, 1.3 g/kg/day of amino acids, and 0.8 g/kg/day of lipids (i.e. 2.8:1.3:0.8) for adult horses have been suggested. Other ratios are possible to meet specific nutritional requirements (see Parenteral nutrition and *Tables 15.9* and *15.10*).
- Calculate the total number of grams per day of each component (i.e. dextrose, amino acids, or lipids) by multiplying the g/kg/day value by the body weight in kilograms (kg) (15.4, B).
- To determine the volume in ml per day of each component, multiply the grams per day value by 2 for a 50% solution, 5 for a 20% solution, or 10 for a 10% solution (15.4, C). There is a wide range of concentrations of the various components, particularly in Europe and Australia, and these calculations need to be adjusted accordingly.
- Add the total volume of KCl, multivitamins, and trace minerals per day (15.4, D).
- Calculate the total volume of parenteral nutrition to be administered per day (ml/day) (15.4, E).

15.4 Example of a parenteral nutrition form that can be used to prepare parenteral nutrition.

- Decide what size fluid bag is needed (e.g. 1 liter, 3 liter, or 4 liter). If >1 bag, divide the total for each component by the number of bags to determine the volume per bag (**15.4, F**).
- Divide by 24 hours to calculate the rate of administration in ml per hour (**15.4, G**).

Complications

See Parenteral nutrition.

NUTRITIONAL SUPPORT

Nutritional requirements

Key points

- Provision of calories sufficient to meet resting energy requirements (RER) is recommended.
- Patients should receive maintenance crude protein.
- Hyperalimentation can be detrimental and even partial supplementation may be beneficial.
- Static equations should be used to estimate initial energy and protein requirements and adjustments made on the basis of careful monitoring.

Energy requirements

If insufficient calories are provided by dietary carbohydrate or fat, endogenous protein is used to meet the body's energy needs. The primary goal of nutritional support, therefore, is to limit the use of endogenous protein as an energy source and conserve body mass. *Table 15.3* shows the energy and nitrogen contents of carbohydrates, proteins, and fats.

Energy requirements are determined by a range of factors including sex, age, lean body mass, body surface area, reproductive status, activity level, and ambient temperature. Nutritionists divide energy requirements based on the level of metabolism that is to be supported (*Table 15.4*). Calculated basal energy requirements, RER, and maintenance energy requirements for adult horses weighing between 200 and 800 kg

---

Table 15.3 Approximate values for calculating energy and nitrogen contents of diets

- Carbohydrate provides 3.4 kcal/g.
- Protein provides 4 kcal/g.
- Lipid provides 11 kcal/g.
- 1 g protein contains 0.16g nitrogen.
- 6.25 g protein provides 1 g nitrogen.

Table 15.4 Definitions of energy requirements and formulae commonly used for adult horses

TYPE	DEFINITION	BODY WEIGHT	ENERGY REQUIREMENT (MCAL/DAY)[1]
Basal energy requirements (BER)	Energy for maintenance of body function in resting animals in a thermoneutral environment		$0.070(BW)^{0.75}$
Resting energy requirements[2] (RER)	BER plus the energy for thermogenesis and thermoregulation		$0.975 + 0.021(BW)$
Maintenance energy requirements (MER)	Energy required for zero body weight change during normal activity in non-working horses (also termed true maintenance)	200–600 kg	$1.4 + 0.03(BW)$
		>600 kg	$1.82 + 0.0383(BW) - 1.5 \times 10^{-5}(BW)^2$

BW, body weight in kilograms (1 kg = 2.2 lb).

RER (or stall maintenance) provide ~70% of the maintenance energy needs for an idle horse. Resting energy requirements are generally used to calculate the energy needs for ill horses.

[1] Energy requirements may be expressed in Joules by using the conversion factor 1 calorie is equivalent to 4.184 Joules (1 Mcal = 4.184 MJ).

[2] Calculated from horses weighing between 125 and 856 kg.

(440 and 1,760 lb) are shown in *Table 15.5*. Energy requirements of foals are considerably higher than those of adults and the RER for foals has been estimated as 45–50 kcal/kg/day (approximately twice that of mature horses).[4] Furthermore, healthy foals increase their body weight by ~2% daily during the first weeks of life and may consume 120–145 kcal/kg/day.

Some disease states (e.g. burns, neoplasia, severe sepsis) result in increased energy requirements. Multiplying factors have been developed to calculate energy requirements for these conditions in humans. However, the validity of these has been questioned and the provision of excessive calories (hyperalimentation) can be detrimental:[5,6]

- Current recommendations suggest provision of sufficient calories initially to meet RER (*Tables 15.4* and *15.5*).
- Even partial supplementation can have a sparing effect on tissue catabolism.
- Large differences in energy requirements exist between individual animals.
- Static equations should be used initially and adjustments made on the basis of careful and repeated monitoring of body weight, as well as blood glucose and serum triglyceride concentrations.

Protein requirements

Protein deficiency in sick animals is most often the result of inadequate food (energy) intake. Healthy adult horses require 0.7–1.5 g/kg/day of protein. Healthy nursing foals consume ~5–6 g/kg/day. It is recommended that patients receiving nutritional support receive maintenance crude protein levels (*Table 15.5*).

Patient monitoring

Careful and repeated monitoring is required to ensure the adequacy of a nutritional program. In addition to body weight and condition (see Body condition scoring), the following parameters should be checked frequently:

- Electrolyte concentrations, particularly potassium, calcium, magnesium, and phosphorous.
- Serum triglyceride concentration, especially in patients predisposed to hyperlipidemia/hyperlipemia (ponies, donkeys, miniature breeds). Pregnancy and pituitary pars intermedia dysfunction (equine Cushing's disease) exacerbates insulin resistance and increases the risk of hyperlipidemia/hyperlipemia.
- Glucose concentration; although hypoglycemia is commonly observed in malnourished foals, it occurs infrequently in malnourished adults.

Table 15.5 **Calculated energy and maintenance protein requirements for adult horses of various weights**

	BODY WEIGHT (KG)							
	200	300	400	450	500	600	700	800
Energy requirement (Mcal/day)								
Basal energy requirements	3.7	5.0	6.3	6.8	7.4	8.5	9.5	10.5
Resting energy requirements	5.2	7.3	9.4	10.4	11.5	13.6	15.7	17.8
Maintenance energy requirements	7.4	10.4	13.4	14.9	16.4	19.4	21.3	22.9
Maintenance protein requirements (g/day)[1]	296	416	536	596	656	776	852	916

[1] Maintenance crude protein requirements (g) = 40 × maintenance energy requirements.

Excessive or prolonged hyperglycemia and glucosuria should be avoided in both foals and adults.

- Measurement of serum urea nitrogen concentration may provide some information on protein metabolism.

Enteral nutrition
Key points
- Horses receiving enteral nutrition via a nasogastric or esophagostomy tube should be fed small meals frequently.
- Changes in diet should be made gradually over several days.
- Horses and foals should be checked for reflux prior to each meal.
- Water intake (and hydration status) must be closely monitored, particularly in adult horses.

Definition/overview
Enteral nutrition is defined as delivery of nutrients directly into the stomach, duodenum, or jejunum. Enteral diets developed for use in the horse include:
- Blender diets. Finely ground feed (most commonly a complete pelleted diet) suspended in water.
- Compositional diets. Liquid formulations designed for human patients comprised of highly digestible carbohydrates, fat, and protein (usually casein or soy).
- Elemental diets. Formulations containing amino acids and peptides rather than whole protein. These diets are expensive and there are few indications for their use in equine medicine.

Indications
If the GI tract is functional and accessible, enteral feeding is physiologically more appropriate and less expensive than parenteral nutrition. Enteral feeding is thought to maintain GI tract function better and may help prevent bacterial translocation.[7]

Animals with poor appetites should be offered a variety of palatable feeds and forages. The appetite of many hospitalized horses will improve if they are allowed to graze or offered fresh grass. Foals receiving enteral nutrition may be taught to drink from a bottle or bucket; bucket feeding is often preferred as it is less labor intensive and the risk of aspiration is reduced. Animals that are unable or unwilling voluntarily to consume sufficient calories may be fed via a nasogastric or nasoesophageal tube. Dysphagic animals that are at risk of aspiration or foals with a poorly developed suck reflex (e.g. foals with hypoxic–ischemic encephalopathy) may also be fed in this manner. Small diameter (12–18 French [4–6 mm internal diameter] 108–250 cm length) feeding tubes are available (**15.5**) for adult

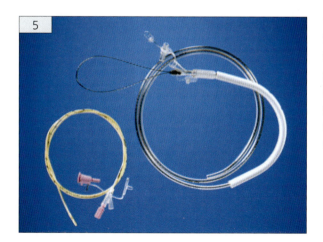

5

15.5 Examples of 6 French (90 cm in length) and 14 French (125 cm in length) nasogastric tubes suitable for use as indwelling feeding tubes. Longer tubes of greater diameter are also available (see text). Fluids and liquid diets may be administered via these tubes and patients are able to eat and drink around them. The tubes are easily secured to the muzzle using tape or suture.

horses and foals and are suitable for liquid diets. Placement of these thin feeding tubes can be difficult, but is aided by use of an endoscope. The tubes can be left in place and patients are able to eat and drink around them; however, they can be regurgitated and the lumen is too small for blender type diets. Diets containing pulverized pellets or a source of fiber require a nasogastric tube with a larger bore (e.g. 12.7 mm internal diameter). Tubes should be open ended rather than fenestrated to prevent clogging. A technique has been described for placement of an esophagostomy tube if nasogastric intubation is not possible (see Placement of an esophagostomy feeding tube).

Technique

Adult horses: A number of diets have been designed that can be fed via a nasogastric or esophagostomy tube for patients unable to ingest sufficient calories voluntarily (*Tables 15.6, 15.7,* and *15.8*).[8,9] Enteral meals should be small and fed frequently (every 4–6 hours). Most horses will tolerate ~6–8 liters per feeding, but this may be reduced in chronically anorectic animals. Feed should be introduced gradually starting at ~25% of the target allowance and reaching 100% of allowance over 4–7 days. It may be possible to increase the amount administered more quickly to patients that have only recently become anorectic. When the patient is able to voluntarily consume 75% of its maintenance energy requirements, it should be weaned off nutritional support.

Blender diets (*Table 15.6*): Blender diets made from complete pelleted rations are inexpensive and the ingredients are readily available. Two to three liters of water must be added to each pound (500 g) of feed prior to grinding; this allows swelling, eases administration, and reduces the workload of the blender. Blender diets made from complete pelleted rations generally provide a source of fiber, which can make them difficult to administer; larger bore nasogastric tubes are usually required.

The addition of 1–2 cups of vegetable oil (~1.6 Mcal per cup or 240 ml) increases the energy content without increasing bulk. Supplemental fat should not be given to animals with hyperlipemia.

Compositional diets (*Tables 15.7* and *15.8*): Commercially available human liquid diets have been used in equine medicine[10] and several diets that can be administered as a liquid have been specifically developed for horses. A home-made compositional diet for horses has also been designed (*Table 15.7*).

Table 15.6 Example of a blender diet using a complete pelleted feed and recommended tube feeding schedule for a 450 kg horse. (Modified from Fascetti and Stratton-Phelps, 2003.[9])

	DAY[1]			
	1 AND 2	3 AND 4	5 AND 6	7 AND 8
Water (liters/day)	8	16	24	24
Percentage full allowance (%)	25	50	75	100
Pelleted feed (g/day)[2]	1,000	2,100	3,200	4,400
Vegetable oil (ml/day)[3]	100	200	300	400
Digestible energy (Mcal/day)	3.4	7.0	10.7	14.6

[1] The day's ration should be administered in a minimum of four meals. If the horse has become acutely anorectic, the full allowance may be reached in less than 8 days.

[2] Equine Senior® provides ~2.7 Mcal/kg. Other commercial complete pelleted feeds are available and may be used for this type of meal.

[3] Vegetable oil contains ~0.67 Mcal/100 ml. The use of vegetable oil increases the caloric content without increasing bulk, but may be associated with some side-effects including diarrhea, steatorrhea, and lipemia.

Table 15.7 Example of a liquid compositional diet developed for enteral feeding. (Modified from Naylor _et al.,_ 1984[8])

	DAY[1]						
	1	**2**	**3**	**4**	**5**	**6**	**7**
Water (liters/day)	21	21	21	21	21	21	21
Electrolyte mix (g/day)[2]	230	230	230	230	230	230	230
Dextrose (g/day)	300	400	500	600	700	800	900
Caesin (g/day)[3]	300	450	600	750	900	900	900
Dehydrated alfalfa meal (g/day)	2,000	2,000	2,000	2,000	2,000	2,000	2,000
Digestible energy (Mcal/day)	7.4	8.4	9.4	10.4	11.8	11.8	12.2

[1] Each day's allowance should be divided and administered as 3 or 4 meals.

[2] Composition of electrolyte mix: sodium chloride (NaCl) 10g; sodium bicarbonate (NaHCO$_3$) 15g; potassium chloride (KCl) 75g; potassium phosphate (K$_2$HPO$_4$) 60g; calcium chloride (CaCl$_2$) 45g; magnesium oxide (MgO) 25g.

[3] For example, Casein or Edible Acid Casein-90.

Table 15.8 Examples of human liquid enteral products and a liquid diet designed specifically for horses (Critical Care Meals®)

	OSMOLITE[1,2]	OSMOLITE 1.2 CAL[1,2]	VITAL HN[1]	JEVITY 1.5 CAL[1,2,3]	CRITICAL CARE MEALS[4]
Calories (kcal/l)	1060	1200	1000	1500	1066
Carbohydrate (g/l)[% of diet]	151.1 [57.0%][5]	157.5 [52.5%][5]	185.0 [73.8%][5,6]	215.7 [53.6%][5]	[73%]
Protein (g/l))[% of diet]	37.1 [14.0%][7]	55.5 [18.5%][8]	41.7 [16.7%][9]	63.8 [17.0%][7]	[12%]
Fat (g/l))[% of diet]	34.7 [29.0%]	39.3 [29.0%]	10.8 [9.5%]	49.8 [29.4%]	[1%]
Non-protein calorie:N ratio (kcal:g)	153:1	110:1	125:1	122:1	
Osmolarity (mOsmol/l)	252	295	386	477	

Although convenient and easy to administer, the products designed for human use may contain excessive fat, very little or no fiber, and insufficient protein. Note that approximately 10 liters of the human products will be required to provide resting energy requirements for a 450 kg horse.

[1] Ross Products Division, Abbott Laboratories.

[2] Other combinations available with higher energy or protein contents.

[3] Contains 22 g/l of dietary fiber.

[4] MD's Choice Inc.; supplied as 340 g packet of dried powered; caloric content is per 340 g. Manufacturer recommends that horses be fed a maximum of 6 packets per day as 3 meals. Additional supplements, which contain a source of dietary fiber, are available from the same manufacturer.

[5] Corn maltodextrin.

[6] Sucrose; only diets containing a limited amount of sucrose should be used for horses.

[7] Caseinates and soy protein.

[8] Caseinates.

[9] Whey, meat, and soy protein.

Human diets are relatively expensive, lack fiber, and provide insufficient protein; however, they require little effort to prepare and may be administered through a small nasogastric tube.

A slurry of alfalfa meal or other forage-based feed may be added to provide fiber, but will necessitate a larger bore nasogastric tube. Some of the commercially available equine-specific liquid diets may be tailored to meet individual needs and can provide considerable roughage (fiber).

Foals: Mare's milk is the ideal feed for foals if available and if the GI tract will tolerate enteral feeding. Commercially produced milk replacers are widely available and these may be fed at the same rate if mare's milk is unavailable. Although very good, these products often contain high concentrations of sodium and other electrolytes when compared with mare's milk and can cause problems with water balance. Goat's milk may be used as a temporary feed if nothing else is available and pasteurized cow's milk (2% fat with ~6 g of dextrose added per liter) has been used by the author without apparent problem.

Neonates should initially be fed 10% of their body weight (i.e. 100 ml/kg) daily divided into 12 meals. The volume fed may be increased to 20% of their body weight (200 ml/kg) daily over several days if tolerated. The frequency of meals may be slowly decreased (to every 4–8 hours) in foals aged 2 weeks or older. Smaller starting volumes (e.g. 1–5% of body weight daily) may be required in some foals, especially those with hypoxic–ischemic injury to the GI tract.

Complications

Low-fiber diets in adult horses are frequently associated with GI tract disturbances, usually a low-volume self-limiting diarrhea. Colic, ileus, abdominal and gastric distension, and laminitis may occur in some adult horses on some enteral diets. Indigestion and mild colic are relatively common in foals fed mare's milk substitutes; if indigestion occurs, the frequency and/or volume of meals should be decreased.

Parenteral nutrition
Key points
- Diets should be introduced gradually and administration rates increased as tolerated.
- Blood glucose concentration should be measured frequently (every 3–6 hours) initially until it has stabilized.
- Serum triglyceride concentrations should be monitored daily.
- Increases in administration rates above the suggested guidelines should be based on continued body weight losses. Care must be taken to avoid hyperalimentation, as this is associated with a high incidence of complications.
- Meticulous preparation of solutions and catheter care is essential to avoid complications associated with infection.

Definition/overview
Parenteral nutrition is defined as the provision of nutrition by means of IV feeding, thus completely bypassing the alimentary canal. Total parenteral nutrition (TPN) (theoretically) provides all the carbohydrates, proteins, fats, water, electrolytes, and minerals needed by an animal. Partial parenteral nutrition (PPN) provides some portion or selected components of an animal's nutritional requirements.

Indications
Parenteral nutrition should be considered in the following situations:
- GI tract dysfunction where prolonged recovery is anticipated or in animals with limited reserves.
- Pharyngeal or esophageal disease that precludes use of a nasogastric or esophagostomy tube.
- Recumbent patients.
- Animals with markedly increased nutritional needs (e.g. pregnancy and lactation) but limited ability to increase intake.
- Severely malnourished animals in which immediate nutritional support is required.

Technique

Dextrose: In its most basic form, parenteral nutrition simply provides carbohydrate in the form of intravenous dextrose (or glucose).

Dextrose (or glucose) administered at a rate of 2 mg/kg/minute to an average sized horse (i.e. 5% dextrose solution at ~1 liter/hour) provides ~4 Mcal/day or ~45% of RER. IV dextrose (or glucose) may be used when intake reduction is only partial or for a short duration of time. Horses may not tolerate high dextrose (or glucose) infusion rates initially and administration should begin at 25–50% of the target rate and increased gradually (e.g. by 25% every 6–24 hours) if blood glucose concentrations remain within normal limits.

Partial parenteral nutrition: To avoid the complications associated with lipid administration and to reduce the expense of TPN, dextrose (or glucose) and amino acid combinations can be used to supply PPN to adults and may provide some benefits (e.g. protein sparing) over dextrose (or glucose) alone. Some manufacturers produce pre-mixed dextrose/amino acid combinations, but they can also be prepared from individual components by the clinician. Solutions should be administered to provide the desired carbohydrate load.

Total parenteral nutrition: TPN formulations contain a combination of carbohydrate, lipid, and amino acids designed to meet energy and protein requirements. Optimal ratios for glucose, lipid, and protein for the critically ill horse have not been established and formulations are based on information from human medicine.[6]

It should be recognized that enterocytes obtain the nutrients they require for normal function from the bowel lumen. If possible, animals receiving parenteral nutrition should be administered small enteral meals to provide for enterocyte nutrition. These 'trophic feedings' have been shown to encourage GI tract development, help maintain normal GI tract function, and improve immune function.

Carbohydrates (dextrose or glucose): The low caloric density and high osmolarity of dextrose (or glucose) solutions make it difficult to provide adequate energy using dextrose alone. Carbohydrates should provide 50–70% of non-protein calories.

Lipids: Lipids are added to increase caloric density and reduce the osmolarity of parenteral nutrition solutions. Lipids are provided in emulsions most commonly consisting of long-chain fatty acids derived from safflower, canola, or soybean oil. The combination of lipid and glucose appears to confer a metabolic advantage over administration of glucose alone. Lipids generally provide 15–30% of total caloric intake or 30–50% of non-protein calories in human clinical practice.[11] Formulations containing >15% of calories derived from fats are contraindicated in hyperlipemic patients. There is some concern that long-chain fatty acids may impair immune function and contribute to the pathogenesis of inflammatory conditions.[11]

Protein (amino acids): Amino acids are provided in a range of concentrations from 8 to 20% solutions. The ideal ratio of non-protein calories to nitrogen for horses is unclear; ratios of 120:1 to 150:1 (kcal:g) have been suggested for healthy humans with lower ratios ~80:1 to 90:1 (kcal:g) recommended for acutely ill human patients.[6]

Rates of 1–2 g/kg/day of amino acids have been suggested for adult equine patients; this rate approximates to calculated maintenance needs. Rates of 2–3 g/kg/day of amino acids are commonly used in hospitalized neonates.

Non-protein calorie to nitrogen ratios of 80:1 to 100:1 (kcal:g) are probably appropriate for critically ill veterinary patients provided that protein supplementation is not contraindicated (i.e. in patients with renal failure or liver disease).

Vitamins and trace minerals: The vitamin and trace element requirements for critically ill adult horses and foals are not known. Multivitamin and trace mineral mixtures are empirically added to parenteral nutrition formulations.

Formulating parenteral nutritional solutions: When formulating a parenteral nutrition solution, the aim should be to meet maintenance protein requirements and then provide the remaining calories (up to RER) with carbohydrates and lipids. Solutions composed of 2.8–8 g/kg/day of dextrose, 1.3–2 g/kg/day of amino acids, and 0.8–1 g/kg/day of lipid have been suggested for adult horses (*Table 15.9*).[12,13] Formulations for adult horses should contain relatively less energy when compared with parenteral nutrition formulations for foals. **Note:** The formulations providing 5–8 g/kg/day dextrose will likely provide too much energy for most adult patients, but may be required for animals in highly catabolic states.

A parenteral formula commonly used in neonates at the author's hospital provides dextrose at 10 g/kg/day, amino acids at 2 g/kg/day, and lipids at 1 g/kg/day (i.e. a dextrose:amino acid:lipid ratio of 10:2:1). This formulation provides ~53 kcal/kg/day. Other formulations, which provide more energy by increasing the content of dextrose and lipid (*Table 15.10*), have been suggested.[3]

Parenteral nutrition should be administered using an infusion pump to ensure accurate delivery. Infusions should begin at 25–50% of the calculated target rate and the rate increased by 25% every 6–24 hours if tolerated. Increases above the final calculated rate should be based on continued weight loss and other measured parameters. Once enteral feeding is tolerated and the animal is consuming 75% of MER, the rate of parenteral nutrition administration is decreased by half every 6–8 hours.

Parental nutrition solutions should be prepared under sterile conditions and preferably in a laminar

---

Table 15.9 Examples of parenteral nutrition formulation for adult horses (450 kg)

Dextrose:amino acid:lipid composition (g/kg/day)	2.8:1.3:0.8	5:2:1	8:2:1
50% dextrose (ml) [% non-protein calories]	2520 [52]	4500 [61]	7200 [71]
10% amino acids (ml)[1]	5850	9000	9000
10% lipids (ml) [% non-protein calories][2]	3600 [48]	4500 [39]	4500 [29]
Osmolarity (mOsm/l)[3]	1038.9	1134.8	1317.9
Protein (g)	93.6	144	144
Non-protein calorie:nitrogen (kcal:g) ratio	88.1:1	87.5:1	119.4:1
Target rate (ml/hour)[4]	500	750	860
Mcal/day	10.6	16.2	20.7
kcal/kg/day	24	36	46

Note that the formulations with dextrose:amino acid:lipid compositions of 5:2:1 and 8:2:1 g/kg/day provide too much energy in most cases, but may be required in highly catabolic patients.

[1] Available as Aminosyn II®, Travasol, or Aminoven.

[2] Available as Liposyn II or Intralipid.

[3] Calculations were made using values from Aminosyn II® 10% (870 mOsmol/l) and Liposyn II 10% (258 mOsmol/l).

[4] If no additional fluids are added.

flow hood. The dextrose and amino acids should be mixed first and lipids added last to avoid instability of the lipids as a result of the low pH of dextrose. Prepared bags may be refrigerated and stored for 24 hours prior to use. If the lipid component separates and does not mix, the solution should be discarded. Parenteral nutrition solutions are hypertonic and should be administered into a central vein in foals. Administration into the jugular vein in adults is well tolerated.

Meticulous attention to sterility is required when placing IV catheters for use with parenteral nutrition. Long-term catheters made of non-thrombogenic material with a double lumen are preferred, with one port dedicated to the parenteral nutrition. Parenteral nutrition IV lines should be changed every 24–72 hours and should not be disconnected between changes. The catheter site must be monitored closely and checked at least twice daily. Inline filters (20 μm) should be used if lipids are not administered; however, the inclusion of lipids in parenteral nutrition solutions precludes

their use. The injection ports on parenteral nutrition IV lines should not be used for administration of other drugs and blood should not be drawn through parenteral nutrition lines.

Complications

Hyperglycemia: The risk of hyperglycemia is reduced by gradual introduction of parenteral nutrition, but remains the most common complication. Mild hyperglycemia may be tolerated provided that glucose concentration does not exceed the renal threshold (~10 mmol/l [180 mg/dl]). Blood glucose concentrations should be measured every 3–6 hours initially and urine checked frequently for the presence of glucose. Blood glucose monitoring can be less frequent once the patient's blood glucose concentration has stabilized. Hypergylcemia may be controlled with exogenous insulin administered either as single injections of ultralente insulin (0.2–0.3 IU/kg SC q12–24h) or as a continuous infusion of regular insulin (0.002–0.02 IU/kg/hour).

Table 15.10 Examples of parenteral nutrition formulations for foals (45 kg)

Dextrose:amino acid:lipid composition (g/kg/day)	10:2:1	10:3.5:2	12:3:2	15:3:3
50% dextrose (ml) [% non-protein calories]	900 [76]	900 [61]	1,080 [65]	1,350 [61]
10% amino acids (ml)[1]	900	1575	1,350	1,350
10% lipids (ml) [% non-protein calories][2]	450 [24]	900 [39]	900 [35]	1,350 [39]
Osmolarity (mOsm/l)[3]	1,412.4	1,164.6	1,238.6	1,210.8
Nitrogen (g)	14.4	25.2	21.6	21.6
Non-protein calorie:nitrogen (kcal:g) ratio	140.6:1	100:1	130.8:1	175:1
Target rate (ml/hour)[4]	94	141	139	169
Mcal/day	2.39	3.15	3.37	4.32
kcal/kg/day	53	70	76	96

[1] Available as Aminosyn® II, Travasol®, or Aminoven®.

[2] Available as Liposyn® II or Intralipid®.

[3] Calculations made using values from Aminosyn® II 10% (870 mOsmol/l) and Liposyn® II 10% (258 mOsmol/l).

[4] If no additional fluids are added.

If hyperglycemia is persistent, the rate of administration or dextrose content of the solution may have to be slowed.

Abrupt cessation of IV glucose administration can lead to a profound hypoglycemia because of increased endogenous insulin activity.

Electrolyte abnormalities: The most common electrolyte abnormality experienced by horses on parenteral nutrition is hypokalemia, but hypomagnesemia, hypocalemia, and hypophosphatemia are not uncommon. Hypophosphatemia may be potentiated by exogenous insulin therapy.

Hypertriglyceridemia: Hypertriglyceridemia (serum triglyceride concentration >1.1 mmol/l [100 mg/dl]) may occur in some patients, particularly neonates or those with severe sepsis. Serum triglyceride concentration should be measured every 24 hours. The rate of administration or the lipid content of the solution may have to be decreased if hyperlipemia persists.

Heparin (40 IU/kg SC q12h) has been suggested as a means of increasing lipoprotein lipase activity and might be of some benefit in controlling hypertriglyceridemia. Exogenous lipids should probably not be given to patients with existing hyperlipemia and hepatic lipidosis.

Infection: Infection of the catheter site and thrombophlebitis are common complications of parenteral feeding. These may be avoided by meticulous catheter placement and care, the use of a large (central) vein, and by reducing the osmolarity of infused solutions as much as possible.

CHAPTER 16

ANTIMICROBIAL DRUGS

James A. Orsini

GENERAL CONSIDERATIONS FOR ANTIMICROBIAL DRUG USE

- Antimicrobial drugs may be indicated in the critical care patient for prophylaxis or for the treatment of an existing infection.
- Overuse of antimicrobial drugs is an increasing concern in both human and veterinary medicine because it can accelerate the development of bacterial resistance to commonly used antimicrobial drugs.
- The goal should be to maximize efficacy while minimizing cost and adverse effects both at the patient and population level.
- Wherever possible, antimicrobial therapy in the critically ill patient should be targeted and should comprise bactericidal drugs and dosages.
- Pharmacokinetics may be different from expected because of:
  - Disorders of fluid balance or systemic circulation (e.g. dehydration or endotoxemia).
  - Organ failure (especially hepatic or renal).
  - Severe or widespread edema.
  - Ongoing fluid or plasma protein losses, which may not be readily apparent, predictable, or calculable (e.g. in patients with severe enterocolitis or extensive burns).
  - Alteration in metabolic rate associated with catabolism, hypo- or hyperthermia, or extensive tissue repair.
  - Pharmacokinetics in neonates are not always the same as in adults; prematurity may compound this difference.

- Pharmacodynamics may be different from expected because:
  - Inflammation, purulent material, fibrosis, ischemia, or necrosis at the site of infection can interfere with drug delivery to the infected tissue or decrease efficacy once at the site.
  - Drugs that are usually efficacious for the pathogen or circumstance may perform poorly with multidrug-resistant pathogens.
- There is increased opportunity for infection because:
  - Catheters and other implants can serve as reservoirs for infection.
  - There is a greater need for human handling, which increases the risk for iatrogenic infections.
  - There is an increased risk for nosocomial infections, especially with enteric organisms, some of which are multidrug resistant.
  - The nature of the presenting or complicating problem may render the patient more vulnerable to its own microflora (e.g. breaks in the skin or mucosal barrier).
- There is increased susceptibility to infection in critically ill patients, particularly:
  - Neonates (especially if there is inadequate passive transfer of maternal antibodies).
  - Immunocompromised patients (e.g. patients with leukopenia or hypercortisolemia associated with pituitary pars intermedia dysfunction).
  - Patients receiving immunosuppressive therapy (e.g. corticosteroids).

- There is an increased potential for drug interactions in critically ill patients because other drugs used in patient care may interact or compete with the antimicrobial drug, affecting the efficacy of one or both drugs and increasing the potential for toxicity and toxic effects of each drug used may be cumulative.
- Routes of administration may be limited by the patient's clinical condition (e.g. oral administration is contraindicated in patients with nasogastric reflux).
- Stressed or critically ill patients may be at risk for enterocolitis with antimicrobial drugs.

GENERAL APPROACH TO ANTIMICROBIAL DRUG USE

Prophylactic antimicrobial drug use

Prophylaxis is a legitimate reason for antimicrobial use in the critically ill patient. However, rational and responsible use of antimicrobial drugs for this purpose is encouraged because the emergence of multidrug-resistant strains of bacteria in veterinary medicine has already begun to parallel the situation in human medicine.[1–6] Pathogens resistant to multiple commonly used antimicrobial drugs are increasingly being cultured from hospitalized horses. They include methicillin-resistant *Staphylococcus aureus*[7–9] methicillin-resistant *S. epidermidis*[10], penicillin-resistant *Actinobacillus* spp.[11], and aminoglycoside-resistant *Escherichia coli*.[6,12,13]

The following guidelines are proposed for prophylactic antimicrobial use:

- Use based on risk: use only in patients at significant risk for infection or when infection would have catastrophic consequences.
- Selection based on likelihood: base drug choice(s) on the type of infection most likely to occur in the particular patient or circumstance.
- Administration only through risk period: use for only as long as necessary to protect the patient during the period of highest risk.

Use based on risk

Determining a patient's risk for infection beforehand is generally based on clinical judgment. Certain types of patients, procedures, and problems are inherently associated with a high risk for potentially serious bacterial infections:

- Breaks in the natural barriers to bacteria, including the skin, mucosa, and cornea/sclera (e.g. wounds, extensive burns, open fractures; severe inflammatory or ischemic bowel disease; esophageal rupture; patent umbilical remnant in neonatal foals; dystocia requiring manual exploration beyond the vaginal vault and/or involving severe trauma to the reproductive tract; any clean-contaminated or contaminated surgical procedure; and aspiration of substances that are irritating to the airways such as gastric contents).
- Impeded clearance mechanisms (e.g. aspiration of substances that are not readily cleared from the airways, such as mineral oil, food, milk, meconium; recumbency for more than a few hours; patients that must remain standing with the head held above chest height for more than a few hours; and structural damage such as cervical laceration).
- Immunocompromise (e.g. neonates with partial or complete FPT of maternal antibodies; patients with hypercortisolemia caused by pituitary pars intermedia dysfunction [equine Cushing's disease]; any patient with marked leukopenia, especially neutropenia; and any patient with marked hypoproteinemia).
- Other situations (e.g. use of surgical implants, such as screws, plates, pins, or mesh; extensive soft tissue trauma causing ischemia or necrosis; severe lymphedema, particularly of the distal limb(s); severe circulatory compromise; and any other circumstance when infection would be catastrophic).

Selection based on likelihood

While broad-spectrum aerobic coverage is common both for prophylaxis and for initial antimicrobial therapy, a more targeted approach, based on the type(s) of bacteria most likely to be involved, may lessen the development of antimicrobial drug resistance. Bacterial culture and antimicrobial susceptibility testing in the individual patient is not relevant for guiding prophylactic use because by definition prophylactic antimicrobial use is administration in advance of bacterial infection. However, drug selection can be guided by culture and susceptibility data accumulated for the patient population and by the types of bacteria most likely to cause infection in the particular patient or circumstance.[14,15]

The most likely bacterial isolates in horses and foals by site or lesion type are listed in *Table 16.1*. Antimicrobial susceptibility data for various pathogens isolated from horses at one large veterinary hospital in the USA

Table 16.1 Most common bacterial isolates in horses and foals by site or lesion type

SITE OR LESION TYPE	MOST COMMON ISOLATES
Normal equine skin	*Bacillus* spp., non-hemolytic *Staphylococcus* spp., *Micrococcus* spp.
	Less often or in lower numbers: *Corynebacterium* spp. (varies by geographic region), *Streptomyces* spp., non-hemolytic *Streptococcus* spp., other non-enteric genera
Cellulitis/lymphangitis	Coagulase-positive *Staphylococcus* spp.
	Less often: β-hemolytic *Streptococcus* spp., coagulase-negative *Staphylococcus* spp., gram-negative aerobic bacteria, anaerobes
Synovial infections (joints, tendon sheaths, bursae)	Traumatic*: gram-negative enteric organisms, anaerobes, *Staphylococcus* spp., *Streptococcus* spp.; polymicrobial infections are common.
	Post-surgical: *Staphylococcus* spp., *Enterobacter* spp., *Pseudomonas* spp.
Digit (including the hoof)	Polymicrobial infection with gram-negative enteric bacteria and, with penetrating wounds, anaerobes such as *Bacteroides* spp.
Bone, physeal cartilage	Traumatic*: *Enterobacter* spp., *Streptococcus* spp., *Staphylococcus* spp.
	Post-surgical: *Streptococcus equi* subsp. *zooepidemicus*, *Staphylococcus aureus*, α-*Streptococcus* spp.
	Young foals: gram-negative organisms
Respiratory tract, oropharynx	Traumatic*: combinations of gram-positive aerobes (especially *Streptococcus equi* subsp. *zooepidemicus)*, gram-negative aerobes (e.g. *Actinobacillus* spp., *Pasteurella* spp., *Escherichia coli*, *Klebsiella pneumoniae)*, and anaerobes (e.g. *Bacteroides* spp., *Fusobacterium* spp., and *Peptostreptococcus* spp.)
Gastrointestinal tract, peritoneal cavity	Compromised bowel: gram-negative enteric organisms, especially *Escherichia coli* and *Klebsiella pneumoniae*, and anaerobes.
	Intra-abdominal abscess: *Streptococcus equi* subsp. *equi* and *zooepidemicus*, *Corynebacterium pseudotuberculosis*
Muscle	*Clostridium* spp., *Corynebacterium pseudotuberculosis*
Blood (i.e. septicemia) in neonates	Most often single infection with *E. coli*, *Actinobacillus equuli*, or non-hemolytic *Streptococcus* spp.. Less often, mixed infection or single infection with other *Actinobacillus* spp. or *Enterococcus* spp., *Klebsiella* spp., *Bacillus* spp., *Corynebacterium* spp., *Acinetobacter* spp., *Pseudomonas* spp., *Staphylococcus* spp., or *Enterbacter* spp.

* Secondary to penetrating wound.

Adapted from Schneider *et al.*, 1992[29]; MacDonald *et al.*, 1994[30]; Hague *et al.*, 1997[31]; Galuppo *et al.*, 1999[34]; Cruz *et al.*, 2006[33]; Corley *et al.*, 2007.[32]

is summarized in *Table 16.2*. This information must serve as a guide only. Sensitivity patterns vary among geographic areas and over time, being influenced by the type and extent of antimicrobial use in a particular population.[6,14]

As a general rule, the older, more widely used drugs (e.g. penicillin G, gentamicin) should be used for prophylaxis, leaving the newer or less commonly used drugs (e.g. cephalosporins, fluoroquinolones) for the treatment of infections with bacteria of known susceptibility to these antimicrobial drugs. This approach is aimed at preserving antimicrobial susceptibility in common equine pathogens.

Administration only through risk period

Antimicrobial drug administration should be limited to the period during which the patient is at greatest risk for infection. For example, for prophylaxis in surgical patients, the recommendation is to begin antimicrobial administration within 1 hour before the surgical incision and discontinue use by 24 hours after the end of surgery, unless there is a clear clinical reason to continue administration.[16]

In other circumstances, the duration of prophylactic use similarly is dictated by the duration of risk. A recumbent horse or foal, for example, may remain on prophylactic antimicrobial drugs until it is able to stand. If at any time the patient shows signs of infection (e.g. fever, malaise, neutrophilia or neutropenia, or hyperfibrinogenemia), then antimicrobial administration becomes therapeutic in purpose, and treatment is adjusted accordingly.

Therapeutic antimicrobial drug use

Whenever possible, the choice of antimicrobial drug(s) should be guided by bacterial culture and antimicrobial susceptibility testing when treating bacterial infections. Appropriate tissue and/or fluid samples should be carefully collected using aseptic techniques. These samples should be collected before antimicrobial therapy is initiated or, if the horse is already receiving antimicrobial drugs, before the regimen is changed. In the latter instance, it is usually best to discontinue antimicrobial drug administration for 24–72 hours before sample collection (depending on the dosing interval being used) provided that the patient is clinically stable. In patients suspected of being bacteremic or septicemic, blood culture should be performed on blood collected aseptically. Multiple blood samples for culture is often necessary.

Samples for microbiologic testing should be sent to the laboratory in appropriate shipping containers and media. Unless a particular type of aerobic organism is strongly suspected, both aerobic and anaerobic bacterial culture and antimicrobial susceptibility testing should be requested. Anaerobes should be suspected particularly when routine aerobic culture results are negative and in patients with osteomyelitis, abscessation, deep puncture wounds, draining tracts, infection involving gas formation within the tissues, strongly malodorous necrotic tissue or discharges, or infection involving a body cavity or hollow organ (GI, respiratory, or urogenital tract).

In patients that have responded poorly to initial antimicrobial therapy or in which infection recurs once treatment is discontinued, multidrug-resistant bacteria should also be considered, and the laboratory staff notified of the horse's recent antimicrobial history.

Table 16.2 *In-vitro* sensitivity of equine pathogens to various antimicrobial drugs at a university hospital*

ORGANISM	DRUG TESTED (PERCENTAGE OF SUSCEPTIBLE ISOLATES)
Gram-positive bacteria	
Enterococcus faecalis	Ampicillin (100%), amoxicillin/clavulanic acid (100%), chloramphenicol (90%), tetracycline (90%), erythromycin (40%)
Enterococcus faecium	Ampicillin (90%), amoxicillin/clavulanic acid (90%), chloramphenicol (80%), tetracycline (70%), erythromycin (10%)
Rhodococcus equi	Ceftiofur (100%), ceftizoxime (100%), gentamicin (100%), trimethoprim-sulfonamide (100%), rifampin (88%), amikacin (87%), chloramphenicol (63%), erythromycin (63%), cephalothin (39%), tetracycline (25%)
Staphylococcus aureus	Chloramphenicol (97%), amikacin (94%), enrofloxacin (94%), rifampin (94%), cephalothin (91%), amoxicillin/clavulanic acid (88%), erythromycin (76%), ceftiofur (69%), oxacillin (67%), trimethoprim-sulfonamide (55%), gentamicin (45%), ceftizoxime (36%), tetracycline (36%), penicillin G (30%)
Coagulase-negative *Staphylococcus* spp.	Amikacin (100%), amoxicillin/clavulanic acid (100%), cephalothin (97%), rifampin (97%), enrofloxacin (96), chloramphenicol (94%), tetracycline (81%), ceftiofur (77%), oxacillin (77%), ceftizoxime (74%), gentamicin (74%), trimethoprim-sulfonamide (74%), erythromycin (61%), penicillin G (13%)
Streptococcus zooepidemicus	Amoxicillin/clavulanic acid (100%), ampicillin (100%), ceftiofur (100%), ceftizoxime (100%), cephalothin (100%), cefquinome (100%), chloramphenicol (100%), erythromycin (100%), penicillin G (100%), trimethoprim-sulfonamide (100%), rifampin (71%), gentamicin (7%), amikacin (0%)
Gram-negative bacteria	
Actinobacillus spp. (*A. suis*-like, *A. equuli*, *A. ligniersii*)	Amikacin (100%), amoxicillin/clavulanic acid (100%), ceftiofur (100%), ceftizoxime (100%), cephalothin (100%), chloramphenicol (100%), gentamicin (100%), penicillin G (100%), ampicillin (89–100%), trimethoprim-sulfonamide (86–100%), tetracycline (86–100%), erythromycin (0–30%)
Escherichia coli	Amikacin (100%), enrofloxacin (100%), ceftizoxime (97%), ceftiofur (94%), ticarcillin (94%), amoxicillin/clavulanic acid (93%), chloramphenicol (91%), gentamicin (86%), cephalothin (73%), tetracycline (71%), ampicillin (68%), trimethoprim-sulfonamide (60%)
Klebsiella pneumoniae	Amikacin (100%), ceftiofur (100%), ceftizoxime (100%), enrofloxacin (100%), ticarcillin (87%), chloramphenicol (80%), amoxicillin/clavulanic acid (79%), gentamicin (67%), trimethoprim-sulfonamide (67%), cephalothin (66%), tetracycline (54%), ampicillin (14%)
Pasteurella spp.	Amikacin (100%), amoxicillin/clavulanic acid (100%), ampicillin (100%), cephalothin (100%), chloramphenicol (100%), gentamicin (100%), penicillin G (100%), tetracycline (100%), trimethoprim-sulfonamide (100%), ceftiofur (83%), ceftizoxime (83%), enrofloxacin (83%), erythromycin (33%)
Salmonella spp. (*S. agona, S. typhimurium*)	Amikacin (100%), amoxicillin/clavulanic acid (100%), ceftiofur (100%), ceftizoxime (100%), cephalothin (100%), enrofloxacin (100%), tetracycline (73–92%), ticarcillin (54–91%), gentamicin (49–82%), trimethoprim-sulfonamide (15–82%), ampicillin (0–82%), chloramphenicol (0–82%)
Serratia marcescens	Ceftizoxime (100%), enrofloxacin (100%), ceftiofur (75%), tetracycline (50%), amikacin (0%), amoxicillin/clavulanic acid (0%), cephalothin (0%), chloramphenicol (0%), gentamicin (0%), ticarcillin (0%), trimethoprim-sulfonamide (0%)

* Organisms isolated from horses presented for treatment at the University of California, Davis during 1998. Adapted from Wilson, 2001.[14]

While awaiting culture and sensitivity testing results, empiric antimicrobial therapy can be initiated, provided all samples for culture and cytology have been collected. In-house cytologic examination using Gram's stain greatly facilitates the selection of drugs for this interim therapy. The site of infection can also be used as a general guide (*Table 16.3*). In many cases, broad-spectrum antimicrobial therapy is the best approach while awaiting culture and sensitivity results. The combination of penicillin G and gentamicin has been the mainstay of broad-spectrum systemic antimicrobial therapy in adult horses for many years. However, penicillin G may not be the most appropriate choice in some circumstances.

Several common equine pathogens produce β-lactamases, which inactivate penicillin G; they include many *Staphylococcus* spp., most gram-negative enteric organisms, and many *Bacteroides* spp. (including *Bacteroides fragilis*).[14] In cases where these organisms are likely to be involved (*Table 16.1*), a penicillinase-resistant or potentiated penicillin or a cephalosporin should be used in place of penicillin G. Metronidazole may be added if *Bacteroides fragilis* or clostridial enterocolitis is suspected.

Monitoring response to therapy

Critical care patients with serious infections should be monitored frequently until the infection is resolved. Physical examination should be performed at least twice a day initially and WBC count and fibrinogen or serum amyloid A concentration repeated every 2–3 days until the patient's condition stabilizes. Provided an appropriate treatment plan is implemented, a positive response to therapy (e.g. improvement in attitude and appetite; resolution of fever; reduction in local or regional signs of inflammation; improvement in WBC count and fibrinogen concentration) should be seen within a couple of days.

If there is no improvement within 2–3 days of starting or changing treatment, the case should be reviewed. Depending on the circumstances, physical examination and WBC count and fibrinogen

---

Table 16.3 **Empirical antimicrobial choices for interim treatment* based on the affected tissue(s)**

TISSUE OR LESION INVOLVED	EMPIRIC ANTIMICROBIAL DRUG OPTIONS
Cellulitis/lymphangitis	Ceftiofur + gentamicin/amikacin; or enrofloxacin (adult horses only)
Synovial structures (joint, tendon sheath, bursa)	Ceftiofur + gentamicin/amikacin; or enrofloxacin (adult horses only)
Distal limb, foot	Penicillin G/ceftiofur + gentamicin/amikacin + metronidazole
Bone or physeal cartilage	As for synovial structures
Respiratory tract (e.g. penetrating neck or chest wound)	Penicillin G or ampicillin + gentamicin + metronidazole; ceftiofur and amikacin can be substituted for penicillin/ampicillin and gentamicin, respectively
Bowel (e.g. penetrating abdominal wounds, open drainage for septic peritonitis)	Penicillin G or ampicillin + gentamicin; ceftiofur and amikacin can be substituted for penicillin/ampicillin and gentamicin, respectively
Internal abscess	Penicillin G or ampicillin ± rifampin
Muscle	Penicillin G or ampicillin ± metronidazole (for *Clostridium* spp.)
Blood (i.e. septicemia) in neonates	Ampicillin/ceftiofur + amikacin. Concurrent treatment for endotoxemia is advised in foals with gram-negative sepsis treated with β-lactam drugs

* Empirical antimicrobial therapy instituted while awaiting bacterial culture and antimicrobial susceptibility testing results.

Note: Enrofloxacin and other fluoroquinolones are not recommended for use in foals.

concentration are repeated, any wounds are further explored and debrided, and bacterial culture and antimicrobial sensitivity testing is repeated. The treatment plan is then adjusted accordingly with a change of drug, dosage, and/or delivery route. Such changes may also be necessary if signs of drug toxicity develop during treatment.

Even when the patient responds well to the chosen antimicrobial drug(s), it is wise to repeat culture and sensitivity testing at least once during prolonged antimicrobial therapy (i.e. treatment continuing for 3 weeks or more) and within a week of discontinuing treatment for polymicrobial infections or infections involving multidrug-resistant organisms.

Monitoring antimicrobial drug resistance and responsible antimicrobial drug use

It is recommended that hospitals establish a biosecurity program whereby trends in resistance of particular bacteria to commonly used antimicrobial drugs for both therapeutic and prophylactic use is monitored. Monitoring for methicillin-resistant *S. aureus* (MRSA) and extended-spectrum β-lactamase bacteria is important. It is recommended that patients infected with these types of bacteria are isolated from the general hospital population. At a minimum, wearing gloves and appropriate hand washing is critical to prevent the spread of resistant bacteria and to prevent nosocomial infection.

Use of highly effective antimicrobial drugs such as imipenem (p. 725) and vancomycin (p. 731) should be reserved for patients with an infection that is caused by bacteria that are resistant to other antimicrobial drugs and documented sensitivity to these antimicrobial drugs. Use of such antimicrobial drugs should be monitored by a hospital biosecurity committee to ensure appropriate use of these drugs in large hospitals.

Adjunctive immunotherapy

Antimicrobial therapy is most effective in patients with a competent immune system. In fact, immunocompromise presents a great challenge in the management of serious infections. With the exception of hyperimmune plasma for FPT, treatment of endotoxemia, or prevention of specific infections (e.g. *Rhodococcus equi*),

immunotherapy is not widely used nor extensively studied in the horse. Two strategies that are used in other species to augment the patient's own immune resources in the face of overwhelming bacterial infection are described below. Other immunotherapeutic strategies in horses and foals requiring emergency or critical care are less well supported at this time.

Supplemental immunoglobulins

A strategy that is used in human medicine to treat serious bacterial infections is to combine IV administration of pooled human immunoglobulins with IV antimicrobial drugs. Clinically, this combination has been shown to have a synergistic effect, greatly improving treatment efficacy over antimicrobial drug use alone.[17]

Commercial equine immunoglobulin products are widely available for parenteral use in adult horses and foals. Examples include Seramune®, Immuno-Glo™ and High-Glo™, and Hypermune. Although not yet studied in horses, this treatment approach may prove clinically valuable and cost-effective in the management of severe bacterial infections in critically ill patients.

Granulocyte colony-stimulating factor

Recombinant granulocyte colony-stimulating factor (G-CSF) is used in severely leukopenic patients, as it stimulates neutrophil and monocyte production and enhances the bacterial killing capacity of neutrophils.[18,19] It also inhibits the expression of tumor necrosis factor-α (TNF-α), which may limit the extension of tissue destruction without impairing bacterial killing capacity.[18] However, not all studies show a clear survival benefit of using G-CSF. One group of authors stated that this strategy may simply 'buy time' in severely septic patients, survival being primarily contingent on the management of associated metabolic abnormalities and organ dysfunction.[20]

Recombinant canine or bovine G-CSF has been studied to a limited extent in horses and foals.[21–23] Based on clinical experience with human recombinant G-CSF (filgrastim [Neupogen®]), a dosage of 5 μg/kg given slowly IV over 30 minutes and repeated every 24 hours as needed is recommended. Failure to respond is considered a very poor prognostic sign.

Alternative modes of delivery

In the majority of critically ill patients with documented bacterial infections, parenteral systemic antimicrobial therapy is indicated. Local or regional modes of delivery may also be advantageous in individual cases, based on the site of infection, the antimicrobial drug(s) chosen, and even the pathogen(s) involved.

Intrathecal injection

For infections involving a joint, tendon sheath, or bursa, injection of an appropriate antimicrobial drug into the synovial space following lavage can be a very effective adjunct to systemic antimicrobial therapy. At the dosages given in *Table 16.4*, supratherapeutic concentrations of drug are delivered directly to the synovial space. If the synovial membrane is largely intact, the structure acts as a temporary reservoir for the drug, thereby maximizing antimicrobial efficacy at the infection site. The dosages listed appear to be effective and well tolerated, causing minimal damage to the synovial membrane or articular cartilage. (See also Chapter 2.)

Regional perfusion

Regional perfusion involves IV or IO (intramedullary) delivery of the antimicrobial drug distal to a tourniquet. Dosages are given in *Table 16.4*. Efficacy is maximized with low doses of drug because local tissue levels 5–50 times higher than the MIC for susceptible pathogens are achieved through diffusion down a concentration

---

Table 16.4 Dosages for antimicrobial drugs administered locally or regionally in horses

ROUTE AND DRUG	DOSAGE
Intrathecal injection (joint, tendon sheath, bursa)	
Amikacin	500–1000 mg
Cefazolin	250–500 mg
Ceftiofur	150 mg
Gentamicin	150–500 mg
Na- or K-penicillin	2–5 million units
Regional perfusion of the distal limb (IV or IO [intramedullary])	
Amikacin	125–500 mg (up to 1 gram has been used safely)
Ampicillin	10–20 million units
Gentamicin	100–300 mg (up to 1 gram has been used safely)
Na- or K-penicillin	10–20 million units
Vancomycin	300 mg
Antimicrobial-impregnated PMMA beads	
Aminoglycosides, cephalosporins, penicillins, or vancomycin	1–4 grams per 20 grams of PMMA powder (use only one antimicrobial drug per batch of beads)

PMMA, polymethylmethacrylate.

Adapted from Whitehair *et al.*, 1992a, b[25,26]; Santschi *et al.*, 1998[35]; Anderson and Ethell, 1999[27], Scheuch *et al.*, 2002.[24]

gradient from the vasculature to the interstitial space.[24] Compared with systemic administration of an equal or higher dose of the drug, regional perfusion achieves much higher tissue and synovial fluid concentrations of drug at the site.[24–26] Therapeutic concentrations of antimicrobial drug can even be achieved in poorly vascularized or necrotic tissue.[27]

Regional perfusion is primarily used for infections at or below the level of the carpus or tarsus, as venous outflow proximal to the infected area must be occluded during the procedure. (See also Chapter 2.)

Antimicrobial-impregnated implants

Various materials may be combined with antimicrobial drugs to create an antimicrobial-impregnated implant; they include polymethylmethacrylate (PMMA) beads, cancellous bone, collagen sponges, plaster of Paris, and other polymers. These implants are another means of effectively delivering therapeutic concentrations of antimicrobial drug to the site of infection while minimizing systemic concentrations and thus drug cost and toxicity. Higher local tissue concentrations of the drug can be achieved with this method than with systemic administration at recommended dosages.[27,28]

Antimicrobial-impregnated implants are of particular value in the treatment of infected wounds that have a poor blood supply or contain surgical implants that must remain in place. By implanting the antimicrobial-impregnated material in the wound, therapeutic concentrations of the antimicrobial drug are delivered directly to the target tissues. Continuous release of the drug from the implant sustains therapeutic concentrations in surrounding tissues for several days and in some cases for weeks or months, depending on the elution characteristics of the antimicrobial-implant combination.[27,28] The use of antimicrobial-impregnated implants also allows the use of drugs that would be cost-prohibitive for systemic administration in the horse.[28] The antimicrobial drugs that have been used with good effect in polymethylmethacrylate implants are listed in *Table 16.4*. (See also Chapter 2.)

ANTIMICROBIAL DRUGS

Antimicrobial drugs are discussed in alphabetical order.

Aminoglycosides

Key points

- Aminoglycosides are active against some gram-positive bacteria, including some staphylococci, and many gram-negative bacteria.
- They are concentration-dependent drugs and have a post-antibiotic effect, so once a day dosing can be used.
- Aminoglycosides are well distributed in the extracelluar fluid, including synovial fluid, but they do not penetrate most tissues well and are less effective in hypoxic or inflamed tissues.
- Aminoglycosides are potentially nephrotoxic, so they should be avoided or used with caution in hypovolemic or hypotensive patients and those in renal failure.
- Fluid support should be provided and serum creatinine and (if possible) drug concentrations monitored in at-risk patients

Definition/mechanism of action

Aminoglycosides are glycosides with an amino substituent. They work by binding to the bacterial 30S ribosomal subunit (some work by binding to the 50S subunit), inhibiting the translocation of the peptidyl-tRNA from the A-site to the P-site and also causing misreading of mRNA, leaving the bacterium unable to synthesize proteins vital to its growth.

Aminoglycosides include amikacin, gentamicin, kanamycin, neomycin, streptomycin, tobramycin, and a few others. At recommended dosages, they are bactericidal drugs, which all have similar antimicrobial, pharmacokinetic, and toxic profiles.

Indications

With the exception of streptomycin (which is mostly active against gram-negative bacteria), aminoglycosides are active against some gram-positive bacteria, including some staphylococci, and many gram-negative bacteria. Susceptible organisms include *Escherichia coli* and *Acinetobacter*, *Enterobacter*, *Klebsiella*, *Proteus*, and *Salmonella* spp. Amikacin, gentamicin, and tobramycin also are active against *Pseudomonas aeruginosa*. Anaerobes generally are resistant to the aminoglycosides, but aminoglycosides are synergistic with β-lactam drugs (penicillins, cephalosporins, imipenem).[36] However, aminoglycosides should not be mixed in the same syringe or solution with β-lactam drugs.

Clinical use

Aminoglycosides are concentration-dependent antimicrobial drugs; they need only a short contact time to kill susceptible bacteria, provided that the dose given yields drug levels 10–12 times higher than the MIC for the target pathogen at the site of infection. Aminoglycosides also have a post-antibiotic effect, so extended dosing intervals (e.g. every 24 hours) can be used with good clinical effect and less risk of toxicity. Recommended dosages are given in *Table 16.5*.

Aminoglycosides are well distributed in the extracelluar fluid. Following systemic administration, therapeutic levels generally are achieved in synovial, pleural, and peritoneal fluids, especially if inflammation is present. However, aminoglycosides do not penetrate well into CSF, ocular fluids, milk, intestinal fluids, fetal tissues, or amniotic fluid. Neither do they penetrate most tissues well, except for the kidneys where they accumulate in the renal cortex. Aminoglycosides are rendered less effective in hypoxic tissues and in acidic environments such as sites of circulatory compromise or inflammation.[36]

Changes in extracellular fluid volume or distribution can affect the pharmacokinetics, increasing the potential for toxicity or decreasing drug efficacy. Aminoglycosides are eliminated by the kidney via glomerular filtration. A variable amount is resorbed by the renal tubule cells and excessive accumulation can lead to renal tubular necrosis. Aminoglycosides must, therefore, be avoided or used with caution in hypovolemic or hypotensive patients and those in renal failure. Fluid support should be provided concurrently in at-risk patients.[36]

Neonates: Neonates require special consideration. The extracellular fluid compartment relative to body weight is greater in neonates than in adults, so higher initial doses of aminoglycosides may be required in neonates to achieve target plasma concentrations (see Monitoring). At the same time, renal elimination rates may be lower in neonates, making toxicity more likely at the dosing intervals commonly used in adults.[36]

Based on serum drug monitoring, underdosing with amikacin is common in critically ill neonatal foals, particularly hypoxic premature foals and any neonatal foal receiving aggressive fluid therapy. Increasing both the dose and the dosing interval may be needed in these patients.[37,38] While there does not appear to

---

Table 16.5 Recommended systemic dosages for the aminoglycosides in horses and foals

DRUG	DOSAGE	COMMENTS
Amikacin	15–25 mg/kg IV or IM q24h	IV route is preferred.
Gentamicin	6.6 mg/kg IV or IM q24h	Maintain hydration throughout treatment.
		Avoid if possible in patients with renal compromise.
		Monitor BUN and creatinine in systemically compromised patients.
		DO NOT USE in patients with neuromuscular weakness (e.g. botulism).
		Amikacin is preferred over gentamicin in foals
Neomycin	8–20 mg/kg PO q8h, q12h, or q24h	Used primarily to decrease enteric ammonia production.
		Prolonged administration (>3 doses) or higher doses may cause diarrhea

Adapted from Spurlock and Hanie, 1989[39] and Wilson, 2001.[14]

be an association between sepsis score and amikacin pharmacokinetics in neonatal foals, concurrent hypoxia and azotemia decrease amikacin clearance and thus increase both peak and trough serum concentrations in these patients.[37]

Monitoring: Serum creatinine concentrations and, where possible, peak and trough aminoglycoside concentrations should be monitored in susceptible patients and drug dosages adjusted accordingly. Recommended peak serum concentrations for patients with severe gram-negative infections are >40 µg/ml for gentamicin and >60 µg/ml for amikacin (30 minutes post administration); trough serum concentrations for either drug should be <2 µg/ml (8–12 hours post administration).

Complications

Owing to their potential nephrotoxicity, aminoglycosides can cause renal failure. In addition to dosage, factors that predispose to aminoglycoside nephrotoxicosis include: age (young foals and geriatric patients are at high risk); renal insufficiency; prolonged duration of treatment; dehydration or hypovolemia from other causes (e.g. sepsis and endotoxemia); acidosis; and concurrent administration of other potentially nephrotoxic drugs or furosemide.[36] If aminoglycoside therapy must be used or continued in a patient with renal compromise, the guidelines given in *Table 16.6* are suggested when therapeutic drug monitoring is not available.

Aminoglycosides are also ototoxic (both auditory and vestibular dysfunction are possible) and they can cause neuromuscular blockade when used concurrently with skeletal muscle relaxants or gaseous anesthetics.[36] These toxic effects appear to be uncommon in horses.

Cephalosporins
Key points
- Cephalosporins are similar to penicillins in many respects, including spectrum of activity, susceptibility to bacterial β-lactamases, and incompatibility with other drugs.
- Cephalosporins are widely distributed in most body fluids and tissues, including joints and bone.
- The gram-negative spectrum is wider with the newer generation cephalosporins, but at the expense of the gram-positive spectrum.
- Ceftiofur is a third-generation drug, but it has a gram-negative spectrum more like the first-generation drugs and activity against *Staphylococcus* species is unpredictable.
- Ceftiofur dosages 2–5 times higher than the label recommendations are frequently used in critically ill equine patients.
- Adverse effects are uncommon, although ceftiofur has been implicated as a cause of diarrhea in horses.

Table 16.6 Guidelines for use of aminoglycosides in patients with renal failure based on plasma creatinine concentration

PLASMA CREATININE (µmol/l) (mg/dl)	DOSE AND DOSING INTERVAL
≤88.4 (1)	Full dose at usual dosing interval
176.8 (2)	Full dose but double the usual dosing interval
265.2 (3)	Full dose but triple the usual dosing interval
353.6 (4)	Halve the dose and double the usual dosing interval
≥442 (5)	*Do not use aminoglycosides*

Note: Aminoglycosides are usually avoided in horses with signs of renal failure and monitoring of peak and trough aminoglycoside concentrations is recommended.

Definition/mechanism of action

Cephalosporins are a large class of β–lactam antimicrobial drugs that are similar to the penicillins in many respects, including spectrum and susceptibility to bacterial β-lactamases. Cephalosporins act by disrupting the synthesis of the peptidoglycan layer of bacterial cell walls, which is important for cell wall structural integrity.

Indications

Individual cephalosporins have been grouped by generation, reflecting their evolution. In general, the gram-negative spectrum is wider with the newer generations than with the older cephalosporins, but at the expense of the gram-positive spectrum. Resistance to β-lactamases also tends to increase from one generation to the next. Owing to their cost, only a few of the cephalosporins are used in equine medicine.

First-generation cephalosporins: First-generation cephalosporins include cefazolin, cephalexin, cephalothin, and cephapirin. This group of cephalosporins is active against most gram-positive aerobes, but only moderately active against gram-negative organisms. Enteric streptococci (enterococci) and some staphylococci may be resistant, while some strains of *Escherichia coli* and *Proteus*, *Klebsiella*, *Salmonella*, and *Enterobacter* spp. are susceptible. Like penicillin G, these cephalosporins are susceptible to β-lactamases, but unlike the penicillins they are not very effective against anaerobes, including *Bacteroides fragilis*.[36]

Second-generation cephalosporins: Second-generation cephalosporins include cefoxitin, cefuroxime, and several others. Compared with the first-generation drugs, they have greater activity against gram-negative bacteria, but are less active against gram-positive bacteria. They are ineffective against enterococci, *Pseudomonas aeruginosa*, and many obligate anaerobes. They are, however, relatively resistant to β-lactamases.[36]

Third-generation cephalosporins: Third-generation cephalosporins include cefoperazone, cefotaxime, ceftazidime, ceftiofur, and ceftriaxone. In general, they have only moderate activity against gram-positive bacteria, but they are active against a wide variety of gram-negative bacteria, including some strains of *Pseudomonas*, *Proteus*, *Enterobacter*, and *Citrobacter* spp. They usually are highly resistant to β-lactamases and some (notably cefotaxime) readily penetrate the blood–brain barrier.[36]

Ceftiofur is the cephalosporin that is most widely used in horses. It is a third-generation drug, but it has a gram-negative spectrum that is more like the first-generation drugs, and activity against *Staphylococcus* spp. is unpredictable.[36] Dosages 2–5 times higher than the label recommendations are frequently used in critically ill equine patients. Cefoperazone, in contrast, has gram-positive activity similar to the first-generation drugs with the extended gram-negative activity of the third-generation drugs. It is one of the only cephalosporins that are routinely effective against *Pseudomonas* spp.

Fourth-generation cephalosporins: Fourth-generation cephalosporins used in horses include cefquinome and cefepime. Cefquinome has been developed for veterinary use and is approved in horses to treat respiratory infections caused by *Streptococcus equi* subsp. *zooepidemicus* and to treat foals with *Escherichia coli* sepsis. It has an extended spectrum of activity with improved inhibition of gram-positive bacteria and improved β-lactamase stability. It has excellent *in-vitro* activity against most *Enterobacteriaceae* and hemolytic streptococci, good activity against methicillin-sensitive *Staphylococcus aureus*, moderate to low activity against MRSA and *Pseudomonas aeruginosa*; and almost no activity against gram-negative anaerobes.[40]

Cefepime has a broad spectrum of activity against gram-positive and gram-negative bacteria. It is a poor inducer of and has increased stability from β-lactamases.[41] Cefepime is effective against many gram-negative bacteria and *Pseudomonas aeruginosa*. It has variable activity against anaerobic bacteria and is not effective against methicillin-resistant staphylococci and enterococci.[41]

Clinical use

In general, cephalosporins are bactericidal against susceptible bacteria at the recommended dosages (*Table 16.7*).

Cephalosporins are widely distributed in most body fluids and tissues, including joints and bone, and are particularly useful for treating septic arthritis or osteomyelitis caused by susceptible organisms. However, with the exception of some of the third- and fourth-generation drugs, penetration into the CSF is poor, even when inflammation compromises the blood–brain barrier.[36]

Most cephalosporins are excreted by renal tubular secretion, although glomerular filtration is important with some (e.g. cephalexin and cefazolin). Thus, dosages should be reduced in patients with renal failure. Dosage modifications may also be required in patients with hepatic disease. Incompatibilities with other drugs and solutions are similar to those described for the penicillins.[36]

Complications

Cephalosporins are relatively non-toxic. Laboratory aberrations that may occur with their use variably include increases in serum ALP, AST, LDH, and BUN concentrations compared with normal, glucosuria, and a false-positive Coombs test.[36] IM injections can be painful. Ceftiofur has been implicated in the development of diarrhea in horses.

Table 16.7 Recommended systemic dosages for the cephalosporins in horses and foals

DRUG	DOSAGE	COMMENTS
Cefazolin	11–22 mg/kg IV q6h, q8h, or q12h	First-generation
Cefepime	11 mg/kg IV q8h (foals)	Fourth-generation
Cefoperazone	30 mg/kg IV q8h	Third-generation
Cefotaxime	40–50 mg/kg IV q6h or q8h	Third-generation
Cefquinome	1.0–2.5 mg/kg IV q12h (MIC<0.125 µg/ml). 4.5 mg/kg IV q12h (MIC 0.125–0.5 µg/ml)	Fourth-generation
Ceftazidime	20–40 mg/kg IV or IM q6h, q8h, or q12h	Third-generation
Ceftiofur	2.2–4.4 mg/kg IM q24h (label dose). 5–10 mg/kg IV or IM q12h or 1–5 mg/kg q6h, q8h, or q12h for gram-negative infections. Dosages up to 8 mg/kg IV q8h used in critical care patients	Third-generation. Label dose based on studies using highly susceptible ß-hemolytic streptococci. Higher dose (2–5 times label dose) recommended for other susceptible pathogens (e.g. *Escherichia coli*). Kinetic profile slightly better for IM than for IV, but high IM doses are irritating. Diarrhea is more likely with higher-than-label doses. Unstable in solution, so use within 12 hours or refrigerate unused portion and use within 7 days.
Excede®	6.6 mg/kg 1M or SC q4days (foals)	DO NOT give IV
Ceftriaxone	25–50 mg/kg IV or IM q12h	Third-generation
Cephalexin	25 mg/kg PO q6h	First-generation. **Note**: Oral route of administration
Cephalothin	20 mg/kg IV or IM q6h	First-generation
Cephapirin	20–30 mg/kg IV or IM q4h, q6h, or q8h	First-generation. Diarrhea and anaphylaxis have been reported

Note: Cephalosporins are compatible with aminoglycosides in the patient, but they **must not be mixed** in the same solution or syringe.

Adapted from Spurlock and Hanie, 1989[39], Wilson, 2001[14], Smiet *et al.*, 2012.[40]

Chloramphenicol

Key points

- Chloramphenicol is rarely used in equine emergency and critical care; however, it can be useful when long-term oral antimicrobial therapy is needed.
- Chloramphenicol can be used to treat *Lawsonia intracellularis*, the agent that causes proliferative enteropathy in foals.

Definition/mechanism of action

Chloramphenicol is a bacteriostatic antimicrobial drug that acts by inhibiting bacterial protein synthesis.

Indications

Chloramphenicol has a very broad spectrum of activity. It is active against gram-positive bacteria (including most strains of MRSA), gram-negative bacteria, and anaerobes. It is not active against *Pseudomonas aeruginosa* or *Enterobacter* spp.

Chloramphenicol is seldom used in equine practice. It is included here because it is one of the few drugs that is effective against *Bacteroides fragilis* and against many strains of *Salmonella* species.[36] It also appears to be effective against *Lawsonia intracellularis*, the agent that causes proliferative enteropathy in foals.[42] While merely bacteriostatic at recommended dosages, it is effective against intracellular organisms. However, resistance to chloramphenicol is often accompanied by resistance to tetracyclines, erythromycin, ampicillin, and several other antimicrobial drugs.[36]

Clinical use

The recommended dosage of chloramphenicol is 40–60 mg/kg PO q6–8h.[14,39] Chloramphenicol is poorly absorbed orally and has a very short half-life when given intravenously.

Complications

Complications associated with chloramphenicol use in horses are rare. However, care should be taken when administering chloramphenicol and gloves worn because it has been associated with aplastic anemia in humans. This effect is rare and is generally fatal.

Enrofloxacin

Key points

- Enrofloxacin is rapidly bactericidal and has a post-antibiotic effect.
- It is active against a wide range of gram-negative bacteria and several gram-positive aerobes, including some staphylococci and streptococci.
- It is effective against most enteric pathogens except obligate anaerobes and most group D enterococci (e.g. *Enterococcus faecalis* and *Enterococcus faecium*).
- Enrofloxacin penetrates tissues (including bone) well and can be administered PO and by IV or IM injection.
- Fluoroquinolones should be avoided in pregnant or lactating mares and in horses under 18 months of age.

Definition/mechanism of action

Enrofloxacin is a synthetic chemotherapeutic agent and a member of the fluoroquinolone group of antimicrobial drugs. Its mechanism of action is thought to be inhibition of bacterial DNA-gyrase (a type-II topoisomerase) and subsequent prevention of DNA supercoiling and synthesis.

Indications

Enrofloxacin is active against a wide range of gram-negative bacteria and several gram-positive aerobes, including some staphylococci and streptococci. It is considered highly effective against most enteric pathogens, with the exception of obligate anaerobes and most group D enterococci (e.g. *Enterococcus faecalis* and *Enterococcus faecium*). It is, however, synergistic with the β-lactam drugs, aminoglycosides, and metronidazole.[36]

Clinical use

Enrofloxacin is rapidly bactericidal at dosages of 5–7.5 mg/kg IV or PO q24h and has a significant post-antibiotic effect against susceptible organisms, including *Escherichia coli*, *Klebsiella pneumoniae*, and *Pseudomonas aeruginosa*.[14,39] Enrofloxacin should be reserved for treatment of gram-negative or staphylococcal infections that are resistant to other antimicrobial drugs.

Interestingly, fluoroquinolones often have a significant antibacterial effect at very low concentrations (often at <1 µg/ml), but efficacy tends to diminish at concentrations >10 µg/ml.[36]

Enrofloxacin is well absorbed following oral administration, although the presence of food in the stomach may delay absorption and concurrent use of antacids may interfere with absorption. Enrofloxacin may also be administered IV, IM, or SC. Regardless of the route of administration, it penetrates all tissues well, including bone and CSF.

Enrofloxacin is excreted primarily via the kidneys; both glomerular filtration and tubular secretion are involved. Clearance is thus impaired in patients in renal failure, so a reduction in dosage is needed in these patients.[36]

Complications

As it can cause cartilage erosions in immature animals, enrofloxacin should be avoided in horses <18 months of age. For the same reason, it should also be avoided in pregnant or lactating mares, as it readily crosses the placental and mammary barriers. Embryonic loss is another possibility in pregnant animals treated with high doses of quinolones.[36] Possible alterations in laboratory indices with use in any patient include increases in serum ALP, AST, and BUN concentrations compared with normal.[36]

Imipenem (with cilastatin)

Key points

- Imipenem is bactericidal against a wide range of aerobic and anaerobic gram-positive and gram-negative organisms, including several multidrug-resistant enteric pathogens.
- Even so, its use should be limited to cases of documented infection with multidrug-resistant organisms, to avoid the development of imipenem resistance in equine pathogens.
- Dosage adjustments may be needed in neonates and patients with renal compromise.
- Imipenem may worsen endotoxemia in patients with gram-negative sepsis, so concurrent treatment for endotoxemia is advised.

Definition/mechanism of action

Imipenem (with cilastatin) is a β-lactam antimicrobial drug of the carbapenem group. Its mechanism of action is through inhibiting cell wall synthesis of various gram-positive and gram-negative bacteria. It remains very stable in the presence of β-lactamase (both penicillinase and cephalosporinase) produced by some bacteria, and is a strong inhibitor of beta-lactamases from some gram-negative bacteria that are resistant to most β-lactam antimicrobial drugs. Because it is rapidly degraded by the renal enzyme dehydropeptidase when administered alone, imipenem is always co-administered with cilastatin to prevent inactivation.

Indications

Imipenem is bactericidal against a wide range of aerobic and anaerobic gram-positive and gram-negative organisms, including multidrug-resistant enteric pathogens (*Escherichia coli*, *Klebsiella* spp., *Salmonella* spp.), *Pseudomonas aeruginosa*, and *Bacteroides fragilis*. Some strains of MRSA, *Enterococcus faecium*, and *Clostridium difficile* are naturally resistant, but so far the development of resistance to imipenem is very limited and is mostly confined to strains of *Pseudomonas aeruginosa*.[36,43]

Because of its potency and broad spectrum of activity, imipenem is widely used in human critical care, especially in patients with immunocompromise, severe burns, polymicrobial infections, infections caused by unidentified bacteria, or infections caused by multidrug-resistant bacteria. It is even used as empiric monotherapy in these patients. However, overuse of imipenem and the subsequent development of drug resistance in currently imipenem-susceptible pathogens is of real concern in human medicine.

Imipenem use should be limited to cases with documented infections with multidrug-resistant organisms.

Clinical use

The recommended dosage for imipenem (with cilastatin) is 10–15 mg/kg IV q6–8h. Imipenem (with cilastatin) should be given slowly and diluted in fluids. It is a time-dependent antimicrobial drug. A dosing interval of 6 hours is recommended based on pharmacokinetic studies in horses.[43] When the MIC for a specific pathogen is very low, less frequent dosing may be effective. For susceptible pathogens in which the MIC is >1 µg/ml, CRI may be superior, in both efficacy and cost, to periodic dosing. An infusion rate of 16 µg/kg/minute is suggested, for a total daily dose of 23 mg/kg.[43]

Imipenem cannot be used with penicillins or cephalosporins, but can be used with amikacin.

While toxicity is low, imipenem is eliminated primarily via the kidneys, so the dosing interval should be increased to 8–12 hours (depending on the severity of renal compromise) in patients with renal insufficiency.[43]

Although not yet studied in foals, the pharmacokinetics of imipenem in humans is different in neonates than in adults because of the greater volume of distribution and the lower renal clearance rate in neonates compared with adults. Dosages may need to be adjusted accordingly in neonates.

The pharmacokinetics may be different from expected in critically ill horses, both adults and neonates. In critically ill human patients, such as those with severe hypovolemia, endotoxemia, serious infections, multiorgan failure, or extensive severe burns, imipenem pharmacokinetics are highly variable among individuals and are unpredictable.

Complications

In an *in-vitro* study of equine neonatal gram-negative sepsis it was found that imipenem induced a greater degree of endotoxin production and synthesis of TNF-α than did amikacin. Concurrent treatment for endotoxemia is recommended when using imipenem to treat gram-negative sepsis in foals.[12]

Macrolides

Key points

- Macrolides are used most often in combination with rifampin for the treatment of *Rhodococcus equi* infection in foals.
- Macrolides are also used for treatment of proliferative enteropathy (enteric infection with *Lawsonia intracellularis*) in foals and weanlings.
- Adverse effects associated with macrolide antimicrobial use include potentially fatal enterocolitis in adults and hyperthermia in foals.

Definition/mechanism of action

The macrolides are a group of antimicrobial drugs whose activity stems from the presence of a macrolide ring. The mechanism of action of the macrolides is inhibition of bacterial protein biosynthesis by binding irreversibly to the subunit 50S of the bacterial ribosome, thus inhibiting translocation of peptidyl tRNA.

Indications

Macrolides generally are active against most aerobic and anaerobic gram-positive bacteria. They are not active against most gram-negative bacteria, although gram-negative organisms without cell walls usually are sensitive. *Bacteroides fragilis* is moderately susceptible. Cross-resistance among macrolides is common.[36]

Macrolides are used most often in equine practice for the treatment of *Rhodococcus equi* infection in foals (in combination with rifampin). A second emerging use is for proliferative enteropathy (enteric infection with *Lawsonia intracellularis*) in foals and weanlings.[42] Use of the macrolides in equine medicine is otherwise limited by their activity, spectrum, and potential for adverse effects.

Clinical use

Macrolides used in horses and foals include erythromycin, azithromycin, and clarithromycin. Dosages are listed in *Table 16.8*. These drugs are bacteriostatic in action, although at high concentrations erythromycin may be bactericidal.

Complications

Adverse effects associated with macrolide antimicrobial use include potentially fatal enterocolitis in adults and hyperthermia in foals.

Metronidazole

Key points

- Metronidazole is active against both protozoa and bacteria, especially obligate anaerobes.
- It is not active against most facultative anaerobes or aerobes.

Definition/mechanism of action

Metronidazole is a nitroimidazole antimicrobial drug used mainly in the treatment of infections caused by susceptible organisms, particularly anaerobic bacteria and protozoa. Metronidazole is a prodrug. It is converted in anaerobic organisms by the redox enzyme pyruvate-ferredoxin oxidoreductase. The nitro group of metronidazole is chemically reduced by ferredoxin and the products disrupt the DNA helical structure and inhibit nucleic acid synthesis.

Indications

Metronidazole is active against both protozoa and bacteria, especially obligate anaerobes, although it is not active against most facultative anaerobes or aerobes. It is bactericidal against *Bacteroides fragilis*, *Fusobacterium* spp., and clostridia, including *Clostridium perfringens* and most strains of *Clostridium difficile*.[36] However, metronidazole-resistant strains of pathogenic *Clostridium difficile* have recently been reported in horses in an intensive care facility.[44]

Clinical use

Metronidazole is administered at a dosage of 15–25 mg/kg PO q6–8h or 15–20 mg/kg IV q8–12h. Dosing intervals should be extended in patients with hepatic insufficiency and foals <1 week of age.[36]

Metronidazole is rapidly absorbed following oral administration, although bioavailability is variable (60–100%). It is widely distributed in all tissues, even penetrating the blood–brain barrier and reaching therapeutic concentrations in abscesses.[36] Metronidazole can be administered per rectum if the oral route is contraindicated, although bioavailability reportedly is only 50% of that for oral administration.

Complications

Adverse effects are uncommon, although inappetence or anorexia occurs in some patients. In these patients, metronidazole can be given rectally using the oral dosage. Neurologic signs have been reported when recommended dosages are exceeded or with rapid IV administration. Diarrhea has also been observed in some horses.

Table 16.8 Recommended dosages for macrolides used systemically in horses and foals

DRUG	DOSAGE	COMMENTS
Azithromycin	10 mg/kg PO q24h for 5 days then q48h	Better bioavailability and longer half-life than erythromycin
Clarithromycin	7.5 mg/kg PO q12h	Risk of colitis in adults
Erythromycin	25–30 mg/kg PO q6h, q8h, or q12h	Use with caution in patients older than 5 months of age (risk of drug-induced enterocolitis). May increase serum theophylline concentrations to toxic levels with concurrent administration

Adapted from Spurlock and Hanie, 1989[39] and Wilson, 2001.[14]

Penicillins

Key points

- Penicillins are frequently indicated in equine patients.
- Penicillin G is active against many aerobic and anaerobic gram-positive bacteria, but only a few gram-negative bacteria.
- Ampicillin and amoxicillin are active against many gram-positive and gram-negative bacteria, but they are readily inactivated by β-lactamases unless potentiated with clavulanate or sulbactam.
- Penicillins are time-dependent antimicrobial drugs, so the dosing interval is important in clinical efficacy.
- Most penicillins are unstable in solution and they should not be mixed with other drugs (aminoglycosides) or added to acidic or basic solutions.

Definition/mechanism of action

Penicillins are a large group of β-lactam antimicrobial drugs that act by inhibiting the formation of peptidoglycan cross-links in the bacterial cell wall. They can be categorized according to their spectrum and susceptibility to bacterial enzymes (i.e. β-lactamases) as narrow-spectrum, broad-spectrum, or potentiated penicillins.

Indications

Narrow-spectrum penicillins: Narrow-spectrum, β-lactamase-susceptible penicillins include penicillin G (benzylpenicillin) and penicillin V. These penicillins are active against many aerobic and anaerobic gram-positive bacteria, but only a few gram-negative bacteria. Despite its good anaerobic spectrum, penicillin G is not effective against most strains of *Bacteroides fragilis*. Organisms of clinical relevance in equine practice that are usually susceptible *in vitro* to penicillin G include streptococci, penicillin-sensitive staphylococci, and clostridia.[36]

The narrow-spectrum, β-lactamase-resistant penicillins include oxacillin, methicillin, and several others. They are more resistant to β-lactamases than penicillin G, making them active against many (but not all) penicillin-resistant staphylococci, including *Staphylococcus aureus* and *Staphylococcus epidermidis*. However, they are less active against many other gram-positive bacteria and they are inactive against almost all gram-negative bacteria.[36]

Broad-spectrum penicillins: Broad-spectrum, β-lactamase-susceptible penicillins include ampicillin and amoxicillin. They are active against many gram-positive and gram-negative bacteria, but they are readily inactivated by β-lactamases (unless potentiated). Susceptible genera include *Clostridium, Corynebacterium, Escherichia, Klebsiella, Pasteurella, Proteus, Salmonella, Staphylococcus,* and *Streptococcus*. Carbenicillin, ticarcillin, and piperacillin are examples of other penicillins in this group that have extended spectra, being also active against *Pseudomonas aeruginosa* and certain resistant strains of *Proteus, Klebsiella,* and *Enterobacter*.[36]

Potentiated penicillins: Potentiated penicillins have the broadest gram-positive and gram-negative spectra of the penicillins because of the addition and protection of β-lactamase-inhibiting compounds such as clavulanate or sulbactam. These penicillins include amoxicillin-clavulanate, ticarcillin-clavulanate, and ampicillin-sulbactam. Ticarcillin-clavulanate has been used to treat bacteremia in foals, either alone or in combination with amikacin. However, it does not have as broad a spectrum as imipenem or some of the third- or fourth-generation cephalosporins.

Clinical use

At the dosages recommended in *Table 16.9*, penicillins are generally bactericidal against susceptible bacteria. Penicillins are time-dependent antimicrobial drugs, meaning that their efficacy is linked to the amount of time that plasma/tissue drug concentrations remain above the MIC for the infecting bacteria. Therefore, the dosing interval is important in clinical efficacy.

Penicillins are widely distributed in body fluids and tissues, although concentrations tend to be low in poorly perfused areas such as the cornea, bronchial secretions, cartilage, and bone. Penicillins do not readily cross the blood–brain, placental, or mammary barrier unless there is inflammation present. Inflammation also allows effective concentrations of penicillins to be reached in abscesses.[36]

The main route of elimination is the kidney. Broad-spectrum penicillins may also be excreted via the biliary pathway. About 20% of renal excretion occurs by glomerular filtration and the remaining 80% by tubular secretion. Thus, oliguric or anuric renal failure increases the plasma half-life. Also, clearance may be considerably lower in neonates than in adults.[36]

Penicillins are somewhat unstable in solution, so most require reconstitution with a diluent just before administration. They are also sensitive to extremes in pH, which should be borne in mind when administering with acidic or basic solutions. In fact, several of the penicillins are physically incompatible with many different drugs and solutions, including aminoglycosides, so penicillins should be administered separately.

Potassium penicillin G should be given slowly when administered IV, particularly in hyperkalemic patients.[36]

Complications

Adverse effects to penicillins are uncommon in horses, with the exception of procaine penicillin G, which can cause CNS excitation. However, alterations in some laboratory indices may occur with penicillin administration. They variably include increases in serum ALP and AST, eosinophilia, glucosuria, proteinuria, and a false-positive Coombs test.[36]

Rifampin
Key points
- Rifampin is effective against susceptible intracellular organisms such as *Rhodoccocus equi* and probably *Lawsonia intracellularis*.
- Rifampin resistance can develop rapidly, so it should always be used in combination with another antimicrobial drug.

Definition/mechanism of action
Rifampin is a bactericidal antibiotic drug of the rifamycin group that inhibits DNA-dependent RNA polymerase in bacterial cells by binding to its beta-subunit and preventing transcription to RNA and subsequent translation to proteins.

Indications
Rifampin is active against gram-positive organisms, a few gram-negative cocci, and some anaerobes. It has excellent tissue and cell membrane penetration, so it is effective against susceptible intracellular organisms such as *Rodoccocus equi* and probably *Lawsonia intracellularis*.[42]

Table 16.9 Recommended systemic dosages for the penicillins in horses and foals

DRUG	DOSAGE	COMMENTS
Ampicillin sodium	15–20 mg/kg IV q6h, q8h, or q12h	Reconstitute with sterile water or saline (not dextrose) and use immediately.
Ampicillin trihydrate	11–22 mg/kg IV or IM q8h or q12h	
Na- or K-penicillin G (crystalline penicillin)	22,000–44,000 IU/kg IV or IM q4h, q6h, q8h, or q12h 4–11 IU/Kg/hour CRI	Give K-pen SLOWLY (over 15 minutes) when using IV route.
Oxacillin	20–40 mg/kg IV q6h or q8h	
Procaine penicillin G	15,000–44,000 IU/kg IM q12h	DO NOT GIVE IV. Potential for CNS excitation even with IM administration. Give no more than 15 ml per site per dose
Ticarcillin	50–100 mg/kg IV or IM q6h or q8h	
Ticarcillin-clavulanate	50–200 mg/kg IV q6h or q8h or 100 mg/kg IV loading dose, then 50 mg/kg IV q6h	Irritating if given IM

Note: Penicillis are compatible with aminoglycosides in the patient, but DO NOT MIX in the same solution or syringe.

Adapted from Spurlock and Hanie, 1989[39] and Wilson, 2001.[14]

Clinical use

The recommended dosage of rifampin is 5–10 mg/kg PO q12h.[14,39] It is active even at low pH and in the presence of purulent material. However, resistance can develop rapidly, so rifampin should always be used in combination with another antimicrobial drug such as penicillin or a macrolide.[36]

Complications

Rifampin is neither practical to use nor well accepted by horses. It may cause inappetence and in adults diarrhea. Rifampin can increase the rate of elimination of theophylline and diazepam in foals.

Tetracycline

Key points

- Tetracyclines are active against both aerobic and anaerobic gram-positive and gram-negative bacteria, mycoplasmae, rickettsiae, chlamydiae, and some protozoa.
- Tetracyclines are primarily used in equine practice to treat rickettsial infections.
- Oxytetracycline is potentially nephrotoxic at high doses in hypovolemic patients and in patients with renal failure.

Definition/mechanism of action

Tetracycline is a broad-spectrum polyketide antibiotic produced by *Streptomyces* bacteria and indicated for use against many bacterial infections. It works by inhibiting action of the prokaryotic 30S ribosome, by binding aminoacyl-tRNA.

Indications

Tetracyclines all have a similar broad-spectrum profile, being active against both aerobic and anaerobic gram-positive and gram-negative bacteria, mycoplasmae, rickettsiae, chlamydiae, and some protozoa. However, they are merely bacteriostatic at the recommended dosages, and a number of important equine pathogens are resistant, including pathogenic strains of *Escherichia coli*, *Pseudomonas aeruginosa*, and *Proteus*, *Serratia*, *Klebsiella*, and *Corynebacterium* spp.[36]

Tetracyclines are primarily used in equine practice to treat rickettsial infections such as *Neorickettsia* (formerly *Ehrlichia*) *risticii*, which is the causal agent of Potomac horse fever, and *Anaplasma phagocytophilum* (formerly *Ehrlichia equi*).

A common non-antimicrobial use of oxytetracycline is the treatment of flexor deformity/contracture in neonatal foals, where doses as high as 3 grams per foal are used. However, care must be taken with this use as oxytetracycline is potentially nephrotoxic at high doses.

Oxytetracycline has begun to be used by practitioners as a matrix metalloproteinase inhibitor in horses with laminitis. Further study is required to validate its safety and efficacy for this purpose.

Clinical use

Oxytetracycline can be administered at a dosage of 6.6 mg/kg IV q12h. It must be given slowly IV and preferably diluted in fluids.[14,39] It cannot be given in fluids containing bicarbonate, magnesium, or calcium. Doxycycline can be administered at a dosage of 5–10 mg/kg PO q12h.

The dosage for oxytetracycline used to treated flexor contracture in foals is 30–60 mg/kg IV. The drug should be used only in foals that are well hydrated and have normal renal function, and it must first be diluted in fluids that do not contain bicarbonate, magnesium, or calcium. Subsequent doses, if needed, should be spaced at least 24 hours and preferably 48 hours apart, preceded by re-evaluation of renal function (BUN and creatinine concentrations), and limited to a total of three doses.

Complications

Oxytetracycline is potentially nephrotoxic at high doses in hypovolemic patients and in patients with renal failure. Oxytetracycline can cause hemolysis and hypotension (which can lead to collapse) when administered undiluted as an IV bolus.[36]

Trimethoprim-sulfonamides (potentiated sulfonamides)

Key points

- Use of trimethoprim-sulfonamide (potentiated sulfonamide) is not recommended for critically ill patients or patients with more serious conditions requiring emergency attention.
- Diarrhea can be a major complication associated with use of trimethoprim-sulfonamide.

Definition/mechanisms of action

Trimethoprim is a bacteriostatic antibiotic that acts by interfering with the action of bacterial dihydrofolate reductase, inhibiting synthesis of tetrahydrofolic acid. Tetrahydrofolic acid is an essential precursor in the *de novo* synthesis of the DNA nucleotide thymidine. Bacteria are unable to take up folic acid from the environment and are dependent on their own *de novo* synthesis. Inhibition of the enzyme starves the bacteria of nucleotides necessary for DNA replication.

Sulfonamides are synthetic bacteriostatic antimicrobial drugs that contain the sulfonamide group and act as competitive inhibitors of the enzyme dihydropteroate synthetase, which catalyses the conversion of para-aminobenzoate to dihydropteroate, a key step in folate synthesis. Folate is necessary for the cell to synthesize nucleic acids for DNA replication.

Indications

Potentiated sulfonamides are widely used in equine practice and often used as a broad-spectrum antimicrobial in emergency cases such as horses with minor lacerations or wounds. Other than silver sulfadiazine (used topically for control of infection in burn patients), these drugs have limited application in equine critical care.

Clinical use

At recommended dosages, potentiated sulfonamides are generally bacteriostatic. There is a variable lag period between onset of therapy and antibacterial action, and bacterial resistance in equine pathogens is widespread.[36] The recommended dosage is 20–30 mg/kg IV or PO q12h. They should not be given IV following administration of detomidine.

Complications

Trimethoprim-sulfonamides should not be used in patients with ileus. Oral administration has been associated with diarrhea in adult horses, particularly if other risk factors are present (e.g. transport stress, systemic illness, surgery, pain, high-grain diet).

Vancomycin

Key points

- Vancomycin is active against most gram-positive bacteria, but it is ineffective against gram-negative organisms.
- It is one of the few antimicrobial drugs that are effective against multidrug-resistant strains of MRSA, methicillin-resistant *Staphylococcus epidermidis*, and enterococci.
- Its use in horses and foals should be limited to life-threatening staphylococcal or enterococcal infections when culture and sensitivity results clearly indicate that vancomycin is likely to be effective and for which there are no other reasonable alternatives.

Definition/mechanism of action

Vancomycin is a glycopeptide antibiotic used in the prophylaxis and treatment of infections caused by gram-positive bacteria. Vancomycin acts by inhibiting proper cell wall synthesis.

Indications

Vancomycin is active against most gram-positive bacteria, but is ineffective against gram-negative organisms. In human medicine, vancomycin remains one of the few antimicrobial agents that are effective against multidrug-resistant strains of MRSA, methicillin-resistant *Staphylococcus epidermidis*, and enterococci. Vancomycin, either alone or in combination with an aminoglycoside, has also been shown to be safe and effective in horses and foals with serious staphylococcal and enterococcal infections that are resistant to other antimicrobial drugs.[45]

Vancomycin resistance in MRSA and enterococci is an increasing concern in human medicine. Vancomycin-intermediate *Staphylococcus aureus* strains have been reported in humans and vancomycin-resistant enterococci are widely reported in humans and in fecal samples from farm animals, including horses. Of even greater concern, vancomycin-resistant strains of *Staphylococcus aureus* have begun to emerge in human hospitals.[45]

To date, no clinical cases involving confirmed isolates of vancomycin-intermediate *Staphylococcus aureus*, vancomycin-resistant strains of *Staphylococcus aureus*, or vancomycin-resistant enterococci in horses have been reported. Nevertheless, veterinarians should be mindful of the existence of these pathogens and of their increasing prevalence in the human population.

It is recommended that vancomycin use in horses be limited to life-threatening staphylococcal or enterococcal infections when culture and sensitivity results clearly indicate that vancomycin is likely to be effective and for which there are no other reasonable alternatives. Infection with metronidazole-resistant *Clostridium difficile* may be another legitimate use of vancomycin in horses.

Clinical use

Therapeutic concentrations can be achieved and maintained in plasma and synovial fluid at a dosage of 7.5 mg/kg IV q8h.[46] Vancomycin should be given slowly over 30 minutes and diluted in fluids. Clinical experience indicates that systemic administration may need to be supplemented with local or regional delivery for cases of chronic, severe infection involving a joint, physeal cartilage, or bone.[45]

Regional limb perfusion with vancomycin, either IV or IO, may help ameliorate concerns about bacterial resistance and toxicity, at least for infections confined to regions or tissues amenable to this approach. Studies in horses showed that vancomycin (300 mg as a 0.5% solution in sterile isotonic saline), administered by IV or IO regional limb perfusion, was well tolerated and achieved therapeutic concentrations in the synovial fluid and medullary sinusoidal plasma of the distal limb.[47,48] Vancomycin-impregnated polymethylmethacrylate beads have also been used with good clinical effect in horses.[10,45] (See Alternative modes of delivery, Regional perfusion, and Antimicrobial-impregnated implants.)

Complications

Adverse effects of vancomycin in humans include nephrotoxicity and ototoxicity (neurotoxicity of the auditory nerve). They are seen primarily at high dosages, when peak serum concentrations exceed 80 µg/ml or trough concentrations exceed 10 µg/ml. The dosage recommended for horses maintains peak and trough concentrations well below these putative thresholds.[45] While synergism between vancomycin and aminoglycosides is reported against enterococci and against vancomycin-intermediate *Staphylococcus aureus*, concurrent use of these potentially nephrotoxic drugs increases the risk for renal damage.

Vancomycin is excreted primarily via the kidneys, so renal failure can result in marked accumulations of the drug and an increased risk for toxicity. Vancomycin should thus be used with caution, and with appropriate fluid therapy, in patients with renal compromise. As with aminoglycoside use, monitoring the serum creatinine concentration and, if available, peak and trough serum vancomycin concentrations, is recommended during therapy in at-risk patients. Suggested peak and trough serum concentrations of vancomycin are in the range of 25–40 µg/ml and 2–5 µg/ml, respectively.[46]

THE SYSTEMIC INFLAMMATORY RESPONSE

Michelle H. Barton and
K. Gary Magdesian

GENERAL APPROACH TO THE SYSTEMIC INFLAMMATORY RESPONSE

- The systemic inflammatory response is the body's reaction to a septic or non-septic inflammatory condition.
- Endotoxemia is probably the most common cause of a systemic inflammatory response in horses.
- The response may be mild with signs such as fever, tachypnea, and tachycardia. In severe cases, shock, coagulopathy, and multiple organ dysfunction can develop.
- Management is predominantly supportive with fluid therapy (see Chapter 12) and anti-inflammatory drugs (see Chapter 14) and treatment of the specific underlying cause.
- The progression of sepsis includes severe sepsis and septic shock. Septic shock represents a vasopressor dependent state. Sepsis is managed with supportive care, including fluid therapy (see Chapter 12), and antimicrobial drugs (see Chapter 16) to treat the underlying infection.
- Other forms of shock include distributive, cardiogenic, hypovolemic, obstructive and hypoxic shock.

SYSTEMIC INFLAMMATORY RESPONSE

Endotoxemia

Key points

- Endotoxemia refers to endotoxin in the bloodstream.
- The presence of endotoxin in the bloodstream can lead to SIRS, MODS, and DIC.
- Management involves treatment of the underlying disease, as well as anti-endotoxin and supportive therapy.

Definition/overview

Endotoxemia refers to the systemic condition varying from malaise to shock that is caused by the presence of endotoxin in the bloodstream.

Etiology/pathogenesis

Endotoxin, a lipopolysaccharide that is an essential component of the outer cell wall of gram-negative bacteria (**17.1A**), is spontaneously released during logarithmic bacterial growth or bacteriolysis. Therefore, endotoxemia can become the sequela to any locally extensive or systemic invasion with gram-negative bacteria such as septicemia in neonates, pleuropneumonia, peritonitis, salmonella-associated colitis, or metritis. In addition to its release during gram-negative sepsis, an endogenous source of endotoxin is contained in the lumen of the intestinal tract. Normally, endotoxin released by the resident enteric flora is restricted to the intestinal lumen by a healthy mucosal barrier. However, if the intestinal wall becomes severely inflamed or ischemic, luminal endotoxin will translocate to the peritoneal cavity, portal circulation, and, eventually, the general circulation. In mature horses, acute intestinal disease is the most common cause of endotoxemia, while in neonatal foals, endotoxemia most commonly is a consequence of gram-negative bacterial septicemia.[1]

Once endotoxin gains access to the general circulation, intense activation of the innate immune defense system ensues. Since it is a lipopolysaccharide with amphiphilic properties, in the blood, the toxic hydrophobic lipid A portion of the molecule is directed centrally in a micelle-like aggregate. Lipopolysaccharide-binding protein, a glycoprotein whose concentration increases in the acute phase response, acts as a transport molecule, effectively plucking endotoxin molecules from the circulating aggregates.[2] Subsequently, the endotoxin–lipopolysaccharide-binding protein complex is shuttled to the surface of host defense cells, principally monocytes and macrophages, where the membrane receptors for endotoxin, CD14, Toll-like receptor 4 (TLR4), and MD2 reside. Activation of the CD14/TLR4/MD2 complex plays a pivotal role in endotoxemia, as it initiates a series of complex intracellular signaling cascades that culminate in the transcription of genes encoding a vastly diverse array of inflammatory molecules, such as cytokines including IL-1 and TNF-α (**17.1B**).[3–5] Furthermore, cell-signaling-induced

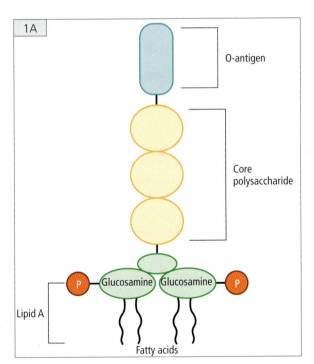

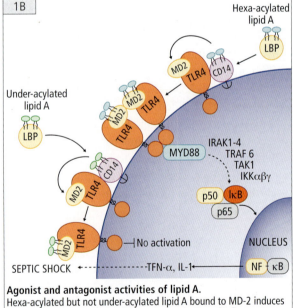

Agonist and antagonist activities of lipid A.
Hexa-acylated but not under-acylated lipid A bound to MD-2 induces oligomerization of TLR4, leading to the production of inflammatory cytokines.

17.1A, B Schematic illustration of the endotoxin (lipopolysaccharide) molecule (A) and the interaction of endotoxin with lipopolysaccharide-binding protein (LBP) and cell surface molecules MD2, CD14, and Toll-like receptor 4 (TLR4). Interaction with TLR4 causes intracellular signaling, leading to transcription of proinflammatory cytokines (tumor necrosis factor-α (TNF-α) and interleukin-1 (IL-1) via NF-κB (B).

synthesis and activation of enzymes and proteases promote tissue damage, eicosanoid synthesis, and free radical production. Ultimately, it is the actions of endotoxin-induced, host-generated inflammatory mediators that are responsible for the clinical signs of endotoxemia and endotoxic shock.

Clinical features

Because endotoxemia is a manifestation of acute inflammatory or ischemic diseases of the intestinal tract or a consequence of gram-negative bacterial sepsis, the clinical signs of endotoxemia may be initially overshadowed by the primary event generating its release. Through experimental infusion studies, the clinical response to endotoxin is well characterized in horses.[6,7] Within the first 30–60 minutes of a sublethal IV challenge with endotoxin, horses yawn frequently, have mucous membrane pallor, become dull, anorectic, tachypneic,

tachycardic, and restless, develop fasciculations and mild to moderate signs of colic, and pass loose feces. This period is the early hyperdynamic phase of endotoxemia that is characterized by pulmonary hypertension (increased pulmonary arterial and wedge pressures and increased pulmonary vascular resistance) and ileus. By 1–2 hours after endotoxin challenge, dullness and anorexia continue and are affiliated with the onset of fever and hypotension. This hypodynamic phase of endotoxemia is due to decreased SVR from the release of prostaglandins. Mucous membranes and unpigmented skin are often hyperemic (**17.2**), CRT is prolonged, and sclerae become injected. With reduced tissue perfusion, the classic 'toxic line' develops as a red to blue-purple line at the periphery of the gums, particularly notable above the upper incisors of mature horses (**17.3**). If hypotension advances, mucous membranes become diffusely congested with poorly oxygenated

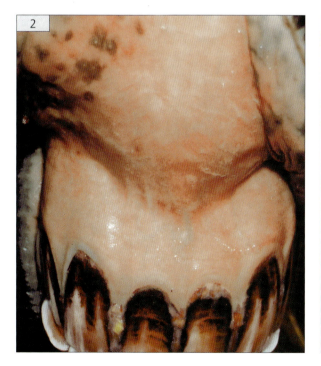

17.2 Hyperemic oral mucous membranes.

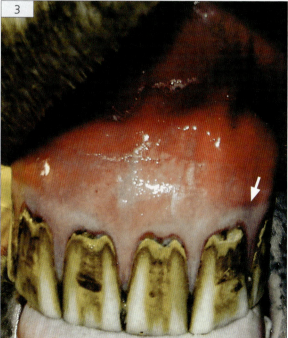

17.3 The classic 'toxic line'. A red to blue–purple line at the periphery of the gums, particularly notable above the upper incisors (arrow).

blood and progress to a cyanotic-like blue to purple color (**17.4**) and then to a grayish-purple pallor.

When the inflammatory response to endotoxin is uncontrolled and malignant, the clinical stage known as the SIRS (p. 737) may develop. Any of the clinical signs discussed above may be present and intensify dynamically. In addition, with loss of immunologic homeostasis, subsequent alterations in hemodynamics, the production of proinflammatory mediators, and unregulated coagulation, clinical signs of septic shock (p. 747), DIC (p. 752), and MODS (p. 740) may arise.

Differential diagnosis
- **General**. Hypovolemic shock; septic shock; hemorrhagic shock; cardiogenic shock.
- **Specific**. Intestinal strangulation or ischemia; proximal enteritis; colitis; GI tract rupture; septic peritonitis; pleuropneumonia; RFM (postpartum mare); metritis (postpartum mare).

Diagnosis
Although the limulus amebocyte lysate assay is a highly specific test for the detection of endotoxin, its tedious nature makes it impractical as a routine diagnostic test. Likewise, quantification of specific endotoxin-induced inflammatory mediators can provide a presumptive diagnosis, as well as prognostic information, though again, these types of assays are rarely available in clinical settings.[1] Therefore, the diagnosis of endotoxemia relies heavily on identification of clinical signs and diagnostic markers in diseases known to be associated with the release of endotoxin. One cardinal diagnostic marker of endotoxemia and/or acute overwhelming bacterial infection is profound neutropenia with toxic neutrophil morphology (**17.5**). Other diagnostic markers typically reflect non-specific secondary changes from stress (hyperglycemia), hypovolemia, (relative polycythemia, hyperproteinemia, azotemia, metabolic acidosis, increased anion gap, lactic acidosis), and specific organ damage from decreased perfusion (azotemia, increased creatine kinase, liver enzyme, or cardiac troponin activities).

Management/treatment
Considering the pathophysiology of endotoxemia, a logical treatment plan would ideally be directed at controlling three main targets: (1) preventing the release of endotoxin; (2) neutralizing free endotoxin; and (3) controlling the cellular response and the biological actions of endogenous mediators.

Preventing the release of endotoxin: When endotoxemia is the result of acute intestinal inflammation or ischemia, translocation of luminal endotoxin might be abated by administration of di-tri-octahedral smectite (0.45 kg in water PO q8–12h), which absorbs bacteria and bacterial toxins, and by specific treatment directed

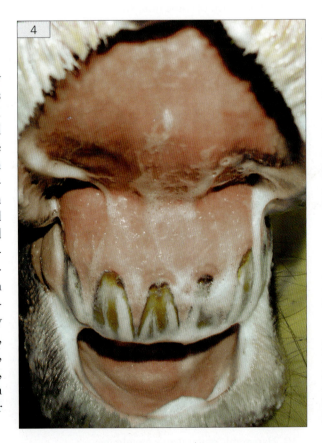

17.4 Cyanotic-like blue to purple colored oral mucous membranes.

towards the underlying disease, such as surgical excision of the ischemic intestine. If endotoxemia is due to gram-negative sepsis, tissue debridement and lavage should be undertaken where possible. Caution should be exercised when antimicrobials are used, as the bacteriocidal actions of certain drug classes may in fact increase the release of endotoxin.[8]

Neutralizing free endotoxin: Once endotoxin is released, drugs that directly bind to it can be a highly effective means of neutralization and prevention of cellular interaction if given prophylactically or early in the course of endotoxemia. Both polymyxin B (1,000–6,000 IU/kg IV q8–12) and plasma or serum containing core endotoxin antibodies are effective in neutralizing endotoxin.[9–11] Unfortunately, once endotoxin is bound to membrane receptors and cell signaling is initiated, the immense diversity of mediator synthesis and actions diminishes the likelihood that any single therapy or anti-inflammatory agent will be of significant benefit. Although numerous drugs have been tested in the later stages of endotoxemia, none has been shown to dramatically improve survival in the clinical setting. Hyperimmune equine plasma did not alter the clinical signs but did decrease TNF-α bioactivity compared with saline in a low-dose endotoxin model.[12]

Controlling the cellular response and the biological actions of endogenous mediators: The mainstays of treatment that are most commonly employed are general supportive fluid therapy and the use of the NSAID flunixin meglumine (0.25 mg/kg IV q8h to 1.1 mg/kg IV q12h).[13] At the lower dose range, flunixin meglumine will inhibit eicosanoid synthesis, but is less likely to provide significant analgesia and, therefore, is unlikely to mask signs of pain that may provide guidance in the diagnosis of the underlying cause of endotoxemia.

IV lidocaine (1.3 mg/kg over 5 minutes followed by a 0.05 mg/kg/minute CRI) decreased clinical scores and serum and peritoneal fluid TNF-α activity compared with saline following intraperitoneal administration of endotoxin to horses.[14] These findings suggest its use may be beneficial in clinical cases; however, clinical studies are necessary.

Therapy directed specifically against shock (p. 749), SIRS, MODS (p. 740), or DIC (p. 752) should be addressed if these complications develop in cases with advanced endotoxemia.

The prognosis for horses with endotoxemia is highly variable and often depends on the ability to control the underlying cause and the degree and duration of endotoxin release. Common complications of endotoxemia are SIRS, MODS (renal dysfunction, laminitis), DIC, and secondary sepsis.

Systemic inflammatory response syndrome
Key points

- SIRS is a systemic inflammatory response to a septic or non-septic inciting cause.
- Patients are exhibiting signs of SIRS if at least two of the following are present: fever/hypothermia, tachycardia, tachypnea and/or altered WBC count.
- Management is primarily supportive with identification and treatment of the underlying disease.

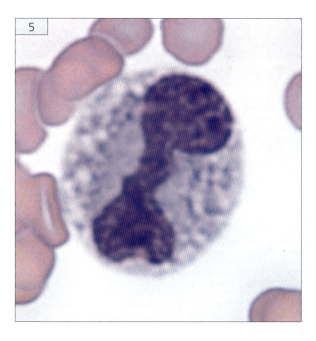

17.5 A toxic neutrophil characterized by basophilic cytoplasm, vacuolization, and presence of Döhle bodies.

Definition/overview

SIRS is a complex clinical syndrome resulting from systemic activation of the innate immune system by localized or systemic infection (see Sepsis and severe sepsis). A number of non-septic conditions, such as severe thermal injury, acute pancreatitis, and trauma, are clinically indistinguishable from sepsis when triggering this same systemic immune reaction. Patients with sterile inflammation can thus mimic those with sepsis. In 1991, the American College of Chest Physicians and Society of Critical Care Medicine developed a consensus defining the systemic response to infection, namely sepsis.[15] This conference introduced the acronym 'SIRS' (systemic inflammatory response syndrome) to describe this systemic reaction to both septic and non-septic insults and described clinical features to define the syndrome (*Table 17.1*). They defined SIRS as being present when patients have more than one of the following: body temperature >38°C or <36°C; heart rate >90 bpm; hyperventilation evidenced by respiratory rate >20 breaths/minute or $PaCO_2$ <32 mmHg; and a WBC count of >12 × 10^9 cells/l (12 × 10^3 cells/µl) or <4 × 10^9 cells/l (4 × 10^3 cells/µl) or >10% bands. In effect, a patient should be considered to have SIRS if at least two of the following signs are present in response to septic or non-septic triggers: fever/hypothermia, tachycardia, tachypnea, and/or altered WBC count. While definitions for SIRS criteria have not been well accepted for the equine species, SIRS was defined in neonatal foals as meeting two or more of the following criteria: (1) leukocytosis or leukopenia (peripheral WBC count >12.5 × 10^9 cells/l [12.5 × 10^3 cells/µl] or <4 × 10^9 cells/l [4 × 10^3 cells/µl], or >10% immature ['band'] neutrophils); (2) hyper- or hypothermia (rectal temperature >39.2°C or <37.2°C); (3) tachycardia (heart rate >120 bpm), or (4) tachypnea (respiratory rate >30 breaths/minute) and evidence of sepsis, cerebral ischemia or hypoxia, or trauma.[16,17]

Table 17.1 Clinical definition of SIRS and severe SIRS

SYNDROME	CLINICAL DEFINITION
SIRS	≥ 2 of the following: • Pyrexia or hypothermia. • Tachycardia. • Tachypnea. • Leukocytosis, leukopenia, or >10% bands.
Severe SIRS	SIRS in addition to organ hypoperfusion or dysfunction, for example: • Acute changes in demeanor. • Oxygenation disturbances (hypoxemia). • Metabolic acidemia and hyperlactatemia. • Oliguria/anuria. • Coagulation disturbances. • Hyperbilirubinemia.

SIRS, systemic inflammatory response syndrome.

Etiology/pathogenesis

The pathophysiology of SIRS begins with a trigger of reticuloendothelial cells and a cascade of inflammation that follows. Examples of triggers include endotoxin, exotoxins, intact infectious agents, or tissue trauma. Once activated, cytokines (IL-1, IL-6, IL-10, TNF-α) are released and stimulate activation of neutrophils, platelets, endothelial cells, and other secondary inflammatory cells. ILs and other cytokines, prostaglandins, thromboxanes, platelet activating factor, tissue factor, C-reactive protein, procalcitonin, and other inflammatory mediators are released. The result of this progressive and exuberant inflammatory response is increased endothelial permeability, inappropriate vasodilation, myocardial depression, hypovolemia, and coagulopathies (**17.6**). Microvascular malperfusion is the end result, with reduced oxygen delivery and resultant cytopathic hypoxia and eventual multiple organ dysfunction.

A common cause of SIRS in horses is the endotoxemia that occurs with gram-negative sepsis such as colitis, enteritis, peritonitis, pleuropneumonia, and metritis. Septicemia, severe tissue hypoxia, GI strangulation or ischemia, thermal injury, heat exhaustion, pancreatitis, and severe trauma are additional examples of SIRS states in horses.

Clinical features

Fever or hypothermia, tachycardia, tachypnea, and leukocytosis or leukopenia are, by definition, the clinical features of SIRS. Specific clinical features will vary depending on the underlying disease process as well as the age of the patient (i.e. neonate versus adult).

Differential diagnosis

Proximal enteritis; colitis; peritonitis; pleuropneumonia; metritis; septicemia; strangulating intestinal lesion; severe trauma; thermal injury; heat exhaustion; tissue hypoxia.

Diagnosis

SIRS is a clinical diagnosis. Hematology should be performed to identify the presence of a leukocytosis or leukopenia or left shift. A thorough physical examination should be performed to identify the inciting cause of SIRS. Once a diagnosis of an underlying cause is made, diagnostic tests should be pursued for the specific disease. Blood culture and antimicrobial susceptibility testing may be performed to identify bacteremia.

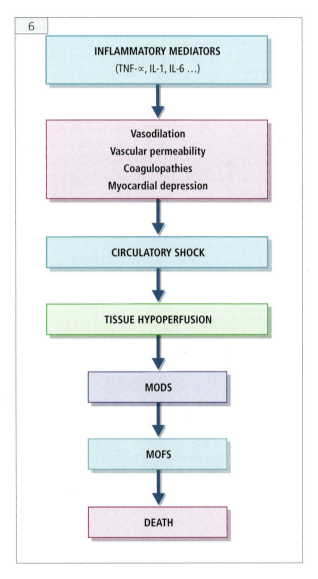

17.6 Schematic illustration of the effect of systemic inflammatory response syndrome on the cardiovascular system. MODS, multiple organ dysfunction syndrome; MOFS, multiple organ failure syndrome.

Management/treatment

Treatment of horses with SIRS is primarily directed at the underlying cause. Because sepsis is the most common cause of SIRS, antimicrobial drug administration is at the cornerstone of therapy whenever infection is documented or suspected. IV fluid support is critical to combat the hemodynamic derangements present with SIRS. Combinations of hypertonic saline, isotonic crystalloids, and colloids are used in the volume resuscitation phase in attempts to restore perfusion (see Chapter 12). Additional support measures include vasopressor therapy (see Chapter 13), nutritional support (see Chapter 15) and controversial anti-endotoxin treatment, such as the use of hyperimmune plasma, flunixin meglumine, pentoxyfylline, and polymyxin B (Neutralizing free endotoxin). Low molecular weight heparin can be given (50 IU/kg SC q24h of dalteparin), in addition to plasma transfusions, for the treatment of coagulopathies.

The prognosis of horses with SIRS depends on the underlying disease and the initial response to therapy.

Multiple organ dysfunction syndrome

Key points

- MODS refers the presence of organ dysfunction or failure that develops subsequent to a systemic inflammatory response that ultimately affects organs at remote sites from the initial insult.
- The respiratory, renal, hemostatic, cardiovascular, GI, nervous, hepatic, musculoskeletal, and adrenal systems are the organs most commonly affected by MODS.
- Identification and treatment of the primary initiating cause should be undertaken, with particular attempts to control the proinflammatory response and to maintain adequate hydration, tissue perfusion, oxygenation, and nutrition.

Definition/overview

MODS is the presence of altered organ function in an acutely ill patient such that homeostasis cannot be maintained without intervention.[18]

Etiology/pathogenesis

Primary MODS refers to the presence of organ dysfunction that is the direct result of a primary insult or disease process affecting that organ, whereas secondary MODS develops subsequent to any disease process that provokes a systemic response that ultimately affects organs at remote sites from the initial insult.

The synthesis and release of the proinflammatory cytokines, TNF-α, IL-1, and IL-6 are key events that drive both SIRS and, subsequently, MODS.[19] A variety of conditions can evoke SIRS including sepsis, endotoxemia, DIC, massive trauma, thermal injury, ischemia, and anaphylaxis. The common theme in these conditions is inflammatory injury coupled with altered hemodynamics and reduced tissue perfusion. Because appropriate function of one organ often depends on adequate function of another, the systemic effects of a single organ failure can contribute to a self-perpetuating cycle of multiple organ failure.

The respiratory, renal, hemostatic, cardiovascular, GI, nervous, hepatic, musculoskeletal, and adrenal systems are the organs most commonly affected by MODS.[19] ARDS, AKI, and DIC are described in more detail elsewhere. Briefly, ARDS develops when injury to the alveoli and pulmonary endothelium causes thromboembolism and protein-rich pulmonary edema.[20] Subsequently, type II pneumocytes and fibroblasts are recruited to replace damaged areas in the alveoli. Collectively, these injuries severely impair gas exchange. AKI is defined as the presence of azotemia and/or oliguria in a normovolemic patient.[21] Acute tubular necrosis with subsequent luminal obstruction and decreased glomerular filtration are the main events leading to acute renal dysfunction. The major event triggering DIC is the expression of tissue factor that is upregulated by proinflammatory cytokines.[22] The microvascular thrombosis that occurs in the hyper-coagulative phase of DIC impedes tissue perfusion, further amplifying the crisis of MODS.

The exact mechanism for cardiac failure in MODS is not entirely understood, as myocardial perfusion appears to remain relatively unaffected.[23] However, the systemic release of inflammatory mediators can cause myocardial damage. Furthermore, electrolyte distur-bances that may be present as the result of the primary insult or subsequent to renal or GI failure can also affect myocardial function. Reduced cardiac output, arrhyth-mias, and hypotension ensue, further compromising hemodynamic homeostasis.

Reduced tissue perfusion, increased systemic sym-pathetic tone, and inflammation contribute to GI failure, manifested principally by ileus[24], GI reflux, diarrhea, and mucosal ulceration. Protein losing enter-opathy will compromise oncotic pressure and elec-trolyte derangements can further affect distal organ function, especially cardiac, muscular, and neural. Mucosal damage enhances the translocation of luminal bacteria and endotoxin with subsequent septicemia and endotoxemia.

Overt hepatic failure is not commonly recognized in horses with MODS; however, bombardment of the liver by endotoxin in the portal circulation, coupled with reduced hepatic perfusion, contributes to hepatic injury. If ileus and GI reflux are present, bile flow may be hindered and lead to pressure necrosis around the bile cannaliculi. If hepatic injury is significant, protein, carbohydrate, and lipid metabolism are altered, leading to HE, hypoglycemia, and hyperlipidemia. Since the liver is the site of synthesis of the majority of proteins involved in hemostasis, severe hepatic injury will per-petuate coagulopathy.

Hypoxia, electrolyte derangements, alterations in glucose homeostasis, HE, and microthrombosis all affect neural function. Encephalopathy of MODS could be easily overlooked when it may simply manifest as dullness or altered behavior. In severe cases, stupor and coma may develop.

A musculoskeletal manifestation of MODS that is unique to the horse is laminitis. The etiology of lamini-tis is complex, though it can be viewed as a form of sec-ondary MODS that commonly develops as a sequela to systemic disease such as endotoxemia, acute GI disease, sepsis, or AKI. Although intensely studied, the exact pathophysiology of laminitis is incompletely under-stood.[25] In general terms, laminitis is most similar to a compartment syndrome wherein postcapillary bed venoconstriction in the digit increases blood pressure in the foot. The non-compliant hoof wall restricts edema in the extravascular space of the foot, further constrict-ing capillary blood flow. In addition to the alteration in local hemodynamics, there appear to be important inflammatory and enzymatic components to laminitis. (See also Chapter 2.)

The term relative adrenal insufficiency is used to describe the scenario in which the adrenal glands response is insufficient for the degree of stress imposed by acute systemic illness, resulting in transient hypo-corticoidism. Mechanisms that have been proposed for relative adrenal insufficiency are cytokine-induced inhibition of ACTH release from the anterior pitui-tary gland and hypoxic damage to its target organ, the adrenal gland. Relative adrenal insufficiency has been recently described in septicemic foals.[26]

Clinical features

Any single organ or combination of organs can be affected in MODS. The most common clinical signs associated with individual organ dysfunction in the horse are summarized in *Table 17.2*.

Diagnosis

Multiple organ dysfunction is a syndrome that is definition-dependent and, unfortunately, a consensus definition has not yet been proposed for horses. In humans, the syndrome is defined by criteria for

Table 17.2 Clinical signs and diagnostic findings suggestive of organ failure in the horse

ORGAN SYSTEM	CLINICAL SIGNS OR PHYSICAL FINDINGS OF FAILURE	DIAGNOSTIC CRITERIA FOR DYSFUNCTION
Respiratory	Tachypnea Labored breathing Nasal flare Cough Pulmonary crackles	Diffuse interstitial pattern radiographically; PaO_2/FIO_2 ratio ≤ 300 (if FIO_2 is unknown, assume a value of 0.21) Hypercapnea Proteinacious fluid in the conducting airways, transtracheal aspirate, or bronchoalveolar aspirate demonstrating neutrophilic inflammation
Renal	Decreased urine output Subcutaneous and pulmonary edema	Increased serum creatinine concentration Increased central venous pressure
Hemostasis	Thrombi, petechiae, ecchymoses, or any sign of excessive hemorrhage at sites of trauma, at mucocutaneous orifices, or compartmentally	Thrombocytopenia Prolonged prothrombin or activated partial thromboplastin time Decreased fibrinogen concentration or prolonged thrombin time Increased fibrin degradation products or D dimer concentrations Decreased antithrombin III activity
Cardiovascular	Tachycardia Arrhythmia Prolonged capillary refill time Overt heart failure (dependent edema, jugular pulsation, cough, pulmonary crackles, syncope) Hypothermia	Hypotension Unexplained metabolic acidosis Lactic acidosis Reduced fractional shortening Reduced cardiac output Chamber dilation Increased serum cardiac troponin concentration
Gastrointestinal	Diagnosis is mostly dependent on the clinical signs of ileus including colic, decreased borborygmi, abdominal distension, gastrointestinal reflux, and/or diarrhea	
Hepatic	Icterus Hepatic encephalopathy	Increased serum sortibol dehydrogenase or gamma glutamyl transferase activities Increased serum bilirubin and serum bile acid concentrations Hypertriglyceridemia Hyperammonemia Hypoglycemia
Neurologic	Diagnosis is mostly dependent on the presence of clinical signs of alteration in behavior, dullness, and stupor progressing to coma	
Musculoskeletal	Weakness. Recumbency Reluctance to move Clinical signs of laminitis	Increased serum creatine kinase activity if muscular involvement. For laminitis, hoof tester positive, pain eliminated by abaxial nerve block, radiographic evidence of laminar edema or separation of the hoof wall from the coffin bone (rotation or sinking)

identification of individual organ dysfunction in combination with numerical scoring systems in which higher scores prompt clinicians to be alerted that multiple organ failure and poor outcome are highly probable.[27,28] Two common scoring systems currently used to identify MODS in human patients are summarized in *Table 17.3*. Until a consensus definition is proposed for use in horses, MODS should be suspected when there is clinical or diagnostic information supporting the failure of more than one organ system in any patient with a condition known to trigger SIRS or MODS. Some diagnostic features of organ dysfunction in the horse are summarized in *Table 17.2*.

Management/treatment

Identification and treatment of the primary initiating cause should be undertaken, with particular attempts to control the proinflammatory response and to maintain adequate hydration, tissue perfusion, oxygenation, and nutrition. Specific therapy for individual organ failure is addressed elsewhere, but briefly, the mainstay therapy for ARDS is positive end-expiratory pressure ventilation (see Chapter 3). When ventilation is not possible, NO insufflation should be considered. Inhaled or parenterally administered corticosteroids may also provide benefit.[20] If AKI is present, hydration and blood pressure should be addressed with fluids. If hypotension per-

Table 17.3 Diagnostic criteria and the MODS and SOFA scoring systems for identification of multiple organ dysfunction syndrome in human patients

ORGAN SYSTEM	SCORE SYSTEM	SCORE				
		0	1	2	3	4
Respiratory	MODS score (1)	>300	226–300	151–225	75–150	≤75
(PaO_2/FIO_2 ratio)	SOFA score (2)	>400	≤400	≤300	≤200 with ventilation	≤100 with ventilation
Renal: serum creatinine (µmol/l [mg/dl])	MODS score	≤100 [≤1.1]	101–200 [1.2–2.2]	201–350 [2.3–3.9]	351–500 [4–5.6]	≥501 [≥5.7]
	SOFA score	≤105 [≤1.2]	106–169 [1.2–1.9]	170–300 [2.0–3.4]	301–439 [3.5–4.9] with <500 ml urine/day	≥440 ≥5.0 with <200 ml urine/day
Hepatic: bilirubin (µmol/l [mg/dl])	MODS score	≤20 [≤1.2]	21–60 [1.3–3.5]	61–120 [3.6–7]	121–240 [7.1–14]	>240 [>14]
	SOFA score	≤20 [≤1.2]	21–33 [1.2–1.9]	34–100 [2–5.9]	101–204 [6–11.9]	≥205 [≥12]
Cardiovascular	MODS score	≤10 PAR	10.1–15 PAR	15.1–20 PAR	20.1–30 PAR	>30 PAR
	SOFA score	No hypotension	MAP <70 mmHg	Dopamine ≤5 µg/kg/minute or dobutamine at any dose	Dopamine >5 µg/kg/minute or epinephrine ≤0.1 µg/kg/minute	Dopamine >15 µg/kg/minute or epinephrine >0.1 µg/kg/minute

(continued overleaf)

Table 17.3 *(continued)*

ORGAN SYSTEM	SCORE SYSTEM	SCORE				
		0	1	2	3	4
Hematologic: platelet count ($\times 10^9/l$ [$\times 10^3/\mu l$])	MODS score	>120 [>120]	81–120 [81–120]	51–80 [51–80]	21–50 [21–50]	<20 [<20]
	SOFA score	>150 [>150]	≤150 [≤150]	≤100 [≤100]	≤50 [≤50]	≤20 [≤20]
Neurologic (Glasgow coma scale score) (4)	MODS score	15	13–14	10–12	7–9	<7
	SOFA score	15	13–14	10–12	6–9	<6

(1) A MODS (multiple organ dysfunction syndrome) score of at least 4 represents marked functional derangement and a mortality rate of ≥50%.[27]

(2) SOFA = sequential organ function assessment.[28]

(3) PAR = pressure adjusted heart rate (heart rate × ratio of the right atrial pressure to the MAP).

(4) The Glasgow coma scale score is derived by measuring three types of responses and adding them together to give an overall score: (1) eye opening (1, no eye opening; 2, eye opening to pain; 3, eye opening to verbal command; 4, eyes open spontaneously); (2) best verbal response (1, no verbal response; 2, incomprehensible sounds; 3, inappropriate word; 4, confused; 5, orientated); and (3) best motor response (1, no motor response; 2, extension to pain; 3, flexion to pain; 4, withdrawal from pain; 5, localizing pain; 6, obeys commands).

sists in the face of rehydration, particularly in neonatal foals, then norepinephrine can be tried (0.1–1 µg/kg/ minute). If anuria or oliguria is still present after these are addressed, diuretics (furosemide 0.12 mg/kg followed by 0.12 mg/kg/hour or 0.5–1 mg/kg q2–12h; mannitol 0.25–1 g/kg IV over 30 minutes followed by 1–2 mg/kg/minute if some urine is produced after initial bolus) can be given. Dopamine (2–3 µg/kg/minute) can also be tried to initiate or increase urine production. Aminophylline (0.5 mg/kg IV over 30 minutes q8–12h) can also be tried (see Chapter 5). Special attention to electrolyte derangements and fluid balance should be addressed. In general, in the hemorrhagic phase of DIC, fresh (when thrombocytopenic) or frozen plasma and heparin therapy are recommended. If hypotension exists from reduced cardiac output, vasopressors and inotropes are indicated (see Septic shock). Use of antiarrhythmic drugs is dictated by the specific arrhythmia. Ileus may necessitate no oral intake of feed or water, frequent gastric decompression, use of prokinetics, especially lidocaine (1.3 mg/kg loading dose over 10 minutes, followed by a CRI at 0.05 mg/kg/minute)[24] and partial to total parenteral nutrition (see Chapter

15). NSAIDs, particularly phenylbutazone (2.2–4.4 mg/ kg IV q12h), and frog support are the most commonly used treatments for laminitis (see Chapter 2). Icing of the limbs may be preventive of laminitis.

Perhaps the most difficult aspect of managing MODS is being mindful of the numerous treatments necessary to maintain multiple failing organs and their potential negative interactions (i.e. treatment for one failing organ may be contraindicated for another).

As one might logically assume, as the number of organ systems failing increases, the likelihood of death increases. Mortality typically reaches nearly 100% in human patients with four failing organ systems.[29]

Sepsis and severe sepsis
Key points
- Sepsis is localized or generalized infection with SIRS and severe sepsis is infection with MODS or fluid-responsive hypotension.
- Antimicrobial drugs and hemodynamic support are the most important components of treatment.
- Treatment of the underlying disease is critical for a favorable outcome.

Definition/overview

Sepsis is SIRS associated with a localized or generalized infection (*Table 17.4*). Specifically, sepsis is defined as the presence of concurrent infection and SIRS (more than one of hypothermia or pyrexia, tachycardia, tachypnea, leukocytosis, leukopenia, or >10% bands) in human critical care. The definition of sepsis has been expanded to include clinical criteria beyond these four clinical features.[15] The current definition is more flexible and meant to provide practical bedside criteria for the clinician to use in the diagnosis and prognosis of sepsis. These criteria fall into five categories: (1) general; (2) inflammatory; (3) hemodynamic; (4) organ dysfunction; and (5) tissue perfusion variables (see below).

Severe sepsis refers to sepsis complicated by organ dysfunction, hypoperfusion, or arterial hypotension. The hypotension with severe sepsis, in contrast to that observed with septic shock, is responsive to fluid therapy.

Etiology/pathogenesis

The pathophysiology of sepsis is that of SIRS, with the inciting cause being an infection. Sepsis begins with a trigger of reticuloendothelial cells (such as Kupffer cells, dendritic cells, glial cells, mesangial cells, monocytes, or macrophages) by the presence of bacteria, viruses, fungi, and exotoxins or endotoxins. Cytokines (IL-1, IL-6, IL-10, TNF-α) are released in response to the pathogens, and these stimulate neutrophils, lymphocytes, macrophages, platelets, endothelial cells, and other secondary inflammatory cells. ILs and other cytokines, prostaglandins, thromboxanes, platelet activating factor, tissue factor, C-reactive protein, procalcitonin, and other mediators are released. The result of this progressive and exuberant inflammatory response is increased endothelial permeability, inappropriate vasodilation, myocardial depression, hypovolemia, and coagulopathies. Microvascular malperfusion is the end result, with reduced oxygen delivery and eventual cytopathic hypoxia, and finally multiple organ dysfunction, as with other forms of unchecked SIRS. The pathophysiology of severe sepsis ('sepsis syndrome') is similar to sepsis, with the addition of organ dysfunction or fluid-responsive hypotension (**17.7**).

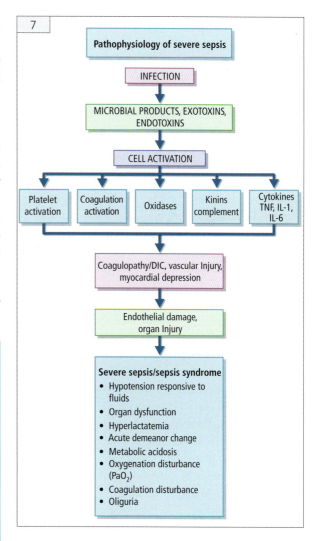

17.7 Schematic illustration of the pathophysiology of severe sepsis.

Table 17.4 **Clinical definition of sepsis, severe sepsis, and septic shock**	
SYNDROME	**CLINICAL DEFINITION**
Sepsis	SIRS with concurrent presumed or confirmed infection
Severe sepsis (sepsis syndrome)	Sepsis plus fluid-responsive hypotension or organ hypoperfusion/dysfunction
Septic shock	Sepsis with vasopressor dependency (hypotension despite adequate fluid resuscitation)

SIRS, systemic inflammatory response syndrome.

Common examples of sepsis in adult horses include enterocolitis, pleuritis/pneumonia, peritonitis, mastitis, phlebitis, and metritis. Septicemia, associated with bacteremia without a specific localized infection, is one of the leading causes of morbidity and mortality in neonatal foals. Gram-negative sepsis is very common in horses and is particularly devastating due to the associated endotoxemia. In the literature, 50% of foals and 30–40% of acute colic cases were reported to have detectable endotoxemia. Gram-positive infections, including those with *Streptococcus* spp., *Staphylococcus* spp., *Corynebacterium pseudotuberculosis*, and *Rhodococcus equi*, are also common. In neonatal foals, gram-negative bacteria, especially *E. coli*, *Klebsiella* spp., *Actinobacillus* spp., and *Enterobacter* spp., are the primary causes, although concurrent infections with gram-positive microbes are also common.

Clinical features

Sepsis: By definition, sepsis is a localized or generalized infection associated with signs of SIRS. The clinical signs of sepsis have been categorized as:

- General. Variables include fever/hypothermia, tachypnea, tachycardia, altered mental status, hyperglycemia, and positive fluid balance or edema. Although these clinical findings are also present in many septic equine patients, it should be noted that tachycardia is not a reliable or consistent finding in septic neonatal foals. In addition, hypoglycemia is more common than hyperglycemia in newborns because of a lack of nursing and paucity of body glycogen and adipose reserves.
- Inflammatory. Criteria include leukocytosis or leukopenia, immature neutrophilia (presence of bands), and increased circulating concentrations of procalcitonin and C-reactive protein.
- Hemodynamic. Variables that are used to define sepsis in human patients include arterial hypotension, increased central venous oxygen saturation (except in neonates), and increased cardiac index (except in neonates).
- Organ dysfunction. Variables include arterial hypoxemia, oliguria, azotemia, ileus, thrombocytopenia and coagulation disorders, and hyperbilirubinemia.

- Tissue perfusion variables for human patients. Tissue perfusion variables have the fewest criteria and include hyperlactatemia (plasma lactate >1 mmol/l) and prolonged CRT or mottling. Though not all of these criteria are easily obtained or commercially available in equine practice, most of them are applicable to horses. Further study and work towards consensus statements on diagnostic criteria for sepsis are needed in equine veterinary medicine.

Severe sepsis: Severe sepsis, by definition, is sepsis associated with organ dysfunction, hypoperfusion, or arterial hypotension (**17.7, 17.8,** *Table 17.4*).[15] The hypotension is reversible with fluid volume loading; septic shock differs in that the hypotension is fluid refractory and is dependent on vasopressor therapy (see Septic shock). Organ dysfunction includes: arterial hypoxemia; oliguria; high serum creatinine concentration; ileus and colic; thrombocytopenia and coagulation disorders; hyperbilirubinemia; myocardial failure; altered demeanor; endocrine disorders (hypocalcemia, hyperglycemia, hypertriglyceridemia); and laminitis. It seems intuitive that horses or foals with these complications have a poorer prognosis than those with uncomplicated sepsis.

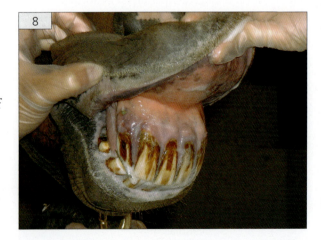

17.8 Oral mucous membranes from a horse with severe sepsis due to colitis.

Differential diagnosis

Septicemia; FPT transfer (neonates); hypoxic–ischemic syndrome (neonates); enterocolitis; pleuritis/pneumonia; peritonitis; mastitis; phlebitis; metritis; myositis; cholangiohepatitis/hepatitis (uncommon); pancreatitis (uncommon).

Diagnosis

The importance of establishing uniform guidelines for clinical diagnosis of sepsis lies in the fact that microbiologic confirmation is not always possible and is often delayed. The sensitivity of blood cultures and culture of body fluids is far from 100%, which prevents documentation of infection in all cases. In one study, the sensitivity of blood cultures in foals was estimated to be close to 50% compared with cultures of postmortem tissues.[30]

Hematology should be performed to identify the presence of a leukocytosis or leukopenia and immature neutrophils. Serum or plasma biochemistry should be used to measure glucose, creatinine, bilirubin, and lactate concentrations. Blood glucose can be monitored on a glucometer and lactate on a hand-held lactate analyzer. A coagulation profile should be performed. A sample of blood should be aseptically collected for bacterial culture and sensitivity testing. If a CVP catheter is placed, a sample of blood can be collected for measurement of central venous oxygen saturation. Procalcitonin and C-reactive protein are not routinely measured in equine patients; however, fibrinogen or serum amyloid A concentration can be used. Arterial blood pressure can be measured directly or indirectly. Cardiac output (or cardiac index) is not routinely measured in equine patients; however, with the development of more practical means for measuring cardiac output, this may become available in the near future. (See also Chapter 11.)

Management/treatment

The basis of treatment of sepsis includes antimicrobial drugs and hemodynamic support. Broad-spectrum and bactericidal antimicrobial drugs, such as aminoglycoside-β lactam combinations or third-generation cephalosporins, should be instituted early. More specific antimicrobial drug therapy can target microbiologic results if and when they become available. Early and appropriate use of antimicrobial drugs is critical. In human medicine, timing of antimicrobial drug use is associated with survival in patients with pneumonia and septic shock.[31,32] Survival decreased with each hour of delay in the administration of antimicrobial drugs after the onset of hypotension in septic patients.[32]

Hemodynamic support is in the form of fluid volume (see Chapter 12) and inotrope and vasopressor therapy (see Chapter 13). Adjunctive therapies include nutritional support (see Chapter 15), anti-endotoxin treatments (p. 736), plasma and low molecular weight heparin for coagulopathies (p. 754), and laminitis prevention (see Chapter 2).[33]

Novel treatments that have demonstrated benefit in human patients in recent years include moderate glucose regulation, low-dose (physiologic) corticosteroids in patients on vasopressor therapy, early goal-directed therapy for hemodynamic optimization, and activated protein C in high-risk patients.[34–37] These therapies require study in horses, but they may have applications to the equine sector. (**Note:** Subsequent studies failed to show any benefit of activated protein C and it has since been withdrawn from the market.)

The prognosis for horses with sepsis is variable, depending on site of infection, offending agent, and host response. Reported survival rates for neonatal foals with septicemia include 21.4–57%.[38–45] Severe sepsis is the most common cause of death in human non-coronary critical care units and is a frequent cause of death in horses.

Septic shock

Key points

- Septic shock is a state of sepsis with vasopressor-dependent hypotension.
- The hypotension in horses and foals with septic shock is no longer responsive to fluid administration.
- Septic shock represents the final stage in the progression of sepsis.

Definition/overview

Septic shock is defined by arterial hypotension despite adequate fluid resuscitation. It is a state of circulatory failure associated with sepsis that represents the next step in progression after 'severe sepsis'. In human patients, hypotension is categorized as systolic blood pressure <90 mmHg (or for children <2 SD below the normal for their age) or MAP <60 mmHg. A reduction in systolic blood pressure of >40 mmHg from baseline, despite appropriate fluid volume administration, is also considered hypotension consistent with septic shock. Another perspective on septic shock is vasopressor dependency.

Etiology/pathogenesis

A number of pathophysiologic processes contribute to septic shock. Myocardial depression and vasodilation are prominent among these. Myocardial depression occurs in response to release of cytokines, especially TNF-α, IL-1, IL-2, and IL-6. The mechanism behind this cytokine-mediated depression of contractility is due, at least in part, to nitric oxide and formation of peroxynitrite radical, in addition to direct effects of increased amounts of adrenomedullin and lactate with sepsis, among other mediators (**17.9**).

Vasodilation is a complex disorder, representing failure of vascular smooth muscle to contract appropriately to increased plasma catecholamines (**17.10**). This occurs due to a number of pathophysiologic processes, including increased nitric oxide from endothelial cells and reduced affinity of alpha-adrenergic receptors for norepinephrine caused by peroxynitrite. Increased atrial natriuretic peptide also contributes to vasodilation through increasing intracellular cGMP. Decreased circulating concentrations of vasopressin play a role in inappropriate vasodilation. Vasopressin is a potent vasoconstrictor acting through V1 receptors, and human septic patients have reduced vasopressin as compared with healthy controls. This is believed to be due in part to exhaustion of vasopressin stores in the neurohypophysis, as well as hypothalamic dysfunction. Relative adrenal insufficiency may also play a role in sepsis-induced vasodilation, as corticosteroids sensitize the vasculature to the pressor effects of catecholamines. Adenosine triphosphate [ATP]-sensitive potassium channels on the membrane of vascular smooth muscle cells may also play a role. These channels open in response to reduced cytosolic pH, decreased ATP concentrations, or increased lactate concentrations,

9

Causes of myocardial depression in septic shock
– TNF-α — Leukotrienes
– IL-1β — Prostaglandins
– IL-2 — Lysozyme C
– IL-6 — Bacterial nucleic acid
– PAF — Adrenomedullin

↓

Changes of cellular level in myocardium:
– Nitric oxide
– Calcium derangements
– Oxygen radicals
– Altered beta-adrenergic signal transduction
– Lactate

↓

Clinical myocardial depression:
– Decreased ejection fraction
– Ventricular dilatation
– Decreased ventricular compliance

17.9 Schematic illustration of the causes of myocardial depression in septic shock.

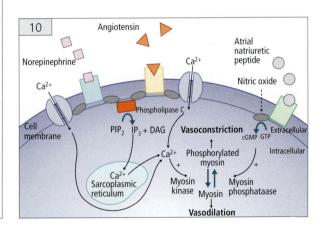

17.10 Schematic illustration of the causes of vasodilation in septic shock.

and serve to hyperpolarize the cell membrane potential through the efflux of potassium ions. Hyperpolarization reduces calcium entry, which is necessary for smooth muscle contraction. Finally, adrenomedullin is also vasodilatory.

Clinical features

Horses with septic shock have a suspected or documented infection. Hypotension is, by definition, a clinical feature of horses with septic shock. Clinical signs shown by horses with hypotension include obtundation, poor pulse quality, prolonged CRT, cold extremities, tachycardia (variable in foals), pale to muddy mucous membranes, prolonged jugular refill time, and oliguria or anuria. Horses with myocardial depression have reduced ventricular compliance, ventricular dilatation, and a decreased ejection fraction.

Differential diagnosis

Septicemia; FPT (neonates); hypoxic–ischemic syndrome (neonates); enterocolitis; pleuritis/pneumonia; peritonitis; mastitis; phlebitis; metritis; myositis; cholangiohepatitis/hepatitis (uncommon); pancreatitis (uncommon); other forms of shock including heart failure, marked hypoxemia, hypovolemic shock, anaphylaxis, obstructive shock.

Diagnosis

Diagnosis of septic shock is contingent on documenting vasopressor dependency; this is manifest by a lack of blood pressure response to fluid loading in the face of sepsis. Additional diagnostics are the same as for sepsis (p. 744), including culture of blood and body fluids, and hematology and serum chemistry analyses.

Management/treatment

Treatment of septic shock is difficult, owing to the severity of the hemodynamic and inflammatory compromise already in place. Reversal of shock can be attempted with vasopressors, catecholamines, and non-catecholamines, as well as drugs that increase vascular responsiveness (see Chapter 13). Catecholamines include norepinephrine, phenylephrine, and epinephrine. Because of concerns over splanchnic perfusion, norepinephrine is the first-line choice. Dobutamine is not a vasopressor, but is commonly used in conjunction

with vasopressors because it increases myocardial contractility and helps in countering the effects of increased SVR on cardiac output. Non-catecholamine pressors include vasopressin and terlipressin. Corticosteroids increase the sensitivity of the vascular smooth muscle to catecholamines.

Early and appropriate antimicrobials, early hemodynamic optimization through early-goal directed therapy, low-dose corticosteroids in patients on vasopressor therapy, low tidal volume mechanical ventilation, and glucose control are all relatively new treatment modalities used in human patients with severe sepsis and septic shock.

Currently, the prognosis for foals and horses with septic shock is poor; however, it is dependent on the underlying disease and the initial response to therapy.

Shock
Key points
- Shock can be defined as inadequate ATP production leading to cellular dysfunction and ultimately organ failure and death.
- Forms of shock include distributive, hypovolemic, cardiogenic, obstructive, and hypoxic shock.
- Management is different for the various forms of shock and for different etiologies.

Definition/overview

Shock can be defined as inadequate ATP production leading to cellular dysfunction and ultimately organ failure and death. Forms of shock include distributive, hypovolemic, cardiogenic, obstructive, and hypoxic shock. The first four categories are examples of circulatory shock. Circulatory shock can be further broken down into two broad categories, hypodynamic (hypovolemic, cardiogenic, and obstructive) and hyperdynamic shock (distributive).

Etiology/pathogenesis

Distributive shock: Examples of distributive shock include sepsis, anaphylaxis, spinal shock, adrenal insufficiency, and drug intoxication. The hemodynamic characteristics of these forms of shock include increased cardiac index and reduced peripheral vascular resistance associated with vasodilation, leading to a hyperdynamic state. The net effect of these hemodynamic alterations includes maldistribution of blood flow and compromised microvascular perfusion. In this case, the oxygen extraction ratio is usually normal or decreased despite evidence of hypoperfusion. This occurs because of inflammatory mediators, coupled with hypoperfusion, resulting in cellular injury, cytopathic hypoxia, and organ dysfunction.

Hypovolemic shock: The hypodynamic forms of shock result in reduced cardiac index and a high-resistance vasoconstricted state, with hypotension resulting. Increased oxygen extraction, resulting in reduced SvO_2, and a high blood lactate concentration are present and reflect global hypoperfusion. Organ dysfunction is a common sequela. Hypovolemic shock may result from hemorrhage, third space loss of fluids due to burns, GI or urinary losses, and increased vascular permeability. Filling pressures, including CVP and pulmonary arterial wedge pressure (PAWP), are reduced. In contrast, these filling pressures are high with cardiogenic shock.

Cardiogenic shock: Examples of cardiogenic shock include cardiomyopathy, severe valvular lesions, and myocardial infarction. Some forms of septic shock, which result in severe myocardial depression, demonstrate cardiogenic shock.

Obstructive shock: Obstructive shock may be difficult to differentiate clinically from cardiogenic shock in that increased CVP and normal to high PAWP predominate. Examples of obstructive shock include pericardial tamponade, tension pneumothorax, and pulmonary embolism. Filling pressures are high with obstructive shock due to outflow obstruction, impaired ventricular filling, and decreased ventricular compliance.

It should be noted that there is considerable overlap among these forms of shock (**17.11**). For example, hypovolemia accompanies most of the other types of shock, and patients with sepsis may develop a hypodynamic profile due to myocardial failure and low cardiac output. As shock progresses, the primary hypodynamic forms will develop vasomotor failure and terminal vasodilation.

Hypoxic shock: Hypoxic shock includes hypoxemia and cellular hypoxia. Sepsis induces derangements in cellular respiration, leading to a state of cytopathic hypoxia. Cytopathic hypoxia occurs with mitochondrial dysfunction secondary to prolonged hypoperfusion, persistent hyperglycemia, and inflammatory cytokines. Cyanide toxicity is another cause of hypoxic shock.

11	MAP	PAWP	CO	SVR	SvO$_2$	Lactate
Hypodynamic:						
Hypovolemic	↓	↓	↓	↑	↓	↑
Cardiogenic	↓	↑	↓	↑	↓	↑
Obstructive	↓	N to ↑	↓	↑	↓	↑
Hyperdynamic:						
Distributive	↓	N to ↓	N to ↑	↓	N to ↑ to ↓	↑

MAP, mean arterial pressure; PAWP, pulmonary arterial wedge pressure; CO, cardiac output; SVR, systemic vascular resistance; SvO$_2$, venous oxygen saturation.

17.11 Hemodynamic profiles of the different forms of circulatory shock.

Clinical features

Distributive shock: Typically, this form of shock manifests with hyperemic mucous membranes and shortened CRTs, particularly in the early stages. Later signs include muddy or toxic mucous membranes. Depending on the underlying etiology, horses with distributive shock might demonstrate clinical features of sepsis, anaphylaxis (respiratory distress, pulmonary edema, colic, loose feces, angioedema, or urticaria), spinal shock (neurologic signs, weakness), or adrenal shock (weakness, obtundation).

Hypovolemic shock: Clinical features of hypovolemic shock are abnormalities in the perfusion parameters. These include prolonged CRT, pale mucous membranes, poor pulse quality, poor jugular refill, obtundation, and tachycardia.

Cardiogenic shock: Clinical features of cardiogenic shock include signs of heart failure. Horses with left-sided heart failure demonstrate coughing, tachypnea, respiratory distress, and pulmonary edema (pink-tinged froth at the nares). Right-sided heart failure leads to distended jugular veins with pulsations, peripheral edema, and pleural and peritoneal effusions. Ultrasound examination may demonstrate hepatomegaly.

Obstructive shock: Clinical features of horses with obstructive shock are nondescript. Horses with pneumothorax have signs of respiratory distress and tachypnea, as well as quiet lung sounds in the dorsal lung fields. Horses with tamponade may show signs of weakness, obtundation, hypoperfusion, and right-sided heart failure. Horses with pulmonary embolism may be the most elusive, often showing minimal signs acutely. Those with significant pulmonary infarction demonstrate clinical signs similar to pleuropneumonia, often with sanguineous to hemorrhagic nasal discharge and pleural effusions. Thoracic ultrasonography and radiography are diagnostic of these conditions.

Hypoxic shock: Horses with significant hypoxemia may demonstrate cyanosis if PaO_2 is <40 mmHg. Those with pulmonary origin hypoxemia present with respiratory distress. Those with cytopathic hypoxia often have concurrent septic shock or endotoxemia, and the clinical feature indicating abnormal oxygen utilization is a decrease in calculated oxygen consumption or an increase in central or mixed venous oxygen saturation (on room air). Cyanide toxicity has occurred with ingestion of wild cherry (*Prunus* spp.) leaves, saplings, or bark. Clinical signs of cyanide toxicity include seizures, apnea, cardiac arrest, and sudden death. Blood may appear cherry red.

Differential diagnosis

See Etiology/pathogenesis.

Diagnosis

Distributive shock: Diagnosis of distributive shock depends on the etiology (see Sepsis). Diagnosis of anaphylactic shock rests largely on clinical signs and history of recent exposure to drugs or potential allergens. Spinal shock should be suspected in the hypotensive patient with acute neurologic signs, especially associated with trauma. Adrenal insufficiency is diagnosed with an ACTH stimulation test, but should be suspected as a rule out with hyponatremia, hypochloremia, hyperkalemia, and possibly hypoglycemia.

Hypovolemic shock: Hypovolemic shock is diagnosed with clinical signs of hypovolemia. Signs or history of acute hemorrhage may be present. CVP measurements can aid in the diagnosis of hypovolemia, as it is low or even negative.

Cardiogenic shock: Echocardiography is the diagnostic tool of choice. Additional diagnostics include measurement of CVP (high) and cardiac pressures. Electrocardiography and measurement of cardiac troponin I or C are additional diagnostics.

Obstructive shock: Diagnosis of obstructive shock is dependent on thoracic and cardiac ultrasound examination and radiography.

Hypoxic shock: Hypoxemia is diagnosed using ABG analysis and pulse oximetry. Cytopathic hypoxia is more difficult to diagnose, but should be suspected with an increased (supranormal) central or mixed venous oxygen saturation on room air. Documentation of decreased oxygen consumption in the face of adequate perfusion and arterial oxygenation is strong evidence.

Management/treatment

Management of the various forms of shock is dependent on the etiology. Distributive shock should be treated by addressing the underlying cause, for example by administering antimicrobial drugs for sepsis. Fluid therapy is an important component of the management of hypotension associated with distributive shock. Vasopressors may be indicated.

Anaphylaxis is treated with epinephrine (0.01–0.02 mg/kg slow IV or IM of 1:1,000), corticosteroids (parenteral prednisolone succinate or dexamethasone), and antihistamines (diphenhydramine, 0.5–1 mg/kg IM or slow IV; hydroxyzine, 1 mg/kg PO). Furosemide (1 mg/kg IV) and oxygen insufflation are indicated for pulmonary edema.

Hypovolemic shock is addressed with fluid volume loading. Crystalloids, colloids, or a combination can be used. The fluid challenge method of fluid administration is a rapid and safe means of fluid replacement. For crystalloids, a dose of 10–20 ml/kg is bolused over 15–30 minutes with subsequent reassessment of perfusion parameters (i.e. CRT, pulse quality) and blood lactate concentration. Because colloids are usually limited to the intravascular space, the dose is smaller (3–10 ml/kg), with the total dose for hetastarch not exceeding 10 ml/kg (see Chapter 12). The safety of collsids in humans has been called into question because of some preliminary evidence of increased renal injury and mortality.

Treatment of cardiogenic shock is multifaceted. Pulmonary edema is treated with furosemide and oxygen insufflation. For CHF, inotropic drugs (usually digoxin) and vasodilators (ACE inhibitors) are indicated. Arrhythmias may need to be addressed (see Chapter 4).

Treatment of obstructive shock should be directed at the underlying cause. For example, cardiac tamponade requires pericardiocentesis. Hypoxic shock due to hypoxemia is treated with oxygen insufflation. Cytopathic hypoxia is difficult to treat and may represent irreversible cellular changes.

Disseminated intravascular coagulation
Key points

- DIC is an acquired syndrome of dyshemostasis that is initiated by excessive thrombi formation, culminating terminally in unregulated hemorrhage, shock, and multiple organ hypoxia.
- DIC should be suspected if any three of the following diagnostic criteria are present in an 'at-risk' patient: thrombocytopenia, prolonged PT, prolonged aPTT, hypofibrinogenemia or a prolonged thrombin time, decreased antithrombin III activity, or increased fibrin degradation product or D dimer concentrations.
- Treatment of DIC should be directed at identification and treatment of the underlying initiating cause. Judicial use of plasma and heparin may be warranted.

Definition/overview

DIC is an acquired syndrome of dyshemostasis that is initiated by excessive thrombi formation, especially in the microvasculature. Subsequently, platelets and coagulation, anticoagulant, and fibrinolytic factors are consumed and the normally regulated balance between clot formation and dissolution is lost, culminating terminally in unregulated hemorrhage, shock, and multiple organ hypoxia.

Etiology/pathogenesis

The hypercoagulative phase of DIC is initiated when another primary disease process excessively activates the coagulation cascade. In the horse, diseases that are most commonly reported with DIC are sepsis, endotoxemia, and metastatic neoplasia.

Current evidence indicates that the most direct mechanism responsible for the procoagulative state of DIC is activation of the extrinsic coagulation cascade via enhanced membrane tissue factor expression (**17.12**). In the most common scenario, it is the evolutionary link between the hemostatic and immune systems that is responsible for triggering DIC. Constitutively expressed membrane tissue factor on monocytes, endothelial cells, and macrophages can be directly upregulated by the innate immune system's recognition of certain microbial products, such as lipopolysaccharide (endotoxin), or indirectly upregulated by cytokines that are generated in the process of recognition of 'non-self'.[22,46] In addition to promoting expression of tissue factor, cytokines inactivate tissue factor pathway inhibitor. Direct activation of the intrinsic coagulation cascade appears to be of minor importance, although indirectly, the role of intrinsic coagulation is amplified by connections between coagulation pathways (**17.12**).

In addition to events that activate coagulation, failure of appropriate fibrinolysis and consumption of anticoagulant factors further promote clot formation. In horses, endotoxin and endotoxin-induced cytokines favor activation of plasminogen activator inhibitor over tissue plasminogen activator, a response that would be expected to enhance clot formation (**17.12**).[47,48] The

natural anticoagulants antithrombin III and protein C are rapidly consumed in sepsis, as they combine with activated clotting factors.[48–50] In addition to their anti-coagulant effects (**17.12**), antithrombin III and protein C possess several anti-inflammatory effects. Ultimately, the consequence of insufficient antithrombin III and protein C is two-fold: increased clot formation and an increased inflammatory response, the latter effect serving to 'fuel the fire' of driving more coagulation.

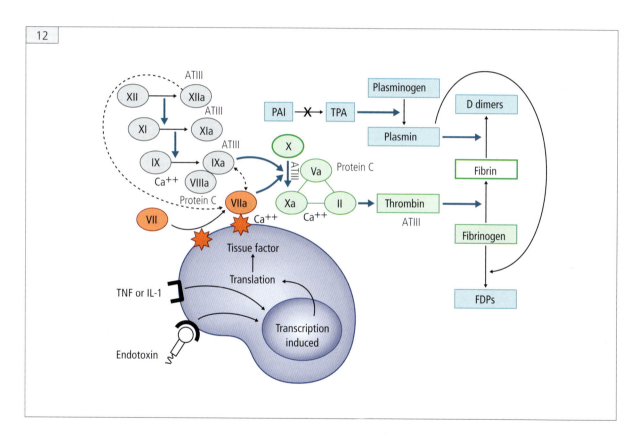

17.12 The role of the proinflammatory response in activation of the coagulation and fibrinolytic cascades. Endotoxin can enhance tissue factor expression directly by inducing transcription or indirectly by inducing the synthesis of cytokines, such as TNF and IL-1, which in turn, activate *de novo* expression of tissue factor. The intrinsic coagulation cascade components are in black, the extrinsic coagulation cascade components are in red, the common coagulation cascade is in green, and the fibrinolytic pathway is depicted in blue. Interactions between the intrinsic and extrinsic pathways are shown by dashed lines. ATIII and protein C are depicted at their respective sites of inhibition. TNF, tumor necrosis factor; IL-1, interleukin 1; PAI, plasminogen activator inhibitor; TPA, tissue plasminogen activator; FDPs, fibrin degradation products; ATIII, antithrombin III.

Clinical features

Apart from the overshadowing signs of the primary initiating disease process, there are few to no direct overt clinical signs of the hypercoagulative phase of DIC. In the horse, the laminae of the digit and the kidneys are common sites of microthrombosis, therefore signs of laminitis and renal insufficiency might be apparent. Large vessel thrombi occasionally form at venipuncture sites. When DIC advances to a consumptive coagulopathy stage, additional clinical signs of loss of control of primary and secondary hemostasis ensue and may include mucosal or dermal petechiae (**17.13**) or ecchymoses (**17.14**), or any sign of excessive hemorrhage at mucocutaneous orifices (epistaxis, melena, hematuria), at sites of vascular access, minor invasion, or trauma (**17.15**), or compartmentally, such as hematoma formation, hyphema, hemarthrosis, hemothorax, or hemoperitoneum. As hemorrhage continues, most patients will demonstrate signs of shock and end-organ hypoxia.

Differential diagnosis

Primary or immune-mediated thrombocytopenia; acquired soluble factor deficiency (consumptive DIC phase); warfarin toxicity, liver failure.

Diagnosis

Diagnosis of DIC is confounded by several factors: it is a dynamic and complex process that lacks a universal diagnostic definition; testing is not standardized; and some tests are not routinely available in clinical settings.[51,52] Testing is recommended in any patient that has an underlying disorder known to be associated with DIC. In general, DIC should be suspected if any three of the following diagnostic criteria are present in an 'at-risk' patient: thrombocytopenia; prolonged PT; prolonged aPTT; hypofibrinogenemia or a prolonged thrombin time; decreased antithrombin III activity; or increased fibrin degradation products or D dimer concentrations. In neonatal foals, coagulation tests should be compared against age-related references.[48]

Management/treatment

The cardinal rule for the treatment of DIC is to identify and treat the underlying initiating cause. For horses, this would entail identifying and treating underlying sepsis, endotoxemia, or neoplasia. Antimicrobial therapy and treatments specifically directed against sepsis (p. 744) or endotoxemia (p. 736) would be indicated. In patients with shock or organ hypoxia, circulatory support should be instituted (see Shock).

Controversy still prevails with regard to therapy directed specifically at dyshemostasis[53], especially in the lesser studied equine species. In human patients, replacement therapy (frozen plasma or platelet rich fresh plasma if thrombocytopenia is present) with concurrent administration of heparin is generally recommended for patients in DIC with significant bleeding.[53] Whether such treatment is beneficial in the horse is not conclusively known, as combination therapy has not been studied. Meta-analysis on septic human patients supports the prophylactic use of heparin without replacement therapy in patients that are not bleeding.[54]

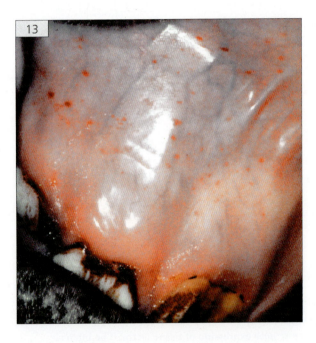

17.13 Petechial hemorrhages are present on the oral mucous membranes and are indicative of the presence of thrombocytopenia in disseminated intravascular coagulation.

In one study on DIC in equine colic patients, the survival rate was better for horses that were treated with heparin (40–90 units/kg SC q8h).[55] Colicky horses treated with low molecular weight heparin (dalteparin 50 IU/kg SC q24h) had fewer side-effects than those treated with unfractionated heparin.[33] The effect on survival was not reported. Epsilon-aminocaproic acid (20–80 mg/kg diluted 1:9 in saline given IV over 30–60 minutes) has been used to block fibrinolysis; however, its effectiveness in equine DIC is unknown and it would be contraindicated during the hypercoagulable stages of DIC. If used, heparin should be given concurrently. For patients in hemorrhagic shock, whole blood transfusion might be indicated and, like plasma replacement therapy, should be accompanied by the use of heparin.

The prognosis for horses with DIC depends on both the ability to control the underlying primary disease process and the stage of DIC. In general, the risk for death is considerably greater in horses with inflammatory conditions and concurrent overt DIC.[52]

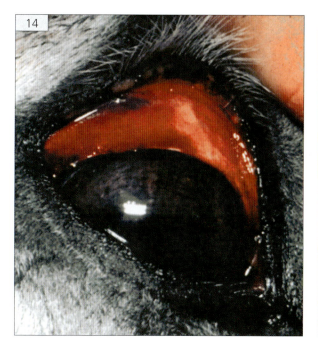

17.14 Ecchymotic hemorrhages in the sclera are indicative of extensive loss of primary (i.e. platelets) and/or secondary (coagulation proteins) hemostasis in the overt hemorrhagic phase of disseminated intravascular coagulation.

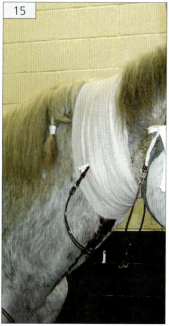

17.15 This horse was in the overt bleeding stage of disseminated intravascular coagulation as evidenced by excessive hemorrhage at the catheter site in the jugular vein, despite application of a pressure wrap.

POSTOPERATIVE COLIC PATIENT

Louise L. Southwood

GENERAL APPROACH TO THE POSTOPERATIVE COLIC PATIENT

- Many postoperative colic patients require minimum postoperative care (e.g. horses with non-strangulating large colon lesions [see Chapter 1]).
- The minimum treatment generally includes:
  - Flunixin meglumine (1.1 mg/kg IV q12h for 2–3 days followed by 0.5 mg/kg IV q12h for 1–2 days).
  - IV maintenance polyionic isotonic crystalloid fluids supplemented with 20 mEq/l potassium chloride (2 ml/kg/hour) for 6–12 hours (see Chapter 12).
- A COX-1 sparing NSAID, such as firocoxib (0.27 mg/kg loading dose IV followed by 0.09 mg/kg IV q24h for 3–4 days) or meloxicam (0.6 mg/kg IV for 3–4 days), may be used as an alternative to flunixin meglumine.
- Oral fluids can be used in place of IV fluids if borborygmi are present and the horse has no reflux following nasogastric tube passage.
- Antimicrobial drugs (penicillin and gentamicin) should be given preoperatively. Postoperative administration is unnecessary in most cases and should only be used for up to 24 hours except in cases with pre-existing infection.

- Feed can generally be introduced 3–6 hours after surgery and the amount of feed given increased to full feed over 36–72 hours in uncomplicated cases.
- Horses with strangulating lesions (see Chapter 1) often require more intensive monitoring and treatment because they are predisposed to postoperative complications.
- Postoperative colic patients are at a high risk of developing nosocomial infections (e.g. salmonellosis). Biosecurity procedures include hand cleansing between patients, wearing disposable gloves and gowns, and foot disinfection when entering and leaving the stall.
- Most surgeons are currently using absorbable suture material for skin apposition. Staples or non-absorbable suture material is removed 10–14 days after surgery.
- Following hospital discharge, horses should be confined to a stall for 4 weeks, then a stall and run for 4 weeks, followed by pasture turn out or light exercise for 4 weeks. The horse can be returned to its intended use after this time.

MONITORING

Patient observation
Key points
- Patient observation is critical during the early postoperative period and a great deal of information regarding patient well being can be obtained from simply observing patient behavior.

Pain scores
Pain scoring systems have been established for the postoperative colic patient[1] and are based on posture and socialization:
- Gross pain behavior: pawing, sweating, flank staring, flehmen, lying down.
- Head position: above withers (non-painful), at withers, below withers (painful).
- Ear position: forward and frequent movement (non-painful), slightly back and little movement (painful).
- Location in stall: at door watching environment (non-painful) to standing in middle and facing back of stall (painful).
- Spontaneous locomotion: moves freely (non-painful) to no movement (painful).
- Responds to open door: moves to door (non-painful) to no response (painful).
- Responds to approach: moves towards observer with ears forward (non-painful) to does not move and with ears back (painful).
- Lifting feet: freely lifts feet when asked (non-painful) to extremely unwilling to lift feet (painful).
- Response to grain: moves to door and reaches for grain (non-painful), looks at door, no response (painful) (see Attitude and appetite).

While these scoring systems are mostly used for comparison of treatment groups in experimental studies, such observations can also be used to monitor the clinical patient and to direct the use of additional analgesia (see Chapter 14). Horses may show some signs of pain in the early postoperative period (i.e. 3–6 hours); however, they should display non-painful behavior after about 6 hours. Persistent indications of pain warrant close monitoring and possibly further diagnostic tests to determine the reason (see below for differential diagnoses of pain).

Attitude and appetite
The postoperative colic patient should be observed for appropriateness of attitude and appetite. While some horses will be dull immediately following abdominal surgery (i.e. initial 3–6 hours), horses should have a good appetite when offered feed and have a bright attitude upon refeeding. Postoperative colic patients that do not become bright when hand walked outside and are not interested in grazing require a thorough examination and, in general, this is not associated with a good prognosis. Common reasons for persistent dull demeanor and inappetence in the postoperative period include:
- Gastric dilation necessitating passage of a nasogastric tube and checking for reflux.
- Functional or mechanical intestinal obstruction.
- Enterocolitis caused by *Salmonella* spp., a tentative diagnosis of which can be made based on fever, leukopenia, and/or accumulation of liquid in the colon observed on ultrasonographic examination. Reflux following nasogastric tube passage is also a clinical feature in some horses with salmonellosis. PCR or bacterial culture of serial fecal and/or reflux samples for *Salmonella* spp. can be used to confirm the diagnosis.
- Non-viable or leaking intestine.
- Metabolic alterations such as hypertriglyceridemia (p. 764).
- Oral, pharyngeal, esophageal, or gastric lesions/ulceration, especially with repeated nasogastric tube passage. It is not recommended routinely to leave a nasogastric tube in place postoperatively because of trauma and the possibility of inducing reflux.

Colic, abdominal distension, and fecal production

The horse should be observed for signs of colic, abdominal distension, and fecal production. Any horse that is painful postoperatively, particularly in combination with abdominal distension and a lack of fecal production, should have a thorough examination, as this is often indicative of a functional or mechanical obstruction. Causes for signs of colic, abdominal distension, and lack of fecal production include:

- Gastric dilation secondary to a small intestinal functional or mechanical obstruction and necessitating nasogastric tube passage for decompression.
- Severe postoperative ileus.
- Complications with an anastomosis (e.g. intraluminal obstruction with ingesta or adhesions).
- Ongoing intestinal ischemia or ischemia-reperfusion injury.
- Reimpaction of the small colon or cecum.
- Failure to remove an enterolith at surgery.
- Reimpaction of the colon with sand.
- Redisplacement.

Any horse that is dull or inappetent, tachycardic, or showing signs of colic postoperatively should have a nasogastric tube passed to check for reflux and an abdominal palpation performed per rectum. Abdominal ultrasonographic examination can be performed to determine the cause of the clinical signs. If the pain is persistent, repeat celiotomy may be necessary.

If there is insufficient fecal production, no nasogastric reflux, and the signs of abdominal pain are not severe, enteral water and electrolytes can be given via a nasogastric tube (e.g. 4–6 liters q6–12h for 24–48 hours) to ensure adequate hydration and assist with defecation.

Water consumption and urination

Water consumption and urination should be monitored closely. Horses on IV fluids generally do not drink large volumes of water. Normal urine production in an adult horse is 0.6–1.25 ml/kg/hour (i.e. 300–625 ml/hour or 7.2–15 liters/day for a 500 kg horse). Fluid 'ins and outs' are not usually measured in adult horses and urine production is subjectively assessed by observing actual urination and the amount of urine in the stall. A horse should produce a good stream of urine every few hours and the stall should have several wet areas (**18.1**) but not be soaking wet. Urine SG in a horse on IV fluids should be 1.010–1.020.

Physical examination

Key points
- Physical examination should be performed often as part of the management strategy of postoperative colic patients.
- Physical examination can provide information regarding cardiovascular status, pain level, and early postoperative complications such as infection.
- As with any monitoring, it is important to consider trends over time and use a combination of observational, physical examination, and laboratory findings when assessing the postoperative colic patient.

Procedure
Postoperative colic patients should be examined every 3–6 hours depending on the severity of illness and

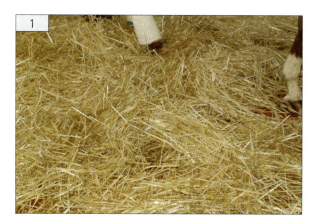

18.1 There should be several wet areas within the stall indicating that the horse is urinating.

duration of time since surgery (**18.2**). The heart rate should be within normal limits within 24–36 hours postoperatively. Persistent tachycardia is associated with pain (e.g. colic, laminitis) or cardiovascular compromise (e.g. hypovolemia, endotoxemia, hemorrhage). Persistent unexplained tachycardia should be investigated further with an ECG and if any murmurs are ausculted, an echocardiographic examination is indicated (see Chapter 4).

Oral mucous membranes should be pink and moist and the CRT <2 seconds. Injected or toxic mucous membranes indicate endotoxemia and pale mucous membranes in combination with tachycardia may indicate hemorrhage. Pulse quality should be good and the extremities warm. Tachypnea can be an indication of pain (e.g. colic, laminitis), shock, underlying respiratory tract disease, high ambient temperature, or fever. A mild fever may be present within 12–24 hours of surgery; however, a persistent or high fever necessitates a thorough examination (see Fever). Borborygmi may be decreased compared with normal immediately postoperatively, but should improve with reintroduction of feed. Absent borborygmi in combination with other clinical signs may indicate ongoing GI disease (e.g. ischemic intestine, ileus, re-obstruction) or endotoxemia (see Endotoxemia).

2	ICU FLOW SHEET				
Case #: _____ Owner: _____ Stall #: _____					
Date					
Time					
Temp (°F)					
Pulse (/min) and character					
Respiratory rate (/min)					
Mucous membranes					
CRT					
GI motility					
Abdominal distention					
Digital pulses					
Heat in feet					
Urine (vol/character)					
Feces (vol/character)					
PCV (%)					
T.S. (g/dl)					
Oral fluid intake					
Comments*					
Signature					

*Additional comments need to be entered in the case record; please asterisk if comments are made.

18.2 An example of a physical examination sheet for postoperative colic patients.

Incisional care
Key points
- A celiotomy incision does not require any specific postoperative treatment.
- Horses are confined to a stall then stall and run for the early postoperative period to allow for body wall healing.
- A postoperative fever may be an early sign of an incisional infection and the incision should be monitored for signs of infection (edema and drainage).

Procedure
The incision can be covered during recovery from general anesthesia using an iodine-impregnated adhesive drape (**18.3**) or stent bandage (**18.4**). There is some clinical evidence that a stent bandage may increase incisional infection rate[2]; however, in the author's experience if the stent bandage is removed immediately when the horse stands following recovery from general anesthesia, incisional infection does not appear to be a problem. A more recent report suggested that a stent bandage was protective and decreased incisional infection. It is recommended to remove either a stent or iodine-impregnated adhesive drape immediately following recovery from general anesthesia. An abdominal support bandage should be applied during the initial 24–48 hour period until the celiotomy wound has a fibrin seal and can be used for a more extended period (e.g. 5–14 days) postoperatively to decrease peri-incisional edema and protect the incision in horses showing signs of colic or lying down excessively (**18.5A, B**). Studies

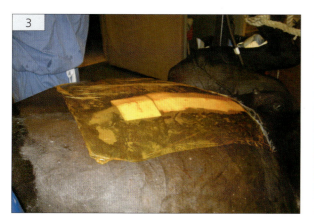

18.3 Iodine-impregnated adhesive drape.

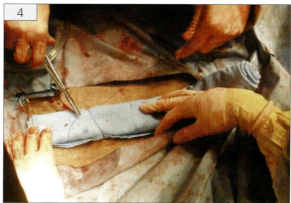

18.4 Stent bandage.

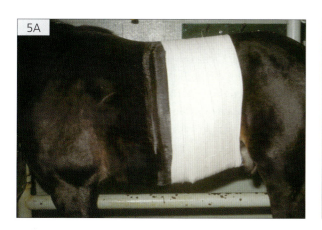

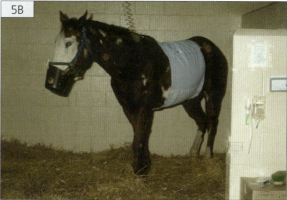

18.5A, B Abdominal support-bandage. (A) Elastic adhesive dressing; (B) re-usable elastic bandage.

have shown a decrease in incisional complication rate with the use of an abdominal bandage.[3] If it is necessary to palpate the incision during the postoperative period, sterile gloves should be worn. The incision does not require cleaning or topical treatment during the postoperative period unless the wound becomes soiled.

Horses should be confined to a stall with hand walking for 4 weeks postoperatively followed by a stall and small run for 4 weeks, then turned out to pasture for 4 weeks, after which normal activity can be resumed. If an incisional infection develops, this recovery period should be longer and the horse should be confined to a stall with hand walking until signs of infection have abated and any cutaneous and subcutaneous wound dehiscence healed. The duration of confinement in cases with an incisional infection depends on the severity of the infection and the degree of cutaneous wound dehiscence. Skin staples should be removed 10–14 days postoperatively. Most surgeons have discontinued the use of staples and appose the subcuticular layer only or the subcutaneous layer and then appose the skin with glue or a synthetic absorbable suture material in a simple continuous pattern. (See also Incisional infection.) Skin glue should not be used if a repeat caliotomy may become necessary because it is difficult to remove during surgical site preparation.

Intravenous catheter
Key points
- The IV catheter and catheterized vein should be monitored closely for any signs of catheter-related problems.
- If any complications are identified, the catheter should be removed and replaced if necessary.

Procedure
Most colic patients have an IV catheter placed in a jugular vein for administration of fluids, NSAIDs, antimicrobials, and other medication. (See Chapter 12.) Any IV catheter should be placed and maintained aseptically and be well secured in place. Bandaging of the catheter site is unnecessary and generally not recommended. If a short-term (polytetrafluoroethylene or Teflon®) catheter is used, the catheter should be changed every 72 hours. Long-term (polyurethane or Silastic®) catheters can be used for several weeks without replacement (**18.6A, B**). The catheter should be checked and flushed regularly and should not be left in place longer than necessary. The catheter should be monitored for:
- Loosening between the catheter and extension set or injection cap.
- Kinking (**18.7**), which can lead to breaking and leakage of fluids and other treatments administered via the catheter into the subcutaneous tissue.
- Thrombus formation (**18.8**).
- Heat, pain, swelling, or drainage indicating septic thrombophlebitis or cellulitis (**18.9**).

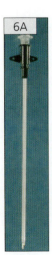
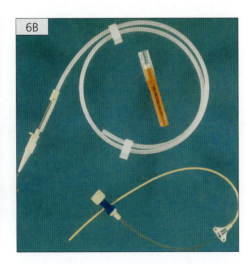

18.6A, B Long-term catheters inserted using the over-the-needle (A) or over-the-wire (Seldinger) (B) techniques. Using the over-the-wire technique, the needle is inserted into the vein. The wire is fed through the needle into the vein; the needle is removed and the catheter is placed over the wire into the vein. The wire is then removed. The catheter is sutured in place.

The patient should be monitored for signs of a fever and if there is a persistent unexplained fever or any abnormal findings with the catheter, it should be removed and replaced only if necessary. If infection is suspected, the tip of the catheter should be submitted for bacterial culture and sensitivity testing. A lateral thoracic catheter (**18.10**) can be placed in patients that develop complications with a jugular vein and require ongoing IV catheterization. Lateral thoracic catheters are somewhat more difficult to place and ultrasonographic guidance may be necessary in some cases.

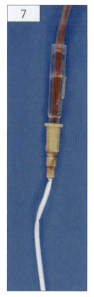

18.7 Catheter kinking. (Courtesy Dr Josie Traub-Dargatz)

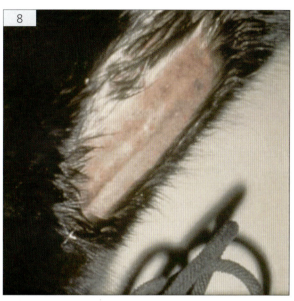

18.8 Jugular vein thrombosis. (Courtesy Dr Josie Traub-Dargatz)

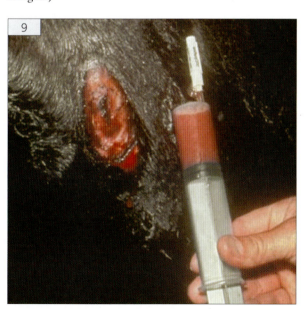

18.9 Septic thrombophlebitis. (Courtesy Dr Josie Traub-Dargatz)

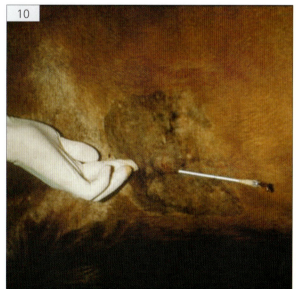

18.10 Lateral thoracic catheter. Cranial is to the left. (Courtesy Dr Josie Traub-Dargatz)

Laboratory data

Key points

- Laboratory data can complement findings on patient observation and physical examination, particularly with regard to cardiovascular and metabolic status.
- Trends over time are often more useful than a single measurement at one point in time.

Packed cell volume and total plasma protein

PCV and TPP should be monitored every 6–24 hours in postoperative colic patients depending on patient stability, severity of the disease, and duration of time since surgery. While PCV and TPP are not the 'gold standard' for assessing hydration status, they can be used as a rough guideline for adjusting the rate of fluid administration as well as the need for other fluids, such as colloids, in a horse with hypoproteinemia. Horses that are accumulating fluid within the GI tract (i.e. postoperative ileus or colitis) often have a rapid increase in PCV, with the TPP also increasing or remaining the same. An increase in the PCV with a concurrent decrease in the TPP is a poor prognostic indicator and is associated with severe endotoxemia, ischemic intestine, intestinal perforation, or colitis (see Chapter 17). PCV can also be used to monitor horses for blood loss during the postoperative period.

Leukocyte count and fibrinogen concentration

Leukocyte count and fibrinogen concentration should be measured in any patient with a postoperative fever, showing signs of colic, or with diarrhea. Horses with abnormal values preoperatively should also be monitored postoperatively. Postoperative colic patients without complications should have a leukocyte count within normal limits (5,500–12,500 cells/μl) and a fibrinogen concentration of less than 5–7 g/l (500–700 mg/dl).

Leukopenia is an indication of endotoxemia, which may be associated with colitis, severely damaged or non-viable intestine, or intestinal leakage and septic peritonitis. Some horses with strangulating lesions or inflammatory disease may have a mild to moderate leukopenia (2,500–4,500 cells/μl) in the early (i.e. 1–2 days) postoperative period. These horses should be monitored closely for other clinical signs indicating complications (e.g. inappetence, colic, tachycardia, fever) and serial leukocyte counts measured to monitor resolution.

Hyperfibrinogenemia (>8 g/l [800 mg/dl]), particularly with a fever, may indicate an infection site (see Fever). Hypofibrinogenemia (absolute or relative; i.e. <3 g/l [300 mg/dl]) in the postoperative period may be an indication of a coagulopathy (see Coagulation and Chapter 11). Serum amyloid A is likely a more sensitive and specific indicator of postoperative infection following colic surgery.

Plasma creatinine concentration

Plasma creatinine concentration can be measured to assess organ and tissue perfusion as well as renal function. If a postoperative colic patient has persistent azotemia (creatinine concentration >160 μmol/l [1.8 mg/dl]), either the IV fluid rate is inadequate (prerenal azotemia) or the horse is in renal failure. Renal failure can be diagnosed using urinalysis (isosthenuria, urinary casts) and urinary fractional excretion of sodium (see Chapter 11).

Blood and urine glucose and serum or plasma triglyceride concentration

Blood and urine glucose should be monitored, particularly in patients on dextrose-containing fluids. An insulin IV CRI (regular insulin starting rate 0.01 IU/kg/hour[4]) or intermittent administration (regular insulin 0.02–0.2 IU/kg SC or IV q6–24h) should be considered in some patients with persistent hyperglycemia and glucosuria (see Chapter 15). Blood glucose should probably be maintained between 4.44 and 6.66 mmol/l (80 and 120 mg/dl). The renal threshold for glucose is 8.88–10.0 mmol/l (160–180 mg/dl) and if blood glucose concentration is above this value, horses will become glucosuric and this may have an osmotic diuretic effect with excessive loss of water into the urine.

Serum or plasma triglyceride concentration should be monitored in patients at high risk for hyperlipidosis and hyperlipemia (triglyceride concentration >0.57 mmol/l [50 mg/dl] and >5.65 mmol/l [500 mg/dl], respectively), particularly ponies. Importantly, horses often have mild to moderate hypertriglyceridemia (0.57–3.39 mmol/l [50–300 mg/dl]) 24–36 hours postoperatively, which usually decreases to within normal limits following reintroduction of feed.[5] Patients with persistent or severe hypertriglyceridemia should be supported with enteral or parenteral nutrition and, in some cases, with insulin.[6–9] (see Chapter 11 and Chapter 15.)

Blood lactate concentration

Lactate is produced as the end product of anaerobic glycolysis and is a marker of peripheral perfusion and oxygen delivery. While there are several metabolic causes of hyperlactatemia (lactate concentration >1 mmol/l [9 mg/dl]), tissue hypoxia from hypovolemia, hypoxemia, hypotension, or a hypermetabolic state is the most common cause of hyperlactatemia. Hyperlactatemia in the postoperative colic patient represents inadequate tissue perfusion and, most likely, an inadequate IV fluid rate. Postoperative colic patients receiving apparently adequate IV fluids with a lactate concentration >1 mmol/l (9 mg/dl) should be examined carefully because it generally indicates development of a complication (e.g. postoperative reflux, colitis, nonviable bowel). (See also Chapter 11 and Chapter 17.)

Central venous oxygen tension and central venous oxygen saturation

$PcvO_2$ and $ScvO_2$ reflect tissue oxygen delivery relative to consumption and can be measured by collecting blood from the cranial vena cava through a CVP catheter. Low $PcvO_2$ (<45 mmHg) and $ScvO_2$ (<65%) is an indication of inadequate tissue oxygen delivery (perfusion), particularly with concurrent hyperlactatemia (see Shock). (See also Chapter 11 and Chapter 17.)

Coagulation

Coagulopathies are relatively common in critically ill postoperative colic patients (e.g. large colon volvulus patient or horse with colitis). A coagulation profile (platelet count, fibrinogen, fibrin degradation products, APTT, PT, and antithrombin III activity) can be performed on any patient suspected of having a coagulopathy (i.e. overt clinical signs, hypofibrinogenemia, or thrombocytopenia). Current treatment of coagulopathy involves plasma and possibly heparin administration). (See also Chapter 11 and Chapter 17.)

Colloid osmotic pressure

COP is the osmotic force exerted by intravascular macromolecules, particularly albumin, and is important for retaining fluid within the vascular space. In most postoperative colic patients, measurement of TPP (albumin, globulin, and fibrinogen; total solids) provides a useful estimation of COP (indirect measurement). However, in critically ill hypoproteinemic patients or if a synthetic colloid such as hetastarch is used, the TPP may no longer accurately estimate COP.[10] The serum albumin:globulin ratio may be altered in hypoproteinemic patients and the TPP measured on the refractometer does not reflect the COP of synthetic colloids, making indirect measurements of COP potentially less accurate.[10] The median total solids measurement of hetastarch, for example, was 39 g/l (3.9 g/dl) and the COP 31 mmHg.[11] COP can be measured directly using a COP analyzer. In practice, however, horses with a low TPP, even following hetastarch administration, generally have a low COP. A low COP (<15 mmHg), TPP (<40 g/l [4 g/dl]), or albumin (<20 g/l [2 g/dl]) indicates the need for either synthetic colloids or plasma to maintain an appropriate circulating volume for tissue perfusion (see Chapter 12).

Hemodynamic monitoring
Key points

- Observation of the patient's attitude, appetite, and fecal and urine production provides a general overview of well being and any abnormalities observed necessitate further investigation.
- Physical examination provides an early indication of postoperative complications such as infection.
- Hemodynamic monitoring in conjunction with some laboratory data can be used to guide fluid therapy.

Arterial blood pressure

Arterial pressure, particularly MAP, can be used to estimate organ and tissue perfusion. Postoperative colic patients may have a decreased MAP compared with normal (hypotension) as a result of hypovolemia or the systemic inflammatory response syndrome (see Chapter 17) secondary to endotoxemia.

However, values are often within normal limits even in critically ill patients because of endogenous compensatory mechanisms. Arterial blood pressure can be measured directly or indirectly. Arterial pressure is measured directly using an arterial catheter (**18.11A**), a pressure transducer, and a continuous recorder. Indirect arterial pressure is most commonly measured using the oscillometric method (**18.11B**) with an occlusion cuff over the coccygeal (tail) (**18.11C**), dorsal metatarsal, median, or palmar digital (limb) artery. The internal inflatable bladder length should be 80% of the tail or limb circumference and the width 20–25% and 40–50% of the tail and limb circumference, respectively.[12] The oscillometric method provides a heart rate that should be the same as that obtained on physical examination for measured pressures to be considered reliable. The accuracy of indirect blood pressure measurements can be improved by taking serial repeat measurements, using minimal restraint in a quiet environment, and maintaining the head in a resting position.[10] (See also Chapter 11.)

Central venous pressure

CVP is the venous pressure in the intrathoracic cranial vena cava and is a measure of blood volume, venous tone, and cardiac function. CVP can be useful to guide fluid therapy in postoperative colic patients that have vascular leakage, hypoproteinemia, and hypotension. CVP measurements may be useful in severely endotoxemic horses (e.g. patients with colitis or a postoperative large colon volvulus) and horses that are refluxing large volumes of fluid. The goal of CVP monitoring is to treat hypovolemia without causing fluid overload. CVP is measured using a jugular catheter that terminates in the intrathoracic cranial vena cava (**18.12A**).

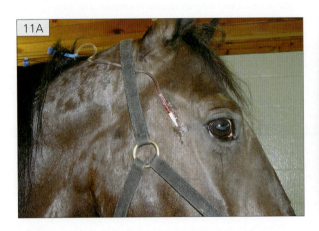

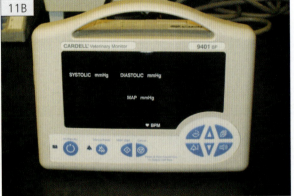

18.11A–C **Arterial blood pressures measured using the direct (A) or indirect (B, C) method. The direct method involves catheterization of a peripheral artery such as the transverse facial artery (A) and a transducer. Indirect pressure can be measured using the oscillometric method (B) with an occlusion cuff over the coccygeal artery (C).**

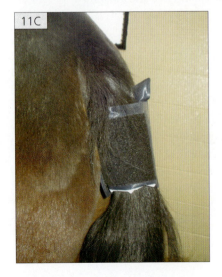

The catheter should not be intracardiac. The catheter is attached to a water manometer, which is zeroed at the base of the heart or the point of the shoulder (**18.12B**). The water manometer should be attached to a fluid stand to ensure zero reference consistency with repeated measurements. The catheter, extension sets, and water manometer should be checked for air bubbles with each measurement. The meniscus should oscillate slightly with respiration if the catheter terminates correctly in the thorax. CVP in normal adult standing horses is 7.5 ± 0.9 to 12 ± 6 cmH$_2$O[13] and in severely ill patients an attempt should be made to maintained it above 5 cmH$_2$O. (See also Chapter 11.)

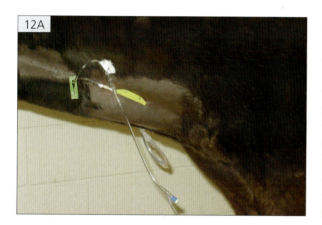

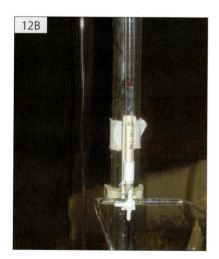

18.12A, B Central venous pressures measured using a water manometer. Central venous catheter (A) and water manometer (B). The white tape around the fluid stand indicates the point of the horse's shoulder and is used for consistency between readings.

BASIC MANAGEMENT

Fluid and electrolyte therapy
Crystalloids
Key points

- Hydration and intravascular volume is maintained with polyionic isotonic crystalloid fluids.
- Horses that are receiving a fluid volume greater than that required for maintenance, and have signs of dehydration or hypovolemia, should be thoroughly examined for the source of fluid loss (e.g. reflux, diarrhea).

Polyionic isotonic crystalloids

Polyionic isotonic crystalloid fluids are usually administered IV in the postoperative colic patient. Because the crystalloid fluids that are available in 5 liter bags are resuscitation or replacement and not maintenance fluids (i.e. high sodium and low potassium concentration such as lactated Ringer's solution, Normasol-R, Plasmalyte), potassium chloride (20 mEq/l) should be added to the fluids. Calcium borogluconate (100 ml per 5 liter bag) is also often added in hypocalcemic patients. Maintenance fluid rates are 1–2 ml/kg/hour (0.5–1 liters/hour for a 500 kg horse). Horses with a simple large colon displacement or impaction often do not need postoperative IV fluids. If there is concern about water intake and hydration status and the horse has normal borborygmi, the oral route of water and electrolyte administration can be used.

Horses with nasogastric reflux and diarrhea require maintenance fluids plus replacement of fluid losses. Reflux should be quantified in liters per hour and the losses replaced. Fluid therapy in these patients can be monitored using physical examination (mucous membrane moistness, CRT, and jugular filling), PCV and TPP, urine SG (maintain between approximately 1.010 and 1.020), blood lactate and plasma creatinine concentration, and CVP. (See also Chapter 12.)

In patients that are not receiving enteral nutrition, dextrose can be added to the fluids at a final concentration of 2.5–5.0%. (See also Chapter 15.)

Hypertonic saline

Hypertonic saline (7% sodium chloride) is occasionally necessary in the postoperative colic patient showing signs of shock. Hypertonic saline can be administered at 4 ml/kg (2 liters for a 500 kg horse) and should be followed by 20 liters of polyionic isotonic crystalloid fluids. (See also Chapter 12.)

Colloids
Key points

- Maintenance of COP with synthetic colloids and plasma is important in postoperative colic patients with SIRS secondary to endotoxemia and protein losing enteropathy.
- The use of dextran-70 is not recommended in these patients because of the complications associated with coagulation.

Synthetic colloids

Synthetic colloids and plasma are necessary in some hypoproteinemic/hypoalbuminemic or endotoxemic patients to maintain oncotic pressure and maintain or expand plasma volume. Hydroxyethyl starch (6%) is the only synthetic colloid used in the author's hospital because of a lack of availability of pentastarch and the complications associated with 6% Dextran-70 (i.e. inhibition of platelet and leukocyte aggregation and histamine release with anaphylactoid reactions[14]). While hetastarch can cause coagulopathy associated with a dose-dependent decrease in von Willebrand factor antigen and factor VIII:C, in one study there was no increase in bleeding time at a rate of 10 ml/kg and so this dose is thought to be safe in normal patients.[14,15] While there may be some concerns with its use in colic patients with a pre-existing coagulopathy, these patients often need colloids to maintain their intravascular volume. The main advantages of hetastarch over plasma are: (1) the molecules are larger and less likely to leak from the vessels into the subcutaneous tissue or into the colonic wall or lumen; (2) the COP of hetastarch is higher than that of plasma; (3) hetastarch does not require thawing; (4) hetastarch is less expensive; and (5) hetastarch has not been associated with anaphylactic reaction. Hetastarch can be given at 10 ml/kg/day (5 liters for a 500 kg horse). (See also Chapter 12.)

Plasma

Plasma can be given as a colloid as well as to provide active proteins, such as acute-phase proteins, complement, clotting factors, and antithrombin III, and to provide antiendotoxin antibodies. Plasma is not an ideal colloid for raising the COP in patients with endotoxemia, for example, because albumin is the principle colloid in plasma and is lost from the vascular space and the COP of plasma (20 mmHg) is lower than that of the synthetic colloids (30–60 mmHg); 1 liter of plasma raises the TPP by 0.5–1.00 g/l (0.05–0.1 mg/dl). Albumin, however, has other important functions besides maintenance of COP. Other disadvantages with the use of plasma are the risk of anaphylactic reaction, time taken to thaw frozen plasma, and expense. Plasma is commonly administered in boluses of 2–10 liters or more to critically ill postoperative colic patients. Plasma should be administered through a blood administration set and patients monitored closely during administration for signs of anaphylaxis (fever, tachycardia, tachypnea, uticaria). (See also Chapter 12.)

Antimicrobial drugs
Key points

- Antimicrobial drugs should be administered immediately prior to colic surgery.
- Postoperative antimicrobial drugs are unnecessary in the majority of patients following colic surgery.
- Horses undergoing an enterotomy or intestinal resection and anastomosis are unlikely to require postoperative antimicrobial drugs and do not need antimicrobial drugs beyond 24 hours postoperatively.
- Horses with existing infection require a therapeutic antimicrobial drug regimen, ideally based on culture and sensitivity results.

Administration

Antimicrobial drugs should be administered preoperatively immediately before induction of general anesthesia or <60 minutes prior to beginning surgery. While some colic surgeries are clean, in most cases the surgeon cannot be sure that the surgery will not become a clean-contaminated procedure. The surgical site infection rate when antimicrobial drugs are administered following surgery only is no different to that when antimicrobial drugs are not used.[16] Antimicrobial drugs should be readministered intraoperatively during prolonged procedures (i.e. >2 hours). Penicillin and gentamicin are the most commonly used perioperative antimicrobial drugs in colic patients. (See also Chapter 16.)

Postoperative antimicrobial drugs are not necessary in the vast majority of colic patients. Horses that had a clean surgical procedure (e.g. simple colonic displacement) do not require postoperative antimicrobial drugs. Information from the human literature strongly suggests that when there is contamination only and no pre-existing infection, postoperative antimicrobial drugs are unnecessary in patients undergoing abdominal surgery. The results of these studies in human patients would suggest that horses undergoing enterotomy or intestinal resection and anastomosis do not require postoperative antimicrobial drugs.[17,18] However, there have been no studies in equine patients evaluating the necessity of postoperative antimicrobial drugs following such clean-contaminated procedures. The author currently uses penicillin and gentamicin for 24 hours postoperatively in horses that have undergone an enterotomy or intestinal resection and anastomosis. The main reasons for not using antimicrobial drugs for a period beyond 24 hours are: (1) higher risk for developing enterocolitis (e.g. *Salmonella* spp. and *Clostridium* spp.) in patients administered antimicrobial drugs compared with patients not administered antimicrobial drugs[19]; (2) emergence of bacteria with antimicrobial drug resistance[20]; (3) studies in human patients have shown a higher risk of nosocomial infections, particularly with resistant microorganisms, in patients that are treated with antimicrobial drugs compared with patients that are not[21,22]; and (4) based on clinical experience to date antimicrobial drug administration beyond 24 hours and probably beyond the preoperative dose is unnecessary.

Some clinicians are concerned that not having the horse on antimicrobial drugs for 2–5 days postoperatively may result in a high incisional infection rate. In the author's hospital, enteric microorganisms (e.g. *Escherichia coli*, *Enterobacter cloacae*, and *Enterococcus faecium* and *faecalis*) are most commonly isolated from incisional infections following colic surgery and hospital-acquired infections with enteric bacteria are frequently multidrug resistant and culture and sensitivity testing is necessary (Dr Helen Aceto, personal communication). Therefore, routinely used antimicrobial drugs, such as penicillin and gentamicin, are often ineffective against these infecting bacteria regardless of the duration used.

The benefit of antimicrobial drugs in critically ill postoperative colic patients (e.g. a horse with a large colon volvulus) is unknown. Horses with SIRS or MODS may be immunocompromised. The effect of leukopenia on the ability of the immune system to manage contamination is unknown. The effect on immune function of inadequate nutrition in inappetent horses should also be considered.

Anti-inflammatory drugs and analgesics
Key points
- Flunixin meglumine is the mainstay anti-inflammatory analgesic drug used in postoperative colic patients. The horse's renal function should be considered when using flunixin meglumine postoperatively and prolonged use should be avoided because of the potential for intestinal mucosal injury.
- Firocoxib or meloxicam can also be used as postoperative anti-inflammatories/analgesics and may have a less negative impact on intestinal mucosal healing.

Administration
Analgesia is an important component of postoperative medical management of the colic patient. Flunixin meglumine is used in most cases (e.g. 1.1 mg/kg IV q12h for 2–3 days then 0.5 mg/kg IV or PO q12h for another 1–2 days). Flunixin meglumine should be used with caution or its use avoided in horses with a high plasma creatinine concentration. Flunixin meglumine should not be used for prolonged periods of time because of the risk of right dorsal colitis (see Chapter 1). More recently, firocoxib, a COX-1 sparing NSAID, can be used at a loading dose of 0.27 mg/kg IV followed by 0.09 mg/kg IV q24h. Firocoxib precipitates with crystalloid fluids and must be given either directly IV or through a catheter injection cap (i.e. no extension), with a DMSO flush solution, or by withdrawing patient's blood into the catheter extension then injecting the firocoxib, followed by use of a routine heparinized catheter flush solution.

Lidocaine (loading dose of 1.3 mg/kg, followed by a CRI of 0.05 mg/kg/minute) is anecdotally thought to provide postoperative analgesia and is reported to have anti-inflammatory properties (see Postoperative ileus).

Butorphanol can also be used as an analgesic following abdominal surgery. Horses treated with butorphanol (13 μg/kg/hour) following colic surgery had a lower plasma cortisol concentration, less weight loss, and a shorter hospital stay compared with horses not treated with butorphanol.[23]

Ketamine is an anti-inflammatory drug that provides analgesia.[24] It also has been used at a dose of 0.4–0.8 mg/kg/hour as an analgesic for horses with colic, with equivocal results.[25] Ketamine inhibited lipopolysaccharide-induced TNF-α and IL-6 in an equine macrophage cell line.[26] Ketamine has been used as a CRI at 1.5 mg/kg/hour for 6 hours without side-effects.[24]

Xylazine (0.2–0.4 mg/kg IV) and butorphanol (0.01–0.02 mg/kg IV), or detomidine (0.01–0.02 mg/kg IV) can be administered as needed. Alpha$_2$-agonists should be avoided where possible because of their negative effects on intestinal motility; however, clinically appreciable complications associated with their use are not often observed. In postoperative colic patients showing signs of mild colic, acepromazine, a motility stimulant, can be used as a sedative, although it is not an analgesic.

Postoperative feeding

Key points

- Feeding is a critical component of postoperative patient care and should be tailored for the individual patient.
- Enteral nutrition is important for maintaining intestinal motility and mucosal health and calories and protein are important for healing. Therefore, at least small amounts of feed should be offered during the early postoperative period.
- Horses with a simple obstruction of the large colon can tolerate rapid refeeding; however, horses recovering from cecal and small colon impactions and small intestinal strangulating obstructions likely benefit from a slower refeeding regimen.

Procedure

Postoperative feeding is a critical part of patient care following colic surgery. Enteral nutrition is important for GI mucosal healing and adequate protein and caloric intake is necessary for wound healing. Complications can occur, however, if feed is reintroduced inappropriately. The lesion severity, type, and location should be taken into consideration when planning a refeeding regimen. The postoperative clinical appearance of the horse, including the amount and duration of reflux following nasogastric tube passage, amount of fecal production, intestinal borborygmi, and appetite should also be used to determine the type of feed as well as the frequency and amount of feed offered. Parenteral nutrition should be considered in cases where refeeding is not possible (see Chapter 15).

Hand grazing is probably the ideal early postoperative feed. In the author's hospital, postoperative colic patients are hand walked and grazed 2–4 times daily, beginning 3–6 hours after surgery (**18.13**).

Feed should be withheld for 3–6 hours after surgery and then gradually reintroduced over a period of 24–72 hours in uncomplicated cases. A typical postoperative feeding regimen would be to offer the horse a handful of hay (**18.14**) every 3–4 hours for 12–24 hours, then a quarter flake of hay every 3–4 hours for 12–24 hours, then one flake of hay every 6 hours for 12–24 hours, then *ad libitum* hay.

In horses with small intestinal disease and/or horses undergoing small intestinal resection and anastomosis, feed should be withheld for 6–12 hours. While it is not recommended to leave a nasogastric tube in place postoperatively, the horse should be checked for reflux if there are signs of dull demeanor, inappetence, tachycardia, or colic. In some cases, it may be beneficial to check for reflux a few times prior to reintroducing feed and water. Allowing the horse to graze small amounts of fresh grass is probably the best way to reintroduce feed. The horse can be walked and allowed to graze a few mouthfuls of grass several times a day or fresh grass can be picked for the horse and fed every 3–6 hours depending on the severity of the intestinal injury and procedure performed. If grazing is tolerated, feed (pelleted feed or hay) can be gradually reintroduced over a period of 48–72 hours. A complete feed (e.g. Equine

Senior®) can be used as an alternative to hay (**18.15**). A typical regimen would be 115 g (4 oz) every 3–4 hours for 12–24 hours, then 225 g (8 oz) every 3–4 hours for 12–24 hours, then 455 g (1 lb) every 3–4 hours for 12–24 hours, then maintenance requirements based on the manufacturer's recommendations. Horses may not eat this type of feed after 1–2 days because of its apparent poor palatability. A typical regimen for refeeding hay would be to feed a small handful of hay (**18.14**) every 3–6 hours for 24 hours, then a large handful or a quarter flake every 3–4 hours for 12–24 hours, then half a flake every 3–4 hours for 12–24 hours, then one flake every 3–4 hours for 12–24 hours, then *ad libitum* hay. A combination of pelleted feed and hay can be used. It is important to ascertain from the owner the horse's regular feeding regimen and have a plan to get the horse onto a feed that is acceptable to the owner and appropriate for the clinical condition of the horse. Water should be reintroduced slowly, particularly in horses that have been refluxing, because these horses tend to drink large volumes of water if given unrestricted access. It is recommended to leave only 1–2 liters of water in the bucket initially and then if the horse does not drink it all, it is probably safe to fill the bucket.

Horses with cecal and small colon impactions are prone to reimpaction and feed should be reintroduced over a period of 5–7 days. Feed should be withheld for 12–24 hours. Initial feeding with fresh grass or a complete feed (**18.15**) should be considered for the first 2–4 days. If the horse has good borborygmi and is producing feces, hay can be reintroduced over the next 2–4 days.

All postoperative colic patients should be monitored closely during the refeeding period for signs of inappetence, colic, tachycardia, lack of defecation, abdominal distension, or poor borborygmi. If any of these clinical signs of GI tract disturbance are identified, feed should be reduced or withheld and the horse thoroughly evaluated.

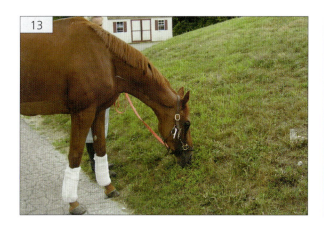

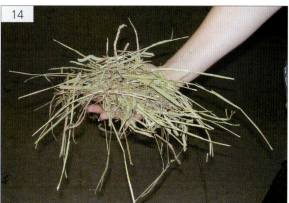

18.13 Grazing is a critical part of postoperative colic patient care. Postoperative colic patients should be grazed on a hill to lower the risk of contamination of the area with fecal material from defecation and from their hooves.

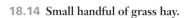

18.14 Small handful of grass hay.

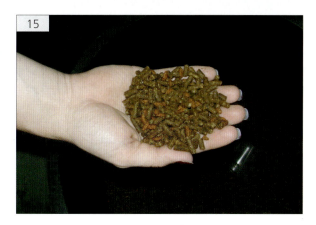

18.15 Complete pelleted feed.

POSTOPERATIVE COMPLICATIONS

Fever
Key points
- Empirically selected antimicrobial drugs should not be used routinely in horses with a postoperative fever.
- The source of a persistent fever should be determined and treatment directed at the identified infection site.
- Sample collection for bacterial culture and sensitivity testing is important for treatment and monitoring of postoperative complications.

Definition/overview
An adult horse with a rectal temperature >38.3°C (101°F) or a foal with a rectal temperature >38.9°C (102°F).

Etiology/pathogenesis
Fever can be associated with inflammation with or without an infection. Common sources of postoperative infection are incisional infection, colitis, salmonellosis, pneumonia/pleuropneumonia, and catheter site infection. Septic peritonitis is an uncommon postoperative complication and often occurs with other complications such as intestinal leakage, severe colitis, or incisional infection. Surgical trauma can cause inflammation and endotoxemia can be associated with a systemic inflammatory response, either of which could cause a fever in the early postoperative period.

The presence of a high rectal temperature (i.e. fever or hyperthermia) does not necessarily mean that the horse has an infection. In a study of human patients undergoing abdominal surgery, 38% developed a postoperative fever, but only 16% of the febrile patients had a bacterial infection.[27] Bacterial infection was associated with: (1) leukocyte count <5,000 or >10,000 cells/μl; (2) blood urea nitrogen ≥5.35 mmol/l (15 mg/dl); and (3) onset of fever after the second postoperative day.[27] When these index factors were used to assess the likelihood of a patient having a bacterial infection, there was an increase in the likelihood of bacterial infection related to the increase in the number of index factors identified (i.e. zero, one, two, or three index factors was associated with a 2, 14, 45, and 100% infection rate, respectively). Similarly, 62% of horses developed a fever following exploratory celiotomy, but only 29% of febrile horses developed an incisional infection.[28] However, a positive association was found between fever and surgical site infection.[28] An association was also found between a high number of non-segmented neutrophils (left shift) preoperatively and surgical site infection.[28] In another study, 87% of horses developed a postoperative fever and only 37% had an infection (incisional, salmonellosis, pneumonia, catheter-associated, peritonitis).[29] Time to peak fever greater than 48 hours after surgery, duration of fever longer than 48 hours, and peak temperature higher than 38.9°C (102°F) were associated with the presence of an infection. These findings can be used to determine whether further diagnostic tests are warranted.

Clinical features
Horses with a mild fever (38.3–39.2°C [101–102.5°F]) may show no clinical signs other than the presence of a fever. Horses with a marked fever (>39.7°C [103.5°F]) may show signs of dull demeanor and inappetence depending on the underlying cause. Localized clinical signs specific to the cause of the fever are often observed (e.g. high respiratory rate and effort with pneumonia, diarrhea with colitis, or peri-incisional swelling and drainage with an incisional infection).

Differential diagnosis
Endotoxemia and a systemic inflammatory response; incisional (surgical site) infection; septic jugular thrombophlebitis (catheter-associated infection); pneumonia/pleuropneumonia; peritonitis; enteritis; colitis; reproductive tract (periparturient mares).

Diagnosis
Hematology and measurement of plasma fibrinogen or serum amyloid A concentrations should be performed on any postoperative colic patient with a persistent fever (i.e. >24 hours duration). Leukopenia can be an early indication of colitis, non-viable intestine, or septic peritonitis associated with leakage from an anastomosis site.

Postoperative colic patients usually have a fibrinogen concentration of 5–7 g/l (500–700 mg/dl); a concentration of >8 g/l (800 mg/dl) likely indicates an infection. Serum amyloid A may be more beneficial than plasma fibrinogen because of its high specificity and sensitivity and correlation with the degree of inflammatory response.

A thorough physical examination should always be performed on any horse with a postoperative fever including examination of the incision, IV catheter site, and a rebreathing examination. Ultrasonographic examination can be used to evaluate the peritoneal fluid for higher than normal volume or echogenicity (septic peritonitis), as well as the cecal and large colon contents for an abnormal volume of fluid or wall thickening (typhlocolitis). The incision site, catheterized vein, and thorax can also be evaluated ultrasonographically. The reproductive tract should be evaluated in periparturient mares.

Samples of any possible infection site should be taken and submitted for cytology (including a Gram's stain) and culture and sensitivity testing.

Management/treatment

Routinely treating patients with a postoperative fever with an empirical antimicrobial drug regimen is not recommended. It is critical to determine whether or not an infection is likely present, identify the site of infection, and obtain fluid or tissue samples for antimicrobial culture and sensitivity testing. Common causes of postoperative fever in horses include SIRS, viral or bacterial respiratory tract infection, enterocolitis, IV catheter site infection, and superficial and deep surgical site infection. The best approach to patients with a postoperative fever is to sequentially consider and rule out each potential site of infection. On rare occasions, a horse may develop a fever and the source cannot be identified. If the fever is persistent (>48–72 hours) and the horse is ill, the horse can be treated with empirically selected antimicrobial drugs.

Incisional infection

Key points

- Incisional infection is a relatively common complication following abdominal surgery.
- Adequate drainage should be provided and the incision cleaned several times a day.
- The benefit of managing incisional infections with antimicrobial drugs is unknown. Systemic antimicrobial drug therapy should be selected based on bacterial culture and sensitivity testing.
- Horses with an incisional infection should be confined to a stall with hand walking for an extended period of time.

Definition/overview

Incisional infection is a superficial surgical site infection and is usually defined as drainage of serous, serosanguineous, or purulent material from the celiotomy incision. Drainage of serosanguineous fluid during the initial 24–36 hours after surgery is not necessarily associated with an incisional infection. A positive bacterial culture confirms the presence of an infection in most cases.

Etiology/pathogenesis

Superficial surgical site infection rates following abdominal exploration are reported to range from 24 to 37%.[28,30–32] Predisposing factors for surgical site infection include cecum/large colon obstruction, repeat celiotomy during the early healing period, duration of surgery >2 hours, patients older than 1 year or more than 300 kg, and near-far-far-near suture pattern.[28,30–32] Horses undergoing repeat celiotomy during the early healing period are reported to have had a surgical site infection rate of 60–88%.[30–32] Incisional trauma was proposed to be a major contributing factor for surgical site infection in horses with cecum/large colon obstruction and repeat celiotomy. Multiple studies have indicated that clean-contaminated surgeries are not predisposed to developing a surgical site infection[28,31,32], supporting the notion that trauma and surgical technique rather than contamination at the time of surgery may be a major contributing factor to surgical site infection post celiotomy.

Bacteria can contaminate the incision during prolonged surgical procedures, during recovery from general anesthesia, or in the immediate postoperative period. Interestingly, in the majority of cases, the bacteria cultured at the completion of exploratory celiotomy were different to the bacteria cultured from a surgical site infection post celiotomy; however, there was an association between positive bacterial culture and subsequent incisional drainage.[28] It is possible that the contaminating bacteria are sensitive to routine antimicrobial drug prophylaxis, but the resistant bacteria proliferate and cause a surgical site infection if in sufficient numbers at the completion of surgery. Alternatively, contamination can occur in the immediate postoperative period during recovery from general anesthesia. In a more recent study, intraoperative bacterial culture did not typically yield any growth; however, postoperative incisional infections were more likely to occur in horses that had bacterial growth after recovery and 24 hours after surgery. These results emphasize the importance of incisional care during the early postoperative period.[33]

Clinical features

Horses with a surgical site infection post celiotomy may have a fever, which is usually mild to moderate (38.3–39.5°C [101–103°F]) or, rarely, severe (>40°C [104°F]). Often horses do not have a fever associated with an incisional infection. Local signs of edema or cellulitis (**18.16**), pain on palpation, and drainage (**18.17**) are seen in horses with a post-celiotomy surgical site infection. The fever often abates once incisional drainage is established. Incisional drainage most often begins between 3 and 14 days postoperatively and drainage may persist for several weeks. Peri-incisional edema also occurs in patients that do not have a surgical site infection because of surgical trauma and the dependent location of the surgical site. Occasionally, the infection is severe and the skin and subcutaneous tissue layers of the incision will dehisce, exposing the linea alba and the sutures holding the abdominal wall together (**18.18**).

Differential diagnosis

Edema only; suture sinus formation; body wall dehiscence and herniation; hemoabdomen (drainage serosanguineous fluid); peritonitis (drainage purulent fluid).

Diagnosis

Ultrasonographic evaluation can be used to assess areas of fluid accumulation that may require drainage and that can be used to obtain a sample for culture and sensitivity testing. The sample is collected by aseptically preparing the skin surrounding the incisional drainage site and then expressing a sample of the drainage fluid onto a culture swab or into a culture vial or small syringe. Aerobic and anaerobic bacterial culture should be performed. Common bacterial isolates from celiotomy incisional infections in the author's hospital are *Escherichia coli*, *Enterobacter cloacae*, and *Enterobacteriacea faecium* or *fecalis*. In one study the most common isolates were *Streptococcus* spp., *Staphylococcus* spp., and *E. coli*.[28] Often, multiple bacteria are isolated from an incisional infection. Enteric bacteria are characteristically resistant and common antimicrobial drug sensitivity includes amikacin, chloramphenicol, and occasionally enrofloxacin (Dr Helen Aceto, personal communication). Because of the high percentage of resistant organisms associated with a surgical site infection, bacterial culture and sensitivity testing is strongly recommended. Antimicrobial drug selection should be based on the results of these tests or the most likely antimicrobial drug effective against the common infecting bacteria for the hospital. The latter requires diligent surveillance of hospital surgical site infections.

Management/treatment

If incisional drainage is present, the incision should be cleaned several times a day using a chlorhexidine- or povidone–iodine-based surgical scrub and wiping thoroughly with sterile saline. Gloves should be used when examining or cleaning the incision. If skin staples or sutures were used to appose the skin, they should be removed adjacent to the area of infection to facilitate wound drainage. Topical antimicrobial drugs can be used and some surgeons like to place antimicrobial-impregnated collagen sponges in the subcutaneous tissue adjacent to the site of drainage. The author does not usually use topical treatments. The association between topical antimicrobial drug use and emergence of resistant bacteria is unknown for equine patients. If an abdominal support bandage is used, it should be changed frequently to avoid having copious amounts of purulent material adjacent to the incision and it is recommended to leave the wound exposed with the bandage off for a period of time during the day. Horses should be confined to a stall with hand walking for at least 4 weeks following complete healing of the skin wound to minimize the risk of evisceration and hernia formation. Stall confinement can be followed

by 4 weeks in a stall and small run and then pasture turn-out for 4 weeks prior to gradual return to exercise. Hand walking and grazing during periods of stall confinement is recommended.

The use of systemic antimicrobials for management of celiotomy incisional infections is controversial. There have been no studies to date demonstrating a benefit of systemic antimicrobial drug use with regard to duration of time that the incision drains, hernia formation, or adhesion of abdominal contents to the incision. It is possible that the incision will continue to drain until suture resorption occurs (polyglactin 910 (Vicryl®) takes 56–70 days), regardless of antimicrobial drug use. If antimicrobial drugs are used, selection should be based on bacterial culture and sensitivity testing.

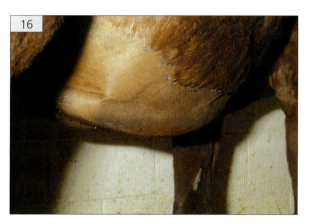

18.16 Edema associated with a celiotomy incision.

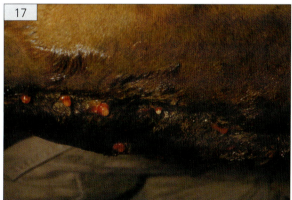

18.17 Drainage from a celiotomy incision. (Courtesy Colorado State University)

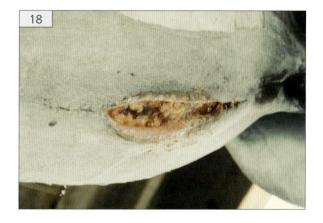

18.18 Severe incisional infection with dehiscence of the subcutaneous tissue and exposure of the body wall sutures.

Hernia formation is not uncommon following a post-celiotomy surgical site infection (**18.19A, B**), with a reported incidence of 9–16% following celiotomy.[28,31] There was a significant association between incisional drainage and hernia formation, with the odds of herniation being 62.5 times greater in horses with incisional drainage compared with horses that did not have incisional drainage.[28] The use of a hernia belt (**18.20**) is recommended in horses with a severe incisional infection to prevent hernia formation.[33] The belt is custom fit to the horse and requires measurements (1) around the girth 5–10 cm caudal to the withers, (2) around the part of the abdomen with the greatest circumference (it is recommended to add 5 cm to the measured length for a pad and the pad should be at least 2.5 cm thick), and (3) of the length of the abdominal incision.[33] The use of a hernia belt may have decreased the need for hernioplasty. Hernioplasty is usually not performed until at least 3–4 months and usually longer following surgical site infection resolution. The necessity for hernioplasty depends on the hernia size and the use of the horse.

Occasionally, repeat celiotomy is necessary in horses with a surgical site infection. In these cases, an approach can be made through a paramedian incision or through the infected incision. The approach selected depends on the anticipated lesion type and location and surgical procedures to be performed, as well as surgeon preference. If an approach is made through the infected incision and the body wall integrity is in question, the body wall incision can be apposed using monofilament stainless steel wire in an interrupted vertical mattress pattern supported with hard rubber tubing stents.[34]

Shock
(See also Chapter 17.)

Key points
- Early recognition and aggressive treatment of shock is necessary for a favorable outcome.

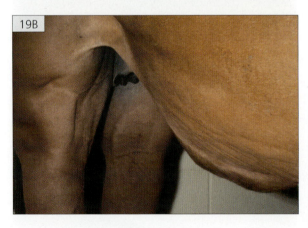

18.19A, B Abdominal hernia formation. (Courtesy Colorado State University)

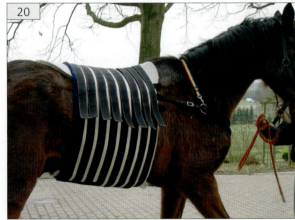

18.20 A horse with severe incisional infection wearing a CM™ Heal Hernia Belt to prevent hernia formation. (Courtesy CM Equine Products, Norco, CA. Note: The belt and the theory on which it is based is patient protected.)

Definition/overview
Shock is defined as inadequate tissue oxygen delivery leading to insufficient ATP production to maintain cell integrity.

Etiology/pathogenesis
Shock in the postoperative colic patient can occur most commonly as a result of hypovolemia, endotoxemia, sepsis, or hemorrhage.

Clinical features
Horses with shock are generally tachycardic and tachypneic and have discolored oral mucous membranes (**18.21, 18.22A, B**) and a prolonged

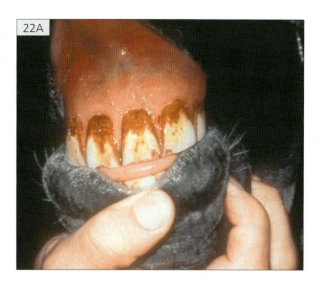

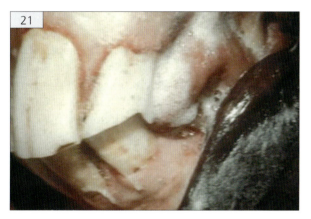

18.21 Pale mucous membranes associated with hemorrhagic shock. (Courtesy Colorado State University)

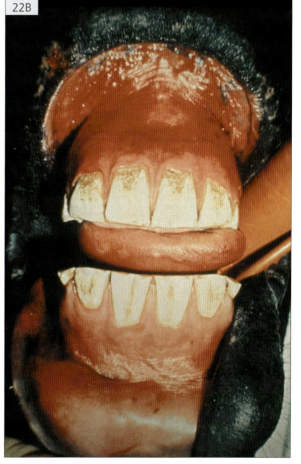

18.22A, B Injected (A) and brick-red (B) mucous membranes in two horse with endotoxemic shock.

CRT (**18.23**). Horses with hemorrhagic shock often have pale mucous membranes (**18.21**) and horses with endotoxemic shock may have injected or brick red mucous membranes (**18.22A, B**). Borborygmi are generally decreased compared with normal or are absent. The horse may also show non-specific signs of dull demeanor and inappetence.

Differential diagnosis
Hypovolemia; endotoxemia; non-viable bowel; enteritis/colitis; septic peritonitis; hemorrhage.

Diagnosis
Basic monitoring procedures should be used and include physical examination, arterial blood pressure, CVP, serum or plasma creatinine and blood lactate concentrations, and central venous oxygen tension and saturation (if a central venous catheter is placed). Hemorrhagic shock is diagnosed based on a rapid decrease in the PCV and TPP. Other specific causes of shock should be identified.

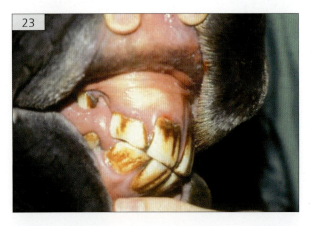

18.23 Prolonged capillary refill time.

Management/treatment
The major clinical problems to address in these patients are hypovolemia, hypoperfusion, hypotension, and hypoproteinemia. Other likely problems are endotoxemia and coagulopathy. IV fluid therapy to increase the intravascular volume is the first part of the approach. Hypertonic saline (7%) can be given (2–4 ml/kg), if not given preoperatively, to increase the intravascular volume. Hypertonic saline also has immune modulating effects that may protect tissues from oxidative injury and enhance cell-mediated immune function. Every liter of hypertonic saline should be followed with 10 liters of isotonic fluids. Isotonic polyionic crystalloids can be given as 20 ml/kg (10 liters for a 500 kg horse) boluses up to 60 ml/kg (30 liters for a 500 kg horse). It should be anticipated that the TPP will decrease to <40 g/l (4 mg/dl). Plasma can be given to provide albumin to maintain oncotic pressure; approximately 10 liters of plasma are necessary to increase the TPP by 5–10 g/l (0.5–1 g/dl) in an adult horse. Plasma is also used to manage endotoxemia (see below) and coagulopathy. Hydroxyethyl starch (6%) at a dose of 10 ml/kg (5 liters/day for a 500 kg horse) can also be given to maintain COP and at this dose is associated with minimal coagulopathies in normal horses. The effect of this in horses with an underlying coagulopathy is unknown. The COP should be measured using colloid osmometery following hydroxyethyl starch administration.

The goals of therapy following the initial resuscitation should be to maintain mean arterial blood pressure (direct) at >65 mmHg, CVP at >5 cmH$_2$O, COP at >15 mmHg, blood lactate concentration at <1.0 mmol/l, PcvO$_2$ at >35 mmHg and ScvO$_2$ at >65%, serum or plasma creatinine concentration at <132.6 μmol/l (1.5 mg/dl), and urine production within normal limits (see above). This is important to maintain intestinal perfusion. IV crystalloid fluid rates of 6–10 ml/kg/hour (3–5 liters/hour for a 500 kg horse) plus several units of plasma may be necessary to accomplish these goals. Inotropes and vasopressors may be necessary in some cases (see Chapter 13).

Endotoxemia
(See also Chapter 17.)

Key points
- Endotoxemia is one of the most common and most difficult to manage postoperative complications, particularly in horses with strangulating intestinal lesions.
- Supportive care is probably the most important component of treatment.
- Identification and treatment of the underlying disease (e.g. colitis, non-viable intestine) is critical for a favorable outcome.

Definition/overview
Endotoxemia refers to the presence of endotoxin (lipopolysaccharide) in the blood.

Etiology/pathogenesis
Endotoxin is the lipopolysaccharide layer of gram-negative bacteria cell wall. During bacterial cell death or rapid proliferation, endotoxin is released into the systemic circulation. Any disturbance in GI tract motility or mucosal integrity can cause an increase in absorption of luminal endotoxin compared with normal. Endotoxemia causes a SIRS, which is defined by having any two of the following: (1) tachycardia, (2) tachypnea, (3) fever (or hypothermia), (4) leukocytosis or leukopenia, and (5) a marked left shift (>10% immature neutrophils) (see Chapter 17). Severe endotoxemia can progress to MODS.

Clinical features
The classical clinical signs of endotoxemia in horses are inappetence, dull demeanor, muscle fasciculations, colic, tachycardia, tachypnea, fever, injected to brick red to purple oral mucous membranes, initially rapid (hyperdynamic phase) followed by prolonged (hypodynamic phase) CRT, decreased to absent borborygmi, and leukopenia. Horses may also have diarrhea or semiformed feces. The hyperdynamic phase of endotoxic shock is characterized by a high cardiac output and low peripheral vascular resistance and the hypodynamic phase by low cardiac output, hypotension, and high peripheral vascular resistance. Signs of endotoxic and hypovolemic shock include marked tachycardia, weak pulses, hypothermia, cool extremities, and dry purple or pale mucous membranes.

Differential diagnosis
Expected postoperative response in a horse with a strangulating lesion (mild endotoxemia); non-viable intestine remaining in the abdomen; septic peritonitis enteritis; colitis; salmonellosis.

Diagnosis
A tentative diagnosis of endotoxemia is made based on clinical signs of dull demeanor, colic, tachycardia, tachypnea, fever, and injected oral mucous membranes, particularly in a horse that has been treated for an intestinal strangulating lesion. A leukocyte count should be performed and the presence of leukopenia supports the diagnosis of endotoxemia.

Management/treatment
Supportive care is the most important treatment for horses with endotoxemia and mostly consists of fluid and electrolyte therapy with both crystalloids and colloids. Treatment includes:
- Flunixin meglumine (0.25 to 1.1 mg/kg IV q6–12h), a COX inhibitor that suppresses the increase in prostaglandin F_1 and thromboxane B2 and prevents the clinical signs, cardiovascular and hemodynamic alterations, arterial hypoxemia, and lactic acidosis after endotoxin administration.[35–38]
- Plasma containing antibodies to endotoxin (e.g. J5 plasma); plasma from horses vaccinated against mutant rough strains of either J5 *Escherichia coli* or the Re mutant of *Salmonella* spp., which have lost their ability to attach O-specific side chains and have the core polysaccharide exposed, has antibodies directed against the core polysaccharide component of endotoxin. J5 plasma has been shown to improve clinical signs and reduce hospitalization time and mortality in endotoxemic horses.[39]

- Polymixin B (1,000–5,000 U/kg IV q8–12h) is a cyclic cationic polypeptide that has a high affinity to the lipid A portion of endotoxin. Lipid A is the toxic portion of the endotoxin molecule. Polymixin B has been shown to improve clinical signs following endotoxin administration and reduce TNF and IL responses in a dose-dependent manner.[40,41] Polymixin B should be administered in 500–1,000 ml of saline.
- Pentoxifylline (10 mg/kg PO q12h), a methylxanthine derivative that improves red and white cell deformability and blood viscosity, decreases platelet aggregation, enhances chemotaxis, decreases neutrophil adherence, causes vasodilation, and may improve microcirculation.[42–44] It also inhibits TNF production and its effects on leukocytes and decreases thromboxane B2 concentration and tissue thromboplastin activity.[44]
- Lidocaine (1.3 mg/kg slow IV bolus followed by 0.05 mg/kg/minute IV CRI) is proposed to have anti-inflammatory effects and may improve clinical signs in patients with endotoxemia.[45]
- Laminitis prevention (applying ice to the feet).

Postoperative ileus and motility modification

Key points

- Horses with small intestinal lesions should be monitored closely in the postoperative period for signs of ileus.
- Maintenance of intravascular volume and hydration and motility stimulants are important for management of horses with postoperative ileus.
- Other differential diagnoses should always be considered in horses showing signs of colic, nasogastric reflux, and dilated small intestine on palpation per rectum during the postoperative period.
- A repeat celiotomy may be indicated to obtain a definitive diagnosis and for decompression.

Definition/overview

Postoperative ileus is defined as a functional inhibition of aboral transit of intestinal contents following abdominal surgery.[46] In human patients, adynamic ileus is defined as a short-term alteration in GI motility and paralytic ileus a loss of motility for >72 hours. In the horse, postoperative ileus has been defined by >20 liters of reflux following nasogastric tube passage during a 24 hour period or >8 liters at a single time after surgery.[47,48] Postoperative ileus is one of the most common reasons for euthanasia following colic surgery.[49]

Etiology/pathogenesis

Propulsion of ingesta along the GI tract is dependent on contraction of enteric smooth muscle in response to generation of an action potential (spiking activity) (**18.24**).[46] Enteric smooth muscle generates slow waves (spontaneous oscillations of the membrane potential), which are inadequate to generate an action potential. Input from the enteric (intrinsic) and autonomic (extrinsic), namely sympathetic (adrenergic) and parasympathetic (cholinergic, vagus), nervous systems is required for sufficient depolarization to reach the threshold potential and generate an action potential.[46] The enteric nervous system consists of ganglia in the myenteric (Auerbach's) and submucosal (Meissner's) plexuses and uses neuropeptides and nitric oxide as neurotransmitters. Sympathetic hyperactivity results in splanchnic vasoconstriction and decreased propulsive motility; therefore, α-adrenergic agonists impair motility and α-adrenergic antagonists enhance intestinal motility. Parasympathetic hypoactivity causes a reduction in motility and decrease in intestinal secretion. Cholinomimetics should, therefore, promote intestinal motility.[46] Importantly, complete severance of the autonomic nervous system has little effect on intestinal motility.[46] This emphasizes the importance of the enteric nervous system and smooth muscle cells on maintenance of propulsive intestinal motility and the impact that damage to these cells has in the role of postoperative ileus.

Intestinal ischemia and reperfusion injury, prolonged intestinal distension, intestinal inflammation, postoperative pain, drugs administered, endotoxemia, and shock can cause an imbalance between the sympathetic and parasympathetic nervous input to the intestine, impairment of enteric nervous system function, and injury to the enteric smooth muscle cells, leading to accumulation of ingesta, liquid, and gas within the stomach and small intestine and signs of postoperative ileus.

General categories of causes of ileus include shock, electrolyte abnormalities, hypoalbuminemia, peritonitis, endotoxemia, intestinal distension, ischemia, and inflammation.[47,50,51] Horses undergoing small intestinal resection and anastomosis were found to have a neutrophilic infiltration at the oral resection margin and evidence of leukocyte activation, indicating that inflammation may play a critical role in postoperative ileus.[52] Horses with small intestinal lesions appear to be predisposed, particularly those with strangulating lesions and undergoing a jejunocecostomy.[53] Admission PCV, heart rate, and blood glucose concentration, prolonged CRT and >8 liters of reflux at admission, type and location of the lesion, and length of intestine resected and increasing age were associated with the risk of postoperative ileus development.[48,50]

Clinical features

In equine patients, postoperative ileus is generally used to describe a syndrome with signs of persistent nasogastric reflux with or without signs of inappetence, dull demeanor, colic, tachycardia, decreased compared with normal borborygmi, and dilated small intestine on palpation per rectum or abdominal ultrasonographic examination. Often the signs of colic will abate following gastric decompression with a nasogastric tube. Horses generally produce a mild to moderate amount of reflux fluid (i.e. 1–3 liters/hour). The CRT may be prolonged and the PCV and TPP may also begin to increase as the horse becomes hemoconcentrated because of the large volume of fluid accumulating in the GI tract. The oral mucous membranes may be injected or bright pink. Abdominal distension is not a clinical feature of postoperative ileus involving the small intestine. Other differential diagnoses, particularly a mechanical obstruction associated with the anastomosis site, should always be considered in these cases.

Horses with a large colon volvulus, for example, can also develop postoperative ileus involving the small intestine or large intestine. Signs consistent with large intestinal ileus are abdominal distension, lack of fecal production, colic, and dilated large colon or cecum on abdominal palpation per rectum. In the author's experience, large intestinal ileus in horses with a large colon volvulus is not associated with a favorable outcome.

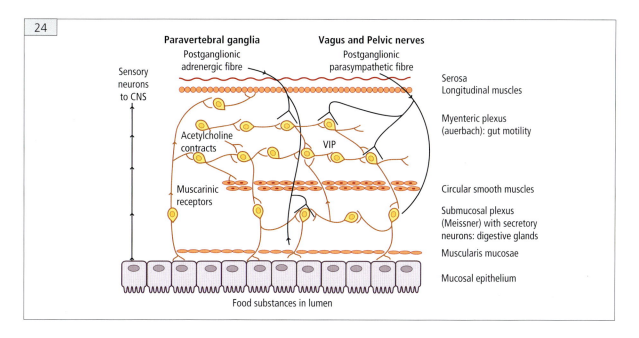

18.24 Physiology of intestinal motility.

Differential diagnosis

Impaction with ingesta at the anastomosis site; hematoma at the anastomosis site causing obstruction; intussusception or small intestinal volvulus at the anastomosis site; enteritis; peritonitis; intestinal nonviability associated with the primary disease; kinking at a jejunocecostomy site; adhesions.

Diagnosis

A tentative diagnosis of postoperative ileus can be made based on the clinical signs (inappetence, dull demeanor, colic, nasogastric reflux, dilated small intestine on abdominal palpation per rectum) occurring during the immediate postoperative period in a horse with small intestinal disease or having undergone a small intestinal resection and anastomosis. It can be challenging, however, to differentiate ileus from a mechanical obstruction.

Abdominal ultrasonographic examination can be used to differentiate postoperative ileus from a mechanical obstruction; however, prospective studies on the accuracy of ultrasonographic examination for this purpose have not been performed.

Repeat celiotomy is the most reliable method to diagnose postoperative ileus; horses with postoperative ileus have dilated and fluid-filled small intestine with no apparent mechanical obstruction. Laparoscopy can also be used in some cases.

Management/treatment

Management of horses with postoperative ileus involves maintaining hydration with IV polyionic isotonic crystalloid fluids at a maintenance plus loss rate (see Chapter 12), NSAIDs, and supportive care. The horse should be decompressed via a nasogastric tube frequently (i.e. every 2–6 hours depending on the volume of reflux obtained). Electrolytes should be monitored, particularly chloride, sodium, potassium, and calcium, and any deficits corrected. The PCV and TPP should also be measured every 6 hours and can be used as a crude assessment of intravascular volume and hydration status. Urine production should also be monitored closely and CVP can be measured to assess the patients fluid requirements (see Chapter 11).

Commonly used motility stimulants are IV lidocaine hydrochloride (HCl), metoclopramide HCl, erythromycin lactobionate, acepromazine maleate, neostigmine methylsulfate, and bethanechol hydrochloride. *Table 18.1* shows the mechanism of action, dose rates, and complications.

Intravenous lidocaine HCl: IV lidocaine is reported to decrease postoperative ileus in colic patients.[54–56] In a controlled prospective study evaluating the use of IV lidocaine in horses with postoperative ileus or enteritis, 65% of horses treated with lidocaine stopped refluxing within 30 hours compared with 27% of horses in the saline control group, and lidocaine-treated horses had a shorter duration of hospitalization compared with horses in the saline control group.[55] While there are some concerns regarding the risk of incisional infection with lidocaine use, there was no difference in the rate of incisional infection, jugular thrombosis, laminitis, or diarrhea in horses treated with lidocaine compared with the saline control group.[55] Muscle fasciculations (and ataxia or weakness) have been observed with lidocaine use and were reported to occur in 18% of horses.[55] Lidocaine should not be used with cimetidine or metronidazole because it can potentiate the toxic effects[46] (*Table 18.1*) and should be administered using a fluid pump to be sure that the appropriate dose is administered. Collapse and seizure may occur if CNS toxic levels are reached. Horses generally recover rapidly once the lidocaine infusion is stopped; however, injury can occur. More recent findings with regards to the beneficial role of IV lidocaine for treating postoperative colic cases include attenuation of ischemia-reperfusion injury in an *in-vivo* jejunal model[57] and improvement in smooth muscle contractility and basic cell function following ischemia-reperfusion injury.[58]

Metoclopramide HCl: Metoclopramide clinically and experimentally has been shown to improve intestinal motility and ingesta transit. Metoclopramide restored coordinated gastroduodenal motility and ingesta transit in an equine postoperative ileus model[59] and horses treated with metoclopramide prophylactically following small intestinal resection and anastomosis had a lower total volume, duration, and rate of nasogastric reflux compared with horses that were not treated with metoclopramide.[60] Metoclopramide also improved gastric emptying in horses given endotoxin.[61] Importantly, metoclopramide HCl can cross the blood–brain barrier and also suppress the central dopamine (D2) receptor, which can cause extrapyramidal side-effects such as tremor, agitation, excitement, and aggression. The author currently uses metoclopramide in cases of postoperative ileus that are non-responsive to IV lidocaine and begins treating horses with 0.02 mg/kg/hour and then gradually increases the rate over several hours to reach the therapeutic dose rate of 0.04 mg/kg/hour if no side-effects are observed.

Erythromycin lactobionate: Erythromycin is most commonly used in horses with postoperative ileus and cecal impactions. In one study, erythromycin decreased contractile amplitude of the equine pyloric antrum circular smooth muscle and increased contractile amplitude of the longitudinal smooth muscle *in vitro*[62], which may explain its role in accelerating the rate of gastric emptying in horses *in vivo*. Erythromycin improves motility (gastric and cecal emptying) in normal experimental horses; however, it may not be as effective in clinical cases. Jejunal contraction in response to erythromycin *in vitro* is weaker following jejunal distension. While binding of erythromycin to the motilin receptor does not appear to be affected by ischemia or distension, jejunal distension causes a decrease in the number

Table 18.1 Drugs used to stimulate gastrointestinal motility

DRUG	MECHANISM OF ACTION	DOSE	SIDE-EFFECTS
Lidocaine hydrochloride	↓ afferent neuron activity in intestinal wall associated with sympathetic inhibition of motility Anti-inflammatory: ↓ prostaglandin, ↓ neutrophil migration, ↓ lysosomal enzyme release Stimulates enteric smooth muscle	1.3 mg/kg slow IV bolus. 0.05 mg/kg/minute	Muscle fasciculations, ataxia, collapse, seizure
Metoclopramide hydrochloride	Substituted benzamide Dopamine receptor antagonist ↑ acetylcholine from intrinsic cholinergic neurons Adrenergic blockade	0.04 mg/kg/hour IV CRI* 0.25 mg/kg in 500 ml saline given over 0.5–1 hour	Excitement, restlessness, colic, sweating
Erythromycin lactobionate	Macrolide antibiotic Motilin agonist Stimulates acetylcholine through serotonin receptors	1–2 mg/kg diluted in 1 liter saline given IV over 1 hour q6h	Colic, diarrhea, tachyphylaxis
Acepromazine maleate	α-adrenergic antagonists Inhibit sympathetic activity	0.01 mg/kg IM q4h	Peripheral vasodilation, priapism
Neostigmine methylsulfate	Cholinesterase inhibitor Prolongs acetylcholine activity by inhibiting its breakdown at synapses	0.0044 mg/kg SC or IV every 30–60 minutes Up to 0.02 mg/kg	Colic
Bethanechol	Muscarinic cholinergic agonist Stimulates acetylcholine receptors on GI smooth muscle causing contraction Parasympathomimetic	0.025 mg/kg SC or PO q3–4h	Colic, diarrhea, salivation, gastric secretion

*Recommended

of motilin receptors compared with normal, which is most likely associated with a decrease in motilin receptor synthesis.[51,63] Motilin receptors may also be downregulated with prolonged erythromycin use (tachyphylaxis).[64] The availability of injectable erythromycin is currently limited within the US.

Acepromazine maleate: Acepromazine has been used to manage horses that are refluxing and/or showing mild signs of colic following small intestinal resection and anastomosis. Acepromazine does not provide analgesia, but its sedative effect in combination with its potential motility enhancing effect may be beneficial in some cases. Acepromazine causes peripheral vasodilation and should be used with caution in horses with signs of shock. Care should be taken when using acepromazine in stallions because of the potential for priapism. Yohimbine HCl acts similarly to acepromazine; however, it is a specific α_2-adrenergic antagonist and does not cause peripheral vasodilation. Slow IV infusion of yohimbine (cumulative close of 0.075 mg/kg) attenuated the inhibitory effects of endotoxin on cecal motility[65] and, at a dose of 0.15 mg/kg every 3 hours in combination with bethanechol, decreased the severity of postoperative ileus in an equine model.[59] Yohimbine is not commonly used to treat horses with postoperative ileus.

Neostigmine methylsulfate: Neostigmine was shown to increase the amplitude of rhythmic contractions in normal and distended small intestine and improved myoelectric activity in the ileum, cecum, and right ventral colon and increased cecal emptying[66]; however, in earlier studies, while it stimulated propulsive pelvic flexure motility, it delayed gastric emptying and decreased jejunal motility.[67] Neostigmine has been used in horses with large intestinal motility disorders, including colitis, and cecal, large colon, and small colon impactions.[46] Signs of colic can occur with its use and it is recommended to start at the lowest dose rate and increase gradually to effect (*Table 18.1*).

Bethanechol HCl: In an equine postoperative ileus model, bethanechol in combination with yohimbine shortened GI tract transit time; however, it was less effective than metoclopramide.[59] While bethanechol could be used to manage gastric and cecal impactions,

its use in the management of postoperative ileus requires further investigation.[46] Bethanechol is not commonly used for prevention or treatment of postoperative ileus because of data showing that it does little to restore coordinated intestinal motility and has side-effects including abdominal pain, diarrhea, salivation, and gastric secretion.[46]

Postoperative intra-abdominal adhesions
Key points
- Prevention of postoperative intra-abdominal adhesion formation is critical because treatment is often unsuccessful.
- Early referral and surgical intervention as well as aseptic and atraumatic surgical techniques are most important in prevention of postoperative intra-abdominal adhesion formation.

Definition/overview
Postoperative intra-abdominal adhesions are defined as fibrinous or fibrous adhesions involving adjacent intestine, mesentery, omentum, or body wall. Adhesions can form between adjacent loops of intestine (**18.25**), mesentery and intestine (**18.26**), omentum and intestine (**18.27**), or body wall and intestine. Adhesions can be focal or diffuse affecting multiple areas of bowel (**18.28**). Clinical signs of colic occur when the adhesions cause luminal obstruction or intestinal strangulation.

Etiology/pathogenesis
The principal causes of adhesions are trauma, inflammation, and ischemia. Adhesion formation is the body's response to injury to heal and revascularize injured tissue by providing cellular and vascular support. Intestinal distension, drying and abrasion of serosal surfaces, surgical manipulation, infection, bacterial contamination, foreign material such as suture, glove powder, and lint, and ischemia associated with a strangulating lesion, vascular compromise, tight suture placement, or intestinal distension are all potential causes of postoperative intra-abdominal adhesion formation.

Factors that have been shown to predispose horses to adhesions include small intestinal lesions, small intestinal resection and anastomosis, repeat celiotomy, peritonitis, and prolonged postoperative ileus.[31,68,69] Adhesions appear to cause more problems in foals than adult horses and this may be because plasma antithrombin III concentrations are lower in foals than in adult horses and the concentrations of other coagulation or fibrinolytic factors may also vary with age.[70] Alternatively, foals may be predisposed to adhesion formation because of enhanced healing capabilities and higher occurrence of small intestinal disease. Miniature horses are also reported to be predisposed to adhesion formation[71]; however, this may be associated with the high incidence of small colon obstruction in this breed.

In patients with intestinal lesions and undergoing abdominal surgery, there is thought to be an imbalance within the peritoneal cavity between fibrin formation and fibrinolysis, with persistence of fibrin on serosal surfaces. Plasminogen activator converts plasminogen to plasmin, which is important in fibrinolysis. Plasminogen activator inhibitor is increased compared with normal in inflammatory and ischemic conditions. Low intraperitoneal tissue plasminogen activator is thought to be important in adhesion formation and the degree of reduction in tissue plasminogen concentrations correlated with the severity of adhesions in human patients.[72]

Phospholipases are surface active materials that have a hydrophobic and hydrophilic component. Phospholipids adhere to the negatively charged peritoneum by their positively charged component, with

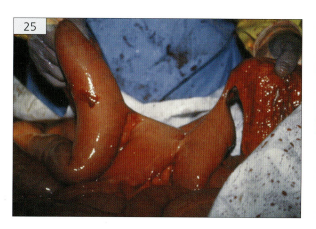

18.25 Adhesions between adjacent loops of jejunum.

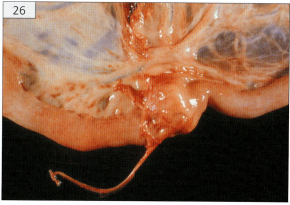

18.26 A focal adhesion between the mesentery and adjacent jejunum.

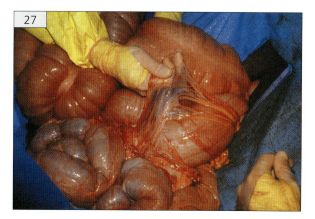

18.27 An omental adhesion.

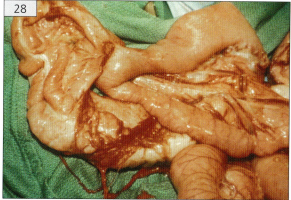

18.28 Diffuse jejunal adhesions.

the hydrophobic component exposed to the abdominal cavity. Phospholipids are thought to cause lubrication between intestinal loops and prevent close and prolonged contact between serosal and peritoneal surfaces. Loss of the phospholipid layer through trauma could predispose to adhesion formation. Phospholipase A2 is increased in ischemia and inflammation and hydrolyzes phospholipids.[73,74] Mast cells[75] and neutrophils[76] are also likely to play a role in intra-abdominal adhesion formation.

Adhesions can also form between the bowel and the body wall. Incisional infection may predispose to this type of adhesion.

The occurrence of postoperative intra-abdominal adhesions may have decreased over the past 15 years, which is likely an example of the impact of early referral and surgical intervention. Early return of intestinal function is also likely to be a key factor in adhesion prevention.

Clinical features

Horses with adhesions generally begin to show signs of colic as early as 3–4 days to several months to years postoperatively. Horses that show clinical signs within the first 2 months reportedly have a less favorable prognosis than horses with a longer duration of time between surgery and the onset of clinical signs.[68] Signs of colic may be mild (e.g. inappetence and occasional flank staring and pawing that is responsive to treatment with flunixin meglumine and dietary modification) to moderate (persistent signs of colic with rolling). Adhesions can form without causing clinical signs; however, these usually remain undiagnosed. Horses with small intestinal adhesions generally have reflux following nasogastric tube passage and distended loops of small intestine on palpation per rectum. Tachycardia and tachypnea as well as a prolonged CRT may occur in horses with prolonged obstruction and/or copious reflux. Mucous membranes may appear injected in horses with a strangulating lesion associated with a lesion.

Differential diagnosis

Postoperative ileus (early postoperative period); intraluminal obstruction at the anastomosis with ingesta or a hematoma; intussusception or segmental volvulus at the anastomosis; anastomosis stomal stricture or stenosis.

Diagnosis

Adhesions should be suspected in any horse having undergone a small intestinal resection and anastomosis that shows signs of colic postoperatively, reflux following nasogastric tube passage, and/or dilated small intestine on abdominal palpation per rectum. Clinical signs associated with adhesion formation do not usually appear until a few days postoperatively.

A tentative diagnosis of adhesions can be made based on ultrasonographic examination where a segment of bowel does not move in relation to adjacent structures along with an obstructive pattern (i.e. dilated small intestine of normal mural thickness, as well as normal collapsed and contracting small intestine). Laparoscopy or repeat celiotomy is necessary to obtain a definitive diagnosis.

Management/treatment

Prevention of adhesions is critical. Early referral and surgical intervention and meticulous surgical technique are probably the most important factors in preventing adhesions. Additional techniques that are currently used to prevent adhesions include:

- Perioperative treatment with flunixin meglumine and antimicrobial drugs.[77]
- Intraperitoneal fucoidan solution (Peridan™ Concentrate), which is administered as a 50 ml concentrate diluted in 5 liters of lactated Ringer's solution (LRS) at the completion of surgery (5 ml in 500 ml LRS for foals). The solution can be administered directly into the abdomen by opening the bag or by using a 4-prong irrigation set (**18.29A, B**).[78,79]
- Intraoperative sodium carboxymethylcellulose to facilitate intestinal manipulation and instillation of 1–2 liters intraperitoneally at the completion of surgery.[80]
- Hyaluronate-carboxymethylcellulose membrane (e.g. Seprafilm®, **18.30A, B**) to cover the anastomosis or focal sites predisposed to adhesion formation.[80] The membrane may be effective but is expensive and can be difficult to apply.
- IV lidocaine as an anti-inflammatory drug and to improve intestinal motility (see Postoperative ileus).
- Heparin (40 IU/kg IV during surgery and then SC q12h for 48 hours).[81] IV heparin during surgery may increase surgical site bleeding.

- Dimethylsulphoxide (20 mg/kg as a 10% solution IV q12h for 48 hours).[77]
- Postoperative abdominal lavage using 10 liters of isotonic polyionic crystalloid fluids every 8 hours for 36–48 hours.[82] This technique is somewhat labor intensive and in the author's hospital is generally reserved for patients with a particular predisposition to adhesions (e.g. abdominal abscesses, post adhesiolysis).
- Omentectomy.[83]

Management of horses with adhesions is challenging. While some horses with adhesions can be managed with dietary modification (e.g. pelleted feed or pasture),

repeat celiotomy or laparoscopy is necessary for diagnosis and treatment in many cases. Surgical options to treat adhesions include adhesiolysis, intestinal resection and anastomosis, or surgical bypass of the affected intestine. In horses or foals predisposed to adhesion formation, laparoscopy can be performed within 3–5 days of celiotomy to identify fibrinous adhesions and perform adhesiolysis before they become fibrous and cause clinical signs of colic. This is particularly useful when adhesions form between the small intestine and the body wall and the adhesions are identified early during the postoperative period.

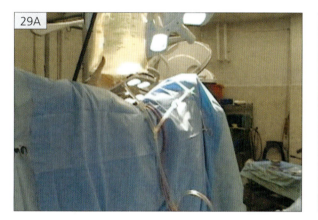
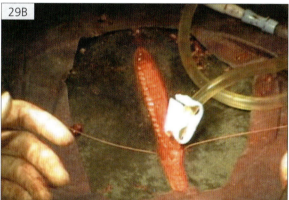

18.29A, B Administration of intraperitoneal Peridan™ solution using a 4-prong irrigation set. A 5-liter bag containing lactated Ringer's solution with Peridan™ is hung from a hoist (A) and then the solution is placed into the abdomen immediately prior to body wall closure (B)

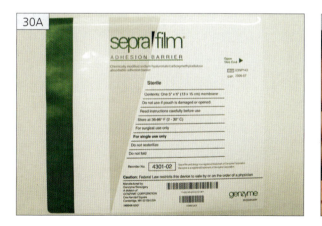
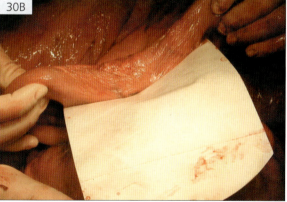

18.30A, B (A) Seprafilm® used to prevent intra-abdominal adhesions. (B) Application of Seprafilm® to the serosal surface of the jejunum at a site of a previous adhesion between the jejunum and the ventral body wall.

INTRODUCTION

Emergency presentation of the peripartum mare presents a diagnostic challenge with problems ranging from those associated with the pregnancy itself up to and including critical illness not directly associated with, but impacted by, pregnancy.[1–3] Management is complicated by consideration for the well being of the fetus or neonate. Some commonly encountered problems of the peripartum mare are presented here, but any emergency problem of the adult horse can be present in the pregnant mare.

PREPARTUM PROBLEMS

Placentitis
Etiology/pathogenesis
Placentitis is primarily caused by ascending bacterial or fungal infections that originate in the region of the cervix (**19.1**). These infections can cause *in-utero* sepsis or compromise the fetus by local elucidation of inflammatory mediators or altered placental function.

Clinical features
Premature udder development and vaginal discharge are common clinical signs of placentitis.[2–4]

19.1 Placenta from a mare with placentitis showing an erythematous, thickened region surrounding the cervical star. Note that the cervical star has not ruptured in this case. The mare experienced premature placental separation and the foal had evidence of perinatal asphyxia.

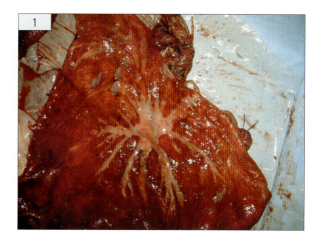

Management/treatment

Treatment primarily consists of administration of broad-spectrum antimicrobials, NSAIDs, and tocolytics:

- Trimethoprim-sulfa drugs are the antimicrobials of choice in many practices. They reach higher concentrations in fetal fluids compared with penicillin and gentamicin. Treatment should be directed by culture and sensitivity results if available.
- NSAIDs, such as flunixin meglumine, are administered in an effort to combat alterations in prostaglandin balance that may develop in association with infection and inflammation.
- Tocolytic agents and agents that promote uterine quiescence have been used and include altrenogest (0.044–0.088 mg/kg PO q24h), isoxuprine, and clenbuterol (0.8–1.6 µg/kg PO q12h).
  - Altrenogest is usually administered, although its usefulness in late gestation can be challenged.
  - The efficacy of isoxuprine as a tocolytic in the horse is unproven, and bioavailability of orally administered isoxuprine appears to be highly variable.
  - Long-term administration of clenbuterol as a tocolytic is inadvisable because of receptor population changes associated with long-term use and the unknown effects on the fetus. Administration of clenbuterol may be indicated during management of dystocia in preparation for assisted delivery or cesarean section. (**Note:** The IV form of clenbuterol is not available in the USA.)
  - Pentoxifylline (8.4 mg/kg PO q12h or q8h) has been used for its rheologic effect, which could potentially improve blood flow in the placenta, and also for its general anti-inflammatory effects.

Other treatments that should be considered:

- Intranasal oxygen supplementation at 10–15 liters/minute can be provided in the hope of improving oxygen delivery to the fetus.
- Vitamin E (tocopherol) can be administered orally at 5,000 IU/day to high-risk mares as an antioxidant.
- Mares that are inappetent or withheld from feed because of their medical condition are at particularly high risk for fetal loss because low or absent feed intake alters prostaglandin metabolism. Dextrose (as a 2.5–5% solution in 0.45% saline or water) can be administered at maintenance fluid rates in these patients to support energy metabolism.

Body wall hernia and prepubic tendon rupture[1,2,5,6]

Definition/overview

Body wall hernias and prepubic tendon rupture are usually detected by the owner as an abrupt change in the contour of the abdominal wall with concurrent lethargy and inappetence in the mare. Catastophic body wall tears can develop in mares at any time and can be life-threatening.

Etiology/pathogenesis

The most common reasons for presentation are abdominal discomfort or colic and ventral edema. Other reasons include abdominal enlargement, reluctance to move, tachycardia, and lameness. Although body wall tears are frequently anecdotally associated with hydrops, twinning, advanced maternal age, draft breed, and multiparous state, results of a recent study[6] suggested that none of these predisposing conditions may be present.

Clinical features

Clinical signs include ventral edema, softening or pain on palpation of the abdominal wall, particularly in the flank region (**19.2**), colic, tachycardia, hemorrhagic mammary secretions, flattened mammary glands, unwillingness to walk, abdominal enlargement, and sudden-onset lordosis.

Diagnosis

The body wall defect can be difficult to identify because of edema. Transabdominal sonographic examination can be helpful in making a definitive diagnosis, although the edema may again limit examination.

Management/treatment

Effective treatment most often is conservative, with enforced strict stall rest, placement of large abdominal support wraps (**19.3**), and analgesics administered as needed. Some mares initially require IV fluid support. The best outcome for both mare and foal is achieved with conservative management of parturition, suggesting that close monitoring for parturition and provision of assistance if necessary constitute the most effective approach, and that induction of parturition or elective cesarean section is not necessary in most instances and may even be harmful.

Mares with body wall tears and hydrops appear to have the worst prognosis for a good outcome for both mare and foal, and induction of parturition prior to final fetal maturation may be required to save the mare. Mares for which the breed registry permits assisted reproductive technologies may go on to become embryo donors, but rebreeding and permitting the mare to carry a foal to term is generally not recommended.

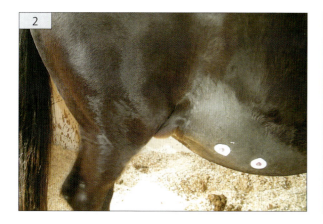

19.2 Late pregnant mare with a body wall tear in the flank region. Note the accumulation of edema in the flank fold, which is characteristic in the early stages.

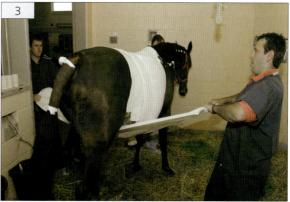

19.3 Placing an abdominal support wrap on a late pregnant mare with bilateral body wall tears. (Courtesy Dr Julie Ross)

Hydrops conditions

Definition/overview

Hydrops allantois is an emergency condition for which prompt action in a short time interval is needed to ensure the health of the mare, as secondary complications, such as respiratory compromise, hypovolemic shock at delivery, and body wall hernia, may develop.

Clinical features

This condition is often detected by the owner as a sudden onset of abdominal distension with progressive lethargy and inappetence, and possibly dyspnea associated with intra-abdominal hypertension (abdominal compartment syndrome).

Diagnosis

Diagnosis is made on the basis of rectal palpation, which reveals an enlarged, fluid-filled uterus. Hydrops is confirmed by sonographic examination per rectum, in which an excessive volume of allantoic and, less commonly, amnionic, fluid is observed. Affected mares are at risk of body wall tear secondary to the increased weight of the abdominal contents and rapid abdominal distension.

Management/treatment

Induction of parturition and controlled removal of uterine fluid and contents is usually performed. Complications during induction include hypovolemic collapse and dystocia. An IV catheter should be placed prior to induction of parturition, and fluid should then be siphoned with a large-bore drainage tube once the fetal membranes are ruptured. As the fluid is removed, IV fluids may be administered to combat hypovolemia. Close monitoring of the heart rate and measurement of arterial blood pressure may be beneficial. There is one report of a foal surviving following a pregnancy afflicted with hydrops.[7]

Future breeding soundness may not be compromised in mares with uncomplicated resolution of a hydrops condition.

PERIPARTUM PROBLEMS

Bleeding

Etiology/pathogenesis

Urogenital hemorrhage ('bleeding') is generally thought of as an episode of acute shock associated with massive blood loss within hours of parturition, although uterine vessel trauma during pregnancy has also been reported and may present as intermittent or low-grade chronic colic. Blood loss may occur secondary to rupture of the middle uterine artery or utero-ovarian artery, secondary to uterine rupture involving a vessel, or from severe vaginal trauma with tearing of a vaginal artery.

Clinical features

Clinical signs include abdominal pain, manifest by pawing and rolling. Flehman behavior, excessive sweating, tachycardia, lethargy, and anorexia have also been seen with uterine hemorrhage. Fever is common in mares that survive and may not be infectious in origin.

Diagnosis

Clinicopathologic evidence of substantial blood loss, such as anemia, hypoproteinemia, and hypofibrinogenemia, may or may not be detected, depending on the acuity of the blood loss. Abdominal palpation per rectum may reveal a soft fluctuant mass (a hematoma) in the broad ligament of the uterus, which may contain a palpable pulse. Other diagnostic findings may include hemoperitoneum, and sonographic examination may reveal a hematoma in the broad ligament or blood in the uterine lumen or peritoneal space.

Management/treatment

Treatments vary and are administered primarily on the basis of the veterinarian's experience and clinical impression of efficacy, as no reports have been published, to the author's knowledge, in which treatments and outcomes of various treatment regimens were rigorously compared.

Mares should be kept as calm and quiet as possible. Many mares receive IV fluids during the suspected acute bleeding phase. Anti-inflammatory treatment generally consists of administration of flunixin meglumine at various dosages. Alpha-2 agonists (e.g. xylazine and detomidine) are sometimes used for pain management, but carry a risk of transient hypertension. Naloxone (0.01–0.02 U/kg IV or IM q12h), an opioid antagonist, has been used for analgesia. Acepromazine has been used both as an anxiolytic and to decrease arterial pressure in the hope of decreasing bleeding.

Mares that survive the initial bleeding episode generally receive antimicrobials; penicillin and gentamicin in combination, ceftiofur, or trimethoprim sulfa are commonly used.

Because large-volume blood loss can result in coagulopathy associated with loss of clotting factors, fresh frozen plasma, a fresh whole blood transfusion, or both, can be administered. Anecdotally, dilute formalin (10–30 ml 10% formalin in 1 liter isotonic crystalloid fluids) solution added to an isotonic crystalloid fluid has been administered IV to initiate clot formation and hemostasis at the site of bleeding.

One study of 32 bleeding mares referred for treatment revealed a higher than anticipated survival rate of up to 84%.[1] This was a self-selected population of mares that survived both the initial acute episode of hemorrhage and transport and is likely not fully representative of all bleeding mares.

Mares that have hemorrhaged previously can be successfully rebred and may produce foals in subsequent years but should be monitored carefully for recurrence of hemorrhage. Clinical experience suggests that in future years it might be difficult to find an appropriate blood donor for many of these mares because of cross-match incompatibility.

GASTROINTESTINAL PROBLEMS

Rectal prolapse
Etiology/pathogenesis
Rectal prolapse may occur in any animal species in association with prolonged periods of tenesmus and may occur during parturition in the mare.

Rectal prolapse is graded as follows: type I, only mucosa is prolapsed; type II, full-thickness rectum is prolapsed; type III, some length of small colon intussusception into the rectum develops; and type IV, both small colon and rectum are involved in the prolapse.

Diagnosis
Diagnosis is straightforward, as the prolapse is visible.[1–3] The severity of type III and type IV prolapse warrants exploration of the abdomen to evaluate the integrity of the affected bowel and mesocolon.

Management/treatment
Low-grade prolapses may be reduced manually, depending on the severity of swelling in the affected tissues. Severe prolapse may require amputation of the affected segment and carries a poorer prognosis for life.

Small colon trauma
Etiology/pathogenesis
The small colon is another section of the GI tract that is vulnerable to injury during parturition. Injury may involve the bowel wall itself or, as is more common, may involve the mesocolon, leading to ischemic necrosis of the bowel. Mares with small colon injury may have a history of normal parturition with no complications or may have had dystocia with or without subsequent development of type III or IV rectal prolapse.[1–3]

Clinical features

Clinical signs in mares with this complication include: gradual onset of depression after parturition; moderate to mild colic; signs consistent with peritonitis, including fever, ileus, and gastric distension with reflux fluid; depression, tachycardia, and signs of mild discomfort.

Rectal examination findings can be unremarkable; conversely small colon impaction may be present. Serosal roughening and pneumoperitoneum may be detected if small colon rupture has occurred.

Diagnosis

Analysis of fluid obtained via abdominocentesis may be suggestive of either septic or non-septic peritonitis, with a high nucleated cell count (sometimes >100,000 cells/μl) and TPP concentration. Clinicopathologic data may be normal or inflammatory. Fndings consistent with the latter include leukopenia, leukocytosis, hyperfibrinogenemia, hemoconcentration, azotemia, and hypoproteinemia. A definitive diagnosis is made by exploratory celiotomy or laparoscopy.

Management/treatment

Outcome is variable and depends on the duration and degree of bowel wall necrosis and secondary peritoneal contamination. The rate of survival to discharge is low, with 36–50% short-term survival rates reported.

Small intestine trauma

Etiology/pathogenesis

Similar in etiology and presentation to traumatic injury of the small colon, trauma of the small intestine may also occur and may involve direct injury to the bowel or mesenteric trauma with subsequent bowel necrosis.

Clinical features

Physical examination findings are often suggestive of small bowel obstruction, with gastric reflux, signs of severe abdominal pain, and small intestinal distension (palpable on rectal examination).

Diagnosis

Exploratory celiotomy is indicated for definitive diagnosis.

Management/treatment

Treatment, if possible, is by resection of the affected bowel segment.[1-3] This can be done when a diagnostic exploratory celiotomy is performed.

Large colon volvulus

Etiology/pathogenesis

Large colon volvulus has been anecdotally associated with broodmares, occurring during both gestation and the postpartum period, but is typically not directly related to parturition.

Clinical features

Mares with large colon volvulus usually have signs of severe, acute, abdominal pain.

Management/treatment

The decision to proceed with surgical intervention is often made on the basis of unrelenting pain. A complete discussion of large colon volvulus is available elsewhere in this book (see Chapter 1).[1-3]

PROBLEMS AT PARTURITION

Dystocia
Definition/overview
Dystocia in mares is a true emergency and threatens survival of both fetus and dam (**19.4**). (See also Chapter 5.)

Clinical features
The period from onset of stage II parturition to delivery has important effects on outcome for mare and foal. It is clear that the duration of stage II labor directly impacts fetal survival, with an increased risk of non-survival for each 10-minute increase in stage II labor duration beyond 30 minutes. Few foals are delivered alive or survive if delivered alive after approximately 100 minutes.[8]

Management/treatment
Factors associated with good outcome include a well-coordinated approach to dystocia and a well-defined protocol to minimize the time spent non-productively. Both these factors should be designed specifically for the hospital in question, utilizing their personnel and equipment to their best advantage. Examples of protocols may be found in the veterinary literature.[8,9] Because outcome is improved for both mare and foal with rapid resolution, undue delays in resolution should be minimized, including consideration of rapid referral once it is recognized that the dystocia will not be easily corrected. If the fetal nares are palpable, blind intrapartum nasotracheal intubation of the fetus and hand ventilation with a re-inflating bag device can be attempted. This intervention has been referred to as EXIT (extrauterine intrapartum technique) (**19.5**).

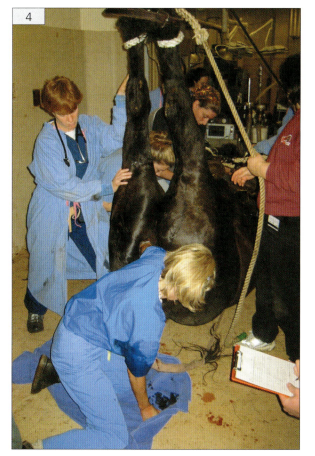

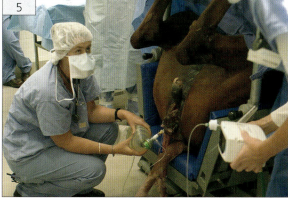

19.5 The extrauterine intrapartum technique (EXIT). The mare is in dorsal recumbency under general anesthesia being prepared for a cesarean section. The foal has been nasotracheally intubated and is being ventilated manually using a self-inflating bag device. Fetal end-tidal carbon dioxide is being monitored using capnography via tubing attached to the nasotracheal tube and self-inflating bag.

19.4 Mare with dystocia. This mare has been entered to an organized dystocia management protocol and in undergoing controlled vaginal delivery. (Courtesy Dr Jane Axon)

POSTPARTUM PROBLEMS

Metritis–laminitis syndrome
Definition/overview
Postparturient metritis can develop with varying degrees of severity, and many cases do not warrant emergency intervention. In a small number of mares, however, septic metritis can become life-threatening as a result of subsequent development of laminitis.

Clinical features
The history often includes dystocia or assisted delivery, with or without placental retention, and development of fever within 48 hours after parturition. Sometimes, the condition is so acute that laminitis is evident at the time of initial examination for suspected uterine infection.

Diagnosis
Diagnosis is made by examination of the reproductive tract via rectal and vaginal palpation and observation of the uterine discharge. Clinical pathology often reveals leukopenia and hyperfibrinogenemia, but findings may also be unremarkable.

Management/treatment
Management/treatment of postparturient metritis includes:
- Local treatment with uterine lavage, with or without infusion of antimicrobial solutions.
- Systemic treatment including IV antimicrobials and anti-inflammatory treatment.
- Anti-endotoxin therapy.
- Equine plasma.
- Polymyxin B (3,000–6,000 IU/kg IV in 1 liter of isotonic crystalloid fluid q12h).
- Pentoxifylline.

Outcome is dependent on the development and severity of complications such as laminitis.

CHAPTER 20

THE NEONATE

Jane E. Axon and
Pamela A. Wilkins

INTRODUCTION

The ongoing critical care of the neonate is as crucial to its survival as the initial emergency treatment and stabilization. To improve the neonate's chance of survival and reduce secondary complications, it is critical to provide continuous monitoring to detect subtle changes and trends, excellent nursing care, and ongoing therapies for specific problems.

NURSING CARE

Nursing is an extremely important facet of neonatal critical care. A busy neonatal ICU relies on the skills of the nursing staff for ongoing treatment and monitoring of the neonate. Attention to detail is required to detect subtle changes in the foal. The general cleanliness of the hospital and foal are also important to ensure minimal stress, cross contamination, nosocomial infections, and secondary complications.

Restraint of the foal

Working quietly and gently with proper restraint will minimize stress and injury to both handler and foal. Foals can be caught by using the mare to corner the foal or by creeping up on the foal with the handler's head height below that of the foal. The foal is caught and subsequently restrained (**20.1**). For longer procedures, the foal is 'folded' and laid down in lateral recumbency (**20.2**). To stimulate a recumbent foal to stand up, scratching along the spine, often vigorously, will help wake the foal up. Ensure that the forelimbs are out in front of the foal and, if needed, lift using the sternum/elbows and pelvis; do not use the tail or put pressure on the abdomen.

Care of the recumbent foal

Bedding

The recumbent foal should be kept clean and dry in order to avoid urine and fecal scalding and decubital ulcers. Urinary catheters can be used; however, there is an increased risk of ascending infections.[1] The foal is turned every 2 hours and the wet side is dried off with towels and talcum powder.

Respiratory care

The INO_2 tube needs to be cleaned at least once a day. The most common complications with INO_2 therapy are nasal irritation and airway drying resulting in excessive discharge.[2] Maintaining the foal in sternal recumbency and alternating the side of recumbency every 2 hours assists with improving oxygenation. Coupage, nebulizing with saline, and ensuring the foal is hydrated will assist with loosening secretions. When standing the foal can be coupaged with its head lowered.

Umbilical care

2.5% iodine solution is applied to the external stump twice daily for the first 3 days after birth. Recumbent foals are at increased risk of developing a patent urachus or umbilical infection.

Eye care

Recumbent foals are at increased risk of developing corneal ulcers. Artificial tears/lubricant should be placed in the eyes every 6–12 hours in foals with decreased eyelid tone and tear production. If the foal is thrashing, protective foam helmets can be made to encircle and protect the eye socket.

Temperature control

Premature foals have poor thermoregulation. Hypothermic foals should be gradually warmed with water bottles, blankets, heated water mats, air blankets, or heat lamps, ensuring scalding and secondary burning of the underlying skin does not occur. Hyperthermic foals can be cooled with cold water and alcohol baths, and fans.

Care of the standing foal

Deep dry bedding should be provided as pressure sores can develop with increased recumbency, muscle weakness, and struggling to stand. Straw bedding is preferred over shavings. If the foal is nursing, the mare's udder should be checked frequently to ensure the foal is nursing well. The foal's urine SG is monitored to ensure it is maintaining hydration (SG <1.008). Foals usually urinate just after standing or nursing.

Foals with diarrhea need frequent cleaning and applications of emollients to prevent scalding of the perineum and vulva.

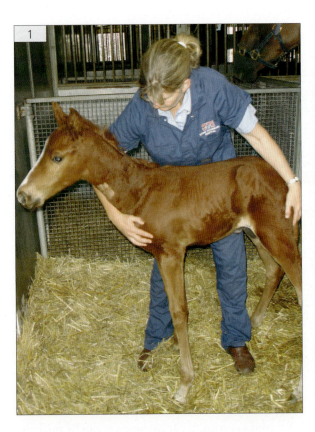

20.1 A foal is easily restrained in this position and a physical examination or short procedure can be performed. If further restraint is required, the hand around the shoulder moves to the base of the foal's ear and the other hand moves to around the tail. The ear and tail can be held if further restraint is required.

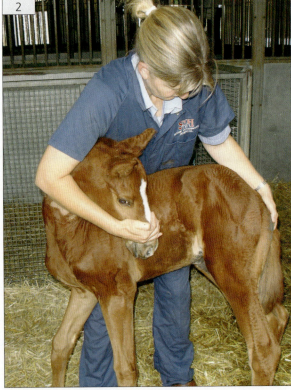

20.2 The foal is 'folded' by pointing the muzzle towards the hind end, curling the hind end towards the muzzle, and, when the foal is relaxed, taking a few steps back to lie the foal down. The holder sits down behind the foal's wither with one leg under the foal's neck and other leg over, but not on, the foal's abdomen/thorax.

Feeding the foal

Foals that are nursing from the mare should have their nursing observed to ensure that they are actually nursing and there are no signs of aspiration. Mares whose foals are not nursing are milked out every 2 hours; the milk is stored and frozen for future use. Foals with a functional GI tract but no suckle or swallow reflex are fed via an indwelling nasogastric tube. Complications that can occur with indwelling nasogastric tubes are pharyngeal and esophageal irritation (most common; oral sucralfate helps with alleviating discomfort), aspiration pneumonia, or an inflow of air into the stomach through an uncapped tube. The position of the tube should be checked prior to each feeding by feeling the tube in the esophagus above the pharynx. The tube is checked for reflux by applying gentle suction. Feeding is by gravity flow. Recumbent foals should be maintained in a sternal position during and for 10 minutes after feeding (**20.3**). Standing foals are fed near the mare to encourage bonding.

The mare

It is very important to ensure that the bond with the mare is maintained (**20.4**). Once the foal is being assisted to stand, the mare is brought over to the foal. Vigorously scratching the mare's withers often starts grooming behavior towards the foal. Taking the mare and foal outside on warm sunny days helps improve their (and the staff's) attitude. Warm compresses should be applied to the udder if swollen and edematous and to assist with milk let down.

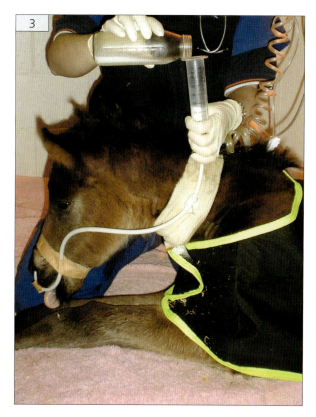

20.3 The foal is kept in sternal recumbency with its head elevated above the level of the stomach while being fed via a nasogastric tube. Milk is gravity fed.

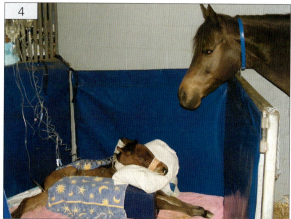

20.4 The foal is kept in the same stall as the mare to try and maintain the bond. Note the sternal support keeping the foal in sternal recumbency, and bedding and diapers to assist with keeping the foal dry.

MONITORING

Monitoring clinical signs, clinicopathologic values, and results of ancillary testing is important when assessing the neonate's response to therapy and clinical progression. Detection of subtle changes is important to allow early instigation of treatment and modifications to therapy. The frequency of monitoring depends on the severity of illness and the stability of the patient. Record keeping and observation of trends are essential (*Table 20.1*). The abnormal findings may be a single event; however, a trend of repeated abnormalities is indicative of possible deterioration of the foal.

Weight

Daily weighing of the foal is important in monitoring fluid therapy, nutrition, and efficacy of sepsis treatment. A healthy foal should gain 1–1.5 kg/day. Lack of weight gain is a sign of ongoing sepsis or inadequate nutrition.

Body temperature

Critically ill neonates should have their temperature monitored regularly until stable. Fevers are often present in the evening.

Body systems

Examination of the foal should be methodical so no abnormalities are missed. Ancillary tests such as ultrasonography, radiography, ECG, urine analysis, fluid culture, and cytology are all utilized where necessary to further evaluate the different organ systems.

Attitude and nervous system

A change in the foal's attitude is often the first sign of a problem and can be seen before vital parameters have changed. Changes include a reduction in nursing, less responsive when stimulated, and reluctance to stand. Intermittent nystagmus, becoming stiff with stimulation, and gentle forelimb 'marching' are signs of impending seizure activity. Signs of improvement include becoming more aware and responsive, more easily aroused, standing more easily and with less assistance, developing an affinity for the mare, and finally, becoming inquisitive and playing.

Cardiovascular system

Mucous membranes are examined for color, CRT, moisture, and presence of petechiae. Heart rate, rhythm, and presence or change in character of murmurs should

---

Table 20.1 An abbreviated hourly monitoring intensive care flow sheet. Extra comments concerning subjective observations such as the foal's attitude are written in the patient's comment sheets

NAME:................................

DATE:................................

SCONE EQUINE HOSPITAL
24-HOUR FOAL INTENSIVE CARE FLOW SHEET

TIME	T°	HR	PULSE QUALITY	m/m COLOR	CRT	RR	LUNGS L	LUNGS R	GIT SOUNDS	GI INTAKE SOURCE	GI INTAKE METH	GI INTAKE AMT	GI INTAKE TOTAL	URINE AMT/DESC.	URINE TOTAL	S.G.	FECES DESCRIBE
8 am																	
9 am																	
↓																	
7 am																	

be monitored. The great metatarsal artery is the usual place for assessment of peripheral pulses. The temperature of the distal extremities is monitored to assist with assessing perfusion. Blood pressure is usually measured by indirect methods and is monitored frequently until the patient has stabilized.[3] CVP can be measured to assist with monitoring fluid therapy.[4] Catheterized veins should be examined daily for evidence of heat, pain, or swelling associated with infection.

Respiratory system

The foal's auscultation findings, respiratory rate, pattern, and effort are monitored. Changes in pattern or an increased effort are often the first signs of deterioration. ABG analyses are used to monitor respiratory function and assist with interpretation of clinical signs. A decrease in effort may be a sign of improvement. However, if seen with an increasing $PaCO_2$, it may be a sign of respiratory failure.

Gastrointestinal system

The tongue is examined for the presence of *Candida* spp. (**20.5**). Foals should be regularly evaluated for the presence of gastric reflux when ileus is present and before each feed if feeding via a nasogastric tube. The character of borborygmi should be noted. A measuring tape is used to more accurately measure abdominal circumference to monitor for distension. Fecal volume and consistency should be recorded. It is usually difficult to find feces in a stall, therefore both nursing and abdominal size are monitored in ambulatory foals.

Urinary system

Urine SG is measured frequently to assess hydration. Urine output should be monitored in relation to fluid intake; however, a lack of urine production over a 4-hour period requires further evaluation.[5] If renal dysfunction is suspected, urine output should be monitored by using a closed urine collection system. The area along the ventral midline, axilla region, and around the tail should be palpated for signs of edema.

The umbilicus should be monitored for any signs of bleeding, infection, or patency.

Ocular

The eyes are monitored for development of corneal ulcers, entropion, or hypopion. Sclera are evaluated for injection or development of petechiae.

Musculoskeletal system

Ambulatory foals should have their gait examined daily for any signs of lameness. Conformation should also be monitored for development of ALD. Joints, physes, and limbs should be palpated in recumbent and standing neonates for any heat or swelling that can be associated with infectious orthopedic disease or cellulitis. Edema that develops under the axilla region may be associated with fractured ribs.

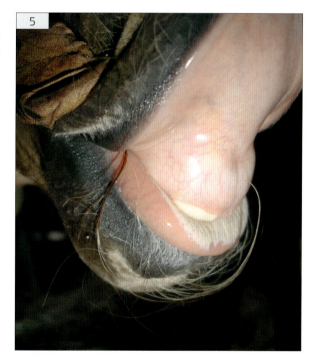

20.5 The tongue is examined for the presence of *Candida* spp.

Integument

The skin is examined for development of decubital sores (**20.6**).

Laboratory data

Hematology and biochemistry values are monitored until the foal has stabilized and are re-evaluated if the foal deteriorates. Glucose is monitored frequently in foals on parenteral nutrition or that are not appropriately regulating blood glucose concentrations. Lactate concentrations are used to assist with evaluating tissue perfusion and metabolic homeostasis. Electrolytes are re-evaluated frequently if the foal is on parenteral nutrition, diuretic therapy, or has GI tract or renal disease. WBC count and fibrinogen concentration are used to assess response to antimicrobial therapy. RBC count is monitored if hemolysis, bleeding, or anemia of chronic disease is suspected.

The mare

The mare, the reproductive tract, and the udder need to be monitored closely for post-partum complications.

FLUID AND ELECTROLYTE THERAPY

The volume and type of fluid used in the young neonate requires understanding of their physiology.[6,7] Critically ill neonates are likely have increased vascular permeability and capillary filtration rate and increased interstitial compliance.[8] An increase in systemic blood pressure results in increased capillary pressure and filtration and increased shifting of fluid into the interstitium at the expense of the plasma volume.[8] Foals that have undergone *in-utero* stress can be born overhydrated because of compensatory intrauterine fluid shifts, which overload the interstitial space.

The neonate's ability to handle sodium is also different from an adult.[8] As the foal has a low sodium diet (1–3 mEq/kg/day from mare's milk), renal mechanisms have been developed to conserve sodium. Thus the neonate is prone to sodium overloading as 1 liter of sodium-based crystalloids or 1 liter of plasma contains the daily sodium requirement of the foal. If, however, there is renal tubular damage, such as with HIS, there may be excessive sodium loss, so deciding which fluid to give the foal becomes difficult unless urinary excretion of sodium is evaluated. Sodium overloading can result in edema and sodium wasting can result in hyponatremia (**20.7**).

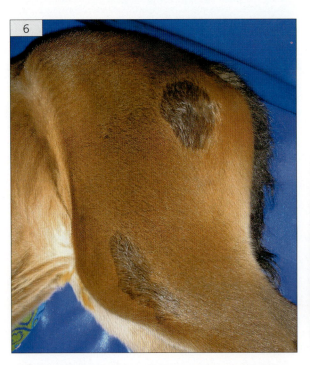

20.6 The skin is examined for the presence of decubiti.

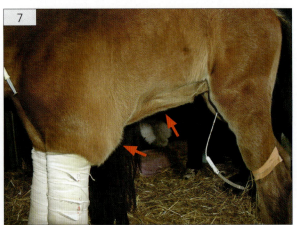

20.7 Subcutaneous edema apparent in axillary, ventral abdomen and flank skin folds (arrows). These foals are colloquially referred to as 'jelly-belly' foals.

The initial fluid therapy plan is designed to replace fluid deficits and stabilize the neonate and then is tailored to meet the individual's requirements as the neonate's specific responses and renal function are unknown.

Fluid therapy in the first 24 hours

After the neonate has been stabilized (see Chapter 12), glucose supplemented fluids are used to provide both blood glucose and fluid support. Sodium-sparing fluids are used as the foal is sodium loaded during stabilization. One approach is to initially start on 5% dextrose providing 4 mg glucose/kg/minute and the concentration of dextrose increased to provide 8 mg glucose/kg/minute according to the foal's glucose tolerance.[8] This does have the potential to fluid overload the neonate; however, rates can be decreased if renal dysfunction is suspected. The authors begin with 10% dextrose at 5 mg/kg/minute (150 ml/50 kg/hour) or 5% dextrose at 4 mg/kg/minute (~240 ml/hour for a 50 kg foal) (*Table 20.2*). If the neonate is immediately started on parenteral nutrition, a maintenance fluid formulation and rate are begun. IV plasma is given if further colloid or passive immune therapies are required.

Fluid therapy after the first 24 hours
Volume and rate

The daily fluid requirements of the neonate will vary depending on oral intake, water losses, systemic disease, and renal function. There are currently two approaches (*Table 20.2*):

- Higher rates: 3–5 ml/kg/hour[9] or 4–6 ml/kg/hour.[10] These rates may predispose to overhydration and edema formation if there is poor renal function. The authors use 2–4 ml/kg/hour.
- A 'dry' fluid rate (Holliday–Segar formula), which calculates a base volume and rate to formulate the maintenance plan around.[8] This formula estimates the fluid requirement from the basal metabolic rate to provide the maintenance needs of the neonate and avoids overhydration.

Table 20.2 Fluid therapy rates after stabilization of the neonate

Fluid therapy for the first 24 hours

1. 4 mg/kg/minute = 240 ml/50 kg/hour of 5% dextrose
   6 mg/kg/minute = 240 ml/50 kg/hour of 7.5% dextrose
   8 mg/kg/minute = 240 ml/50 kg/hour of 10% dextrose

2. 150 ml/50 kg/hour of 10% dextrose

Base fluid rate for maintenance after 24 hours

1. 2–4 ml/kg/hour (starting at 3 ml/kg/hour)

2. Holliday–Segar formula ('dry' maintenance formula)
   100 ml/kg/day for first 10 kg of body weight = 100 ml/kg/day
   + 50 ml/kg/day for second 10 kg of body weight = 50 ml/kg/day
   + 25 ml/kg/day for the remainder of the body weight.

Thus for a 50 kg foal: (100 ml/kg x 10) + (50 ml/kg x 10) + (25 ml/kg x 30)/day
Rate = 94 ml/hour

The authors use the Holliday–Segar formula in neonates that have poor renal function or initially in neonates <3 days of age where renal function is not known. A higher fluid rate of 2–4 ml/kg is used in neonates with adequate renal function as determined by appropriate urine SG (<1.008), urine volume, lack of edema formation, and normal renal laboratory values. Estimated ongoing losses of fluid that occur are then added to the maintenance volume.

Type of fluid

The type of fluid used is important to ensure that sodium overloading is avoided. Most commercially available fluids are replacement, not maintenance, fluid formulations. Several crystalloid fluid formulations do have low sodium concentrations (*Table 20.3*). A combination of dextrose and lactated Ringer's solution (LRS) can also be used to decrease the concentration of sodium provided by LRS.

Foals with suspected sodium losses, such as with diarrhea, should initially not be sodium restricted and are started on balanced electrolyte replacement solutions.

Electrolyte therapy

Electrolyte concentrations, if abnormal on presentation, should be re-evaluated. If acid–base abnormalities are present, an ABG analysis should be performed to assist with interpretation. Electrolytes need to be closely monitored in foals receiving diuretic therapy, as well as those with renal dysfunction, ileus, or diarrhea.

Potassium supplementation needs to be considered in foals that are not being fed and are not hyperkalemic. It is difficult to estimate total body potassium deficits; however, if plasma concentrations are low, it is usually a reflection of a total body potassium deficit, and once a deficit occurs it is difficult to normalize without oral supplementation (5 g oral KCl q6–12h). Foals that are begun on parenteral nutrition (*Table 20.4*) need to have the potassium concentration monitored closely.

IV sodium supplementation needs to be administered carefully to avoid complications associated with rapid correction of the serum sodium concentration. Oral sodium chloride or sodium bicarbonate (5 g q6–12h) may be needed in foals with GI losses due to diarrhea.

Table 20.3 **Commonly used sodium sparing intravenous fluids.**

	SODIUM	POTASSIUM	CHLORIDE	CALCIUM	MAGNESIUM
Normosol M	40	13	40	0	3
Plasma-Lyte 56	40	13	40	0	3
5% Dextrose	0	0	0	0	0

Table 20.4 **Parenteral nutrition formulation guidelines**

Parenteral nutrition formulation:

Glucose	10 g/kg/day	So for a 50 kg foal	500 g/day
Amino acids	2 g/kg/day		100 g/day
Lipids	1 g/kg/day		50 g/day

Products used:

50% Dextrose (50 g/100 ml)

10% Amino acids (10 g/100 ml)

10% Lipids (10 g/100 ml)

For 50 kg foal:

Glucose	500 g/day = 1,000 ml of 50% Dextrose
Amino acids	100 g/day = 1,000 ml of 10% Amino acids
Lipids	50 g/day = 500 ml of 10% Lipids

If foals are on parenteral nutrition (PN) for longer than 3 days, pediatric trace mineral and vitamins are added. If not available, 1 ml of vitamin B complex is added every second day.

Compounding and infusion of solution:

Fluids are made up into a bag with transfer leads. Mixing of solutions should be as aseptic as possible, ideally under a laminar flow hood or more practically a closed system with transfer leads, with sterile gloves and mask in a dust-free environment. Add glucose, then amino acids, then lipids. A fluid line should be dedicated for PN and not be used for medication infusion or blood collections. Lines should be changed daily. PN is administered by a fluid infusion pump.

Infusion rate:

1,000 + 1,000 + 500 ml per day = 2,500 ml/day or target rate of 104 ml/hour for a 50 kg foal.

Begin at ¼ the hourly infusion rate and increase by ¼ every 4 hours until the target rate is reached.

Monitoring:

Blood and urine glucose are monitored every 4 hours. If the foal become hyperglycemic, turn rate back down and consider insulin therapy.

Catheter sites need to be monitored frequently because of the increased risk of thrombophlebitis.

Insulin therapy:

Insulin therapy: begin at 0.05 IU/kg/hour. Ensure line is attached to PN line. Use glass bottles. Prime lines with insulin for 20 minutes.

Weaning off:

To wean off total PN, decrease the run rate by ¼ every 4 hours. If the catheter becomes blocked and the foal is not receiving any glucose supplementation, hypoglycemia can occur, therefore catheter replacement needs to be considered an emergency.

ANTIMICROBIAL THERAPY

The neonate has different absorption, metabolism, and excretion of antimicrobial drugs compared with an adult.[11] There is increased absorption from the GI tract, a higher percentage of body water, decreased protein binding, and often immature hepatic function. Also, many disease processes can affect the pharmacokinetics of antimicrobials.[11]

Instigation of antimicrobial therapy

Antimicrobial therapy often has to be initiated prior to culture and sensitivity results becoming available, therefore an empirical antimicrobial choice has to be made. The choice is based on sensitivity of isolates from the surrounding geographical area and the clinician's experience. Therapy can then be altered according to culture and sensitivity results and clinical response.

The most common bacteria isolated from septic foals are enteric gram-negative bacteria; however, gram-positive organisms can also be involved. Thus, a recommended initial treatment plan for a septic foal with normal renal function involves the combination of an aminoglycoside (e.g. gentamicin or amikacin) with a β-lactam (e.g. penicillin, ampicillin, or a first-generation cephalosporin such as cephazolin). In cases where renal function is not normal or unknown, high-dose ceftiofur, trimethoprim-sulfonamides, ticarcillin/clavulanic acid, or a third-generation cephalosporin can be used. Clinical experience will determine selection as there is variability among the effectiveness of these antimicrobials and the isolates from different locations.[12,13]

Route of administration

IV administration is the ideal and most effective route in the <7-day-old foal. IM administration is practical in the field setting; however, repeated injections cause muscle swelling and pain. Oral administration is easy and convenient and is suitable for older foals.

Length of treatment

A minimum of 10–14 days of treatment is recommended for bacteremic foals without localizing signs. If used prophylactically, treatment for 3–5 days is recommended. When localizing signs are present, therapy should be continued until all signs of infection are resolved and temperature, WBC count, and fibrinogen concentration have been normal for 72 hours. WBC count and fibrinogen concentration are measured 7 days after discontinuation of therapy to ensure there is no recurrence of infection.

Once the disease is in the subacute and chronic stages, oral formulations can be considered for long-term therapy when susceptibility patterns indicate their use.[11] Oral therapies include cefpodoxime, cefuroxime, cephalexin, trimethoprim-sulfonamide, doxycycline, chloramphenicol, and rifampin.

Classes of commonly used antimicrobials

β-lactam group

Penicillins are bactericidal and have a good gram-positive spectrum, good soft tissue penetration, low toxicity, and are inexpensive. There is a synergy between the β-lactams and aminoglycosides. Ampicillin has an extended spectrum; however, it should not be used alone if gram-negative coverage is needed. Ticarcillin–clavulanic acid has an extended activity against β-lactamase-producing bacteria.

Cephalosporins are broad-spectrum antimicrobials that vary widely in their spectrum of activity, resistance to β-lactamases, penetration into the CNS, and elimination half-life.[14] They have a relatively low toxicity.

Carbapenem β-lactams such as imipenem and the newer fourth-generation cephalosporins have good broad-spectrum coverage; however, their use should be restricted to aminoglycoside-resistant gram-negative microbes to avoid the development of resistance.[11]

Aminoglycosides

Aminoglycosides have an excellent gram-negative spectrum; however, they are associated with nephrotoxicity. Amikacin is slightly less nephrotoxic than gentamicin. Therapeutic drug monitoring (TDM), serum creatinine concentrations, and urinalysis should be monitored. TDM is recommended so that if prolonged clearance occurs, doses can be altered before renal toxicity occurs (*Table 20.5*).[15] Serum creatinine, BUN concentration, and urinalysis are not as sensitive as TDM because significant renal damage can occur before changes in values are detected.

Other antimicrobials

Other antimicrobial that can be used are:

- Trimethoprim-sulfonamides. Bacteriocidal, but are not recommended in some geographic locations due to resistance.[11]
- Tetracyclines. Broad spectrum and bacteriostatic, therefore are not recommended in septic neonates. The authors have found tetracycline an effective antimicrobial for treatment of osteomyelitis in older foals.
- Metronidazole. Indicated in foals with clostridial enterocolitis. There may be increased intestinal absorption in neonates, with subsequent side-effects, so a lower dose rate is recommended.[11]
- Enrofloxacin. Has been associated with arthropathy, therefore its routine use is not recommended.[18]
- Chloramphenicol. Used with caution as it has potential human toxicity; however, it is a useful oral broad-spectrum bacteriostatic antimicrobial with good tissue penetration.
- Fluconazol and amphocetericin B. Used to treat candidiasis; the former has less side-effects.[19]
- Acyclovir. Has been used in EHV-1 infection with varied success.[20]

Table 20.5 Recommended antimicrobial drug dosages for foals.[15–17]

DRUG	DOSE, ROUTE, FREQUENCY	COMMENTS
Acyclovir	16 mg/kg PO q8h	
Amikacin sulfate	<1wk old: 25–30 mg/kg IV q24h	Nephrotoxic
	2–4wk old: 20–25 mg/kg IV q24h	TDM: 30 minute peak >45 µg/ml
		8 hour trough: <15 µg/ml
		12 hour trough: <5 µg/ml
Ampicillin sodium	50–100 mg/kg IV q6h	
Azithromycin	10 mg/kg PO q24h for 5 days then every other day	Hyperthermia, diarrhea in foal and mare
Cefazolin	25 mg/kg IM q6–8h	First-generation cephalosporin
Cephalexin	30 mg/kg PO q8h	First-generation cephalosporin
Cefuroxime	30 mg/kg/day PO q6–12h	Second-generation cephalosporin
	50–100 mg/kg/day IV q6–8h	
Cefotaxime	50–100 mg/kg IV q6h	Third-generation cephalosporin
Ceftazidime	40 mg/kg IV q6–8h	Third-generation cephalosporin
Ceftiofur	5 mg/kg IV q12h	Third-generation cephalosporin
	10 mg/kg IV q6h	No CNS penetration
	CRI: 1.5 mg/kg/hour	Ideally given over 20 mins
	Nebulized: 1 mg/kg as 25 mg/ml solution q8–12h	Higher doses: broader gram-negative spectrum
Cefpodoxime	10 mg/kg PO q6–12h	Third-generation cephalosporin
Ceftriaxone	25 mg/kg IV q12h	Third-generation cephalosporin
Cefepime	11 mg/kg IV/IM q8h	Fourth-generation cephalosporin
Chloramphenicol	50 mg/kg PO q6h	Public health concerns

(continued overleaf)

Table 20.5 *(continued)*

DRUG	DOSE, ROUTE, FREQUENCY	COMMENTS
Clarithromycin	7.5 mg/kg PO q12h	Hyperthermia, diarrhea in foal and mare
Doxycycline	10 mg/kg PO q12h	
Enrofloxacin	5 mg/kg PO q24h	Chondropathy and arthropathy
Erythromycin stearate	25 mg/kg PO q8h	Hyperthermia, diarrhea in foal and mare
Fluconazole	8 mg/kg loading then 4 mg/kg PO q12h	
Gentamicin sulfate	<7 days old: 11–13 mg/kg IV q24h Older foals: 6.6 mg/kg IV q24h Nebulized: 2.2 mg/kg as 50 mg/ml solution q24h	Nephrotoxic TDM: 30 minute peak >25 µg/ml 8 hour trough: <5 µg/ml 12 hour trough: <2 µg/ml
Imipenem	10–20 mg/kg IV q6h	
Metronidazole	10–15 mg/kg PO or IV q8h	10 mg/kg q12h if increased GI tract absorption may occur
Oxytetracycline	10 mg/kg IV q12h	Nephrotoxic, give slowly
Na or K penicillin	20,000–50,000 IU/kg IV q6h	Use upper dose in severe infections
Procaine penicillin	20,000–50,000 IU/kg IM q12h	
Rifampin	5 mg/kg PO q12h	Use with other antimicrobials
Ticarcillin and clavulanic acid	50–100 mg/kg IV q6h CRI: 2–4 mg/kg/hour	
Trimethoprim-sulfonamide	30 mg/kg PO, IM, or IV q12h	Dose/kg is combined trimethoprim and sulfonamide

CHAPTER 21

THE RECUMBENT HORSE

Pamela A. Wilkins

GENERAL CONSIDERATIONS

The recumbent horse is one of the greatest challenges faced by the equine veterinarian. For either the adult horse or the foal there is no simple, efficient, or low-cost way of managing these patients. Care must be continued 24 hours per day and potentially for days to weeks, depending on the disease process that resulted in the recumbency. There are many diseases that can result in a foal or adult horse becoming recumbent and many body systems that may be primarily or secondarily affected. While neurologic diseases are common, neuromuscular disease (e.g. botulism), systemic disease (e.g. severe sepsis), and muscular (e.g. rhabdomyolysis) and musculoskeletal problems (e.g. laminitis) can all result in prolonged recumbency in the affected patient. This chapter is by no means intended as an exhaustive review of diseases that result in recumbency, but rather an introduction to the challenges of management, monitoring, and nursing care.

Horses with a disease that predisposes them to recumbency present unique problems related to safety, of both themselves and their caretakers, and efficacy. In addition, the disease process may require specific management modalities that vary from case to case.

Safety is a paramount concern. Stall size must be adequate and should have more than one exit in order to provide room for caretakers' movement around the patient and ready egress should the horse become manic, attempt to stand without support, or develop seizures when being handled or undergoing treatment. Padding in the stalls is beneficial as horses may need to lean against walls and may fall. Rough surfaces (concrete block, raw wood) can contribute to skin abrasions and ocular complications.

Flooring is a consideration as weak horses are at increased risk of slipping and serious to catastrophic injuries may result. A floor that retains traction even when wet, has some degree of padding, and is easily cleaned and disinfected is ideal. However, rough flooring surfaces can contribute to recumbency-associated morbidity including the aforementioned integument and ocular problems, myopathy, bruising, and serious pressure necrosis of skin and underlying structures leading to extensive decubiti.

Slings can be useful in caring for recumbent horses of all sizes but are not necessarily appropriate for all patients. Slings are most useful in cases where the patient can almost stand but has difficulty supporting itself (i.e. the patient who requires the sling for stability or uses the sling episodically for period of 'rest' (**21.1**). The sling should not be expected to support the entire weight of the patient except when being used to transport a patient (anesthetized or not). There are many slings commercially available for use in both adult

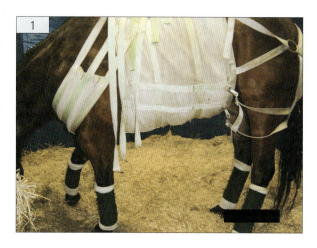

21.1 An adult horse using a sling well. Note that the horse is supporting its own weight and is only episodically using the sling for stabilization. (Courtesy Equine Medicine and Surgery, University of Illinois)

horses and foals. Preference is generally based on building design, ease of use, and financial consideration, although investment in a good quality useful sling with an appropriate overhead pulley or winch is essential for a high-quality equine hospital.

Horses that use the sling to support their entire weight do not survive and 'hanging' in the sling results in significant respiratory compromise to the patient (**21.2**). The receptivity of the patient to being managed in a sling may preclude use of the sling in horses that are temperamentally unsuited (**21.2**).

Ideally, stalls designed for recumbent and/or weak horses should either be equipped, or be capable of being equipped, with an electric overhead pulley or winch system rated to carry the weight of the intended patient population (plus a large margin of safety) and having a rapid rate of travel/ascent/descent. Slow moving devices are of no assistance and old-fashioned 'block and tackle' pulley systems are also generally too slow or are more than a hindrance.

It is important to maintain a quiet and calm environment with recumbent horses as overstimulation may result in additional self-trauma. Padded head covers, while useful, should be checked frequently for slippage, as the head covers can also contribute to additional eye trauma.

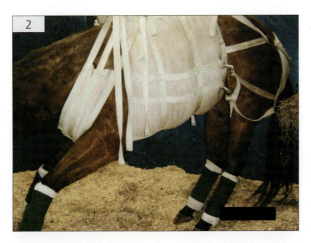

21.2 An adult horse not using a sling well. Note that the horse has dropped back in the sling and is supporting the majority of its weight on the sling. (Courtesy Equine Medicine and Surgery, University of Illinois)

MONITORING AND NURSING CARE

Almost all body systems must be monitored in recumbent horses; the intensity and frequency of monitoring will depend on the initiating cause. Complications of recumbency should be expected and include ocular and head trauma, decubital ulceration, colic, pneumonia, and peripheral neuropathies.

Decubital ulcers begin over bony prominences and are usually observed within 2 days in adults (**21.3**). Diligent and appropriate care can prevent them almost entirely in young foals. Both pressure and movement abrasion play important roles in the development of decubital ulcers as does excessive moisture at contact points that allows for integument maceration.

Prevention of decubital ulcers centers on frequent changes of recumbency (turning), ideally at 2-hour intervals, followed by drying of the skin that is now on the 'up' side of the patient. This 'turning' of adult horses may only be possible 2–4 times daily, but nonetheless should still be done. Towel drying, use of blow dryers on a 'low' or 'air' setting, and liberal application of cornstarch, talc, or baby powder are all useful.

Padding should be used under recumbent horses. Thick mats (30 cm [12 in] in depth) covered with a moisture impermeable material that can be disinfected are ideal (**21.4**). Waterbeds can be used for foals and smaller adults if king sized, with the additional benefit of improved comfort if a waterbed heater is used. For adult horses, the bed should be placed under the horse while empty and then filled until the lowest point of the horse is 2.5–7.5 cm (1–3 in) off the ground.

Recumbent horses are frequently unable to micturate normally, either due to the primary complaint or associated with an inability to position themselves properly. This is a more acute problem in the adult male because of the long narrow urethra presenting increased resistance to urine flow. Placement of indwelling urinary catheters in recumbent patients will keep bladder fill to a minimum and allow for monitoring of urine production and repeat urinalysis to monitor renal function and adequacy of fluid therapy. Patients with indwelling urinary catheters should be on appropriate prophylactic antimicrobial treatment to prevent ascending urinary tract infection. Frequent urinalyses should be performed, as should creatinine concentration measurements, as recumbent horses are frequently receiving treatments with the potential for inducing renal disease.

Recumbency increases the risk of all patients for developing respiratory disease. Eating and drinking fluids in an abnormal position may contribute to aspiration pneumonia, while abnormal thoracic pressure causes atelectasis of the down lung and may impair normal gas exchange. Monitoring for respiratory tract infection may include frequent fibrinogen concentration determinations, periodic ultrasonographic examination of the thorax, and ABG analyses as indicated. Some disease processes that induce recumbency, such as botulism, directly impact respiratory function, with respiratory failure a potential cause of the demise of the patient.

All recumbent foals should be fed ONLY in a sternal position and should be maintained there for at least 10 minutes once feeding is complete in order to prevent aspiration. Feeding through an indwelling nasoesophogeal tube is the ideal and carries a reduced risk of aspiration over bottle feeding in these cases. Adult horses should be held in sternal recumbency while being fed or drinking water for similar reasons.

Altered diet, antimicrobial treatment, lack of activity, and the primary disease process all contribute to problems associated with the GI tract. Decreased GI motility can result in impaction or gas colic. Diarrhea is not uncommon in these cases due to altered GI flora, altered GI motility, and antimicrobial treatment. Infectious and zoonotic causes for diarrhea should be ruled out in these cases and appropriate therapy instituted.

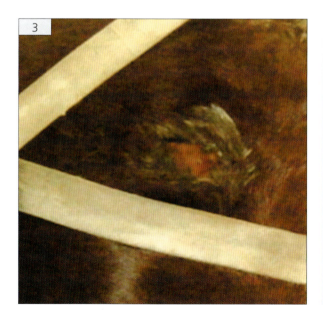

21.3 Early decubital ulcer located over the point of the hip in an adult horse. Also visible are the straps of the sling supporting the horse. (Courtesy Equine Medicine and Surgery, University of Illinois)

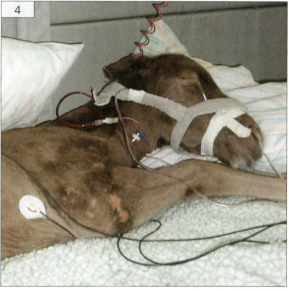

21.4 A recumbent foal being maintained on a mattress with protective soft coverings. Despite intensive nursing care and frequent turning, this foal has developed a decubital ulcer of the right point of the elbow.

SPECIAL CONSIDERATIONS

Recumbency in horses may be due to infectious diseases. These diseases include, but are not limited to, the neurologic form of EHV-1 and rabies. The possibility of infectious and communicable causes must always be considered and biosecurity concerns must be considered in the management of these cases.

APPENDIX: RESOURCES FOR DEVICES FOR MOVING, LIFTING, AND 'SLINGING' RECUMBENT HORSES (USA ONLY)

Glides

Most horses will require sedation using this method. The Rescue Glide can be used to transport horses from the pasture to a safe place out of the weather in the barn, or even to a veterinary facility via an ambulance trailer or from a trailer to a stall once at a referral facility. B&M Plastics in Greenville, South Carolina (www.rescueglides.com) make a recycled plastic glide and accessories to strap the patient down for transport.

Slings

There are several versions of equine slings for the purpose of lifting a recumbent horse:
- One of the best known is the Anderson Sling, made for the purpose of medical support, and the industry standard for helicopter lifts. The Anderson Sling is an excellent sling to maintain horses suspended for prolonged (days or weeks) periods of time, but it may be cost-prohibitive for some practices (www.andersonsling.com/anderson_sling.html).

- The University of California, Davis, has introduced a short-term lift sling-like device (www.largeanimallift.com).
- The Becker sling is a simple vertical lift sling (www.hast.net/rescue-equipment.htm).
- A variety of slings for large animals can be found at the Springwater Animal Supply website (www.springwateranimalsupply.com).

ADDITIONAL READING

1. Corley K, Stephen J (2008) (eds) *The Equine Hospital Manual*. Wiley-Blackwell, Ames.
2. Russell CM, Wilkins PA (2006) Evaluation of the recumbent neonate. *Clin Tech Equine Pract* **5**:161–171.
3. Wilkins PA (2007) Botulism. In: *Equine Infectious Diseases*. (eds D Sellon, M Long) Saunders-Elsevier, Philadelphia, pp. 372–375.
4. Wilkins PA, Del Piero F (2007) Rabies. In: *Equine Infectious Diseases*. (eds D Sellon, M Long) Saunders-Elsevier, Philadelphia, pp.185–190.

CHAPTER 1: DIGESTIVE SYSTEM AND PERITONEAL DISEASE

1   Delesalle C, Dewulf J, Lefebvre RA *et al.* (2007) Determination of lactate concentrations in blood plasma and peritoneal fluid in horses with colic by an Accusport Analyzer. *J Vet Int Med* **21**:293–301.

2   Latson KM, Nieto JE, Beldomenico PM *et al.* (2005) Evaluation of peritoneal fluid lactate as a marker of intestinal ischaemia in equine colic. *Equine Vet J* **37**:342–346.

3   Peloso JG, Cohen ND (2012) Use of serial measurement of peritoneal fluid lactate concentration to identify strangulating intestinal lesions in referred horses with signs of colic. *J Am Vet Med Assoc* **240**:1208–1217.

3a Slack J (2012) Abdominal sonographic evaluation. In: *Practical Guide to Equine Colic.* (ed LL Southwood) Wiley-Blackwell, Ames, pp. 116–148.

4   Pease AP, Scrivani PV, Erb HN *et al.* (2004) Accuracy of increased large-intestine wall thickness during ultrasonography for diagnosing large-colon torsion in 42 horses. *Vet Radiol Ultrasound* **45**:220–224.

5   Abutarbush SM, Carmalt JL, Shoemaker RW (2005) Causes of gastrointestinal colic in horses in western Canada: 604 cases (1992 to 2002). *Can Vet J* **46**:800–805.

6   Epstein K, Short D, Parente E *et al.* (2008) Gastrointestinal ultrasonography in normal adult ponies. *Vet Radiol Ultrasound* **49**:282–286.

7   Busoni V, DeBusscher V, Lopez D *et al.* (2011) Evaluation of a protocol for fast localized abdominal sonography of horses (FLASH) admitted for colic. *Vet J* **188**:77–82.

8   Fischer AT Jr. (1997) Advances in diagnostic techniques for horses with colic. *Vet Clin N Am Equine Pract* **13**:203–219.

8a Epstein KL, Fehr J (2012) Colic surgery. In: *Practical Guide to Equine Colic.* (ed LL Southwood) Wiley-Blackwell, Ames, pp. 173–203.

9   Feige K, Schwarzwald C, Fürst A *et al.* (2000) Esophageal obstruction in horses: a retrospective study of 34 cases. *Can Vet J* **41**:207–210.

10 Chiavaccini L, Hassel DM (2010) Retrospective review of clinical features and prognostic variables in 109 horses with esophageal obstruction (1992–2009). *J Vet Int Med* **24**:1147–1152.

11 Duncanson GR (2006) Equine oesophageal obstruction: a long-term study of 60 cases. *Equine Vet Educ* **18**:262–265.

12 Fielding CL, Magdesian KG, Rhodes DM *et al.* (2009) Clinical and biochemical abnormalities in endurance horses eliminated from competition for medical complications and requiring emergency medical treatment: 30 cases (2005–2006). *J Vet Emerg Crit Care* **19**:473–478.

13 Meyer GA, Rashmir-Raven A, Helms RJ *et al.* (2000) The effect of oxytocin on contractility of the equine oesophagus: a potential treatment for oesophageal obstruction. *Equine Vet J* **32**:151–155.

14 Todhunter RJ, Stick JA, Trotter GW (1984) Medical management of esophageal stricture in seven horses. *J Am Vet Med Assoc* **185**:784–787.

15 Knottenbelt DC, Harrison LJ, Peacock PJ (1992) Conservative treatment of oesophageal stricture in five foals. *Vet Rec* **131**:27–30.

15a Anon (1999) Equine Gastric Ulcer Council recommendations for the diagnosis and treatment of equine gastric ulcer syndrome (EGUS). *Equine Vet Educ* **11**:262–272.

15b Merritt AM (2009) Appeal for proper usage of the term 'EGUS': equine gastric ulcer syndrome. *Equine Vet J* **41**:616.

16 Nadeau JA, Andrews FM (2008) Gastric ulcer syndrome. In: *Current Therapy in Equine Medicine 6.* (eds NE Robinson, KA Sprayberry) Saunders Elsevier, St. Louis, pp. 366–371.

17 Nadeau JA, Andrews FM, Patton CS *et al.* (2003) Effects of hydrochloric, valeric, and other volatile fatty acids on pathogenesis of ulcers in the nonglandular portion of the stomach of horses. *Am J Vet Res* **64**:413–417.

18 Nadeau JA, Andrews FM, Patton CS *et al.* (2003) Effects of hydrochloric, acetic, butyric, and propionic acids on pathogenesis of ulcers in the nonglandular portion of the stomach of horses. *Am J Vet Res* **64**:404–412.

19 Nadeau JA, Andrews FM (2009) Equine gastric ulcer syndrome: the continuing conundrum. *Equine Vet J* **41**:611–615.

19a Andrews FM, Sifferman RL, Bernard W *et al.* (1999) Efficacy of omeprazole paste in the treatment and prevention of gastric ulcers in horses. *Equine Vet J Suppl* **29**:81–86.

20 Zedler S, Embertson R, Barr B *et al.* (2009) Surgical treatment of gastric outflow obstruction in 40 foals: 1986–2004 *Vet Surg* **38**:623–630.

21 Coleman MC, Slovis NM, Hunt RJ (2009) Long-term prognosis of gastrojejunostomy in foals with gastric outflow obstruction: 16 cases (2001–2006). *Equine Vet J* **41**:653–657.

22 Dukti SA, Perkins S, Murphy J *et al.* (2006) Prevalence of gastric squamous ulceration in horses with abdominal pain. *Equine Vet J* **38**:347–349.

23   Hewetson M, Cohen ND, Love S
et al. (2006) Sucrose concentration
in blood: a new method for assessment of gastric permeability in horses
with gastric ulceration. *J Vet Int Med*
20:388–394.

24   Merritt AM, Sanchez LC, Burrow JA
et al. (2003) Effect of GastroGard and
three compounded oral omeprazole
preparations on 24 h intragastric
pH in gastrically cannulated mature
horses. *Equine Vet J* **35**:691–695.

25   Lester GD, Smith RL, Robertson
ID (2005) Effects of treatment with
omeprazole or ranitidine on gastric
squamous ulceration in racing
Thoroughbreds. *J Am Vet Med Assoc*
227:1636–1639.

26   Barclay WP, Phillips TN, Foerner
JJ (1982) Intussusception associated
with *Anoplocephalal perfoliata* infection
in five horses. *J Am Vet Med Assoc*
180:752–753.

27   Doxey DL, Milne EM, Rowland AC
et al. (1987) Equine gastric primary
impaction. *Vet Rec* **121**:263–264.

28   Owen RA, Jagger DW, Jagger
F (1987) Two cases of equine
primary gastric impaction. *Vet Rec*
121:102–105.

29   Blikslager AT, Wilson DA (2006)
Stomach and spleen. In: *Equine
Surgery*, 3rd edn. (JA Auer, JA Stick)
Saunders Elsevier, St Louis, pp.
374–386.

29a   Bird AR, Knowles EJ, Sherlock CE
et al. (2012) The clinical and pathological features of gastric impaction in
twelve horses. *Equine Vet J* **44(Suppl
43)**:105–110.

30   Honnas CM, Schumacher J (1985)
Primary gastric impaction in a pony.
J Am Vet Med Assoc **187**:501–502.

31   Cummings CA, Copedge KJ, Confer
AW (1997) Equine gastric impaction,
ulceration, and perforation due to persimmon (*Diospyros virginiana*) ingestion. *J Vet Diagn Invest* **9**:311–313.

32   Kellam LL, Johnson PJ, Kramer J
et al. (2000) Gastric impaction and
obstruction of the small intestine
associated with persimmon phytobezoar in a horse. *J Am Vet Med Assoc*
216:1279–1281.

33   McGorum BC, Murphy D, Love
S et al. (1999) Clinicopathological
features of equine primary hepatic

disease: a review of 50 cases. *Vet Rec*
145:134–139.

34   Arzt J, Mount ME (1999)
Hepatotoxicity associated with pyrrolizidine alkaloid (*Crotalaria* spp.)
ingestion in a horse on Easter Island.
Vet Hum Toxicol **41**:96–99.

35   Milne EM, Pogson DM, Doxey DL
(1990) Secondary gastric impaction
associated with ragwort poisoning in
three ponies. *Vet Rec* **126**:502–504.

36   Tennant B, Keirn DR, White KK
et al. (1982) Six cases of squamous cell
carcinoma of the stomach of the horse.
Equine Vet J **14**:238–243.

37   Olsen SN (1992) Squamous cell carcinoma of the equine stomach: a report
of five cases. *Vet Rec* **131**:170–173.

38   Taylor SD, Haldorson GJ, Vaughan
B et al. (2009) Gastric neoplasia in
horses. *J Vet Int Med* **23**:1097–1102.

39   Boy MG, Palmer JE, Heyer G et al.
(1992) Gastric leiomyosarcoma
in a horse. *J Am Vet Med Assoc*
200:1363–1364.

40   McKenzie EC, Mills JN, Bolton
JR (1997) Gastric squamous cell
carcinoma in three horses. *Aust Vet J*
75:480–483.

41   Foreman JH (2004) Changes in body
weight. In: *Equine Internal Medicine*,
2nd edn. (eds SM Reed, WM Bayly,
DC Sellon) Saunders Elsevier, St
Louis, pp. 124–129.

42   Keirn JM, White KK, King JM (1982)
Endoscopic diagnosis of squamous
cell carcinoma of the equine stomach.
J Am Vet Med Assoc **180**:940–942.

43   Ford TS, Vaala WE, Sweeney CR
et al. (1987) Pleuroscopic diagnosis
of gastroesophageal squamous cell
carcinoma in a horse. *J Am Vet Med
Assoc* **190**:1556–1558.

44   Todhunter RJ, Erb HN, Roth L
(1986) Gastric rupture in horses:
a review of 54 cases. *Equine Vet J*
18:288–293.

45   Kiper ML, Traub-Dargatz J, Curtis
CR (1990) Gastric rupture in horses:
50 cases (1979–1987) *J Am Vet Med
Assoc* **196**:333–336.

46   Pratt SM, Hassel DM, Drake C et al.
(2003) Clinical characteristics of
horses with gastrointestinal ruptures
revealed during initial diagnostic
evaluation: 149 cases (1990–2002).

*Proc 49th Ann Conv Am Assoc Equine
Practnrs*, pp. 366–370.

47   Morris DD, Moore JN, Ward S (1989)
Comparison of age, sex, breed, history
and management in 229 horses with
colic. *Equine Vet J Suppl* **7**:129–132.

48   Steenhaut M, Vlaminck K, Gasthuys F
(1986) Surgical repair of a partial
gastric rupture in a horse. *Equine Vet J*
18:331–332.

49   Hogan PM, Bramlage LR, Pierce
SE (1995) Repair of a full-thickness
gastric rupture in a horse. *J Am Vet
Med Assoc* **207**:338–340.

49a   Epstein KL, Fehr J (2012) Colic
surgery. In: *Practical Guide to Equine
Colic.* (ed LL Southwood) Wiley-
Blackwell, Ames, pp. 173–203.

50   Archer DC, Freeman DE, Doyle
AJ et al. (2004) Association between
cribbing and entrapment of the small
intestine in the epiploic foramen in
horses: 68 cases (1991–2002). *J Am Vet
Med Assoc* **224**:562–564.

51   Archer DC, Pinchbeck GK, French
NP et al. (2008) Risk factors for
epiploic foramen entrapment colic:
an international study. *Equine Vet J*
40:224–230.

52   Archer DC, Pinchbeck GL, French
NP et al. (2008) Risk factors for
epiploic foramen entrapment colic in
a UK horse population: a prospective case-control study. *Equine Vet J*
40:405–410.

53   Freeman DE, Schaeffer DJ (2001) Age
distributions of horses with strangulation of the small intestine by a lipoma
or in the epiploic foramen: 46 cases
(1994–2000). *J Am Vet Med Assoc*
219:87–89.

53a   Freeman DE, Schaeffer DJ (2005)
Short-term survival after surgery for
epiploic foramen entrapment compared with other strangulating diseases
of the small intestine in horses. *Equine
Vet J* **37**:292–295.

54   Archer DC, Pinchbeck GL, Proudman CJ et al. (2006) Is equine colic
seasonal? Novel application of a model
based approach. *BMC Vet Res* **2**:1–11.

55   Proudman CJ, Edwards GB, Barnes
J et al. (2005) Factors affecting long-term survival of horses recovering
from surgery of the small intestine.
Equine Vet J **37**:360–365.

56 Jenei TM, García–López JM, Provost PJ *et al.* (2007) Surgical management of small intestinal incarceration through the gastrosplenic ligament: 14 cases (1994–2006). *J Am Vet Med Assoc* **231**:1221–1224.

57 Ford TS, Freeman DE, Ross MW *et al.* (1990) Ileocecal intussusception in horses: 26 cases (1981–1988). *J Am Vet Med Assoc* **196**:121–126.

58 Cribb NC, Cote NM, Boure LP *et al.* (2006) Acute small intestinal obstruction associated with *Parascaris equorum* infection in young horses: 25 cases (1985–2004). *New Zeal Vet J* **54**:338–343.

59 Edwards GB (1986) Surgical management of intussusception in the horse. *Equine Vet J* **18**:313–321.

60 Southwood LL, Cohen J, Busschers E *et al.* (2010) Acquired jejunal pseudo-diverticula in a yearling Arabian filly. *Vet Surg* **39**:101–106.

61 Lowe JE (1968) Intussusception in three ponies following experimental enterotomy. *Cornell Vet* **58**:288–292.

62 Frankeny RL, Wilson DA, Messer NT *et al.* (1995) Jejunal intussusception: a complication of functional end-to-end stapled anastomoses in two ponies. *Vet Surg* **24**:515–517.

63 Boswell JC, Schramme MC, Gains M (2000) Jejunojejunal intussusception after an end-to-end jejunojejunal anastomosis in a horse. *Equine Vet J* **12**:303–306.

64 Dean PW, Robertson JT, Jabobs RM (1985) Comparison of suture materials and suture patterns for inverting intestina anastomosis of the jejunum in the horse. *Am J Vet Res* **46**:2072–2077.

65 Huskamp B (1982) The diagnosis and treatment of acute abdominal conditions in the horse; the various types and frequency as seen at the Animal Hospital in Hochmoor. *Proc 1st Equine Colic Res Symp*, pp. 261–272.

66 Freeman DE (2006) Small intestine. In: *Equine Surgery*, 3rd edn. (eds JA Auer, JA Stick) WB Saunders, Philadelphia, pp. 401–436.

67 Cable CS, Fubini S L, Erb HN *et al.* (1997) Abdominal surgery in foals: a review of 199 cases (1977–1994). *Equine Vet J* **29**:257–261.

68 Ford TS, Freeman DE, Ross MW *et al.* (1990) Ileocecal intussusception in horses: 26 cases (1981–1988). *J Am Vet Med Assoc* **196**:121–126.

69 Greet TRC (1992) Ileal intussusception in 16 young Thoroughbreds. *Equine Vet J* **24(2)**:81–83.

70 Beard WL, Byrne BA, Henninger RW (1992) Ileocecal intussusception corrected by resection within the cecum in two horses. *J Am Vet Med Assoc* **200**:1978–80.

71 Gayle JM, Blikslager AT, Bowman KF (2000) Mesenteric rents as a source of small intestinal strangulation in horses: 15 cases (1990–1997). *J Am Vet Med Assoc* **216**:1446–1449.

72 Sutter WW, Hardy J (2004) Laparoscopic repair of a small intestinal mesenteric rent in a broodmare. *Vet Surg* **33**:92–95.

73 Garcia-Seco E, Wilson DA, Kramer J *et al.* (2005) Prevalence and risk factors associated with outcome of surgical removal of pedunculated lipomas in horses: 102 cases (1987–2002). *J Am Vet Med Assoc* **226**:1529–1537.

74 Abutarbush SM, Naylor JM (2005) Comparison of surgical versus medical treatment of nephrosplenic entrapment of the large colon in horses: 19 cases (1992–2002). *J Am Vet Med Assoc* **227**:603–605.

75 Downes EE, Ragle CA, Hines MT (1994) Pedunculated lipoma associated with recurrent colic in a horse. *J Am Vet Med Assoc* **204**:1163–1164.

76 Jansson N (2000) Spontaneous correction of a nonstrangulating ileal obstruction caused by a pedunculated lipoma in a 14-year-old pony. *Equine Vet Educ* **12**:147–149.

77 Edwards GB, Proudman CJ (1994) An analysis of 75 cases of intestinal obstruction caused by pedunculated lipomas. *Equine Vet J* **26**:18–21.

78 Brosnahan MM, Paradis MR (2003) Demographic and clinical characteristics of geriatric horses: 467 cases (1989–1999). *J Am Vet Med Assoc* **223**:93–98.

79 Blikslager AT, Bowman KF, Haven ML *et al.* (1992) Pedunculated lipomas as a cause of intestinal obstruction in horses 17 cases (1983–1990). *J Am Vet Med Assoc* **201**:1249–1252.

80 Moll HD, Juzwiak JS, Santschi EM *et al.* (1991) Small-intestinal volvulus as a complication of acquired inguinal hernia in two horses. *J Am Vet Med Assoc* **198**:1413–1414.

81 Freeman DE, Koch DB, Boles CL (1979) Mesodiverticular bands as a cause of small intestinal strangulation and volvulus in the horse. *J Am Vet Med Assoc* **175**:1089–1094.

82 Grant BD, Tennant B (1973) Volvulus associated with Meckel's diverticulum in the horse. *J Am Vet Med Assoc* **162**:550–551.

83 Rooney JR (1965) Volvulus, strangulation, and intussusception in the horse. *Cornell Vet* **55**:644–653.

84 Vatistas NJ, Snyder JR, Wilson WD *et al.* (1996) Surgical treatment for colic in the foal (67 cases): 1980–1992. *Equine Vet J* **28**:139–145.

85 Stephen JO, Corley KTT, Johnston JK *et al.* (2004) Small intestinal volvulus in 115 horses: 1988–2000. *Vet Surg* **33**:333–339.

86 Stephen JO, Corley KTT, Johnston JK *et al.* (2004) Factors associated with mortality and morbidity in small intestinal volvulus in horses. *Vet Surg* **33**:340–348.

87 Rakestraw PC (1998) Modulation of intestinal motility. In: *Current Techniques in Equine Surgery and Lameness*, 2nd edn. (eds NA White, JN Moore) WB Saunders, Philadelphia, pp. 303–307.

88 Wylie CE, Proudman CJ (2009) Equine grass sickness: epidemiology, diagnosis, and global distribution. *Vet Clin N Am Equine Pract* **25**:381–399.

89 Hunter LC, Miller JK, Poxton IR (1999) The association of *Clostridium botulinum* type C with equine grass sickness: a toxicoinfection? *Equine Vet J* **31**:492–499.

90 Hunter LC, Poxton IR (2001) Systemic antibodies to *Clostridium botulinum* type C: do they protect horses from grass sickness (dysautonomia)? *Equine Vet J* **33**:547–553.

91 Garrett LA, Brown R, Poxton IR (2002) A comparative study of the intestinal microbiota of healthy horses and those suffering from equine grass sickness. *Vet Microbiol* **87**:81–88.

92 Newton JR, Wylie CE, Proudman CJ *et al.* (2010) Equine grass sickness: are we any nearer to answers on cause and prevention after a century of research. *Equine Vet J* **42**:477–481.

93 Gilmour JS, Jolly GM (1974) Some aspects of the epidemiology of equine grass sickness. *Vet Rec* **95**:77–81.

94 Doxey DL, Gilmour JS, Milne EM (1991) A comparative study of normal equine populations and those with grass sickness (dysautonomia) in eastern Scotland. *Equine Vet J* **23**:365–369.

95 Wood JL, Milne EM, Doxey DL (1998) A case-control study of grass sickness (equine dysautonomia) in the United Kingdom. *Vet J* **156**:7–14.

96 Pirie RS (2006) Grass sickness. *Clin Tech Equine Pract* **5**:30–36.

97 Milne EM, Pirie RS, McGorum BC *et al.* (2010) Evaluation of formalin-fixed ileum as the optimum method to diagnose equine dysautonomia (grass sickness) in simulated intestinal biopsies. *J Vet Diagns Invest* **22**:248–252.

98 Cottrell DR, McGorum BC, Pearson GT (1999) The neurology and enterology of equine grass sickness: a review of basic mechanisms. *Neurogastroent Motil* **11**:79–92.

99 Freeman DE (1999) Small intestine. In: *Equine Surgery*, 2nd edn. (eds JA Auer, JA Stick) WB Saunders, Philadelphia, pp. 232–257.

100 Little D, Blikslager AT (2002) Factors associated with development of ileal impaction in horses with surgical colic: 78 cases (1986–2000). *Equine Vet J* **34**:464–468.

101 Mueller POE, Fleming K (2009) Ileal impaction. In: *Current Therapy in Equine Medicine*, 6th edn. (eds E Robinson, KA Sprayberry) Saunders Elsevier, St. Louis, pp. 402–404.

102 Embertson RM, Colahan PT, Brown MP *et al.* (1985) Ileal impaction in the horse. *J Am Vet Med Assoc* **186**:570–572.

103 Hanson RR, Wright JC, Schumacher J *et al.* (1998) Surgical reduction of ileal impactions in the horse: 28 cases. *Vet Surg* **27**:555–560.

104 Proudman CJ, French NP, Trees AJ (1998) Tapeworm infection is a significant risk factor for spasmodic colic and ileal impaction colic in the horse. *Equine Vet J* **30**:194–199.

105 Proudman CJ, Holdstock NB (2000) Investigation of an outbreak of tapeworm-associated colic in a training yard. *Equine Vet J Suppl* **32**:37–41.

106 Parks AH, Doran RE, White NA *et al.* (1989) Ileal impaction in the horse: 75 cases. *Cornell Vet* **79**:83–91.

107 Hanson RR, Schumacher J, Humburg J *et al.* (1996) Medical treatment of horses with ileal impactions: 10 cases (1990–1994). *J Am Vet Med Assoc* **208**:898–900.

107a Fleming K, Mueller POE (2011) Ileal impaction in 245 horses: 1995–2007. *Can Vet J* **52**:759–763.

108 Lindsay WA, Confer AW, Ochoa R (1981) Ileal smooth muscle hypertrophy and rupture in a horse. *Equine Vet J* **13**:66–67.

109 Chaffin MK, Fuenteabla IC, Schumacher J *et al.* (1992) Idiopathic muscular hypertrophy of the equine small intestine: 11 cases (1980–1991). *Equine Vet J* **24**:372–378.

110 Mair TS, Lucke VM (2000) Ileal muscular hypertrophy and rupture in a pony three years after surgery for ileocecal intussusception. *Vet Rec* **146**:472–473.

111 Blennerhassett MG, Vignjevic P, Vermillion DL *et al.* (1992) Inflammation causes hyperplasia and hypertrophy in smooth muscle of rat small intestine. *Am J Physiol* **262**:G1041–G1046.

112 Robertson JT (1990) Diseases of the small intestine. In: *The Equine Acute Abdomen.* (ed NA White) Lea & Febiger, Philadelphia, pp. 347–368.

113 Edwards GB (1999) The role of tapeworms in equine colic. *Pferdeheilkunde* **15**:309–312.

114 Southwood LL (2008) Gastrointestinal tract diverticula: what, when, and why? *Equine Vet Educ* **20**:572–574.

115 Sprinkle TP, Swerczek TW, Crowe MW (1984) Meckel's diverticulum in the horse. *J Equine Vet Sci* **4**:175–179.

116 Assenza M, Ricci G, Antoniozzi A *et al.* (2007) Perforated jejunal diverticulosis. Case report and review of literature. *Ann Ital Chir* **78**:247–250.

117 Southwood LL, Ragle CA, Snyder JR *et al.* (1996) Surgical treatment of ascarid impactions in horses and foals. *Proc 42nd Ann Conv Am Assoc Equine Practnrs*, pp. 258–263.

118 Clayton HM (1986) Ascarids. Recent advances. *Vet Clin N Am Equine Pract* **2**:313–328.

119 Southwood LL, Baxter GM, Ragle CA *et al.* (1998) Ascarid impaction in young horses. *Comp Contin Educ Pract Vet* **20**:100–110.

120 Taylor SD, Pusterla N, Vaughan B *et al.* (2006) Intestinal neoplasia in horses. *J Vet Int Med* **20**:1429–1436.

121 Seahorn TL, Cornick JL, Cohen ND (1992) Prognostic indicators for horses with duodenitis-proximal jejunitis: 75 horses (1985–1989). *J Vet Int Med* **6**:307–311.

122 Underwood C, Southwood LL, McKeown LP *et al.* (2008) Complications and survival associated with surgical compared with medical management of horses with duodenitis-proximal jejunitis. *Equine Vet J* **40**:373–378.

123 Arroyo LG, Stampfli HR, Weese JS (2006) Potential role of *Clostridium difficile* as a cause of duodenitis-proximal jejunitis in horses. *J Med Microbiol* **55**:605–608.

124 White NA, Tyler DE, Blackwell RB *et al.* (1987) Hemorrhagic fibrinonecrotic duodenitis-proximal jejunitis in horses: 20 cases (1977–1984). *J Am Vet Med Assoc* **190**:311–315.

125 Jones RL, Shideler RK, Cockerell GL (1988) Association of *Clostridium difficile* with foal's diarrhea. In: *Equine Infectious Disease V.* University Press of Kentucky, Lexington, pp. 236–240.

126 Schumacher J, Mullen J, Shelby R *et al.* (1995) An investigation of the role of *Fusarium moniliforme* in duodenitis/proximal jejunitis of horses. *Vet Hum Toxicol* **37**:39–45.

127 Goel S, Schumacher J, Lenz SD *et al.* (1996) Effects of *Fusarium moniliforme* isolates on tissue and serum sphingolipid concentrations in horses. *Vet Hum Toxicol* **38**:265–270.

128 Cohen ND, Toby E, Roussel AJ *et al.* (2006) Are feeding practices associated with duodenitis-proximal jejunitis? *Equine Vet J* **38**:526–531.

129 Cohen ND, Brumbaugh GW, Faber NA *et al.* (1993) Duodenitis/proximal jejunitis: review and role of prokinetic drugs. *Proc 39th Ann Conven Am Assoc Equine Practnrs*, San Antonio, **39**:201–202.

130 Johnston JK, Morris DD (1987) Comparison of duodenitis/proximal jejunitis and small intestinal obstruction in horses: 68 cases (1977–1985). *J Am Vet Med Assoc* **191:**849–854.

131 Malone E, Ensink J, Turner T *et al.* (2006) Intravenous continuous infusion of lidocaine for treatment of equine ileus. *Vet Surg* **35:**60–66.

132 Cohen ND, Carter GK, Mealey RH *et al.* (1995) Medical management of right dorsal colitis in 5 horses: a retrospective study (1987–1993). *J Vet Int Med* **9:**272–276.

133 Cohen ND, Parson EM, Seahorn TL *et al.* (1994) Prevalence and factors associated with development of laminitis in horses with duodenitis/proximal jejunitis: 33 cases (1985–1991). *J Am Vet Med Assoc* **204:**250–254.

134 Fernandes WR, Coelho CS, Marques MS *et al.* (2003) A retrospective analysis of duodenitis-proximal jejunitis: 26 horses (1996–2000). *Cienc Rural* **33:**97–102.

135 Mair T, Pearson GR, Divers TJ (2006) Malabsorption syndromes in the horse. *Equine Vet Educ* **18:**383–392.

136 Divers T, Pelligrini-Masini A, McDonough S (2006) Diagnosis of inflammatory bowel disease in a Hackney pony by gastroduodenal endoscopy and biopsy and successful treatment with corticosteroids. *Equine Vet Educ* **18:**368–371.

137 Kalck KA (2009) Inflammatory bowel disease in horses. *Vet Clin N Am Equine Pract* **25:**303–315.

138 Schumacher J, Edwards JF, Cohen ND (2000) Chronic idiopathic inflammatory bowel diseases of the horse. *J Vet Intern Med* **14:**258–265.

139 Southwood LL, Kawcak CE, Trotter GW *et al.* (2000) Idiopathic focal eosinophilic enteritis associated with small intestinal obstruction in 6 horses. *Vet Surg* **29:**415–419.

140 Scott EA, Heidel JR, Snyder SP *et al.* (1999) Inflammatory bowel disease in horses: 11 cases (1988–1998). *J Am Vet Med Assoc* **214:**1527–1530.

141 Roberts M (2004) Proliferative and inflammatory intestinal diseases associated with malabsorption and maldigestion. In: *Equine Internal Medicine*, 2nd edn. (eds S Reed, WM Bayly, DC Sellon) WB Saunders, St. Louis, pp. 878–884.

142 Barr BS (2006) Infiltrative intestinal disease. *Vet Clin N Am Equine Pract* **22:**e1–7.

143 Lindberg R, Nygren A, Persson SGB (1996) Rectal biopsy diagnosis in horses with clinical signs of intestinal disorders: a retrospective study of 116 cases. *Equine Vet J* **28:**275–284.

143a Southwood LL (2012) Gastrointestinal parasitology and anthelmintics. In: *Practical Guide to Equine Colic.* (ed LL Southwood) Wiley-Blackwell, Ames, pp. 316–324.

144 Cooper DM, Gebhart CJ (1998) Comparative aspects of proliferative enteritis. *J Am Vet Med Assoc* **212:**1446–1451.

145 Wuersch K, Huessy D, Koch C *et al.* (2006) *Lawsonia intracellularis* proliferative enteropathy in a filly. *J Vet Med* **53:**17–21.

146 Lavoie JP, Drolet R, Parsons D *et al.* (2000) Equine proliferative enteropathy: a cause of weight loss, colic, diarrhoea and hypoproteinaemia in foals on three breeding farms in Canada. *Equine Vet J* **32:**418–425.

147 McClintock SA, Collins AM (2004) *Lawsonia intracellularis* proliferative enteropathy in a weanling foal in Australia. *Aust Vet J* **82:**750–752.

148 Sampieri F, Hinchcliff KW, Toribio RE (2006) Tetracycline therapy of *Lawsonia intracellularis* enteropathy in foals. *Equine Vet J* **38:**89–92.

149 Feary DJ, Hassel DM (2002) Enteritis and colitis in horses. *Vet Clin N Am Equine Pract* **22:**437–479.

150 Lawson GH, Gebhart CJ (2000) Proliferative enteropathy. *J Comp Path* **122:**77–100.

150a Epstein KL, Fehr J (2012) Colic surgery. In: *Practical Guide to Equine Colic.* (ed LL Southwood) Wiley-Blackwell, Ames, pp. 173–203

151 Blikslager AT (2008) Cecal impaction. In: *Current Therapy in Equine Medicine*, 6th edn. (NE Robinson, KA Sprayberry) Saunders Elsevier, St. Louis, pp. 405–406.

152 Campbell ML, Colahan PC, Brown MM *et al.* (1984) Cecal impaction in the horse. *J Am Vet Med Assoc* **184:**950–952.

153 Plummer AE, Rakestraw PC, Hardy J (2007) Outcome of medical and surgical treatment of cecal impaction in horses: 114 cases (1994–2004). *J Am Vet Med Assoc* **231:**1378–1385.

154 Hackett R (1990) Cecal impaction. In: *Current Practice of Equine Surgery.* (eds N White, J Moore) JB Lippincott, Philadelphia, pp. 331–334.

155 Smith LC, Payne RJ, Boys Smith SJ *et al.* (2010) Outcome and long-term follow-up of 20 horses undergoing surgery for caecal impaction: a retrospective study (2000–2008). *Equine Vet J* **42:**388–392.

156 Lester GD, Bolton JR, Cullen LK *et al.* (1992) Effects of general anesthesia on myoelectric activity of the intestine in horses. *Am J Vet Res* **53:**1553–1557.

157 Dabareiner RM, White NA (1995) Large colon impaction in horses: 147 cases (1985–1991). *J Am Vet Med Assoc* **206:**679–685.

158 Dart A, Hodgson D, Snyder J (1997) Caecal disease in equids. *Aust Vet J* **75:**552–557.

159 Voss JL (1969) Rupture of the cecum and ventral colon of mares during parturition. *J Am Vet Med Assoc* **155:**745–747.

160 Rakestraw PC, Hardy J (2006) Large intestine. In: *Equine Surgery*, 3rd edn. (eds JA Auer, JA Stick) WB Saunders, Philadelphia, pp. 436–478.

161 Huscamp B, Scheideman W (2000) Diagnosis and treatment of chronic recurrent caecal impaction. *Equine Vet J Suppl* **32:**65.

161a Aitken MR, Southwood LL, Kraus BM *et al.* (2012) Surgical and non-surgical management of cecal impaction in 150 horses (1991–2011). *Proc Am Coll Vet Surg, National Harbor.* (**Note**: Meeting was cancelled due to Hurricane Sandy, but abstracts still online.)

162 Barclay WP, Foerner JJ, Phillips TN *et al.* (1982) Primary gastric impaction in the horse. *J Am Vet Med Assoc* **181:**682–683.

163 Gaughan EM, Hackett RP (1990) Cecocolic intussusception in horses: 11 cases (1979–1989). *J Am Vet Med Assoc* **197:**1373–1375.

164 Martin BB Jr, Freeman DE, Ross MW et al. (1999) Cecocolic and cecocecal intussusception in horses: 30 cases (1976–1996). *J Am Vet Med Assoc* **214:**80–84.

165 Gaughan EM, van Harreveld P (2000) Cecocecal and cecocolic intussusception in horses. *Comp Contin Educ Pract Vet* **22:**616–621.

166 Mair TS, Sutton DGM, Love S (2000) Caecocaecal and caecocolic intussusceptions associated with larval cyathostomosis in four young horses. Equine *Vet J Suppl* **32:**77–80.

167 Hubert JD, Hardy J, Holcombe SJ et al. (2000) Cecal amputation within the right ventral colon for surgical treatment of nonreducible cecocolic intussusception in 8 horses. *Vet Surg* **29:**317–325.

168 Boussaw BH, Domingo R, Wilderjans H (2001) Treatment of irreducible caecocolic intussusception in horses by jejuno(ileo-)colostomy. *Vet Rec* **149:**16–18.

169 Lores M, Ortenburger AI (2008) Use of cecal bypass via side-to-side ileocolic anastomosis without ileal transection for treatment of cecocolic intussusception in three horses. *J Am Vet Med Assoc* **232:**574–577.

170 Embertson RM, Cook G, Hance SR et al. (1996) Large colon volvulus: surgical treatment of 204 horses (1986–1995). *Proc 42nd Ann Conven Am Assoc Equine Practnrs*, pp. 254–255.

171 Southwood LL, Bergslien K, Jacobi A et al. (2002) Large colon displacement and volvulus in horses: 495 cases (1987–1999). *Proc 7th Int Equine Colic Res Symp*, pp. 32–33.

172 Dolente BA, Sullivan EK, Boston R et al. (2005) Mares admitted to a referral hospital for postpartum emergencies: 163 cases (1992–2002). *J Vet Emerg Crit Care* **15:**193–200.

173 Abutarbush SM (2006) Use of ultrasonography to diagnose large colon volvulus in horses. *J Am Vet Med Assoc* **228:**409–413.

174 Moore RM, Hance SR, Hardy J et al. (1996) Colonic luminal pressure in horses with strangulating and non-strangulating obstruction of the large colon. *Vet Surg* **25:**134–141.

175 Van Hoogmoed L, Snyder JR (1998) Intestinal viability. In: *Current Techniques in Equine Surgery and Lameness.*

(eds NA White, JN Moore) WB Saunders, Philadelphia, pp. 273–279.

176 Driscoll N, Baia P, Fischer AT et al. (2008) Large colon resection and anastomosis in horses: 52 cases (1996–2006). *Equine Vet J* **40:**342–347.

177 Ellis CM, Lynch TM, Slone DE et al. (2008) Survival and complications after large colon resection and end-to-end anastomosis for strangulating large colon volvulus in seventy–three horses. *Vet Surg* **37:**786–790.

178 Mathis SC, Slone DE, Lynch TM et al. (2006) Use of colonic luminal pressure to predict outcome after surgical treatment of strangulating large colon volvulus in horses. *Vet Surg* **35:**356–360.

179 Southwood LL (2004) Postoperative management of the large colon volvulus patient. *Vet Clin N Am Equine Pract* **20:**167–197.

180 Johnston K, Holcombe SJ, Hauptman JG (2007) Plasma lactate as a predictor of colonic viability and survival after 360 degrees volvulus of the ascending colon in horses. *Vet Surg* **36:**563–567.

181 Cohen ND, Peloso JG (1996) Risk factors for history of previous colic and for chronic, intermittent colic in a population of horses. *J Am Vet Med Assoc* **208:**697–703.

182 Cohen ND, Gibbs PG, Woods AM (1999) Dietary and other management factors associated with colic in horses. *J Am Vet Med Assoc* **215:**53–60.

183 Hudson JM, Cohen ND, Gibbs PG et al. (2001) Feeding practices associated with colic in horses. *J Am Vet Med Assoc* **219:**1419–1425.

184 Hillyer MH, Taylor FGR, Proudman CJ et al. (2002) Case control study to identify risk factors for simple colonic obstruction and distention colic in horses. *Equine Vet J* **34:**455–463.

185 Tinker MK, White NA, Lessard P et al. (1997) Prospective study of equine colic incidence and mortality. *Equine Vet J* **29:**448–453.

186 Kristula M, McDonnell S (1994) Effect of drinking water temperature on consumption and preference of water during cold weather in ponies. *Proc 40th Ann Conv Am Assoc Equine Practnrs* **40:**95.

187 Sullins KE (1990) Diseases of the large colon. In: *The Equine Acute Abdomen.*

(ed NA White) Lea & Febiger, Philadelphia, pp. 375–391.

188 Roberts MC, Argenzio RA (1986) Effects of amitraz, several opiate derivatives and anticholinergic agents on intestinal transit in ponies. *Equine Vet J* **18:**256.

189 Auer DE, Seawright AA, Pollitt CC et al. (1984) Illness in horses following spraying with amitraz. Aust *Vet J* **61:**257–259.

190 Hallowell GD (2008) Retrospective study assessing efficacy of treatment of large colonic impactions. *Equine Vet J* **40:**411–413.

191 Lopes MA, Walker BL, White NA 2nd et al. (2002) Treatments to promote colonic hydration: enteral fluid therapy versus intravenous fluid therapy and magnesium sulphate. *Equine Vet J* **34:**505–509.

192 Southwood LL, Dolente BA, Lindborg S et al. (2009) Survival rate of horses admitted on an emergency basis to a university referral hospital. *Equine Vet J* **41:**1–6.

193 Ruohoniemi M, Kaikkonen R, Raekallio M et al. (2001) Abdominal radiography in monitoring the resolution of sand accumulations from the large colon of horses treated medically. *Equine Vet J* **33:**59–64.

194 Kendall A, Ley C, Egenvall A et al. (2008) Radiographic parameters for diagnosing sand colic in horses. *Acta Vet Scand* **50:**17.

195 Keppie NJ, Rosenstein DS, Holcombe SJ et al. (2007) Objective radiographic assessment of abdominal sand accumulation in horses. *Vet Radiol Ultrasound* **49:**122–128.

196 Korolainen R, Ruohoniemi M (2002) Reliability of ultrasonography compared to radiography in revealing intestinal sand accumulations in horses. *Equine Vet J* **34:**499–504.

197 Specht TE, Colahan PT (1988) Surgical treatment of sand colic in equids: 48 cases (1978–1985). *J Am Vet Med Assoc* **193:**1560–1564.

198 Ragle CA, Meagher DM, Lacroix CA et al. (1989) Surgical treatment of sand colic. Results in 40 horses. *Vet Surg* **18:**48–51.

199 Hassel DM, Langer DL, Snyder JR et al. (1999) Evaluation of enterolithiasis in equids: 900 cases (1973–1996). *J Am Vet Med Assoc* **214:**233–237.

199a Hassel DM, Rakestraw PC, Gardner IA *et al.* (2004) Dietary risk factors and colonic pH and mineral concentrations in horses with enterolithiasis. *J Vet Int Med* **18**:346–349.

199b Maher O, Puchalski SM, Drake C *et al.* (2011) Abdominal computed radiography for diagnosis of enterolithiasis in horses: 142 cases (2003–2007). *J Am Vet Med Assoc* **239**:1483–1485.

200 Yarbrough TB, Langer DL, Snyder JR *et al.* (1994) Abdominal radiography for diagnosis of enterolithiasis in horses: 141 cases (1990–1992). *J Am Vet Med Assoc* **205**:592–595.

201 Livesey MA, Arighi M, Ducharme NG *et al.* (1988) Equine colic: seventy-six cases resulting from incarceration of the large colon by the suspensory ligament of the spleen. *Can Vet J* **29**:135–141.

202 Röcken M, Schubert C, Mosel G *et al.* (2005) Indications, surgical technique, and long-term experience with laparoscopic closure of the nephrosplenic space in standing horses. *Vet Surg* **34**:637–641.

203 Burba DJ, Moore RM (1997) Renosplenic entrapment: a review of clinical presentation and treatment. *Equine Vet Educ* **9**:180–184.

204 Mariën T, Adriaenssen A, von Hoeck F *et al.* (2001) Laparoscopic closure of the renosplenic space in standing horses. *Vet Surg* **30**:559–563.

205 Moll HE, Schumacher J, Dabareiner RM (1993) Left dorsal displacement of the colon with splenic adhesions in three horses. *J Am Vet Med Assoc* **203**:425–427.

206 Hardy J, Minton M, Robertson JT *et al.* (2000) Nephrosplenic entrapment in the horse: a retrospective study of 174 cases. *Equine Vet J Suppl* **32**:95–97.

207 Santschi EM, Slone DE, Frank WM (1993) Use of ultrasound in horses for diagnosis of left dorsal displacement of the large colon and monitoring its nonsurgical correction. *Vet Surg* **22**:281–284.

208 Hardy J, Bednarski RM, Biller DS (1994) Effect of phenylephrine on hemodynamics and splenic dimensions in horses. *Am J Vet Res* **55**:1570–1578.

209 Frederick J, Giguère S, Butterworth K *et al.* (2010) Severe phenylephrine-associated hemorrhage in five aged horses. *J Am Vet Med Assoc* **237**:830–834.

210 van Harreveld PD, Gaughan EM, Valentino LW (1999) A retrospective analysis of left dorsal displacement of the large colon treated with phenylephrine hydrochloride and exercise in 12 horses (1996–1998). *New Zeal Vet J* **47**:109–111.

210a Baker WT, Frederick J, Giguere S *et al.* (2011) Reevaluation of the effect of phenylephrine on resolution of nephrosplenic entrapment by the rolling procedure in 87 horses. *Vet Surg* **40**:825–829.

210b Lindegaard C, Ekstrøm CT, Wulf SB *et al.* (2011) Nephrosplenic entrapment of the large colon in 142 horses (2000–2009): analysis of factors associated with decision of treatment and short-term survival. *Equine Vet J Suppl* **39**:63–68.

211 Busschers E, Parente EJ, Southwood LL (2007) Laparoscopic diagnosis and correction of a nephrosplenic ligament entrapment of the large colon in a horse. *Equine Vet Educ* **19**:60–63.

212 Farstvedt E, Hendrickson D (2005) Laparoscopic closure of the nephrosplenic space for prevention of recurrent nephrosplenic entrapment of the ascending colon. *Vet Surg* **34**:642–645.

213 Epstein KL, Parente EJ (2006) Laparoscopic obliteration of the nephrosplenic space using polypropylene mesh in five horses. *Vet Surg* **35**:431–437.

214 Brounts SH, Kooreman KM (2004) Risk factors for right dorsal displacement of the large colon in horses: 67 cases (1990–2000). *Proc 14th Ann Meeting Am Coll Vet Surg*, pp. 12–13.

215 Gardner RB, Nydam DV, Mohammed HO *et al.* (2005) Serum gamma glutamyl transferase activity in horses with right or left dorsal displacements of the large colon. *J Vet Int Med* **19**:761–764.

216 Whitcomb MB (2005) Advanced abdominal ultrasound for chronic colic. *Proc 15th Ann Meeting Am Coll Vet Surg*, pp. 39–44.

217 Carter JD, Hird DW, Farver TB *et al.* (1986) Salmonellosis in hospitalized horses: seasonality and case fatality rates. *J Am Vet Med Assoc* **188**:163–167.

218 Hird DW, Casebolt DB, Carter JD *et al.* (1986) Risk factors for salmonellosis in hospitalized horses. *J Am Vet Med Assoc* **188**:173–177.

219 Traub-Dargatz JL, Salman MD, Jones RL (1990) Epidemiologic study of salmonellae shedding in the feces of horses and potential risk factors for development of the infection in hospitalized horses. *J Am Vet Med Assoc* **196**:1617–1622.

220 House JK, Mainar-Jaime RC, Smith BP *et al.* (1999) Risk factors for nosocomial Salmonella infection among hospitalized horses. *J Am Vet Med Assoc* **214**:1511–1516.

221 Schott HC 2nd, Ewart SL, Walker RD *et al.* (2001) An outbreak of salmonellosis among horses at a veterinary teaching hospital. *J Am Vet Med Assoc* **218**:1152–1159.

222 Ernst NS, Hernandez JA, MacKay RJ *et al.* (2004) Risk factors associated with fecal *Salmonella* shedding among hospitalized horses with signs of gastrointestinal tract disease. *J Am Vet Med Assoc* **225**:275–81.

223 Ekiri AB, MacKay RJ, Gaskin JM *et al.* (2009) Epidemiologic analysis of nosocomial *Salmonella* infections in hospitalized horses. *J Am Vet Med Assoc* **234**:108–19.

224 Weese JS, Staempfli HR, Prescott JF (2001) A prospective study of the roles of *Clostridium difficile* and enterotoxigenic *Clostridium perfringens* in equine diarrhoea. *Equine Vet J* **33**:403–409.

225 Båverud V, Gustafsson A, Franklin A *et al.* (2003) *Clostridium difficile*: prevalence in horses and environment, and antimicrobial susceptibility. *Equine Vet J* **35**:465–471.

226 East LM, Dargatz DA, Traub-Dargatz JL *et al.* (2000) Foaling-management practices associated with the occurrence of enterocolitis attributed to *Clostridium perfringens* infection in the equine neonate. *Prev Vet Med* **46**:61–74.

227 MacKay RJ (2001) Equine neonatal clostridiosis: treatment and prevention. *Comp Contin Educ Pract Vet* **23**:280–285.

228 Herholz C, Miserez R, Nicolet J et al. (1999) Prevalence of beta2-toxigenic *Clostridium perfringens* in horses with intestinal disorders. *J Clin Microbiol* **37**:358–361.

229 Schotte U, Truyen U, Neubauer H (2004) Significance of β2-toxigenic *Clostridium perfringens* infections in animals and their predisposing factors: a review. *J Vet Med B, Infect Dis Vet Public Health* **51**:423–426.

230 Madigan JE, Pusterla N, Johnson E et al. (2000) Transmission of *Ehrlichia risticii*, the agent of Potomac horse fever, using naturally infected aquatic insects and helminth vectors: preliminary report. *Equine Vet J* **32**:275–279.

231 Mair T (2002) Chronic diarrhea. In: *Manual of Equine Gastroenterology.* (eds T Mair, T Divers, N Ducharme) WB Saunders, London, pp. 427–428.

232 Hyatt DR, Weese JS (2004) *Salmonella* culture: sampling procedures and laboratory techniques. *Vet Clin N Am Equine Pract* **20**:577–585.

233 Van Duijkeren E, Flemming C, Sloet van Oldruitenborgh-Oosterbaan M et al. (1995) Diagnosing salmonellosis in horses: culturing of multiple versus single fecal samples. *Vet Quart* **17**:63–66.

234 Medina-Torres CE, Weese JS, Staempfli HR (2010) Validation of a commercial enzyme immunoassay for detection of *Clostridium difficile* toxins in feces of horses with acute diarrhea. *J Vet Int Med* **24**:628–632.

235 Biswas B, Mukherjee D, Mattingly-Napier BL et al. (1991) Diagnostic application of polymerase chain reaction for detection of *Ehrlichia risticii* in equine monocytic ehrlichiosis (Potomac horse fever). *J Clin Microbiol* **29**:2228–2233.

236 Mott J, Rikihisa Y, Zhang Y et al. (1997) Comparison of PCR and culture to the indirect fluorescent-antibody test for diagnosis of Potomac horse fever. *J Clin Microbiol* **35**:2215–2219.

237 Weese JS, Cote NM, deGannes RV (2003) Evaluation of in vitro properties of di-tri-octahedral smectite on clostridial toxins and growth. *Equine Vet J* **35**:638–641.

238 Hassel DM, Smith PA, Nieto JE et al. (2009) Di-tri-octahedral smectite

for the prevention of post-operative diarrhea in equids with surgical disease of the large intestine: results of a randomized clinical trial. *Vet J* **182**:210–214.

239 Desrochers AM, Dolente BA, Roy MF et al. (2005) Efficacy of *Saccharomyces boulardii* for treatment of horses with acute enterocolitis. *J Am Vet Med Assoc* **227**:954–959.

240 Jang SS, Hansen LM, Breher JE et al. (1997) Antimicrobial susceptibilities of equine isolates of *Clostridium difficile* and molecular characterization of metronidazole-resistant strains. *Clin Infect Dis 25 Suppl* **2**:S266–S267.

241 Cohen ND, Woods AM (1999) Characteristics and risk factors for failure of horses with acute diarrhea to survive: 122 cases (1990–1996). *J Am Vet Med Assoc* **214**:382–390.

242 Hough ME, Steel CM, Bolton JR et al. (1999) Ulceration and stricture of the right dorsal colon after phenylbutazone administration in four horses. *Aust Vet J* **77**:785–788.

243 Jones SL, Davis J, Rowlingson K (2003) Ultrasonographic findings in horses with right dorsal colitis: five cases (2000–2001). *J Am Vet Med Assoc* **222**:1248–1251.

244 Cohen ND (2002) Right dorsal colitis. *Equine Vet Educ* **14**:212–219.

245 Karcher LF, Dill SG, Anderson WI et al. (1990) Right dorsal colitis. *J Vet Int Med* **4**:247–253.

246 McConnico RS, Morgan TW, Williams CC et al. (2008) Pathophysiologic effects of phenylbutazone on the right dorsal colon in horses. *Am J Vet Res* **69**:1496–1505.

247 East LM, Trumble TN, Steyn PF et al. (2000) The application of technetium-99m hexamethylpropyleneamine oxime (99mTc-HMPAO) labeled white blood cells for the diagnosis of right dorsal ulcerative colitis in two horses. *Vet Radiol Ultrasound* **41**:360–364.

248 Cook VL, Shults JJ, McDowell M et al. (2008) Attenuation of ischaemic injury in the equine jejunum by administration of systemic lidocaine. *Equine Vet J* **40**:353–357.

249 Simmons TR, Gaughan EM, Ducharme NG et al. (1990) Treatment

of right dorsal ulcerative colitis in a horse. *J Am Vet Med Assoc* **196**:455–458.

250 Lane JK, Cohen JM, Zedler ST et al. (2010) Right dorsal colon resection and bypass for treatment of right dorsal colitis in a horse. *Vet Surg* **39**:879–883.

250a de Bont MP, Proudman CJ, Archer DC (2013) Surgical lesions of the small colon and post operative survival in a UK hospital population. *Equine Vet J* **45**:460–464.

251 Ruggles AJ, Ross MW (1991) Medical and surgical management of small colon impaction in horses: 28 cases (1984–1989). *J Am Vet Med Assoc* **199**:1762–1766.

252 Rhoads WS, Barton MH, Parks AH (1999) Comparison of medical and surgical treatment for impaction of the small colon in horses: 84 cases (1986–1996) *J Am Vet Med Assoc* **214**:1042–1046.

253 Frederico LM, Jones SL, Blikslager AT (2006) Predisposing factors for small colon impaction in horses and outcome of medical and surgical treatment: 44 cases (1999–2004). *J Am Vet Med Assoc* **229**:1612–1616.

254 Reeves MJ, Gay JM, Hilbert BJ et al. (1989) Association of age, sex and breed factors in acute equine colic: a retrospective study of 320 cases admitted to a veterinary teaching hospital in the USA. *Prev Vet Med* **7**:149–160.

255 Dart AJ, Snyder JR, Pascoe JR et al. (1992) Abnormal conditions of the equine descending (small) colon: 102 cases (1979–1989). *J Am Vet Med Assoc* **200**:971–978.

256 Archer RM, Parsons JC, Lindsay WA et al. (1988) A comparison of enterotomies through the antimesenteric band and the sacculation of the small (descending) colon of ponies. *Equine Vet J* **20**:406–413.

257 McClure JT, Kobluk C, Voller K et al. (1992) Fecalith impaction in four miniature foals. *J Am Vet Med Assoc* **200**:205–207.

258 Ragle CA, Snyder JR, Meagher DM et al. (1992) Surgical treatment of colic in American miniature horses: 15 cases (1980–1987). *J Am Vet Med Assoc* **201**:329–331.

259 Gay CC, Speirs VC, Christie BA *et al.* (1979) Foreign body obstruction of the small colon in six horses. *Equine Vet J* **11**:60–63.

260 Schumacher J, Mair T (2002) Small colon obstruction in the mature horse. *Equine Vet Educ* **14**:17–18.

261 Prange T, Holcombe SJ, Brown JA *et al.* (2010) Resection and anastomosis of the descending colon in 43 horses. *Vet Surg* **39**:748–753.

262 Southwood LL, Gassert T, Lindborg S (2010) Colic in geriatric compared to mature nongeriatric horses. Part 2: Treatment, diagnosis and short-term survival. *Equine Vet J* **42**:628–635.

263 Alexander GR, Gibson KT (2002) Non-surgical management of rectal tears in two mares. *Aust Vet J* **80**:137–139.

264 Welland LM (2003) Transmural rectal intestinal evisceration associated with parturition in a primiparous mare. *Can Vet J* **44**:470–472.

265 Arnold JS, Meacher DM, Lohse CL (1978) Rectal tears in the horse. *J Equine Med Surg* **2**:55–61.

266 Kay AT, Spirito MA, Rodgerson DH *et al.* (2005) How to repair grade IV rectal tears in post-parturient mares. *Proc 51st Ann Meeting Am Assoc Equine Practnrs*, pp. 487–489.

267 Claes A, Ball BA, Brown JA *et al.* (2008) Evaluation of risk factors, management, and outcome associated with rectal tears in horses: 99 cases (1985–2006). *J Am Vet Med Assoc* **233**:1605–1609.

268 Slone DE, Humburg JM, Jagar JE *et al.* (1982) Noniatrogenic rectal tears in three horses. *J Am Vet Med Assoc* **180**:750–751.

269 Guglick MA, MacAllister CG, Ewing PJ *et al.* (1996) Thrombosis resulting in rectal perforation in a horse. *J Am Vet Med Assoc* **209**:1125–1127.

270 Stauffer VD (1981) Equine rectal tears: a malpractice problem. *J Am Vet Med Assoc* **178**:798–799.

271 Freeman DE (2006) Rectum and anus. In: *Equine Surgery*, 3rd edn. (eds JA Auer, JA Stick) WB Saunders, Philadelphia, pp. 479–491.

272 Watkins JP, Taylor TS, Schumacher J *et al.* (1989) Rectal tears in the horse:

an analysis of 35 cases. *Equine Vet J* **21**:186–188.

273 Eastman TG, Taylor TS, Hooper RN *et al.* (2000) Treatment of rectal tears in 85 horses presented to the Texas Veterinary Medical Center. *Equine Vet Educ* **12(5)**:236–266.

274 Baird AN, Freeman DE (1997) Management of rectal tears. *Vet Clin N Am Equine Pract* **13**:377–392.

275 Sanders-Shamis M (1985) Perirectal abscesses in six horses. *J Am Vet Med Assoc* **187**:499–500.

276 Magee AA, Ragle CA, Hines MT *et al.* (1997) Anorectal lymphadenopathy causing colic, perirectal abscesses, or both in five young horses. *J Am Vet Med Assoc* **210**:804–807.

277 Stick JA (2006) Abdominal hernias. In: *Equine Surgery*, 3rd edn. (eds JA Auer, JA Stick) WB Saunders, Philadelphia, pp. 491–499.

278 Schneider RK, Milne DW, Kohn CW (1982) Acquired inguinal hernia in the horse: a review of 27 cases. *J Am Vet Med Assoc* **180**:317–320.

279 Blackford JT, Toal RL, Latimer FG *et al.* (1993) Percutaneous ultrasonographic diagnosis of suspected acquired inguinal and scrotal herniation in horses. *Proc Ann Conven Am Assoc Equine Practnrs* **38**: 357–374.

279a Caron JP, Brakenhoff J (2008) Intracorporeal suture closure of the internal inguinal and vaginal rings in foals and horses. *Vet Surg* **37**:126–131.

279b Rossignol F, Perrin R, Boening KJ (2007) Laparoscopic hernioplasty in recumbent horses using transposition of a peritoneal flap. *Vet Surg* **36**:557–562.

280 Tulleners EP (1999) Disease of the abdominal wall. In: *Equine Medicine and Surgery*, 5th edn. (eds PT Colahan, AM Merritt, JN Moore *et al.*) Mosby, St. Louis, pp. 808–816.

281 Freeman DE, Spencer PA (1991) Evaluation of age, breed, and gender as risk factors for umbilical hernia in horses of a hospital population. *Am J Vet Res* **52**:637–639.

282 Bristol DG (1986) Diaphragmatic hernias in horses and cattle. *Comp Contin Educ Pract Vet* **8**:S407–S412.

283 Collobert C, Gillet JP, Esling W (1988) A case of congenital diaphragmatic hernia in a foal. *Equine Pract* **10**:43–46.

284 Schambourg MA, Laverty S, Mullim S *et al.* (2003) Thoracic trauma in foals: post-mortem findings. *Equine Vet J* **35**:78–81.

285 Hart SK, Brown JA (2009) Diaphragmatic hernia in the horse: 44 cases (1986–2006). *J Vet Emerg Crit Care* **19**:357–362.

286 Santschi EM, Juzwiak JS, Moll HD *et al.* (1997) Diaphragmatic hernia repair in three young horses. *Vet Surg* **26**:242–245.

287 Malone ED, Farnsworth K, Lennox T *et al.* (2001) Thoracoscopic-assisted diaphragmatic hernia repair using a thoracic rib resection. *Vet Surg* **30**:175–178.

288 Barton MH (2010) Disorders of the liver. In: *Equine Internal Medicine*, 3rd edn. (eds SM Reed, WM Bayly, DC Sellon) WB Saunders, St. Louis, pp. 939–975.

289 Dyson S (1983) Review of 30 cases of peritonitis in the horse. *Equine Vet J* **15**:25–30.

290 Mair TS, Hillyer MH, Taylor FGR (1990) Peritonitis in adult horses: a review of 21 cases. *Vet Rec* **126**:567–570.

291 Hawkins JF, Bowman KF, Roberts MC *et al.* (1993) Peritonitis in horses: 67 cases (1985–1990). *J Am Vet Med Assoc* **203**:284–288.

292 Southwood LL, Russell G (2007) The use of clinical findings in the identification of equine peritonitis cases that respond favorably to medical therapy. *J Vet Emerg Crit Care* **17**:382–390.

293 Golland LC, Hodgson DR, Hodgson JL *et al.* (1994) Peritonitis associated with *Actinobacillus equuli* in horses: 15 cases (1982–1992). *J Am Vet Med Assoc* **205**:340–343.

294 Henderson ISF, Mair TS, Keen JA *et al.* (2008) Study of the short- and long-term outcomes of 65 horses with peritonitis. *Vet Rec* **163**:293–297.

295 Dechant JE, Nieto JE, LeJeune S (2006) Hemoperitoneum in horses: 67 cases (1989–2004). *J Am Vet Med Assoc* **229**:253–258.

CHAPTER 2: MUSCULOSKELETAL SYSTEM

1 Wright IM, Smith MWR, Humphrey DJ *et al.* (2003) Endoscopic surgery in the treatment of contaminated and infected synovial cavities. *Equine Vet J* **35**:613–619.

2 Trotter GW, McIlwraith CW (1996) Clinical features and diagnosis of equine joint disease In: *Joint Disease in the Horse.* (eds CW McIlwraith, GW Trotter) WB Saunders, Philadelphia, pp. 120–145.

3 Schneider RK, Bramlage LR, Moore RM *et al.* (1992) A retrospective study of 192 horses affected with septic arthritis/tenosynovitis. *Equine Vet J* **24**:436–442.

4 McIlwraith CW, Nixon AJ, Wright IM *et al.* (2005) Tenoscopy. In: *Diagnostic and Surgical Arthroscopy in the Horse,* 3rd edn. (eds CW McIlwraith, AJ Nixon, IM Wright *et al.*) Mosby, New York, pp. 365–408.

5 Bertone AL (1994) Management of orthopedic emergencies. *Vet Clin N Am Equine Pract* **10**:603–625.

6 Bramlage LR (1996) First aid and transportation of fracture patients. In: *Equine Fracture Repair.* (ed AJ Nixon) WB Saunders, Philadelphia, pp. 36–42.

7 Furst AE (2006) Emergency treatment and transportation of equine fracture patients. In: *Equine Surgery,* 3rd edn. (eds JA Auer, JA Stick) WB Saunders, St. Louis, pp. 972–981.

8 Mudge MC, Bramlage LR (2007) Field fracture management. *Vet Clin N Am Equine Pract* **23**:117–133.

9 Schneider RK (2006) Synovial and osseous infections. In: *Equine Surgery,* 3rd edn. (eds JA Auer, JA Stick) WB Saunders, St. Louis, pp. 1121–1130.

10 Goodrich LR (2006) Osteomyelitis in horses. *Vet Clin N Am Equine Pract* **22**:389–417, viii–ix.

11 Ivester KM, Adams SB (2007) Orthopedic infection: the use of local antimicrobial therapy. *Comp Contin Ed Pract Vet: Equine Edition* **2**:82–90.

12 Scheuch BC, Van Hoogmoed LM, Wilson WD (2002) Comparison of intraosseous and intravenous infusion for delivery of amikacin sulfate to the tibiotarsal joint of horses. *Am J Vet Res* **63**:374–380.

13 Whitehair KJ, Blevins WE, Fesler JR *et al.* (1992) Regional perfusion of the equine carpus for antibiotic delivery. *Vet Surg* **21**:279–285.

14 Werner LA, Hardy J, Bertone AL (2003) Bone gentamicin concentration after intra-articular or regional intravenous perfusion in the horse. *Vet Surg* **32**:559–565.

15 Boothe DM (2001) Antimicrobial drugs. In: *Small Animal Clinical Pharmacology and Therapeutics.* (ed DM Boothe) WB Saunders, Philadelphia, pp. 150–174.

16 Rubio-Martinez L, Lopez-Sanroman J, Cruz AM *et al.* (2005) Evaluation of safety and pharmacokinetics of vancomycin after intravenous regional limb perfusion in horses. *Am J Vet Res* **66**:2107–2113.

17 Pille F, DeBaere S, Ceelen L *et al.* (2005) Synovial fluid and plasma concentrations of ceftiofur after regional intravenous perfusion in the horse. *Vet Surg* **34**:610–617.

18 Parra-Sanchez A, Lugo J, Boothe DM (2006) Pharmacokinetics and pharmacodynamics of enrofloxacin and a low dose of amikacin administered via regional intravenous limb perfusion in standing horses. *Am J Vet Res* **67**:1687–1695.

19 Baxter GM (1996) Instrumentation and techniques for treating orthopedic infections in horses. *Vet Clin N Am Equine Pract* **12**:303–335.

20 Holcombe SJ, Schneider RK, Bramlage LR *et al.* (1997) Use of antibiotic-impregnated polymethyl methacrylate in horses with open or infected fractures or joints: 19 cases (1987–1995). *J Am Vet Med Assoc* **211**:889–893.

21 Henry SL, Hood GA, Seligson D (1993) Long-term implantation of gentamicin-polymethylmethacrylate antibiotic beads. *Clin Orthop Relat Res* **295**:47–53.

22 Henry SL, Seligson D, Mangino P *et al.* (1991) Antibiotic-impregnated beads. Part 1: Bead implantation versus systemic therapy. *Orthop Rev* **20**:242–247.

23 Phillips H, Boothe DM, Shofer F *et al.* (2007) In-vitro elution studies of amikacin and cefazolin from polymethyl-methacrylate. *Vet Surg* **36**:272–278.

24 Ramos JR, Howard RD, Pleasant RS *et al.* (2003) Elution of metronidazole and gentamicin from polymethylmeth-acrylate beads. *Vet Surg* **32**:251–261.

25 Farnsworth KD, White NA 2nd, Robertson J (2001) The effect of implanting gentamicin-impregnated polymethylmethacrylate beads in the tarsocrural joint of the horse. *Vet Surg* **30**:126–131.

26 Scott EA, McDole M, Shires MH (1979) A review of third phalanx fractures in the horse: sixty-five cases. *J Am Vet Med Assoc* **174**:1337–1343.

27 Honnas CM, O'Brien TR, Linford RL (1988) Distal phalanx fractures in horses: a survey of 274 horses with radiographic assessment of healing in 36 horses. *Vet Radiol* **29**:98–107.

28 Bertone AL (1996) Fractures of the distal phalanx. In: *Equine Fracture Repair.* (ed AJ Nixon) WB Saunders, Philadelphia, pp. 146–152.

29 Yovich JV, Stashak TS, DeBowes RM *et al.* (1986) Fractures of the distal phalanx of the forelimb in eight foals. *J Am Vet Med Assoc* **189**:550–554.

30 Watkins JP (1996) Fractures of the middle phalanx. In: *Equine Fracture Repair.* (ed AJ Nixon) WB Saunders, Philadelphia, pp. 129–145.

31 Rose PL, Seeherman H, O'Callaghan M (1997) Computed tomographic evaluation of comminuted middle phalangeal fractures in the horse. *Vet Radiol Ultrasound* **38**:424–429.

32 Nixon AJ (2006) Phalanges and the metacarpophalangeal and meta-tarsophalangeal joints. In: *Equine Surgery,* 3rd edn. (eds JA Auer, JA Stick) WB Saunders, St. Louis, pp. 1217–1238

33 Joyce J, Baxter GM, Sarrafian TL *et al.* (2006) Use of transfixation pin casts to treat adult horses with comminuted phalangeal fractures: 20 cases (1993–2003). *J Am Vet Med Assoc* **229**:725–730.

34 Lescun TB, McClure SR, Ward MP *et al.* (2007) Evaluation of transfixation casting for treatment of third metacarpal, third metatarsal, and phalangeal fractures in horses: 37 cases (1994–2004). *J Am Vet Med Assoc* **230**:1340–1349.

35 Richardson DW (1996) Fractures of the proximal phalanx. In: *Equine Fracture Repair*. (ed AJ Nixon) WB Saunders, Philadelphia, pp. 117–128.

36 Holcombe SJ, Schneider RK, Bramlage LR *et al.* (1995) Lag screw fixation of noncomminuted sagittal fractures of the proximal phalanx in racehorses: 59 cases (1973–1991). *J Am Vet Med Assoc* **206:**1195–1199.

37 Markel MD, Richardson DW (1985) Noncomminuted fractures of the proximal phalanx in 69 horses. *J Am Vet Med Assoc* **186:**573–579.

38 Kraus BM, Richardson DW, Nunamaker DM *et al.* (2004) Management of comminuted fractures of the proximal phalanx in horses: 64 cases (1983–2001). *J Am Vet Med Assoc* **224:**254–263.

39 Schneider RK, Jackman BR (1996) Fractures of the third metacarpus and metatarsus. In: *Equine Fracture Repair*. (ed AJ Nixon) WB Saunders, Philadelphia, pp. 179–194.

40 McClure SR, Watkins JP, Glickman NW *et al.* (1998) Complete fractures of the third metacarpal or metatarsal bone in horses: 25 cases (1980–1996). *J Am Vet Med Assoc* **213:**847–850.

41 Zekas LJ, Bramlage LR, Embertson RM *et al.* (1999) Characterisation of the type and location of fractures of the third metacarpal/metatarsal condyles in 135 horses in central Kentucky (1986–1994). *Equine Vet J* **31:**304–308.

42 Richardson DW (2006) Metacarpal and metatarsal bones. In: *Equine Surgery*, 3rd edn. (eds JA Auer, JA Stick) WB Saunders, St. Louis, pp. 1238–1253.

43 Norrdin RW, Kawcak CE, Capwell BA *et al.* (1998) Subchondral bone failure in an equine model of overload arthrosis. *Bone* **22:**133–139.

44 McIlwraith CW (1996) Fractures of the carpus. In: *Equine Fracture Repair*. (ed AJ Nixon) WB Saunders, Philadelphia, pp. 208–221.

45 Ruggles AJ (2006) Carpus. In: *Equine Surgery*, 3rd edn. (eds JA Auer, JA Stick) WB Saunders, St. Louis, pp. 1253–1266.

46 Tapprest J, Audigie F, Radier C *et al.* (2003) Magnetic resonance imaging for the diagnosis of stress fractures in a horse. *Vet Radiol Ultrasound* **44:**438–442.

47 Getman M, Southwood LL, Richardson DW (2006) Palmar carpal osteochondral fragments in racehorses: 31 cases (1994–2004). *J Am Vet Med Assoc* **228:**1551–1558.

48 Kraus BM, Ross MW, Boston RC (2005) Surgical and nonsurgical management of sagittal slab fractures of the third carpal bone in racehorses: 32 cases (1991–2001). *J Am Vet Med Assoc* **226:**945–950.

49 Nixon AJ (1996) Fractures and luxations of the hock. In: *Equine Fracture Repair*. (ed AJ Nixon) WB Saunders, Philadelphia, pp. 259–272.

50 Davidson EJ, Ross MW, Parente EJ (2005) Incomplete sagittal fracture of the talus in 11 racehorses: outcome. *Equine Vet J* **37:**457–461.

51 Auer JA (2006) Tarsus. In: *Equine Surgery*, 3rd edn. (eds JA Auer, JA Stick) WB Saunders, St. Louis, pp. 1288–1307.

52 Nixon AJ (1996) Fractures of the ulna. In: *Equine Fracture Repair*. (ed AJ Nixon) WB Saunders, Philadelphia, pp. 231–241.

53 Watkins JP (2006) Radius and ulna. In: *Equine Surgery*, 3rd edn. (eds JA Auer, JA Stick) WB Saunders, St. Louis, pp. 1267–1279.

54 Swor TM, Watkins JP, Bahr A *et al.* (2003) Results of plate fixation of type 1b olecranon fractures in 24 horses. *Equine Vet J* **35:**670–675.

55 Swor TM, Watkins JP, Bahr A *et al.* (2006) Results of plate fixation of type 5 olecranon fractures in 20 horses. *Equine Vet J* **38:**30–34.

56 Auer JA (1996) Fractures of the radius. In: *Equine Fracture Repair*. (ed AJ Nixon) WB Saunders, Philadelphia, pp. 222–230.

57 Matthews S, Dart AJ, Dowling BA *et al.* (2002) Conservative management of minimally displaced radial fractures in three horses. *Aust Vet J* **80:**44–47.

58 Watkins JP (1996) Fractures of the tibia. In: *Equine Fracture Repair*. (ed AJ Nixon) WB Saunders, Philadelphia, pp. 273–283.

59 O'Sullivan CB, Lumsden JM (2003) Stress fractures of the tibia and humerus in Thoroughbred racehorses: 99 cases (1992–2000). *J Am Vet Med Assoc* **222:**491–498.

60 Verheyen KL, Newton JR, Price JS *et al.* (2006) A case-control study of factors associated with pelvic and tibial stress fractures in Thoroughbred racehorses in training in the UK. *Prev Vet Med* **74:**21–35.

61 Bramlage LR (2006) Tibia. In: *Equine Surgery*, 3rd edn. (eds JA Auer, JA Stick) WB Saunders, St. Louis, p. 1308.

62 Ramzan PH, Newton JR, Shepherd MC *et al.* (2003) The application of a scintigraphic grading system to equine tibial stress fractures: 42 cases. *Equine Vet J* **35:**382–388.

63 Nixon AJ, Watkins JP (1996) Fractures of the humerus. In: *Equine Fracture Repair*. (ed AJ Nixon) WB Saunders, Philadelphia, pp. 242–253.

64 Fortier LA (2006) Shoulder. In: *Equine Surgery*, 3rd edn. (eds JA Auer, JA Stick) WB Saunders, St. Louis, pp. 1280–1288.

65 Carter BG, Schneider RK, Hardy J *et al.* (1993) Assessment and treatment of equine humeral fractures: retrospective study of 54 cases (1972–1990). *Equine Vet J* **25:**203–207.

66 Hance SR, Bramlage LR (1996) Fractures of the femur and patella. In: *Equine Fracture Repair*. (ed AJ Nixon) WB Saunders, Philadelphia, pp. 284–293.

67 Richardson DW (2006) Femur and pelvis. In: *Equine Surgery*, 3rd edn. (eds JA Auer, JA Stick) WB Saunders, St. Louis, pp. 1334–1340.

68 Hance SR, Bramlage LR, Schneider RK *et al.* (1992) Retrospective study of 38 cases of femur fractures in horses less than one year of age. *Equine Vet J* **24:**357–363.

69 McClure SR, Watkins JP, Ashman RB (1998) In-vivo evaluation of intramedullary interlocking nail fixation of transverse femoral osteotomies in foals. *Vet Surg* **27:**29–36.

70 Radcliffe RM, Lopez MJ, Turner TA *et al.* (2001) An in-vitro biomechanical comparison of interlocking nail constructs and double plating for fixation of diaphyseal femur fractures in immature horses. *Vet Surg* **30:**179–190.

71 Turner AS, Milne DW, Hohn RB *et al.* (1979) Surgical repair of fractured capital femoral epiphysis in three foals. *J Am Vet Med Assoc* **175**:1198–1202.

72 Ducharme NG (1996) Pelvic fracture and coxofemoral luxation. In: *Equine Fracture Repair*. (ed AJ Nixon) WB Saunders, Philadelphia, pp. 294–298.

73 Rutkowski JA, Richardson DW (1989) A retrospective study of 100 pelvic fractures in horses. *Equine Vet J* **21**:256–259.

74 Pierce KN, Gerard MP (2006) What is your diagnosis? Pelvic fracture detected by ultrasonography. *J Am Vet Med Assoc* **229**:37–38.

75 Barrett EL, Talbot AM, Driver AJ *et al.* (2006) A technique for pelvic radiography in the standing horse. *Equine Vet J* **38**:266–270.

76 DeBowes RM (1996) Fractures of the cranium. In: *Equine Fracture Repair*. (ed AJ Nixon) WB Saunders, Philadelphia, pp. 313–322.

77 DeBowes RM (1996) Fractures of the mandible and maxilla. In: *Equine Fracture Repair*. (ed AJ Nixon) WB Saunders, Philadelphia, pp. 323–336.

78 Auer J (2006) Craniomaxillofacial disorders. In: *Equine Surgery*, 3rd edn. (eds JA Auer, JA Stick) WB Saunders, St. Louis, pp. 1341–1362.

79 Holcombe SJ (2006) Physiologic response to trauma: evaluating the trauma patient. In: *Equine Surgery*, 3rd edn. (eds JA Auer, JA Stick) WB Saunders, St. Louis, pp. 88–95.

80 Richardson DW, Ahern BJ (2012) Synovial and osseous infections. In: *Equine Surgery*, 3rd edn. (eds JA Auer, JA Stick) WB Saunders, St. Louis, pp. 1189–1201.

81 Gaughan EM, Rendano VT, Ducharme NG (1999) Surgical treatment of septic pedal osteitis in horses: nine cases (1980–1987). *J Am Vet Med Assoc* **195**:1131–1134.

82 Cauvin ER, Monroe GA (1998) Septic osteitis of the distal phalanx: findings and surgical treatment in 18 cases. *Equine Vet J* **30**:512–519.

83 Linford S, Embertson R, Bramlage L (1994) Septic osteitis of the third phalanx: a review of 63 cases. *Proc Am Assoc Equine Practnrs* **40**:103.

84 Neil KM, Axon JE, Todhunter PG *et al.* (2007) Septic osteitis of the distal phalanx in foals: 22 cases (1995–2002). *J Am Vet Med Assoc* **230**:1683–1690.

85 Bertone AL (1996) Fractures of the proximal sesamoid bones. In: *Equine Fracture Repair*. (ed AJ Nixon) WB Saunders, Philadelphia, pp. 163–171.

86 Parkin TD, Clegg PD, French NP *et al.* (2004) Risk of fatal distal limb fractures among Thoroughbreds involved in the five types of racing in the United Kingdom. *Vet Rec* **154**:493–497.

87 Anthenill LA, Stover SM, Gardner IA *et al.* (2006) Association between findings on palmarodorsal radiographic images and detection of a fracture in the proximal sesamoid bones of forelimbs obtained from cadavers of racing Thoroughbreds. *Am J Vet Res* **67**:858–868.

88 Foland JW, Trotter GW, Stashak TS *et al.* (1991) Traumatic injuries involving tendons of the distal limbs in horses: a retrospective study of 55 cases. *Equine Vet J* **23**:422–425.

89 Bertone AL (1995) Tendon lacerations. *Vet Clin N Am Equine Pract* **11**:293–314.

90 Fraser BS, Bladon BM (2004) Tenoscopic surgery for treatment of lacerations of the digital flexor tendon sheath. *Equine Vet J* **36**:528–531.

91 Jann H, Pasquini C (2005) Wounds of the distal limb complicated by involvement of deep structures. *Vet Clin N Am Equine Pract* **21**:145–165, viii.

92 Davis CS, Smith RKW (2006) Diagnosis and management of tendon and ligament disorders. In: *Equine Surgery*, 3rd edn. (eds JA Auer, JA Stick) WB Saunders, St. Louis, pp. 1086–1111.

93 Belknap JK, Baxter GM, Nickels FA (1993) Extensor tendon lacerations in horses: 50 cases (1982–1988). *J Am Vet Med Assoc* **203**:428–431.

94 Semevolos SA, Nixon AJ, Goodrich LR *et al.* (1998) Shoulder joint luxation in large animals: 14 cases (1976–1997). *J Am Vet Med Assoc* **213**:1608–1611.

95 Bailey JV, Barber SM, Fretz PB *et al.* (1984) Subluxation of the carpus in thirteen horses. *Can Vet J* **25**:311–314.

96 Reeves MJ, Trotter GW (1991) Tarsocrural joint luxation in a horse. *J Am Vet Med Assoc* **199**:1051–1053.

97 Dowling BA, Dart AJ, Hodgson DR (2000) Surgical treatment of tarsometatarsal joint luxation in a miniature horse foal. *Aust Vet J* **78**:683–684.

98 Yovich JV, Turner AS, Stashak TS *et al.* (1987) Luxation of the metacarpophalangeal and metatarsophalangeal joints in horses. *Equine Vet J* **19**:295–298.

99 McIlwraith CW, Goodman NL (1989) Conditions of the interphalangeal joints. *Vet Clin N Am Equine Pract* **5**:161–178.

100 Schneider RK, Bramlage LR, Hardy J (1993) Arthrodesis of the distal interphalangeal joint in two horses using three parallel 5.5-mm cortical screws. *Vet Surg* **22**:122–128.

101 Schneider RK, Bramlage LR, Moore RM *et al.* (1992) A retrospective study of 192 horses affected with septic arthritis/tenosynovitis. *Equine Vet J* **24**:436–442.

102 Smith LJ, Marr CM, Payne RJ *et al.* (2001) What is the likelihood that Thoroughbred foals treated for septic arthritis will race? *Equine Vet J* **36**:452–456.

103 Palmer JL, Bertone AL (1994) Joint structure, biochemistry and biochemical disequilibrium in synovitis and equine joint disease. *Equine Vet J* **26**:263–277.

104 Curtiss PH Jr (1973) The pathophysiology of joint infections. *Clin Orthop Relat Res* **96**:129–135.

105 Bertone AL (1996) Infectious arthritis. In: *Joint Disease in the Horse*. (eds CW McIlwraith, GW Trotter) WB Saunders, Philadelphia, pp. 397–409.

106 Tulamo RM, Bramlage LR, Gabel AA (1989) Sequential clinical and synovial fluid changes associated with acute infectious arthritis in the horse. *Equine Vet J* **21**:325–331.

107 Schneider RK, Bramlage LR (1991) Recommendations for the clinical management of septic arthritis in horses. *Proc 36th Ann Conv Am Assoc Equine Practnrs*, pp. 551–556.

108 Meijer MC, van Weeren PR, Rijken-huizen AB (2000) Clinical experiences of treating septic arthritis in the equine by repeated joint lavage: a series of 39 cases. *J Vet Med – Series* A **47**:351–365.

109 Honnas CM, Schumacher J, Cohen ND *et al.* (1991) Septic tenosynovitis in horses: 25 cases (1983–1989). *J Am Vet Med Assoc* **199**:1616–1622.

110 Bertone AL (1995) Infectious tenosynovitis. *Vet Clin N Am Equine Pract* **11**:163–176.

111 Snyder JR, Pascoe JR, Hirsch DC (1987) Antimicrobial susceptibility of microorganisms isolated from equine orthopedic patients. *Vet Surg* **16**:197–201.

112 Waguespack RW, Burba DJ, Moore RM (2006) Surgical site infection and the use of antimicrobials. In: *Equine Surgery*, 3rd edn. (eds JA Auer, JA Stick) WB Saunders, St. Louis, pp. 70–87.

113 Smith CS, Smith RK (2006) Diagnosis and management of tendon and ligament disorders. In: *Equine Surgery*, 3rd edn. (eds JA Auer, JA Stick) WB Saunders, St. Louis, pp. 1086–1111.

114 Wereszka MM, White NA, Furr MO (2007) Factors associated with outcome following treatment of horses with septic tenosynovitis: 51 cases (1986–2003). *J Am Vet Med Assoc* **230**:1195–1200.

115 Frees KE, Lillich JD, Gaughan EM *et al.* (2002) Tenoscopic-assisted treatment of open digital flexor tendon sheath injuries in horses: 20 cases. *J Am Vet Med Assoc* **220**:1823–1827.

116 Celeste CJ, Szoke MO (2005) Management of equine hoof injuries. *Vet Clin N Am Equine Pract* **21**:167–190, viii.

117 Furst AE, Lischer CJ (2006) Foot. In: *Equine Surgery*, 3rd edn. (eds JA Auer, JA Stick) WB Saunders, St. Louis, pp. 1184–1217.

118 Wright IM, Phillips TJ, Walmsley JP (1999) Endoscopy of the navicular bursa: a new technique for the treatment of contaminated and septic bursae. *Equine Vet J* **31**:5–11.

119 Wright IM (2002) Endoscopy in the management of puncture wounds to the foot. *Proc Europ Coll Vet Surg* **11**:107–108.

120 Hood DM (1999) The mechanisms and consequences of structural failure of the foot. *Vet Clin N Am Equine Pract* **15**:437–461.

121 Hood DM (1999) Laminitis in the horse. *Vet Clin N Am Equine Pract* **15**:287–294, v.

122 Hood DM (1999) The pathophysiology of developmental and acute laminitis. *Vet Clin N Am Equine Pract* **15**:321–343.

123 Herthel D, Hood DM (1999) Clinical presentation, diagnosis, and prognosis of chronic laminitis. *Vet Clin N Am Equine Pract* **15**:375–394, vii.

124 Morgan SJ, Grosenbaugh DA, Hood DM (1999) The pathophysiology of chronic laminitis. Pain and anatomic pathology. *Vet Clin N Am Equine Pract* **15**:395–417, vii.

125 Van Eps AW, Pollitt CC (2004) Equine laminitis: cryotherapy reduces the severity of the acute lesion. *Equine Vet J* **36**:255–260.

126 Peek SF, Semrad SD, Perkins GA (2003) Clostridial myonecrosis in horses (37 cases 1985–2000). *Equine Vet J* **35**:86–92.

127 Jeanes LV, Magdesian KG, Madigan JE *et al.* (2001) Clostridial myositis in horses. *Comp Contin Educ Pract Vet* **23**:577–587.

128 Brown CM, Kaneene JB, Walker RD (1988) Intramuscular injection techniques and the development of clostridial myositis or cellulitis in horses. *J Am Vet Med Assoc* **193**:668–670.

129 Owen J, Bevins GA (1998) Gas gangrene in a horse. *Vet Rec* **142**:555–556.

130 Stewart AJ (2006) Clostridial myositis and collapse in a standardbred filly. *Vet Clin N Am Equine Pract* **22**:127–143.

131 Stevens DL, Maier KA, Mitten JE (1987) Effect of antibiotics on toxin production and viability of *Clostridium perfringens*. *Antimicrob Agents Chemother* **31**:213–218.

132 MacLeay JM, Sorum SA, Valberg SJ *et al.* (1999) Epidemiologic analysis of factors influencing exertional rhabdomyolysis in Thoroughbreds. *Am J Vet Res* **60**:1562–1566.

133 MacLeay JM, Valberg SJ, Sorum SA *et al.* (1999) Heritability of recurrent exertional rhabdomyolysis in Thoroughbred racehorses. *Am J Vet Res* **60**:250–256.

134 Valberg SJ, Macleay JM, Billstrom JA *et al.* (1999) Skeletal muscle metabolic response to exercise in horses with 'tying–up' due to polysaccharide storage myopathy. *Equine Vet J* **31**:43–47.

135 McKenzie EC, Valberg SJ, Pagan JD (2003) Nutritional management of exertional rhabdomyolysis. In: *Current Therapy in Equine Medicine*, 5th edn. (ed NE Robinson) WB Saunders, St Louis, pp. 727–734.

136 Dranchak PK, Valberg SJ, Onan GW *et al.* (2005) Inheritance of recurrent exertional rhabdomyolysis in thoroughbreds. *J Am Vet Med Assoc* **227**:762–767.

137 McGowan CM, Fordham T, Christley RM (2002) Incidence and risk factors for exertional rhabdomyolysis in Thoroughbred racehorses in the United Kingdom. *Vet Rec* **151**:623–626.

138 Valberg S, Jonsson L, Lindholm A *et al.* (1993) Muscle histopathology and plasma aspartate aminotransferase, creatine kinase and myoglobin changes with exercise in horses with recurrent exertional rhabdomyolysis. *Equine Vet J* **25**:11–16.

139 MacLeay (2010) Inborn errors of metabolism. In: *Equine Internal Medicine*. (eds SM Reed, WM Bayly, DC Sellon) WB Saunders, St Louis, pp. 503–512.

140 Spier S, Valberg S, Carr E *et al.* (1995) Update on hyperkalemic periodic paralysis. *Proc 41st Ann Conv Am Assoc Equine Practnrs*, pp. 231–233.

CHAPTER 3: RESPIRATORY TRACT

1　Wilkins PA, Seahorn TL (2000) Intranasal oxygen therapy in adult horses. *J Vet Emerg Crit Care* **10**:221.

2　Stewart JH, Rose RJ, Barco AM (1984) Response to oxygen administration in foals: effect of age, duration and method of administration on arterial blood gas values. *Equine Vet J* **16**:329–331.

3　Wilson DV, Schott HC 2nd, Robinson NE *et al.* (2006) Response to nasopharyngeal oxygen administration in horses with lung disease. *Equine Vet J* **38**:219–223.

4　Hoffman AM, Viel L (1992) A percutaneous transtracheal catheter system for improved oxygenation in foals with respiratory distress. *Equine Vet J* **24**:239–241.

5　Wilkins PA (2003) Lower respiratory problems of neonates. *Vet Clin N Am Equine Pract* **19**:19-34.

6　Wilkins PA (2003) Lower airway disease of adult horses. *Vet Clin N Am Equine Pract* **19**:101–122.

7　Wilkins PA (2000) Arterial blood gas analysis in foals. *Proc 18th Am Coll Vet Intern Med* 195–197.

8　Wilkins PA (2008) Diagnostic procedures for the respiratory system. In: *Large Animal Internal Medicine*, 4th edn. (ed BP Smith) Mosby Inc, Philadelphia, pp. 490–500.

9　Hoffman AM, Viel L (1997) Techniques for sampling the respiratory tract of horses. *Vet Clin N Am Equine Pract* **13**:463–475.

10　Giguere S (2008) Bacterial pneumonia and pleuropneumonia in adult horses. In: *Large Animal Internal Medicine*, 4th edn. (ed BP Smith) Mosby Inc, Philadelphia, pp. 500–510.

11　Chaffin MK, Carter GK, Dabareiner RM (2000) How to place an indwelling chest tube for drainage and lavage of the pleural cavity in horses affected with pleuropneumonia. *Proc Ann Conven Am Assoc Equine Practnrs* **26**:145–149.

12　Chaffin MK, Carter GK, Relford RL (1994) Equine bacterial pleuropneumonia. Part II. Clinical signs and diagnostic evaluation. *Compend Contin Educ Pract Vet* **16**:363–379.

13　Chaffin MK, Carter GK, Byars TD (1994) Equine bacterial pleuropneumonia. Part III. Treatment, sequelae, and prognosis. *Compend Contin Educ Pract Vet* **16**:1585–1596.

14　Schott HC III, Mannsman RA (1990) Thoracic drainage in horses. *Compend Contin Educ Pract Vet* **12**:251–261.

15　Holcombe SJ, Ducharme NG (2004) Abnormalities of the upper airway. In: *Equine Sports Medicine and Surgery*. (eds KW Hinchcliff, AJ Kaneps, RG Geor) Saunders, New York, pp. 559–598.

16　Parente EJ (2003) Arytenoid chondrosis. In: *Current Therapy in Equine Medicine* 5. (ed EW Robinson) Saunders, St Louis, pp. 381–383.

17　Chalmers HJ, Cheetham J, Yeager AE *et al.* (2006) Ultrasonography of the equine larynx. *Vet Radiol Ultrasound* **47**:476–481.

18　Hay WP, Tulleners E (1993) Excision of intralaryngeal granulation tissue in 25 horses using a neodymium:YAG laser (1986–1991). *Vet Surg* **22**:129–134.

19　Sullins KE (2002) Minimally invasive laser treatment of arytenoid chondritis in horses. *Clin Tech Equine Pract* **1**:13–16.

20　Rakestraw PC, Eastman TG, Taylor PS *et al.* (2000) Long-term outcome of horses undergoing permanent tracheostomy: 42 cases. *Proc Ann Conven Am Assoc Equine Practnrs* **46**:111–112.

21　Schumacher J, Hanselka DV (1987) Nasopharyngeal cicatrices in horses: 47 cases (1972–1985). *J Am Vet Med Assoc* **191**:239–242.

22　McClure SR, Schumacher J, Snyder JR (1994) Transnasal incision of restrictive nasopharyngeal cicatrix in three horses. *J Am Vet Med Assoc* **205**:461–463.

23　Dixon PM, McGorum BC, Railton DI *et al.* (2001) Laryngeal paralysis: a study of 375 cases in a mixed-breed population of horses. *Equine Vet J* **33**:452–458.

24　Southwood LL, Gaynor JS (2003) Postanesthetic upper respiratory tract obstruction. In: *Current Therapy in Equine Medicine* 5. (ed NE Robinson) Saunders, St Louis, pp. 391–393.

25　McGorum BC, Murphy D, Love S *et al.* (1999) Clinicopathological features of equine primary hepatic disease: a review of 50 cases. *Vet Rec* **145**:134–139.

26　Rose RJ, Hartley WJ, Baker W (1981) Laryngeal paralysis in Arabian foals associated with oral haloxon administration. *Equine Vet J* **13**:171–176.

27　Slocombe RF, Huntington PJ, Friend SC *et al.* (1992) Pathological aspects of Australian Stringhalt. *Equine Vet J* **24**:174–183.

28　Mair TS, Lane JG (1996) The differential diagnosis of sudden onset respiratory distress. *Equine Vet Educ* **8**:131–136.

29　Sweeney CR, Timoney JF, Newton JR *et al.* (2005) *Streptococcus equi* infections in horses: guidelines for treatment, control, and prevention of strangles. *J Vet Intern Med* **19**:123–134.

30　Spoormakers TJP, Ensink JM, Goehring LS *et al.* (2003) Brain abscesses as a metastatic manifestation of strangles: symptomatology and the use of magnetic resonance imaging as a diagnostic aid. *Equine Vet J* **35**:146–151.

31　Newton JR, Wood JL, Dunn KA *et al.* (1997) Naturally occurring persistent and asymptomatic infection of the guttural pouches of horses with *Streptococcus equi. Vet Rec* **25**:84–90.

32　Golland LC, Hodgson DR, Davis RE *et al.* (1995) Retropharyngeal lymph node infection in horses: 46 cases (1977–1992). *Aust Vet J* **72**:161–164.

33　Waller AS, Jolley KA (2007) Getting a grip on strangles: recent progress towards improved diagnostics and vaccines. *Vet J* **173**:492–501.

34　De Clercq D, van Loon G, Nollet H *et al.* (2003) Percutaneous puncture technique for treating persistent retropharyngeal lymph node infections in seven horses. *Vet Rec* **152**:169–172.

35　Newton JR, Verheyen K, Talbot NC *et al.* (2000) Control of strangles outbreaks by isolation of guttural pouch carriers identified using PCR and culture of *Streptococcus equi. Equine Vet J* **32**:515–526.

36 Hardy J, Leveile R (2003) Diseases of the guttural pouches. *Vet Clin N Am Equine Pract* **19**:123–158.

37 Blazyczek I, Hamann H, Deegen E *et al.* (2004) Retrospective analysis of 50 cases of guttural pouch tympany in foals. *Vet Rec* **28**:261–264.

38 Freeman DE (1980) Diagnosis and treatment of diseases of the guttural pouch (part 1). *Compend Contin Educ Pract Vet* **II**:S3–S11.

39 Tate LP Jr, Blikslager AT, Little ED (1995) Transendoscopic laser treatment of guttural pouch tympanites in eight foals. *Vet Surg* **24**:367–372.

40 Schambourg MA, Marcoux M, Celeste C (2006) Salpingoscopy for the treatment of recurrent guttural pouch tympany in a filly. *Equine Vet Educ* **18**:298–302.

41 Dickinson CE, Traub-Dargatz JL, Dargatz DA *et al.* (1996) Rattlesnake venom poisoning in horses: 32 cases (1973–1993). *J Am Vet Med Assoc* **208**:1866–1871.

42 Seahorn TL, Divers TJ (2003) Respiratory system. In: *Manual of Equine Emergencies: Treatment and Procedures*, 2nd edn. (eds JA Orsini, TJ Divers) Saunders, Philadelphia, pp.501–528.

43 Landolt GA (2007) Management of equine poisoning and envenomation. *Vet Clin N Am Equine Pract* **23**:31–47.

44 Mirtschin PJ, Masci P, Paton DC *et al.* (1998) Snake bites recorded by veterinary practices in Australia. *Aust Vet J* **76**:195–198.

45 Jeanes LV, Magdesian KG, Madigan JE *et al.* (2001) Clostridial myositis in horses. *Compend Contin Educ Pract Vet* **23**:577–587.

46 Peek SF, Semrad SD, Perkins GA (2003) Clostridial myonecrosis in horses (37 cases 1985–2000). *Equine Vet J* **35**:86–92.

47 Brown CM, Kaneene JB, Walker RD (1988) Intramuscular injection techniques and the development of clostridial myositis or cellulitis in horses. *J Am Vet Med Assoc* **193**:668–670.

48 Adam EN, Southwood LL (2006) Surgical and traumatic wound infections, cellulitis, and myositis in horses. *Vet Clin N Am Equine Pract* **22**:335–361.

49 Stewart AJ (2006) Clostridial myositis and collapse in a standardbred filly. *Vet Clin N Am Equine Pract* **22**:127–143.

50 Barber SM (2005) Management of neck and head injuries. *Vet Clin N Am Equine Pract* **21**:191–215.

51 Fubini SL, Todhunter RJ, Vivrette SL *et al.* (1985) Tracheal rupture in two horses. *J Am Vet Med Assoc* **187**:69–70.

52 Freeman DE (1989) Wounds of the esophagus and trachea. *Vet Clin N Am Equine Pract* **5**:683–693.

53 Kirker-Head CA, Jakob TP (1990) Surgical repair of ruptured trachea in a horse. *J Am Vet Med Assoc* **196**:1635–1638.

54 Saulez MN, Slovis NM, Louden AT (2005) Tracheal perforation managed by temporary tracheostomy in a horse. *J S Afr Vet Assoc* **76**:113–115.

55 Sweeney CR, Freeman DE, Sweeney RW *et al.* (1993) Hemorrhage into the guttural pouch (auditory tube diverticulum) associated with rupture of the longus capitis muscle in three horses. *J Am Vet Med Assoc* **202**:1129–1131.

56 Knight AP (1977) Dysphagia resulting from unilateral rupture of the rectus capitis ventralis muscles in a horse. *J Am Vet Med Assoc* **170**:735–738.

57 Freeman DE (2003) Sinus disease. *Vet Clin N Am Equine Pract* **19**:209–243.

58 Howard RD, Stashak TS (1993) Reconstructive surgery of selected injuries of the head. *Vet Clin N Am Equine Pract* **9**:185–198.

59 Dowling BA, Dart AJ, Trope G (2001) Surgical repair of skull fractures in four horses using cuttable bone plates. *Aust Vet J* **79**:324–327.

60 Urquhart KA, Gerring EL, Shepherd MP (1981) Tracheobronchial foreign body in a pony. *Equine Vet J* **13**:262–264.

61 Brown CM, Collier MA (1983) Tracheobronchial foreign body in a horse. *J Am Vet Med Assoc* **182**:280–281.

62 Mair TS, Lane JG (1990) Tracheal obstructions in two horses and a donkey. *Vet Rec* **31**:303–304.

63 Mellins RB, Stalcup SA (1983) Pulmonary edema. In: *Disorders of the Respiratory Tract in Children*, 4th edn. (eds EL Kendig, V Chernick) WB Saunders, Philadelphia, pp. 458–475.

64 Kollias-Baker CA Pipers FS, Heard D *et al.* (1993) Pulmonary edema associated with transient airway obstruction in three horses. *J Am Vet Med Assoc* **202**:116–118.

65 Tute A, Wilkins PA, Gleed RD *et al.* (1996) Negative pressure pulmonary edema (NPE) as a post-anesthetic complication associated with upper airway obstruction in a horse. *Vet Surg* **25**:519–523.

66 Kaartinen MJ, Pang DS, Cuvelliez SG (2010) Post-anesthetic pulmonary edema in two horses. *Vet Anaesth Analg* **37**:136–143.

67 Wilkins PA, Otto CM, Dunkel B *et al.* (2007) Acute lung injury (ALI) and acute respiratory distress syndromes (ARDS) in veterinary medicine: consensus definitions. Special commentary. *J Vet Emerg Crit Care* **17**:333–339.

68 Dunkel B, Wilkins PA (2008) Acute respiratory distress syndrome. In: *Large Animal Internal Medicine*, 4th edn. (ed BP Smith) Mosby Inc, Philadelphia, pp. 536–538.

69 Wilkins PA (2008) Pulmonary edema. In: *Large Animal Internal Medicine*, 4th edn. (ed BP Smith) Mosby Inc, Philadelphia, pp. 554–555.

70 Tobin T, Roberts BL, Swerczek TW *et al.* (1978) The pharmacology of furosemide in the horse. III: Dose and time response relationships, effects of repeated dosing, and performance effects. *J Equine Med Surg* **2**:216–226.

71 Geor RJ, Ames TR (1991) Smoke inhalation injury in horses. *Compend Contin Educ Pract Vet* **13**:1162–1168.

72 Kirkland KD, Goetz TE, Foreman JH *et al.* (1992) Smoke inhalation injury in a pony. *J Vet Emerg Crit Care* **3**:83–89.

73 Kemper T, Spier S, Barratt-Boyes SM *et al.* (1993) Treatment of smoke inhalation in five horses. *J Am Vet Med Assoc* **202**:91–94.

74 Marsh PS (2007) Fire and smoke inhalation injury in horses. *Vet Clin N Am Equine Pract* **23**:19–30.

75 Murakami K, Tabor DL (2003) Pathophysiological basis of smoke inhalation injury. *News Physiol Sci* **18**:125–129.

76 Seltzer KL, Byars TD (1996) Prognosis for return to racing after recovery from infectious pleuropneumonia in Thoroughbred racehorses: 70 cases (1984–1989). *J Am Vet Med Assoc* **208**:1300–1301.

77 Racklyeft DJ, Raidal S, Love DN (2000) Towards an understanding of equine pleuropneumonia: factors relevant for control. *Aust Vet J* **78**:334–338.

78 Oikawa M, Takagi S, Anzai R *et al.* (1995) Pathology of equine respiratory disease occurring in association with transport. *J Comp Pathol* **113**:29–43.

79 Raidal SL, Love DN, Bailey GD (1995) Inflammation and increased numbers of bacteria in the lower respiratory tract of horses within 6 to 12 hours of confinement with the head elevated. *Aust Vet J* **72**:45–50.

80 Austin SM, Foreman JH, Hungerford LL (1995) Case-control study of risk factors for development of pleuropneumonia in horses. *J Am Vet Med Assoc* **207**:325–328.

81 Feige K, Schwarzwald C, Fürst A *et al.* (2000) Esophageal obstruction in horses: a retrospective study of 34 cases. *Can Vet J* **41**:207–210.

82 Scarratt WK, Moon ML, Sponenberg DP *et al.* (1998) Inappropriate administration of mineral oil resulting in lipoid pneumonia in three horses. *Equine Vet J* **30**:85–88.

83 Carr EA, Carlson GP, Wilson WD *et al.* (1997) Acute hemorrhagic pulmonary infarction and necrotizing pneumonia in horses: 21 cases (1967–1993). *J Am Vet Med Assoc* **210**:1774–1778.

84 Murray MJ, Del Piero F, Jeffrey SC *et al.* (1998) Neonatal equine herpesvirus type 1 infection on a Thoroughbred breeding farm. *J Vet Intern Med* **12**:36–41.

85 Peek SF, Landolt G, Karasin AI *et al.* (2004) Acute respiratory distress syndrome and fatal interstitial pneumonia associated with equine influenza in a neonatal foal. *J Vet Intern Med* **18**:132–134.

86 Vachon AM, Fischer AT (1998) Thoracoscopy in the horse: diagnostic and therapeutic indications in 28 cases. *Equine Vet J* **30**:467–475.

87 Freeman DE (1991) Standing surgery of the neck and thorax. *Vet Clin N Am Equine Pract* **7**:603–626.

88 Boy MG, Sweeney CR (2000) Pneumothorax in horses: 40 cases (1980–1997). *J Am Vet Med Assoc* **216**:1955–1959.

89 Perkins G, Ainsworth DM, Yeager A (1999) Hemothorax in 2 horses. *J Vet Intern Med* **13**:375–378.

90 Hance SR, Robertson JT (1992) Subcutaneous emphysema from an axillary wound that resulted in pneumomediastinum and bilateral pneumothorax in a horse. *J Am Vet Med Assoc* **200**:1107–1110.

91 Klein LV, Wilson DV (1989) An unusual cause of increasing airway pressure during anesthesia. *Vet Surg* **18**:239–241.

92 Spurlock SL, Spurlock GH, Donaldson LL (1988) Consolidating pneumonia and pneumothorax in a horse. *J Am Vet Med Assoc* **192**:1081–1082.

93 Lowe JE (1967) Pneumothorax in a horse from a puncture wound. A case report. *Cornell Vet* **57**:200–204.

94 Axon JA (2008) Thoracic trauma. In: *Large Animal Internal Medicine*, 4th edn. (ed BP Smith) Mosby Inc, Philadelphia, pp. 551–554.

95 Savage CJ, Traub-Dargatz JL, Mumford EL (1998) Survey of the large animal diplomates of the American College of Veterinary Internal Medicine regarding percutaneous lung biopsy in the horse. *J Vet Intern Med* **12**:456–464.

96 Peroni JF, Robinson NE, Stick JA *et al.* (2000) Pleuropulmonary and cardiovascular consequences of thoracoscopy performed in healthy standing horses. *Equine Vet J* **32**:280–286.

97 Rozenman J, Yellin A, Simansky DA *et al.* (1996) Re-expansion pulmonary oedema following spontaneous pneumothorax. *Resp Med* **90**:235–238.

98 Robinson NE (2000) International workshop on equine chronic airway disease, Michigan State University, June 16–18, 2000. *Equine Vet J* **33**:5–19.

99 Seahorn T, Beadle R (1993) Summer pasture-associated obstructive pulmonary disease in horses: 32 cases (1983–1991). *J Am Vet Med Assoc* **202**:779–782.

100 Ainsworth DM (2008) Recurrent airway obstruction. In: *Large Animal Internal Medicine*, 4th edn. (ed BP Smith) Mosby Inc, Philadelphia, pp. 556–563.

101 Williams KJ, Maes R, Del Piero F *et al.* (2007) Equine multinodular pulmonary fibrosis: a newly recognized herpesvirus-associated fibrotic lung disease. *Vet Pathol* **44**:849–862.

102 Wong DM, Belgrave RL, Williams KJ *et al.* (2008) Multinodular pulmonary fibrosis in five horses. *J Am Vet Med Assoc* **232**:898–905.

103 Niedermaier G, Poth T, Gehlen H (2010) Clinical aspects of multinodular pulmonary fibrosis in two warmblood horses. *Vet Rec* **166**:426–430.

104 Priester WA, McKay FW (1980) *The Occurrence of Tumors in Domestic Animals, Monograph 54*. National Cancer Institute, Washington DC, pp. 56–57.

105 Cotchin E, Baker-Smith J (1975) Tumours in horses encountered in an abattoir survey. *Vet Rec* **97**:339 (Correspondence).

106 Sweeney CR, Gillette DM (1989) Thoracic neoplasia in equids: 35 cases (1967–1987). *J Am Vet Med Assoc* **195**:374–377.

107 Scarratt WK, Crisman MV (1998) Neoplasia of the respiratory tract. *Vet Clin N Am Equine Pract* **14**:451–473.

108 Steinman A, Sutton G A, Lichawski D *et al.* (2002) Osteoma of paranasal sinuses in a horse with inspiratory dyspnoea. *Aust Vet J* **80**:140–142.

109 Henson FMD, Dixon K, Dobson JM (2004) Treatment of 4 cases of equine lymphoma with megavoltage radiation. *Equine Vet Educ* **16**:312–314.

110 Walker MA, Schumacher J, Schmitz DG *et al.* (1998) Cobalt 60 radiotherapy for treatment of squamous cell carcinoma of the nasal cavity and paranasal sinuses in three horses. *J Am Vet Med Assoc* **212**:848–851.

CHAPTER 4: CARDIOVASCULAR SYSTEM

1 Kraus MS, Jesty SA, Gelzer AR *et al.* (2010) Measurement of plasma cardiac troponin I concentration by use of a point-of-care analyzer in clinically normal horses and horses with experimentally induced cardiac disease. *Am J Vet Res* **71**:55–59.

2 Patteson M (1999) Electrophysiology and arrhythmogenesis. In: *Cardiology of the Horse*. (ed C Marr) WB Saunders, London, pp. 51–69.

3 Divers TJ (2003) Monitoring tissue oxygenation in the ICU patient. *Clin Tech Equine Pract* **2**:138–143.

4 Heidmann P, Tornquist SJ, Qu A *et al.* (2005) Laboratory measures of hemostasis and fibrinolysis after intravenous administration of epsilon-aminocaproic acid in clinically normal horses and ponies. *Am J Vet Res* **66**:313–318.

5 Ross J, Dallap BL, Dolente BA *et al.* (2007) Pharmacokinetics and pharmacodynamics of epsilon–aminocaproic acid in horses. *Am J Vet Res* **68**:1016–1021.

6 Sellon DC (2004) Disorders of the hematopoietic system. In: *Equine Internal Medicine.* (eds SM Reed, WM Bayly, DC Sellon) WB Saunders, St. Louis, pp. 721–768.

6a Martens RJ (1982) Pediatrics. In: *Equine Medicine and Surgery*, 3rd edn., Vol 1. (eds RA Mansmann, ES McAllister, PW Pratt) American Veterinary Publications, Santa Barbara, pp. 301–355.

7 Jesty SA, Reef V (2008) Cardiovascular system. In: *Equine Emergencies*. (eds JA Orsini, TJ Divers) Saunders Elsevier, St. Louis, pp. 60–100.

8 Hubbell JA, Muir WW, Gaynor JS (1993) Cardiovascular effects of thoracic compression in horses subjected to euthanasia. *Equine Vet J* **25**:282–284.

9 Frauenfelder HC, Fessler JF, Latshaw HS *et al.* (1981) External cardiovascular resuscitation of the anesthetized pony. *J Am Vet Med Assoc* **179**:673–676.

10 Sage A (2002) Cardiac disease in the geriatric horse. *Vet Clin N Am Equine Pract* **18**:575–589.

11 Davis JL, Gardner SY, Schwabenton B *et al.* (2002) Congestive heart failure in horses: 14 cases (1984–2001). *J Am Vet Med Assoc* **220**:1512–1515.

12 Sage AM, Valberg S, Hayden DW *et al.* (2006) Echocardiography in a horse with cor pulmonale from recurrent airway obstruction. *J Vet Int Med* **20**:694–696.

13 Marr C (2010) Heart failure. In: *Cardiology of the Horse*, 2nd edn. (eds C Marr, IM Bowen) Saunders Elsevier, Philadelphia, pp. 239–252.

14 Hall JE (2011) Role of the kidneys in long-term control of arterial pressure and in hypertension: the integrated system for arterial pressure regulation. In: *Textbook of Medical Physiology*, 12th edn. (ed JE Hall) Saunders Elsevier, Philadelphia, pp. 213–228.

15 Mann DL (2008) Pathophysiology of heart failure. In: *Braunwald's Heart Disease*, 8th edn. (eds P Libby, RO Bonow, DL Mann *et al.*) Saunders Elsevier, Philadelphia, pp. 541–560.

16 Elliott J, Bowen M (2010) Neuroendocrine control of cardiovascular function: physiology and pharmacology. In: *Cardiology of the Horse*, 2nd edn. (eds C Marr, IM Bowen) Saunders Elsevier, Philadelphia, pp. 21–33.

17 Reef VB, Bain FT, Spencer PA (1998) Severe mitral regurgitation in horses: clinical, echocardiographic and pathological findings. *Equine Vet J* **30**:18–27.

18 Marr C (2010) Cardiac murmurs: valvular regurgitation and insufficiency. In: *Cardiology of the Horse*, 2nd edn. (eds C Marr, IM Bowen) Saunders Elsevier, Philadelphia, pp. 207–216.

19 Bonagura JD, Reef V, Schwarzwald CC (2010) Cardiovascular diseases. In: *Equine Internal Medicine*, 3rd edn. (eds SM Reed, WM Bayly, DC Sellon) Saunders Elsevier, St. Louis, pp. 372–487.

20 Herndon WE, Kittleson MD, Sanderson K *et al.* (2002) Cardiac troponin I in feline hypertrophic cardiomyopathy. *J Vet Int Med* **16**:558–564.

21 Oyama MA, Sisson DD (2004) Cardiac troponin-I concentration in dogs with cardiac disease. *J Vet Int Med* **18**:831–839.

22 Sweeney RW, Reef VB, Reimer JM (1993) Pharmacokinetics of digoxin administered to horses with congestive heart failure. *Am J Vet Res* **54**:1108–1111.

23 Mogg T (1999) Equine cardiac disease: clinical pharmacology and therapeutics. *Vet Clin N Am Equine Pract* **15**:523–534.

24 Muir WW, McGuirk SM (1985) Pharmacology and pharmacokinetics of drugs used to treat cardiac disease in horses. *Vet Clin N Am Equine Pract* **1**:335–352.

25 Parraga ME, Kittleson MD, Drake CM (1995) Quinidine administration increases steady state serum digoxin concentration in horses. *Equine Vet J Suppl* **19**:114–119.

26 Gehlen H, Vieht JC, Stadler P (2003) Effects of the ACE inhibitor quinapril on echocardiographic variables in horses with mitral valve insufficiency. *J Vet Med Series A* **50**:460–465

27 Muir III WW, Sams RA, Hubbell JAE *et al.* (2001) Effects of enalaprilat on cardiorespiratory, hemodynamic, and hematologic variables in exercising horses. *Am J Vet Res* **62**:1008–1013.

28 Gardner SY, Atkins CE, Sams RA *et al.* (2004) Characterization of the pharmacokinetic and pharmacodynamic properties of the angiotensin-converting enzyme inhibitor, enalapril, in horses. *J Vet Int Med* **18**:231–237.

29 Sleeper MM, McDonnell SM, Ely JJ *et al.* (2008) Chronic oral therapy with enalapril in normal ponies. *J Vet Cardiol* **10**:111–115.

30 Sage A, Mogg T (2010) Pharmacology of drugs used to treat cardiac disease. In: *Cardiology of the Horse*, 2nd edn. (eds C Marr, IM Bowen) Saunders Elsevier, Philadelphia, pp. 75–87.

31 Muir WW, Milne DW, Skarda RT (1976) Acute hemodynamic effects of furosemide administered intravenously in the horse. *Am J Vet Res* **37**:1177–1180.

32 Freestone JF, Carlson GP, Harrold DR *et al.* (1988) Influence of furosemide treatment on fluid and electrolyte balance in horses. *Am J Vet Res* **49**:1899–1902.

33 Sage A (2010) Fever: endocarditis and pericarditis. In: *Cardiology of the Horse*, 2nd edn. (eds C Marr, IM Bowen) Saunders Elsevier, Philadelphia, pp. 217–225.

34 Maxson AD, Reef VB (1997) Bacterial endocarditis in horses: ten cases (1984–1995). *Equine Vet J* **29**:394–399.

35 Porter SR, Saegerman C, van Galen G *et al.* (2008) Vegetative endocarditis in equids (1994–2006). *J Vet Int Med* **22**:1411–1416.

36 Nilsfors L, Lombard CW, Weckner D *et al.* (1991) Diagnosis of pulmonary valve endocarditis in a horse. *Equine Vet J* **23**:479–482.

37 Buergelt CD, Cooley AJ, Hines SA *et al.* (1985) Endocarditis in six horses. *Vet Path*ol **22**:333–337.

38 Aalbaek B, Ostergaard S, Buhl R *et al.* (2007) *Actinobacillus equuli* subsp. *equuli* associated with equine valvular endocarditis. *Acta Path Micro Im* **115**:1437–1442.

39 Ewart S, Brown C, Derksen F *et al.* (1992) *Serratia marcescen*s endocarditis in a horse. *J Am Vet Med Assoc* **200**:961–963.

40 Travers CW, van den Berg JS (1995) *Pseudomona*s spp. associated vegetative endocarditis in two horses. *J S Afr Vet Assoc* **66**:172–176

41 Pace LW, Wirth NR, Foss RR *et al.* (1994) Endocarditis and pulmonary aspergillosis in a horse. *J Vet Diagn Invest* **6**:504 506.

42 Jesty SA, Reef VB (2006) Septicemia and cardiovascular infections in horses. *Vet Clin N Am Equine Pract* **22**:481–495.

43 Worth LT, Reef VB (1998) Pericarditis in horses: 18 cases (1986–1995). *J Am Vet Med Assoc* **212**:248–253.

44 Reef V, McGuirk SM (1996) Diseases of the cardiovascular system. In: *Large Animal Internal Medicine*, 2nd edn. (ed B Smith) Mosby, St Louis, pp. 507–549.

45 Seahorn JL, Slovis NM, Reimer JM *et al.* (2003) Case control study of factors associated with fibrinous pericarditis among horses in central Kentucky during spring 2001. *J Am Vet Med Assoc* **223**:832–838.

46 Vachon AM, Fischer AT (1998) Thoracoscopy in the horse: diagnostic and therapeutic indications in 28 cases. *Equine Vet J* **30**:467–475.

47 Machida N, Taniguchi T, Nakamura T *et al.* (1997) Cardio-histopathological observations on aborted equine fetuses infected with equid herpesvirus 1 (EHV 1). *J Comp Pathol* **116**:379–385.

48 Dolente BA, Seco OM, Lewis ML (2000) Streptococcal toxic shock in a horse. *J Am Vet Med Assoc* **217**:64–67, 30.

49 Cranley JJ, McCullagh KG (1981) Ischaemic myocardial fibrosis and aortic strongylosis in the horse. *Equine Vet J* **13**:35–42.

50 Peet RL, McDermott J, Williams JM *et al.* (1981) Fungal myocarditis and nephritis in a horse. *Aust Vet J* **57**:439–440.

51 Divers TJ, Kraus MS, Jesty SA *et al.* (2009) Clinical findings and serum cardiac troponin I concentrations in horses after intragastric administration of sodium monensin. *J Vet Diagn Invest* **21**:338–343.

52 Helman RG, Edwards WC (1997) Clinical features of blister beetle poisoning in equids: 70 cases (1983–1996). *J Am Vet Med Assoc* **211**:1018–1021.

53 Dickinson CE, Traub-Dargatz JL, Dargatz DA *et al.* (1996) Rattlesnake venom poisoning in horses: 32 cases (1973–1993). *J Am Vet Med Assoc* **208**:1866–1871.

54 Lawler JB, Frye MA, Bera MM *et al.* (2008) Third-degree atrioventricular block in a horse secondary to rattlesnake envenomation. *J Vet Int Med* **22**:486–490.

55 Reef VB (1985) Cardiovascular disease in the equine neonate. *Vet Clin N Am Equine Pract* **1**:117–129.

56 Southwood LL, Schott HC, 2nd, Henry CJ *et al.* (2000) Disseminated hemangiosarcoma in the horse: 35 cases. *J Vet Int Med* **14**:105–109.

57 Sugiyama A, Takeuchi T, Morita T *et al.* (2008) Mediastinal lymphoma with complete atrioventricular block in a horse. *J Vet Med Sci* **70**:1101–1105.

58 Slack JA, McGuirk SM, Erb HN *et al.* (2005) Biochemical markers of cardiac injury in normal, surviving septic, or nonsurviving septic neonatal foals. *J Vet Int Med* **19**:577–580.

59 Nostell K, Brojer J, Hoglund K *et al.* (2011) Cardiac troponin I and the occurrence of cardiac arrhythmias in horses with experimentally induced endotoxaemia. *Vet J* **192**:171–175.

60 Schwarzwald CC, Hardy J, Buccellato M (2003) High cardiac troponin I serum concentration in a horse with multiform ventricular tachycardia and myocardial necrosis. *J Vet Int Med* **17**:364–368.

61 Serra M, Papakonstantinou S, Adamcova M *et al.* (2010) Veterinary and toxicological applications for the detection of cardiac injury using cardiac troponin. *Vet J* **185**:50–57.

62 Holbrook TC, Birks EK, Sleeper MM *et al.* (2006) Endurance exercise is associated with increased plasma cardiac troponin I in horses. *Equine Vet J Suppl* **36**:27–31.

63 Nostell K, Haggstrom J (2008) Resting concentrations of cardiac troponin I in fit horses and effect of racing. *J Vet Cardiol* **10**:105–109.

64 Kraus MS, Kaufer BB, Damiani A *et al.* (2013) Elimination half–life of intravenously administered equine cardiac troponin I in healthy ponies. *Equine Vet J* **45**:56–59.

65 Kiryu K, Nakamura T, Kaneko M *et al.* (1987) Cardiopathology of sudden cardiac death in the race horse. *Heart Vessels Suppl* **2**:40–46.

66 Reef V, Marr C (2010) Dysrhythmias: assessment and medical management. In: *Cardiology of the Horse*, 2nd edn. (eds C Marr, IM Bowen) Saunders Elsevier, Philadelphia, pp. 159–178.

67 Reef VB, Reimer JM, Spencer PA (1995) Treatment of atrial fibrillation in horses: new perspectives. *J Vet Int Med* **9**:57–67.

68 Young L (2004) Diseases of the heart and vessels. In: *Equine Sports Medicine and Surgery*. (eds K Hinchcliff, A Kaneps, R Geor *et al.*) WB Saunders, Edinburgh, pp. 728–767.

69 Knottenbelt D (2006) *Equine Formulary*. WB Saunders, Edinburgh.

70 Morris DD, Fregin GF (1982) Atrial fibrillation in horses: factors associated with response to quinidine sulfate in 77 clinical cases. *Cornell Vet* **72**:339–349.

71 Muir WW, 3rd, McGuirk S (1987) Cardiovascular drugs. Their pharmacology and use in horses. *Vet Clin N Am Equine Pract* **3**:37–57.

72 De Clercq D, van Loon G, Baert K *et al.* (2006) Intravenous amiodarone treatment in horses with chronic atrial fibrillation. *Vet J* **172**:129–134.

73 De Clercq D, van Loon G, Baert K et al. (2007) Effects of an adapted intravenous amiodarone treatment protocol in horses with atrial fibrillation. *Equine Vet J* **39**:344–349.

74 McGurrin MK, Physick-Sheard PW, Kenney DG (2008) Transvenous electrical cardioversion of equine atrial fibrillation: patient factors and clinical results in 72 treatment episodes. *J Vet Int Med* **22**:609–615.

75 McGurrin MK, Physick-Sheard PW, Kenney DG (2005) How to perform transvenous electrical cardioversion in horses with atrial fibrillation. *J Vet Cardiol* **7**:109–119.

76 van Loon G, De Clercq D, Tavernier R et al. (2005) Transient complete atrioventricular block following transvenous electrical cardioversion of atrial fibrillation in a horse. *Vet J* **170**:124–127.

77 Cornick JL, Seahorn TL (1990) Cardiac arrhythmias identified in horses with duodenitis/proximal jejunitis: six cases (1985–1988). *J Am Vet Med Assoc* **197**:1054–1059.

78 Whitton DL, Trim CM (1985) Use of dopamine hydrochloride during general anesthesia in the treatment of advanced atrioventricular heart block in four foals. *J Am Vet Med Assoc* **187**:1357–1361.

79 Pibarot P, Vrins A, Salmon Y et al. (1993) Implantation of a programmable atrioventricular pacemaker in a donkey with complete atrioventricular block and syncope. *Equine Vet J* **25**:248–251.

80 van Loon G (2010) Dysrhythmias: cardiac pacing and electrical cardioversion. In: *Cardiology of the Horse*, 2nd edn. (eds C Marr, IM Bowen) Saunders Elsevier, Philadelphia, pp. 179–192.

81 Reimer JM, Reef VB, Sweeney RW (1992) Ventricular arrhythmias in horses: 21 cases (1984–1989). *J Am Vet Med Assoc* **201**:1237–1243.

82 Olgin JE, Zipes DP (2008) Specific arrhythmias: diagnosis and treatment. In: *Braunwald's Heart Disease*, 8th edn. (eds P Libby, RO, DL Mann et al.) Saunders Elsevier, Philadelphia, pp. 863–931.

83 Wijnberg ID, Ververs FF (2004) Phenytoin sodium as a treatment for ventricular dysrhythmia in horses. *J Vet Int Med* **18**:350–353.

84 Garber JL, Reef VB, Reimer JM et al. (1992) Postsurgical ventricular tachycardia in a horse. *J Am Vet Med Assoc* **201**:1038–1039.

85 Leroux AJ, Schott HC, 2nd, Hines MT (1995) Ventricular tachycardia associated with exhaustive exercise in a horse. *J Am Vet Med Assoc* **207**:335–337.

86 MacLeay JM, Wilson JH (1998) Type-II renal tubular acidosis and ventricular tachycardia in a horse. *J Am Vet Med Assoc* **212**:1597–1599.

87 Traub-Dargatz JL, Schlipf JW, Boon J et al. (1994) Ventricular tachycardia and myocardial dysfunction in a horse. *J Am Vet Med Assoc* **205**:1569–1573.

88 Gonzalez ER (1993) Pharmacologic controversies in CPR. *Ann Emerg Med* **22**:317–323.

89 De Clercq D, van Loon G, Baert K et al. (2007) Treatment with amiodarone of refractory ventricular tachycardia in a horse. *J Vet Int Med* **21**:78–880.

90 Kiryu K, Machida N, Kashida Y et al. (1999) Pathologic and electrocardiographic findings in sudden cardiac death in racehorses. *J Vet Med Sci* **61**:921–928.

91 Gaynor JS, Bednarski RM, Muir WW 3rd (1993) Effect of hypercapnia on the arrhythmogenic dose of epinephrine in horses anesthetized with guaifenesin, thiamylal sodium, and halothane. *Am J Vet Res* **54**:315–321.

92 Robertson SA, Malark JA, Steele CJ et al. (1996) Metabolic, hormonal, and hemodynamic changes during dopamine infusions in halothane anesthetized horses. *Vet Surg* **25**:88–97.

93 Steffey EP, Kelly AB, Farver TB et al. (1985) Cardiovascular and respiratory effects of acetylpromazine and xylazine on halothane–anesthetized horses. *J Vet Pharmacol Ther* **8**:290–302.

94 Hubbell JA, Muir WW, Gaynor JS (1993) Cardiovascular effects of thoracic compression in horses subjected to euthanasia. *Equine Vet J* **25**:282–284.

95 Kellagher RE, Watney GC (1986) Cardiac arrest during anaesthesia in two horses. *Vet Rec* **119**:347–349.

96 McGoldrick TM, Bowen IM, Clarke KW (1998) Sudden cardiac arrest in an anaesthetised horse associated with low venous oxygen tensions. *Vet Rec* **142**:610–611.

97 Robertson SA (2010) Cardiovascular emergencies associated with anesthesia. In: *Cardiology of the Horse*, 2nd edn. (eds C Marr, IM Bowen) Saunders Elsevier, Philadelphia, pp. 253–266.

98 Hall TL, Magdesian KG, Kittleson MD (2010) Congenital cardiac defects in neonatal foals: 18 cases (1992–2007). *J Vet Int Med* **24**:206–212.

99 Waguespack R, Belknap J, Williams A (2001) Laparoscopic management of postcastration haemorrhage in a horse. *Equine Vet J* **33**:510–513.

100 Trumble TN, Ingle-Fehr J, Hendrickson DA (2000) Laparoscopic intra-abdominal ligation of the testicular artery following castration in a horse. *J Am Vet Med Assoc* **216**:1596–1598, 1569.

101 Auer J (2006) Surgical techniques. In: *Equine Surgery*, 3rd ed. (eds JA Auer, JA Stick) WB Saunders, St Louis, pp. 151–161

102 Erne JB, Mann FA (2003) Surgical hemostasis. *Comp Contin Educ Pract Vet* **25**:732–740.

103 Ludwig A, Gatineau S, Reynaud MC et al. (2005) Fungal isolation and identification in 21 cases of guttural pouch mycosis in horses (1998–2002). *Vet J* **169**:457–461.

104 Sweeney CR, Freeman DE, Sweeney RW et al. (1993) Hemorrhage into the guttural pouch (auditory tube diverticulum) associated with rupture of the longus capitis muscle in three horses. *J Am Vet Med Assoc* **202**:1129–1131.

105 Woodie JB, Ducharme NG, Gleed RD et al. (2002) In horses with guttural pouch mycosis or after stylohyoid bone resection, what arterial ligation(s) could be effective in emergency treatment of a hemorrhagic crisis. *Vet Surg* **31**:498–499.

106 Caron JP, Fretz PB, Bailey JV et al. (1987) Balloon-tipped catheter arterial occlusion for prevention of hemorrhage caused by guttural pouch mycosis: 13 cases (1982–1985). *J Am Vet Med Assoc* **191**:345–349.

107 Freeman DE, Ross MW, Donawick WJ et al. (1989) Occlusion of the external carotid and maxillary arteries in the horse to prevent hemorrhage from guttural pouch mycosis. *Vet Surg* **18**:39–47.

108 Cheramie HS, Pleasant RS, Robertson JL *et al.* (1999) Evaluation of a technique to occlude the internal carotid artery of horses. *Vet Surg* **28**:83–90.

109 Leveille R, Hardy J, Robertson JT *et al.* (2000) Transarterial coil embolization of the internal and external carotid and maxillary arteries for prevention of hemorrhage from guttural pouch mycosis in horses. *Vet Surg* **29**:389–397.

110 Bacon Miller C, Wilson DA, Martin DD *et al.* (1998) Complications of balloon catheterization associated with aberrant cerebral arterial anatomy in a horse with guttural pouch mycosis. *Vet Surg* **27**:450–453.

111 Freeman DE, Staller GS, Maxson AD *et al.* (1993) Unusual internal carotid artery branching that prevented arterial occlusion with a balloon-tipped catheter in a horse. *Vet Surg* **22**:531–534.

112 Lepage OM, Piccot-Crezollet C (2005) Transarterial coil embolisation in 31 horses (1999–2002) with guttural pouch mycosis: a 2-year follow-up. *Equine Vet J* **37**:430–434.

113 Dolente BA, Sullivan EK, Boston R *et al.* (2005) Mares admitted to a referral hospital for postpartum emergencies: 163 cases (1992–2002). *J Vet Emerg Crit Care* **15**:193–200.

114 Arnold CE, Payne M, Thompson JA *et al.* (2008) Periparturient hemorrhage in mares: 73 cases (1998–2005). *J Am Vet Med Assoc* **232**:1345–51.

115 Ueno T, Nambo Y, Tajima Y *et al.* (2010) Pathology of lethal peripartum broad ligament haematoma in 31 Thoroughbred mares. *Equine Vet J* **42**:529–533.

116 Stowe HD (1968) Effects of age and impending parturition upon serum copper of Thoroughbred mares. *J Nutr* **95**:179–183.

117 Taylor EL, Sellon DC, Wardrop KJ *et al.* (2000) Effects of intravenous administration of formaldehyde on platelet and coagulation variables in healthy horses. *Am J Vet Res* **61**:1191–1196.

118 Weld JM, Kamerling SG, Combie JD *et al.* (1984) The effects of naloxone on endotoxic and hemorrhagic shock in horses. *Res Commun Chem Pathol Pharmacol* **44**:227–238.

119 Marr CM, Reef VB, Brazil TJ *et al.* (1998) Aorto-cardiac fistulas in seven horses. *Vet Radiol Ultrasound* **39**:22–31.

120 Rooney JR, Prickett ME, Crowe MW (1967) Aortic ring rupture in stallions. *Vet Pathol* **4**:268–274.

121 Roby KW, Reef VB, Shaw DP *et al.* (1986) Rupture of an aortic sinus aneurysm in a 15-year old broodmare. *J Am Vet Med Assoc* **189**:305–308.

122 Sleeper MM, Durando MM, Miller M *et al.* (2001) Aortic root disease in four horses. *J Am Vet Med Assoc* **219**:491–496.

123 Bonagura JD, Reef VB (2004) Disorders of the cardiovascular system. In: *Equine Internal Medicine.* (eds SM Reed, WM, DC Sellon) WB Saunders, Philadelphia, pp. 355–459

124 Ploeg M, Saey V, de Bruijn CM *et al.* (2013) Aortic rupture and aortopulmonary fistulation in the Friesian horse: characterisation of the clinical and gross post mortem findings in 24 cases. *Equine Vet J* **45**:101–106.

125 Marino PL (2006) *The ICU Book,* 3rd edn. Lippincott, Williams, and Wilkins, Philadelphia.

126 Ettlinger JJ, Palmer JE, Benson C (1992) Bacteria found on intravenous catheters removed from horses. *Vet Rec* **130**:248–249.

127 Dolente BA, Beech J, Lindborg S *et al.* (2005) Evaluation of risk factors for development of catheter-associated jugular thrombophlebitis in horses: 50 cases (1993–1998). *J Am Vet Med Assoc* **227**:1134–1141.

128 Gardner SY, Reef VB, Spencer PA (1991) Ultrasonographic evaluation of horses with thrombophlebitis of the jugular vein: 46 cases (1985–1988). *J Am Vet Med Assoc* **199**:370–373.

129 Cotovio M, Monreal L, Navarro M *et al.* (2007) Detection of fibrin deposits in tissues from horses with severe gastrointestinal disorders. *J Vet Int Med* **21**:308–313.

130 Duncan SG, Meyers KM, Reed SM *et al.* (1985) Alterations in coagulation and hemograms of horses given endotoxins for 24 hours via hepatic portal infusions. *Am J Vet Res* **46**:1287–1293.

131 Dallap BL, Boston R (2003) Coagulation profiles in 27 horses with large colon volvulus. *J Vet Emerg Crit Care* **13**:215–225.

132 Dolente BA, Wilkins PA, Boston RC (2002) Clinicopathologic evidence of disseminated intravascular coagulation in horses with acute colitis. *J Am Vet Med Assoc* **220**:1034–1038.

133 Saville WJ, Hinchcliff KW, Moore BR *et al.* (1996) Necrotizing enterocolitis in horses: a retrospective study. *J Vet Int Med* **10**:265–270.

134 Brianceau P, Divers TJ (2001) Acute thrombosis of limb arteries in horses with sepsis: five cases (1988–1998). *Equine Vet J* **33**:105–109.

135 Feige K, Schwarzwald CC, Bombeli T (2003) Comparison of unfractioned and low molecular weight heparin for prophylaxis of coagulopathies in 52 horses with colic: a randomised double-blind clinical trial. *Equine Vet J* **35**:506–513.

CHAPTER 5: UROGENITAL SYSTEM

1 Byron CR, Embertson RM, Bernhard WV *et al.* (2002) Dystocia in a referral hospital setting: approach and results. *Equine Vet J* **35**:82–85.

2 McCue PM, Ferris RA (2012) Parturition, dystocia and foal survival: a retrospective study of 1047 births. *Equine Vet J* **44(Suppl 41)**:22–25.

3 Christensen BW (2011) Parturition. In: *Equine Reproduction,* 2nd edn. (eds AO McKinnon, EL Squires, WE Vaala *et al.*) Wiley-Blackwell, Ames, pp. 2268–2276.

4   Embertson RM (1999) Dystocia and caesarean sections: the importance of duration and good judgement. *Equine Vet J* **31**:179–180.

5   Norton JL, Dallap BL, Johnston JK *et al.* (2007) Retrospective study of dystocia in mares at a referral hospital. *Equine Vet J* **39**:37–41.

6   Abernathy-Young KK, LeBlanc MM *et al.* (2012) Survival rates of mares and foals and postoperative complications and fertility of mares after cesarean section: 95 cases (1986–2000). *J Am Vet Med Assoc* **241**:927–934.

7   Frazer G (2011) Dystocia management. In: *Equine Reproduction*, 2nd edn. (eds AO McKinnon, EL Squires, WE Vaala *et al.*) Wiley-Blackwell, Ames, pp. 2479–2496.

8   Embertson RM (2006) Ovaries and uterus. In: *Equine Surgery*, 3rd edn. (eds JA Auer, JA Stick) Saunders-Elsevier, St Louis, pp. 855–864.

9   Carluccio A, Contri A, Torsi U *et al.* (2007) Survival rate and short-term fertility rate associated with the use of fetotomy for resolution of dystocia in mares: 72 cases (1991–2005). *J Am Vet Med Assoc* **230**: 1502–1505.

10 Nimmo MR, Slone DE, Hughes FE *et al.* (2007) Fertility and complications after fetotomy in 20 brood mares. *Vet Surg* **36**:771–774.

11 Dolente BA (2004) Critical peripartum disease in the mare. *Vet Clin N Am Equine Pract* **20**:151–165.

12 Otero RM, Nguyen HB, Huang DT *et al.* (2006) Early goal-directed therapy in severe sepsis and septic shock revisited: concepts, controversies, and contemporary findings. *Chest* **130**:1579–1595.

13 Dolente BA, Sullivan EK, Boston R *et al.* (2005) Mares admitted to a referral hospital for postpartum emergencies: 163 cases. *J Vet Emerg Crit Care* **15**:193–200.

14 Threlfall WR (2011) Retained fetal membranes. In: *Equine Reproduction*, 2nd edn. (eds AO McKinnon, EL Squires, WE Vaala) Wiley-Blackwell, Ames, pp. 2521–2529.

15 Perkins NR, Robertson JT, Colon LA (1992) Uterine torsion and uterine tear in a mare. *J Am Vet Med Assoc* **1**:92–94.

16 Honnas CM, Spensley MS, Laverty S *et al.* (198) Hydramnios causing uterine rupture in a mare. *J Am Vet Med Assoc* **193**:334–336.

17 Javsicas LH, Giguere S, Freeman DE *et al.* (2010) Comparison of surgical and medical treatment of 49 postpartum mares with presumptive or confirmed uterine tears. *Vet Surg* **39**:254–260.

18 Mogg TD, Hart J, Wearn J (2006) Postpartum hemoperitoneum and septic peritonitis in a Thoroughbred mare. *Vet Clin N Am Equine Pract* **22**:61–71.

19 Sutter WW, Hopper S, Embertson RM *et al.* (2003) Diagnosis and surgical treatment of uterine lacerations in mares (33 cases). *Proc 49th Ann Conv Am Assoc Equine Practnrs*, New Orleans, pp. 357–359.

20 Hassel DM, Ragle CA (1994) Laparoscopic diagnosis and covservative treatment of uterine tear in a mare. *J Am Vet Med Assoc* **205**:1531–1533.

21 Frazer GS, Embertson RM, Perkins NR (2002) Complications of late gestation in the mare. *Equine Vet Educ* **5**:16–21.

22 Chaney KP, Holcomve SJ, LeBlanc MM *et al.* (2007) The effect of uterine torsion on mare and foal survival: a retrospective study, 1985–2005. *Equine Vet J* **39**:33–36.

23 Pascoe JR, Meagher DM, Wheat JD (1981) Surgical management of uterine torsion in the mare. *J Am Vet Med Assoc* **179**:351–354.

24 Jung C, Hospes R, Bostedt H *et al.* (2008) Surgical treatment of uterine torsion using a ventral midline laparotomy in 19 mares. *Aust Vet J* **86**:272–276.

25 Frazer GS (2003) Postpartum complications in the mare. Part 2: Fetal membrane retention and conditions of the gastrointestinal tract, bladder, and vagina. *Equine Vet Educ* **15**:91–100.

26 Tulleners EP, Richardson DW, Reid BW (1985) Vaginal evisceration of the small intestine in three mares. *J Am Vet Med Assoc* **186**:385–387.

27 Gomez JH, Rodgerson DH (2008) How to repair cranial vaginal and caudal uterine tears in mares. *Proc 54th Ann Conv Am Assoc Equine Practnrs* **54**:295–297.

28 Perkins NR, Frazer GS (1994) Reproductive emergencies in the mare. *Vet Clin N Am Equine Pract* **10**:643–670.

29 Lillich JF, Fischer AT, DeBowes RM (2006) Bladder. In: *Equine Surgery*, 3rd edn. (eds JA Auer, JA Stick) Saunders-Elsevier, St Louis, pp. 877–887.

30 Rodgerson DH, Spirito MA, Thorpe PE *et al.* (1999) Standing surgical repair of cystorrhexis in two mares. *Vet Surg* **28**:113–116.

31 Ross J, Palmer JE, Wilkins PA (2008) Body wall tears during late pregnancy in mares: 13 cases (1995–2006). *J Am Vet Med Assoc* **232**:257–261.

32 Wilson JF, Quist CF (1992) Professional liability in equine surgery. In: *Equine Surgery*, 2nd edn. (eds JA Auer, JA Stick) Saunders-Elsevier, St Louis, pp.13–35.

33 May KA, Moll DH (2002) Recognition and management of equine castration complications. *Comp Contin Educ Pract Vet* **24**:150–162.

34 Moll HD, Pelzer KD, Pleasant RS *et al.* (1995) A survey of equine castration complications. *J Equine Vet Sci* **15**:522–526.

35 Shoemaker R, Bailey J, Janzen E *et al.* (2004) Routine castration in 568 draught colts: incidence of evisceration and omental herniation. *Equine Vet J* **36**:336–340.

36 Schumacher J (2006) Testis: postoperative complications of testicular surgery. In: *Equine Surgery*, 3rd edn. (eds JA Auer, JA Stick) Saunders-Elsevier, St Louis, pp. 775–810.

37 Trumble TN, Ingle-Fehr J, Hendrickson DA (2000) Laparoscopic intraabdominal ligation of the testicular artery following castration in a horse. *J Am Vet Med Assoc* **216**:1596–1598, 1569.

38 Feary DJ, Moffett PD, Bruemmer JE *et al.* (2005) Chemical ejaculation and cryopreservation of semen from a breeding stallion with paraphimosis secondary to priapism and haemorrhagic colitis. *Equine Vet Educ* **17**:299–304.

39 Driessen B, Zarucco L, Kalir D *et al.* (2011) Contemporary use of acepromazine in the anaesthetic management of male horses and ponies: a retrospective study and opinion poll. *Equine Vet J* **43**:88–98.

40 Threlfell WR, Carleton CL, Robertson J *et al.* (1990) Recurrent torsion of the spermatic cord and scrotal testis in a stallion. *J Am Vet Med Assoc* **196:**1641–1643.

41 Perkins NR, Frazer GS (1994) Reproductive emergencies in the stallion. *Vet Clin N Am Equine Pract* **10:**671–683.

42 Laverty S, Pascoe JR, Ling GV *et al.* (1992) Urolithiasis in 68 horses. *Vet Surg* **21:**56–62.

43 Neumann RD, Ruby AL, Ling GV *et al.* (1994) Ultrastructure and mineral composition of urinary calculi from horses. *Am J Vet Res* **55:**1357–1367.

44 Sertich PL, Pozor MA, Meyers SA *et al.* (1998) Medical management of urinary calculi in a stallion with breeding dysfunction. *J Am Vet Med Assoc* **213:**843–846.

45 Röcken M, Stehle C, Mosel G *et al.* (2006) Laparoscopic-assisted cystotomy for urolith removal in geldings. *Vet Surg* **35:**394–397.

46 Lillich JD, Fischer AT, Debower RM (2006) Kidneys and ureters. In: *Equine Surgery*, 3rd edn. (eds JA Auer, JA Stick) Saunders-Elsevier, St Louis, pp. 870–877.

47 Bayly WM (2004) Acute renal failure. In: *Equine Internal Medicine*, 2nd edn. (eds SM Reed, WM Bayly, DC Sellon) Saunders, St. Louis, pp. 1221–1230.

48 Divers TJ, Whitlock RH (1987) Acute renal failure in six horses resulting from haemodynamic causes. *Equine Vet J* **19:**178–184.

49 Bartol JM, Divers TJ, Perkins GA (2000) Nephrotoxicant-induced acute renal failure in five horses. *Comp Contin Educ Pract Vet* **22:**870–876.

50 Divers TJ, Timoney JF, Lewis RM *et al.* (1992) Equine glomerulonephritis and renal failure associated with complexes of Group-C streptococcal antigen and IgG antibody. *Vet Immunol Immunopathol* **32:**93–102.

51 van den Ingh TS, Hartman EG, Bercovich Z (1989) Clinical *Leptospira interrogans* serogroup *Australis* serovar *lora* infection in a stud farm in The Netherlands. *Vet Quart* **11:**175–82.

52 Grossman BS, Brobst DF, Kramer JW *et al.* (1982) Urinary indices for differentiation of prerenal azotemia and renal azotemia in horses. *J Am Vet Med Assoc* **180:**284–288.

53 Tyner GA, Nolen-Walston RD, Hall T *et al.* (2011) A multicenter retrospective study of 151 renal biopsies in horses. *J Vet Intern Med* **25:**532–539.

CHAPTER 6: SKIN

1 Stashak TS (1991) Principles of wound management and selction of approaches to wound closure. In: *Equine Wound Management*. (ed TS Stashak) Lea & Febiger, Baltimore, pp. 36–50.

2 Stashak TS (1991) Wound management and reconstructive surgery of problems associated with the distal limbs. In: *Equine Wound Management*. (ed TS Stashak) Lea & Febiger, Baltimore, pp. 163–217.

3 Knottenbelt DC (2002) Basic wound management. In: *Handbook of Equine Wound Management*. (ed DC Knottenbelt) WB Saunders, Philadelphia, pp. 39–77.

4 Hendrickson DA (2006) Management of superficial wounds. In: *Equine Surgery*, 3rd edn. (eds JA Auer, JA Stick) Saunders, St. Louis, pp. 288–298.

5 Stashak TS (1991) Management of wounds associated with tendons, paratendons, and tendon sheaths. In: *Equine Wound Management*. (ed TS Stashak) Lea & Febiger, Baltimore, pp. 238–257.

6 Knottenbelt DC (2002) Complicated wounds. In: *Handbook of Equine Wound Management*. (ed DC Knottenbelt) WB Saunders, Philadelphia, pp. 95–126.

7 Jann H, Pasquini C (2005) Wounds of the distal limb complicated by involvement of deep structures. *Vet Clin N Am Equine Pract* **21:**145–165.

8 Hendrickson DA (2006) Management of deep and chronic wounds. In: *Equine Surgery*, 3rd edn. (eds JA Auer, JA Stick) Saunders, St. Louis, PP. 299–305.

9 Stashak TS (1991) Wounds of the body. In: *Equine Wound Management*. (ed TS Stashak) Lea & Febiger, Baltimore, pp. 145–162.

10 Barber SM (2005) Management of neck and head injuries. *Vet Clin N Am Equine Pract* **21:**191–215.

11 Stashak TS (1991) Wound management and reconstructive surgery of the head region. In: *Equine Wound Management*. (ed TS Stashak) Lea & Febiger, Baltimore, pp. 89–144.

12 Adam EN, Southwood LL (2006) Wound infection, cellulitis, and myositis. *Vet Clin N Am Equine Pract* **22:**335–361.

13 Adam EN, Southwood LL (2007) Primary and secondary limb cellulitis in horses: 44 cases. *J Am Vet Med Assoc* **231:**1696–1703.

14 Baxter GM (1999) Management of burns. In: *Equine Medicine and Surgery*, 5th edn. (eds PT Colahan, IG Mayhew, AM Merritt *et al.*) American Veterinary Publications, Goleta, pp. 1843–1847.

15 Hanson RR (2005) Management of burn injuries in the horse. *Vet Clin N Am Equine Pract* **21:**105–123.

16 Knottenbelt DC (2003) Management of burn injuries. In: *Current Therapy in Equine Medicine* 5. (ed NE Robinson) WB Saunders, Philadelphia, pp. 220–225.

17 Fox SM, Cooper RC, Gillis JP *et al.* (1988) Management of a large thermal burn in a horse. *Comp Contin Educ Pract Vet* **10:**88–95.

18 Gieser DR, Walker RD (1984) Management of thermal injuies in large animals. *Vet Clin N Am Large Anim Pract* **6**:91–105.

19 Gieser DR, Walker RD (1985) Management of large animal thermal injuries. *Comp Contin Educ Pract Vet* **7**:S69–S78.

20 Stashak TS (1991) Principles of free skin grafting. In: *Equine Wound Management*. (ed TS Stashak) Lea & Febiger, Baltimore, pp. 218–237.

21 Rees CA (2010) Disorders of the skin. In: *Equine Internal Medicine*, 3rd edn. (eds SM Reed, WM Bayly, DC Sellon) Saunders Elsevier, St. Louis, pp. 682–729.

22 Knight AP, Walter RG (2001) *A Guide to Plant Poisoning of Animals in North America*. Teton New Media, Jackson.

23 Rowe LD (1989) Photosensitization problems in livestock. *Vet Clin N Am Food Animal Pract* **5**:301–323.

24 Burrows GE, Tyrl RJ (2001) *Toxic Plants of North America*, 1st edn. Iowa State University Press, Ames.

25 Rees CA (2004) Disorders of the skin. In: *Equine Internal Medicine*, 2nd edn. (eds SM Reed, WM Bayly, DC Sellon) Saunders Elsevier, St. Louis, pp. 667–720.

26 Wolkenstein P, Revuz J (2000) Toxic epidermal necrolysis. *Dermatol Clin* **18**:485–495.

27 Harr T, French LE (2010) Toxic epidermal necrolysis and Stevens-Johnson syndrome. *Orphanet J Rare Dis* **5**:39–50.

28 Pereira FA, Mudgil AV, Rosmarin DM (2007) Toxic epidermal necrolysis. *J Am Acad Dermatol* **56**:181–199.

29 Rajaratnam R, Mann C, Balasubramaniam P *et al.* (2010) Toxic epidermal necrolysis: retrospective analysis of 21 consecutive cases managed at a tertiary centre. *Clin Exp Dermatol* **35**:853–862.

CHAPTER 7: NEUROLOGY

1 DeLahunta A (1978) Diagnosis of equine neurologic problems. *Cornell Vet* **68**:122–132.

2 Adams R, Mayhew IG (1985) Neurologic diseases. *Vet Clin N Am Equine Pract* **1**:209–234.

3 Blythe LL (1987) Neurologic examination of the horse. *Vet Clin N Am Equine Pract* **3**:255–281.

4 Mayhew IG (1988) Neurological and neuropathological observations on the equine neonate. *Equine Vet J Suppl* **5**:28–33.

5 Reed S (1992) The neurologic examination of the horse for purchase. *Vet Clin N Am Equine Pract* **8**:377–386.

6 McCue M, Davis EG, Rush BR (2004) Diagnostic evaluation, clinical management and transport of recumbent horses. *Comp Contin Educ Pract Vet* **26**:138–148.

7 MacKay RJ (2005) Neurologic disorders of neonatal foals. *Vet Clin N Am Equine Pract* **21**:387–406.

8 Cohen ND (1993) Neurologic evaluation of the equine head and neurogenic dysphagia. *Vet Clin N Am Equine Pract* **9**:199–212.

9 Mayhew IG (1975) Collection of cerebrospinal fluid from the horse. *Cornell Vet* **65**:500–511.

10 Jackson C, deLahunta A, Divers TJ *et al.* (1996) The diagnostic utility of measurements of cerebrospinal fluid creatine kinase activity in the horse. *J Vet Intern Med* **10**:246–251.

11 Miller MM, Sweeney CR, Russell GE *et al.* (1999) Effects of blood contamination of cerebrospinal fluid on western blot analysis for detection of antibodies against *Sarcocystis neurona* and on albumin quotient and immunoglobulin G index in horses. *J Am Vet Med Assoc* **215**:67–71.

12 Finno CJ, Packham AE, Wilson DW *et al.* (2007) Effects of blood contamination of cerebrospinal fluid on results of indirect fluorescent antibody tests for detection of antibodies against *Sarcocystis neurona* and *Neospora hughesi*. *J Vet Diagn Invest* **19**:286–289.

13 Aleman M, Borchers A, Kass PH *et al.* (2007) Ultrasound-assisted collection of cerebrospinal fluid from the lumbosacral space in equids. *J Am Vet Med Assoc* **230**:378–84.

14 Gollob E, Edinger H, Stanek C *et al.* (2002) Ultrasonographic investigation of the atlanto-occipital articulation in the horse. *Equine Vet J* **34**:44–50.

15 Audigié F, Tapprest J, Didierlaurent D *et al.* (2004) Ultrasound-guided atlanto-occipital puncture for myelography in the horse. *Vet Radiol Ultrasound* **4**:340–344.

16 Sweeney CR, Russell GE (2000) Differences in total protein concentration, nucleated cell count, and red blood cell count among sequential samples of cerebrospinal fluid from horses. *J Am Vet Med Assoc* **217**:54–57.

17 Wamsley HL, Alleman AR, Porter MB *et al.* (2002) Findings in cerebrospinal fluids of horses infected with West Nile virus: 30 cases (2001). *J Am Vet Med Assoc* **221**:1303–1305.

18 Furr M (2007) Humoral immune responses in the horse after intrathecal challenge with ovalbumin. *J Vet Intern Med* **21**:806–811.

19 Wilson WD (1997) Equine herpesvirus 1 myeloencephalopathy. *Vet Clin N Am Equine Pract* **13**:53–72.

20 Henninger RW, Reed SM, Saville WJ *et al.* (2007) Outbreak of neurologic disease caused by equine herpesvirus-1 at a university equestrian center. *J Vet Intern Med* **21**:157–165.

21 Allen GP (2007) Development of a real-time polymerase chain reaction assay for rapid diagnosis of neuropathogenic strains of equine herpesvirus-1. *J Vet Diagn Invest* **19**:69–72.

22 Pelligrini-Massini A, Livesay LC (2006) Meningitis and encephalitis in horses. *Vet Clin N Am Equine Pract* **22**:553–589.

23 Bentz BG, Maxwell LK, Erkert RS *et al.* (2006) Pharmacokinetics of acyclovir after single intravenous and oral administration to adult horses. *J Vet Intern Med* **20**:589–594.

24 Wilkins PA, Papich M, Sweeney RW (2005) Acyclovir pharmacokinetics in adult horses. *J Vet Emerg Crit Care* **15**:174–178.

25 Snook CS, Hyman SS, Del Piero F *et al.* (2001) West Nile virus encephalomyelitis in eight horses. *J Am Vet Med Assoc* **218**:1576–1579.

26 Ostlund EN, Crom RL, Pedersen DD *et al.* (2001) Equine West Nile encephalitis, United States. *Emerg Infect Dis* **7**:665–669.

27 Wilkins PA, Del Piero F (2004) West Nile virus: lessons from the 21st century. *J Vet Emerg Crit Care* **14**:2–14

28 Long MT, Jeter W, Hernandez J *et al.* (2006) Diagnostic performance of the equine IgM capture ELISA for sero-diagnosis of West Nile virus infection, *J Vet Intern Med* **20**:608–13.

29 Long MT, Gibbs EP, Mellencamp MW *et al.* (2007) Efficacy, duration, and onset of immunogenicity of a West Nile virus vaccine, live Flavivirus chimera, in horses with a clinical disease challenge model. *Equine Vet J* **39**:491–497.

30 Tanner JM, Traub-Dargatz JL, Hill AE *et al.* (2006) Evaluation of factors associated with positive IgM capture ELISA results in equids with clinical signs compatible with West Nile virus infection: 1,017 cases (2003). *J Am Vet Med Assoc* **228**:414–21.

31 Smith JJ, Provost PJ, Paradis MR (2004) Bacterial meningitis and brain abscesses secondary to infectious disease processes involving the head in horses: seven cases (1980–2001). *J Am Vet Med Assoc* **224**:739–742.

32 Dowling PM (1999) Clinical pharmacology of nervous system diseases. *Vet Clin N Am Equine Pract* **15**:575–588.

33 Wilkins PA, Del Piero F (2007) Rabies. In: *Equine Infectious Diseases.* (eds D Sellon, M Long) Elsevier Saunders, Philadelphia, pp. 185–190.

34 Dubey JP, Lindsay DS, Saville WJ *et al.* (2001) A review of *Sarcocystis neuron*a and equine protozoal myeloencephalitis (EPM). *Vet Parasitol* **95**:89–131.

35 MacKay RJ, Granstrom DE, Saville WJ *et al.* (2000) Equine protozoal myeloencephalitis. *Vet Clin N Am Equine Pract* **16**:405–425.

36 Saville WJ, Sofaly CD, Reed SM *et al.* (2004) An equine protozoal myeloen-cephalitis challenge model testing a second transport after inoculation with *Sarcocystis neurona* sporocysts. *J Parasitol* **90**:1406–1410.

37 Furr M, MacKay R, Granstrom D *et al.* (2002) Clinical diagnosis of equine protozoal myeloencephalitis (EPM). *J Vet Intern Med* **16**:618–621.

38 MacKay RJ (2004) Brain injury after head trauma: pathophysiology, diagnosis, and treatment. *Vet Clin N Am Equine Pract* **20**:199–221.

39 Barber SM (2005) Management of neck and head injuries. *Vet Clin N Am Equine Pract* **21**:191–215.

40 Feary DJ, Magdesian KG, Aleman MA *et al.* (2007) Traumatic brain injury in horses: 34 cases (1194–2004). *J Am Vet Med Assoc* **231**:259–266.

41 Hardy J, Leveile R (2003) Diseases of the guttural pouches. *Vet Clin N Am Equine Pract* **19**:123–158.

42 Walker AM, Sellon DC, Cornelisse CJ *et al.* (2002) Temporohyoid osteoar-thropathy in 33 horses (1993–2000). *J Vet Intern Med* **16**:697–703.

43 Hughes KJ, Hodgson DR (2006) Unilateral ataxia and head tilt in a 7-year-old Thoroughbred stallion: temporohyoid osteoarthropathy. *Aust Vet J* **84**:136–137, 141–142.

44 Blythe LL (1997) Otitis media and interna and temporohyoid osteoar-thropathy. *Vet Clin N Am Equine Pract* **13**:21–42.

45 Pease AP, van Biervliet J, Dykes NL *et al.* (2004) Complication of partial stylohyoidectomy for treatment of temporohyoid osteoarthropathy and an alternative surgical technique in three cases. *Equine Vet J* **36**:546–550.

46 Smith MR, Stevens KB, Durham AE *et al.* (2003) Equine hepatic disease: the effect of patient- and case-specific variables on risk and prognosis. *Equine Vet J* **35**:549–552.

47 Johns IC, Del Piero F, Wilkins PA (2007) Hepatic encephalopathy in a pregnant mare: identification of histopathological changes in the brain of the mare and the fetus. *Aust Vet J* **85**:337–340.

48 Durham AE, Smith KC, Newton JR (2003) An evaluation of diagnostic data in comparison to the results of liver biopsies in mature horses. *Equine Vet J* **35**:554–559.

49 Peek SF, Divers TJ, Jackson CJ (1997) Hyperammonaemia associated with encephalopathy and abdominal pain without evidence of liver disease in four mature horses. *Equine Vet J* **29**:70–74.

50 Wilkins PA, Wacholder S, Detrisac C *et al.* (2001) Evidence for transmission of *Halicephalobus deletrix* (H gingivalis) from dam to foal. *J Vet Intern Med* **15**:412–417.

51 Tennent-Brown BS (2007) Trauma with neurologic sequelae. *Vet Clin N Am Equine Pract* **23**:81–101.

52 Whitlock RH, Buckley C (1997) Botulism. *Vet Clin N Am Equine Pract* **13**:107–28.

53 Shapiro RL, Hatheway C, Swerdlow DL (1998) Botulism in the United States: a clinical and epidemiologic review. *Ann Intern Med* **129**:221.

54 Galey FD (2001) Botulism in the horse. *Vet Clin N Am Equine Pract* **17**:579.

55 Wilkins PA, Palmer JE (2003) Botulism in foals less than 6 months of age: 30 cases (1989–2002). *J Vet Intern Med* **17**:702–707.

56 Wilkins PA (2007) Botulism. In: *Equine Infectious Diseases.* (eds D Sellon, M Long) Elsevier Saunders, Philadelphia, pp. 372–375.

57 Humeau Y, Doussau F, Grant NJ *et al.* (2000) How botulinum and tetanus neurotoxins block neurotransmitter release, *Biochimie* **82**:427–446.

58 Wilkins PA, Palmer JE (2003) Mechanical ventilation in foals with botulism: 9 cases (1989–2002). *J Vet Intern Med* **17**:708–711.

59 Green SL, Little CB, Baird JD *et al.* (1994) Tetanus in the horse: a review of 20 cases (1970 to 1990). *J Vet Intern Med* **8**:128–132.

60 Markel MD, Madigan JE, Lichten-steiger CA *et al.* (1986) Vertebral body osteomyelitis in the horse. *J Am Vet Med Assoc* **188**:632–634.

61 Prescott JF (1994) *Rhodococcus equi* vertebral osteomyelitis in foals. *Equine Vet J* **26**:1–2.

62 Tyson R, Graham JP, Roberts GD *et al.* (2004) What is your diagnosis? Osteomyelitis of a vertebral body. *J Am Vet Med Assoc* **225**:515–516.

63 Paradis MR (1998) Tumors of the central nervous system. *Vet Clin N Am Equine Pract* **14**:543–561.

64 Tietje S, Becker M, Böckenhoff G (1996) Computed tomographic evaluation of head diseases in the horse: 15 cases. *Equine Vet J* **28**:98–105.

CHAPTER 8: EYE AND ASSOCIATED STRUCTURES

1   Giulinao EA, Maggs DJ, Moore CP *et al.* (2000) Inferomedial placement of a single-entry subpalpebral lavage tube for treatment of equine eye disease. *Vet Ophthalmol* **3**:153–156.

2   Clode AB (2011) Diseases and surgery of the cornea. In: *Equine Ophthalmology*, 2nd edn. (ed BC Gilger) Elsevier Saunders, Maryland Heights, pp. 181–266.

3   Giuliano EA (2011) Equine ocular adnexal and nasolacrimal disease. In: *Equine Ophthalmology*, 2nd edn. (ed BC Gilger) Elsevier Saunders, Maryland Heights, pp. 133–180.

4   Hewes CA, Keoughan GC, Gutierrez-Nibeyro S (2007) Standing enucleation in the horse: a report of 5 cases. *Can Vet J* **48**:512–514.

5   Pollock PJ, Russell T, Hughes TK *et al.* (2008) Transpalpebral eye enucleation in 40 standing horses. *Vet Surg* **37**:306–309.

6   Utter ME, Wotman KL, Covert KR (2010) Return to work following unilateral enucleation in 34 horses (2000–2008). *Equine Vet J* **42**:156–160.

7   Hamor RE, Roberts SM, Severin GA (1993) Use of orbital implants after enucleation in dogs, horses, and cats: 161 cases (1980–1990). *J Am Vet Med Assoc* **203**:701–706.

8   Michau TM, Gilger BC (2004) Cosmetic globe surgery in the horse. *Vet Clin N Am Equine Pract* **20**:467–84, viii–ix.

9   Brooks DE, Clark CK, Lester GD (2000) Cochet-Bonnet aesthesiometer-determined corneal sensitivity in neonatal foals and adult horses. *Vet Ophthalmol* **3**:133–137.

10 Kalf KL, Utter ME, Wotman KL (2008) Evaluation of duration of corneal anesthesia induced with ophthalmic 0.5% proparacaine hydrochloride by use of a Cochet-Bonnet aesthesiometer in clinically normal horses. *Am J Vet Res* **69**:1655–1658.

11 Utter ME, Wotman KL (2012) Distichiasis causing recurrent corneal ulceration in two Friesian horses. *Equine Vet Educ* **24**:556–560

12 Hurn S, Turner A, McCowan C (2005) Ectopic cilium in seven horses. *Vet Ophthalmol* **8**:199–202.

13 Brooks DE (2006) Orbit. In: *Equine Surgery*, 3rd edn. (eds JE Auer, JE Stick) Saunders Elsevier, St. Louis, pp. 755–766.

14 Nasisse MP, Nelms S (1992) Equine ulcerative keratitis. *Vet Clin N Am Equine Pract* **8**:537–555.

15 Ollivier FJ, Brooks DE, Kallberg ME *et al.* (2003) Evaluation of various compounds to inhibit activity of matrix metalloproteinases in the tear film of horses with ulcerative keratitis. *Am J Vet Res* **64**:1081–1087.

16 Ledbetter EC, Patten VH, Scarlett JM *et al.* (2007) In vitro susceptibility patterns of fungi associated with keratomycosis in horses of the northeastern United States: 68 cases (1987–2006). *J Am Vet Med Assoc* **231**:1086–1091.

17 Pearce JW, Giuliano EA, Moore CP (2009) In vitro susceptibility patterns of *Aspergillus* and *Fusarium* species isolated from equine ulcerative keratomycosis cases in the midwestern and southern United States with inclusion of the new antifungal agent voriconazole. *Vet Ophthalmol* **12**:318–324.

18 Wotman KL, Utter ME, Rankin SC (2008) Antifungal susceptibility testing of *Aspergillus* species isolated from horses with keratomycosis in Southeast Pennsylvania: 10 cases (2006–2007). *Proc Ann Meeting Am Coll Vet Ophthalmol*, Boston.

19 Lassaline ME, Brooks DE, Ollivier FJ *et al.* (2005) Equine amniotic membrane transplantation for corneal ulceration and keratomalacia in three horses. *Vet Ophthalmol* **8**:311–317.

20 Plummer CE, Ollivier F, Kallberg M *et al.* (2009) The use of amniotic membrane transplantation for ocular surface reconstruction: a review and series of 58 equine clinical cases (2002–2008). *Vet Ophthalmol* **12(Suppl 1)**:17–24.

21 Chmielewski NT, Brooks DE, Smith PJ *et al.* (1997) Visual outcome and ocular survival following iris prolapse in the horse: a review of 32 cases. *Equine Vet J* **29**:31–39.

22 Lavach JD, Severin GA, Roberts SM (1984) Lacerations of the equine eye: a review of 48 cases. *J Am Vet Med Assoc* **184**:1243–1248.

23 Gilger BC (2011) Diseases and surgery of the globe and orbit. In: *Equine Ophthalmology*, 2nd edn. (ed BC Gilger) Elsevier Saunders, Maryland Heights, pp. 93–132.

24 Hendrix DV, Brooks DE, Smith PJ *et al.* (1995) Corneal stromal abscesses in the horse: a review of 24 cases. *Equine Vet J* **27**:440–447.

25 Rebhun WC (1982) Corneal stromal abscesses in the horse. *J Am Vet Med Assoc* **181**:677–679.

26 Andrew SE, Willis AM (2005) Diseases of the cornea and sclera. In: *Equine Ophthalmology*, 2nd edn. (ed BC Gilger) Elsevier Saunders, Maryland Heights, pp. 157–252.

27 Lassaline ME, Brooks DE, Andrew SE *et al.* (2002) Histology of equine stromal abscesses excised during corneal transplantation. *Proc Ann Meeting Am Coll Vet Ophthalmol*, Denver.

28 Andrew SE, Brooks DE, Biros DJ *et al.* (2000) Posterior lamellar keratoplasty for treatment of deep stromal abesses in nine horses. *Vet Ophthalmol* **3**:99–103.

29 Brooks DE, Plummer CE, Kallberg ME *et al.* (2008) Corneal transplantation for inflammatory keratopathies in the horse: visual outcome in 206 cases (1993–2007). *Vet Ophthalmol* **11**:123–133.

30 Plummer CE, Kallberg ME, Ollivier FJ *et al.* (2008) Deep lamellar endothelial keratoplasty in 10 horses. *Vet Ophthalmol* **11(Suppl 1)**:35–43.

31 Gilger BC, Michau TM, Salmon JH (2005) Immune-mediated keratitis in horses: 19 cases (1998–2004). *Vet Ophthalmol* **8**:233–239.

32 Matthews A, Gilger BC (2009) Equine immune-mediated keratopathies. *Vet Ophthalmol* **12(Suppl 1)**:10–16.

33 Gilger BC, Malok E, Cutter KV *et al.* (1999) Characterization of T-lymphocytes in the anterior uvea of eyes with chronic equine recurrent uveitis. *Vet Immunol Immunopathol* **71**:17–28.

34 Dwyer AE, Crockett RS, Kalsow CM (1995) Association of leptospiral seroactivity and breed with uveitis and blindness in horses: 372 cases (1986–1993). *J Am Vet Med Assoc* **207**:1327–1331.

35 Gilger BC, Salmon JH, Yi NY *et al.* (2008) Role of bacteria in the pathogenesis of recurrent uveitis in horses from the southeastern United States. *Am J Vet Res* **69**:1329–1335.

36 Gilger BC, Deeg C (2011) Equine recurrent uveitis. In: *Equine Ophthalmology*, 2nd edn. (ed BC Gilger) Elsevier Saunders, Maryland Heights, pp. 317–349.

37 Utter ME, Brooks DE (2011) Glaucoma. In: *Equine Ophthalmology*, 2nd edn. (ed BC Gilger) Elsevier Saunders, Maryland Heights, pp. 350–366.

38 Brem S, Gerhards H, Wollanke B *et al.* (1999) 35 leptospira isolated from the vitreous body of 32 horses with recurrent uveitis (ERU). *Berl Munch Tierarzt Wochenschr* **112**:390–393.

39 Faber NA, Crawford M, LeFebvre RB *et al.* (2000) Detection of *Leptospira* spp. in the aqueous humor of horses with naturally acquired recurrent uveitis. *J Clin Microbiol* **38**:2731–2733.

40 Wollanke B, Rohrbach BW, Gerhards H (2001) Serum and vitreous humor antibody titers in and isolation of *Leptospira interrogans* from horses with recurrent uveitis. *J Am Vet Med Assoc* **219**:795–800.

41 Gilger BC, Wilkie DA, Clode AB *et al.* (2010) Long-term outcome after implantation of a suprachoroidal cyclosporine drug delivery device in horses with recurrent uveitis. *Vet Ophthalmol* **13**:294–300.

42 Nell B, Walde I (2010) Posterior segment diseases. *Equine Vet J Suppl* **37**:69–79.

43 Strobel BW, Wilkie DA, Gilger BC (2007) Retinal detachment in horses: 40 cases (1998–2005). *Vet Ophthalmol* **10**:380–385.

44 Knollinger AM, La Croix NC, Barrett PM *et al.* (2005) Evaluation of a rebound tonometer for measuring intraocular pressure in dogs and horses. *J Am Vet Med Assoc* **227**:244–248.

45 Komaromy AM, Garg CD, Ying GS *et al.* (2006) Effect of head position on intraocular pressure in horses. *Am J Vet Res* **67**:1232–1235.

46 Smith PJ, Gum GG, Whitley RD *et al.* (1990) Tonometric and tonographic studies in the normal pony eye. *Equine Vet J* **10(Suppl)**:36–38.

47 van der Woerdt A, Gilger BC, Wilkie DA *et al.* (1995) Effect of auriculopalpebral nerve block and intravenous administration of xylazine on intraocular pressure and corneal thickness in horses. *Am J Vet Res* **56**:155–158.

48 Germann SE, Matheis FL, Rampazzo A *et al.* (2008) Effects of topical administration of 1% brinzolamide on intraocular pressure in clinically normal horses. *Equine Vet J* **40**:662–665.

49 van Der Woerdt A, Wilkie DA, Gilger BC *et al.* (2000) Effect of single- and multiple-dose 0.5% timolol maleate on intraocular pressure and pupil size in female horses. *Vet Ophthalmol* **3**:165–168.

50 Willis AM, Robbin TE, Hoshaw-Woodard S *et al.* (2001) Effect of topical administration of 2% dorzlamide hydrochloride or 2% dorzlamide hydrochloride-0.5% timolol maleate on intraocular pressure in clinically normal horses. *Am J Vet Res* **62**:709–713.

51 Studer ME, Martin CL, Stiles J (2000) Effects of 0.005% latanoprost solution on intraocular pressure in healthy dogs and cats. *Am J Vet Res* **61**:1220–1224.

52 Willis AM, Diehl KA, Hoshaw-Woodard S *et al.* (2001) Effects of topical administration of 0.005% latanoprost solution on eyes of clinically normal horses. *Am J Vet Res* **62**:1945–1951.

53 Herring IP, Pickett JP, Champagne ES *et al.* (2000) Effect of topical 1% atropine sulfate on intraocular pressure in normal horses. *Vet Ophthalmol* **3**:139–143.

54 Mughannam AJ, Buyukmihci NC, Kass PH (1999) Effect of topical atropine on intraocular pressure and pupil diameter in the normal horse eye. *Vet Ophthalmol* **2**:213–215.

55 Annear MI, Wilkie DA, Gemensky-Metzler AJ (2008) Diode laser transscleral cyclophotocoagulation for treatment of equine glaucoma: a retrospective study of 42 eyes of 36 horses. *Proc Ann Meeting Am Coll Vet Ophthalmol*, Boston.

56 Miller TL, Willis AM, Wilkie DA *et al.* (2001) Description of ciliary body anatomy and identification of sites for transscleral cyclophotocoagulation in the equine eye. *Vet Ophthalmol* **4**:183–190.

57 Morreale RJ, Wilkie DA, Gemensky-Metzler AJ *et al.* (2007) Histologic effect of semiconductor diode laser transscleral cyclophotocoagulation on the normal equine eye. *Vet Ophthalmol* **10**:84–92.

58 Wilkie DA (2011) Disease of the ocular posterior segment. In: *Equine Ophthalmology*, 2nd edn. (ed BC Gilger) Elsevier Saunders, Maryland Heights, pp. 367–396.

59 McMullen RJ Jr, Utter ME (2010) Current developments in equine cataract surgery. *Equine Vet J Suppl* **37**:38–45.

60 Ben-Shlomo G, Plummer C, Barrie K *et al.* (2012) Characterization of the normal dark adaptation curve of the horse. *Vet Ophthalmol* **15**:42–45.

61 Komaromy AM, Andrew SE, Sapp HL Jr *et al.* (2003) Flash electroretinography in standing horses using the DTL microfiber electrode. *Vet Ophthalmol* **6**:27–33.

62 Scotty NC, Cutler TJ, Brooks DE *et al.* (2004) Diagnostic ultrasonography of equine lens and posterior segment abnormalities. *Vet Ophthalmol* **7**:127–139.

63 Dwyer AE (2011) Practical management of blind horses. In: *Equine Ophthalmology*, 2nd edn. (ed BC Gilger) Elsevier Saunders, Maryland Heights, pp. 470–481.

CHAPTER 9: NEONATOLOGY

1 Axon JE (2006) Assessment of the critically-ill neonate. *Proc 28th Bain Fallon Memorial Lectures*, Coffs Harbour, **28**:97–110.

2 Palmer JE (2005) Ventilatory support of the critically ill foal. *Vet Clin N Am Equine Pract* **21**:457–486

3 Wong DM, Alcott CJ, Wang C *et al.* (2010) Physiologic effects of nasopharyngeal administration of supplemental oxygen at various flow rates in healthy neonatal foals. *Am J Vet Res* **9**:1081–1088.

4 Giguère S, Sanchez LC, Shih A *et al.* (2007) Comparison of the effects of caffeine and doxapram on respiratory and cardiovascular function in foals with induced respiratory acidosis. *Am J Vet Res* **12**:1407–1416

5 Giguère S, Slade JK, Sanchez LC (2008) Retrospective comparison of caffeine and doxapram for the treatment of hypercapnia in foals with hypoxic-ischemic encephalopathy. *J Vet Intern Med* **22**:401–405.

6 Axon JE (2006) Treatment of the critically-ill neonate. *Proc 28th Bain Fallon Memorial Lectures*, Coffs Harbour, **28**:112–134.

7 Palmer JE (2004) Fluid therapy in the neonate: not your mother's fluid space. *Vet Clin N Am Equine Pract* **20**:63–75.

8 Magdesian KG (2010) Update on fluid therapy in horses. *Proc Central Veterinary Conference*, Kansas.

9 Magdesian KG, Madigan JE (2003) Volume replacement in the neonatal ICU: crystalloids and colloids. *Clin Tech Equine Pract* **2**:20–30.

10 Hollis A, Wilkins PA, Tennent-Brown B *et al.* (2010) The effect of intravenous plasma administration on fibrinogen concentration in sick neonatal foals. *J Vet Intern Med* **24**:786. (abstract)

11 Wotman K, Palmer JE, Boston RC *et al.* (2005) Lactate concentration in foals presenting to a neonatal intensive care unit: association with outcome. American College Veterinary Internal Medicine Scientific Forum. *J Vet Intern Med* **19**:409.

12 Henderson ISF, Franklin RP, Boston RC *et al.* (2007) Association of hyperlactatemia with age, diagnosis and survival in equine neonates. *Proc Am Assoc Equine Practnrs* **53**:354–355.

13 Borchers A, Wilkins PA, Marsh PM *et al.* (2012) Admission L-lactate concentration in hospitalized equine neonates: a prospective multicenter study. *Equine Vet J* **41**:57–63.

14 Corley KTT (2004) Inotropes and vasopressors in adults and foals. *Vet Clin N Am Equine Pract* **20**:77–106.

15 Palmer JE (2002) When fluids are not enough - inopressor therapy. *8th International Emergency and Critical Care Symposium*, San Antonio, pp. 669–673.

16 Giguère S, Knowles HA Jr, Valverde A *et al.* (2005) Accuracy of indirect measurement of blood pressure in neonatal foals. *J Vet Intern Med* **19**:571–576.

17 Russell CM, Axon JE, Blishen A *et al.* (2008) Blood culture isolates and antimicrobial sensitivities from 427 critically ill neonatal foals. *Aust Vet J* **86**:266–271.

18 Russell C, Palmer JE, Boston RC *et al.* (2007) Agreement between point-of-care glucometry, blood gas and laboratory based measurement of glucose in an equine neonatal intensive care unit. *J Vet Emerg Crit Care* **17**:236–242.

19 Hackett ES, McCue PM (2010) Evaluation of a veterinary glucometer for use in horses. *J Vet Intern Med* **24**:617–621.

20 Wilkins PA (2004) Disorders of foals. In: *Equine Internal Medicine*, 2nd edn. (eds SM Reed, WM Bayly, DC Sellon) Saunders, St. Louis, pp. 1381–1431.

21 Spurlock SL, Furr M (1990) Fluid therapy. In: *Equine Clinical Neonatology*. (eds AM Koterba, WH Drummond, PC Kosch) Lea and Febiger, Philadelphia, pp. 671–700.

22 Corley KTT (2002) Fluid therapy for horses with gastrointestinal disease. In: *Large Animal Internal Medicine*, 2nd edn. (ed BP Smith) Mosby Year Book, St. Louis, pp. 682–694.

23 Olsson AM, Persson S, Schöder R (1978) Effects of terbutaline and isoproterenol on hyperkalemia in nephrectomized rabbits. *Scand J Urol Nephrol* **12**:35–38.

24 Magdesian KG (2005) Neonatal foal diarrhea. *Vet Clin N Am Equine Pract* **21**:295–312.

25 Giguere S, Polkes AC (2005) Immunologic disorders in neonatal foals. *Vet Clin N Am Equine Pract* **21**:241–272.

26 Sellon DC, Wilkins PA (2010) Failure of passive transfer. In: *Equine Internal Medicine*, 3rd edn. (eds SM Reed, WM Bayly, DC Sellon) Saunders, St. Louis, pp. 1335–1336.

27 LeBlanc MM (1990) Immunological considerations. In: *Equine Clinical Neonatology*. (eds AM Koterba, WH Drummond, PC Kosch) Lea and Febiger, Philadelphia, pp. 55–70.

28 Davis R, Giguere S (2005) Evaluation of five commercially available assays and measurement of serum total protein concentration via refractometry for diagnosis of failure of passive transfer of immunity in foals. *J Am Vet Med Assoc* **227**:640–645.

29 Holmes MA, Lunn DP (1991) A study of bovine and equine immunoglobulin levels in pony foals fed bovine colostrum. *Equine Vet J* **23**:116–118.

30 Vivrette SL (2001) Colostrum and oral immunoglobulin therapy in newborn foals. *Comp Contin Educ Pract Vet* **23**:286–291.

31 Wilkins PA, Dewan-Mix S (1994) Efficacy of intravenous plasma therapy for treatment of failure of passive transfer in normal and clinically ill equine neonates. *Cornell Vet* **84**:7–14.

32 Chavatte P, Clement F, Cash R *et al.* (1998) Field determination of colostrum quality by using a novel, practical method. *Proc 44th Ann Conven Am Assoc Equine Practnrs* **44**:206–209.

33 Vaala WE (1990) Neonatal anemia. In: *Equine Clinical Neonatology*. (eds AM Koterba, WH Drummond, PC Kosch) Lea and Febiger, Philadelphia, pp. 571–588.

34 Sellon DC, Wilkins PA (2010) Neonatal isoerythrolysis. In: *Equine Internal Medicine*, 3rd edn. (eds SM Reed, WM Bayly, DC Sellon) Saunders, St. Louis, pp. 1336–1337.

35 McClure J (1997) Strategies for prevention of neonatal isoerythrolysis in horses and mules. *Equine Vet Educ* **9**:118–122.

36 Polkes AC, Giguère S, Lester GD *et al.* (2008) Factors associated with outcome in foals with neonatal isoerythrolysis (72 cases, 1988–2003). *J Vet Intern Med* **5**:1216–1222.

37 Bailey E, Conboy HS, McCarthy PF (1987) Neonatal isoerythrolysis of foals: an update on testing. *Proc 3rd Ann Conven Am Assoc Equine Practnr*s **33**:341–355.

38 Divers TJ (2003) Liver failure and hemolytic anemia. In: *Manual of Equine Emergencies*, 2nd edn. (eds. JA Orsini, TJ Divers) Saunders, Philadelphia, pp.315–338.

39 Elfenbein JR, Giguère S, Meyer SK *et al.* (2010) The effects of deferoxamine mesylate on iron elimination after blood transfusion in neonatal foals. *J Vet Intern Med* **24**:1475–1482.

40 Paradis MR (2005) Neonatal septicemia. In: *Current Therapy in Equine Medicine*. (ed NE Robinson) Saunders, St Louis, pp. 656–662.

41 Sanchez LC (2005) Equine neonatal sepsis. *Vet Clin N Am Equine Pract* **21**:273–293.

42 Hollis AR, Wilkins PA, Palmer JE *et al.* (2008) Bacteremia in equine neonatal diarrhea: a retrospective study (1990–2007). *J Vet Intern Med* **22**:1203–1209.

43 Marsh PS, Palmer JE (2001) Bacterial isolates from blood and their susceptibility patterns in critically ill foals: 543 cases (1991–1998). *J Am Vet Med Assoc* **218**:1608–1610.

44 Corley KT, Pearce G, Magdesian KG *et al.* (2007) Bacteraemia in neonatal foals: clinicopathological differences between gram-positive and gram-negative infections, and single organism and mixed infections. *Equine Vet J* **39**:84–89.

45 Sanchez LC, Giguère S, Lester GD (2008) Factors associated with survival of neonatal foals with bacteremia and racing performance of surviving Thoroughbreds: 423 cases (1982–2007). *J Am Vet Med Assoc* **233**:1446–1452.

46 Roy M-F (2004) Sepsis in adults and foals. *Vet Clin N Am Equine Pract* **20**:41–61.

47 Wilkins PA (2003) Lower respiratory problems of the neonate. *Vet Clin N Am Equine Pract* **19**:19–33

48 Wilkins PA, Otto CM, Dunkel B *et al.* (2007) Acute lung injury (ALI) and acute respiratory distress syndromes (ARDS) in veterinary medicine: consensus definitions. Special commentary. *J Vet Emerg Crit Care* **17**:333–339.

49 Labelle AL, Hamor RE, Townsend WM *et al.* (2011) Ophthalmic lesions in neonatal foals evaluated for non-ophthalmic disease at referral hospitals. *J Am Vet Med Assoc* **239**:486–492.

50 Brewer BD, Koterba AM (1988) Development of a scoring system for the early diagnosis of equine neonatal sepsis. *Equine Vet J* **20**:18–22.

51 Corley KT, Furr M (2003) Evaluation of a score to predict sepsis in foals. *J Vet Emerg Crit Care* **13**:149–153.

52 Trumble TN (2005) Orthopedic disorders in neonatal foals. *Vet Clin N Am Equine Pract* **21**:357–385.

53 Lester GD (2005) Maturity of the neonatal foal. *Vet Clin N Am Equine Pract* **21**:333–355.

54 Jeffcott LB, Rossdale PD, Leadon DP (1982) Haematological changes in the neonatal period of normal and induced premature foals. *J Reprod Fert Suppl* **32**:537–544.

55 Ousey JC, Kölling M, Kindahl H *et al.* (2011) Maternal dexamethasone treatment in late gestation induces precocious fetal maturation and delivery in healthy Thoroughbred mares. *Equine Vet J* **43**:424–429.

56 Jellyman JK, Allen VL, Forhead AJ *et al.* (2012) Hypothalamic-pituitary-adrenal axis function in pony foals after neonatal ACTH-induced glucocorticoid overexposure. *Equine Vet J* **44(Suppl 41)**:38–42.

57 Lester GD (1997) Prematurity. In: *Current Therapy in Equine Medicine*. (ed NE Robinson) Saunders, St Louis, pp. 641–644.

58 Chaney KP, Holcombe SJ, Schott HC 2nd *et al.* (2010) Spurious hypercreatininemia: 28 neonatal foals (2000–2008). *J Vet Emerg Crit Care* **20**:244–249.

59 Wilkins PA (2010) Persistent pulmonary hypertension. In: *Equine Internal Medicine*, 3rd edn. (eds SM Reed, WM Bayly, DC Sellon) Saunders, St. Louis, pp. 1319–1320.

60 Kosch PC, Koterba AM, Coons TJ *et al.* (1984) Developments in management of the newborn foal in respiratory distress. **1:** Evaluation. *Equine Vet J* **16**:312–318.

61 Adams R (1990) Noninfectious orthopedic problems. In: *Equine Clinical Neonatology*. (eds AM Koterba, WH Drummond, PC Kosch) Lea and Febiger, Philadelphia, pp. 333–366

62 Auer JA, von Rechenberg B (2006) Treatment of angular limb deformities in foals. *Clin Tech Equine Pract* **5**:270–281.

63 Hardy J (1998) Uroabdomen in foals. *Equine Vet Educ* **10**:1021–1025.

64 Dunkel B, Palmer JE, Olson KN *et al.* (2005) Uroperitoneum in 32 foals: influence of intravenous fluid therapy, infection, and sepsis. *J Vet Intern Med* **19**:889–893.

65 Kablack KA, Embertson RM, Bernard *et al.* (2000) Uroperitoneum in the hospitalised equine neonate: retrospective study of 31 cases, 1988–1997. *Equine Vet J* **32**:505–508.

66 Vander Werf KA, Beard LA, McMurphy RM (2010) Urinothorax in a Quarter Horse filly. *Equine Vet Educ* **22**:239–243.

67 Wilkins PA (2004) Respiratory distress in foals with uroperitoneum: possible mechanisms. *Equine Vet Educ* **16**:377–380.

68 Adams R (1990) Urinary tract disruption. In: *Equine Clinical Neonatology*. (eds AM Koterba, WH Drummond, PC Kosch) Lea and Febiger, Philadelphia, pp. 464–481.

69 Vaala WE (1994) Peripartum asphyxia. *Vet Clin N Am Equine Pract* **10**:187–218.

70 Wilkins PA (2010) Perinatal asphyxia syndrome. In: *Equine Internal Medicine*, 3rd edn. (eds SM Reed, WM Bayly, DC Sellon) Saunders, St. Louis, pp.1324–1328.

71 Rossdale PD (2004) The maladjusted foal. *Proc 50th Ann Conven Am Assoc Equine Practnrs* **50**:75–126.

72 Palmer JE (2005) Neonatal diseases in foals. In: *Havemeyer Foundation Workshop, Uterine Infection in Mares and Women: a Comparative Study II*. South Carolina

73 Bain FT (2004) Management of the foal from the mare with placentitis: a clinician's approach. *Proc 50ᵗʰ Ann Conven Am Assoc Equine Practnrs* **50**:162–164.

74 Wilkins PA (2005) How to use midazolam to control equine neonatal seizures. *Proc 51ˢᵗ Ann Conven Am Assoc Equine Practnrs* **51**:279–280.

75 Papazian L, Albanese J, Thirion X *et al.* (1993) Effect of bolus doses of midazolam on intracranial pressure and cerebral perfusion pressure in patients with severe head injury *Br J Anaesth* **71**:267–271.

76 Akman M, Akbal H, Emir H *et al.* (2000) The effects of sucralfate and selective intestinal decontamination on bacterial translocation. *Pediatr Surg Int* **16**:91–93.

77 Colak T, Ipek T, Paksoy M *et al.* (2001) The effects of cefephim, G-CSF, and sucralfate on bacterial translocation in experimentally induced acute pancreatitis. *Surg Today* **31**:502–506.

78 Wilson WD (2003) Foal pneumonia. In: *Current Therapy in Equine Medicine*, 5ᵗʰ edn. (ed NE Robinson) Saunders, St. Louis, pp. 666–674.

79 Giguere S, Prescott JF (1997) Clinical manifestations, diagnosis, treatment and prevention of *Rhodococcus equi* infections in foals. *Vet Microbiol* **56**:313–334.

80 Slovis NM, McCracken JL, Mundy G (2005) How to use thoracic ultrasound to screen foals for *Rhodococcus equi* at affected farms. *Proc 51ˢᵗ Ann Conven Am Assoc Equine Practnrs* **51**:274–278.

81 McKenzie HC (2006) Treating foal pneumonia. *Comp Cont Educ Pract Vet: Equine Edition* **Spring**:47–53.

82 Jean D, Laverty S, Halley J *et al.* (1999) Thoracic trauma in newborn foals. *Equine Vet J* **31**:149–152.

83 Bellazzo F, Hunt RJ, Provost P *et al.* (2004) Surgical repair of fractures in 14 neonatal foals: case selection, surgical technique and results. *Equine Vet J* **36**:557–562.

84 Sprayberry KA, Fairfield FT, Seahorn TL *et al.* (2001) 56 cases of rib fractures in neonatal foals hospitalized in a referral center intensive care unit from 1997–2001. *Proce 47ᵗʰ Ann Conven Am Assoc Equine Practnrs* **47**:395–399.

85 Schambourg MA, Laverty S, Mullim S (2003) Thoracic trauma in foals: post mortem findings. *Equine Vet J* **35**:78–81.

86 Kraus BM, Richardson DW, Sheridan G *et al.* (2005) Multiple rib fractures in a neonatal foal using a nylon strand suture repair technique. *Vet Surg* **34**:399–404.

87 Pusterla N, Magdesian KG, Maleski K *et al.* (2004) Retrospective evaluation of the use of acetylcysteine enemas in the treatment of meconium retention in foals: 44 cases (1987–2002). *Equine Vet Educ* **16**:133–136.

88 Fischer AT, Yarbrough TY (1995) Retrograde contrast radiography of the distal portions of the intestinal tract in foals. *J Am Vet Med Assoc* **207**:734–737.

89 Axon JE (2006) Medical treatment of abdominal pain in the neonatal foal. *Proc 28ᵗʰ Bain Fallon Memorial Lecture Series*, Coffs Harbour, pp. 152–157.

90 Ryan CA, Sanchez C (2005) Nondiarrheal disorders of the gastrointestinal tract in neonatal foals. *Vet Clin N Am Equine Pract* **21**:313–332.

91 Cohen ND, Snowden K (1996) Cryptosporidial diarrhea in foals. *Comp Contin Educ Pract Vet* **18**:298–306.

92 Dunkel B, Wilkins PA (2004) Infectious foal diarrhoea: pathophysiology, prevalence and diagnosis. *Equine Vet Educ* **16**:94–101.

93 Lester GD (2003) Foal diarrhea. In: *Current Therapy in Equine Medicine*, 5ᵗʰ edn. (ed NE Robinson) Saunders, St Louis, pp. 677–680.

94 Furr M, Cohen ND, Axon JE *et al.* (2012) Treatment with histamine-type 2 receptor antagonists and omeprazole increase the risk of diarrhoea in neonatal foals treated in intensive care units. *Equine Vet J* **41**:80–86.

95 Auer JA (2006) Diagnosis and treatment of flexural deformities in foals. *Clin Tech Equine Pract* **5**:282–295.

96 Hunt RJ (1997) Noninfectious musculoskeletal disorders of foals. In: *Current Therapy in Equine Medicine*, 5ᵗʰ edn. (ed NE Robinson) Saunders, St Louis, pp. 623–627.

97 Bramlage LR, Auer JA (2006) Diagnosis, assessment and treatment strategies for angular limb deformities in the foal. *Clin Tech Equine Pract* **5**:259–269.

CHAPTER 10: TOXICOLOGY

1 Beasley VR, Dorman DC (1990) Management of toxicoses. *Vet Clin N Am Small Anim Pract* **20**:307–337.

2 Landolt GA (2007) Management of equine poisoning and envenomation. *Vet Clin N Am Equine Pract* **23**:31–47.

3 Shannon MW, Haddad LM (1998) The emergency management of poisoning. In: *Clinical Management of Poisoning and Drug Overdose*, 3ʳᵈ edn. (eds LM Haddad, MW Shannon, JF Winchester) WB Saunders, Philadephia, pp. 2–31.

4 Poppenga RH (2004) Treatment. In: *Clinical Veterinary Toxicology*. (ed KH Plumlee) Mosby, St. Louis, pp. 13–21.

5 Winchester JF (2005) Extracorporeal removal of toxic substances. In: *Critical Care Toxicology: Diagnosis and Management of the Critically Poisoned Patient*. (eds J Brent, KL Wallace, KK Burkhart *et al.*) Elsevier Mosby, Philadelphia, pp. 65–71

6 Proudfoot AT, Krenzelok EP, Vale JA (2004) Position paper on urine alkalinization. *J Toxicol Clin Toxicol* **42**:1–26.

7 Seger DL (2005) Common complications in the critically poisoned patient. In: *Critical Care Toxicology: Diagnosis and Management of the Critically Poisoned Patient*. (eds J Brent, KL Wallace, KK Burkhart *et al.*) Elsevier Mosby, Philadelphia, pp. 73–86.

8   Howland MA (2006) Antidotes in depth: activated charcoal. In: *Goldfrank's Toxicologic Emergencies*. (eds NE Flomenbaum, MA Howland, LR Goldfrank *et al.*) McGraw-Hill, New York, pp. 128–134.

9   Levy G (1982) Gastrointestinal clearance of drugs with activated charcoal. *N Engl J Med* **307:**676–678.

10 Krenzelok EP, Vale JA (2005) Gastrointestinal decontamination. In: *Critical Care Toxicology: Diagnosis and Management of the Critically Poisoned Patient*. (eds J Brent, KL Wallace, KK Burkhart *et al.*) Elsevier Mosby, Philadelphia, pp. 53–60.

11 Stewart J (1983) Effects of emetics and cathartic agents on the gastrointestinal tract and the treatment of toxic ingestions. *J Toxicol Clin Toxicol* **20:**199–253.

12 Perry H, Shannon M (1996) Emergency department gastrointestinal decontamination. *Pediatr Ann* **25:**19–26.

13 Christopherson AJ, Hoegberg LCG (2006) Techniques used to prevent gastrointestinal absorption. In: *Goldfrank's Toxicologic Emergencies*. (eds NE Flomenbaum, MA Howland, LR Goldfrank *et al.*) McGraw-Hill, New York, pp. 109–123

14 Barr AC, Reagor JC (2001) Toxic plants: what the horse practitioner needs to know. *Vet Clin N Am Equine Pract* **17:**529–546.

15 Panter KE, Gardner DR, Lee ST *et al.* (2007) Important poisonous plants of the United States. In: *Veterinary Toxicology: Basic and Clinical Principles*. (ed RC Gupta) Elsevier Academic Press, Amsterdam, pp. 825–872.

16 Knight AP, Walter RG (2001) *A Guide to Plant Poisoning of Animals in North America*. Teton New Media, Jackson.

17 Ames T, Angelos J, Gould S *et al.* (1994 Secondary photosensitization in horses eating *Cymodothea trifolli*-infested clover. *Am Assoc Vet Lab Diagnost Proc* p. 45.

18 Casteel SW (2004) Forage-induced photosensitization. In: *Clinical Veterinary Toxicology*. (ed KH Plumlee) Mosby, St. Louis, pp. 427–428.

19 Barton MH (2004) Disorders of the liver. In: *Equine Internal Medicine*, 2nd edn. (eds SM Reed, WM Bayly, DC Sellon) Saunders, Philadelphia, pp. 951–994.

20 Pickrell JA, Oehme F (2004) Cyanogenic glycosides. In: *Clinical Veterinary Toxicology*. (ed KH Plumlee) Mosby, St. Louis, pp. 391–392.

21 Holstedge CP, Isom GE, Kirk MA (2006) Cyanide and hydrogen sulfide. In: *Goldfrank's Toxicologic Emergencies*. (eds NE Flomenbaum, MA Howland, LR Goldfrank *et al.*) McGraw-Hill, New York, pp. 1712–1724

22 Borron SW, Stonebrook M, Reid F (2006) Efficacy of hydroxycobalamin for the treatment of acute cyanide poisoning in adult beagle dogs. *Clin Toxicol* **44(Suppl 1):**5–15.

23 Burrows GE, Tyrl RJ (2001) *Toxic Plants of North America*, 1st edn. Iowa State University Press, Ames.

24 Schmitz DG (2004) Toxicologic Problems. In: *Equine Internal Medicine*, 2nd edn. (eds SM Reed, WM Bayly, DC Sellon) Saunders, Philadelphia, pp. 1441–1512.

25 Galey FD (1990) Effect of an aqueous extract of black walnut (*Juglans nigra*) on isolated equine digital vessels. *Am J Vet Res* **151:**83–88.

26 Galey FD, Whiteley HE, Goetz TE *et al.* (1991) Black walnut (*Juglans nigra*) toxicosis: a model for equine laminitis. *J Comp Pathol* **104:**313–326.

27 Peroni JF, Harrison WE, Moore JN *et al.* (2005) Black walnut extrac-induced laminitis in horses is associated with heterogenous dysfunction of the laminar microvasculature. *Equine Vet J* **37:**546–551.

28 Adair HS, Goble DO, Schmidhammer JL *et al.* (2000) Laminar microvascular flow, measured by means of laser Doppler flowmetry, during prodromal stages of black walnut-induced laminitis in horses. *Am J Vet Res* **61:**862–868.

29 Fontaine GL, Belknap JK, Allen D *et al.* (2001) Expression of interleukin-1 beta in the digital laminae of horses in the prodromal stage of experimentally induced laminitis. *Am J Vet Res* **62:**714–720.

30 Waguespack RW, Cochran A, Belknap JK (2004) Expression of the cyclooxygenase isoforms in the prodromal stage of black walnut-induced laminitis in horses. *Am J Vet Res* **65:**1724–1729.

31 Waguespack RW, Kemppainen RJ, Cochran A *et al.* (2004) Increased expression of MAIL, a cytokine-associated nuclear protein, in the prodromal stage of black walnut-induced laminitis. *Equine Vet J* **36:**285–291.

32 Hurley DJ Parks RJ, Reber AJ *et al.* (2006) Dynamic changes in circulating leukocytes during the induction of equine laminitis with black walnut extract. *Vet Immunol Immunopathol* **110:**195–206.

33 Ralston SL, Rich VA (1983) Black walnut toxicosis in horses. *J Am Vet Med Assoc* **183:**1095.

34 Uhlinger C (1989) Black walnut toxicosis in ten horses. *J Am Vet Med Assoc* **195:**343–344.

35 Galey (2004) Black walnut. In: *Clinical Veterinary Toxicology*. (ed KH Plumlee) Mosby, St. Louis, pp. 425–427.

36 Stokes AM, Eades SC, Moore RM (2004) Pathophysiology and treatment of acute laminitis. In: *Equine Internal Medicine*, 2nd edn. (eds SM Reed, WM Bayly, DC Sellon) Saunders, Philadelphia, pp. 522–531.

37 Knight AP (1987) Locoweed poisoning. *Comp Contin Educ Pract Vet* **9:**F418–F420.

38 Boyer JD, Breeden DC, Brown DL (2002) Isolation, identification, and characterization of compounds from *Acer rubrum* capable of oxidizing equine erythrocytes. *Am J Vet Res* **63:**604–610.

39 Divers TJ, George LW, George JW 1(982) Hemolytic anemia in horses after the ingestion of red maple leaves. *J Am Vet Med Assoc* **180:**300–302.

40 George LW, Divers TJ, Mahaffey EA *et al.* (1982) Heinz body anemia and methemoglobinemia in ponies given red maple (*Acer rubrum*) leaves. *Vet Pathol* **19:**521–533.

41 Tennant B, Glickman LT, Mirro EJ *et al.* (1981) Acute hemolytic anemia, methemoglobinemia, and Heinz body formation associated with ingestion of red maple leaves by horses. *J Am Vet Med Assoc* **179:**143–150.

42 Corriher CA, Gibbons SE, Parviainen AKJ *et al.* (1999) Equine red maple leaf toxicosis. *Comp Contin Educ Pract Vet* **21:**74–80.

43 Stair EL, Edwards WC, Burrows GL *et al.* (1993) Suspected red maple (*Acer rubrum*) toxicosis with abortion in two Percheron mares. *Vet Hum Toxicol* **35**:229–230.

44 Plumlee KH (1991) Red maple toxicity in a horse. *Vet Hum Toxicol* **33**:66–67.

45 McConnico RS, Brownie CF (1992) The use of ascorbic acid in the treatment of 2 cases of red maple (*Acer rubru*m)-poisoned horses. *Cornell Vet* **82**:293–300.

46 Plumb DC (2005) *Plumb's Veterinary Drug Handbook*, 5th edn. PharmaVet, Stockholm pp. 45, 221, 273, 384, 407, 506, 512, 638, 675.

47 Galey FD, Holstedge DM, Plumlee KH *et al.* (1996) Diagnosis of oleander poisoning in livestock. *J Vet Diagn Invest* **8**:358–364.

48 Jortani SA, Helm RA, Valdes Jr R (1996) Inhibition of Na, K-ATPase by oleandrin and oleandrogenin, and their detection by digoxin immunoassays. *Clin Chem* **42**:1654–1658.

49 Siemens LM, Galey FD, Johnson B *et al.* (1995) The clinical, cardiac, and patholo-physiological effect of oleander toxicity in horses. *J Vet Intern Med* **9**:217

50 Smith PA, Aldridge BM, Kittleson MD 2003 Oleander toxicosis in a donkey. *J Vet Intern Med* **17**:111–114.

51 Eddleston M, Rajapakse S, Jayalath S *et al.* (2000) Anti-digoxin Fab fragments in cardiotoxicity induced by ingestion of yellow oleander: a randomized controlled trial. *Lancet* **355**:967–972.

52 Camphausen C, Haas NA, Mattke AC (2005) Successful treatment of oleander intoxication (cardiac glycosides) with digoxin-specific Fab antibody fragments in a 7-year-old child. *Z Kardiol* **94**:817–823.

53 Stegelmeier B (2004) Pyrrolizidine alkaloids. In: *Clinical Veterinary Toxicology*. (ed KH Plumlee) Mosby, St. Louis, pp. 370–377.

54 Lessard P, Wilson WD, Olander HJ *et al.* (1986) Clinicopathologic study of horses surviving pyrrolizidine alkaloid (*Senecio vulgaris*) toxicosis. *Am J Vet Res* **47**:1776–1780.

55 Giles CJ (1983) Outbreak of ragwort (*Senecio jacobea*) poisoning in horses. *Equine Vet J* **15**:248–250.

56 Pearson EG (1991) Liver failure attributable to pyrrolizidine alkaloid toxicosis and associated with inspiratory dyspnea in ponies: three cases (1982–1988). *J Am Vet Med Assoc* **198**:1651–1654.

57 Craig AM, Pearson EG, Meyer C *et al.* (1991) Clinicopathologic studies of tansy ragwort toxicosis in ponies: sequential serum and histopathological changes. *Equine Vet Sci* **11**:261–271.

58 Curran JM, Sutherland RJ, Peet RL (1996) A screening test for subclinical liver disease in horses affected by pyrrolizidine alkaloid toxicosis. *Aust Vet J* **74**:236–240.

59 Smetzer DL, Coppock RW, Ely RW *et al.* (1983) Cardiac effects of white snakeroot intoxication in horses. *Equine Pract* **5**:26–32.

60 Olson CT, Keller WC, Gerken DF *et al.* (1984) Suspected tremetol poisoning in horses. *J Am Vet Med Assoc* **185**:1001–1003.

61 Thompson LJ (1989) Depression and choke in a horse. *Vet Hum Toxicol* **31**:321–322.

62 Craig AM, Blythe LL, Roy DN *et al.* (1994) Detection and isolation of neurotoxins from yellow-star thistle (*Centaurea solstitialis*), the cause of equine nigropallidal encephalomalacia. In: *Plant-Associated Toxins: Agricultural, Phytochemical and Ecological Aspects*. (eds SM Colegate, PR Dorling) CAB International, Wallingford, pp. 257–262.

63 Robles M, Wang N, Choi BH (1997) Cytotoxic effects of repin, a principal sesquiterpene lactone of Russian knapweed. *J Neurosci Res* **47**:90–97.

64 Sanders SG, Tucker RL, Bagley RS *et al.* (2001) Magnetic resonance imaging features of equine nigropallidal encephalomalacia. *Vet Radiol Ultrasound* **42**:291–296.

65 Osweiler GD (2001) Mycotoxins. *Vet Clin N Am Equine Pract* **17**:547–566.

66 Greene HJ, Oehme FW (1976) A possible case of equine aflatoxicosis. *Clin Toxicol* **9**:251–254.

67 Angsubhakorn S, Poomvises P, Romruen K *et al.* (1981) Aflatoxicosis in horses. *J Am Vet Med Assoc* **178**:274–278.

68 Vesonder R, Haliburton J, Stubblefield R *et al.* (1991) *Aspergillus flavu*s and aflatoxins B1, B2 and M1 in corn associated with equine death. *Arch Environ Contam Toxicol* **20**:151–153.

69 Schurg WA, Noon TN (1979) Experimentally induced aflatoxicosis in mature horses fed naturally contaminated cotton products. In: *Proc 6th Equine Nutrition Physiology Symposium*, College Station, pp. 72–73

70 Bortell R, Asquith RL, Edds GT *et al.* (1983) Acute experimentally induced aflatoxicosis in the weanling pony. *Am J Vet Res* **44**:2110–2113.

71 Cysewski SJ, Pier AC, Baetz AL *et al.* (1982) Experimental equine aflatoxicosis. *Toxicol Appl Pharm* **65**:354–365.

72 Casteel SW (2002) Alfatoxicosis. In: *The 5-Minute Veterinary Consult: Equine*. (eds CM Brown, JJ Bertone) Lippincott Williams and Wilkins, Baltimore, pp. 60–61.

73 Divers TJ (2002) Toxic hepatopathy. In: *The 5-Minute Veterinary Consult: Equine*. (eds CM Brown, JJ Bertone) Lippincott Williams and Wilkins, Baltimore, pp. 1062–1063.

74 Witonsky SG (2002) Hepatic encephalopathy. In: *The 5-Minute Veterinary Consult: Equine*. (eds CM Brown, JJ Bertone) Lippincott Williams and Wilkins, Baltimore, pp. 500–501.

75 Evans TJ, Rottinghaus GE, Casteel SW (2004) Ergot. In: *Clinical Veterinary Toxicology*. (ed KH Plumlee) Mosby, St. Louis, pp. 239–243.

76 Cheeke PR (1998) *Natural Toxicants in Feeds, Forages, and Poisonous Plants*, 2nd edn. Interstate Publishers, Danville, pp. 88–92.

77 Evans TJ, Rottinghaus GE, Casteel SW (2004) Fescue. In: *Clinical Veterinary Toxicology*. (ed KH Plumlee) Mosby, St. Louis, pp. 243–250.

78 Stickland JR, Cross DL, Birrenkott GP *et al.* (1994) Effect of ergovaline, loline, and dopamine antagonists on rat pituitary cell prolactin release in vitro. *Am J Vet Res* **55**:716–721.

79 Rowell PP, Larson BT (1999) Ergocryptine and other ergot alkaloids stimulate the release of [3H]dopamine from rat striatal synaptomes. *J Anim Sci* **77**:1800–1806.

80 Blodgett DJ (2001) Fescue toxicosis. *Vet Clin N Am Equine Pract* **17**:567–577.

81 Cross DL (1997) Fescue toxicosis in horses. In: *Neotyphodium/Grass Interactions*. (eds CW Bacon, NS Hill) Plenum Press, New York, pp. 289–309.

82 Lyons PC, Plattner RD, Bacon CW (1986) Occurrence of peptide and clavine ergot alkaloids in tall fescue grass. *Science* **232**:487–489.

83 Boosinger TR, Brendemeuhl JP, Bransby DL *et al.* (1995) Prolonged gestation, decreased triiodothyronine concentration, and thyroid gland histomorphometric features in newborn foals of mares grazing *Acremonium coenophialum*-infected fescue. *Am J Vet Res* **56**:66–69.

84 Riet-Correa F, Mendez MC, Schild AL *et al.* (1988) Agalactia, reproductive problems and neonatal mortality in horses associated with the ingestion of *Claviceps purpurea*. *Aust Vet J* **65**:192–193.

85 Brendenmuehl JP (1997) Reproductive aspects of fescue toxicosis. In: *Current Therapy in Equine Medicine*, 4th edn. (ed NE Robinson) WB Saunders, Philadelphia, pp. 571–573.

86 Green EM, Raisbeck MF (1997) Fescue toxicosis. In: *Current Therapy in Equine Medicine*, 4th edn. (ed NE Robinson) WB Saunders, Philadelphia, pp. 670–673

87 Poppenga RH, Mostrom MS, Hascheck WM *et al.* (1984) Mare agalactia, placental thickening, and high foal mortality associated with the grazing of tall fescue: a case report. *Proc Am Assoc Vet Lab Diagnosticians*, Fort Worth, pp. 325–336.

88 Redmond LM, Cross DL, Strickland JR *et al.* (1994) Efficacy of domperidone and sulpiride as treatments for fescue toxicosis in horses. *Am J Vet Res* **55**:722–729.

89 Bennett-Wimbush K, Loch WE (1998) A preliminary study of the efficacy of fluphenazine as a treatment for fescue toxicosis in gravid pony mares. *J Equine Vet Sci* **18**:169–174.

90 Green EM, Loch WE, Messer NT (1991) Maternal and fetal effects of endophyte fungus-infected fescue. *Proc Am Assoc Equine Practitnrs* **37**:29–44.

91 Marasas WFO, Kellerman TS, Gelderblom WCA *et al.* (1988) Leukoencephalomalacia in a horse induced by fumonisin B1 isolated from *Fusarium moniliforme*. *Onderstepoort J Vet Res* **55**:197–203.

92 Kellerman TS, Marasas WFO, Thiel PG *et al.* (1990) Leukoencephalomalacia in two horses induced by oral dosing of fumonisin B1. *Onderstepoort J Vet Res* **57**:269–275.

93 Smith GW (2007) Fumonisins. In: *Veterinary Toxicology: Basic and Clinical Principles*. (ed RC Gupta) Academic Press, New York, pp. 983–996.

94 Wilson TM, Ross PF, Rice LG *et al.* (1990) Fumonisin B1 levels associated with an epizootic of equine leukoencephalomalacia. *J Vet Diagn Invest* **2**:213–216.

95 Ross PF, Rice LG, Reagor JC *et al.* (1991) Fumonisin B1 concentration in feeds from 45 confirmed equine leukoencephalomalacia cases. *J Vet Diagn Invest* **3**:238–241

96 Ramasamy S, Wang E, Hennig B *et al.* (1995) Fumonisin B1 alters spingolipid metabolism and disrupts the barrier function of endothelial cells in culture. *Toxicol Pharmacol* **133**:343–348.

97 Smith GW, Constable PD, Foreman JH *et al.* (2002) Cardiovascular changes associated with intravenous administration of fumonisin B1 in horses. *Am J Vet Res* **63**:538–545.

98 Ross PF, Ledet AE, Owens DL *et al.* (1993) Experimental equine leukoencephalomalacia, toxic hepatosis, and encephalopathy caused by corn naturally contaminated with fumonisins. *J Vet Diagn Invest* **5**:69–74.

99 Smith GW, Constable PD (2004) Fumonisin. In: *Clinical Veterinary Toxicology*. (ed KH Plumlee) Mosby, St. Louis, pp. 250–254.

100 Wang E, Ross PF, Wilson TM *et al.* (1992) Increases in serum sphingosine and sphinganine and decreases in complex sphingolipids in ponies given feed containing fumonisins, mycotoxins produced by *Fusarium moniliforme*. *J Nut* **122**:1706–1716

101 Carson TL (2002) Leukoencephalomalacia (ELEM). In: *The 5-Minute Veterinary Consult: Equine*. (eds CM Brown, JJ Bertone) Lippincott Williams and Wilkins, Baltimore, pp. 624–625.

102 Sockett DC, Baker JC, Stowe CM (1982) Slaframine (*Rhizotonia leguminicola*) intoxication in horses. *J Am Vet Med Assoc* **181**:606.

103 Hagler WM, Behlow RF (1981) Salivary syndrome in horses: identification of slaframine in red clover hay. *Appl Environ Microbiol* **42**:1067–1073.

104 Hunt LD, Blythe L, Holtan DW (1983) Ryegrass staggers in ponies fed processed ryegrass straw. *J Am Vet Med Assoc* **182**:285–286.

105 Munday BL, Monkhouse IM, Gallagher RT (1985) Intoxication of horses by lolitrem B in ryegrass seed cleanings. *Aust Vet J* **62**:207.

106 Plumlee KH, Galey FD (1994) Neurotoxic mycotoxins: a review of fungal toxins that cause neurological disease in large animals. *J Vet Intern Med* **8**:49–54.

107 Dalziel JE, Finch SC, Dunlop J (2005) The fungal neurotoxin lolitrem B inhibits the functioning of human large conductance calcium-activated potassium channels. *Toxicol Lett* **155**:421–426.

108 Gallagher RT, Hawkes AD (1986) The potent tremorgenic neurotoxins lolitrem B and aflatrem: a comparison of the tremor response in mice. *Experientia* **42**:823–825.

109 Poppenga RH (2002) Blue-green algae toxicosis. In: *The 5-Minute Veterinary Consult: Equine*. (eds CM Brown, JJ Bertone) Lippincott Williams and Wilkins, Baltimore, pp. 184–185.

110 Puschner B, Humbert JF (2007) Cyanobacterial (blue-green algae) toxins. In: *Veterinary Toxicology: Basic and Clinical Principles*. (ed RC Gupta) Academic Press, New York, pp. 714–724.

111 Beasley VR, Cook WO, Dahlem AM *et al.* (1989) Algae intoxication in livestock and waterfowl. *Vet Clin N Am: Food Anim Pract* **5**:345–361.

112 Schoeb TR, Panciera RJ (1978) Blister beetle poisoning in horses. *J Am Vet Med Assoc* **173**:75–76.

113 Ray AC, Kyle ALG, Murphy MJ *et al.* (1989) Etiologic agents, incidence and improved diagnostic methods of catharidin toxicosis in horses. *Am J Vet Res* **50**:187–191.

114 Schmitz DG (1989) Cantharidin toxicosis in horses. *J Vet Intern Med* **3**:208–215.

115 Helman RG, Edwards WC (1997) Clinical features of blister beetle poisoning in equids: 70 cases (1983–1996). *J Am Vet Med Assoc* **211**:1018–1021.

116 Stair EL, Plumlee KH (2004) Blister beetles. In: *Clinical Veterinary Toxicology*. (ed KH Plumlee) Mosby, St. Louis, pp. 101–103.

117 Stair EL (2002) Cantharidin toxicosis. In: *The 5-Minute Veterinary Consult: Equine*. (eds CM Brown, JJ Bertone) Lippincott Williams and Wilkins, Baltimore, pp. 214–215.

118 Peterson ME (2004) Reptiles. In: *Clinical Veterinary Toxicology*. (ed KH Plumlee) Mosby, St. Louis, pp. 104–111.

119 Talcott PA, Peterson M (2002) Snake envenomation. In: *The 5-Minute Veterinary Consult: Equine*. (eds CM Brown, JJ Bertone) Lippincott Williams and Wilkins, Baltimore, pp. 994–997.

120 Dickinson CE, Traub-Dargatz JL, Dargatz DA *et al.* (1996) Rattlesnake venom poisoning in horses: 32 cases (1973–1993). *J Am Vet Med Assoc* **208**:1866–1871.

121 Galey FD (2001) Botulism in the horse. *Vet Clin N Am Equine Pract* **17**:579–588.

122 Simpson LL (2004) Identification of the major steps in botulinum toxin action. *Ann Rev Pharmacol Toxicol* **44**:167–193.

123 Whitlock RH, Adams S (2006) Equine botulism. *Clin Tech Equine Pract* **5**:37–42.

124 Kinde H, Bettey RL, Ardans A *et al.* (1991) *Clostridium botulinum* type-C intoxication associated with consumption of processed alfalfa hay cubes in horses. *J Am Vet Med Assoc* **199**:742–746.

125 Hunter HC, Miller JK, Poxton IR (1999) The association of *Clostridium botulinum* type C with equine grass sickness: a toxicoinfection? *Equine Vet J* **31**:492–499.

126 Bernard W, Divers TJ, Whitlock RH *et al.* (1987) Botulism as a sequel to open castration in a horse. *J Am Vet Med Assoc* **191**:73–74.

127 Mitten LA, Hinchcliff KW, Holcombe SJ *et al.* (1994) Mechanical ventilation and management of botulism secondary to an injection abscess in an adult horse. *Equine Vet J* **26**:420–423.

128 Rocke TE (1993) *Clostridium botulinum* In: *Pathogenesis of Bacterial Infections*, 2nd edn. (eds CL Gyles, CO Thoen) Iowa State University Press, Ames, pp. 86–96.

129 Thomas RJ, Rosenthal DV, Rogers RJ (1988) A *Clostridium botulinum* type B vaccine for the prevention of shaker foal syndrome. *Aust Vet J* **65**:78–80.

130 Wilkins PA, Palmer JE (2003) Mechanical ventilation in foals less than 6 months of age: 30 cases (1989–2002). *J Vet Intern Med* **17**:708–712.

131 Whitlock RH, Buckley C (1997) Botulism. *Vet Clin N Am Equine Pract* **13**:107–128.

132 Albretson JC (2004) Iron. In: *Clinical Veterinary Toxicology*. (ed KH Plumlee) Mosby, St. Louis, pp. 202–204.

133 Divers TJ, Warner A, Vaala WE *et al.* (1983) Toxic hepatic failure in newborn foals. *J Am Vet Med Assoc* **183**:1407–1413.

134 Mullaney TP, Brown CM (1988) Iron toxicity in neonatal foals. *Equine Vet J* **20**:119–124.

135 National Research Council (US) (1989) *Nutrient Requirements of Horses*, 5th edn. National Academy Press, Washington DC, pp. 2–31.

136 LaVoie JP, Teuscher E (1993) Massive iron overload and liver fibrosis resembling haemochromatosis in a racing pony. *Equine Vet J* **25**:552–554.

137 Pearson EG, Hedstrom OR, Poppenga RH (1994) Hepatic cirrhosis and hemochromatosis in three horses. *J Am Vet Med Assoc* **204**:1053–1056.

138 Arnbjerg J (1981) Poisoning of animals due to oral application of iron; with a description of a case in a horse. *Nord Vet Med* **33**:71–76.

139 Edens LM, Robertson JL, Feldman BF (1993) Cholestatic hepatopathy, thrombocytopenia and lymphopenia associated with iron toxicity in a Thoroughbred gelding. *Equine Vet J* **25**:81–84.

140 Pearson EG, Andreason CB (2001) Effect of oral administration of excessive iron in adult ponies. *J Am Vet Med Assoc* **218**:400–404.

141 Elfenbein JR, Giguère S, Meyer SK *et al.* (2010) The effects of deferoxamine mesylate on iron elimination after blood transfusion in neonatal foals. *J Vet Intern Med* **24**:1475–1482

142 Casteel SW (2001) Metal toxicosis in horses. *Vet Clin N Am Equine Pract* **17**:517–527.

143 Plumb DC (2005) Deferoxamine. In: *Plumb's Veterinary Drug Handbook*, 5th edn. PharmaVet, Stockholm, pp. 221–222.

144 Egan DA, O'Cuill T (1970) Cumulative lead poisoning in horses in a mining area contaminated with galena. *Vet Rec* **86**:736–738.

145 Schmitt N, Brown G, Devlin EL *et al.* (1971) Lead poisoning in horses: an environmental health hazard. *Arch Environ Health* **23**:185–195.

146 Aronson AL (1972) Lead poisoning in cattle and horses following long-term exposure to lead. *Am J Vet Res* **33**:627–629.

147 Knight HD, Burau RG (1973) Chronic lead poisoning in horses. *J Am Vet Med Assoc* **162**:781–786.

148 Sojka JE, Hope W, Pearson D (1996) Lead toxicosis in two horses: similarity to equine degenerative lower motor neuron disease. *J Vet Intern Med* **10**:420–423.

149 Kruger K, Saulez MN, Neser JA *et al.* (2008) Acute lead intoxication in a pregnant mare. *J S Afr Vet Assoc* **79**:50–53.

150 Dollahite JW, Younger RL, Crookshank HR *et al.* (1978) Chronic lead poisoning in horses. *Am J Vet Res* **39**:961–964.

151 Garza A, Vega R, Soto E (2006) Cellular mechanisms of lead neurotoxicity. *Med Sci Monit* **12**:RA57–RA65.

152 Mateo R, Beyer WN, Spann JW *et al.* (2003) Relationship between oxidative stress, pathology, and behavioral signs of lead poisoning in mallards. *J Toxicol Environ Health* A **66**:1371–1389.

153 Saxena G, Flora SJS (2004) Lead-induced oxidative stress and hematological alterations and their response to combined administration of calcium disodium EDTA with a thiol chelator in rats. *J Biochem Mol Toxicol* **18**:221–233.

154 Thompson LJ (1992) Heavy metal toxicosis. In: *Current Therapy in Equine Medicine*, 3rd edn. (ed NE Robinson) WB Saunders, Philadelphia, pp. 363–366.

155 Gwaltney-Brant (2004) Lead. In: *Clinical Veterinary Toxicology.* (ed KH Plumlee) Mosby, St. Louis, pp. 204–210.

156 Markel MD, Dyer RM, Hattel AL (1984) Acute renal failure associated with the application of a mercuric blister in a horse. *J Am Vet Med Assoc* **185**:92–94.

157 Guglick MA, MacAllister CG, Chandra Edwards WC *et al.* (1995) Mercury toxicosis caused by ingestion of a blistering compound in a horse. *J Am Vet Med Assoc* **206**:210–214.

158 Chiang WK (2001) Mercury. In: *Clinical Toxicology.* (eds MD Ford, KA Delaney, LJ Ling *et al.*) WB Saunders, Philadelphia, pp. 737–743.

159 Poppenga RH (2002) Mercury toxicosis. In: *The 5-Minute Veterinary Consult: Equine.* (eds CM Brown, JJ Bertone) Lippincott Williams and Wilkins, Baltimore, pp. 662–663.

160 Raisbeck MF (2002) Selenium toxicosis. In: *The 5-Minute Veterinary Consult: Equine.* (eds CM Brown, JJ Bertone) Lippincott Williams and Wilkins, Baltimore, pp. 956–957.

161 Kollias-Baker C, Cox K (2004) Non-steroidal anti-inflammatory drugs. In: *Equine Clinical Pharmacology.* (eds JJ Bertone, LJI Horspool) Saunders, Edinburgh, pp. 247–266.

162 MacAllister GC, Morgan SJ, Borne AT *et al.* (1993) Comparison of adverse effects of phenylbutazone, flunixin meglumine, and ketoprofen in horses. *J Am Vet Med Assoc* **202**:71–77.

163 Roder JD (2004) Analgesics In: *Clinical Veterinary Toxicology.* (ed KH Plumlee) Mosby, St. Louis, pp. 282–284.

164 Murray MJ (2002) Non-steroidal anti-inflammatory drug (NSAID) toxicity. In: *The 5-Minute Veterinary Consult: Equine.* (eds CM Brown, JJ Bertone) Lippincott Williams and Wilkins, Baltimore, pp. 694–697.

165 Snow DH, Douglas TA, Thompson H *et al.* (1981) Phenylbutazone toxicosis in equidae: a biochemical and pathophysiologic study. *Am J Vet Res* **42**:1754–1759.

166 Hall J O 2001 Toxic feed constituents in the horse. *Vet Clin N Am Equine Pract* **17**:479–489

167 Aleman M, Magdesian KG, Peterson TS *et al.* (2007) Salinomycin toxicosis in horses. *J Am Vet Med Assoc* **230**:1822–1826.

168 Van Vleet JF, Amstutz HE, Rebar HA (1985) Effects of pretreatment with selenium-vitamin E on monension toxicosis in cattle. *Am J Vet Res* **46**:2221–2228.

169 Rollinson J, Taylor FGR, Chesney J (1987) Salinomycin poisoning in horses. *Vet Rec* **121**:126–128.

170 Muylle E, Vandenhende C, Oyaert W *et al.* (1981) Delayed monesin sodium toxicity in horses. *Equine Vet J* **12**:107–108.

171 Peek SF, Marques FD, Morgan J *et al.* (2004) Atypical acute monensin toxicosis and delayed cardiomyopathy in Belgian draft horses. *J Vet Intern Med* **18**:761–764.

172 Begg LM, Hoffman KL, Begg AP (2006) Serum and plasma cardiac troponin I concentrations in clinically normal Thoroughbreds in training in Australia. *Aust Vet J* **84**:336–337.

173 Hughes KJ, Hoffmann KL, Hodgson DR (2009) Long-term assessment of horses and ponies post exposure to monensin sodium in commercial feed. *Equine Vet J* **41**:47–52.

174 Plumlee KH (2001) Pesticide toxicosis in the horse. *Vet Clin N Am Equine Pract* **17**:491–500.

175 Talcott PA (2002) Organophosphate (OP) and carbamate insecticide toxicosis. In: *The 5-Minute Veterinary Consult: Equine.* (eds CM Brown, JJ Bertone) Lippincott Williams and Wilkins, Baltimore, pp. 728–729.

176 Meerdink GL (2004) Anticholinesterase insecticides. In: *Clinical Veterinary Toxicology.* (ed KH Plumlee) Mosby, St. Louis, pp. 178–180.

177 Fikes JD (1990) Organophosphorus and carbamate insecticides. *Vet Clin N Am Small Anim Pract* **20**:353–368.

178 Geor RJ, Becker RL, Kanara EW *et al.* (1992) Toxicosis in horses after ingestion of hoary alyssum. *J Am Vet Med Assoc* **201**:63–67.

179 Anderson GA, Mount ME, Vrins AA *et al.* (1983) Fatal acorn poisoning in a horse: pathologic findings and diagnostic considerations. *J Am Vet Med Assoc* **182**:1105–1110.

180 Vetter J (2004) Poison hemlock (*Conium maculatum* L.). *Food Chem Toxicol* **42**:1373–1382.

181 Krook L, Wasserman RH, Shively JN *et al.* (1975) Hypercalcemia and calcinosis in Florida horses: implication of the shrub, *Cestrum diurnum*, as the causative agent. *Cornell Vet* **65**:26–56.

182 Carson TL (2004) Gases. In: *Clinical Veterinary Toxicology.* (ed KH Plumlee) Mosby, St. Louis, pp. 155–161.

183 Brumbaugh GW (2002) Aminoglycoside toxicosis. In: *The 5-Minute Veterinary Consult: Equine.* (eds CM Brown, JJ Bertone) Lippincott Williams and Wilkins, Baltimore, pp. 84–8.

184 Klein L, Hopkins J (1981) Behavioral and cardiorespiratory responses to 4-aminopyridine in healthy awake horses. *Am J Vet Res* **42**:1655–1657.

185 Plumb DC (2005) Amphotericn B. In: *Plumb's Veterinary Drug Handbook*, 5th edn. PharmaVet, Stockholm, pp. 45–50.

186 Kore AM (2002) Anticoagulant rodenticide toxicosis. In: *The 5-Minute Veterinary Consult: Equine.* (eds CM Brown, JJ Bertone) Lippincott Williams and Wilkins, Baltimore, pp. 120–121.

187 Poppenga RH (2002) Arsenic toxicosis. In: *The 5-Minute Veterinary Consult: Equine.* (eds CM Brown, JJ Bertone) Lippincott Williams and Wilkins, Baltimore, pp. 132–133.

188 Pickrell JA Oehme F Mannala SA (2004) Tropane alkaloids. In: *Clinical Veterinary Toxicology.* (ed KH Plumlee) Mosby, St. Louis, pp. 381–382.

189 Phillips SD (2005) Fumigants. In: *Critical Care Toxicology: Diagnosis and Management of the Critically Poisoned Patient.* (eds J Brent, KL Wallace, KK Burkhart *et al.*) Elsevier Mosby, St. Louis, pp. 909–915.

190 Spoo W (2001) Industrial chemicals and the horse. *Vet Clin N Am Equine Pract* **17**:501–516.

191 Osweiler GD Carson TL Buck WB *et al.* (1985) Chlorates. In: *Clinical and Diagnostic Veterinary Toxicology*, 3rd edn. Kendall-Hunt Publishing, Dubuque, pp. 251–252.

192 Ensley S (2004) Organochlorine insecticides. In: *Clinical Veterinary Toxicology.* (ed KH Plumlee) Mosby, St. Louis, pp. 186–188.

193 Thompson LJ (2002) Cyanide toxicosis. In: *The 5-Minute Veterinary Consult: Equine*. (eds CM Brown, JJ Bertone) Lippincott Williams and Wilkins, Baltimore, pp. 304–305.

194 Plumb DC (2005) Docusate sodium. In: *Plumb's Veterinary Drug Handbook*, 5th edn. PharmaVet, Stockholm, pp. 273–274.

195 Osweiler GD Carson TL Buck WB *et al.* (1985) (Fluorides). In: *Clinical and Diagnostic Veterinary Toxicology*, 3rd edn. Kendall-Hunt Publishing, Dubuque, pp. 183–188.

196 Plumb DC (2005) Heparin sodium. In: *Plumb's Veterinary Drug Handbook*, 5th edn. PharmaVet, Stockholm, pp. 384–387.

197 Plumb DC (2005) Protamine sulfate. In: *Plumb's Veterinary Drug Handbook*, 5th edn. PharmaVet, Stockholm, pp. 675–677.

198 Plumb DC (2005) Imidocarb dipropinate. In: *Plumb's Veterinary Drug Handbook*, 5th edn. PharmaVet, Stockholm, pp. 407–408.

199 Morgan SE (2004) Iodine. In: *Plumb's Veterinary Drug Handbook*, 5th edn. PharmaVet, Stockholm, pp. 200–202.

200 Plumb DC (2005) Methocarbamol. In: *Plumb's Veterinary Drug Handbook*, 5th edn. PharmaVet, Stockholm, pp.506–507.

201 Osweiler GC (1996) *Insecticides and Molluscacides. National Veterinary Medical Series: Toxicology*. Williams and Wilkins Philadelphia, pp. 231–255.

202 Poppenga RH (2002) Nitrate/nitrite toxicosis. In: *The 5-Minute Veterinary Consult: Equine*. (eds CM Brown, JJ Bertone) Lippincott Williams and Wilkins, Baltimore, pp. 692–693.

203 Poppenga RH (2002) Pentachlorophenol. In: *The 5-Minute Veterinary Consult: Equine*. (eds CM Brown, JJ Bertone) Lippincott Williams and Wilkins, Baltimore, pp. 764–765.

204 DiPietro JA, Todd KS J (1987) Anthelmintics used in the treatment of parasitic infections of horses *Vet Clin N Am Equine Pract* 3:1–14.

205 Easterwood L, Chaffin MK, Marsh PS *et al.* (2010) Phosphine intoxication following oral exposure of horses to aluminum phosphide-treated feed. *J Am Vet Med Assoc* 236:446–450.

206 Cienki JJ (2004) Non-anticoagulant rodenticides. In: *Clinical Toxicology*. (eds MD Ford, KA Delaney, LJ Ling *et al.*) WB Saunders, Philadelphia, pp. 854–861.

207 Plumb DC (2005) Piperazine. In: *Plumb's Veterinary Drug Handbook*, 5th edn. PharmaVet, Stockholm, pp. 638–640.

208 Dorman DC, Haschek WM (1991) Fatal propylene glycol toxicosis in a horse. *J Am Vet Med Assoc* 198:1643–1644.

209 Lloyd KCK, Harrison I, Tulleners E (1985) Reserpine toxicosis in a horse. *J Am Vet Med Assoc* 186:980–981.

210 Parton KH (2002) Sodium fluoroacetate. In: *Clinical Veterinary Toxicology*. (ed KH Plumlee) Mosby, St. Louis, pp. 451–454.

211 Lilley CW (1985) Strychnine poisoning in a horse. *Equine Pract* 7:7–8.

212 Roder JD (2002) Antimicrobials. In: *Clinical Veterinary Toxicology*. (ed KH Plumlee) Mosby, St. Louis, pp. 293–299.

213 Gunson DE, Kowalczyk DF, Shoop CR *et al.* (1982) Environmental zinc and cadmium pollution associated with generalized osteochondrosis, osteoporosis, and nephrocalcinosis in horses. *J Am Vet Med Assoc* 180:295–299.

214 Messer NT (1981) Tibiotarsal effusion associated with chronic zinc intoxication in three horses. *J Am Vet Med Assoc* 178:294–297.

CHAPTER 11: MONITORING

1 Morris DD (1996) Alterations in the leukogram. In: *Large Animal Internal Medicine*, 2nd edn. (ed BP Smith) Mosby, St. Louis, pp. 480–488.

2 Morris DD (1996) Alterations in the erythron. In: *Large Animal Internal Medicine*, 2nd edn. (ed BP Smith) Mosby, St. Louis, pp. 473–479.

3 Johnston JK, Morris DD (1996) Alterations in blood proteins. In: *Large Animal Internal Medicine*, 2nd edn. (ed BP Smith) Mosby, St. Louis, pp. 489–497.

4 Magdesian KG (2004) Monitoring the critically ill equine patient. *Vet Clin N Am Equine Pract* 20:11–39.

5 Van den Berghe G, Wouters P, Weekers F *et al.* (2001) Intensive insulin therapy in the critically ill patients. *N Engl J Med* 345:1359–1367.

6 Moore JN, Garner HE, Shapland J E *et al.* (1980) Lactic acidosis and arterial hypoxemia during sublethal endotoxemia in conscious ponies. *Am J Vet Res* 41:1696–1698.

7 Magdesian KG, Fielding CL, Rhodes DM *et al.* (2006) Changes in central venous pressure and blood lactate concentration in response to acute blood loss in horses. *J Am Vet Med Assoc* 229:1458–1462.

8 Kitchen H, Rossdale PD (1975) Metabolic profiles of newborn foals. *J Reprod Fertil Suppl* 23:705–707.

9 Grosenbaugh DA, Gadawski JE, Muir WW (1998) Evaluation of a portable clinical analyzer in a veterinary hospital setting. *J Am Vet Med Assoc* 213:691–694.

10 Klein LV, Soma LR, Nann LE (1999) Accuracy and precision of the portable StatPal II and the laboratory-based NOVA Stat Profile 1 for measurement of pH, PCO2 and PO2 in equine blood. *Vet Surg* 28:67–76.

11 Madigan JE, Thomas WP (1984) Cardiopulmonary function in normal neonatal foals from 1–14 days of age. In: *Proc 4th Ann Am Coll Vet Intern Med Forum*, Washington, DC, pp.101–116.

12 Stewart JH, Rose RJ, Barko AM (1984) Respiratory studies in foals from birth to seven days old. *Equine Vet J* 16:323–328.

13 Rose RJ, Rossdale PD, Leadon DP (1982) Blood gas and acid-base status in spontaneously delivered, term-induced and induced premature foals. *J Reprod Fertil Suppl* 32:521–528.

14 Rose RJ, Ilkiw JE, Martin ICA (1979) Blood-gas, acid-base and haematological values in horses during an endurance ride. *Equine Vet J* 11:56–59.

15 Aguilera-Tejero E, Estepa JC, Lopez I *et al.* (1998) Arterial blood gases and acid-base balance in healthy young and aged horses. *Equine Vet J* 30:352–354.

16 Madigan JE, Thomas WP, Backus KQ *et al.* (1992) Mixed venous blood gases in recumbent and upright positions in foals from birth to 14 days of age. *Equine Vet J* **24**:399–401.

17 Morris DD (1996) Collection and submission of samples for cytology and hematology. In: *Large Animal Internal Medicin*e, 2nd edn. (ed BP Smith) Mosby, St. Louis, pp. 470–472.

18 Dallap BD (2004) Coagulation in the equine critical care patient. *Vet Clin N Am Equine Pract* **20**:231–251.

19 Donahue SM, Otto CM (2005) Thromboelastography: a tool for measuring hypercoagulability, hypo-coagulability, and fibrinolysis. *J Vet Emerg Crit Care* **15**:9–16.

20 Knottenbelt DC (2003) Differential diagnosis of polyuria/polydipsia. In: *Current Therapy in Equine Medicine*, 5th edn. (ed NE Robinson WB Saunders, Philadelphia, pp. 828–831.

21 Carlson GP (1996) Clinical chemistry tests. In: *Large Animal Internal Medicin*e, 2nd edn. (ed BP Smith) Mosby, St. Louis, pp. 441–469.

22 Shoemaker WC (2000) Invasive and noninvasive monitoring. In: *Textbook of Critical Care*, 4th edn. (eds WC Shoemaker, SM Ayres, A Grenvik *et al.*) WB Saunders, Philadelphia, pp. 74–92.

23 Franco RM, Ousey JC, Cash RS *et al.* (1986) Study of arterial blood pressure in newborn foals using an electronic sphygmomanometer. *Equine Vet J* **18**:475–478.

24 Vaala WE, House JK (2002) Supportive care of the abnormal newborn. In: *Large Animal Internal Medicine*, 2nd edn. (ed BP Smith) Mosby, St. Louis, pp. 294–302.

25 Holdstock NB, Ousey JC, Rossdale PD (1998) Glomerular filtration rate, effective renal plasma flow, blood pressure and pulse rate in the equine neonate during the first 10 days post partum. *Equine Vet J* **30**:335–343.

26 Thomas WP, Madigan JE, Backus KQ *et al.* (1987) Systemic and pulmonary haemodynamics in normal neonatal foals. *J Reprod Fertil Suppl* **35**:623–628.

27 Johnson JH, Garner HE, Hutcheson DP (1976) Ultrasonic measurement of arterial blood pressure in conditioned Thoroughbreds. *Equine Vet J* **8**:55–57.

28 Reef VB, McGuirk SM (2002) Diseases of the cardiovascular system. In: *Large Animal Internal Medicine*, 2nd edn. (ed BP Smith) Mosby, St. Louis, pp. 443–478.

29 Steffey EP, Dunlop CI, Farver TB *et al.* (1987) Cardiovascular and respiratory measurements in awake and isoflurane-anesthetized horses. *Am J Vet Res* **48**:7–12.

30 Bonagura JD, Muir WW (1991) The cardiovascular system. In: *Equine Anesthesia: Monitoring and Emergency Therapy.* (eds WW Muir, JAE Hubbell) Mosby, St Louis, pp. 39–104.

31 Hall LW, Nigam JM (1975) Papers and articles measurement of central venous pressure in horses. *Vet Rec* **97**:66–69.

32 Hallowell GD, Corley KT (2005) Use of lithium dilution and pulse contour analysis cardiac output determination in anaesthetized horses: a clinical evaluation. *Vet Anaesth Analg* **32**:201–211.

33 Giguere S, Bucki E, Adin DB *et al.* (2005) Cardiac output measurement by partial carbon dioxide rebreathing, 2-dimensional echocardiography, and lithium-dilution method in anesthetized neonatal foals. *J Vet Intern Med* **19**:737–743.

CHAPTER 12: FLUID THERAPY

1 Silverstein DC, Aldrich J, Haskins SC *et al.* (2005) Assessment of changes in blood volume in response to resuscitative fluid administration in dogs. *J Vet Emerg Crit Care* **15**:185–192.

2 Hardy J (2000) Critical care. In: *Equine Internal Medicine*, 2nd edn. (eds SM Reed, WM Bayly, DC Sellon) WB Saunders, Philadelphia, p. 273.

3 DiBartola SP (2000) Introduction to fluid therapy. In: *Fluid Therapy in Small Animal Practice*, 2nd edn. (ed SP DiBartola) WB Saunders, Philadelphia, p. 265.

4 Johansson A M, Gardner S Y, Jones S L *et al.* (2003) Hypomagnesemia in hospitalized horses. *J Vet Intern Med* **17**:860–867.

4a Corley K (2008) Fluid therapy. In: *The Equine Hospital Manual.* (eds K Corley, J Stephen) Blackwell Publishing, Oxford.

5 DiBartola SP (2000) Disorders of sodium and water. In: *Fluid Therapy in Small Animal Practice*, 2nd edn. (ed SP DiBartola) WB Saunders, Philadelphia, p. 45.

6 Sterns RH, Spital A, Clark EC (1996) Disorders of water balance. In: *Fluids and Electrolytes*. (eds JP Kokko, RL Tannen) WB Saunders, Philadelphia, p. 63.

7 Oliveira RP, Velasco I, Soriano F *et al.* (2002) Clinical review: hypertonic saline resuscitation in sepsis. *Crit Care* **6**:418–423.

8 Loomis WH, Namiki S, Hoyt DB *et al.* (2001) Hypertonicity rescues T cells from suppression by trauma-induced anti-inflmmatory mediators. *Am J Physiol-Cell Ph* **281**:C840–848.

9 Lescot T, Degos V, Zouaoui A *et al.* (2006) Opposed effects of hypertonic saline on contusions and noncontused brain tissue in patients with severe traumatic brain injury. *Crit Care Med* **34**:3029–3033.

10 Hallowell GD, Corley KT (2006) Preoperative administration of hydroxyethyl starch or hypertonic saline to horses with colic. *J Vet Intern Med* **20**:980–986.

11 Munar F, Ferrer AM, de Nadal M *et al.* (2000) Cerebral hemodynamic effects of 7.2% hypertonic saline in patients with head injury and raised intracranial pressure. *J Neurotraum* **17**:41–51.

12 van Eijk LT, Nooteboom A, Hendriks T *et al.* (2006) Plasma obtained during human endotoxemia increases endothelial albumin permeability in vitro. *Shock* **25**:358–362.

13 Fishel R S, Are C, Barbul A 2003 Vessel injury and capillary leak. *Crit Care Med* **31(Suppl)**:S502–511.

13a Patel A. Waheed U, Brett SJ (2013) Randomised trials of 6% tetrastarch (hydroxyethyl starch 130/0.4 or 0.42) for severe sepsis reporting mortality: systematic review and meta-analysis. *Intensive Care Med* **39**:811–822.

13b Perel P, Roberts I, Ker K (2013) Colloids versus crystalloids for fluid resuscitation in critically ill patients. *Cochrane Database Syst Rev* Feb 28;2:CD000567.

13c Serpa Neto A, Veelo DP, Peireira VG *et al.* (2013) Fluid resuscitation with hydroxyethyl starches in patients with sepsis is associated with an increased incidence of acute kidney injury and use of renal replacement therapy: a systematic review and meta-analysis of the literature. *J Crit Care* doi:pii: S0883–9441(13)00387-0. 10.1016/j.jcrc.2013.09.031. [Epub ahead of print]

13d Rasmussen KC, Johansson PI, Højskow M *et al.* (2013) Hydroxyethyl starch reduces coagulation competence and increase blood loss during major surgery: results from a randomized controlled trial. *Ann Surg* [Epub ahead of print]

13e Haase N, Wetterlev J, Winkel P *et al.* (2013) Bleeding and risk of death with hydroxyethyl starch in severe sepsis: *post hoc* analyses of a randomized clinical trial. *Intensive Care Med* **39**:2126–2134.

13f Gillies MA, Habicher M, Jhanji S *et al.* (2013) Incidence of postoperative death and acute kidney injury associated with i.v. 6% hydroxyethyl starch use: systematic review and meta-analysis. *Brit J Anaesth* doi:10.1093/bja/aet303.

13g Myburgh JA, Finfer S, Bellomo R *et al.* for the CHEST Investigators and the Australian and New Zealand Intensive Care Society Clinical Trials Group (2012) Hydroxyethyl starch or saline for fluid resuscitation in intensive care *N Engl J Med* **367**:1901–1911.

13h Haase N, Pemer A, Hennings LI *et al.* (2013) Hydroxyethyl starch 130/0.38-0.45 versus crystallioid or albumin in patients with sepsis: systematic review with meta-analysis and trial sequential analysis *BMJ* **346**:f839 doi:10.1136/bmj.f839.

14 Jungheinrich C, Neff TA (2005) Pharmacokinetics of hydroxyethyl starch. *Clin Pharmacokinet* **44**:681–699.

14a Hughes D (2000) Fluid therapy with macromolecular plasma volume expanders. In: *Fluid Therapy in Small Animal Practice*, 2nd edn. (ed SP DiBartola) WB Saunders, Philadelphia, p. 483.

15 Jones PA, Tomasic M, Gentry PA (1997) Oncotic, hemodilutional, and hemostatic effects of isotonic saline and hydroxyethyl starch solutions in clinically normal ponies. *Am J Vet Res* **58**:541–548.

16 Moore LE, Garvey MS (1996) The effect of hetastarch on serum colloid oncotic pressure in hypoalbuminemic dogs. *J Vet Intern Med* **10**:300–303.

17 Marx G, Cobas Meyer M *et al.* (2002) Hydroxyethyl starch and modified fluid gelatin maintain plasma volume in a porcine model of septic shock with capillary leakage. *Intens Care Med* **28**:629–635.

18 Oz MC, FitzPatrick MF, Zikria BA *et al.* (1995) Attenuation of microvascular permeability dysfunction in postischemic striated muscle by hydroxyethyl starch. *Microvasc Res* **50**:71–79.

19 Marx G, Pedder S, Smith L *et al.* (2006) Attenuation of capillary leakage by hydroxyethyl starch (130/0.42) in a porcine model of septic shock. *Crit Care Med* **34**:3005–3010.

20 Bumpus SE, Haskins SC, Kass PH (1998) Effect of synthetic colloids on refractometer readings of total solids. *J Vet Emerg Crit Care* **8**:21–26.

21 Thomas LA, Brown SA (1992) Relationship between colloid osmotic pressure and plasma protein concentration in cattle, horses, dogs, and cats. *Am J Vet Res* **53**:2241–2244.

22 Magdesian KG, Fielding CL, Madigan JE (2004) Measurement of plasma colloid osmotic pressure in neonatal foals under critical care: comparison of direct and indirect methods and the association of COP with selected clinical and clinicopathologic variables. *J Vet Emerg Crit Care* **14**:108–114.

23 Runk DT, Madigan JE, Rahal CJ *et al.* (2000) Measurement of plasma colloid osmotic pressure in normal thoroughbred neonatal foals. *J Vet Intern Med* **14**:475–478.

24 Thyes C, Madjdpour C, Frascarolo P *et al.* (2006) Effect of high- and low-molecular-weight low-substituted hydroxyethyl starch on blood coagulation during acute normovolemic hemodilution in pigs. *Anesthesiology* **105**:1228–1237.

25 Strauss RG, Pennell BJ, Stump DC (2002) A randomized, blinded trial comparing the hemostatic effects of pentastarch versus hetastarch. *Transfusion* **42**:27–36.

26 Treib J, Haass A, Pindur G *et al.* (1996) All medium starches are not the same: influence of the degree of hydroxyethyl substitution of hydroxyethyl starch on plasma volume, hemorrheologic conditions, and coagulation. *Transfusion* **36**:450–455.

27 Schusser GF, Rieckoff K, Ungemach FR *et al.* (2005) Effect of hydroxyethyl starch solution in horses with colic or acute colitis. *Proc 8th International Equine Colic Research Symposium*, pp. 161–162.

28 Mehvar R (2000) Dextrans for targeted and sustained delivery of therapeutic and imaging agents. *J Control Release* **69**:1–25.

29 MacKay RJ, Clark CK, Logdberg L *et al.* (1999) Effect of a conjugate of polymyxin B-dextran 70 in horses with experimentally induced endotoxemia. *Am J Vet Res* **60**:68–75.

30 Glowaski MM, Moon-Massat PF, Erb HN *et al.* (2003) Effects of oxypolygelatin and dextran 70 on hemostatic variables in dogs. *Vet Anaesth Analg* **30**:202–210.

31 Moon PF, Snyder JR, Haskins SC *et al.* (1991) Effects of a highly concentrated hypertonic saline-dextran volume expander on cardiopulmonary function in anesthetized normovolemic horses. *Am J Vet Res* **52**:1611–1618.

32 Corely K (2008) Fluid therapy. In: *The Equine Hospital Manual.* (eds K Corley, J Stephen) Blackwell Publishing, Oxford, pp. 364–387.

33 Kramer GC, Harms BA, Bodai BI *et al.* (1982) Mechanisms for redistribution of plasma protein following acute protein depletion. *Am J Physiol* **243**:H803–809.

34 Mazzaferro EM, Rudloff E, Kirby R (2002) The role of albumin in the critically ill veterinary patient. *J Vet Emerg Crit Care* **12**:113–124.

35 Mathews KA, Barry M (2005) The use of 25% human serum albumin: outcome and efficacy in raising serum albumin and systemic blood pressure in critically ill dogs and cats. *J Vet Emerg Crit Care* **15**:110–118.

36 Bunn F, Lefebvre C *et al.* (2000) Human albumin solution for resuscitation and volume expansion in critically ill patients. The Albumin Reviewers. *Cochrane Database Syst Rev* (2) CD001208.

37 Alderson P, Bunn F, Lefebvre C *et al.* (2002) Human albumin solution for resuscitation and volume expansion in critically ill patients. *Cochrane Database Syst Rev* (1) CD001208.

38 Maxson AD, Giger U, Sweeney CR *et al.* (1993) Use of a bovine hemoglobin preparation in the treatment of cyclic ovarian hemorrhage in a miniature horse. *J Am Vet Med Assoc* **203**:1308–1311.

39 Vin R, Bedenice D, Rentko VT *et al.* (2002) The use of ultrapurified bovine hemoglobin solution in the treatment of two cases of presumed red maple toxicosis in miniature horse and a pony. *J Vet Emerg Crit Care* **12**:169–175.

40 Perkins G, Divers T (2001) Polymerized hemoglobin therapy in a foal with neonatal isoerythrolysis. *J Vet Emerg Crit Care* **11**:141–145.

41 Driessen B, Jahr JS, Lurie F *et al.* (2006) Effects of isovolemic resuscitation with hemoglobin-based oxygen carrier Hemoglobin glutamer-200 (bovine) on systemic and mesenteric perfusion and oxygenation in a canine model of hemorrhagic shock: a comparison with 6% hetastarch solution and shed blood. *Vet Anaesth Analg* **33**:368–380.

42 Belgrave RL, Hines MT, Keegan RD *et al.* (2002) Effects of a polymerized ultrapurified bovine hemoglobin blood substitute administered to ponies with normovolemic anemia. *J Vet Intern Med* **16**:396–403.

43 Mudge MC, Macdonald MH, Owens SD *et al.* (2004) Comparison of 4 blood storage methods in a protocol for equine pre-operative autologous donation. *Vet Surg* **33**:475–486.

44 Monk TG (2005) Acute normovolemic hemodilution. *Anesthesiol Clin N Am* **23**:271–281, vi.

45 Shander A, Rijhwani TS (2004) Acute normovolemic hemodilution. *Transfusion* **44(Suppl)**:26S–34S.

46 Day TK (2003) Current development and use of hemoglobin-based oxygen carrying (HBOC) solutions. *J Vet Emerg Crit Care* **13**:77–93.

CHAPTER 13: INOTROPE AND VASOPRESSOR THERAPY

1 Beale RJ, Hollenberg SM, Vincent JL *et al.* (2004) Vasopressor and inotropic support in septic shock: an evidence based review. *Crit Care Med* **32**:S455–S465.

2 Woolsey CA, Coppersmith CM (2006) Vasoactive drugs and the gut: is there anything new? *Curr Opin Crit Care* **12**:155–159.

3 Hollenberg SM, Ahrens TS, Annane D *et al.* (2004) Practice parameters for hemodynamic support of sepsis in adult patients: 2004 update. *Crit Care Med* **32**:1928–1948.

4 Corley KTT (2004) Inotropes and vasopressors in adults and foals. *Vet Clin N Am Equine Pract* **20**:77–106.

5 MacGregor DA, Smith TE, Prielipp RC *et al.* (2000) Pharmacokinetics of dopamine in healthy male subjects. *Anesthesiology* **92**:338–346.

6 Holmes CL, Patel BM, Russell JA *et al.* (2001) Physiology of vasopressin relevant to management of septic shock. *Chest* **120**:989–1002.

7 Valverde A, Giguere S, Sanchez C *et al.* (2006) Effects of dobutamine, norepinephrine, and vasopressin on cardiovascular function in anesthetized neonatal foals with induced hypotension. *Am J Vet Res* **67**:1730–1737.

8 Dellinger RP (2003) Cardiovascular management of septic shock. *Crit Care Med* **3**:946–955.

9 De Backer D, Creteur J, Silva E *et al.* (2003) Effects of dopamine, norepinephrine, and epinephrine on the splanchnic circulation in septic shock: which is best? *Crit Care Med* **31**:1659–1667.

CHAPTER 14: SEDATION AND ANALGESIA

1 Sellon DC (2006) Pain: the fourth vital sign? *Comp Cont Educ Pract Vet Equine* **1**:205–209.

2 Muir WW, Woolf CJ (2001) Mechanisms of pain and their therapeutic implications. *J Am Vet Med Assoc* **219**:1346–1356.

3 Young SS, Taylor PM (1993) Factors influencing the outcome of equine anaesthesia: a review of 1314 cases. *Equine Vet J* **25**:147–151.

4 Mee AM, Cripps PJ, Jones RS (1998) A retrospective study of mortality associated with general anaesthesia in horses: elective procedures. *Vet Rec* **142**:275–276.

5 Mee AM, Cripps PJ, Jones RS (1998) A retrospective study of mortality associated with general anaesthesia in horses: emergency procedures. *Vet Rec* **142**:307–309.

6 Johnston GM, Eastment JK, Wood JLN *et al.* (2002) The confidential enquiry into perioperative equine fatalities (CEPEF): mortality results of phases 1 and 2. *Vet Anaesth Analg* **29**:159–170.

7 Taylor PM (2002) Editorial. *Vet Anaesth Analg* **29**:157–158.

8 Sysel AM, Pleasant RS, Jacobson JD *et al.* (1997) Systemic and local effects associated with long-term epidural catheterization and morphine-detomidine administration in horses. *Vet Surg* **26**:141–149.

9 Martin CA, Kerr CL, Pearce SG *et al.* (2003) Outcome of epidural catheterization for delivery of analgesics in horses: 43 cases (1998–2001). *J Am Vet Med Assoc* **222**:1394–1398.

10 Hamm D, Jochle W (1991) Sedation and analgesia with Domosedan® (detomidine hydrochloride) or acepromazine for suturing of the vulvar lips in mares (Caslick's surgery). *Equine Vet Sci* **11**:86–88.

11 England, GCW, Clarke KW, Goossens L (1992) A comparison of the sedative effects of three alpha-2 adrenoreceptor agonists (romifidine, detomidine and xylazine) in the horse. *J Vet Pharmacol Ther* **15**:194–201.

12 Browning AP, Collins JA (1994) Sedation of horses with romifidine and butorphanol. *Vet Rec* **134**:90–91.

13 Hamm D, Turchi P, Jochle W (1995) Sedative and analgesic effects of detomidine and romifidine in horses. *Vet Rec* **136**:324–327.

14 England, GCW, Clarke KW (1996) Alpha2-adrenoreceptor agonists in the horse – a review. *Brit Vet J* **152**:641–657.

15 Freeman SK, England GCW (1999) Comparison of sedative effects of romifidine following intravenous, intramuscular and sublingual administration to horses. *Am J Vet Res* **60**:954–959.

16 Freeman SL, England GCW (2000) Investigation of romifidine and detomidine for the clinical sedation of horses. *Vet Rec* **147**:507–511.

17 Moens Y, Lanz F, Doherr MG *et al.* (2003) A comparison of the antinociceptive effects of xylazine, detomidine and romifidine on experimental pain in horses. *Vet Anaesth Analg* **30**:183–190.

18 Spadavecchia C, Arendt–Nielsen L, Andersen OK *et al.* (2005) Effect of romifidine on the nociceptive withdrawal reflex and temporal summation in conscious horses. *Am J Vet Res* **66**:1992–1998.

19 Wilson DV, Bohart GV, Evans AT *et al.* (2002) Retrospective analysis of detomidine infusion for standing chemical restraint in 51 horses. *Vet Anaesth Analg* **29**:54–57.

20 Luna SP, Beale NJ, Taylor PM (1992) Effects of atipamezole on xylazine sedation in ponies. *Vet Rec* **130**:268–271.

21 Kollias-Baker CA, Court MH, Williams LL (1993) Influence of yohimbine and tolazoline on the cardiovascular, respiratory, and sedative effects of xylazine in the horse. *J Vet Pharmacol Ther* **16**:350–358.

22 Carroll GL, Matthews NS, Hartsfield SM *et al.* (1997) The effect of detomidine and its antagonism with tolazoline on stress-related hormones, metabolites, physiologic responses, and behavior in awake ponies. *Vet Surg* **26**:69–77.

23 van Dijk P, Lankveld DPK, Rijkenhuizen ABM *et al.* (2003) Hormonal, metabolic and physiological effects of laparoscopic surgery using a detomidine-buprenorphine combination in standing horses. *Vet Anaesth Analg* **30**:72–80.

24 Hubbell JA, Muir WW (2006) Antagonism of detomidine sedation in the horse using intravenous tolazoline or atipamezole. *Equine Vet J* **38**:238–241.

25 Grubb TL, Riebold TW, Huber MJ (1992) Comparison of lidocaine, xylazine, and xylazine/lidocaine for caudal epidural analgesia in horses. *J Am Vet Med Assoc* **201**:1187–1190.

26 Skarda RT, Muir WW (1994) Caudal analgesia induced by epidural or subarachnoid administration of detomidine hydrochloride solution in mares. *Am J Vet Res* **55**:670–680.

27 Wittern C, Hendrickson DA, Trumble T *et al.* (1998) Complications associated with administration of detomidine into the caudal epidural space in a horse. *J Am Vet Med Assoc* **213**:516–522.

28 Skarda RT, Muir WW (1998) Influence of atipamezole on effects of midsacral subarachnoidally administered detomidine in mares. *Am J Vet Res* **59**:468–477.

29 Skarda RT, Muir WW (1999) Effects of intravenously administered yohimbine on antinociceptive, cardiorespiratory, and postural changes induced by epidural administration of detomidine hydrochloride solution to healthy mares. *Am J Vet Res* **60**:1262–1270.

30 Sellon DC, Monroe VL, Roberts MC *et al.* (2001) Pharmacokinetics and adverse effects of butorphanol administered by single intravenous injection or continuous intravenous infusion in horses. *Am J Vet Res* **62**:183–189.

31 Muir WW (2009) Anxiolytics, nonopioid sedative-analgesics, and opioid analgesics. In: *Equine Anesthesia Monitoring and Emergency Therapy*, 2nd edn. (eds WW Muir, JAE Hubbell) Saunders Elsevier, St. Louis, pp. 185–209.

32 Taylor PM, Bennett RC, Brearley JC *et al.* (2001) Comparison of detomidine and romifidine as premedicants before ketamine and halothane anesthesia in horses undergoing elective surgery. *Am J Vet Res* **62**:359–363.

33 Freeman SL, Bowen IM, Bettschart-Wolfensberger R *et al.* (200) Cardiovascular effects of romifidine in the standing horse. *Res Vet Sci* **72**:123–129.

34 Adams SB, Lamer CH, Masty J (1984) Motility of the distal portion of the jejunum and pelvic flexure in ponies. Effects of six drugs. *Am J Vet Res* **45**:795–799.

35 Roger T, Ruckebusch Y (1987) Colonic alpha 2-adrenoceptor-mediated responses in the pony. *J Vet Pharmacol Ther* **10**:310–318.

36 Rutkowski JA, Ross MW, Cullen K (1989) Effects of xylazine and/or butorphanol or neostigmine on myoelectric activity of the cecum and right ventral colon in female ponies. *Am J Vet Res* **50**:1096–1101.

37 Sutton DG, Preston T, Christley RM *et al.* (2002) The effects of xylazine, detomidine, acepromazine and butorphanol on equine solid phase gastric emptying rate. *Equine Vet J* **34**:486–492.

38 Merritt AM, Campbell-Thompson ML, Lowrey S (1989) Effect of xylazine treatment on equine proximal gastrointestinal tract myoelectrical activity. *Am J Vet Res* **50**:945–949.

39 Nunez E, Steffey EP, Ocampo L *et al.* (2004) Effects of α-2 adrenergic receptor agonists on urine production in horses deprived of food and water. *Am J Vet Res* **65**:1342–1346.

40   Katila T, Oijala M (1988) The effect of detomidine on the maintenance of equine pregnancy and foetal development: ten cases. *Equine Vet J* **20**:323–326.

41   Combie J, Dougherty J, Nugent EC *et al.* (1979) The pharmacology of narcotic analgesics in the horse. Part IV. Dose and time response relationships for behavioral responses to morphine, meperidine, pentazocine, anileridine, methadone, and hydromorphone. *J Equine Med Surg* **3**:377–385.

42   Natalini CC, Robinson EP (2000) Evaluation of the analgesic effects of epidurally administered morphine, alfentanil, butorphanol, tramadol, and U50488H in horses. *Am J Vet Res* **61**:1579–1586.

43   Natalini CC, Robinson EP (2003) Effects of epidural opioid analgesics on heart rate, arterial blood pressure, respiratory rate, body temperature, and behavior in horses. *Vet Ther* **4**:364–375.

44   Natalini CC, Linardi RL (2006) Effects of epidural opioid analgesics on heart rate, arterial blood pressure, respiratory rate, body temperature, and behavior in horses. *Am J Vet Res* **67**:11–15.

45   Skarda RT, Muir WW (200) Analgesic, hemodynamic, and respiratory effects induced by caudal epidural administration of meperidine hydrochloride in mares. *Am J Vet Res* **62**:1001–1007.

46   Olbrich VH, Mosing M (2003) A comparison of the analgesic effects of caudal epidural methadone and lidocaine in the horse. *Vet Anaesth Analg* **30**:156–164.

47   Sheehy JG, Hellyer PW, Sammonds GE *et al.* (2001) Evaluation of opioid receptors in synovial membranes of horses. *Am J Vet Res* **62**:1408–1412.

48   Raekallio M, Taylor PM, Johnson CB *et al.* (1996) The disposition and local effects of intra-articular morphine in normal ponies. *J Vet Anaesth* **23**:23–26.

49   Steffey EP, Eisele JH, Baggot JD (2003) Interactions of morphine and isoflurane in horses. *Am J Vet Res* **64**:166–175.

50   Bennett RC, Steffey EP, Kollias-Baker C *et al.* (2004) Influence of morphine sulfate on the halothane sparing effect of xylazine hydrochloride in horses. *Am J Vet Res* **65**:519–526.

51   Clark L, Clutton RE, Blissitt KJ *et al.* (2005) Effects of peri-operative morphine administration during halothane anaesthesia in horses. *Vet Anaesth Analg* **32**:10–15.

52   Haitjema H, Gibson KT (2001) Severe pruritis associated with epidural morphine and detomidine in a horse. *Aust Vet J* **79**:248–250.

53   Burford JH, Corley KTT (2006) Morphine-associated pruritis after single extradural administration in a horse. *Vet Anaesth Analg* **33**:193–198.

54   Sysel AM, Pleasant RS, Jacobson JD *et al.* (1996) Efficacy of an epidural combination of morphine and detomidine alleviating experimentally-induced hindlimb lameness in horses. *Vet Surg* **25**:511–518.

55   Bennett RC, Steffey EP (2002) Use of opioids for pain and anesthetic management in horses. *Vet Clin N Am Equine Pract* **18**:47–60.

56   Goodrich LR, Nixon AJ, Fubini SL *et al.* (2002) Epidural morphine and detomidine decreases postoperative hindlimb lameness in horses after bilateral stifle arthroscopy. *Vet Surg* **31**:232–239.

57   Van Hoogmoed LM, Galuppo LD (2005) Laraoscopic ovariectomy using the endo-GIA stapling device and endo-catch pouches and evaluation of analgesic efficacy of epidural morphine sulfate in 10 mares. *Vet Surg* **34**:646–650.

58   Clarke KW, Paton BS (1988) Combined use of detomidine with opiates in the horse. *Equine Vet J* **20**:331–334.

59   Taylor PM, Browning AP, Harris CP (1988) Detomidine-butorphanol sedation in equine clinical practice. *Vet Rec* **123**:388–390.

60   Schatzman U, Armbruster S, Stucki F *et al.* (2001) Analgesic effect of butorphanol and levomethadone in detomidine sedated horses. *J Vet Med A Physiol Pathol Clin Med* **48**:337–342.

61   Kalpravidh M, Lumb WV, Wright M *et al.* (1984) Analagesic effects of butorphanol in horses: dose–response studies. *Am J Vet Res* **45**:211–216.

62   Kalpravidh M, Lumb WV, Wright M *et al.* (1984) Effects of butorphanol, flunixin, levorphanol, morphine, and xylazine in ponies. *Am J Vet Res* **45**:217–223.

63   Brunson DB, Majors LJ (1987) Comparative analgesia of xylazine, xylazine/morphine, xylazine/butorphanol, and xylazine/nalbuphine in the horse, using dental dolorimetry. *Am J Vet Res* **48**:1087–1091.

64   Sellon DC, Roberts MC, Blikslager AT *et al.* (2004) Effects of continuous rate intravenous infusion of butorphanol on physiologic and outcome variables in horses after celiotomy. *J Vet Intern Med* **18**:555–563.

65   Nolan AM, Hall LW (1984) Combined use of sedatives and opiates in horses. *Vet Rec* **114**: 63–67.

66   Szoke MO, Blais D, Cuvelliez SG *et al.* (1998) Effects of buprenorphine on cardiovascular and pulmonary function in clinically normal horses and horses with chronic obstructive pulmonary disease. *Am J Vet Res* **59**:1287–1291.

67   Carregaro AB, Teixeira Neto FJ *et al.* (2006) Cardiopulmonary effects of buprenorphine in horses. *Am J Vet Res* **67**:1675–1680.

68   Carregaro AB, Luna SPL, Mataqueiro MI *et al.* (2007) Effects of buprenorphine on nociception and spontaneous locomotor activity in horses. *Am J Vet Res* **68**:246–250.

69   Kamerling SG, DeQuick DJ, Weckman TJ *et al.* (1985) Dose-related effects of fentanyl on autonomic and behavioral responses in performance horses. *Gen Pharmacol* **16**:253–258.

70   Maxwell LK, Thomasy SM, Slovis N *et al.* (2003) Pharmacokinetics of fentanyl following intravenous and transdermal administration in horses. *Equine Vet J* **35**:484–490.

71   Orsini JA, Moate PJ, Kuersten K *et al.* (2006) Pharmacokinetics of fentanyl delivered transdermally in healthy horses – variability among horses and its clinical implications. *J Vet Pharmacol Ther* **29**:539–546.

72   Thomasy SM, Slovis N, Maxwell LK *et al.* (2004) Transdermal fentanyl combined with nonsteroidal anti-inflammatory drugs for analgesia in horses. *J Vet Intern Med* **18**:550–554.

73 Thomasy SM, Mama KR, Whitley K *et al.* (2007) Influence of general anaesthesia on the pharmacokinetics of intravenous fentanyl and its primary metabolite in horses. *Equine Vet J* **39**:54–58.

74 Love EJ, Lane JG, Murison PJ (2006) Morphine administration in horses anaesthetized for upper respiratory tract surgery. *Vet Anaesth Analg* **33**:179–188.

75 Mircica E, Clutton RE, Kyles KW *et al.* (2003) Problems associated with perioperative morphine in horses: a retrospective case analysis. *Vet Anaesth Analg* **30**:147–155.

76 Senior JM, Pinchbeck GL, Dugdale AH *et al.* (2004) Retrospective study of the risk factors and prevalence of colic in horses after orthopaedic surgery. *Vet Rec* **155**:321–325.

77 Andersen MS, Clark L, Dyson SJ *et al.* (2006) Risk factors for colic in horses after general anaesthesia for MRI or nonabdominal surgery: absence of evidence of effect from perianaesthetic morphine. *Equine Vet J* **38**:368–74.

78 Robertson JT, Muir WW, Sams R (1981) Cardiopulmonary effects of butorphanol tartrate in horses. *Am J Vet Res* **42**:41–44.

79 Sojka JE, Adams SB, Lamar CH *et al.* (1988) Effect of butorphanol, pentazocine, meperidine, or metoclopramide on intestinal motility in female ponies. *Am J Vet Res* **49**:527–9.

80 Lemke KA (2007) Anticholinergics and sedatives. In: *Lumb and Jones' Veterinary Anesthesia and Analgesia*, 4th edn. (eds WJ Tranquilli, JC Thurmon, KA Grimm) Blackwell Publishing, Ames, pp. 203–239.

81 Johnston GM, Eastment JK, Wood JLN *et al.* (2002) The confidential enquiry into perioperative equine fatalities (CEPEF): mortality results of phases 1 and 2. *Vet Anaesth Analg* **29**:159–170.

82 Marntell S, Nyman G, Funkquist P *et al.* (2005) Effects of acepromazine on pulmonary gas exchange and circulation during sedation and dissociative anaesthesia in horses. *Vet Anaesth Analg* **32**:83–93.

83 Brown RF, Houpt KA, Schryver HF (1976) Stimulation of food intake in horses by diazepam and promazine. *Pharmacol Biochem Behav* **5**:495–497.

84 Kushiro T, Yamashita K, Umar MA *et al.* (2005) Anesthetic and cardiovascular effects of balanced anesthesia using constant rate infusion of midazolam-ketamine-medetomidine with inhalation of oxygen-sevoflurane in horses. *J Vet Med Sci* **67**:379–384.

85 Muir WW, Sams RA, Huffman RH *et al.* (1982) Pharmacodynamic and pharmacokinetic properties of diazepam in horses. *Am J Vet Res* **43**:1756–1762.

86 Gangl M, Grulke S, Detilleux J *et al.* (2001) Comparison of thiopentone/guaifenesin, ketamine/guaifenesin and ketamine/midazolam for the induction of horses to be anaesthetized with isoflurane. *Vet Rec* **149**:147–151.

87 Kohrs R, Durieux ME (1998) Ketamine: teaching an old drug new tricks. *Anesth Analg* **87**:1186–1193.

88 Lin HC (2007) Dissociative anesthetics. In: *Lumb and Jones' Veterinary Anesthesia and Analgesia*, 4th edn. (eds WJ Tranquilli, JC Thurmon, KA Grimm) Blackwell Publishing, Ames, pp. 301–353.

89 Muir WW, Sams R (1992) Effects of ketamine infusion on halothane minimal alveolar concentration in horses. *Am J Vet Res* **53**:1802–1806.

90 Matthews NS, Fielding CL, Swinebroad E (2004) How to use ketamine CRI in horses for analgesia. *Proc Am Assoc Equine Practnrs* **50**:227–228.

91 Fielding CL, Brumbaugh GW, Matthews NS *et al.* (2006) Pharmacokinetics and clinical effects of a subanesthetic continuous rate infusion of ketamine in awake horses. *Am J Vet Res* **67**:1484–1490.

92 Lankveld DP, Driessen B, Soma LR *et al.* (2006) Pharmacodynamic effects and pharmacokinetic profile of a long-term continuous rate infusion of racemic ketamine in healthy conscious horses. *J Vet Pharmacol Ther* **29**:477–488.

93 Gomez De Segura IA, Rossi RD, Santos M *et al.* (1998) Epidural injection of ketamine for perineal analgesia in the horse. *Vet Surg* **27**:384–391

94 Redua MA, Valadao AA, Duque JC *et al.* (2002) The pre-emptive effect of epidural ketamine on wound sensitivity in horses tested by using von Frey filaments. *Vet Anaesth Analg* **29**:200–206.

95 Doherty TJ, Geiser, DR, Rohrbach BW (1997) Effect of high volume epidural morphine, ketamine and butorphanol on halothane minimum alveolar concentration in ponies. *Equine Vet J* **29**:370–373.

96 Lopez-Sanroman FJ, Cruz JM, Santos M *et al.* (2003) Evaluation of the local analgesic effect of ketamine in the palmar digital nerve block at the base of the proximal sesamoid (abaxial sesamoid block) in horses. *Am J Vet Res* **64**:475–478.

97 Skarda RT, Tranquilli WJ (2007) Local anesthetics. In: *Lumb and Jones' Veterinary Anesthesia and Analgesia*, 4th edn. (eds WJ Tranquilli, JC Thurmon, KA Grimm) Blackwell Publishing, Ames, pp. 395–418.

98 Doherty TJ, Frazier DL (1998) Effect of intravenous lidocaine on halothane minimum alveolar concentration in ponies. *Equine Vet J* **30**:300–303.

99 Dzikiti TB, Hellebrekers LJ, van Dijk P (2003) Effects of intravenous lidocaine on isoflurane concentration, physiological parameters, metabolic parameters and stress-related hormones in horses undergoing surgery. *J Vet Med A Physiol Pathol Clin Med* **50**:190–195.

100 Brianceau P, Chevalier H, Karas A *et al.* (2002) Intravenous lidocaine and small-intestinal size, abdominal fluid, and outcome after colic surgery in horses. *J Vet Intern Med* **16**:736–741.

101 Bidwell LA, Wilson DV, Caron JP (2007) Lack of systemic absorption of lidocaine from 5% patches placed on horses. *Vet Anaesth Analg* **34**:443–446.

102 Dart AJ, Hodgson DR (1998) Role of prokinetic drugs for treatment of postoperative ileus in the horse. *Aust Vet J* **76**:25–31.

103 Lamont LA, Mathews KA (2007) Opioids, nonsteroidal anti-inflammatories, and analgesic adjuvants. In: *Lumb and Jones' Veterinary Anesthesia and Analgesia*, 4th edn. (eds WJ Tranquilli, JC Thurmon, KA Grimm) Blackwell Publishing, Ames, pp. 241–271.

104 Hudson N, Balsitis M, Everitt S *et al.* (1993) Enhanced gastric mucosal leukotriene B4 synthesis in patients taking non-steroidal anti-inflammatory drugs. *Gut* **34**:742–747.

105 Reed SK, Messer NT, Tessman RK *et al.* (2006) Effects of phenylbutazone alone or in combination with flunixin meglumine on blood protein concentrations in horses. *Am J Vet Res* **67**:398–402.

106 Schatzmann U, Gugelmann M, Von Cranach J *et al.* (1990) Pharmacodynamic evaluation of the peripheral pain inhibition by carprofen and flunixin in the horse. *Schweiz Arch Tierheilkd* **132**:497–504.

107 Balmer T, Curwen A (1997) Use of carprofen in racehorses. *Vet Rec* **141**:400–414.

108 Toutain PL, Cester CC (2004) Pharmacokinetic-pharmacodynamic relationships and dose response to meloxicam in horses with induced arthritis in the right carpal joint. *Am J Vet Res* **65**:1542–1547.

109 Toutain PL, Reymond N, Laroute V *et al.* (2004) Pharmacokinetics of meloxicam in plasma and urine of horses. *Am J Vet Res* **65**:1533–1541.

110 Mealey KL, Matthews NS, Peck KE *et al.* (2004) Pharmacokinetics of R(-) and S(+) carprofen after administration of racemic carprofen in donkeys and horses. *Am J Vet Res* **65**:1479–1482.

111 Hubbell JAE (2007) Horses. In: *Lumb and Jones' Veterinary Anesthesia and Analgesia*, 4th edn. (eds WJ Tranquilli, JC Thurmon, KA Grimm) Blackwell Publishing, Ames, pp. 717–729.

112 MacAllister CG, Morgan SJ, Borne AT *et al.* (1993) Comparison of adverse effects of phenylbutazone, flunixin meglumine, and ketoprofen in horses. *J Am Vet Med Assoc* **202**:71–77.

113 Ripamonti C, Dickerson ED (2001) Strategies for the treatment of cancer pain in the new millennium. *Drugs* **61**:955–977.

114 Davis JL, Posner LP, Elce Y (2007) Gabapentin for the treatment of neuropathic pain in a pregnant horse. *J Am Vet Med Assoc* **231**:755–758.

CHAPTER 15: NUTRITIONAL SUPPORT

1 Naylor JM, Kenyon SJ (1981) Effect of total calorific deprivation on host defense in the horse. *Res Vet Sci* **31**:369–372.

2 Henneke DR, Potter GD, Kreider *et al.* (1983) Relationship between condition score, physical measurements and body fat percentage in mares. *Equine Vet J* **15**:371–372.

3 Paradis MR (2001) Nutrition and indirect calorimetry in neonatal foals. In: *Proceedings of the 19th American College of Veterinary Internal Medicine*. (eds DJ Davenport, MJ Paradis) pp. 245–247.

4 Paradis MR (2003) Nutritional support: enteral and parenteral. *Clin Tech Equine Pract* **2**:87–95.

5 Magdesian KG (2003) Nutrition for critical gastrointestinal illness: feeding horses with diarrhea or colic. *Vet Clin N Am Equine Pract* **19**:617–644.

6 Dunkel BM, Wilkins PA (2004) Nutrition and the critically ill horse. *Vet Clin N Am Equine Pract* **20**:107–126.

7 Sweeney RW, Wilkins PA (2002) Nutrition of the sick animal: prevention and therapeutic strategies. In: *Large Animal Internal Medicine*, 3rd edn. (ed B Smith) Mosby, St Louis, pp. 1458–1461.

8 Naylor JM, Freeman DE, Kronfeld DS (1984) Alimentation of hypophagic horses. *Comp Cont Educ Pract Vet* **6**:S93–S99.

9 Fascetti A, Stratton-Phelps M (2003) Clinical assessment of nutritional status and enteral feeding in the acutely ill horse. In: *Current Therapies in Equine Medicine*, 5th edn. (ed NE Robinson) Saunders, Philadelphia, pp. 705–710.

10 Sweeney RW, Hansen TO (1990) Use of a liquid diet as the sole source of nutrition in 6 dysphagic horses and as a dietary supplement in 7 hypophagic horses. *J Am Vet Med Assoc* **197**:1030–1032.

11 Wanten GJ, Calder PC (2007) Immune modulation by parenteral lipid emulsions. *Am J Clin Nutr* **85**:1171–1184.

12 Hardy J (2003) Nutritional support and nursing care of the adult horse in intensive care. *Clin Tech Equine Pract* **2**:193–198.

13 Holcombe SJ (2003) Parenteral nutrition for colic patients. In: *Current Therapies in Equine Medicine*, 5th edn. (ed NE Robinson) Saunders, Philadelphia, pp. 111–115.

CHAPTER 16: ANTIMICROBIAL DRUGS

1 Murtaugh RJ, Mason GD (1989) Antibiotic pressure and nosocomial disease. *Vet Clin N Am Small Anim Pract* **19**:1259–1274.

2 van den Bogaard AE, Stobberingh EE (2000) Epidemiology of resistance to antibiotics. Links between animals and humans. *Int J Antimicrob Ag* **14**:327–335.

3 Johnson JA (2002) Nosocomial infections. *Vet Clin N Am Small Anim Pract* **32**:1101–1126.

4 McEwen SA, Fedorka-Cray PJ (2002) Antimicrobial use and resistance in animals. *Clin Infect Dis* **34(Suppl 3)**:S93–S106.

5 Prescott JF, Hanna BWJ, Reid-Smith R *et al.* (2002) Antimicrobial drug use and resistance in dogs. *Can Vet J* **43**:107–116.

6 Dunowska M, Morley PS, Traub-Dargatz JL *et al.* (2006) Impact of hospitalization and antimicrobial drug administration on antimicrobial sensitivity patterns of commensal *Escherichia coli* isolated from the feces of horses. *J Am Vet Med Assoc* **228**:1909–1917.

7 Hartmann FA, Trostle SS, Klohnen AA (1997) Isolation of methicillin-resistant *Staphylococcus aureus* from a postoperative wound infection in a horse. *J Am Vet Med Assoc* **211**:590–592.

8 Seguin JC, Walker RD, Caron JP (1999) Methicillin-resistant *Staphylococcus aureus* outbreak in a veterinary teaching hospital: potential human-to-animal transmission. *J Clin Microbiol* **37**:1459–1463.

9 Walther B, Friedrich AW, Brunnberg L *et al.* (2006) Methicillin-resistant staphylococcus aureus (MRSA) in veterinary medicine: a "new emerging pathogen"? *Berl Munch Tierarztl Wochenschr* **119**:222–232.

10 Trostle SS, Peavey CL, King DS *et al.* (2001) Treatment of methicillin-resistant *Staphylococcus epidermidis* infection following repair of an ulnar fracture and humeroradial joint luxation in a horse. *J Am Vet Med Assoc* **218**:554–559.

11 Smith MA, Ross MW (2002) Postoperative infection with *Actinobacillus* spp. in horses: 10 cases (1995–2000). *J Am Vet Med Assoc* **221**:1306–1310.

12 Bentley AP, Barton MH, Lee MD *et al.* (2002) Antimicrobial-induced endotoxin and cytokine activity in an *in-vitro* model of septicemia in foals. *Am J Vet Res* **63**:660–668.

13 Jacks SS, Giguere S, Nguyen A (2003) In-vitro susceptibilities of *Rhodococcus equi* and other common equine pathogens to azithromycin, clarithromycin, and 20 other antimicrobials. *Antimicrob Agents Ch* **47**:1742–1745.

14 Wilson WD (2001) Rational selection of antimicrobials for use in horses. In: *Proc 47th Ann Conv Am Assoc Equine Practitnrs*, San Diego, pp. 75–93.

15 Chastre J (2003) Antimicrobial treatment of hospital-acquired pneumonia. *Infect Dis Clin N Am* **17**:727–737.

16 Bratzler DW, Houck PM (2004) Antimicrobial prophylaxis for surgery: an advisory statement from the National Surgical Infection Prevention Project. *Clin Infect Dis* **38**:1706–1715.

17 Felts AG, Grainger DW, Slunt JB (2000) Locally delivered antibodies combined with systemic antibiotics confer synergistic protection against antibiotic-resistant burn wound infection. *J Trauma* **49**:873–878.

18 Simmonds A, LaGamma EF (2006) Toward improving mucosal barrier defenses: rhG-CSF plus IgG antibody. *Ind J Pediatr* **73**:1019–1026.

19 Gurleyik G, Yanikkaya G, Gurleyik E *et al.* (2007) Effects of granulocyte-colony stimulating factor on the polymorphonuclear leukocyte activity and the course of sepsis in rats with experimental peritonitis. *Surg Today* **37**:401–405.

20 Cheng AC, Limmathurotsakul D, Chierakul W *et al.* (2007) A randomized contolled trial of granulocyte colony-stimulating factor for the treatment of severe sepsi due to melioidosis in Thailand. *Clin Infect Dis* **45**:308–314.

21 Sullivan KE, Snyder JR, Madigan JE *et al.* (1993) Effects of perioperative granulocyte colony-stimulating factor on horses with ascending colonic ishemia. *Vet Surg* **22**:343–350.

22 Madigan JE, Zinkl JG, Fridmann DM *et al.* (1994) Preliminary studies of recombinant bovine granulocyte-colony stimulating factor on haematological values in normal neonatal foals. *Equine Vet J* **26**:159–161.

23 Zinkl JG, Madigan JE, Fridmann DM *et al.* (1994) Haematological, bone marrow and clinical chemical changes in neonatal foals given canine recombinant granulocyte-colony stimulating factor. *Equine Vet J* **26**:313–318.

24 Scheuch BC, Van Hoogmoed LM, Wilson WD *et al.* (2002) Comparison of intraosseous or intravenous infusion for delivery of amikacin sulfate to the tibiotarsal joint of horses. *Am J Vet Res* **63**:374–380.

25 Whitehair KJ, Blevins WE, Fessler JF *et al.* (1992) Regional perfusion of the equine carpus for antibiotic delivery. *Vet Surg* **21**:279–285.

26 Whitehair KJ, Bowersock TL, Blevins WE *et al.* (199) Regional limb perfusion for antibiotic treatment of experimentally induced septic arthritis. *Vet Surg* **21**:367–373.

27 Anderson BH, Ethell MT (1999) Modes of local drug delivery to the musculoskeletal system. *Vet Clin N Am Equine Pract* **15**:603–622.

28 Swalec Tobias KM, Schneider RK *et al.* (1996) Use of antimicrobial-impregnated polymethyl methacrylate. *J Am Vet Med Assoc* **208**:841–845.

29 Schneider RK, Bramlage LR, Moore RM *et al.* (1992) A retrospective study of 192 horses affected with septic arthritis/tenosynovitis. *Equine Vet J* **24**:436–442.

30 MacDonald DG, Morley PS, Bailey JV *et al.* (1994) An examination of the occurrence of surgical wound infection following equine orthopaedic surgery (1981–1990). *Equine Vet J* **26**:323–326.

31 Hague BA, Honnas CM, Simpson BR *et al.* (1997) Evaluation of skin bacterial flora before and after aseptic preparation of clipped and nonclipped arthrocentesis sites in horses. *Vet Surg* **26**:121–125.

32 Corley KTT, Pearce G, Magdesian KG *et al.* (2007) Bacteraemia in neonatal foals: clinicopathological differences between gram-positive and gram-negative infections, and single organism and mixed infections. *Equine Vet J* **39**:84–89.

33 Cruz AM, Rubio-Martinez L, Dowling T (2006) New antimicrobials, systemic distribution, and local methods of antimicrobial delivery in horses. *Vet Clin N Am Equine Pract* **22**:297–322.

34 Galuppo LD, Pascoe JR, Jang SS *et al.* (1999) Evaluation of iodophor skin preparation techniques and factors influencing drainage from ventral midline incisions in horses. *J Am Vet Med Assoc* **215**:963–969.

35 Santschi EM, Adams SB, Murphey ED (1998) How to perform equine intravenous digital perfusion. In: *Proc 44th Ann Conv Am Assoc Equine Practitnrs*, Baltimore, pp. 198–201.

36 Aiello SE (1998) Chemotherapeutics. In: *The Merck Veterinary Manual*, 8th edn. (ed SE Aiello) Merck Sharp and Dohme, Whitehouse Station, pp. 1738–1788.

37 Green SL, Conlon PD, Mama K *et al.* (1992) Effects of hypoxia and azotaemia on the pharmacokinetics of amikacin in neonatal foals. *Equine Vet J* **24**:475–479.

38   Green SL, Conlon PD (1993) Clinical pharmacokinetics of amikacin in hypoxic premature foals. *Equine Vet J* **25**:276–280.

39   Spurlock SL, Hanie EA (1989) Antibiotics in the treatment of wounds. *Vet Clin N Am Equine Pract* **5**:465–482.

40   Smiet E, Haritova A, Heil BA *et al.* (2012) Comparing the pharmacokinetics of a fourth generation cephalosporin in three different age groups of New Forest ponies. *Equine Vet J* **44 (Suppl 41)**:52–56.

41   Gardner SY, Papich MG (2001) Comparison of cefepime pharmacokinetics in neonatal foals and adult dogs. *J Vet Pharmacol Ther* **24**:187–192.

42   Atherton RP, McKenzie HC III (2006) Alternative antimicrobial agents in the treatment of proliferative enteropathy in horses. *J Equine Vet Sci* **26**:535–541.

43   Orsini JA, Moate PJ, Boston RC *et al.* (2005) Pharmacokinetics of imipenem-cilastatin following intravenous administration in healthy adult horses. *J Vet Pharmacol Ther* **28**:355–361.

44   Magdesian KG, Dujowich M, Madigan JE *et al.* (2006) Molecular characterization of *Clostridium difficile* isolates from horses in an intensive care unit and association of disease severity with strain type. *J Am Vet Med Assoc* **228**:751–755.

45   Orsini JA, Snooks-Parsons C, Stine L *et al.* (2005) Vancomycin for the treatment of methicillin-resistant staphylococcal and enterococcal infections in 15 horses. *Can J Vet Res* **69**:278–286.

46   Orsini JA, Ramberg CF Jr, Benson CE *et al.* (1992) Vancomycin kinetics in plasma and synovial fluid following intravenous administration in horses. *J Vet Pharmacol Ther* **15**:351–363.

47   Rubio-Martinez L M, Lopez-Sanroman J, Cruz AM *et al.* (2005) Evaluation of safety and pharmacokinetics of vancomycin after intravenous regional limb perfusion in horses. *Am J Vet Res* **66**:2107–2113.

48   Rubio-Martinez L, Lopez-Sanroman J, Cruz AM *et al.* (2005) Medullary plasma pharmacokinetics of vancomycin after intravenous and intraosseous perfusion of the proximal phalanx in horses. *Vet Surg* **34**:618–624.

CHAPTER 17: THE SYSTEMIC INFLAMMATORY RESPONSE

1   Moore JN, Morris DD (1992) Endotoxemia and septicemia in horses: experimental and clinical correlates. *J Am Vet Med Assoc* **200**:1903–1914.

2   Fenton MJ, Golenbock DT (1998) LPS-binding proteins and receptors. *J Leukocyte Biol* **64**:25–32.

3   Antal-Szalmas PA (2000) Evaluation of CD14 in host defense. *Eur J Clin Invest* **30**:167–179.

4   Brightbill HD, Modlin RL (2000) Toll-like receptors: molecular mechanisms of the mammalian immune response. *Immunology* **101**:1–10.

5   Nieto JE, MacDonald MH, Poulin Braim AE *et al.* (2009) Effect of lipopolysaccharide infusion on gene expression of inflammatory cytokines in normal horses in vivo. *Equine Vet J* **41**:717–719.

6   Bottoms GD, Fessler JF, Roesel OF *et al.* (1981) Endotoxin-induced hemodynamic changes in ponies: effects of flunixin meglumine. *Am J Vet Res* **42**:1514–1518.

7   Lavoie JP, Madigan JE, Cullor JS *et al.* (1990) Haemodynamic, pathologic, hematologic, and behavioural changes during endotoxin infusion in equine neonates. *Equine Vet J* **22**:23–29.

8   Bentley AP, Barton MH, Lee MD *et al.* (2002) Antimicrobial-induced endotoxin and cytokine activity in an *in-vitro* model of septicemia in foals. *Am J Vet Res* **63**:660–668.

9   Garner HE, Sprouse RF, Lager K (1988) Cross protection of ponies from sublethal *Escherichia coli* endotoxemia by *Salmonella typhimurium* antiserum. *Equine Pract* **10**:10–17.

10   Durando MM, Mackay RJ, Linda S *et al.* (1994) Effects of polymyxin B and *Salmonella typimurium* antiserum on horses given endotoxin intravenously. *Am J Vet Res* **55**:921–927.

11   Barton MH, Parviainen A, Norton N (2004) Polymyxin B protects horses against induced endotoxaemia in vivo. *Equine Vet J* **36**:397–401.

12   Forbes G, Church S, Savage CJ *et al.* (2012) Effects of hyperimmune equine plasma on clinical and cellular responses in a low-dose endotoxaemia model in horses. *Res Vet Sci* **92**:40–44.

13   Semrad SD, Hardee GE, Hardee MM *et al.* (1987) Low dose flunixin meglumine: effects on eicosanoid production and clinical signs induced by experimental endotoxemia in horses. *Equine Vet J* **19**:201–206.

14   Peiró JR, Barnabé PA, Cadioli FA *et al.* (2010) Effect of lidocaine infusion during experimental endotoxemia in horses. *J Vet Intern Med* **24**:940–948.

15   Levy MM, Fink MP, Marshall JC *et al.* (2003) 2001 SCCM/ESICM/ACCP/ATS/SIS International sepsis definitions conference. *Crit Care Med* **31**:1250–1256.

16   Corley KT, Donaldson LL, Furr MO (2005) Arterial lactate concentration, hospital survival, sepsis and SIRS in critically ill neonatal foals. *Equine Vet J* **37**:53–59.

17   Furr M (2003) Systemic inflammatory response syndrome, sepsis, and antimicrobial therapy. *Clin Tech Equine Pract* **2**:3–8.

18   Bone RC, Balk RA, Cerra FB *et al.* (1992) ACCP/SCCM Consensus Conference: definitions for sepsis and organ failure and guidelines for the use of innovative therapies in sepsis. *Crit Care Med* **2**:862–874.

19   Balk RA (2000) Pathogenesis and management of multiple organ dysfunction or failure in severe sepsis and septic shock. *Crit Care Clin* **16**:337–352.

20   Dunkel B, Dolente B, Boston RC (2005) Acute lung injury/acute respiratory distress syndrome in 15 foals. *Equine Vet J* **37**:435–440.

21   Abernethy VE, Lieberthal W (2002) Acute renal failure in the critically ill patient. *Crit Care Clin* **18**:203–222.

22 Opal SM, Esmon CT (2003) Bench to bedside review: functional relationships between coagulation and the innate immune response and their respective roles in the pathogenesis of sepsis. *Crit Care* **7**:23–38.

23 De Backer D (2006) Hemodynamic management of septic shock. *Curr Infect Dis Rep* **8**:336–372.

24 Koenig J, Cote N (2006) Equine gastrointestinal motility-ileus and pharmacological modification. *Can Vet J* **47**:551–559.

25 Bailey SR, Marr CM, Elliot J (2004) Current research and theories on the pathogenesis of acute laminitis in the horse. *Equine Vet J* **167**:129–142.

26 Gold J, Divers T, Barton MH *et al.* (2007) Plasma adrenocorticotropin, cortisol, and adrenocorticotropin/cortisol ratios in septic and normal-term foals. *J Vet Intern Med* **21**:791–796.

27 Marshall JC, Cook DJ, Christou NV *et al.* (1995) Multiple organ dysfunction score: a reliable descriptor of a complex clinical outcome. *Crit Care Med* **23**:1638–1652.

28 Vincent JL, de Mendonca A, Cantraine F *et al.* (1998) Use of the SOFA score to assess the incidence of organ dysfunction/failure in intensive care units: results of a multicenter, prospective study. *Crit Care Med* **26**:1793–1800.

29 Deitch EA, Goodman ER (1999) Prevention of multiple organ failure. *Surg Clin N Am* **79**:1471–1488.

30 Wilson WD, Madigan JE (1989) Comparison of bacteriologic culture of blood and necropsy specimens for determining the cause of foal septicemia: 47 cases (1978–1987). *J Am Vet Med Assoc* **195**:1759–1763.

31 Houck PM, Bratzler DW, Nsa W *et al.* (2004) Timing of antibiotic administration and outcomes for Medicare patients hospitalized with community-acquired pneumonia. *Arch Intern Med* **164**:637–644.

32 Kumar A, Roberts D, Wood KE *et al.* (2006) Duration of hypotension before initiation of effective antimicrobial therapy is the critical determinant of survival in human septic shock. *Crit Care Med* **34**:1589–1596.

33 Feige K, Schwarzwald CC, Bombeli T (2003) Comparison of unfractioned and low molecular weight heparin for prophylaxis of coagulopathies in 52 horses with colic: a randomized double-blinded clinical trial. *Equine Vet J* **35**:506–513.

34 Van den Berghe G, Wouters P, Weekers F *et al.* (2001) Intensive insulin therapy in critically ill patients. *New Engl J Med* **345**:1359–1367.

35 Rivers E, Nguyen B, Havstad S *et al.* (2001) Early goal-directed therapy in the treatment of severe sepsis and septic shock. *New Engl J Med* **345**:1368–1377.

36 Bernard GR, Vincent JL, Laterre PF *et al.* (2001) Efficacy and safety of recombinant human activated protein C for severe sepsis. *New Engl J Med* **344**:699–709.

37 Annane D, Sebille V, Charpentier C *et al.* (2002) Effect of treatment with low doses of hydrocortisone and fludrocortisone on mortality in patients with septic shock. *J Am Vet Med Assoc* **288**:862–871.

38 Hoffman AM, Staempfli HR, Willan A (1992) Prognostic variables for survival of neonatal foals under intensive care. *J Vet Intern Med* **6**:89–95.

39 Raisis AL, Hodgson JL, Hodgson DR (1996) Equine neonatal septicaemia: 24 cases. *Aust Vet J* **73**:137–140.

40 Gayle JM, Cohen ND, Chaffin MK (1998) Factors associated with survival in septicemic foals: 65 cases (1998–1995). *J Vet Intern Med* **12**:140–146.

41 Roy MF (2004) Sepsis in adults and foals. *Vet Clin N Am Equine Pract* **20**:41–61.

42 Slack JA, McGuirk SM, Erb HN *et al.* (2005) Biochemical markers of cardiac injury in normal, surviving septic, or nonsurviving septic neonatal foals. *J Vet Intern Med* **19**:577–580.

43 Peek SF, Semrad S, McGuirk SM *et al.* (2006) Prognostic value of clinicopathologic variables obtained at admission and effect of antiendotoxin plasma on survival in septic and critically ill foals. *J Vet Intern Med* **20**:569–574.

44 Veronesi MC, Magri M, Villani M *et al.* (2006) Factors associated with survival in pathological neonatal equine foals: preliminary results. *Vet Res Commun* **30(Suppl 1)**:215–217.

45 Corley KT, Pearce G, Magdesian KG *et al.* (2007) Bacteraemia in neonatal foals: clinicopathological differences between gram-positive and gram-negative infections, and single organism and mixed infections. *Equine Vet J* **39**:84–89.

46 Henry MM, Moore JN (1991) Clinical relevance of monocyte procoagulant activity in horses with colic. *J Am Vet Med Assoc* **198**:843–848.

47 Collatos CA, Barton MH, Prasse KW *et al.* (1995) Intravascular and peritoneal coagulation and fibrinolysis in horses with acute gastrointestinal diseases. *J Am Vet Med Assoc* **207**:465–470.

48 Barton MH, Morris DD, Norton N *et al.* (1998) Hemostatic and fibrinolytic indices in neonatal foals with presumed septicemia. *J Vet Intern Med* **12**:26–35.

49 Prasse KW, Topper MJ, Moore JN *et al.* (1993) Analysis of hemostasis in horses with colic. *J Am Vet Med Assoc* **203**:685–693.

50 Welles EG, Prasse KW, Moore JN (1991) Use of newly developed assays for protein C and plasminogen in horses with signs of colic. *Am J Vet Res* **52**:345–351.

51 Bakhtiari K, Meijers JC, de Jonge E *et al.* (2004) Prospective validation of the International Society of Thrombosis and Hemostasis scoring system for disseminated intravascular coagulation. *Crit Care Med* **32**:2416–2421.

52 Dolente BA, Wilkins PA, Boston RC (2002) Clinicopathologic evidence of disseminated intravascular coagulation in horses with acute colitis. *J Am Vet Med Assoc* **220**:1034–1038.

53 Franchini M, Lippi G, Manzato F (2006) Recent acquisitions in the pathophysiology, diagnosis, and treatment of disseminated intravascular coagulation. *Thrombosis J* **4**:4.

54 Trzeciak S, Dellinger RP (2004) Other supportive therapies in sepsis: an evidence-based review. *Crit Care Med* **32(11 Suppl)**:S571–S577.

55 Welch RD, Watkins JP, Tayor TS *et al.* (1992) Disseminated intravascular coagulation associated with colic in 23 horses (1984–1989). *J Vet Intern Med* **6**:29–35.

CHAPTER 18: POSTOPERATIVE COLIC PATIENT

1   Pritchett LC, Ulibarri C, Roberts MC et al. (2003) Identification of potential physiological and behavioral indicators of postoperative pain in horses after exploratory celiotomy for colic. *App Anim Behav Sci* **80:**31–43.

2   Mair TS, Smith LJ (2005) Survival and complication rates in 300 horses undergoing surgical treatment of colic. Part 2: Short-term complications. *Equine Vet J* **37:**303–309.

3   Smith LJ, Mellor DJ, Marr CM et al. (2007) Incisional complications following exploratory celiotomy: does an abdominal bandage reduce the risk? *Equine Vet J* **39:**277–283.

4   Stratton-Phelps M (2008) Nutritional management of the hospitalized horse. In: *The Equine Hospital Manual.* (eds K Corley, J Stephen) Blackwell Publishing, Chichester, pp. 261–311.

5   Underwood C, Southwood LL, Walton RM et al. (2010) Hepatic and metabolic changes in surgical colic patients: a pilot study. *J Vet Emerg Crit Care* **20:**578–586.

6   Moore BR, Abood SK, Hinchcliff KW (1994) Hyperlipemia in 9 miniature horses and miniature donkeys. *J Vet Intern Med* **8:**376–381.

7   Mogg TD, Palmer JE (1995) Hyperlipidemia, hyperlipemia, and hepatic lipidosis in American miniature horses: 23 cases (1990–1994). *J Am Vet Med Assoc* **207:**604–607.

8   Dunkel B, McKenzie HC III (2003) Severe hypertriglyceridaemia in clinically ill horses: diagnosis, treatment and outcome. *Equine Vet J* **35:**590–595.

9   Waitt LH, Cebra CK (2009) Characterization of hypertriglyceridemia and response to treatment with insulin in horses, ponies, and donkeys: 44 cases (1995–2005). *J Am Vet Med Assoc* **234:**915–919.

10   Magdesian KG (2004) Monitoring the critically ill equine patient. *Vet Clin North Am Equine Pract* **20:**11–39.

11   Posner LP, Moon PF, Bliss SP et al. (2003) Colloid osmotic pressure after hemorrhage and replenishment with oxyglobin solution, hetastarch, or whole blood in pregnant sheep. *Vet Anaesth Analg* **30:**30–36.

12   Parry BW, McCarthy MA, Anderson GA et al. (1982) Correct occlusive bladder width for indirect pressure measurement in horses. *Am J Vet Res* **43:**50–54.

13   Hall LW, Nigam JM (1975) Measurement of central venous pressure in horses. *Vet Rec* **97:**66–69.

14   MacFarlane D (1999) Hetastarch: a synthetic colloid with potential in equine patients. *Comp Cont Educ Prac Vet* **21:**867–874.

15   Jones PA, Tomasic M, Gentry PA (1997) Oncotic, hemodilutional, and hemostatic effects of isotonic saline and hydroxyethyl starch solutions in clinically normal ponies. *Am J Vet Res* **58:**541–548.

16   Burke JF (1961) The effective period of preventive antibiotic action in experimental incisions and dermal lesions. *Surgery* **50:**161–168.

17   Aberg C, Thore M (1991) Single versus triple dose antimicrobial prophylaxis in elective abdominal surgery and the impact on bacterial ecology. *J Hosp Infect* **18:**149–154.

18   Schein M, Assalia A, Bachus M (1994) Minimal antibiotic therapy after emergency abdominal surgery: a prospective study. *Brit J Surg* **81:**989–991.

19   Hird DW, Casebolt DB, Carter JD et al. (1986) Risk factors for salmonellosis in hospitalized horses. *J Am Vet Med Assoc* **188:**173–177.

20   Dunowska M, Morley PS, Traub-Dargatz JL et al. (2006) Impact of hospitalization and antimicrobial drug administration on antimicrobial susceptibility patterns of commensal *Escherichia coli* isolated from the feces of horses. *J Am Vet Med Assoc* **228:**1909–1917.

21   Kollef MH, Sherman G, Ward S et al. (1999) Inadequate antimicrobial treatment of infections: a risk factor for hospital mortality among critically ill patients. *Chest* **115:**462–474.

22   Archibald L, Phillips L, Monnet D et al. (1997) Antimicrobial resistance in isolates from inpatients and outpatients in the United States: increasing importance of the intensive care unit. *Clin Infect Dis* **24:**211–215.

23   Sellon DC, Roberts MC, Blikslager AT et al. (2002) Continuous butorphanol infusion for analgesia in the postoperative colic horse. *Proc 48th Ann Conven Am Assoc Equine Practitnrs*, Orlando, pp. 244–246

24   Lankveld DP, Driessen B, Soma LR et al. (2006) Pharmacodynamic effects and pharmacokinetic profile of a long-term continuous rate infusion of racemic ketamine in healthy conscious horses. *J Vet Pharm Ther* **29:**477–488.

25   Matthews NS, Fielding CL, Swinebroad E (2004) How to use a ketamine constant rate infusion in horses for analgesia. *Proc 50th Ann Conven Am Assoc Equine Practitnrs*, Denver, pp. 227–228.

26   Lankveld DP, Bull S, Van Dijk P et al. (2005) Ketamine inhibits LPS-induced tumour necrosis factor-alpha and interleukin-6 in an equine macrophage cell line. *Vet Res* **36:**257–262.

27   Mellors JW, Kelly JJ, Gusberg RJ et al. (1988) A simple index to estimate the likelihood of bacterial infection in patients developing fever after abdominal surgery. *Am Surg* **54:**558–564.

28   Ingle-Fehr JE, Baxter GM, Howard RD et al. (1997) Bacterial culturing of ventral median celiotomies for prediction of postoperative incisional complications in horses. *Vet Surg* **26:**7–13.

29   Freeman KD, Southwood LL, Lane J et al. (2012) Postoperative infection, pynexia and perioperative antimicrobial drug use in surgical colic patients. *Equine Vet J* **44:**476–481.

30   Kobluk CN, Ducharme NG, Lumsden JH et al. (1989) Factors affecting incisional complication rates associated with colic surgery in horses: 78 cases (1983–1985). *J Am Vet Med Assoc* **195:**639–642.

31   Phillips TJ, Walmsley JP (1993) Retrospective analysis of the results of 151 exploratory laparotomies in horses with gastrointestinal disease. *Equine Vet J* **25:**427–431.

32   Wilson DA, Baker GJ, Boero MJ (1995) Complications of celiotomy incisions in horses. *Vet Surg* **24:**506–514.

33 Klohnen A, Lores M, Fischer A (2008) Management of postoperative abdominal incisional complications with a hernia belt: 85 horses (2001–2005). *Proc 9th Int Equine Colic Res Symp*, Liverpool, UK.

34 Stick JA (2006) Abdominal hernias. In: *Equine Surgery*. (eds JA Auer, JA Stick) WB Saunders, Philadelphia, pp. 491–499.

35 Moore JN, Garner HE, Shapland JE *et al.* (1981) Prevention of endotoxin-induced arterial hypoxaemia and lactic acidosis with flunixin meglumine in the conscious pony. *Equine Vet J* **13**:95–98.

36 Bottoms GD, Fessler JF, Roesel OF *et al.* (1981) Endotoxin-induced hemodynamic changes in ponies: effects of flunixin meglumine. *Am J Vet Res* **42**:1514–1518.

37 Fessler JF, Bottoms GD, Roesel OF *et al.* (1982) Endotoxin-induced change in hemograms, plasma enzymes, and blood chemical values in anesthetized ponies: effects of flunixin meglumine. *Am J Vet Res* **43**:140–144.

38 Dunkle NJ, Bottoms GD, Fessler JF *et al.* (1985) Effects of flunixin meglumine on blood pressure and fluid compartment volume changes in ponies given endotoxin. *Am J Vet Res* **46**:1540–1544.

39 Spier SJ, Lavoie JP, Cullor JS *et al.* (1989) Protection against clinical endotoxemia in horses by using plasma containing antibody to an Rc mutant of *E. coli* (J5). *Circ Shock* **28**:235–248.

40 Durando MM, MacKay RJ, Linda S *et al.* (1994) Effects of polymixin B and *Salmonella typhimurium* antiserum on horses given endotoxin intravenously. *Am J Vet Res* **55**:921–927.

41 Barton MH, Parviainen A, Norton N (2002) Polymyxin B protects horses against experimentally-induced endotoxaemia in vivo. In: *Proc 7th Int Equine Colic Research Symp*, Manchester, p. 24.

42 Geor RJ, Weiss DJ, Burris SM *et al.* (1992) Effects of furosemide and pentoxifylline on blood flow properties in horses. *Am J Vet Res* **53**:2043–2049.

43 Weiss DJ, Evanson OA, Geor RJ (1994) The effects of furosemide and pentoxifylline on the flow properties of equine erythrocytes: in vitro studies. *Vet Res Comm* **18**:373–381.

44 Baskett A, Barton MH, Norton N *et al.* (1997) Effect of pentoxifylline, flunixin meglumine, and their combination on a model of endotoxemia in horses. *Am J Vet Res* **58**:1291–1299.

45 Peiró JR, Barnabé PA, Cadioli FA *et al.* (2010) Effects of lidocaine infusion during experimental endotoxemia in horses. *J Vet Intern Med* **24**:940–948.

46 Rakestraw PC (2003) Modulation of intestinal motility and ileus. In: *Current Therapy in Equine Medicine*, 5th edn. (ed NE Robinson) WB Saunders, Philadelphia, pp. 108–111.

47 Roussel AJ Jr, Cohen ND, Hooper RN *et al.* (2001) Risk factors associated with development of postoperative ileus in horses. *J Am Vet Med Assoc* **219**:72–78.

48 Holcombe SJ, Rodriguez KM, Haupt JL *et al.* (2009) Prevalence of and risk factors for postoperative ileus after small intestinal surgery in two hundred and thirty-three horses. *Vet Surg* **38**:368–372.

49 Mair TS, Smith LJ (2005) Survival and complication rates in 300 horses undergoing surgical treatment of colic. Part 1: Short-term survival following a single laparotomy. *Equine Vet J* **37**:296–302.

50 Blikslager AT, Bowman KF, Levine JF *et al.* (1994) Evaluation of factors associated with postoperative ileus in horses: 31 cases (1990–1992). *J Am Vet Med Assoc* **205**:1748–1752.

51 Nieto JE, Van Hoogmoed LM, Spier SJ *et al.* (2002) Use of an extracorporeal circuit to evaluate effects of intraluminal distention and decompression on the equine jejunum. *Am J Vet Res* **63**:267–275.

52 Little D, Tomlinson JE, Blikslager AT (2005) Postoperative neutrophilic inflammation in equine small intestine after manipulation and ischemia. *Equine Vet J* **37**:329–335.

53 Freeman DE, Hammock P, Baker GJ *et al.* (2000) Short- and long-term survival and prevalence of postoperative ileus after small intestinal surgery in the horse. *Equine Vet J* **32(Suppl)**:42–51.

54 Cohen ND, Lester GD, Sanchez LC *et al.* (2004) Evaluation of risk factors associated with development of postoperative ileus in horses. *J Am Vet Med Assoc* **225**:1070–1078.

55 Malone E, Ensink J, Turner T *et al.* (2006) Intravenous continuous infusion of lidocaine for treatment of equine ileus. *Vet Surg* **35**:60–66.

56 Torfs S, Delesalle C, Dewulf J *et al.* (2009) Risk factors for equine postoperative ileus and effectiveness of prophylactic lidocaine. *J Vet Intern Med* **23**:606–611.

57 Cook VL, Jones Shults J, McDowell M *et al.* (2008) Attenuation of ischaemic injury in the equine jejunum by administration of systemic lidocaine. *Equine Vet J* **40**:353–357.

58 Guschlbauer M, Hoppe S, Geburek F *et al.* (2010) In-vitro effects of lidocaine on the contractility of equine jejunal smooth muscle challenged by ischaemia-reperfusion injury. *Equine Vet J* **42**:53–58.

59 Gerring EE, Hunt JM (1986) Pathophysiology of equine postoperative ileus: effect of adrenergic blockade, parasympathetic stimulation and metoclopramide in an experimental model. *Equine Vet J* **18**:249–255.

60 Dart AJ, Peauroi JR, Hodgson DR *et al.* (1996) Efficacy of metoclopramide for treatment of ileus in horses following small intestinal surgery: 70 cases (1989–1992). *Aust Vet J* **74**:280–284.

61 Doherty TJ, Andrews FM, Abraha TW *et al.* (1999) Metoclopramide ameliorates the effects of endotoxin on gastric emptying of acetaminophen in horses. *Can J Vet Res* **63**:37–40.

62 Nieto JE, Rakestraw PC, Snyder JR *et al.* (2000) In-vitro effects of erythromycin, lidocaine, and metoclopramide on smooth muscle from the pyloric antrum, proximal portion of the duodenum, and middle portion of the jejunum. *Am J Vet Res* **61**:413–419.

63 Koenig J, Cote N (2006) Equine gastrointestinal motility – ileus and pharmacological modification. *Can Vet J* **47**:551–559.

64 Bologna SD, Hasler WL, Owyang C (1993) Down-regulation of motilin receptors on rabbit colon myocytes by chronic oral erythromycin. *J Pharm Exp Ther* **266**:852–856.

65 Eades SC, Moore JN (1993) Blockade of endotoxin-induced cecal hypoperfusion and ileus with an alpha 2 antagonist in horses. *Am J Vet Res* **54**:586–590.

66 Lester GD, Merritt AM, Neuwirth L *et al.* (1998) Effect of alpha-2 adrenergic, cholinergic, and non-steroidal anti-inflammatory drugs on myoelectrical activity of ileum, cecum, and right ventral colon and on cecal emptying of radiolabeled markers in clinically normal ponies. *Am J Vet Res* **59**:320–327.

67 Adams SB, Lamar CH, Masty J (1984) Motility of the distal portion of the jejunum and pelvic flexure in ponies: effects of six drugs. *Am J Vet Res* **45**:795–799.

68 Baxter GM, Broome TE, Moore JN (1989) Abdominal adhesions after small intestinal surgery in the horse. *Vet Surg* **18**:409–414.

69 MacDonald MH, Pascoe JR, Stover SM *et al.* (1989) Survival after small intestine resection and anastomosis in horses. *Vet Surg* **18**:415–423.

70 Johnstone IB, Physick-Sheard P, Crane S (1989) Breed, age, and gender differences in plasma antithrombin-III activity in clinically normal young horses. *Am J Vet Res* **50**:1751–1753.

71 Ragle CA, Snyder JR, Meagher DM *et al.* (1992) Surgical treatment of colic in American Miniature Horses: 15 cases (1980–1987). *J Am Vet Med Assoc* **201**:329–331.

72 Drollette CM, Badawy SZ (1992) Pathophysiology of pelvic adhesions. Modern trends in preventing infertility. *J Reprod Med* **37**:107.

73 Snoj M (1993) Intra-abdominal adhesion formation is initiated by phospholipase A2. *Med Hypotheses* **41**:525–528.

74 Snoj M, Ar'Rajab A, Ahren B *et al.* (1993) Phospholipase-resistant phosphatidylcholine reduces intra-abdominal adhesions induced by bacterial peritonitis. *Res Exp Med (Berl)* **193**:117.

75 Liebman SM, Langer JC, Marshal JS *et al.* (1993) Role of mast cells in peritoneal adhesions formation. *Am J Surg* **165**:127–130.

76 Gerard MP, Blikslager AT, Roberts MC *et al.* (1999) The characteristics of intestinal injury peripheral to strangulating obstruction lesions in the equine small intestine. *Equine Vet J* **31**:331–335.

77 Sullins KE, White NA, Lundin CS *et al.* (2004) Prevention of ischaemia-induced small intestinal adhesions in foals. *Equine Vet J* **36**:370–375.

78 Yamout S, Bouré L, Theoret C *et al.* (2007) Evaluation of abdominal instillation of 0.03% fucoidan solution for the prevention of experimentally induced abdominal adhesions in healthy pony foals. *Proc Eur Coll Vet Surg 16th Ann Meeting*, Dublin.

79 Morello SM, Southwood LL, Engiles J *et al.* (2012) Effect of intraperitoneal PERIDAN™ Concentrate adhesion reduction device on clinical findings, infection, and tissue healing in an adult horse jejunojejunostomy model. *Vet Surg* **41**:568–581.

80 Mueller PO, Harmon BG, Hay WP *et al.* (2000) Effect of carboxymethylcellulose and a hyaluronate-carboxymethylcellulose membrane on healing of intestinal anastomosis in horses. *Am J Vet Res* **61**:369–374.

81 Parker JE, Fubini SL, Car BD *et al.* (1987) The use of heparin in preventing intra-abdominal adhesions secondary to experimentally induced peritonitis in the horse. *Vet Surg* **16**:459–462.

82 Hague BA, Honnas CM, Berridge BR *et al.* (1998) Evaluation of postoperative peritoneal lavage in standing horses for prevention of experimentally induced abdominal adhesions. *Vet Surg* **27**:122–126.

83 Kuebelbeck KL, Slone DE, May KA (1998) Effect of omentectomy on adhesion formation in horses. *Vet Surg* **27**:132–137.

CHAPTER 19: THE PREGNANT MARE

1 Dolente BA, Sullivan EK, Boston RC *et al.* (2005) Mares admitted to a referral hospital for postpartum emergencies: 163 cases (1992–2002). *J Vet Emerg Crit Care* **15**:193–200.

2 Wilkins PA (2007) Perinatology. In: *Manual of Equine Emergencies*, 3rd edn. (eds JA Orsini, T Divers) Saunders Elsevier, St. Louis, pp. 486–521.

3 Wilkins PA (2009) Complications of the peripartum mare. In: *Current Therapy in Equine Medicine*, 6th edn. (eds N Robinson, K Sprayberry) Saunders Elsevier, St. Louis, pp. 785–788.

4 Wilkins PA (2006) High-risk pregnancy: case 2-1 '03 vital connection: placentitis in the peripartum mare.

In: *Equine Neonatal Medicine: A Case-Based Approach*. (ed MR Paradis) Elsevier Saunders, Philadelphia, pp 13–21.

5 Wilkins PA, Dolente BA (2006) High-risk pregnancy: case 2-2: poppy-body wall tear in late gestational mare and birth resuscitation of a compromised foal. In: *Equine Neonatal Medicine: A Case-Based Approach*. (ed MR Paradis) Elsevier Saunders, Philadelphia, pp. 22–30.

6 Ross J, Palmer JE, Wilkins PA (2008) Retrospective study of body wall tears in late pregnant mares. *J Am Vet Med Assoc* **232**:257–261.

7 Christensen BW, Troedsson MH, Murchie TA (2006) Management of hydrops amnion in a mare resulting in birth of a live foal. *J Am Vet Med Assoc* **228**:1228–1233.

8 Norton JL, Dallap BL, Johnston JK *et al.* (2007) Retrospective study of dystocia in horses at a referral hospital. *Equine Vet J* **39**:37–41.

9 Byron CR, Embertson RM, Bernard WV *et al.* (2001) Dystocia in a referral hospital setting: approach and results. *Equine Vet J* **35**:82–85.

CHAPTER 20: THE NEONATE

1 McDonald PG, Green MA, Vaala WE *et al.* (1990) Nursing care of the neonatal foal. In: *Equine Clinical Neonatology.* (eds AM Koterba, WH Drummond, PC Kosch) Lea and Febiger, Philadelphia, pp. 625–652.

2 Palmer JE (2005) Ventilatory support of the critically ill foal. *Vet Clin N Am Equine Pract* **21**:457–486.

3 Corley KTT (2002) Monitoring and treating haemodynamic disturbances in critically ill neonatal foals. Part 1: Haemodynamic monitoring. *Equine Vet Educ* **14**:345–358.

4 Magdesian KG (2004) Monitoring the critically ill equine neonate. *Vet Clin N Am Equine Pract* **20**:11–39.

5 Brewer B (1990) Renal conditions of the newborn and older foal. *Equine Vet Educ* **2**:127–129.

6 Palmer JE (2002) When fluids are not enough – inopressor therapy. *Proc 8th Int Emerg Crit Care Symposium*, San Antonio, pp. 669–673.

7 Magdesian KG, Madigan JE (2003) Volume replacement in the neonatal ICU: crystalloids and colloids. *Clin Tech Equine Pract Neonatol* **2**:20–30.

8 Palmer JE (2004) Fluid therapy in the neonate: not your mother's fluid space. *Vet Clin N Am Equine Pract* **20**:63–75.

9 Spurlock SL, Furr M (1990) Nursing care of the neonatal foal. In: *Equine Clinical Neonatology.* (eds AM Koterba, WH Drummond, PC Kosch) Lea and Febiger, Philadelphia, pp. 671–685.

10 Vaala W, House J (2001) Perinatal adaptation, asphyxia and resuscitation. In: *Large Animal Internal Medicine*, 3rd edn. (ed BP Smith) Mosby, Philadelphia, pp. 266–276.

11 Magdesian KG (2003) Neonatal pharmacology and therapeutics. In: *Current Therapy in Equine Medicine*, 5th edn. (ed NE Robinson) Saunders, St Louis, pp. 1–5.

12 Russell CM, Axon JE, Blishen A *et al.* (2008) Blood culture results from 427 critically ill neonatal foals (1999 to 2004). *Aust Vet J* **86**:266–271.

13 Sanchez LC (2005) Equine neonatal sepsis. *Vet Clin N Am Equine Pract* **21**:273–293.

14 Wichtel MEG, Buys E, de Luca J *et al.* (1999) Pharmacologic considerations in the treatment of neonatal septicemia and its complications. *Vet Clin N Am Equine Pract* **15**:725–746.

15 Furr M, Mogg TD (2003) Antimicrobial treatment of neonatal foals. *Comp Contin Educ Pract Vet* **25**:302–308.

16 McKenzie HC (2006) Treating foal pneumonia. *Comp Contin Educ Pract Vet Equine Edition* **Spring**:47–53.

17 Wilkins PA (2004) Disorders of foals. In: *Equine Internal Medicine*, 2nd edn. (eds SM Reed, SM Bayly, DC Sellon) Saunders, St Louis, pp. 1381–1431.

18 Vivrette SL, Bostian A, Bermingham E *et al.* (2001) Quinolone-induced arthropathy in neonatal foals. *Proc 47th Ann Conven Am Assoc Equine Practitnrs, San Diego* **47**:376–377.

19 Reilly LK, Palmer JE (1994) Systemic candidiasis in four foals. *J Am Vet Med Assoc* **205**:464–466.

20 Murray MJ, del Piero F, Jeffrey SC *et al.* (1998) Neonatal equine herpesvirus type 1 infection on a thoroughbred breeding farm. *J Vet Intern Med* **12**:36–41.

21 Giguere S, Jacks S, Roberts GD *et al.* (2004) Retrospective comparison of azithromycin, clarithromycin, and erythromycin for the treatment of foals with Rhodococcus equi pneumonia. *J Vet Intern Med* **18**:568–573.

CHAPTER 21: THE RECUMBENT HORSE

1 Corley K, Stephen J (2008) (eds) *The Equine Hospital Manual.* Wiley-Blackwell, Ames.

2 Russell CM, Wilkins PA (2006) Evaluation of the recumbent neonate. *Clin Tech Equine Pract* **5**:161–171.

3 Wilkins PA (2013) Botulism. In: *Equine Infectious Diseases*, 2nd edn. (eds D Sellon, M Long) Saunders-Elsevier, Philadelphia, pp. 203–209.

4 Wilkins PA, Del Piero F (2013) Rabies. In: *Equine Infectious Diseases*, 2nd edn. (eds D Sellon, M Long) Saunders-Elsevier, Philadelphia, pp. 364–367.

Note: Page references in *italic* refer to tables or boxes

abdomen, surgical exploration 41–6
abdominal distension 104, 759
abdominal lavage 787
abdominal sepsis 38
abdominal support bandage 761–2, 775, 791
abdominal wall
    closure 46
    incision 41
    rupture in pregnancy 386–9
abdominal wounds 432, 433, 435
    management 437
abdominocentesis 35–6, 348
    complications 38
    fluid analysis 37–8
    gastric rupture 62
    indications 35
    intestinal neoplasia 95
    peritonitis 150
    post-partum shock 368
    techniques 35–6
abscesses
    brain 465–6
    perirectal 140–1
    spinal cord 481
    strangles 274, 276
    subsolar 155, 242
acepromazine 251, 481, 692
    clinical use 692
    complications 692
    congestive heart
        failure 319
    dose rates *409*
    hemorrhage 343
    indications 692
    mechanism of action 692
    penile paralysis 395
    peripartum blood loss 793
    postoperative ileus *783*, 784
Acer spp. (maples) *557*, 573–4
acetazolamide 252
N-acetyl-DL-penicillamine 600
acetylcysteine enema 546–7
acid burns, cornea 498
acid–base balance 516, 634, 637–8

metabolic and respiratory
    compensations *638*
acorns *607*
Actinobacillus spp. 320
    antimicrobial sensitivity *715*
Actinobacillus equuli 149, 151, 233, 472
activated charcoal *560*, 563–4
activated partial thromboplastin time
    (aPTT) 355, 639
acute kidney injury (AKI) 404–6
    MODS 740–1, 743–4
acute respiratory distress syndrome
    (ARDS) 540, *541*, 740
acyclovir 296, 301, 462, *807*
adenocarcinoma, intestinal 88–9
adhesions, intra-abdominal 784–7
adrenal insufficiency, relative 741, 748
adrenaline, *see* epinephrine
adsorbents *560*, 563–4
aflatoxins 581–2
airway resuscitation, foals 312, 314
albumin 128, 631–2, 669–70
    concentrated human 670
    CSF 460
    normal adult value *632*
albumin quotient (AQ) 460
albumin:globulin ratio *632*
alfalfa hay 116, 591–2
algal toxins 588–91
alkali burn, cornea 498
alkaline phosphatase (ALP) *633*, 634
alkaloids, ergot 582–5
allantochorion, failure to rupture 360
allergic reactions 328, 448, 449
Allium spp. *608*
allopurinol *538*
α-2 agonists 57, 121, 687–8
    clinical use 687–8
    colic *28*
    complications 688
    dose rates *28*, *687*
    epidural 688
    indications 687
    mechanism of action 687
    spinal injuries 478
α-2 antagonists 687
alphaviruses 460, 463–5
altrenogest 790

alyssum, hoary *607*
Amblyomma spp. 447
amikacin 177, 179, 233, 719–21
    dosages in adults *156*, *409*, *721*
    dosages in foals *721*, *807*
    indications 719–20
    regional/local *718*
    toxicity *610*, 721
amino acids, parenteral 707
ε-aminocaproic acid 312, 349, 755
aminoglycosides 177, 179, 214, 404, 719–21
    clinical use 720–1
    dosages 720
    indications 719–20
    local/regional *718*
    mechanism of action 719
    neonate 720–1, 806, *807*
    toxicity *610*, 721
aminophylline 605, 744
4-aminopyridine *610*
amiodarone 329, 335
amitraz 111, 449
ammonia
    blood concentration 148, 474, 475, *633*, 634
    toxicity *610*
amniotic membrane transplant 497
amphotericin B *611*
ampicillin sodium 729, *807*
ampicillin trihydrate 729
Amsinckia spp. (fiddleneck) 576
Anabaena spp. 589–91
analgesia
    burns 445
    colic *28*, 109
    laminitis 247
    postoperative colic patient 769–70
anaphylactic reactions 272, 273, 674, 752
Anderson Sling 812
anemia 311
anesthesia (general) 315, 337–8
aneurysm, aortic 350–1
angiotensin converting enzyme (ACE)
    inhibitors 319
Anoplocephala perfoliata (tapeworm)
    80–1, 102

anorexia, toxicities *558*
anterior chamber
   blood/RBCs (hyphema) 505–6
   collapse 499, 500
anterior uveitis 499
anthelmintics 81, 87, 95, 103
anti-endotoxin therapy 526
antibody index (AI) 460
antifungal agents
   eye 496
   skin 449
   toxicity *611*
antihistamines 449, 674, 752
antimicrobial drugs
   acute liver disease 148
   adjunctive immunotherapy 717
   clostridial myositis 249, 284
   CNS infection 466
   corneal ulcer 496
   difficulty in achieving effective
      tissue levels 179
   dose rates *156*, *409*
   empirical for interim treatment 716
   endocarditis 321
   enrofloxacin 724–5
   foal diarrhea 550
   foal sepsis 526
   hepatic encephalopathy 475
   impregnated implants 179–80,
      233, 719
   increased risk of infection 711
   intra-articular 233
   intrathecal 718
   joint infections 232–3
   neonate 516–17, 806–8
   pericarditis 324
   pharmacodynamics 711
   pharmacokinetics 711
   placentitis 790
   pleuropneumonia/pneumonia 296
   postoperative colic patient 768–9
   proliferative enteropathy 98
   prophylactic 712–14
   regional limb perfusion 176–8, 233,
     420, 718–19
   resistance 126, 177, 711,
     712, 717
   septic arthritis 214
   septic tenosynovitis 237–8
   strangles 276
   susceptibility data 713–14, *715*
   techniques to improve local
     concentrations 233
   therapeutic use 714–17
   topical 445, 446, 775
   toxicity *610*, *615*, 721
   see also named drugs and drug groups
antioxidants 472, 604–5

antithrombin III (ATIII) 355,
   640, 753
antivenin 281, *561*
antiviral agents 301, 462
aorta, rupture/aneurysm 350–1
aortic valve 310, 320–1
aorto-pulmonary fistulation 350
APGAR score 312–13
Appaloosas 252
appetite 703, 758, 790
aqueous humor 508, 509
Arabian breeds 338
aromatic amino acids (AAAs) 475
arrhythmias, *see* cardiac arrhythmias
arsenic toxicity *561*, *611*
arterial blood gas (ABG) analysis
   635–8
   arterial sampling 260–1, 636
   neonate 511
   normal values *636*
   portable analyzers 305, 636
arterial blood pressure 514, 645–6,
   765–6
   interpretation 646, *647*
   measurement 645–6, 766
arterial catheter 766
arterial puncture 260–1
arthrodesis
   carpus 191
   fetlock 186, 218
   pastern joint 227
arthroscopy 232, 240–1
arytenoid chondritis 267–9
arytenoidectomy 273
ascarid impaction 85–7
ascorbic acid 472, *538*
aspartate aminotransferase (AST) 157,
   251, 280, *633*, 634
Aspergillus spp. 320, 344
Aspergillus flavus 581
Aspergillus fumigatus 344
Aspergillus parasiticus 581
aspiration pneumonia 50, 51
Astragalus molissimus 572
asystole 337–8
ataxia, intoxication 556
atipamezole *687*
atlanto–occipital (AO) tap 456, 458
atopy 448, 449
atrial fibrillation (AF) 326–9
atrioventricular block, third-degree
   329–31
atropine
   cardiac disorders 315, 330, 338
   heaves 299, 300
   in toxicities *560*, *591*, *606*
   ophthalmic 496, 505, 509
   toxicity *612*
attitude

foal 800
   postoperative colic patient 758
auricular artery, caudal 346
auriculopalpebral nerve block 484–5
autologous serum 497
autotransfusion *672*, 673–4
axilla, wounds 434, 435, 436
azithromycin 98, 727, *807*
azotemia 61, 404, 405

bacitracin–neomyin–polymyxin B 496
bacterial infections
   cellulitis 440–1, *713*
   endocarditis 320–1
   isolates by site/lesion type *713*
   meningitis 465–6, 527
   risk factors 712
   skin 448, 449
bacterial toxins 441
Bacteroides spp. 150
Bacteroides fragilis 722
Bahia oppositifolia 588
balance 455
balloon thrombectomy 347
bandages 418–20
   abdominal 761–2, 775
   complications 420
   distal limb 420
   elastic adhesive 418, 419
   head 420
   stent 419, 761
   upper limb/full limb 420
base deficit (BD) 637
basisphenoid/basioccipital bone
   fracture 286–7
bedding, foals 798
benzimidazoles 87, 126
benzodiazepines 474, 692–3
   adverse effects *454*
   antagonist (flumazenil) 539, 693
   dose rates *693*
   seizure control *454*
benztropine mesylate 394
Berteroa incana 607
β-adrenergic agonists 300, 363, 375,
   790
β-blockers 329, 334, 509
β-lactam antibiotics 721–3, 806, *807*
β-lactamase 728
bethanechol *783*, 784
bicarbonate 51
bile acids *633*, 634
biliary dysfunction 450
biochemistry 633–5
   interpretation 634–5
   neonate 802
   normal values *633*
bioimpedance 651
biomaterials 497

bismuth subsalicylate *551*
bisphosphonates *560*
black locust *607*
'black-patch' disease (red clover) 586–7
bladder
    calculi 401
    catheterization 642
    defects in neonate 532–5
    eversion 384–6
    rupture 367, 400
    surgical repair 386
blender diets 704
blindness
    acute 510
    toxicities *556*
blister beetles 591–2
blood collection
    arterial blood 260–1, 636
    blood donor 673
    venous blood 628–9
blood culture 321
blood deposit, preoperative *672, 673*
blood gases, *see* arterial blood gas (ABG) analysis
blood loss 311–12, 471, 792–3
    indicators 671–2
    options for blood replacement 671–4
    transfusion requirements *671*
blood pressure, *see* arterial blood pressure
blood transfusion
    allogenic whole blood 671–2, 673
    autologous *672, 673*–4
    hemolysis 312
    hemorrhage 312
    HIE 539
    neonatal isoerythrolysis 522
    post-partum shock 368
    transfusion reactions 519, 670, 674
    uterine artery rupture 348
blood urea nitrogen (BUN) 147, 251, 405, 634, 660, 662
    normal values *633*
blood volume 311
blood–brain barrier 460
blue-green algae 588–91
body condition scoring 697, *698, 699*
borborygmi 625, 760
botulism 272, 478–80, 594–6
    toxicoinfectious (shaker foal syndrome) 595–6
bracken fern *607*
bradycardia, neonate 315
brain
    abscess 465–6
    injury 470–2
    neoplasia 482

    temperature 470–1
    toxicities 580, 581, 585, 586
branched chain amino acids (BCAAs) 475
bretylium tosylate 336
BRIX 0-50% sugar refractometer 520
broad ligament, hematoma 347, 348, 349, 367
bronchoalveolar lavage (BAL) 299
bronchodilators 298, 299, 300, 606
bronchopneumonia 293
broodmares
    abdominal wall rupture 386–9, 790–1
    'at risk' for neonatal isoerythrolysis 521, 523
    critically ill foal 799, 802
    large colon volvulus 104, 794
    metritis-laminitis syndrome 796
    puerperal metritis 369–73
    rectal prolapse 138, 139
    rectal tears 137
    tall fescue toxicosis (ergot alkaloids) 583–5
    uterine artery rupture 347–9
    uterine prolapse 376–7
    uterine torsion 377–9
    see also pregnant mare
Bullet method (cardiac output estimate) 650
buphthalmos 508
buprenorphine 690, 691
burns 442–6
    classification *443*
Buscopan ® *28*, 32, 81, 109
butorphanol 690–1
    after abdominal surgery 770
    dose rates *28, 156, 409*
    foal 547
    right dorsal colitis 129
    spinal injuries 478
    tracheal wash 263
butterfly catheter 178
N-butylscopolammonium bromide (Buscopan ®) *28*, 32, 81, 109

caffeine 512, *513*
calcaneus, fracture 192, 194
calcite 401
calcitonin *560*
calcium, serum 592, *633, 634*
calcium borogluconate 662
calcium disodium EDTA *560*, 599
calcium gluconate 252, 516
calcium oxalate *609*
calculi, urinary tract 401–3
Candida spp. 801
Candida albicans 523

Candida parapsilosis 320
cantharidin 591–2
capillary refill time (CRT) 60, 424, 777–8
    dehydration percentage *660*
carbamates *560*, 605–6
carbohydrate, energy content *701*
carbon dioxide (CO_2)
    partial pressure ($PaCO_2$) 299, 512, *636*, 637
    total *633*, 634
carbon disulfide *612*
carbon monoxide 292, 293, 442
carbon tetrachloride *612*
carbonic anhydrase inhibitors 509
carboxyhemaglobin 293
cardiac arrhythmias 326–36
    atrial fibrillation 326–9
    fatal 335–6
    in toxicities *557*
    premature ventricular contractions 331–3
    third-degree AV block 329–31
    ventricular fibrillation 335–6
    ventricular tachycardia 333–5
cardiac disease 305
    congenital 338–41
    inflammatory 319–26
    toxicities *557*, 575–6, 578–9, *609*
cardiac glycosides *561*, 574–5
cardiac index 651
cardiac output 648–51
    decreased 316, 404, 651
    improving 319
    measurement 649–51
    shock 750
cardiac troponin I (cTnI) 305, 317, 325, 604
cardiomyopathy, dilated 325
cardiopulmonary resuscitation 338
    adults 315
    foals 313–15
cardiovascular system
    clinical signs of failure *742*
    monitoring 800–1
    support in neonate 513–15, 531
cardioversion 328–9
carotid arteries, common
    ligation 345–6, 510
    mycotic plaque 344
carpal sheath, synoviocentesis 167
carprofen *695*
carpus
    accessory bone fracture 190
    bandages/dressings 420
    fractures and luxations 189–91
    incomplete ossification 530
    partial arthrodesis 191

carpus (*continued*)
  splintage *172*, 174
  synoviocentesis 166
Caslick's procedure 381, 382
casting 170–6, 224, 420
castor bean *607*
castration, complications
  341–2, 390–3
casts (urine) 644
cataract 504
catecholamine drugs *676*
catecholamines, plasma 748
cathartics *561*, 564
caudal splint 174–5, 196
cecocolic ligament 42
cecum 98–103
  identification 42
  impaction 34, 98–100
  intussusception 101–3
  rupture 98, 99
  typhlocolitis 125
cefazolin 179, *723*, *807*
cefepime *723*, *807*
cefoperazone *723*
cefotaxime 177, *723*, *807*
cefpodoxime *807*
cefquinome 722, *723*
ceftazidime *723*, *807*
ceftiofur 177, *409*, 721, 722,
  723, *807*
ceftriaxone *723*, *807*
cefuroxime *807*
celiotomy 65, 73, 773–6
cellulitis 440–1, *713*
Centaurea repens 579–80
Centaurea solstitialis 579–80
central venous pressure (CVP) 317,
  646–8
  interpretation 648, 649
  measurement 647–8, 766–7
  normal values 648, 767
cephalexin *723*, *807*
cephalosporins 179, 721–3, 806, *807*
cephalothin *723*
cephapirin *723*
cerebellar signs *453*, 470, 476
cerebrospinal fluid (CSF) 212, 456
  analysis 459–60
  collection 456–9
  drainage 472
cervix, lacerations 379–81
cesarean section 365–6, 388, 389
Cestrum diurnum 609
chemical injury, cornea 498
chest compressions 314–15
chest tube 265–7, 324
chewing disease *558*, 580–1
chiggers 447
chloramphenicol 98, 249, 724, 807

chlorate salts *612*
chlorhexidine 445, 449
chloride *633*
chlorinated hydrocarbons *613*
chlorophenols *616*
choke 27, 47–51, *555*
chokecherry 568
cholangiohepatitis 148
cholecalciferol, toxicity *560*
cholinesterase-inhibitors (insecticides)
  560, *561*, 605–6
cholinomimetics 76, 77
chondroids 274
chordae tendinae 310, 316
Chorioptes equi 447, 448
chronic obstructive pulmonary disease
  (COPD) 298–300
chrysotherapy 452
cicatrix 270
cimetidine 56, 598
Circuta maculata 572
clarithromycin 727, *808*
Claviceps paspali 588
Claviceps purpurea 582–5
clenbuterol 300, 363, 375, 790
clindamycin *615*
clostridial myositis 247–9, 282–4
Clostridium spp. 354
Clostridium baratii 478
Clostridium botulinum 78, 478–80, 595
Clostridium butyricum 478
Clostridium difficile 90, 124–6, *549*
Clostridium perfringens 124, 125, 247,
  282, *548*, *549*
Clostridium septicum 247, 282
Clostridium tetani 480
clot formation time 641
clovers
  alsike 565–6
  red 586, 587
coagulation cascade 640, 752–3
coagulation index 642
coagulation profile 638–42, 765
coagulopathy 152, 355, 793
Coastal Bermuda grass 80, 99, 100
colic
  abdominal ultrasonography 39–40
  clinical signs 27
  drug dosages *28*
  exploratory surgery 40–6
  gas 109
  indications for referral 28–9
  initial treatment 28
  nasogastric intubation 30–2
  postoperative care
    analgesia 769–70
    antimicrobial therapy 768–9
    feeding 770–1
    fluid therapy 767–8

  postoperative complications
    772–87
    adhesions 784–7
    endotoxemia 779–80
    fever 760, 763, 772–3
    ileus 780–4
    incisional infections 762, 773–6
    shock 776–8
  postoperative monitoring 758–67
  rectal examination 32–5
  thromboembolic 354
colitis 124–6
  right dorsal 39, 127–9
collateral sesamoidean ligament
  164, 165
colloid osmometer 632
colloid osmotic pressure (COP) 292,
  445, 663, 765
  correction/maintenance 664–6, 768
  measurement 631–2, 765
colon, *see* large colon; small colon
Colostrometer 520
colostrum 518
  alloantibodies 521–2
  IgG content 518, 520
  supplementation 519, 526
colotomy 103
common digital extensor tendon
  rupture 222–3, 552, 553
  tendon sheath synoviocentesis 167
compensatory anti-inflammatory
  response syndrome (CARS) 523
compositional diets 704, *705*
computed tomography (CT) 191,
  211–12, 230, 456, 478
condylar fractures (third metacarpal/
  metatarsal bones) 186–7, 188
congestive heart failure
  (CHF) 316–19
Conium maculatum 572, *608*
conjunctiva, anesthesia 484
conjunctival graft 486–7, 497
constipation *555*
contracture 552, 554
contrast fistulography 158–9, 236
Coombs test *522*
Cooperia pedunculata 450
copper 348, *561*, *620*
copperheads 280
cor pulmonale 316
coral snakes (elapids) 280, 281
corn oil 129, 446
cornea
  anesthesia 484
  chemical burns 498
  conjunctival graft 486–7, 497
  edema 503, 504, 506
  fluorescein staining 495, 496
  laceration 499–500

'melting' (keratomalacia) 486, 495, 497
opacity 502, 503
stromal abscess 500–2
ulceration 493, 495–8
corneal reflex 455
coronary band
cleft 246
injury 215, 216
coronitis 524
corpus cavernosum, lavage 394
corticosteroids
allergic reactions 449
brain injury 472
endogenous 52
equine multinodular pulmonary fibrosis 301
inflammatory/infiltrative bowel disease 95
ophthalmic 505
pemphigus foliaceus 452
pneumonia 296
recurrent airway obstruction 300
shock 752
transfusion reaction 670
WNV 463
cortisol 528, 529
coumaphos 448
cow's milk 706
coxofemoral joint
luxation 207–8, 225, 227
radiography 205
cranial nerves (CN)
examination 455–6
injury 210, 212
cranial thyroid artery 346
creatine kinase (CK) 251, 280, 633, 634
creatinine (plasma/serum)
aminoglycosides 721
dehydration 660
normal value 633
premature foal 530
renal function 634, 721, 764
crib-biting 64
cricoarytenoideus dorsalis muscles 271, 272
cross-match 312
Crotalaria spectabilis (rattlebox) 576–7
Crotalidae spp. (pit vipers) 280, 561, 592–4
crotoxyphos 448
cryotherapy, glaucoma 509
Cryptosporidium 548, 549
crystalluria 644
cuboidal bones, ossification 530
cyanide toxicity 561, 568–9, 613, 751
cyanocobalamin 570

cyanogenic glycoside-containing plants 556, 566–70
cyanosis, central 340, 341
cyathostomiasis 124–5
diagnostic tests 549
treatment 126
cyclo-oxygenase (COX) enzymes 127, 695
cyclophotocoagulation, transcleral 509
cyclosporine 505
Cynoglossum officinale (hound's tongue) 576–7
cystoscopy 401
cystotomy 402, 403
cytokines, proinflammatory 734, 739, 745, 752–3

D-penicillamine 561
dalteparin 355, 740, 755
Damalinia equi 447
dantrolene 251
Datura stramonium 607
dead space 415, 416
decubital artery, puncture 260–1
decubital ulcers 802, 810, 811
deferoxamine mesylate 522, 561, 598
defibrillation 336
degloving injuries 422
dehydration
clinical signs/estimation of percentage 660
foal/neonate 514, 525
demodicosis 447, 449
dentition 47
Dermacentor spp. 447
Dermanysus gallinae 447, 449
dermatophilosis 448, 449
dermatophytosis (ringworm) 448, 449
descemetocele 496
Descemet's membrane 496, 508
detomidine 475, 478, 687
dose rates 156, 687
epidural 688
detomidine HCl 28, 409
dexamethasone 273, 300, 301
head injury 472
inflammatory/infiltrative bowel disease 95
pemphigus foliaceus 452
third-degree AV block 330
dextrans 667, 668
dextrose 252, 513, 803, 804
parenteral nutrition 707, 708
di-tri-octahedral smectite 551, 736–7
diaphragmatic hernia 145–6
diarrhea
foal 547–51
in toxicities 555

diastolic arterial pressure (DAP) 646, 647
diazepam 147, 332, 454, 471, 481, 539, 606, 693
diazinon 448
diclofenac 353, 441
digital pulses 243, 246
Digitalis spp. 561
Digitalis pupurea 575
digoxin 319, 329
digoxin Fab fragments 561
dimercaprol 600, 611
dimethyl sulfoxide (DMSO) 273, 353, 441, 449, 472, 787
HIE 538
toxicity 613
dioctyl sodium sulfosuccinate (DSS) 58, 614
disseminated intravascular coagulation (DIC) 740–1, 752–5
clinical features/diagnosis 754–5
definition 752
etiology/pathogenesis 741, 752–3
management 754–5
distal interphalangeal joint
arthrocentesis 161–2
hyperextension 220, 221, 424–5, 553
subluxation 227
distal limb
anatomy 425
dressings/bandages 418–20
fractures 180–9
lacerations and puncture wounds 421–30
nerve blocks 409–11
distal (third) phalanx
fracture 180–2
penetrating injuries 243
rotation/sinking in laminitis 245, 246
septic osteomyelitis 214–16
diuretics 406, 606, 744, 752
diverticula, small intestines 84–5
dobutamine 319, 513, 515, 678–9
Döhle bodies 737
domperidone 585
dopamine 331, 406, 513, 540, 676, 680–1, 744
dopamine D2-receptor antagonists 585
Doppler echocardiography 650–1
dorsal metatarsal artery, puncture 260, 261, 511
dorsal/plantar splint 172–4
dorzolamide 509
doxapram 315, 512, 513
doxycycline, neonate 808

drainage
  CSF 472
  pleural fluid 264–7
  septic joint 232
  wounds 415–16
Draschia megastoma 448
dressings 416–20, 445
'dropped elbow' 174–5, 202
'dropped fetlock' 217, 219
drug reactions 452
ductus arteriosus 340
duodenitis–proximal jejunitis 90–3
duodenum
  distension 33
  exploration 45
  ulcers 51, 53
dysmaturity 528
dysphagia 345, *555*, 595
dystocia 347, 358–66
  clinical signs 360
  etiology 358–60
  management 360–6, 795
  tall fescue toxicosis 584
ear, lacerations 439
ear droop 473
Eastern equine encephalomyelitis
  (EEE) 460, 463–5
ecchymoses 754, 755
echocardiography 308–10, 650–1
  congestive heart failure 318
  endocarditis 320–1
  indications 308
  myocarditis/myocardial
    degeneration 325–6
  pericarditis 323
  ventricular septal defect 339
  volumetric 650
ectropion, cicatricial 444
edema
  celiotomy incision 775
  post-castration 392
  sodium overloading 802
  ventral 316, 317, 387, 791
elapids (coral snakes) 280, 281
elbow, dropped 174–5, 202
elbow lock 359, 361
electrical defibrillation 336
electrocardiography (ECG)
  asystole 337
  atrial fibrillation 327
  base-apex 306–7
  congestive heart failure 317
  indications 306
  pericarditis 323
  premature ventricular complexes
    332
  quinidine toxicity 328
  ventricular fibrillation 336
  ventricular tachycardia 333, 334

electrolyte abnormalities 515, 532–5,
  662, 710
electrolyte therapy 111–12, 550
  neonate 515–16, 804
electroretinography 509, 510
enalaprilat 319
encephalitis
  alphaviruses 463–5
  bacterial 465–6
  parasitic 476
encephalopathy, neonatal ischemic
  536–7
endocarditis 320–1
endophthalmitis 483
endophytes 566, 582–3
endoscopy
  esophageal 49
  guttural pouches 278, 279, 344,
    345
endotoxemia 92, 245, 247, 354, 625,
  733–7
  clinical features 735–6, 779
  diagnosis 736
  etiology/pathogenesis 733–4
  foal 526
  kidney injury 404, 406
  management 736–7
  postoperative colic patient 779–80
  retained fetal membranes 374–5
endotoxin 733–5, 753, 779
endotracheal intubation 256–7, 273
enemas 546–7
energy requirements 701–2
enrofloxacin 177, 724–5, *808*
enteral nutrition 703–6
enteric nervous system 76, 780–1
enteritis
  foal 525, 526
  proximal 90–3
Enterobacter spp. 233, 237, 441
enterocentesis 38
Enterococcus spp. *715*, 724
enterocolitis 547–51
enterocytes 707
enterolithiasis 115–18
enteropathy, proliferative 96–8
enterotomy 44
entropion 492–3, 518
enucleation 488–90
envenomation, viperid 280–2, 592–4
eosinophilic enteritis *93*, 94
Epicauta spp. (blister beetles) 591–2
epidural analgesia
  alpha-2 agonists 688
  catheterization 685–6
  local anesthetics *695*
epinephrine (adrenaline)
  anaphylaxis/transfusion reactions
    273, 519, 674, 752

complications 684
  dose rates *684*
  indications 684
  mode of action *684*
  receptor affinity *676*
  resuscitation 313, 315, 338
epiphora 483
epiphysis, septic 213–14
epiploic foramen entrapment 64–5
epistaxis 32, *253*, 286–90, 344–5, 469
Epsom's salt *561*, 564
equine arteritis virus 523
equine herpes viruses (EHV) 294, 296
  EHV-1 523
  EHV-5 300–1
equine herpesvirus
  myeloencephalomyelitis (EHM)
    460–2
equine multinodular pulmonary
  fibrosis (EMPF) 300–1
equine nigropallidal encephalomalacia
  (chewing disease) *558*, 580–1
equine protozoal myeloencephalitis
  (EPM) 467–8
equine recurrent uveitis (ERU) 504–5
ergot alkaloids 582–5
ergovaline 583
erythromycin 77, 98, 727
erythromycin lactobionate 783–4
erythromycin stearate *808*
eschar, burn injuries 445
Escherichia coli 150, 233, 320, 441, 523,
  548
  antimicrobial sensitivity *715*
esmarch bandage 178
esophageal obstruction (choke) 27,
  47–51, *555*
esophagostomy feeding tube 698–700
Eupatorium rugosum 578–9
Eutrombicula spp. 447
evisceration, post-castration 391–2
exercise intolerance 327, 329, 330
exertional rhabdomyolysis 157, 250–1
exotoxins 441
extensor carpi radialis, tendon sheath
  synoviocentesis 167
extensor tendons, injuries 175, 222–3,
  552, 553
external carotid artery 344
  ligation 346
extracellular fluid space 660–1
extrauterine intrapartum technique
  (EXIT) 364, 795
eye
  clinical signs of intoxication *557*
  nerve blocks 484–5
  removal (enucleation) 488–90
eye care 797, 801
eye injuries 483

cornea 493, 495
definitions 483
neonate 518
orbital fracture 494
eye position 455
eyelid
decreased tone 479
entropion 492–3
inability to close 473
lacerations 439, 490–2
surgical closure 488

facial artery 346
blood collection 260, 261
facial nerve 455
facial paralysis 473
facial swelling 280–1, 593
facial symmetry 455
Fagopyrum esculentum 450
failure of passive transfer 518–20
falls, backward 468–9
fasciotomy 284
fast localized abdominal sonography of
horses (FLASH) 40
fecal occult blood 88
fecal production, after colic surgery
759
fecalith obstruction 132–3
feeding
and colonic impaction 111
enterolithiasis 116, 118
exertional rhabdomyolysis 250
gas/spasmodic colic 109
gastric acid exposure 52
HYPP management 252
inflammatory/infiltrative bowel
disease 95
nasogastric/esophagostomy tube
704–6
neonate 798
postoperative colic patient 770–1
proximal enteritis 90
recumbent horse 811
see also nutritional support
feedstuffs
aflatoxins 582
ionophores 603–4
femur, fractures 203–6
fentanyl 445, 690, 691, 692
ferrous fumurate 597
Festuca arundinacea (tall fescue) 582–3
fetal membranes, retention 369–73
fetlock (metacarpo-/
metatarsophalangeal) joints
arthrodesis 186, 218
'dropped' 217, 219
hyperextension 424–5, 553
injuries involving 229, 230, 426
lavage 231

stabilization 220, 221
synoviocentesis 160, 164–5
fetotomy 364, 366
fetus
death 363–4
hypoxia 362
induction of maturation 389
fibrin
circulation 354
pericardium 322
synovial sepsis 228, 231–2, 234
fibrin degradation products 639
fibrinogen 128, 295, 530, 542, 633,
640, 764, 773, 806
measurement 631
normal adult value *632*
fipronil 448
fires 292–3, 442
firocoxib *28*, *155*, *409*, 695, 769
fistula
guttual pouch/nasopharynx 278,
279
rectovaginal 383
flexor tendon sheath
synoviocentesis 164–5
wounds/sepsis 234–8, 422,
426–7
flexor tendons
disruption 219–21
wounds involving 424–9
flooring, recumbent horse 809
fluconazole, neonate 807, *808*
fluid spaces 660–1
fluid therapy (IV)
acute kidney injury 406
calculation for formulation
660, *661*
fluid overload 648
foal diarrhea 550
hemorrhage 312
hypovolemia 752
intravenous 115, 147
neonate 513–14, 802–4
post-partum shock 368
postoperative colic patient 767–8
proximal enteritis 92
sodium-sparing 804
uterine tear/peritonitis 375
fluids 658
colloids 368, 514, 664–74, 752
crystalloids 514, 658–64, 752
enteral 32, 111–12
hemorrhage 212
flumazenil 539, 693
flunixin meglumine 50, 282, 445
dose rates *28*, *155*, *409*
endotoxemia 374, 737, 779
foal 526, 547
hyperthermia 471

mechanism of action 695
postoperative colic patient 769
fluorescein stain 495, 496
fluoride *614*
foals
arterial puncture 260, 261
ascarid impaction 86–7
body condition scoring *698*
cardiopulmonary resuscitation
313–15
common digital extensor tendon
rupture 222–3, 552, 553
diarrhea/enterocolitis 547–51
enteral diets 706
entropion 493, 518
gastric/duodenal ulcers 51,
52–3, 57
guttural pouch tympany 276–80
inguinal hernias 141–4
intussusception 68
orientation/presentation in birth
canal 358–62
parenteral nutrition *709*
premature 528–32
septic arthritis 227–33
septic physitis/epiphysitis 213–14
strangulating umbilical hernia
144–5
tall fescue toxicosis 584–5
toxicoinfectious botulism 595–6
see also neonate
folliculitis, bacterial 448, 449
foot
heel bulb laceration 426
septic navicular bursitis 238–41
see also hoof
foot cast 182
foot–nape posture 359, 361
forebrain syndrome 470
foreign bodies
metallic 158
small colon 133–4
upper airway 289–90
wounds 434, 440
formalin 312, 349, 793
fractures 156
carpus 189–91
distal phalanx 180–2
facial bones 288–9
femur 203–6
humerus 201–3
middle phalanx 182–3
olecranon 194–6
orbit 494–5
pelvis 207–9
proximal phalanx 173, 184–5
radius 196–8
ribs 314–15, 543–5
Salter–Harris 199, 203, 206

fractures (*continued*)
'screwdriver' 185
skull 210–12
splinting and casting 170–6
tarsal bones 191–4
third metacarpus/
metatarsus 186–9
tibia 198–201
freeze burns 442
fresh frozen plasma 312, 519
friction rub 322
frontal (supraorbital) nerve block
484, 485
frostbite 446
fucoidan solution 786–7
fumonisins 585–6
fungal infections
guttural pouch 343–7
skin 448, 449
furosemide 292, 319, 406, 540, 606,
744, 752
Fusarium moniliforme 90
Fusarium proliferatum 585
Fusarium verticillioides 585–6

GABA/benzodiazepine/chloride
ionophore complex 475
gabapentin 696
gag 257
gag reflex 455
gait abnormalities 456, *556*
gamma glutamyltransferase (GGT)
632, 634
gas colic 109
gas humidifier 254
gastric acid 52
gastric impaction 57–8
gastric lavage 58, 562, 598, *612*, *617*
technique 562
gastric outflow obstruction 51, 53
management 57
gastric rupture 58, 60–2
gastric ulcer syndrome 51–7
gastrointestinal stromal tumor (GIST)
88, 89
gastrointestinal (GI) disease
clinical signs 27
concurrent with uterine torsion
379
history 27
in HIS 536, 537
in toxicities *555*
thromboembolism 354–5
gastrointestinal (GI) tract
decontamination 562–4
monitoring 625, 801
neoplasia 35
NSAID toxicity 602–3
premature foal 531

protectants 129, 550, *551*, 598
trauma in parturition 793–4
gastronasal reflux 58, 62, 78, 81
gastroscopy 53–5
gastrosplenic ligament entrapment 66
gelatins 669
general anesthesia 315, 337–8
gentamicin 179, 296, 324, *610*
dose rate *156*, *409*
gentamicin sulfate 321, *808*
Glauber's salt *561*, 564
glaucoma 506, 508–9
glides 812
globulin 631–2
glomerular filtration rate (GFR) 404,
634
glomerulonephritis 404, 405
glucometers 515
glucose
blood 471, 515, *633*, 634–5,
709–10, 764
urine 644, 764
glucose supplementation 515, 531, 803
glutamate 536
gluteal muscles, atrophy 209
glyceryl trinitrate 571
glycopyrrolate 338, *560*
gold salts 452
granulation tissue, larynx 268, 269
granulocyte colony-stimulating factor
(G-CSF) 717
granulomatous enteritis *93*
grass sickness 78–9, 595
grasses, fungal toxins 582–5, 588
grazing, after colic surgery 770–1
griseofulvin 449
guttural pouch
blood/hematoma 287
mycosis 343–7
normal anatomy 276, 277, 344
strangles 274, 275, 276
temporohyoid osteoarthropathy
473, 474
tympany 276–80

Haab's striae 508
habronemiasis, cutaneous
448, 449
Haematopinus asini 447
Halicephalobus spp. 476
halothane anesthesia 337
harvest mites 447, 448–9
hay
alfalfa 116, 591–2
feeding after colic surgery 770–1
toxic plants 565
head
arterial anatomy 346
bandaging 420

burn injuries 444
neurologic examination 455–6
swelling 281, 282, 593
head pressing behavior 475, *556*
head trauma 468–72
neurologic injury 470–2, 510
sinuses/nasal passages 288–9
skull fractures 210–12
types of injury 468–9
wounds 437–40
healing, secondary intention 435, 436
hearing 455
heart failure
congestive 316–19
right-sided 322
heart rate 624, *660*, 760
heaves *253*, 298–300
heavy metal poisoning 272
heel bulb, laceration 426
Heimlich valve 266
hematochezia *555*
hematocrit tube 628, 629
hematology
monitoring 625, 628–31
neonate 802, 806
normal adult values *630*
postoperative colic patient 764
hematoma
uterine broad ligament 347, 348,
349, 367
vulva 384
hematuria 401
hemicastration 399, 400
hemlock, poison *608*
hemodilution, acute normovolemic
672, 673
hemoglobin 311, 471, 522, *630*
hemoglobin-based oxygen-carrying
(HBOC) solutions 672, 674
hemoglobinuria 644
hemolysis, resuscitation 311–12
hemolytic cross-match 522
hemoperitoneum 37, 152–3
hemorrhage 305
pelvic fractures 208
peripartum 792–3
peripheral artery/vein 342–3
post-castration 341–2, 390–1
post-partum 368
resuscitation 311–12
see also blood loss
hemostatic agents 343
hemothorax 266, 296–8, 543–4
heparin
DIC 754–5
hyperlipemia 148, 710
laminitis prophylaxis 92
SIRS 740
thromboembolic disease 355

toxicity *614*
hepatic encephalopathy (HE) 147, 272, 474–6, 581, 582, 597, 598
hepatotoxins 450, 576–8, 585–6
herbicides 565
hernia belt 776
hernias 141–6
  body wall 790–1
  celiotomy incision 776
  diaphragmatic 145–6
  inguinal and scrotal 141–4
  omental 391–2
  umbilical (strangulating) 144–5
hetastarch 666–7, 768
hindbrain syndrome 470
hindquarters, symmetry 208, 209
histamine (H2) receptor antagonists 56, 550, *551*, 602
Holliday–Segar formula 803–4
hoof
  dystrophic growth in selenosis 601
  hoof wall avulsion 214, 215
  laminitic horse 247
  puncture wounds 236, 242–4
  subsolar abscess 155, 242
  see also foot
Horner's syndrome 272
hospital plate 241, 244
humerus, fracture 201–3
hyaline membrane disease 528–9, 531
hyaluronate-carboxymethylcellulose membrane 786–7
hydralazine 319
hydrocele 399
hydrogel dressings 445
hydrops allantois 386, 388–9, 792
hydroxycobalamin 570
hydroxyethyl starch 666
hydroxyurea 95
hydroxyzine hydrochloride 449
hyoscyamine *612*
hyperammonemia 148, 474, 475, *633*, 634
hypercalcemia *560*
hypercoagulable state 352
hyperextension
  foal 552, 553
  secondary to injury 220, 221, 424–5
hyperglobulinemia 632
hyperglycemia 515, 634–5, 709–10, 764
Hypericum perforatum 450
hyperimmune plasma 463, 526, 737
hyperkalemia 515–16, 533, 534–5
hyperkalemic periodic paralysis (HYPP) 252
hyperlactatemia 125, 311, 368, 765
hyperlipemia 147, 148

hypermetria *556*
hypernatremia 516
hyperproteinemia 632
hypersensitivity 448, 449
hyperthermia 245
  brain injury 470–1
hypertriglyceridemia 147, 148, 710, 764–5
hyperventilation 314
hyphema 483, 499, 505–6
hypoalbuminemia 128, 632, 669–70
hypocalcemia 592
Hypochaeris radicata toxicity 272
hypoglycemia 515, 529, 634–5, 702
hypokalemia 319, 327, 516
hyponatremia 125, 516, 533, 534, 802
hypoproteinemia 128, 129, 445, 602, 632
hypopyon 483
hypotension 311, 471, 743–4, 748
  treatment algorithm 677
hypothalamus–pituitary–adrenal (HPA) axis 528
hypothermia 531, 798
hypovolemia
  hemorrhage 342
  neonate 514
hypovolemic shock 750–2
hypoxemia 297, 471, 525, 750, 751
hypoxic ischemic encephalopathy (HIE) 536, 538–9
hypoxic ischemic syndrome (HIS) 517, 534–40, *548*

i-STAT 1 305, 636
IgG index 460
ileo-/jejunocolostomy 100
ileocecal fold 45
ileocolic artery 43
ileum
  exploration 45
  impaction 34, 80–1
  intussusception 66–9
  muscular hypertrophy 82–3
ileus
  in MODS *742*, 744
  postoperative colic patient 780–4
  primary 76–7
ilium, fracture 207–9
imidacloprid 448
imidocarb dipropionate *614*
imipenem (with cilastatin) 177, 717, 725–6, 806, *808*
immunoglobulin G (IgG) 518, 519, 520
immunohistochemistry 461, 463, 464, 467
immunotherapy 717

incisions
  abdominal wall 41
  infections 762, 769, 773–6
  postoperative care 761–2
indolizidine alkaloids 572
inflammatory bowel disease 93–5
inflammatory mediators 734, 739
infratrochlear nerve block 484
infusion pump 678, 686
inguinal hernias 141–4
inotropes *513*, 514–15, 531
  goals of therapy 676
  indications 675
  preparation and administration 676, 678
  see also named drugs
inpatient treatment record 626–7
insect hypersensitivity 449
insecticide toxicity 605–6, *613*
  decontamination/antidotes *560*, *561*
insulin, exogenous 148, *513*, 515, 709, 764
interferon (IFN) 463
interleukins (IL) 734, 739, 753
internal carotid artery 344
  ligation 346
  mycotic plaque 344
intestines
  motility 76, 780–4
  post-castration herniation 391–2
  prolapse in bladder rupture 385–6
  prolapse through vaginal tear 380–1
  viability assessment 106–7
  see also large colon; small colon; small intestines
intracranial pressure (ICP) 471, 472
intraocular pressure (IOP) 503, 505, 506, 508–9
intraosseous (IO) bone perfusion 527
intravenous catheterization 653–8
  complications 656, 658, 762–3
  long-term 656–7
  postoperative colic patient 762–3
  sites 653–4
intravenous catheters 654
  breakage/kinking 658, 763
  foal 512, 513
  lateral thoracic 763
  parenteral nutrition 709, 710
  thrombophlebitis 351–3, 763
intussusception
  cecocecal/cecocolic 101–3
  small intestinal 66–9
iodine, toxicity *615*
ionophores, toxicity 603–5
iridocorneal angle 506, 508, 509
iridocyclitis 483, 499

iris, prolapse 499, 500
iron, toxicity *561*, 596–8
ischemia, causes in neonate *535*
isoproterenol 331
itraconazole 449, 496
ivermectin 87, 95, 126, 448, 449
Ixodes spp. 447

Jackson–Pratt drain 232
jasmine, wild/day blooming *609*
jaundice 521, 524–5
jaundiced foal agglutination (JFA)
    assay 522
jaw fractures 211–12
jejunocecostomy 65
jejunoileostomy 65
jejunojejunostomy 65, 73
jejunum
    adhesions 784, 785
    distension 33
    diverticula formation 84–5
    exploration 45
    intussusception 66–9
    volvulus 73–5
'jelly-belly' foals 802
jimsonweed *607*
Johnsongrass 568, *609*
Joint Infusion Kit 233, 238
joint injections, infection 228
joint lavage 214, 231
joints
    laxity 532
    septic arthritis 227–33
    wounds involving 227–31
Juglans nigra (black walnut) 570–1
jugular groove 273
    injury/inflammation 272
jugular vein
    catheterization 656–8
    thrombophlebitis 351–3, 763

keratectomy 486
keratitis
    exposure 473
    fungal 497
    immune-mediated 502–3
keratomalacia 483, 486, 495, 497
keratoplasty, lamellar 501–2
ketamine 693–4, 770
ketoprofen *695*
Kimzey Leg Saver Splint 170–1,
    172–4, 221
Klebsiella spp. 233
Klebsiella pneumoniae 715
knapweed, Russian 579–80

lactate
    blood 61, 107, 311, 312, 368, *633*,
        635, 765

peritoneal fluid 38
    synovial fluid 161
lactate dehydrogenase (LDH) 147
lactated Ringer's solution (LRS) 60,
    659, 804
lactic acidosis 635
lactose intolerance *548*
lactulose 475
lameness
    distal limb injuries 424, 425
    physical examination 157–8
laminitis 245–7
    clinical signs/diagnosis 157, 246
    etiology/pathogenesis 245
        infections 92, 126, 373, 796
        MODS 741
        toxicities 328, 557, 570–1
    management 157, 247, 744
Landis–Pappenheimer equation 631
laparoscopy 119, 121, 122, 342, 403
laparotomy, standing flank 379
large colon
    decompression 43
    enterolithiasis 115–18
    exploration 42–4
    impaction 34, 110–15
    infarction 108–9, 354
    nephrosplenic ligament entrapment
        35, 118–21
    right dorsal displacement 34, 122–3
    tympany/spasmodic colic 109
    viability assessment 106–7
    volvulus (LCV) 39, 53, 104–7, 794
laryngeal paresis, bilateral 271–3
laryngoplasty, unilateral 273
larynx, normal endoscopy 267
lasalocid 603–5
latanoprost 509
lateral splint 175–6, 194
Lawsonia intracellularis 94, 96–8, *549*,
    724, 726
laxative therapy 547
lead toxicity *560*, *561*, 598–9
left ventricle
    echocardiography 310
    enlargement 318
Leptospira spp. 405, 504
leukocidin 441
leukoencephalomalacia, equine 585,
    586
leukogram 625
leukopenia 61, 125, 525, 530, 764, 772
lice 447
lidocaine 694–5
    arrhythmias 332, 334, 336, 338
    complications 695
    CRI 686, 694
    endotoxemia 780
    epidural *695*

ileus 782, *783*
    mechanism of action 694
    postoperative analgesia 770
    right dorsal colitis 129
    SIRS 737
lidocaine/xylazine, epidural *688*
limb deformities, foal 551–4
lime sulfur 448, 449
limulus amebocyte lysate assay 736
lincomycin *615*
lindane 449
linea alba 41, 46
linguofacial artery 346
lipids
    energy content *701*
    parenteral 707
lipoma
    small colon 135
    small intestine 71–3
lipopolysaccharide-binding protein
    734
lipoprotein lipase 710
lithium dilution 649, 650
Littre's (parietal) hernia 144
liver, 'dishrag' 476
liver disease
    acute 146–8
    aflatoxicosis 581–2
    algal toxins 588, 590
    hepatic encephalopathy 147, 272,
        474–6
    hypoxic ischemic 538
    iron toxicity 597, 598
    MODS 741, *742*
    plant toxicities 450, 565–6, 577–8
    secondary gastric impaction 58
liver enzymes 147, 317, 578, *633*, 634
locoweeds (locoism) 571–3
lolitrems 588
Lolium perenne 588
longus capitis muscle, rupture 286–7
loperamide *551*
lower limb, *see* distal limb; foot
lumbosacral (LS) puncture 457, 458–9
lung biopsy 301
lung tumors 302
luxations 224–7
    carpal joints 189–91
    coxofemoral joint 207–8, 225, 227
    proximal interphalangeal joint 224,
        226, 227
    scapulohumeral joint 225, 227
    tarsal joints 192, 224
Lyell's syndrome 452
lymphadenopathy, strangles 274, 275
lymphocytes, normal values *630*
lymphocytic/plasmacytic enteritis *93*
lymphocytosis 630
lymphoma, intestinal 88–9, *93*, 94, 95

macrolides 726–7
magnesium, serum 592, *633*, 634
magnesium ammonium phosphate (struvite) 116, 133
magnesium sulfate 111, 115, 212, 334–5, 336, 472, *538*, *561*
magnetic resonance imaging (MRI) 230, 303–4, 456, 478
malathion 448
malnutrition 697
mandible, fracture 211–12
mandibular snare 362, 363
mannitol 406, 471, 472, *538*
maples *557*, 573–4
matamycin 496
maxilla, fracture 212
maxillary artery 344, 346
mean arterial pressure (MAP) 514, 645, 646, *647*, 676, 750
mean corpuscular hemoglobin (MCH) 625, 629, *630*, 631
mean corpuscular hemoglobin concentration (MCHC) 625, 629, *630*, 631
mean corpuscular volume (MCV) 625, 629, *630*, 631
mechanical ventilation 512–13
Meckel's diverticulum 84
meconium, impaction/retention 545–7
medial collateral ligament, laceration 226
meloxicam *28*, *155*, *409*, *695*
menace reflex 455
meningitis, bacterial 465–6, 527
mercury toxicity 600
mesenteric injury 69–70, 152, 153
mesodiverticular band 70
metabolic acidosis 517, *638*
metabolic alkalosis 634, *638*
metacarpal/metatarsal bones (third), fracture 186–9
metal chelators *561*, 598, 599, 600
metal toxicities 596–601
metaldehyde toxicity *615*
metatarsal arteries, puncture 260, 261
methemoglobin 570, 573
methoxychlor 448
methylene blue *616*
methylprednisolone sodium succinate 472
metoclopramide hydrochloride 77, 782–3
metritis, puerperal 369–73
metritis–laminitis syndrome 796
metronidazole 92, 129, 179, 180, 249, 284, 296
    hepatic encephalopathy 475
    neonate 807, *808*
    resistance 126

miconazole 449, 496
microcracks 186
Microcystis aeruginosa 588–91
microhematocrit tube 628–9
Micronema, see Halicephalobus spp.
Microsporum spp. 448
midazolam *454*, 471, 539, 693
midbrain syndrome 470
middle phalanx, fracture 182–3
milk replacers 706
Miller technique 631
mineral oil 28, 32, 58, 111, 115, 475, 564, 596
minimum inhibitory concentration (MIC) 233
miosis 501, 504
misoprostol 129, 598
mites 447, 448–9
mitral valve
    endocarditis 320–1
    evaluation 309–10
monensin 603–5
monitoring
    antimicrobial therapy 716–17
    arterial blood gases 635–8
    arterial blood pressure 645–6
    biochemistry 633–5
    cardiac output 648–51
    central venous pressure 646–8
    coagulation profile 638–42
    drug therapy 806
    general approach 623
    goals 623
    hematology 625, 628–31, 806
    intensive care flow sheet 800
    levels 623
    neonate 800–2, 806
    nutritional program 702–3
    patient examination 624–5
    plasma proteins 631–3
    recumbent horse 810–11
    treatment record sheet 626–7
    urine output/urinalysis 642–5
'moon blindness' (equine recurrent uveitis) 504–5
morphine 689–90
    complications 690–1
    epidural *688*, *690*
morphine/detomidine *688*, *690*
morphine/xylazine *688*, *690*
moxidectin 126
mucolytics 543
mucous membranes (oral) 625
    endotoxemia 625, 735–6
    esophageal obstruction 48
    hyperemic 735
    in DIC 754
    pale icteric 521
    postoperative colic patient 760

sepsis 524–5
shock 777
mule foals 521
multifocal syndrome 470
multiple organ dysfunction syndrome (MODS) 523, 740–4
    score *743–4*
murmurs 316, 320, 338–9, 340
muscle enzymes 280, *633*, 634
muscle fasciculations 250, 252, 556, 782
musculoskeletal emergencies
    drug dose rates *155–6*
    general approach 155–7
muzzle, deviation 473
mycosis, guttural pouch 344–7
mycotoxins 556, 581–8
myeloencephalitis, equine protozoal (EPM) 467–8
myocardial damage
    plant toxicities 575, 578–9
    rib fracture 543
myocarditis 316, 324–6, 330
myofascial fenestration 249
myoglobinuria 250, 251, 405, 644
myonecrosis 281
myopathy 157
myosis 501
myositis, clostridial 247–9, 282–4

naloxone 349, 793
nasal cannulae 255, 512
nasal discharge 48, 274, 277
nasal hemorrhage, *see* epistaxis
nasal passages
    trauma 288–9
    tumor 303–4
nasogastric intubation 30–2
    indications 30, 50, 58, 72
    enteral nutrition 517, 703–6
    fluids 32, 111–12
    neonate 517
nasogastric reflux 58, 62, 78, 81, 517
nasogastric tube, sizes 30
nasopharynx, dorsal collapse 278
nasotracheal intubation 256–7, 273, 513
    'blind' in foals 314
navicular bursa
    septic 238–41
    synoviocentesis 162–3
nebulization 543
neck
    lacerations 440
    neurologic examination 456
    vertebral injuries 477–8
neomycin 475, 598, *610*
neonatal isoerythrolysis (NI) 520–3

neonate 511
  cardiovascular support 513–15
  enteral feeding 706
  failure of passive transfer 518–20
  limb deformities 551–4
  meconium impaction/retention 545–7
  monitoring 800–2
  pneumonia 540–3
  respiratory support 511–13
  restraint 797, 798
  rib fractures 543–5
  sepsis 523–7
neoplasia
  CNS 481–2
  gastric 58–9
  hemoperitoneum 152, 153
  intestines 88
  respiratory tract 302–4
Neorickettsia risticii 124, 126
Neospora hughsei 467
neostigmine 77, *783*, 784
Neotrombicula spp. 447
Neotyphodium coenophialum 582–3
nephrosplenic ligament entrapment (NSLE) 35, 118–21
nephrotoxic drugs 230, 404, 405, 602–3, *610–11*, 721
Nerium oleander 563, 574–6
nerve blocks 409–11
  abaxial sesamoid 409–10
  complications 411
  low 4/6 point 410–11
  ophthalmic 484–5
neurologic examination 455–6
neurologic disease 453–4
  common presenting signs *453*
  diagnostic tests *454*
  differential diagnoses *453*
  indications for referral *454*
  intoxication *556*
  lead toxicity 599
neuroprotective agents 212
neurotoxins 474, 569, 605–6
  Clostridium botulinum 478–9
neutropenia 525, 530, 630, 736
neutrophil, toxic 736, 737
neutrophilia 630
nicotine *615*
nightshades *608*
nigropallidal encephalomalacia (chewing disease) *558*, 580–1
Nikolsky's sign 452
nitrates *616*
nitric oxide (NO) 531
nitrite *616*
nitrofurazone 449
NMDA receptor antagonists 693–4

non-steroidal anti-inflammatory drugs (NSAIDs)
  clinical use 695–6
  COX-1-sparing 112
  dose rates *28, 155, 409, 695*
  endotoxemia 737, 779
  mechanism of action 695
  topical 233, 441
  toxicity 404, 405, 602–3, 696
  see also named drugs
norepinephrine *513*, 515, 677–80
Normosol M *659*, 662, *804*
Normosol R *659*, 660
nostril flare 625, 628
nursing care
  HIS 539
  limb deformities 554
  neonate 797–9
  recumbent horse 810–11
nutritional support 446, 539, 550, 697
  botulism 480, 596
  energy requirements 701–2
  enteral 703–6
  neonate 517
  parenteral 706–10
  patient monitoring 702–3
  protein requirements 702

oaks, toxicity *607*
occipital artery 346
oleander toxicity 574–5
olecranon fractures *172*, 194–6
oliguria 405, 406
omental herniation 38, 391–2
omeprazole 56, *551*, 602
onchocerciasis 447, 449
onions *608*
opioids 478, 689–92
  antagonist 349
  complications 690–2
opossum 467
optic nerve syndrome 470
optic neuropathy, ischemic 510
oral erosions *555*
orbit, fracture 494–5
orchipexy 399
organophosphates 272, *560, 561*, 605–6
orotracheal intubation 256–7
orphan foal *548*
oscillometry 646, 766
oseltamivir phsophate 296
ossification, incomplete 530, 531–2
osteomas 304
osteomyelitis 159, 481, 526–7
osteonecrosis 186
ototoxicity 721
oxacillin *729*

oxalate-containing plants *609*
oxygen
  central venous saturation (ScvO$_2$) 765
  central venous tension (PcvO$_2$) 765
  hyperbaric 284
  intranasal insufflation 254–5, 512, 547, 790, 797
  partial pressure (PaO$_2$) 297, 299, 471, 512, 525, 531, *636, 637*
  saturation (SaO$_2$) 512, *636*, 637
oxygen-carrying solutions, hemoglobin-based 672, 674
oxygen–hemoglobin dissociation curve 637
oxytetracycline 98, 127, 249, 284, *808*
oxytocin 50, 349, 371, 377
Oxyuris equi 448

pacemaker implantation 331
packed cell volume (PCV)
  blood loss 212, 311, 343, 671
  dehydration *660*
  gastric rupture 61
  monitoring 628
  normal value *630*
  peritoneal blood 37
  postoperative colic patient 764
  premature foal 531
  tissue perfusion 522
pain assessment 758
Paint Horses 252
palatine artery, major 346
palatopharyngeal arch 267, 268, 269
palmar pouch 164
palpebral reflex 455
pantoprazole 56
paradoxical respiration 529
paralysis, intoxication *556*
paraphimosis 392, 394–8
Parascaris equorum 86–7
parasitic encephalitis 476
parenteral nutrition 706–10
  complications 709–10
  formulation calculation 700–1
  formulation guidelines *805*
parietal hernia 144
parturition
  bladder eversion, prolapse, rupture 384–6
  dystocia 358–66
  fetal membrane retention 369–73
  perineal lacerations 382–4
  post-partum shock 348, 366–9
  small intestine/small colon trauma 793–4
  uterine artery rupture 347–9
  uterine prolapse 376–7

uterine tear 373–5
    vaginal/cervical tears 379–81
paspalitrems 588
pastern
    fractures 182–6, 428
    wounds 422–3, 427
pastern joint, arthrodesis 227
Pasteurella spp. *715*
patent ductus arteriosus
    (PDA) 340–1
patient observation 758–9
pelvic flexure
    enterotomy 106–7, 112, 113
    impaction 34, 111, 113
pelvis, fractures 207–9
pemphigus foliaceus 451–2
penicillins 296, 728–9
    clinical use 728–9
    complications 729
    dosages *729*
    indications 728
    penicillin-G 249, 728
penis
    paraphimosis 394–8
    priapism 393–4
    support/retention devices 397–8
    trauma 392, 394, 395, 400
Penrose drains 416
pentachlorophenol (PCP) *616*
pentastarch 667–8
pentobarbital 471
pentoxyfylline 148, 780, 790
pericardial fluid 316, 318, 324
pericardiectomy 324
pericardiocentesis 324
pericarditis 316, 322–4
Peridan™ solution 786–7
perineum, lacerations 382–4
perineural anesthesia 409–11
periodic ophthalmia (equine recurrent
    uveitis) 504–5
peritoneal fluid
    analysis 37–8
    intestinal neoplasia 88
    peritonitis 150
    post-partum shock 368
    serosanguineous 37, 62–3, 72–3
peritoneal lavage 152
peritonitis 148–52, 354
    clinical features 149, *151*
    diagnosis 38, 149–51
    post-castration 392
    septic 150, 368
    uterine tear 373
permethrin 448
peroxynitrate 748
petechiae 754
petroleum distillates *616*
petrous temporal bone, fracture 469

phalanges, *see* distal phalanx; middle
    phalanx; proximal phalanx
phalopexy (Boltz procedure) 398
phenobarbital 471, 539
phenothiazine 393, 394, 395, 450, *617*
phenylbutazone 445, 695–6
    dose rates *155, 409, 695*
    laminitis 571
    mechanism of action 695
    right dorsal colitis 127, 128
    toxicity 602–3
phenylephrine 121, 329, *676*, 683–4
phenytoin 251, 333, 335
phosphine *617*
phospholipases 785–6
phosphorus
    plasma/serum *633*, 634
    toxicity *617*
photophobia 483
photosensitization 450–1, *557*, 566,
    567
phoxim 448
phylloerythrin 450, 566
physitis, septic 213–14
phytobezoar 133
phytoconglobate 133
Phytolacca americana 608
pinworms 448, 449
piperazine salts *617*
'pit vipers' (*Crotalidae* spp.) 280, 592–4
pituitary adenoma 482
placentitis 789–90
plant toxicities 565–80, *607–9*
    causing photosensitization 450–1,
        566, 567
    cyanogenic glycosides 566–70
    factors predisposing horses 565
    locoweeds 571–3
    maples 573–4
    oleander 563, 574–6
    oxalate-containing plants *609*
    pyrrolizidine alkaloids 58, 450,
        576–8
plantar pouches 168
plasma osmolality 660, 662
plasma proteins 61, 631–3, *632*
plasma therapy 312, 514, 519, 526,
    669–70
    anti-endotoxin antibodies 779
    postoperative colic patient 768
Plasma-Lyte 56, *804*
Plasma-Lyte A *659*, 660
platelet count 638, 639
pleural fluid
    drainage 264–7
    pneumonia/pleuropneumonia
        295–6
pleuritis, primary 296
pleuropneumonia *253*, 290, 294–6

pleurpneumonia 266
plica salpingopharyngea 276, 279
pneumatosis intestinalis 536
pneumonia 294–6
    aspiration 50, 51
    foal 525, 526
    herpes viral 294, 296
    neonate 540–3
pneumoperitoneum 61
pneumothorax 266, 296–8, 436, 751
pokeweed *608*
polymerase chain reaction (PCR) tests
    97, 276
polymethylmethacrylate (PMMA)
    beads, antimicrobial-impregnated
    179–80, 233, *718*, 719
polymixin B 374–5, 526, 737, 780
polysaccharide storage myopathy 250
positive pressure ventilation (PPV)
    531
posthectomy (reefing) 398
postoperative colic patient,
    examination sheet 760
potassium 515–16, 534–5
    HYPP 252
    normal serum values *633*
    supplementation 662, 804
    whole body deficit 328, 804
potassium penicillin 177, 249, 321,
    409, 729, *808*
potassium permanganate *617*
potassium-binding resins 516
Potomac horse fever 124, 126
poultry mite 447
pralidoxime hydrochloride *561*, 606
praziquantel 95, 103
prednisolone 301, 449, 452, 472
pregnant mare
    abdominal wall rupture 386–9
    bleeding 792–3
    body wall hernia/prepubic tendon
        rupture 387, 388, 790–1
    placentitis 789–90
premature foals 528–32
premature ventricular contractions
    331–3
prepubic tendon, rupture 387, 388,
    790–1
prepuce, trauma 394, 395
priapism 393–4
probiotics 566
procainamide 333
procaine penicillin *156, 409, 729, 808*
prolapse
    bladder 384–6
    intestines 380–1, 385–6
    iris 499, 500
    rectum 138–40
    uterus 376–7

proliferative enteropathy 96–8
propranolol 329, 334
propylene glycol *618*
prostaglandin analogs 56, 509
prostaglandins 51–2, 127–8, 406, 602, 695, 790
protamine sulfate *614*
protein
    energy and nitrogen content *701*
    maintenance requirements 702
    parenteral formulae 707
protein C 753
proteinuria 405, 644
proteoglycan synthesis 228
prothrombin time (PT) 639
proton pump inhibitors 56, 550, *551*, 602
proximal (first) phalanx
    avulsion injury 428
    fracture 173, 184–6
proximal interphalangeal joint
    arthrodesis 227
    subluxation 224, 226, 227
    synoviocentesis 162–3
Prunus serotina (wild black cherry) 568
Prunus virginiana (chokecherry) 568
pruritus 446–9
pseudodiverticula 84
Pseudomonas spp. 233, 237, 320, 441
Psoroptes equi 447, 448
psyllium mucilloid 115, 118, 129
Pteridium aquilinum (bracken) *607*
ptyalism 27, *555*, 586–7
pulmonary arterial wedge pressure (PAWP) 750
pulmonary artery pressure 316, 317
pulmonary capillary pressure 291
pulmonary edema 272, 273, 751, 752
    etiology/pathogenesis 291
    negative pressure (NPPE) 291, 292
pulmonary embolism 750, 751
pulmonary fibrosis, equine multinodular (EMPF) 300–1
pulmonary function testing 299
pulmonary hypertension 316, 529, 735
pulmonary thromboembolism (PTE) 294, 354
pulmonic valve 310, 320, 321
pulse contour analysis 651
pulse quality 624
puncture wounds
    distal limb 422
    foot 236, 238–44
    imaging 158–9
    upper limb/body 432–3
pupil, miotic 501, 504
pupillary light reflex 455, 470
purpura hemorrhagica 272

Pyemotes tritici 447, 448–9
pyloric ulcers 53, 56
pyrantel pamoate 87, 103
pyrantel tartrate 95
pyrethrins 448, 449
pyrrolizidine alkaloids 58, 450, 555–6, 576–8

Quarter Horses 122, 250, 252
quinapril 319
quinidine 328–9, 333, 334

R–on–T phenomenon 331, 332, 334
rabies 453, *454*, 466–7
'racing support' 398
radiocarpal joint, synoviocentesis 166–7
radius, fracture 175, 196–8, 433
ragwort 58, 576–8
rain scald 448, 449
ranitidine 56, *551*, 602
rattlesnake bites 280–2, 325, 330
rebreathing examination 624, 625, 651
rectal biopsy 88, 95
rectal pack 137
rectal palpation 32–5
    cecal impaction 34, 99
    ileal impaction 34, 81
    pelvis 208
    peritonitis 151
    small colon impaction 35, 131
    small intestinal intussusception 68
    uterine torsion 378
rectovaginal laceration/fistula 382–3
rectum 135–41
    perirectal abscess 140–1
    prolapse 138–40, 793
    tears 135–8
rectus capitis muscle, rupture 286–7
recumbent horse 809–12
    devices for moving/lifting/slinging 812
    foal 797–8
    monitoring/nursing 810–11
    safety 809
recurrent airway obstruction (RAO) 298–300
recurrent laryngeal nerve 271, 272, 273, 345
red bag delivery 360
red blood cells (RBCs) 628, *630*
    maple intoxication 573–4
    washed dams' 522
referral
    colic 28–9
    neurologic disease *454*
    respiratory emergencies *254*
refractometer 631

regional limb perfusion 176–8, 233, 420, 718–19
    complications 178
    drug dosages *718*
relative adrenal insufficiency 741, 748
renal function
    aminoglycoside toxicity *610*, 721
    hypoxic ischemic syndrome 536, 537, 540
    monitoring 634
    see also acute kidney injury
renal perfusion 404, 405, 406, 536
Rescue Glide 812
reserpine *618*
respiration
    monitoring 801
    paradoxical 529
respiratory distress 268, 282–4, 540, 541, 628, 740
respiratory emergencies *253–4*
respiratory failure *742*
respiratory function
    premature foal 528–9
    recumbent horse 811
    septic foal 525
respiratory paralysis 479, 480, 596
respiratory rate 625
respiratory stimulants 512, *513*
respiratory support
    intranasal oxygen 254–5, 512, 547, 790, 797
    neonate 312–14, 511–13
    premature foal 531
    recumbent foal 797
respiratory tract neoplasia 302–4
resuscitation
    cardiopulmonary 313–15, 338
    hemorrhage/hemolysis 311–12
retention of fetal membranes (RFM) 369–73
retinal detachment 506–7
rhabdomyolysis 157, 250–1
rhinopharyngoscopy 275
rhinoscopy 289, 303
Rhizoctonia leguminicola 586–7
Rhodococcus equi 94, 149, 233, 294, 481
    antimicrobial sensitivity *715*
    foal pneumonia 540–3
rib fractures 314–15, 543–5
Richter's (parietal) hernia 144
Ricinus communis 607
rifampin 249, 729–30, *808*
ringworm (dermatophytosis) 448, 449
Robert Jones bandage 174, 175, 176, 194
Robinia pseudoacacia 607
rodenticides, anticoagulant *561*, *611*, *618*
rolling of horse 121, 376

romifidine *687*, 688
rotavirus *548*, *549*
routine care, changes in 110
ryegrass, perennial 588

safety, recumbent horse 809
safflower oil 129
St. John's wort 450
saline
    hypertonic 368, 471, *659*, 662–4,
        768, 778
    hypotonic 778
    nebulization 293
salinomyin 603–5
salivation, excessive (ptyalism) 27, *555*,
    586–7
Salmonella spp. 90, 124, 125, 130, 233,
    354, *548*
    antimicrobial sensitivity *715*
    diagnostic tests *549*
Salmonella enterica serovar
    newport 90
salpingoscopy 279
Salter–Harris fractures 199, 203, 206
Sarcocystis neurona 460, 467
Sarcoptes scabiei 447, 448
scabies 447
'scalping' injury 438
scapulohumeral joint, luxation
    225, 227
Schalm technique 631
schwannoma 482
scintigraphy 128, 193, 200, 202,
    207, 209
sclera
    ecchymotic hemorrhages 755
    injected 524
scopolamine *612*
scrotal hernias 141–4
scrotum, swelling/edema 317, 399
'seagull' sign 507
sedation
    dystocia 363
    esophageal obstruction 50
    hepatic encephalopathy 475
    spinal cord injuries 478
    tetanus 481
    wound evaluation 408
sedatives
    α-2 agonists 687–8
    acepromazine 692
    benzodiazepines 692–3
    ketamine 693–4
Seidel test 483, 500
seizures *453*, 470
    control 454, 471, 539, 692–3
    HIE 537, 539
    intoxication *556*
    signs of impending 800

selenium 250, 600–1
selenium sulfide 448
Senecio spp. 576–8
Seprafilm® 786–7
sepsis 744–7
    clinical features 746
    diagnosis 747
    etiology/pathogenesis 745–6
    foals 523–7
    management 747
    severe (sepsis syndrome) 745, 746
sepsis score 525
septic arthritis 227–33
    diagnosis 161, 228–30
    etiology/pathogenesis 227–9
    foal 526–7
    management 231–3
    prognosis 227
    synovial fluid analysis 161, 229–30
septic osteomyelitis 214–16
septic physitis/epiphysitis 213–14
septic shock *745*, 747–9
septic tenosynovitis 234–8
septic thrombophlebitis 351–3
sequential organ function assessment
    (SOFA) score *743–4*
sequestrum 214, 215, 216
Serratia marcescens 320, *715*
serum amyloid A (SAA) 764, 773
sesamoid bones, proximal 217, 218
sesamoidean ligaments
    collateral 164, 165
    distal, disruption 217, 218
shaker foal syndrome 595–6
shock 749–52
    burns 442
    clinical features 751, 777–8
    definition 749
    diagnosis 751
    etiology/pathogenesis 749–50
    hypovolemic 750–1
    management 752
    post-partum 348, 366–9
    postoperative colic patient 776–8
    septic *745*, 747–9
shoes
    heel extension 221, 227, 241
    hospital plate 241, 244
    toe extension 223
sildenfil 531
silver sulfadiazine 445, 446
sinus of Valsalva, aneurysm/rupture
    350
sinuses
    masses 302–4
    trauma 288–9, 437
skeletal maturity, premature foals
    531–2
skeletal ossification index 530

skin biopsy 421
skin scraping 420–1
skin staples 414–15
skull
    decompression 471
    fractures 210–12, 468–9
slaframine 586–7
slings 809–10, 812
slit lamp biomicroscopy 508, 509
'slobbers' 586–7
SLUD 605
small colon 44–5, 129–35
    fecalith obstruction 132–3
    impaction 35, 43, 130–2
    intestinal concretions/foreign body
        obstruction 133–4
    prolapse through vaginal tear
        380–1
    strangulating lipoma 135
    trauma 793–4
small intestines
    adhesions 784–8
    ascarid impaction 86–7
    diverticula 84–5
    epiploic foramen entrapment 64–5
    exploration 45
    gastrosplenic ligament
        entrapment 66
    grass sickness 78–9
    ileal impaction 80–1
    ileal muscular hypertrophy 82–3
    inflammatory/infiltrative
        disease 93–5
    intussusception 66–9
    non-strangulating lesions 75
    pedunculated lipoma 71–3
    primary ileus 76–7
    prolapse in bladder rupture
        385–6
    proliferative enteropathy 96–8
    proximal enteritis 90–3
    strangulating lesions 62–3, 91
    strangulation through mesenteric
        rent 69–70
    surgical disorders 46
    trauma 794
    volvulus 73–5
smoke inhalation 292–3, 442
snake bites 280–2, 325, 330, *557*,
    561, 592–4
snakeroot, white 578–9
sodium
    fractional excretion 405–6,
        643, 645
    mare's milk 802
    overloading 802
    serum/plasma 125, 516, 533,
        534, *633*
    supplementation 804

sodium bicarbonate 252, 328, 338, 550, *551*, 804
sodium carboxymethylcellulose 65, 81, 112
sodium chloride, oral 804
sodium fluoroacetate *618*
sodium iodine 449
sodium nitrite *561*, 570
sodium penicillin 324, *729*, *808*
sodium selenite 600–1
sodium sulfate (Glauber's salt) *561*
sodium thiosulfate *561*, 570
Solanum spp. *608*
sole, penetrating wounds 214
sorbitol 563
sorbitol dehydrogenase (SDH) *633*, 634
Sorghum halepense (Johnsongrass) 568, *609*
Sorghum sudanense (Sudan grass) 569, *609*
spermatic cord, torsion 398–9
spinal cord
    bacterial infection 465, 481
    infarction in EHV-1 461
    injury 477–8
    neoplasia 481–2
spleen, displacement 120, 121
splintage 156, 170–6
    carpal bone fractures 191
    caudal 174–5, 196
    dorsal/plantar 172–4
    double 174, 188
    flexor tendon disruption 220–1
    for specific injuries *702*
    indications 170–2
    lateral 175–6, 198, 200–1
    limb deformities 554
    metacarpal/metatarsal bone fractures 188
    olecranon fracture 196
    radial fracture 198
    tibial fracture 200–1
squamous cell carcinoma (SCC)
    stomach 58–9
    upper respiratory tract 302
stall, recumbent horse 809, 810
stallions 358
    aortic root rupture 350–1
    paraphimosis 394–8
    priapism 393–4
    scrotal/inguinal hernias 141–4
Standardbreds 250
Staphylococcus spp. 179, 233, 237, 352, 441, *715*
Staphylococcus aureus 238, 441, 722
    antimicrobial sensitivity *715*

methicillin-resistant (MRSA) 722
Staphylococcus epidermidis 352
Starling's equation 665
stent bandage 419, 761
sternothyrohyoideus muscles 259
stillbirths 584
stomach disorders
    neoplasia 58–9
    see also entries beginning with 'gastric'
'stove pipe' limb 441
strangles 274–6
straw itch mite 447
'street-nail' procedure 240–1
streptococci, group C 405
Streptococcus spp. 233, 237, 320
    β-hemolytic 441
Streptococcus equi subsp. *equi* 274–6
Streptococcus equi subsp. *zooepidemicus* 294, 540, *715*
Streptomyces cinnamonensis 603
stress fractures
    humerus 201, 202
    pelvix 207–8
    tibia 200
stress radiographs 226
stringhalt, Australian 272
strong ion difference 634
Strongylus vulgaris 108, 124–5, 354
struvite 116, 133
strychnine *619*
stylohyoid bone 275, 277, 344
subcutaneous emphysema 260, 264, 285, 432, 433, 436
subpalpebral lavage 484–5, 497
subsolar abscess 155, 242
substantia nigra, malacia 580, 581
succimer *561*, 599
suckle reflex 536, 537
sucralfate 32, 56, 129, 540, 598, 602
    foals *551*
sucrose, serum 54–5
Sudan grass 569, *609*
sudden death 335, 336, 337, *558*
sulfonamides 450, *619*
    potentiated *409*, 466, 731, 807, *808*
summer pasture-associated obstructive pulmonary disease (SPAOD) 298–300
supraorbital (frontal) nerve block 484, 485
surfactant 528–9, 530
    bovine/synthetic 531
suspensory apparatus, disruption 173, 217–18
swainsonine 572
Swan–Ganz catheter 317

sweating, severe *558*
synechiae, posterior/anterior 483, 504
synovial fluid analysis 160–1, 230, 236–7
synovial structures, wounds involving 159–60, 421–30
synoviocentesis 159–61, 412
    carpal joints/carpal sheath 166–7
    complications 170
    distal interphalangeal joint 161–2
    fetlock joint 160, 164–5
    indications 159–60
    metacarpo-/metatarsophalangeal joints 164–5
    navicular bursa 162–3
    proximal interphalangeal joint 162–3
    septic arthritis 229–30
    sonographic guidance 159
    tarsal joints/tarsal sheath 168–9
    technique 160–1
syringe pump 686
systemic inflammatory response syndrome (SIRS) 404, 523, 634, 737–40
systemic vascular resistance (SVR) 645
systolic arterial pressure (SAP) 646, *647*

tachycardia 60, 311, 322, 424, 624, 760
    supraventricular 329
    ventricular 333–5
tachypnea 625, 628, 760
tail tone 479, 595–6
talus, fracture 193
tapeworm infection 68, 69, 80–1, 82, 102
tarsal sheath, synoviocentesis 168–9
tarsometatarsal joint
    subluxation 224
    synoviocentesis 168–9
tarsorrhaphy 488
tarsus (hock)
    bandages/dressings 420
    fractures and luxations 191–4, 224
    premature foal 530
    synoviocentesis 168–9
    wound 231
Taxus spp. *608*
temperature
    brain 470–1
    infections 772
    monitoring 624, 800
    neonate 517, 531, 798
temporohyoid osteoarthropathy (THO) 469, 470, 472–4
tendon injuries 217–23

extensor tendons 222–3
flexor tendons 219–21
suspensory apparatus 217–18
wounds 234–8, 424–7
tendon laxity 552
tendon sheaths
lavage 237
synoviocentesis 164–5, 168–9
wounds/sepsis 234–8, 422, 426–9
tenorrhaphy 221
tenoscopy 237
tenosynovitis, septic 234–8
testes, trauma 400
testicular artery, hemorrhage 341–2
tetanus 480–1
tetrachlorodibenzodioxin
(TCDD) *619*
tetracyclines 249, 450, 730–1, 807
tetralogy/pentalogy of
Fallot 339–40
Theiler's disease 147–8, 476
therapeutic drug monitoring
(TDM) 806
thermoregulation 531, 798
thiamine *538*, 599
thistle, yellow-star 579–80
thoracocentesis 264, 297, 298
thorax, wounds 431, 434, 436–7
thornapple *607*
Thoroughbreds 250
thrombocytopenia 639
thromboelastography (TEG) 641–2
thromboembolic disease 294, 354–5
thrombophlebitis 351–3, 763
tibia, fracture 198–201, 433
tibiotarsal joint
injuries involving 427
septic arthritis 229
synoviocentesis 168–9
ticarcillin *729*
ticarcillin-clavulanate *729*, 806, *808*
tick infestations 447, 449
timentin 177
timolol 509
tissue factor 752, 753
tissue hypoperfusion
indicators 675
treatment algorithm 677
tobramycin 179
tocolytic agents 790
α-tocopherol (vitamin E) 250, 472,
601
toe, 'flipped up' 220, 235
tolazoline *687*
tongue
lacerations 440
tone 456, 479, 595

Torsade de pointes 334
torsion
spermatic cord 398–9
uterus 367, 377–9
total parenteral nutrition (TPN) 706,
707–8
total plasma protein (TPP) 61, 125,
128, 129, 152
COP estimation 631, 765
dehydration *660*
postoperative colic patient 764, 765
total protein (TP) 631
peritoneal fluid 38, 91, 150
synovial fluid 161, 230, 236
tourniquet 177–8
toxaphene 448
toxic epidermal necrolysis (TEN/
Lyell's syndrome) 452
toxicities
algal toxins 588–91
4-aminopyridine *610*
ammonia *610*
amphotericin B *611*
anticoagulant rodenticides *611*
antimicrobials *610*, *615*, 721
approach to treatment 558–62
arsenic *611*
atropine *612*
carbon disulfide *612*
carbon tetrachloride *612*
chlorates *612*
chlorophenols *616*
clinical signs and common causes
555–8
cyanide *561*, 568–9, *613*, 751
decontamination and antidotal
agents *560–1*
dimethyl sulfoxide *613*
dioctyl sodium succinate *614*
feed additives (ionophores) 603–5
fluoride *614*
gastrointestinal decontamination
562–4
heparin *614*
imidocarb dipropionate *614*
insecticides 605–6, *613*
iodine *615*
metaldehyde *615*
metals 595–601
mycotoxins 581–8
nicotine *615*
nitrate-nitrite *616*
NSAIDs 404, 405, 602, *602–3*
petroleum distillates *616*
phenothiazine *617*
phosphine *617*
phosphorus *6*

piperazine salts *617*
plants 565–80, *607–9*
propylene glycol *618*
protective factors 555
reserpine *618*
sodium fluoroacetate *618*
strychnine *619*
sulfonamides *619*
symptomatic/supportive care 562
tetrachlorodibenzodioxin
(TCDD) *619*
zinc salts *560*, *620*
trachea
ingesta contamination 50
mucosal laceration 264
trauma 284–5
tracheal fluid, collection/analysis
262–4
tracheoscopy 285
tracheostomy
complications 260
permanent 273
temporary 258–60, 268,
273, 285
tranquilizers 251, 393
transfusion reaction 519, 670, 674
transtracheal catheter 254
transtracheal wash *253*, 262–4, 299
technique 262–4
tremetol 578
tremorgenic mycotoxins 587–8
tremors, intoxication *556*, 587–8
triamcinolone 449
trichlorfon 449
trichobezoar 133
Trichophyton spp. 448
tricuspid valve
endocarditis 320, 321
regurgitation 318
Trifolium hybridum (alsike
clover) 565–6
Trifolium pratense 586, 587
triglycerides, serum 147, 148, 702,
710, 764–5
trimethoprim–sulfonamides *409*, 731,
790, 807, *808*
trombiculidiasis 447, 448–9
'trophic feedings' 707
troponin I 604
tuber coxae, fracture 208
tumor necrosis factor-α (TNF-α) 717,
734, 737, 739, 753
tympanocentesis 474
typhlectomy, partial 103
typhlocolitis 125
typhlotomy 69
Tyzzer's disease 147–8

ultrasonography
  abdominal 39–40
  chest tube placement 265
  CSF collection 458, 459
  FLASH 40
  musculoskeltal examination 158–9
  pleural fluid 295
  pneumothorax/hemothorax 297, 544
umbilicus
  hernia 144
  infection 526–7
  treatment 518, 797
upper respiratory tract (URT)
  neoplasia 302–4
  obstruction *253, 258*
    arytenoid chondritis 267–9
    clostridial myositis 282, 284
    snake bites 280–2
urachus, rupture 533–5
urethrotomy, perineal 402
urinalysis 405–6, 642–5
urinary alkalinization/acidification 562
urinary casts 644
urinary catheterization 642, 810
urinary system, monitoring 801
urinary tract
  calculi 401–3
  disruption 532–5
urine, specific gravity (SG) 405, 514, 642, 643–4, 759, 798
urine output 642–3
  after colic surgery 759
  assessment 541
uroperitoneum 533–5
uterine artery rupture 152, 347–9
uterus
  lavage 372
  prolapse 376–7
  tear/laceration 373–5
  torsion 367, 377–9
uveitis 483
  equine recurrent 504–5
  neonate 525

vaccinations 463, 466–7, 480, 481
Vacutainer® tube 628
vagina, lacerations 379–81

valacyclovir 301, 462
vancomycin 126, 177, 717, 731–2
vascular endothelial damage 352
vasodilation, septic shock 748
vasodilators 676
vasopressin 681–2, 748
vasopressor therapy *513, 515, 531*
  monitoring 635
  see also named vasopressors
vegetable oil, feeding 705
Venezuelan equine encephalomyelitis (VEE) 460, 463–5
venous stasis *352*
ventilation, mechanical 512–13, 531
ventral edema 316, 317, 387
ventricular fibrillation 335–6
ventricular septal defect 338–9
ventricular tachycardia 333–5
vertebral body
  osteomyelitis 481
  trauma 477–8
vestibular syndrome 470
Viborg's triangle 274
Virchow's triad 352
vitamin C (ascorbic acid) 472
vitamin E (α-tocopherol) 250, 472, *538*, 601, 790
vitamin K$_1$ *561, 611*
volvulus
  large colon (LCV) 39, 53, 104–7, 794
  small intestinal 73–5
voriconazole 496
vulva
  hematoma 384
  lacerations 382–4

walnut, black 570–1
warming, neonate 517
water intake
  after colic surgery 759
  large colon impaction 111
water manometer 767
weight
  monitoring in neonate 800
  see also body condition scoring
West Nile virus (WNV) 460, 462–3
Western equine encephalomyelitis (WEE) 463–5

wet-to-dry dressing 417
white blood cells (WBC)
  foal pneumonia 542
  monitoring 625, 628
  morphology 625
  neonate 806
  normal values *630*
  postoperative colic patient 764
  SIRS 738
  synovial fluid 161, 230, 236–7
whole blood administration 671–2, 673
windsucking 64
worming 81, 87, 95, 103
wounds
  botulism 595
  burns 442–6
  cleansing/debridement 412
  closure 412–15
  dehiscence 415
  distal limb 421–30
  drains 415–16
  dressings and bandaging 416–20
  exudative 436
  eyelid 490–2
  foot/hoof 236, 238–44
  general approach 407–8
  head and neck 437–40
  hemorrhage 342–3
  history *407*
  imaging 158–9
  infection 414
  involving joints 227–33, 426
  involving tendons/tendon sheaths 234–8, 424–9
  packing 416, 436
  upper limb and body 430–7

xylazine 475, 478, 547, 770
  dose rates *28, 155, 409, 687*
  epidural *688*

yellow-star thistle 579–80
yews (*Taxus* spp.) *608*
yohimbine *687*, 784

zinc salts *560, 620*
zootoxins 591–2
zygomatic nerve block 484